Problem Solving in Neuroradiology

Problem Solving in Neuroradiology

Meng Law, MD, MBBS, FRACR
Professor of Radiology and Neurological Surgery
Director of Neuroradiology
Keck School of Medicine
University of Southern California
Los Angeles, California

Peter M. Som, MD, FACR
Professor of Radiology, Otolaryngology, and Radiation Oncology
Department of Radiology
Mount Sinai School of Medicine
New York, New York

Thomas P. Naidich, MD, FACR
Professor of Radiology and Neurosurgery
Mount Sinai School of Medicine
New York, New York

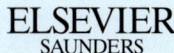

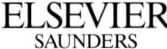

1600 John F. Kennedy Blvd.
Ste 1800
Philadelphia, PA19103-2899

PROBLEM SOLVING IN NEURORADIOLOGY   ISBN: 978-0-323-05929-9
Copyright © 2011 by Saunders, an imprint of Elsevier Inc. All rights reserved.

No part of this publication may be reproduced or transmitted in any form or by any means, electronic or mechanical, including photocopying, recording, or any information storage and retrieval system, without permission in writing from the Publisher. Details on how to seek permission, further information about the Publisher's permissions policies and our arrangements with organizations such as the Copyright Clearance Center and the Copyright Licensing Agency, can be found at our website: www.elsevier.com/permissions.

This book and the individual contributions contained in it are protected under copyright by the Publisher (other than as may be noted herein).

> **Notice**
>
> Knowledge and best practice in this field are constantly changing. As new research and experience broaden our understanding, changes in research methods, professional practices, or medical treatment may become necessary.
>
> Practitioners and researchers must always rely on their own experience and knowledge in evaluating and using any information, methods, compounds, or experiments described herein. In using such information or methods they should be mindful of their own safety and the safety of others, including parties for whom they have a professional responsibility.
>
> With respect to any drug or pharmaceutical products identified, readers are advised to check the most current information provided (i) on procedures featured or (ii) by the manufacturer of each product to be administered to verify the recommended dose or formula, the method and duration of administration, and contraindications. It is the responsibility of practitioners, relying on their own experience and knowledge of their patients, to make diagnoses, to determine dosages and the best treatment for each individual patient, and to take all appropriate safety precautions.
>
> To the fullest extent of the law, neither the Publisher nor the authors, contributors, or editors assume any liability for any injury and/or damage to persons or property as a matter of products liability, negligence or otherwise, or from any use or operation of any methods, products, instructions, or ideas contained in the material herein.

International Standard Book Number: 978-0-323-05929-9

Acquisitions Editor: Rebecca Gaertner
Developmental Editor: Joanie Milnes
Publishing Services Manager: Anne Altepeter
Senior Project Manager: Cheryl A. Abbott
Designer: Steven Stave
Illustrator: Lesley Frazier
Marketing Manager: Radha Mawrie

Printed in China

Last digit is the print number: 9 8 7 6 5 4 3 2 1

To my parents, Lawrence and Sue, for their love and inspiration

ML

To my wife, Judy, for her support and love

PMS

To my dear wife, Michele Levin Naidich, whose love balances my life

TPN

Contributors

Manzoor Ahmed, MBBS, MD
Assistant Professor of Radiology
Lerner College of Medicine
Imaging Institute
Cleveland Clinic, Ohio
Neurodegenerative Disorders

Pascal Bou-Haidar, BMed, MEngSc, FRANZCR
Mount Sinai Hospital
New York, New York
Advanced MR (MR Spectroscopy, Diffusion Imaging, Diffusion Tensor Imaging, and Perfusion Imaging). A Multiparametric Algorithmic Approach to Problem Solving in Neuroradiology
Epilepsy

Alessandro Cianfoni, MD
Assistant Professor of Neuroradiology
Radiology Department
Medical University of South Carolina
Charleston, South Carolina
Brain Trauma
Imaging of Spine Trauma

Cesare Colosimo, MD
Professor of Radiology
Director of Radiology
Department of Bioimages and Radiological Sciences
Policlinico "A. Gemelli"
Catholic University of Rome
Rome, Italy
Brain Trauma
Imaging of Spine Trauma

Marco Essig, MD, PhD
Professor of Radiology
Heidelberg Medical School;
Department of Neuroradiology
University of Erlangen
Erlangen, Germany
Tumor

Girish M. Fatterpekar, MD
Assistant Professor, Radiology
Section Neuroradiology
New York University School of Medicine
New York, New York
Head and Neck Radiology

Julia Frühwald-Pallamar
Department of Radiology
Medical University of Vienna
Vienna General Hospital
Vienna, Austria
Infection/Inflammation

Andre D. Furtado, MD
Clinical Fellow
Department of Radiology
Children's Hospital of Pittsburgh Medical Center
Pittsburgh, Pennsylvania
Intrauterine and Perinatal Infections
Neuroimaging of Pediatric Hypoxic–Ischemic Injury

Rajiv Gupta, MD, PhD
Director, Ultra-High Resolution Volume CT Lab
Department of Radiology
Massachusetts General Hospital
Boston, Massachusetts
Multidetector Computed Tomography as a Problem-Solving Tool in Neuroradiology

Sofia S. Haque, MD
Clinical Assistant Professor of Radiology
New York Presbyterian Hospital
Weill Cornell Medical Center;
Memorial Sloan-Kettering Cancer Center
New York, New York
Metabolic Disorders

Jane J. Kim, MD
Assistant Professor of Clinical Radiology
University of California, San Francisco
San Francisco, California
Magnetic Resonance Imaging as a Problem-Solving Tool

Paul E. Kim, MD
Assistant Professor of Radiology
Director of Spine Imaging and Intervention
Keck School of Medicine
University of Southern California
Los Angeles, California
Spine and Lower Back Pain
Spine: Tumors and Infection

Lale Kostakoglu, MD, MPH
Professor of Radiology
Director, PET/CT Oncology and Research
Department of Radiology
Division of Nuclear Medicine
Mount Sinai School of Medicine
New York, New York
PET/CT Imaging in Squamous Cell Carcinoma of the Head and Neck

Saulo Lacerda, MD
MedImagem-Hospital Beneficencia Portuguesa
Sao Paulo, Brazil
Advanced MR (MR Spectroscopy, Diffusion Imaging, Diffusion Tensor Imaging, and Perfusion Imaging): A Multiparametric Algorithmic Approach to Problem Solving in Neuroradiology
Epilepsy
Intrauterine and Perinatal Infections
Neuroimaging of Pediatric Hypoxic–Ischemic Injury

Meng Law, MD, MBBS, FRACR
Professor of Radiology and Neurological Surgery
Director of Neuroradiology
Keck School of Medicine
University of Southern California
Los Angeles, California
Advanced MR (MR Spectroscopy, Diffusion Imaging, Diffusion Tensor Imaging, and Perfusion Imaging): A Multiparametric Algorithmic Approach to Problem Solving in Neuroradiology
Epilepsy

Michael Lev, MD, FAHA
Director, Emergency Neuroradiology and Neurovascular Lab
Massachusetts General Hospital
Associate Professor of Radiology
Harvard Medical School
Boston, Massachusetts
Multidetector Computed Tomography as a Problem-Solving Tool in Neuroradiology

John K. Lyo, MD
Assistant Professor of Radiology
New York Presbyterian Hospital
Weill Cornell Medical Center;
Memorial Sloan-Kettering Cancer Center
New York, New York
Metabolic Disorders

Sunithi Mani
Assistant Professor
Department of Radiodiagnosis
Christian Medical College
Vellore, India
Multidetector Computed Tomography as a Problem-Solving Tool in Neuroradiology

Stephan Meckel, MD
Consultant Neuroradiologist
Department of Neuroradiology
Neurocenter
University Hospital Freiburg
Freiburg, Germany
Diagnostic Angiography

Amit Mehndiratta, MBBS, MMST, DPhil
Institute of Biomedical Engineering
University of Oxford
Oxford, United Kingdom
Multidetector Computed Tomography as a Problem-Solving Tool in Neuroradiology

Pratik Mukherjee, MD, PhD
Associate Professor of Radiology and Biomedical Imaging, Bioengineering, and Therapeutic Sciences
Department of Radiology and Biomedical Imaging
University of California, San Francisco
San Francisco, California
Magnetic Resonance Imaging as a Problem-Solving Tool

Thomas P. Naidich, MD, FACR
Professor of Radiology and Neurosurgery
Mount Sinai School of Medicine
New York, New York
Intrauterine and Perinatal Infections
Neuroimaging of Pediatric Hypoxic–Ischemic Injury

Danielle Nanigian, MD
University of California at San Diego
Coronado, California
Spine Procedures: Biopsies

Darren B. Orbach, MD, PhD
Assistant Professor of Radiology
Harvard Medical School;
Director of Interventional and Neurointerventional Radiology
Children's Hospital Boston
Boston, Massachusetts
Neurointerventional Radiology

Michael Phillips, MD
Vice Chairman, Research and Academic Affairs
Imaging Institute
Cleveland Clinic Foundation
Cleveland, Ohio
Neurodegenerative Disorders

Stuart Pomerantz, MD
Department of Radiology
Massachusetts General Hospital
Boston, Massachusetts
Multidetector Computed Tomography as a Problem-Solving Tool in Neuroradiology

Stefan B. Puchner, MD
Medical University of Vienna
Department of Radiology
University Hospital Vienna
Vienna, Austria
Infection/Inflammation

Ajit Puri, MD
Clinical Fellow
Interventional Neuroradiology/Endovascular Neurosurgery
Department of Radiology/Neurosurgery
Brigham and Women's Hospital
Boston, Massachusetts
Neurointerventional Radiology

Andrea Rossi, MD
Head, Department of Pediatric Neuroradiology
G. Gaslini Children's Hospital;
Contract Professor of Neuroradiology
University of Genoa
Genoa, Italy
Imaging of Congenital Brain Abnormalities

Peter M. Som, MD, FACR
Professor of Radiology, Otolaryngology, and Radiation Oncology
Department of Radiology
Mount Sinai School of Medicine
New York, New York
Head and Neck Radiology

Ruth Thiex, MD, PhD
Departments of Neurosurgery and Radiology
Brigham and Women's Hospital
Harvard Medical School
Boston, Massachusetts
Neurointerventional Radiology

Majda M. Thurnher, MD
Associate Professor of Radiology
Department of Radiology
Medical University of Vienna
Vienna General Hospital
Vienna, Austria
Infection/Inflammation

Johan W.M. Van Goethem, MD, PhD
Vice-Head of Neuroradiology
Staff Member
University of Antwerp
Antwerp, Belgium
Spine and Lower Back Pain
Spine: Tumors and Infection

Alyssa T. Watanabe, MD
Clinical Associate Professor in Radiology
University of Southern California
 School of Medicine
Los Angeles, California
Spine and Lower Back Pain
Spine: Tumors and Infection

Stephan G. Wetzel, MD
Department of Neuroradiology
Swiss Neuro Institute
Klinik Hirslanden Zürich
Zürich, Switzerland
Diagnostic Angiography

Wade Wong, DO
University of California at San Diego
Coronado, California
Spine Procedures: Biopsies

Robert J. Young, MD
Assistant Professor of Radiology
New York Presbyterian Hospital
Weill Cornell Medical Center;
Memorial Sloan-Kettering Cancer Center
New York, New York
Metabolic Disorders

Foreword

In a departure from commonly constructed textbooks in radiology, three eminent leaders in the field of neuroradiology—Drs. Law, Som, and Naidich—have approached imaging in an original and highly educational manner. With separate sections (each with individual chapters) on advanced imaging, interventional procedures, specific diagnosis, and anatomic considerations, these authors, along with those who have co-authored chapters, bring their material to life with the Socratic method, posing critical questions throughout the book and then answering them.

There are none more qualified than these three primary authors to guide us through the many areas of neuroimaging. Their deep knowledge of the field and their love of teaching—imparting knowledge, combined with a firm foundation of the underlying anatomy of the brain, head and neck, and spine and the associated imaging techniques—results in a textbook that will appeal to all levels of radiologists, from trainee to attending physician. Who better than Tom Naidich to lead us through the intricacies of brain anatomy and to show us how important this knowledge is when applying advanced imaging protocols, or Peter Som to take the reader through the basics of head and neck imaging and address questions of a critical nature related to ENT radiology, or Meng Law to demonstrate the current state-of-the-art of neuroimaging. For years I have learned from them, and to this day I marvel at their command of the intricacies of neuroimaging.

Congratulations to Drs. Law, Som, and Naidich, not only for conceiving this new way of presenting diagnostic imaging but also for offering to the neuroradiology and neuroscience community a book that will provide new insights into diagnosis and intervention in neurological diseases.

Robert M. Quencer, MD

Preface

Neuroradiology is a subspecialty field that has seen exciting advances over the past few decades. The advent of MRI in the 1980s began an era of new techniques for studying the central nervous system. Neurological disorders are often complex, and to make a diagnosis requires knowledge of neuroanatomy, neuropathology, and neurophysiology, as well as knowledge of the tools enabling us to image these entities. As a result, we hope to provide a textbook that describes how to resolve many of the diagnostic problems facing the clinician and diagnostician in a systematic fashion.

We approached this textbook by dividing it into four distinct sections, based in part on the expertise of the editors. The first section provides a state-of-the-art review of advanced imaging modalities available for problem solving, which can help increase the sensitivity and specificity of neurodiagnosis. In this section we review multidetector CT, conventional MRI, advanced MRI (including MR spectroscopy, perfusion, and diffusion), and nuclear medicine, in particular positron emission tomography, as problem-solving tools.

The second section addresses some of the procedures performed in neuroradiology, including diagnostic angiography, interventional neuroradiology or endovascular neurosurgery, and, of course, spine interventional procedures. The third and largest section approaches problem solving in neuroradiology in a disease-based fashion, covering brain and spine neuroradiologic pathology. The fourth section was developed to approach diseases in different anatomic regions, in particular spinal as well as head and neck disorders.

We recognize that to provide a comprehensive textbook in neuroradiology would be a challenge. So rather than covering every aspect of neuroradiology, this textbook serves as a practical approach toward problem solving. Our hope is that this will serve as a reference textbook that will benefit a spectrum of readers, from medical students, radiology residents, and neuroradiology fellows, to the seasoned neuroradiologist. Residents studying for the radiology board certification and fellows preparing for the certificate of added qualification (CAQ) examinations will find the combination of general knowledge and case-based sections to be valuable in a problem-solving approach. It may also be of benefit for students, residents, and practitioners in neurology, neurologic surgery, and the neurosciences.

Meng Law, MD, MBBS, FRACR
Peter M. Som, MD
Thomas P. Naidich, MD

Acknowledgments

I would like to acknowledge the invaluable assistance of my secretary, Ms. Elba Colman, for enabling me to complete this work.

TPN

Contents

SECTION I   ADVANCED MODALITIES: Protocols and Optimization

1. Multidetector Computed Tomography as a Problem-Solving Tool in Neuroradiology   3
   Rajiv Gupta, Sunithi Mani, Amit Mehndiratta, Stuart Pomerantz, and Michael Lev
2. Magnetic Resonance Imaging as a Problem-Solving Tool   61
   Jane J. Kim and Pratik Mukherjee
3. Advanced MR (MR Spectroscopy, Diffusion Imaging, Diffusion Tensor Imaging, and Perfusion Imaging): A Multiparametric Algorithmic Approach to Problem Solving in Neuroradiology   79
   Meng Law, Saulo Lacerda, and Pascal Bou-Haidar
4. PET/CT Imaging in Squamous Cell Carcinoma of the Head and Neck   126
   Lale Kostakoglu

SECTION II   PROCEDURES

5. Diagnostic Angiography   211
   Stephan Meckel and Stephan G. Wetzel
6. Neurointerventional Radiology   276
   Ruth Thiex, Ajit Puri, and Darren B. Orbach
7. Spine Procedures: Biopsies   299
   Wade Wong and Danielle Nanigian

SECTION III   PROBLEM SOLVING: Disease Categories

8. Neurodegenerative Disorders   333
   Manzoor Ahmed and Michael Phillips
9. Infection/Inflammation   361
   Majda M. Thurnher, Julia Frühwald-Pallamar, and Stefan B. Puchner
10. Metabolic Disorders   383
    Robert J. Young, Sofia S. Haque, and John K. Lyo
11. Tumor   412
    Marco Essig
12. Brain Trauma   427
    Alessandro Cianfoni and Cesare Colosimo
13. Imaging of Spine Trauma   473
    Alessandro Cianfoni and Cesare Colosimo
14. Imaging of Congenital Brain Abnormalities   496
    Andrea Rossi
15. Epilepsy   507
    Pascal Bou-Haidar, Saulo Lacerda, and Meng Law

16. Neuroimaging of Pediatric Hypoxic–Ischemic Injury 533
Andre D. Furtado, Saulo Lacerda, and Thomas P. Naidich

17. Intrauterine and Perinatal Infections 547
Andre D. Furtado, Saulo Lacerda, and Thomas P. Naidich

SECTION IV PROBLEM SOLVING: Anatomic Regions

18. Head and Neck Radiology 557
Girish M. Fatterpekar and Peter M. Som

19. Spine: Tumors and Infection 589
Paul E. Kim, Johan W.M. Van Goethem, and Alyssa T. Watanabe

20. Spine and Lower Back Pain 610
Johan W.M. Van Goethem, Paul E. Kim, and Alyssa T. Watanabe

SECTION I

Advanced Modalities: Protocols and Optimization

CHAPTER 1

Multidetector Computed Tomography as a Problem-Solving Tool in Neuroradiology

Rajiv Gupta, Sunithi Mani, Amit Mehndiratta, Stuart Pomerantz, and Michael Lev

■ INTRODUCTION

The concept of x-ray computed tomography (CT) was pioneered by Sir Godfrey Hounsfield at EMI Central Research Laboratories (Middlesex, United Kingdom) and concurrently by Allan McLeod Cormack at Tufts University (Boston, MA, USA). Their main idea of using multiple projections to create tomographic images formed the basis of the EMI scanner, the first clinical brain scanner. Since the days of the first brain scan in the early 1970s, CT has come a long way. Multidetector computed tomography (MDCT) has seen a steady increase in the capabilities, availability, and dedicated protocols for neurologic applications. Although magnetic resonance imaging (MRI) clearly plays an important role in neuroradiology, CT is the main workhorse. Table 1-1 lists a compilation of the main advantages and disadvantages of MDCT and MRI in neurologic applications.

This chapter illustrates how the excellent technical capabilities of a modern MDCT scanner can be put to use for problem solving in neuroradiology. The exposition is example driven. The requirements for the CT protocols for each application domain are summarized and illustrated with the help of clinical examples. Many clinical pearls and pitfalls are presented and illustrated. Guidelines for image acquisition and interpretation are discussed.

■ MDCT IN THE EMERGENCY DEPARTMENT

After a patient has been stabilized in the emergency department, imaging is directed at providing a clearer picture of the extent of injury and information about potential treatments. The ability of CT to rapidly image traumatic conditions has made it invaluable in acute neurotrauma management. CT is the vital imaging modality for determining the full extent and effects of the brain injury. Lesions commonly seen on CT include calvarial fractures, acute intraaxial and extraaxial hemorrhage, hemorrhagic contusions, diffuse axonal injury, and spinal fractures.

For emergent management, the lesions can be broadly classified as traumatic or nontraumatic. MDCT is the main diagnostic tool for both of these conditions. The salient features, protocols, and pitfalls in the use of MDCT for a variety of conditions encountered in the emergency department are summarized here.

Fractures

CT is excellent for showing bony anatomy and far exceeds the capabilities of MRI. With the advent of fast scanning and multiplanar reconstructions, it now is feasible to demonstrate various types of skull fractures in exquisite detail. For example, the various types of Le Fort fractures now can be depicted quickly and easily. Three-dimensional (3-D) renderings of these different fractures are invaluable to ear, nose, and throat (ENT) and plastic surgeons for rendering appropriate therapy. Because of their low sensitivity, skull radiographs have been supplanted by CT, which now is a part of emergency workup in nearly all trauma centers.

The optimal protocol for detecting calvarial and maxillofacial fractures requires thin axial slices constructed using a sharp kernel (e.g., bone kernel for a GE scanner or H50 sharp kernel for a Siemens scanner). The axial slices must be at least 1.25 mm thick with about 50% overlap. These scans may be augmented by coronal, sagittal, multiplanar oblique, or 3-D views to aid in visualization. The reviewing radiologist requires multiplanar reconstructions to assess bony asymmetries and alignment as well as certain structures that are optimally visualized in the coronal or sagittal imaging planes. The referring physicians require 3-D reconstructions for preoperative planning and intraoperative guidance. Figure 1-1 shows selected images from the case of a 45-year-old man who presented after a fall from a 30-foot ladder. The axial CT slices show fractures of the frontal eminence and parietal bone. However, the interrelationship between the fracture fragments is much better appreciated on the 3-D surface-rendered views, which show the extent of fracture from frontal eminence to parietal bone. Use of 3-D views is not limited to trauma cases. Figure 1.2 shows the similar application of the 3-D surface-rendering technique to visualize a congenital cranial malformation.

Table 1-1 Comparison of MDCT and MRI for Neurologic Applications

MDCT	MRI
Fast, more available	Slower, less available
Few contraindications	Multiple contraindications
Radiation exposure	No radiation exposure
Good for acute hemorrhage	Excellent for phases of hemorrhage
Excellent for bone and air–tissue interfaces	Poor visualization of bone, air–tissue interfaces
Poor soft tissue contrast	Great for soft tissues
Higher chance of contrast reaction	Lower chance of contrast reaction
Nephrotoxic contrast	Nephrotoxic contrast (NSF)
Can only measure attenuation	Sensitive to different tissue properties
Excellent contrast-enhanced angiograms	Good contrast-enhanced angiograms
Need contrast for computed tomographic angiography	Noncontrast magnetic resonance angiography (based on flow)

MDCT, Multidetector computed tomography; MRI, magnetic resonance imaging; NSF, nephrogenic systemic fibrosis.

The most common pitfall in evaluating calvarial and skull base fractures is improper protocol. Evaluation of the bony anatomy on slices that are too thick or do not use a sharp kernel can be detrimental. Figure 1-3, which shows thin slices reconstructed using a sharp kernel, demonstrates a subtle right occipital fracture that extends into the skull base. This fracture was missed on the slices acquired at 2.5-mm thickness and standard kernel. Due to the subgaleal hematoma in the vicinity and a high clinical suspicion, retrospective reconstructions at 1.25-mm slice thickness using a sharp kernel demonstrated the nondisplaced fracture shown in the figure.

The scenario described exemplifies a separate but related feature of MDCT. When the projection data are acquired using a helical or spiral protocol, thinner image slices can be retrospectively reconstructed at any user-defined spacing and overlap. This can be done as long as the raw projection data are available. Therefore, operationally it is mandatory for the raw projection data to be saved, at least for a few days after the scanning, while the clinical questions during acute care are still being addressed.

Even though tomographic slices are more sensitive in detecting fractures, scout views sometimes can show linear fractures that may be missed on the tomographic data (Figure 1-4). It is a good practice to always examine the scout view with all CT data. It also is a good practice to review sagittal and coronal views, which can be easily reconstructed on the scanner console. Coronal views are especially helpful because they are more forgiving of side-to-side misregistration, allowing easier comparison between the left and right sides. It is useful to have an individualized checklist of frequent misses, such as fractures of the condylar head, zygoma, around the foramen magnum, pterygoid plates (Le Fort fractures), and nasal bones.

Figure 1-5 shows the case of an 18-year-old man with a history of impaling his face onto the branch of a tree who presented with facial paresthesias. CT scan images show a hypodense foreign body adjacent to the infraorbital nerve that extends into the anterior wall of the left maxillary sinus. Subcutaneous emphysema is present along the entrance track adjacent to the infraorbital foramen. The sagittal and coronal images also demonstrate the foreign body and mucosal thickening in the left maxillary sinus.

Figure 1-6 shows a common pitfall in CT scans of traumatic injury. A CT scan was performed on a 54-year-old man who fell from a tree and complained of irritation in the left eye. Axial CT scan demonstrated proptosis of the left globe with air in the extraconal post-septal region, along the lateral aspect of the orbit, extending posteriorly up to the orbital apex. This was presumed to be posttraumatic air, likely secondary to a fracture. However, a fracture was not identified. The patient returned 2 months later, when MRI scan showed persistent proptosis and extensive inflammatory and phlegmonous changes with enhancement. The central nonenhancing portion was thought to be the necrotic core of an abscess. The patient was emergently taken to the operating room, where a 2-cm wood chip was removed from the left orbit. The take-home point is that wood can have a variety of appearances on CT, with dry wood essentially resembling air in Hounsfield units (HU).

Intracranial Hemorrhage

Hemorrhage due to a direct mechanism, either penetrating or blunt, may be extraaxial (epidural or subdural), intraparenchymal, or associated with a brain contusion. All of these pathologies, with varying degrees of sensitivity and specificity, can be detected and characterized using MDCT. Rotational forces can lead to hemorrhagic shear and diffuse axonal injury at characteristic locations such as the corpus callosum and gray–white junction. CT has relatively low sensitivity for diffuse axonal injury, which is apparent on only 20% to 50% of initial CT scans. Diffuse axonal injury lesions that are visible are commonly found in the subcortical white matter, centrum semiovale, corpus callosum, basal ganglia, brainstem, and cerebellum.

The volume inside the calvaria is limited and fixed. This volume is composed of three components: cerebrospinal fluid, blood, and brain tissue. According to the Monro-Kellie hypothesis, intracranial pressure remains stable as long as the volume added to any one of these components is balanced by the volume displaced. Therefore, a sudden rise in the amount of any one of these components may cause the intracranial pressure to increase if the volume of the other two components remains constant. The greatest risk to a patient with any traumatic injury is a fast-growing intracranial hematoma leading to increased intracranial pressure and

Chapter 1 Multidetector Computed Tomography as a Problem-Solving Tool in Neuroradiology

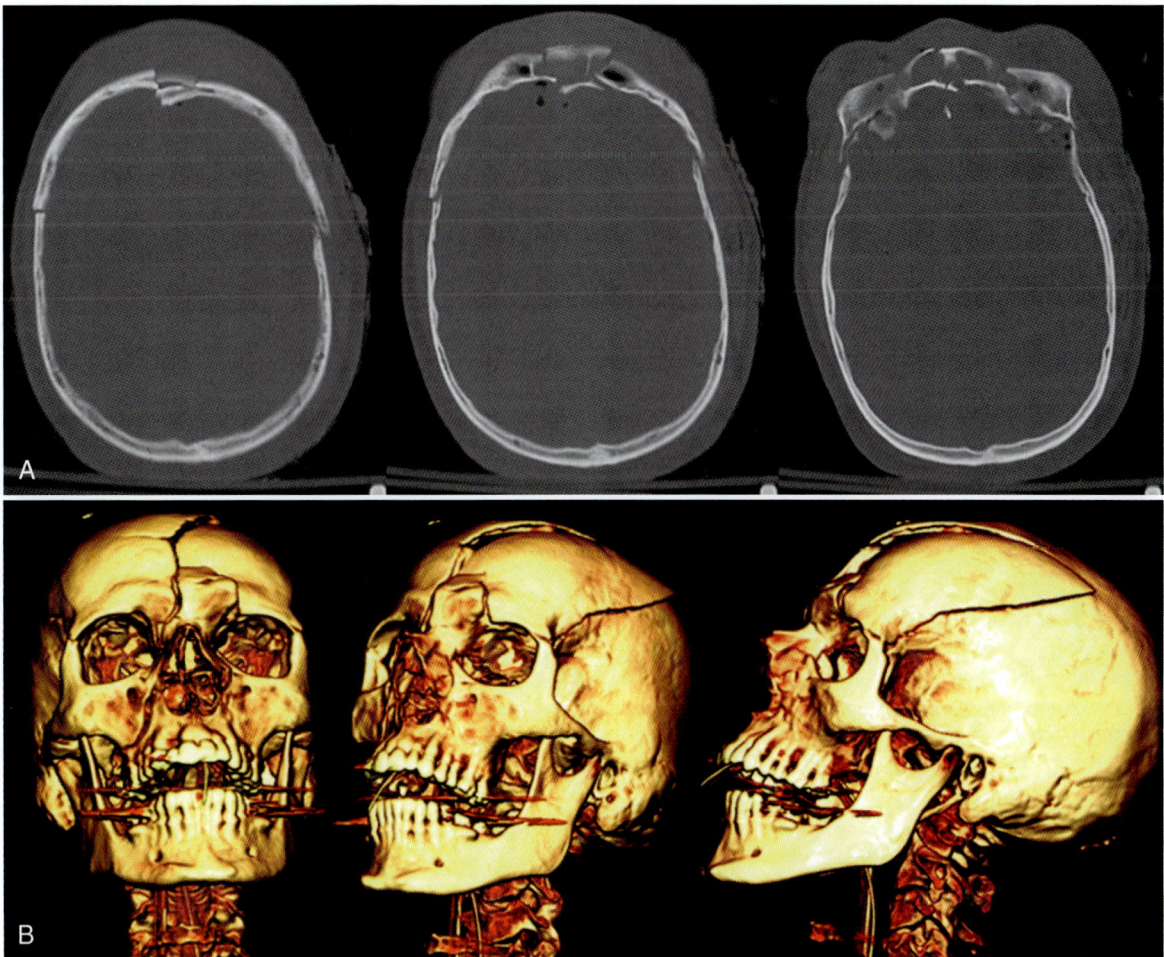

Figure 1-1 Noncontrast maxillofacial multidetector computed tomography of a 45-year-old man who presented with a history of a fall from a 30-foot ladder. **A:** Axial computed tomographic slices showing fracture through the frontal eminence and parietal bone. **B:** The extent of fracture from the frontal eminence to the left parietal bone and the relationship between the various fracture fragments are much better appreciated on these three-dimensional surface-rendered views.

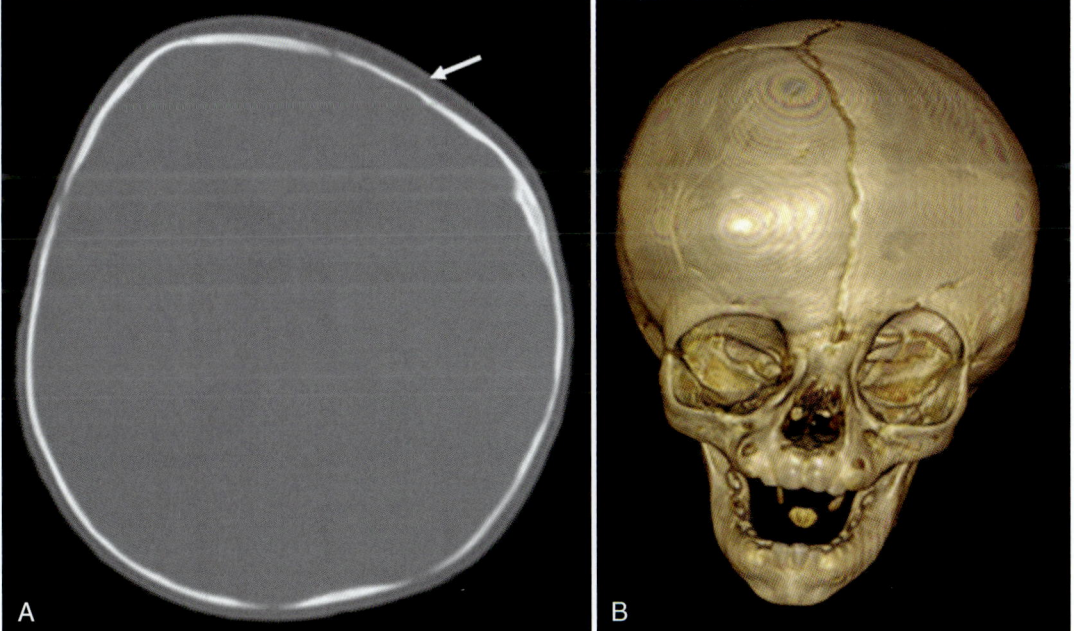

Figure 1-2 Congenital craniofacial malformations are better demonstrated using three-dimensional (3-D) surface-rendered views than routine axial views. Axial **(A)** and 3-D surfaced-rendered **(B)** views of plagiocephaly in a neonatal patient.

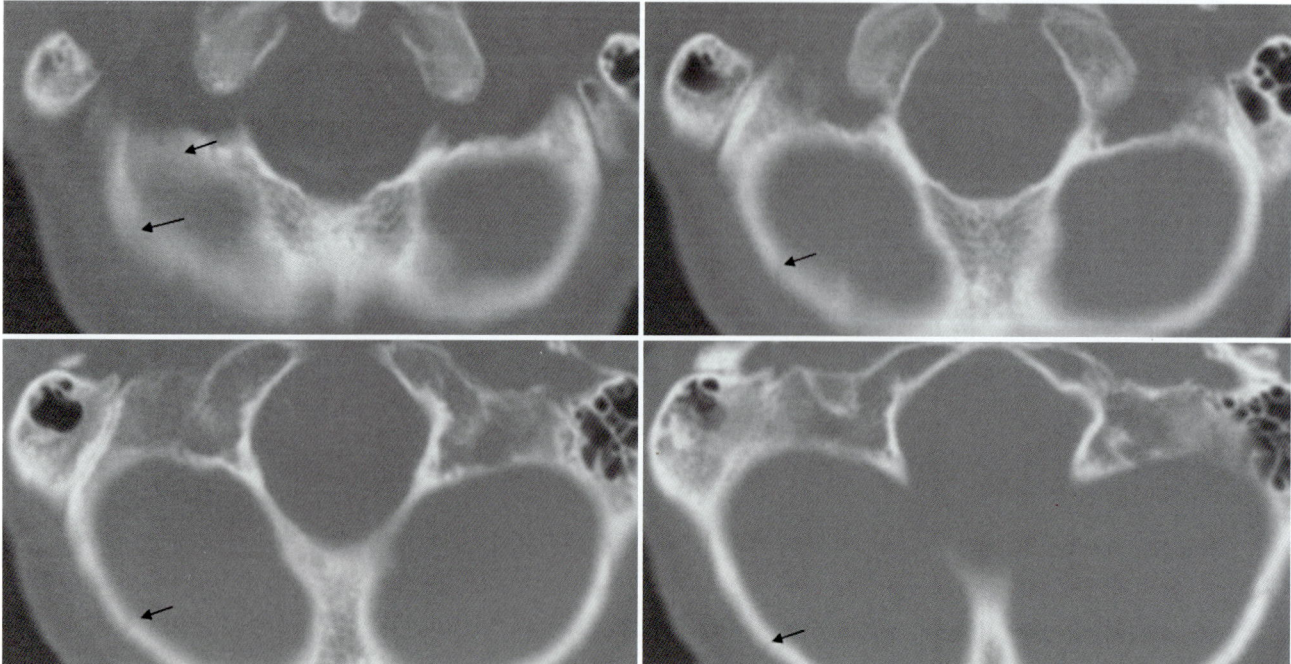

Figure 1-3 Subtle, nondisplaced fracture of the right occipital bone that was not visible on thicker slices. Adjacent subgaleal hematoma overlying the fracture is better seen on the soft tissue windows.

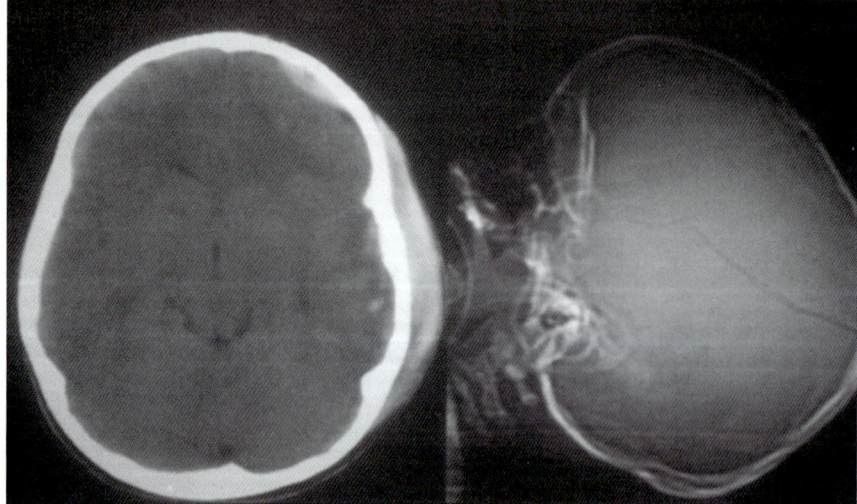

Figure 1-4 Left parietal fracture that is more easily visualized on the scout view.

herniation. The occurrence of this potentially fatal complication is not apparent until clinical deterioration has started and recovery already is endangered.

Intraaxial hematoma may stop because of the tamponade effect from the surrounding brain parenchyma, or it may grow in size over time. It may cause midline shift, herniation, or ventricular entrapment, or it may cross into an adjacent compartment (i.e., become a subarachnoid or intraventricular hemorrhage).

Extraaxial hematoma may be due to an arterial or a venous bleed. Typically, epidural hematomas result from arterial bleeds because arterial pressure is required for the blood to dissect between the outer layer of the dura and the skull. Classically, it presents as a convex hyperdense collection that stops at the sutures. A subdural blood collection in the hemorrhage is generally a result of venous bleed. Subarachnoid hemorrhage is most commonly caused by aneurysmal bleed but also may be posttraumatic.

MDCT is an ideal modality for evaluating intracranial hemorrhage. On a noncontrast CT scan, which is both quite sensitive and specific in detecting hemorrhage, acute blood products appear hyperdense compared with normal brain parenchyma. If intracranial hemorrhage is in the differential, a noncontrast CT scan must be performed before contrast is given. Coronal images have been shown to improve the sensitivity and specificity of detection.

In the emergency department setting, it is important to be aware of many pitfalls in the detection of acute intracranial hemorrhage. First, close attention must be paid to the window-level setting for viewing the images because a subtle hematoma may be missed if an improper window-level setting is used (Figure 1-7). An acute subdural hematoma (SDH) that is less than 72 hours old appears hyperdense compared to brain parenchyma on a CT scan. As the blood products evolve, they progressively become hypodense. A subacute SDH (3 days to 3 weeks old) may appear either isodense or hypodense, whereas a chronic SDH that is more than 3 weeks old is generally always hypodense. An isodense SDH may blend in with the adjacent brain parenchyma, making detection difficult, especially when it is bilateral (Figure 1-8). Medial displacement of the gray–white matter interface and verification that the sulci extend up to the inner table of the calvaria are important radiologic findings when an isodense SDH is present.

Acute ongoing bleeding imparts a complex appearance to otherwise subacute or chronic hemorrhage. Because the morbidity and mortality associated with spontaneous intracerebral hemorrhage are correlated with hematoma progression, early radiologic signs that predict hematoma expansion have been a subject of active research. Patients who present very early to the hospital and those who are taking anticoagulation medications are likely to show hematoma expansion after presentation to the emergency department. Presence of gadolinium-based contrast agent in the hematoma during MRI scanning has been associated with later hematoma expansion. A similar sign for CT scanning has been identified; extravasation of CT contrast agent into the hematoma has been shown to predict hematoma expansion.

Goldstein and colleagues showed that contrast extravasation within the hematoma on computed tomographic angiography (CTA) represents ongoing bleeding. Therefore, this so-called spot sign identifies patients who are at high risk for subsequent hematoma expansion (Figure 1-9) and thus can be used to select patients who are most likely to benefit from interventions aimed at arresting ongoing bleeding. Spot sign, which has a very high negative predictive value, was independently confirmed by Wada and colleagues, who showed that the presence of tiny enhancing foci in the hematoma after administration of contrast is associated with hematoma expansion. They found the sensitivity, specificity, positive predictive value, negative predictive value, and

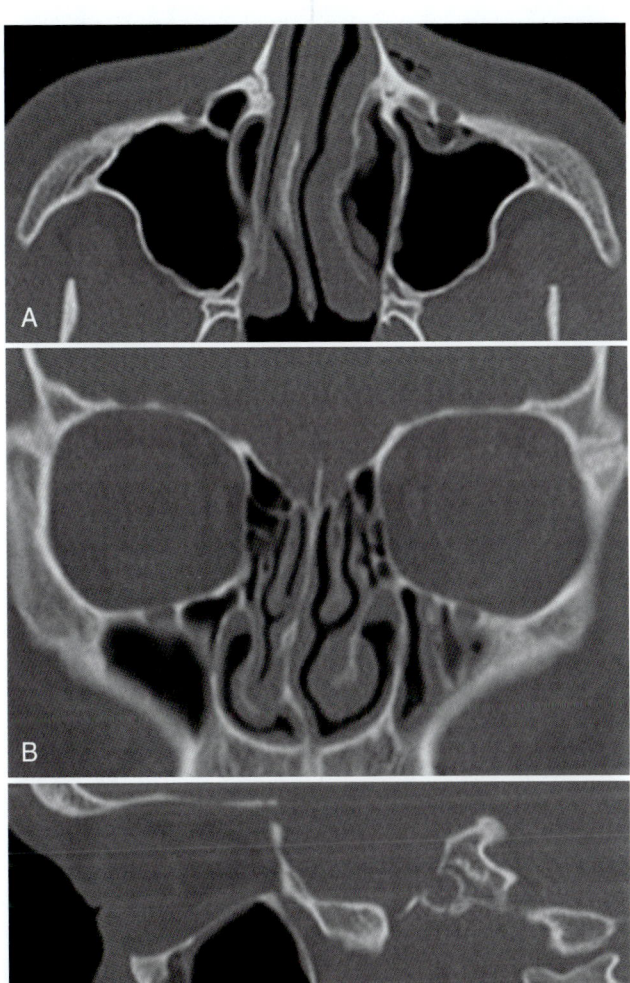

Figure 1-5 Patient with facial paresthesias after being impaled by a tree branch. Triplanar computed tomographic images at the level of the infraorbital foramen show a foreign body adjacent to the infraorbital nerve. **A:** Axial slice showing the foreign body in the anterior wall of the left maxillary sinus. **B, C:** Full extent of the foreign body in sagittal and coronal sections respectively.

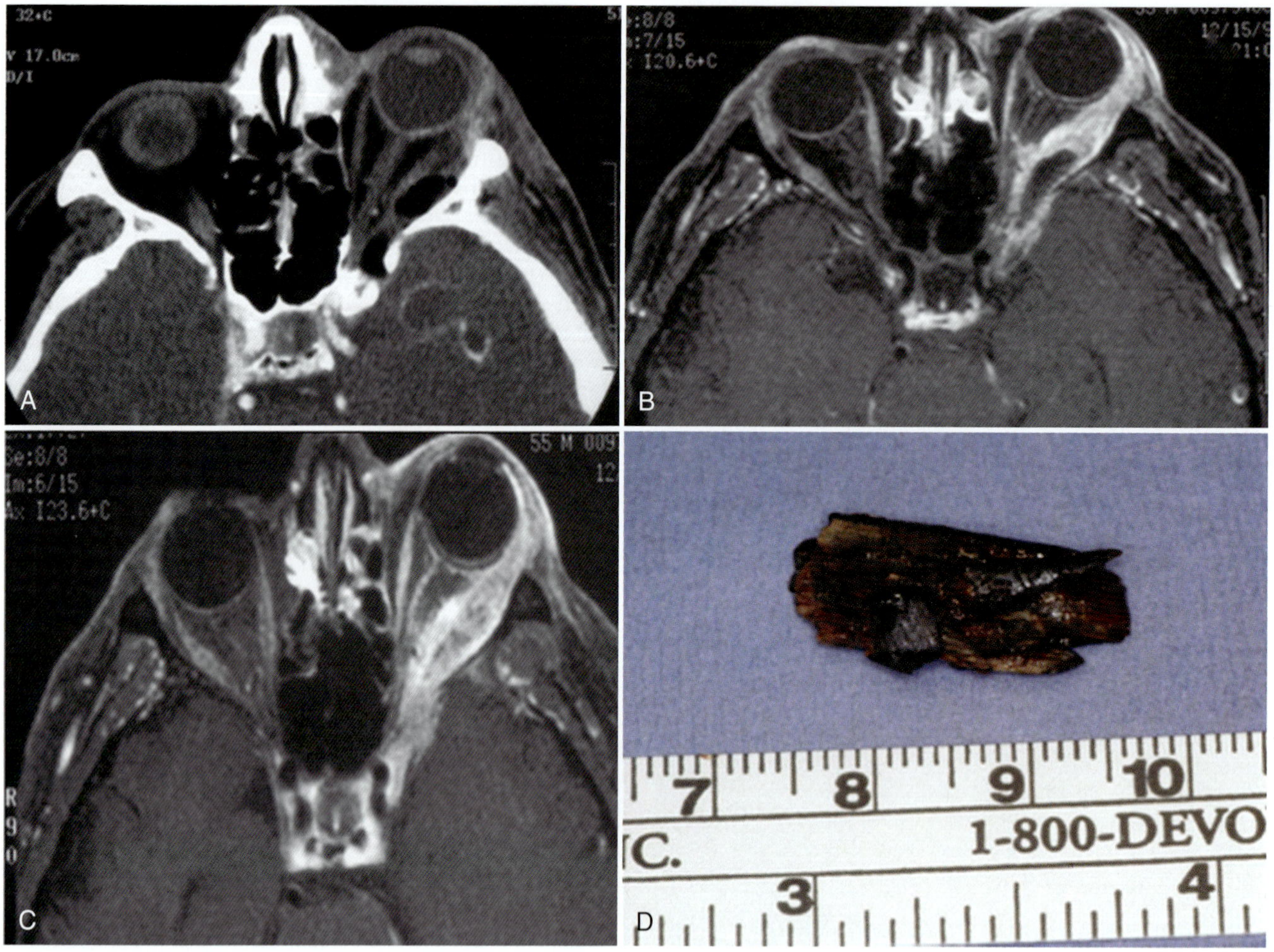

Figure 1-6 Multidetector computed tomography in a patient with pain in the left eye after a fall from a tree. **A:** Axial slice showing a focus of low density lateral to the left lateral rectus muscle that was assumed to be posttraumatic air. **B, C:** Axial postcontrast magnetic resonance images acquired 2 months later showing persistent proptosis, inflammatory changes, and enhancement in the same region with central nonenhancing component. **D:** A 2-cm piece of wood that was removed from the left orbit. (Images courtesy Drs. Huey-Jen Lee, University of Medicine and Dentistry, New Jersey (UMDNJ), and Michelle Rotblat, Massachusetts General Hospital (MGH), Boston.)

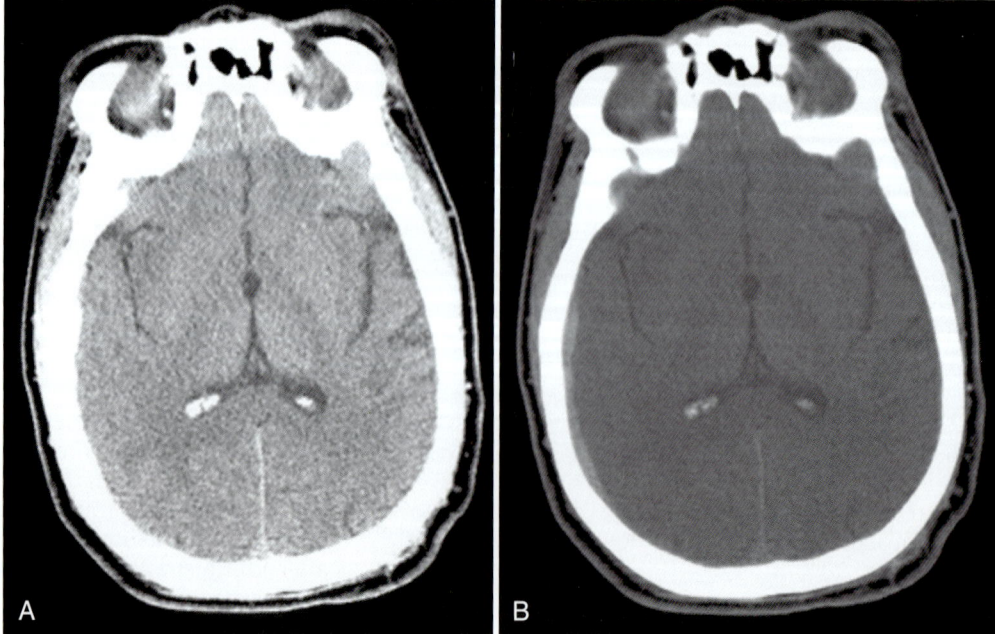

Figure 1-7 Subtle subdural hematoma after traumatic injury, axial brain section view at L = 30 HU, W = 100 HU **(A)** and L = 80 HU, W = 200 HU **(B)**. Note the importance of proper window-level setting for visualization of a small right temporoparietal subdural hematoma.

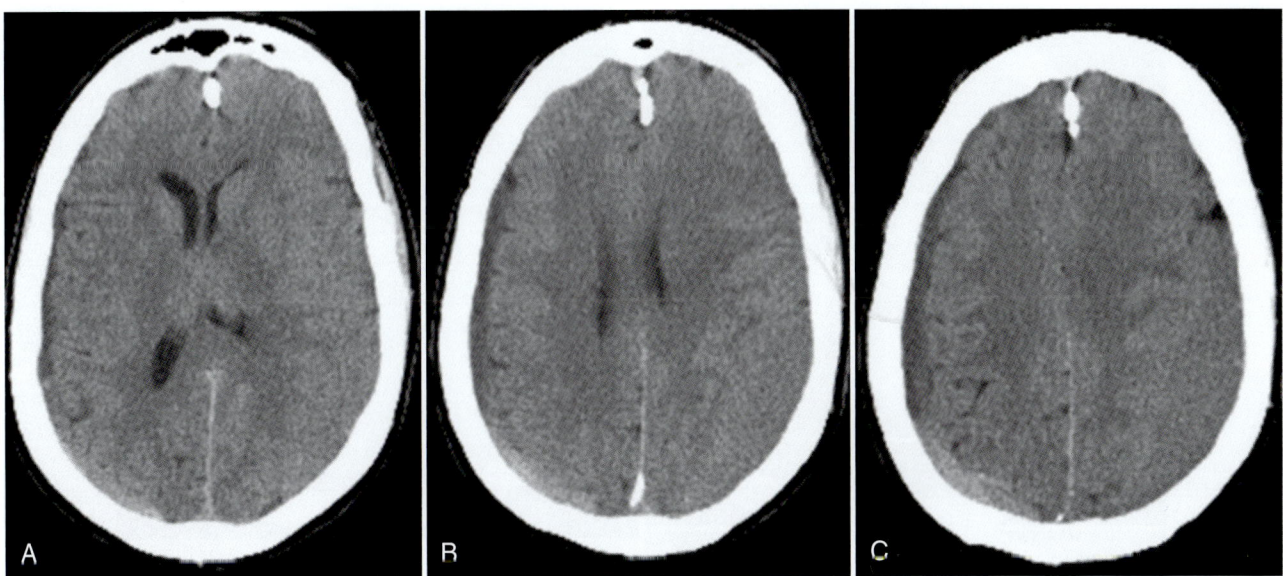

Figure 1-8 Axial brain scans showing isodense subdural hematoma that may be hard to detect because it blends in with brain parenchyma.

likelihood ratio of this finding for expansion were 91%, 89%, 77%, 96%, and 8.5, respectively.

Noncontrast CT is quite sensitive for detecting subarachnoid hemorrhage. If a subarachnoid hemorrhage is detected, contrast-enhanced CTA should be performed next to rule out an aneurysm. Modern scanners cover the entire head in less than 15 seconds after contrast administration. The delay between the start of contrast injection and the start of image acquisition can be varied to image either the arterial or the venous phase of opacification. Therefore, vascular pathologies, such as aneurysm, arteriovenous malformation (AVM), dural arteriovenous fistula, cavernous carotid fistula, and venous sinus thrombosis, can be detected. Although conventional catheter angiography remains the gold standard for aneurysm imaging, CT has replaced it as the first-line modality. The sensitivity of CTA in detecting small aneurysms is only marginally inferior to that of conventional angiography. For example, it can clearly depict any partial thrombosis of the aneurysm, size of the neck, neck-to-dome ratio, small vessels near the base of the aneurysm, and any vessels arising from the aneurysm sac (Figure 1-10). In most situations, CTA provides sufficient information that will guide the staff in making the decision to take the patient directly to the operating room, thus obviating the need for invasive angiography.

■ MDCT IN MANAGEMENT OF ACUTE STROKE

Acute stroke is a clinical syndrome. Approximately 15% of acute strokes are hemorrhagic; the remaining 85% are ischemic. A tally of acute stroke presentations at our institution from 1999 to 2005 revealed that approximately 30% of ischemic strokes were cardioembolic, 30% from large vessels, 20% from small vessels/lacunar, and 20% from other or unknown etiologies. The majority of hemorrhagic strokes were primarily hypertensive. The overall mortality was close to 15%, with no mortality attributable to lacunar infarcts.

CT scanning plays a pivotal role in the management of acute stroke and is the first-line imaging modality when a patient suspected of having acute stroke arrives in the emergency department. A combination of noncontrast CT and CTA provides a quick and noninvasive method for ruling out hemorrhage, detecting regional ischemia, and demonstrating the site of vascular occlusion. In addition, CT perfusion imaging, currently a subject of intense research, has the potential for determining not only the tissue that has progressed to infarction but also the tissue in the ischemic penumbra that is at risk. Major advances in neuroprotective therapeutic regimens in conjunction with such advanced imaging have the potential to limit the ischemic damage beyond the core of the infarct.

Figure 1-11 shows a typical sequence of imaging examinations that are undertaken at a specialized stroke center to manage acute stroke. The sequence is discussed in the following subsections.

Non–Contrast-Enhanced CT

A noncontrast CT scan is the first-line imaging study in patients suspected of having acute stroke. This simple, noninvasive examination reveals a wealth of information that is available immediately and has a direct impact on clinical management. It quickly helps in determining if the signs and symptoms being observed can be attributed to intracranial hemorrhage (i.e., hemorrhagic stroke), hydrocephalus, or a mass lesion. If any of these conditions is determined to be the case, noncontrast CT may be followed by CTA or MRI for further evaluation. In most instances, an acute stroke is quite apparent from the clinical presentation. The biggest contribution of noncontrast CT is ruling out intracranial hemorrhage so that appropriately selected patients

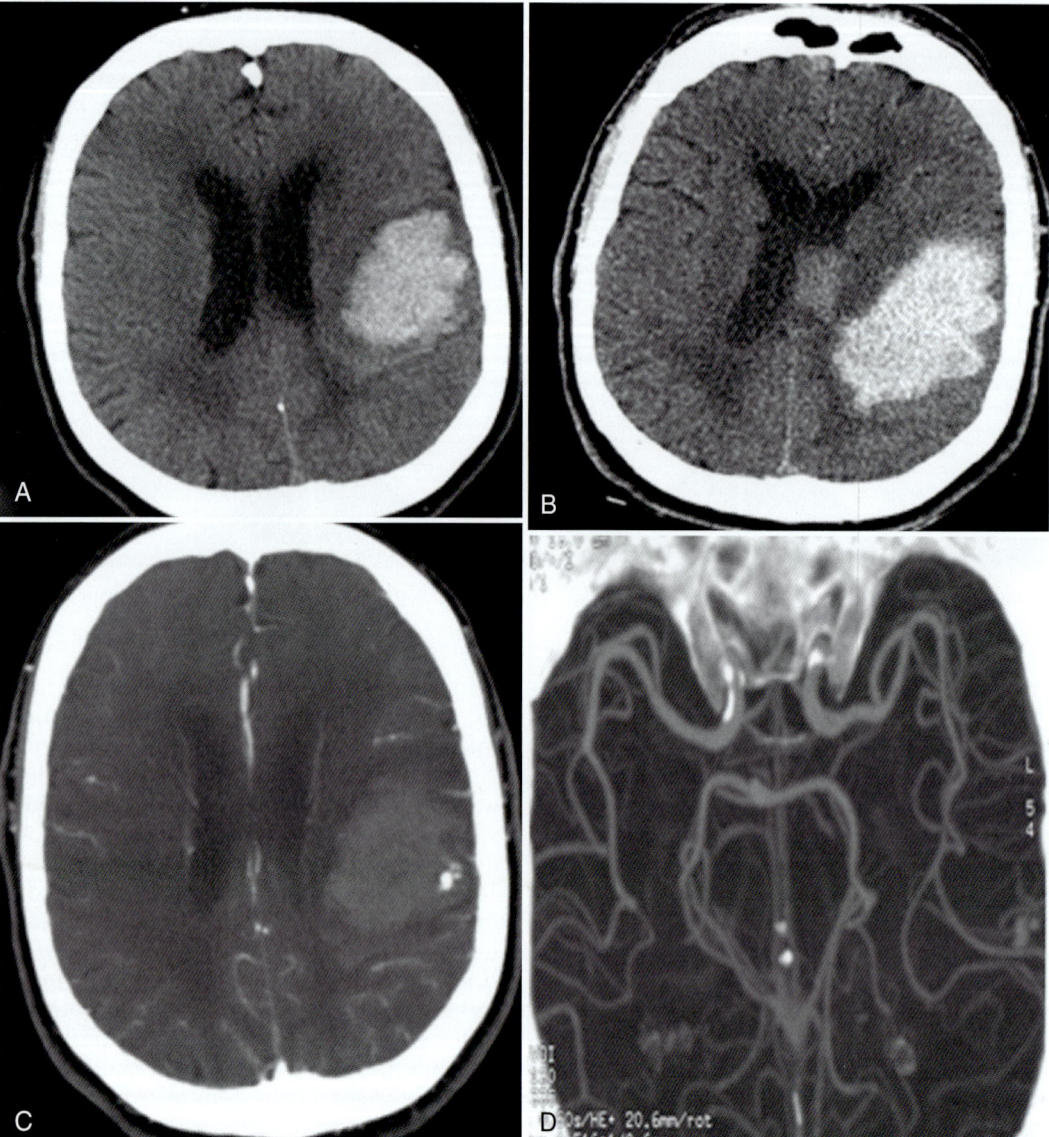

Figure 1-9 Hematoma at presentation (**A**) and 1 day later (**B**) showing interval growth of hematoma. Computed tomographic scan (**C**) after contrast has been administered for acquisition of an angiogram (**D**). Active extravasation of contrast into the hematoma can be readily appreciated in **C** and **D**. This so-called *spot sign* correlates with hematoma expansion.

can be started on intravenous (IV) tissue plasminogen activator (tPA) therapy. For this reason, noncontrast CT is part of the guidelines for management of acute stroke.

The current imaging standard of care in acute stroke is performing an unenhanced CT to rule out hemorrhage and ensuring that the area of infarct at presentation (i.e., the total area of hypodensity in the CT scan) is less than one third of the middle cerebral artery (MCA) territory. If these inclusion criteria are met, the only treatments approved by the US Food and Drug Administration are IV thrombolysis or clot retrieval. IV thrombolysis is recommended only for those cases in which the time of onset of symptoms is known and in which fewer than 3 hours have elapsed from the time of onset to administration of IV tPA. Given these stringent requirements, less than 20% of patients are triaged for evaluation and less than 5% eventually receive IV thrombolysis. The MERCI clot retrieval device (Concentric Medical Inc, Mountain View, CA) is gaining popularity at some centers for patients who do not meet the time window for IV tPA.

In most instances, an acute stroke is quite apparent from the clinical presentation. However, the many mimics of clinical stroke include transient ischemic attacks (TIAs), syncope, dizziness, lightheadedness, seizures, hypoglycemia, tumors, and demyelinating conditions. Similarly, not all new hypodensities on noncontrast CT represent a stroke. Multiple signs point to an acute stroke on a non–contrast-enhanced CT, including (1) a focal area of parenchymal hypoattenuation, (2) cortical swelling resulting in effacement of the normal gyral and sulcal pattern, (3) loss of gray–white differentiation, and (4) a dense vessel sign, typically the MCA or one of its sylvian branches, reflecting thrombus within the lumen of the involved vessel. Some signs of an ischemic stroke on CT can be subtle; however, with proper attention to

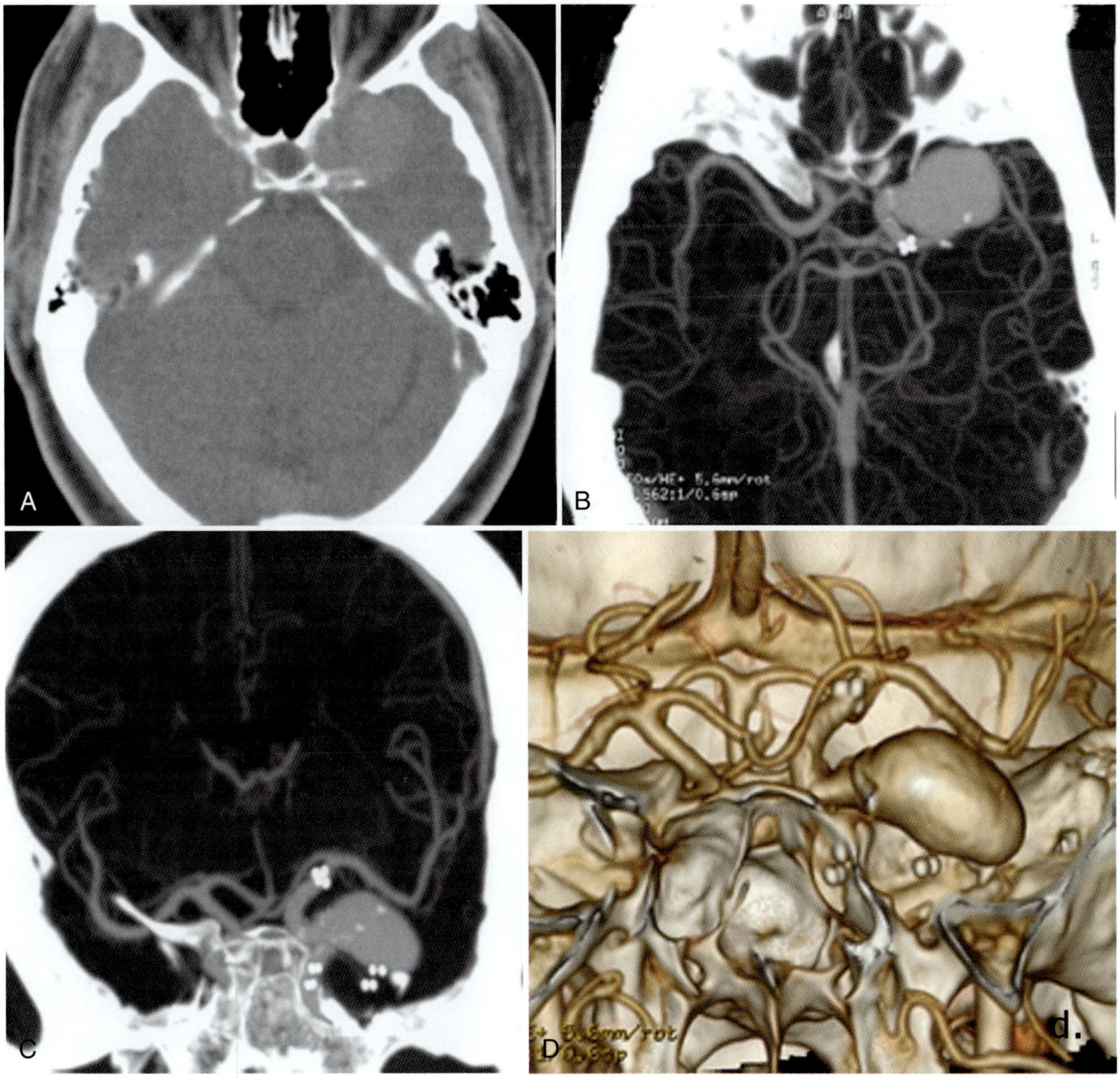

Chapter 1 Multidetector Computed Tomography as a Problem-Solving Tool in Neuroradiology

Figure 1-10 Multidetector computed tomographic images from contrast-enhanced computed tomographic angiography showing an internal carotid artery aneurysm.

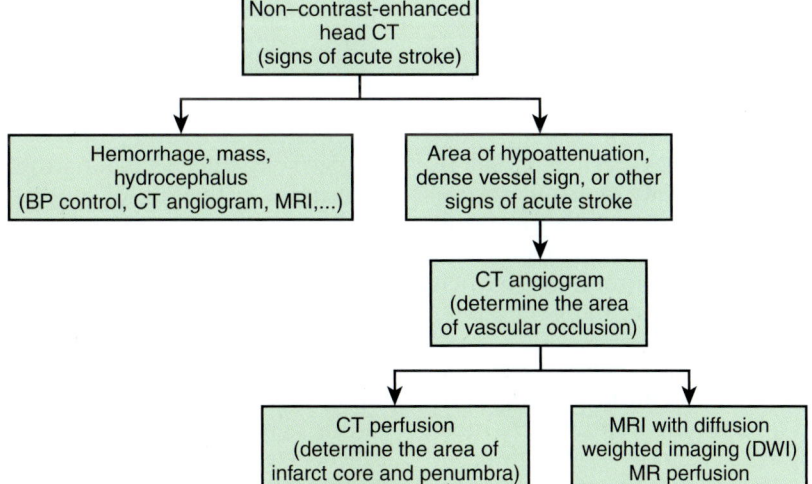

Figure 1-11 Sequence of imaging steps in the management of acute stroke.

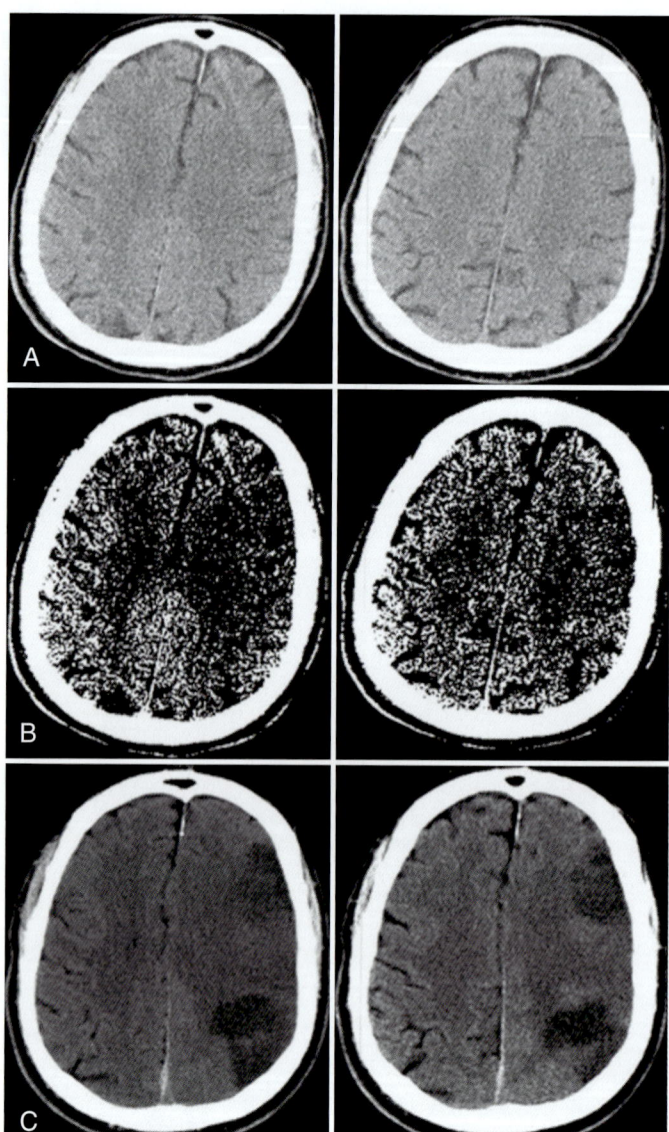

Figure 1-12 A: Pair of contiguous slices displayed using standard window-level setting (L = 80 HU, W = 20 HU) from a patient who presented with acute stroke symptoms. The area of infarction is difficult to discern. **B:** The same slices with a narrow window-level setting (L = 32 HU, W = 8 HU). The subtle areas of loss of gray–white differentiation in left frontal and parietal regions are much more apparent and are concordant with later images showing fully developed infarcted regions (**C**).

detail and window-level settings, in most instances they can be visualized within 6 hours of symptom onset.

Early during an acute stroke, the slight decrease in the CT number of the involved brain parenchyma is thought to be a result of cytotoxic edema, presumably from a failure of energy-dependent cell membrane pumps. Later, vasogenic edema may be responsible for the apparent drop in density. In the evolution of an infarct, a phenomenon called *infarct fogging* has been reported in which the hypoattenuation secondary to the infarct disappears after 2 to 6 weeks. This is thought be the result of higher-density cellular infiltrate in the infarction bed. The infarct reappears in the more chronic stage when the cellular infiltrate clears and cavitary and/or encephalomalacic changes set in.

In order to not miss the subtle changes associated with an acute infarct, it is important to use appropriate window width and level setting. Typically, for most parenchymal pathologies a window-level setting of W = 20 HU and L = 80 HU is used. Lev and colleagues evaluated the use of nonstandard, variable window width and level settings for the detection of acute stroke. Specifically, they determined the sensitivity and specificity of the standard center level and window width settings of 20 and 80 HU. These settings were compared with variable soft-copy settings initially centered at a level of 32 HU and a width of 8 HU. They found that use of variable soft-copy settings improved the sensitivity of stroke detection from 57% to 71% without loss of specificity. The fact that narrow window-level settings help in the evaluation of subtle changes in attenuation is illustrated in Figure 1-12.

Besides ruling out intracranial hemorrhage and demonstrating the areas of infarctions, a noncontrast CT can sometimes show the acute thrombus responsible for the vascular compromise. This finding presents as a hyperdense segment of an intracranial vessel and can involve either an artery or a vein. The most common location of this sign is in the proximal MCA, resulting in the so-called dense MCA sign. In the anterior circulation, the hyperdense vessel sign is highly specific for proximal MCA and its sylvian branches. The sign is not as useful

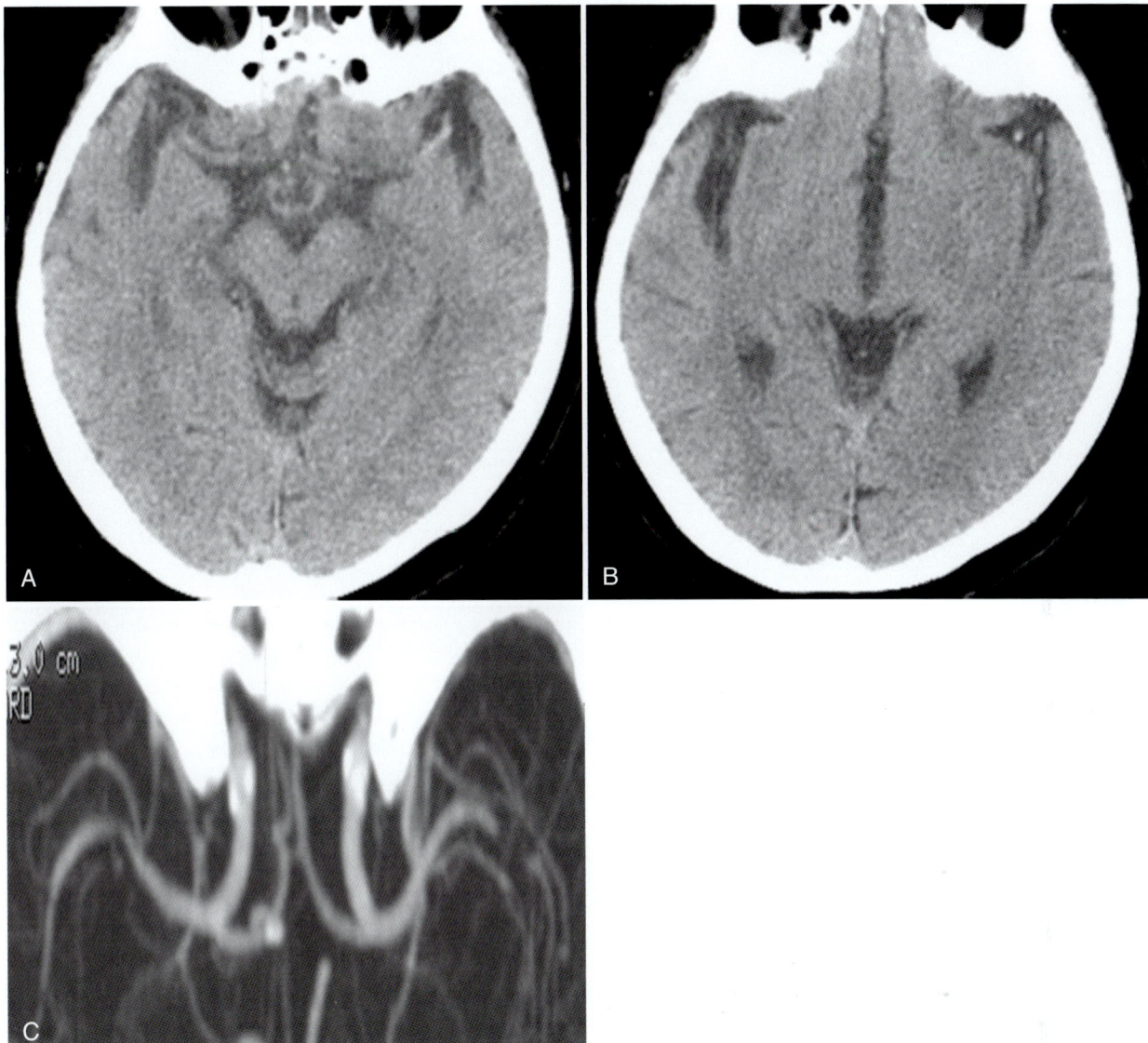

Figure 1-13 Middle cerebral artery (MCA) dot sign. **A, B:** Hyperdense left MCA showing acute thrombus on noncontrast computed tomography. **C:** Computed tomographic angiography showing the corresponding cutoff in the left MCA.

in the posterior circulation. The prognostic value of this sign in predicting thrombolysis efficacy and for differentiating between the so-called red and white clot has been studied. Figure 1-13 shows the presence of hyperdense MCA in an acute stroke setting. Figure 1-14 shows a slightly different and rarer presentation of this sign from thrombosis of a deep vein that resulted in a venous infarct (not shown in figure).

Non contrast CT can suffer from a variety of artifacts that degrade image quality. In order to avoid misinterpretation, it is essential to understand the genesis of these artifacts in order to properly account for them. Beam-hardening artifacts in the posterior fossa are common and somewhat symmetric. The primary concern with so-called spray or metallic artifacts emanating from aneurysm clips, coils, or embolization material, such as Onyx (ev3 Neurovascular, Inc, Irvine, CA), is that they can hide important pathology such as hemorrhage, infarct, or aneurysm neck in their vicinity. Improper positioning of the patient resulting in a tilted reconstruction plane also can introduce asymmetries that can be misinterpreted. The effect of many of these artifacts can be minimized by incorporating coronal images in the reading routine. At our institution, coronal images that correct for head tilt are reconstructed for all noncontrast CT scans performed for the evaluation of head trauma. These views can be constructed directly at the scanner and pushed to the PACS (Picture Archiving and Communication System) along with the axial images. Our experience to date reveals that these views are invaluable for ruling out subtle subarachnoid hemorrhage, small SDHs adjacent to the falx and tentorial leaflets, blowout fractures of the orbital floor, and brain contusions, especially in the anterior temporal and frontal lobes.

CT Angiography

CTA is the study of choice for all emergent and nonemergent neurovascular conditions, including acute stroke. Compared to MRI, it is faster, cheaper, more available,

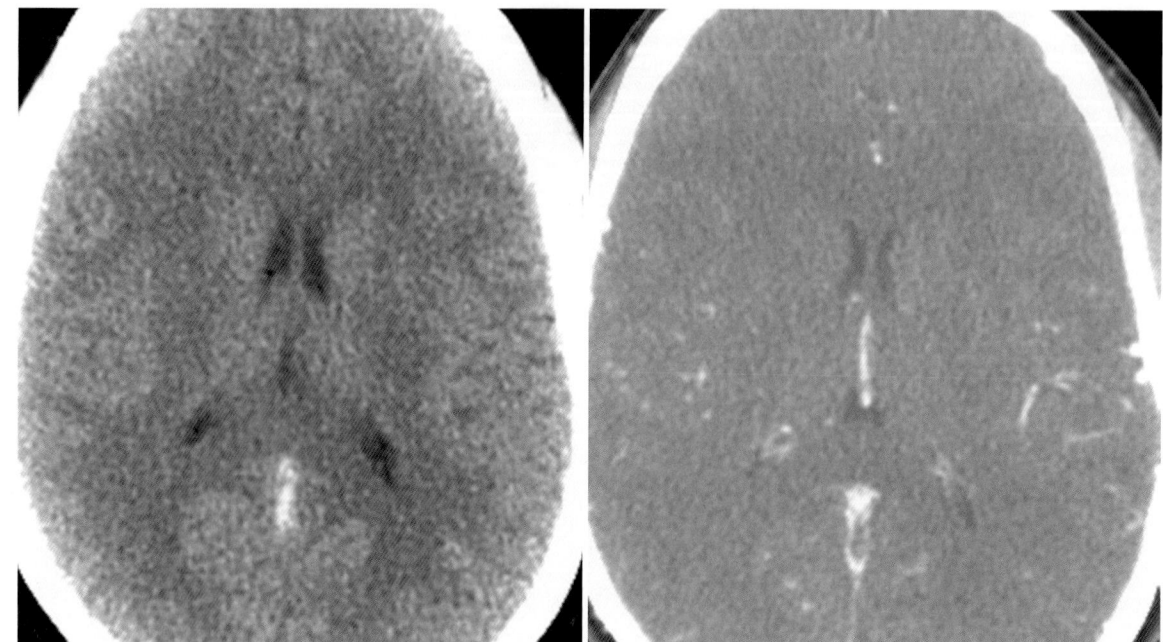

Figure 1-14 Noncontrast computed tomography (CT) showing a linear hyperdensity near the confluence of the vein of Galen and the straight sinus *(left)* that appears as a filling defect on CT venogram *(right)*, consistent with deep venous thrombosis.

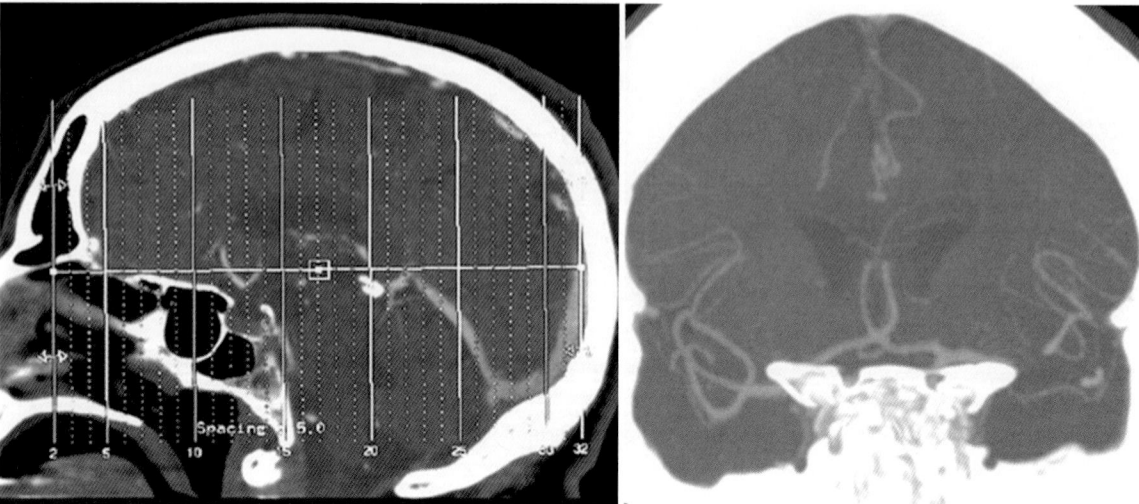

Figure 1-15 Individual 1.25-mm computed tomographic angiographic images can be quite numerous and tedious to go through when the scan is being checked at the scanner. It is possible to generate 30-mm-thick slabs at 5-mm intervals *(left)* (i.e., 25-mm overlap between adjacent slabs) in all three planes. The thick slabs are much easier to review than the individual axial slices *(right)*.

and less prone to artifacts. MRI may be useful as a screening tool, especially when ionizing radiation is a concern (e.g., in pediatric patients). However, CTA is the confirmatory test and is competitive with catheter angiography, the current gold standard for vascular imaging.

In an acute stroke setting, cervical and upper thoracic vasculature should be evaluated in addition to the intracranial vasculature. A combined CTA of the head and neck, from the aortic arch to the cranial vertex, can be obtained with as little as 70 ml of IV contrast in less than 15 seconds. Images should be acquired at slice thickness of at least 1.25 mm, preferably with 50% overlap. In order to facilitate quick visualization of the great arteries, thick 30-mm slabs with a reconstruction interval of 5 mm have proved to be quite effective (Figure 1-15). It is important that slabs overlap with each other so that the vasculature changes slowly as the images are paged through. The technologist can generate these images at the scanner in a matter of minutes, and all three planes can be generated equally easily while correcting for head tilt. The views are extremely useful in providing a quick wet-read in emergent situations and are quite appropriate for making triage decisions before the patient is removed from the CT table. Three-dimensional maximal intensity projection (MIP) images and curved reformats also are useful but require a dedicated core laboratory for generating the views.

An area of hypoattenuation is a nonspecific finding on a noncontrast CT scan and does not necessarily represent an acute stroke. The etiology of this finding may be revealed by CTA. If the hypoattenuation does, in fact, represent an acute stroke, it may be the result of an embolus from a cardiac, carotid, or intracranial arterial source. Arterial atherosclerotic plaque is most often the culprit. Cardiac etiologies include valvular vegetations, tumors, endocarditis, and intracardiac right to left shunts (e.g., patent foramen ovale). A dissection or pseudoaneurysm also may result in an embolic phenomenon. In only a minority of cases does a venous compromise result in an infarction. Most of these etiologies of acute stroke can be directly visualized on CTA of the head and neck (Figures 1-16 through 1-19).

Given the high prevalence of cardiogenic acute strokes, it now is possible to extend the field of coverage of CTA to include the heart in the evaluation. Shapiro, Neilan, and colleagues showed the feasibility of detecting left atrial (LA) appendage thrombus using CT. MDCT has sensitivity of 80%, specificity of 73%, and negative predictive value of 92% for detection of LA appendage thrombus. Therefore, a subgroup of patients at very high risk for LA appendage thrombus may benefit from the high negative predictive value of cardiac MDCT performed in conjunction with a stroke CTA. In this protocol, gated helical cardiac acquisition is performed after a vertex-to-arch CTA is completed. Only 15 ml of additional contrast is needed to complete the additional imaging. Figure 1-20 shows a thrombus in the LA appendage detected using this protocol.

Figure 1-21 shows a computed tomographic venogram (CTV) demonstrating the delta sign from a thrombus in the superior sagittal sinus. The full extent of the dural sinus thrombosis can be appreciated in the 3-D view after automatic bone subtraction.

Figure 1-22 shows an area of hypoattenuation, with internal areas of hyperattenuation, in the left middle and posterior cerebral artery territories. In the absence of a prior history, the differential considerations for these findings include (1) traumatic contusion, (2) hemorrhage from hypertension, bleeding diathesis, amyloid angiopathy, or AVM, (3) infarction from one of many different etiologies, and (4) hemorrhagic tumor. MDCT can help narrow down the differential. Because the area of signal abnormality does not conform to a single vascular territory, an embolic infarct from a purely arterial source is unlikely. In this case, CTA revealed the intracranial arteries to be patent. Because the timing difference between the arterial and venous phases of a contrast bolus is small (intracranial circulation is a low-resistance circuit), most CTAs can be easily converted to combined CTA/CTV by lengthening the duration of the bolus and acquiring the images approximately 10 seconds later than those for CTA. In this case, combined CTA/CTV revealed complete occlusion of the left transverse sinus, confirming a venous infarct.

Occlusion of a venous sinus or cortical vein may be initiated by a partial thrombus or extrinsic compression. This initial insult subsequently progresses to complete occlusion. Once initiated, a thrombus may extend in retrograde fashion into the veins draining into the involved sinus. The resulting lack of venous outflow and the concomitant rise in venous pressure ultimately result in a cortical venous infarction. Venous infarctions are frequently hemorrhagic and are commonly centered in the white matter or at the gray–white matter junction. Sometimes only petechial hemorrhage occurs; however, overtly hemorrhagic venous infarction is not uncommon.

The causes of intracranial venous thrombosis are no different from those occurring elsewhere in the body. They include a hypercoagulable state, dehydration, extrinsic compression, or local invasion of a vein by tumor, an adjacent infectious process (e.g., mastoiditis), a low-flow state within the venous sinus, pregnancy, and the postpartum state. Oral contraceptives also have been associated with increased risk of venous sinus thrombosis. No predisposing risk factors are identified in as many as 25% of patients with demonstrable venous congestion resulting in regional ischemia and infarction. Just as the intracranial arterial beds are well defined, the site of venous thrombosis dictates the part of the brain that will suffer infarction. For example, thrombosis of deep cerebral veins (e.g., basal vein of Rosenthal, internal cerebral veins) typically results in thalamic infarction.

CT Perfusion (CTP)

Millions of neurons and billions of synapses are estimated to be lost per minute during acute stroke. If stretched out, the myelin fibers affected every minute by acute stroke would measure in miles. The saying "time is brain" is clearly apropos in an acute stroke setting. Advanced neuroimaging is attempting to take this concept one step further. Not only can brain tissue that has infarcted be detected, but tissue that is at risk for infarction because of poor cerebral perfusion can be predicted.

The key tasks in an acute stroke setting are to exclude intracranial hemorrhage, define the "core" of infarction, locate the site of intraarterial thrombus responsible for the infarct, and assess the extent of additional brain parenchyma that is threatened if blood flow is not restored.

CT is quite accurate in detecting territorial infarcts; however, diffusion-weighted imaging (DWI) using MRI is more sensitive for detecting small lacunar and distal infarcts. MRI also can detect small, chronic microbleeds that may be missed by CT scan. Despite these limitations, a CT scanner typically is the imaging modality most widely available in an emergency room. Using a CT scanner for processing all aspects of acute stroke management is clearly quite attractive for delivering efficient care.

Noncontrast CT and CTA are helpful in excluding intracranial hemorrhage and locating the site of the thrombus. A CT perfusion scan aims to detect the mismatch between the brain already infarcted at presentation ("core") and that at risk of infarction ("penumbra"). The amount of mismatch, if it can be efficiently derived, then can be factored into patient selection for thrombolysis.

CT perfusion imaging uses the dynamics of first-pass bolus through the brain parenchyma to derive perfusion maps. In its idealized form, CT perfusion is based on administering a short contrast bolus and observing its

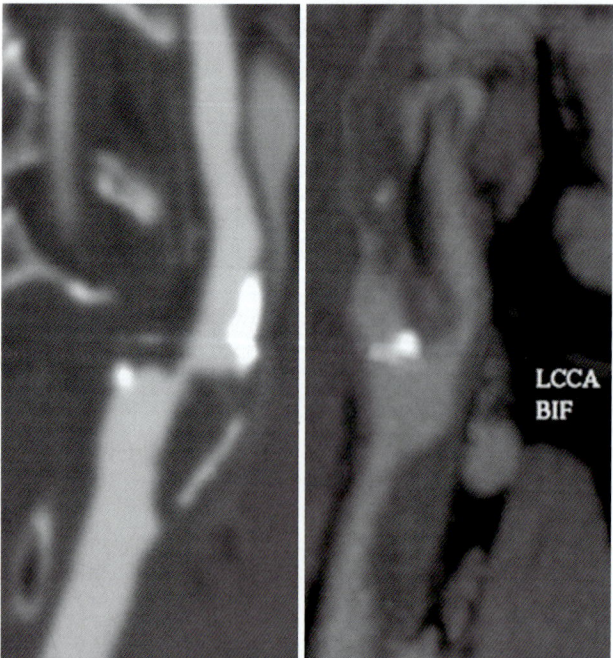

Figure 1-16 Computed tomography angiography of carotid bifurcation in two different patients. *Left:* Extensive noncalicified plaque causing severe stenosis of the proximal left internal carotid artery near the origin. *Right:* Hairline lumen in the proximal external carotid artery. LCCA BIF, left common carotid artery bifurcation).

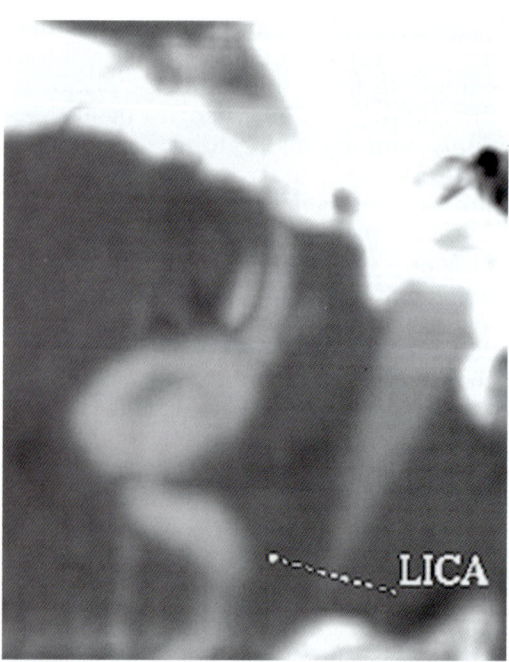

Figure 1-17 Pseudoaneurysm resulting in dilation of the distal left internal carotid artery (LICA) in a three-dimensional maximal intensity projection view.

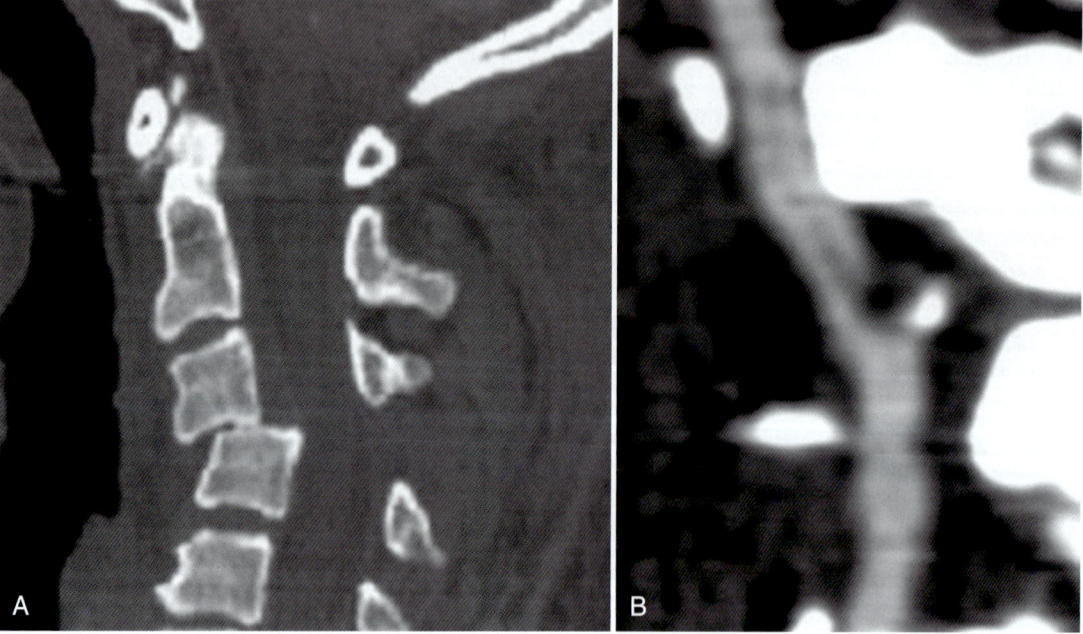

Figure 1-18 Posttraumatic dissection of the vertebral artery. The intimal flap is clearly visualized in the curved reformatted view in A.

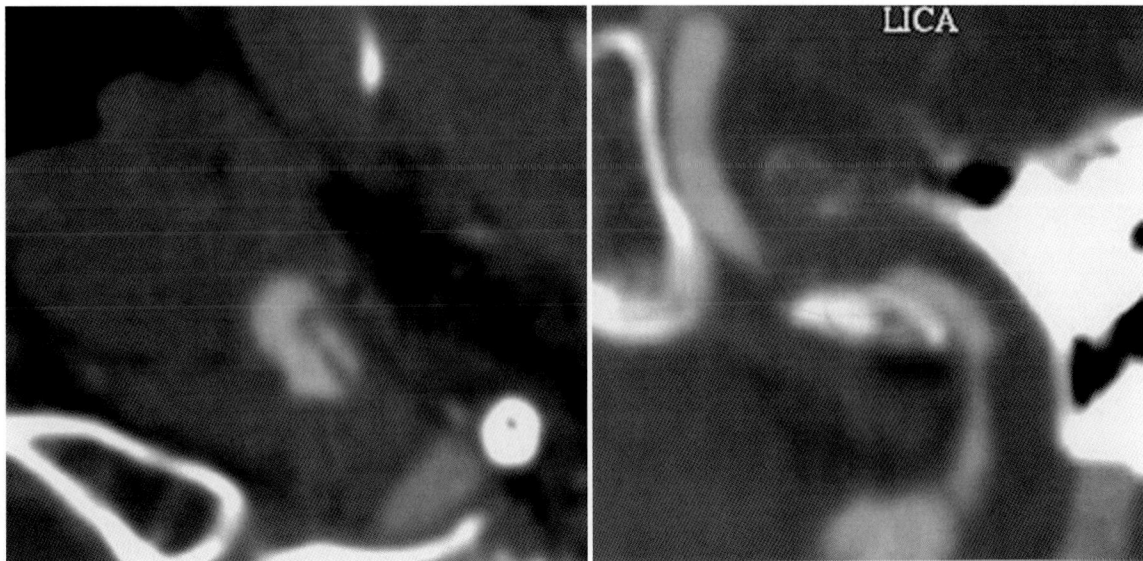

Figure 1-19 Left internal carotid artery *(LICA)* dissection, confirmed by visualization of an intimal flap on an oblique maximal intensity projection image *(left)*, resulting in partial occlusion of the left petrous internal carotid artery distal to the dissection.

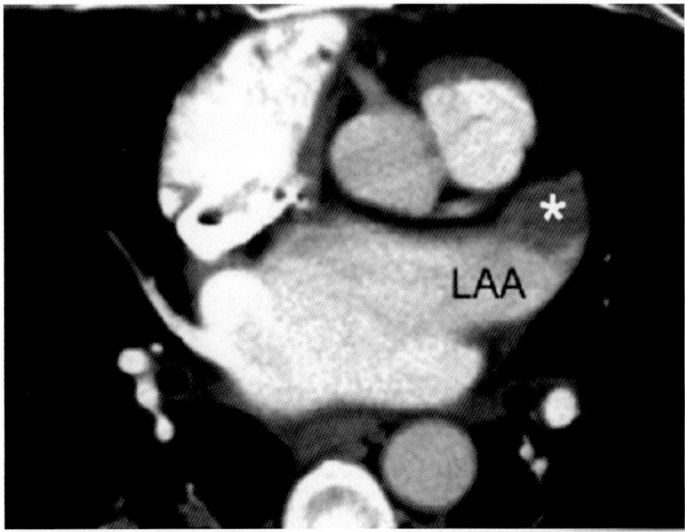

Figure 1-20 Left atrial appendage (LAA) thrombus. Neurologic computed tomographic angiography extended to include the LAA shows a thrombus (asterisk) responsible for acute stroke.

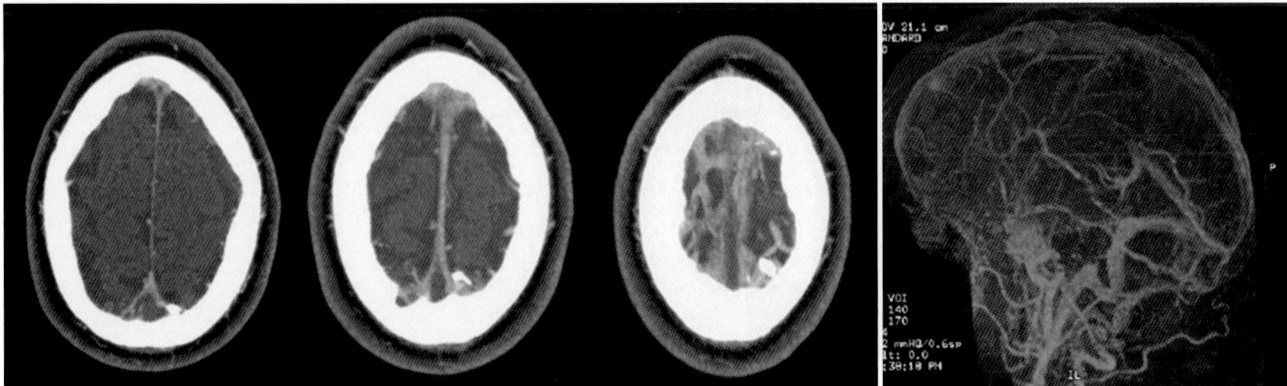

Figure 1-21 Delta sign of venous sinus thrombosis. Axial postcontrast images showing the delta sign from a thrombus in the superior sagittal sinus. The full extent of the thrombus can be appreciated in the three-dimensional view after automatic bone removal.

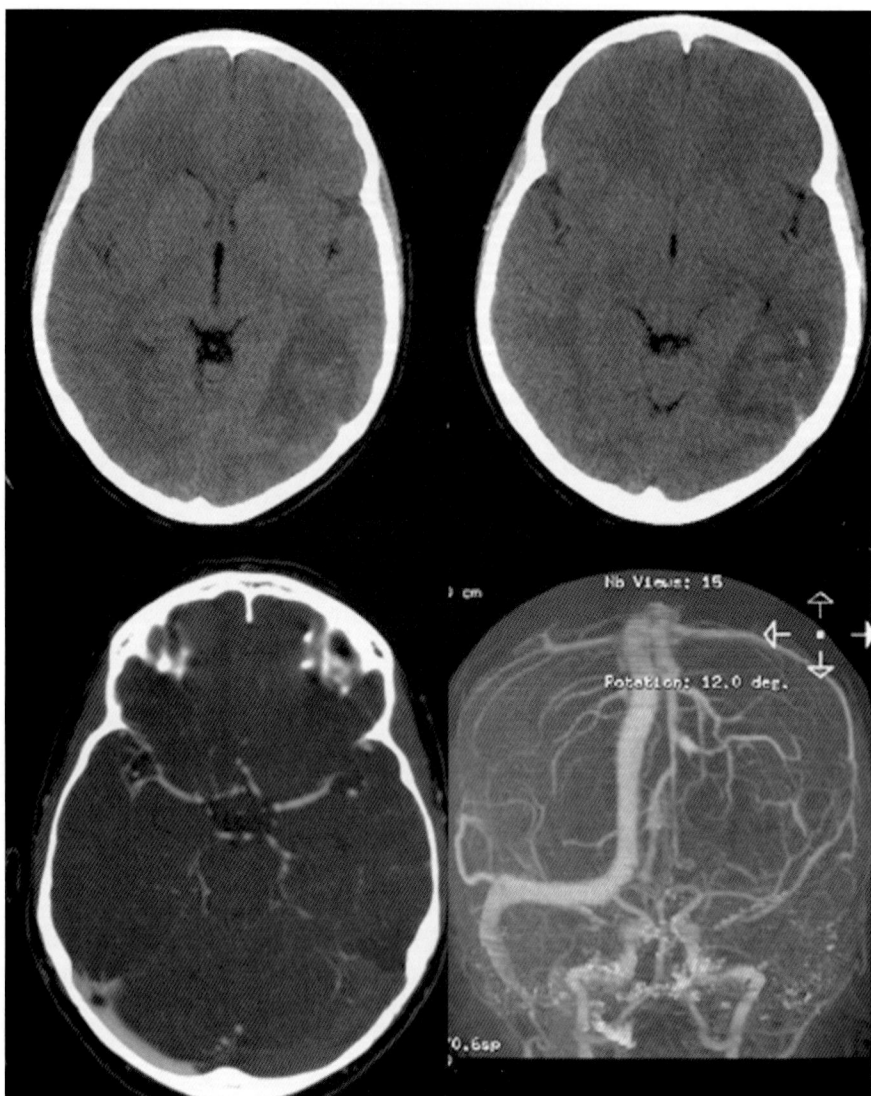

Figure 1-22 Infarct with hemorrhagic conversion that does not fall in a single arterial territory. Computed tomography angiography/computed tomography venography demonstrates patent intracranial arteries and dural venous sinus thrombosis, confirming this infarct to be of venous origin.

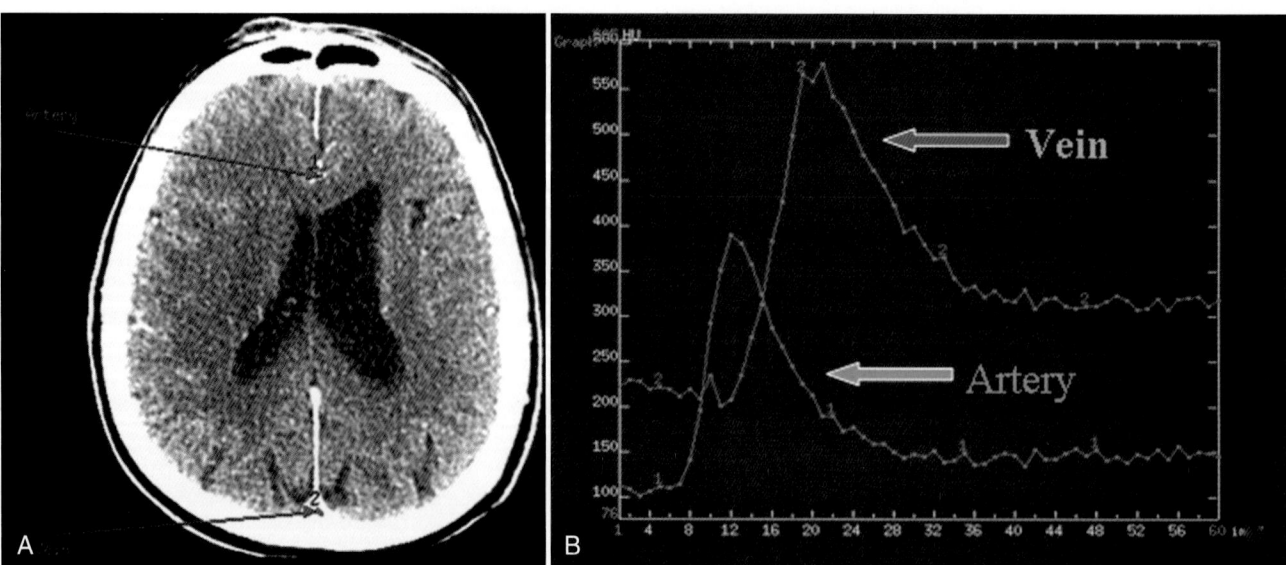

Figure 1-23 Computed tomographic perfusion maps derived from a sequence of images such as that shown in **A**. This sequence documents the temporal evolution of contrast bolus through the brain parenchyma. In one type of processing, arterial input function and venous outflow functions are derived from this sequence (**B**).

evolution in the brain. Repeated CT scans through the brain parenchyma under observation yield a time-attenuation curve for each pixel that documents the changes in tissue contrast during the bolus passage. CT perfusion software is used to process this sequence of images to derive cerebral blood flow (CBF), cerebral blood volume (CBV), mean transit time (MTT), and vascular permeability (kPS) information from dynamic changes in contrast enhancement.

Good histologic evidence exists that the area of restricted diffusion on an MRI scan closely corresponds to the tissue that has infarcted. It is widely believed that in a perfusion scan using MRI, the so-called ischemic penumbra or "at-risk" brain is captured by the MTT and CBF maps. However, because magnetic resonance perfusion is not a quantitative map, it is difficult to set a strict threshold to demarcate the area of "benign oligemia" from those that will proceed to infarction if blood flow is not reestablished.

Unlike MRI, CT provides quantitative maps of CBV, CBF, and MTT. There is growing evidence that CT CBV maps, just like DWI scans, roughly correspond to the brain parenchyma that has already infarcted. MTT and CBF maps describe the area that is at risk or has already infarcted. The difference between the two, therefore, corresponds to the ischemic penumbra that is at risk. The exact threshold for delineating the boundary between these areas is a topic of current active research.

Construction of reliable CT perfusion maps requires delivering a tight bolus and observing an axial slab continuously for about 40 to 60 seconds. Typically, a 40-ml contrast bolus is delivered at 7 ml/s through a peripheral IV line. An 18-gauge or larger-bore IV line is necessary to deliver contrast at such a high rate. Current scanner technology allows a 2- to 4-cm slab to be observed. Generally two such slabs are required to study both the middle and anterior cerebral artery territories. One perfusion slab may suffice if the presentation and symptoms strongly point to one territory over another. Newer scanners also offer a shuttle mode in which the patient table is moved back and forth in order to increase the axial coverage along the Z-direction at the expense of temporal resolution. The exact coverage of a single slab using these newer shuttle modes depends on the equipment vendor and the make and model of the scanner.

Figure 1-23 schematically depicts the set of steps required to make CT perfusion maps. These maps are derived from a sequence of images that documents the temporal evolution of a contrast bolus through the brain parenchyma. A variety of software packages are available to process the perfusion image sequence. In one type of processing, arterial input and venous outflow functions are automatically derived from this sequence. These functions are shown in Figure 1-23B. In addition, the opacification curve for each voxel can be mapped and will have a shape quite similar to that shown in Figure 1-23B. A combination of the arterial input functions and the time-opacification curves is used to derive the perfusion maps (Figure 1-24) that depict CBV, CBF, MTT, and permeability for each voxel in the imaged volume. Generally speaking, CBV corresponds to the area under the time-opacification curve, CBF is proportional to the maximum upslope of the curve, and MTT is proportional to time to peak from the start of bolus arrival.

Excellent software packages that fully automate the generation of perfusion maps are available. The software automatically identifies the arterial input function and the venous outflow (typically using a major venous sinus) required to compute perfusion maps. Clinical studies have shown that the maps generated automatically are essentially identical to those made by experts.

Of note, other perfusion packages that do not rely on the arterial input function are available. A comprehensive discussion of the different algorithms for generation of perfusion maps is beyond the scope of this chapter. Software systems also exist for automatic segmentation of core and penumbra. With the degree of automation that is available, concerns about workflow should not prevent use of CT perfusion for the evaluation of acute stroke patients.

Problem-Solving Tool/Cases in Stroke

Two cases are presented that demonstrate the power of CTP in triaging acute stroke patients based on the size of the tissue at risk. Figure 1-25 shows the case of a patient who presented with acute MCA syndrome. The presentation MRI showed a DWI defect restricted to the insula and frontal operculum. MTT and CBF maps demonstrate that the entire left MCA territory is at risk. This patient was beyond the time window for IV thrombolysis using tPA. She was emergently taken to the neurointerventional suite for catheter-assisted thrombectomy.

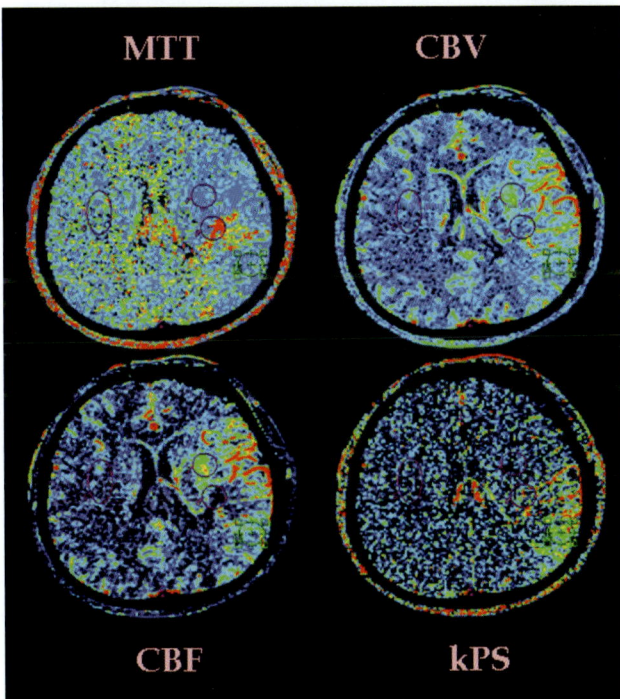

Figure 1-24 Perfusion maps depicting mean transit time (MTT), cerebral blood volume (CBV), cerebral blood flow (CBF), and permeability (kPS) for each voxel in the imaged volume.

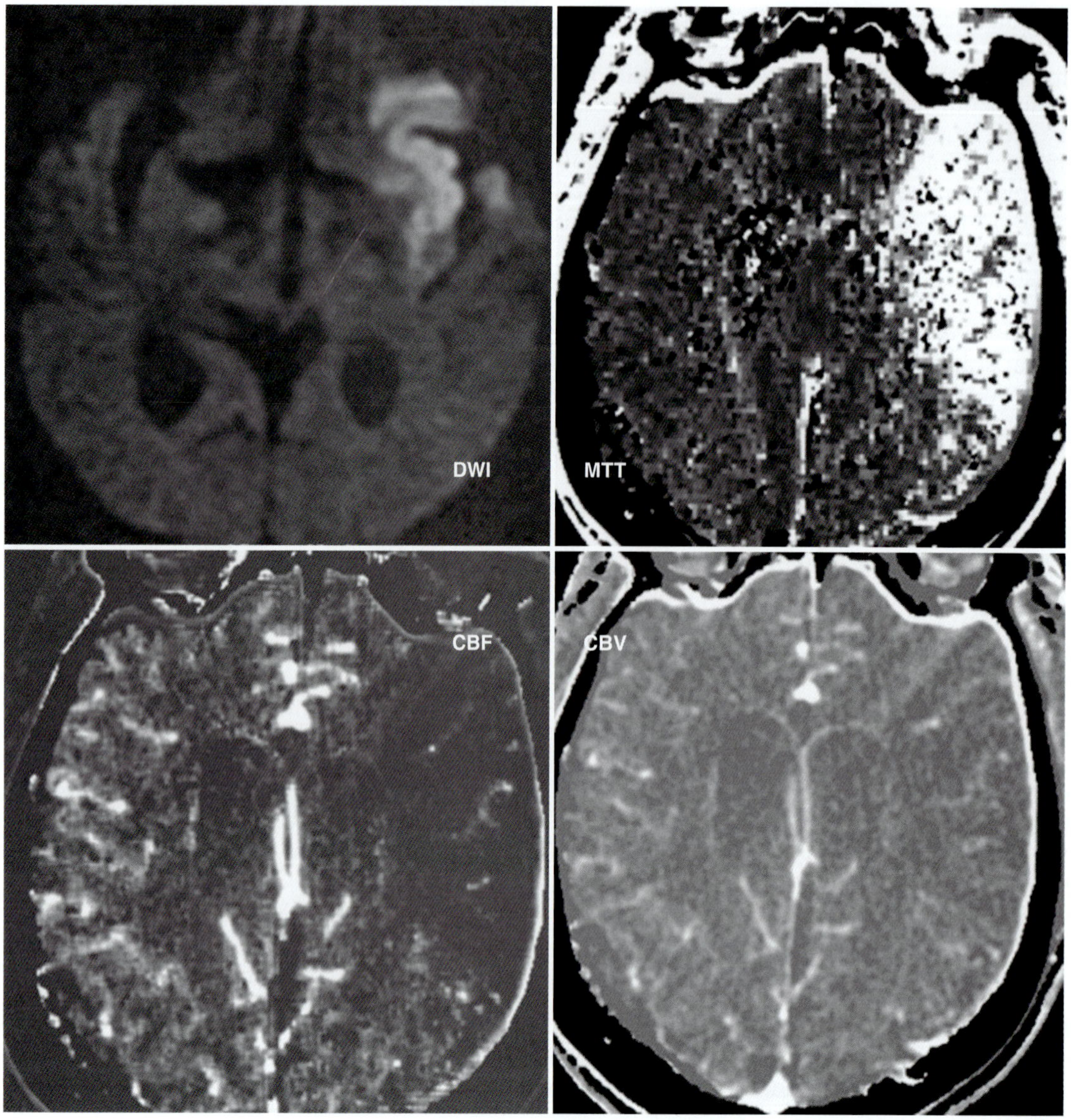

Figure 1-25 Diffusion-weighted images showing the core of the infarct at presentation and the three perfusion maps derived from computed tomography.

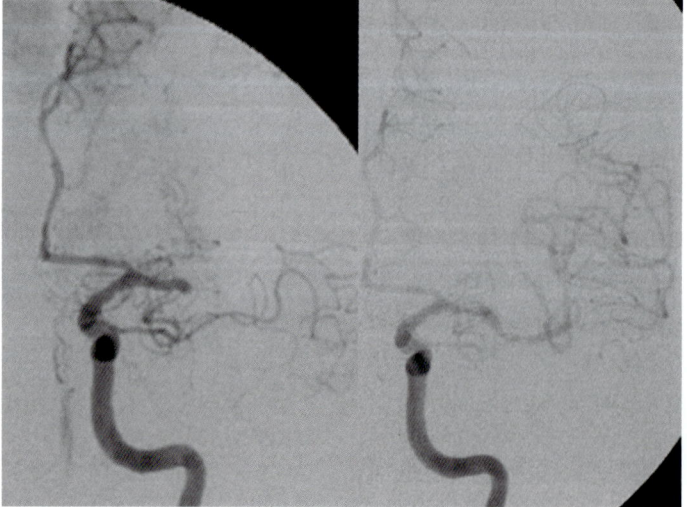

Figure 1-26 Anteroposterior view showing acute occlusion of the left middle cerebral artery stem (**A**) and blood flow after catheter-assisted thrombectomy (**B**).

Figure 1-26 shows the angiogram before and after the procedure. Blood flow to the left MCA territory was fully restored. The discharge DWI scan for this patient was quite similar to that of the core of the infarct, and the procedure was successful in arresting the progression of core into the ischemic penumbra.

Figure 1-27 shows the case of a patient with a perfusion deficit in the posterior left MCA territory. There is a large mismatch between the core and the deficit on CBF and MTT maps. This patient was beyond the window for IV or arterial intervention. On the 48-hour DWI scan, the infarct had grown to involve the additional tissue at risk. The final core of the infarct nearly matched the MTT and CBF abnormality originally seen 2 days earlier.

Derivation of perfusion maps depends on the delivery of contrast to different portions of the brain. If the main arteries supplying a portion of the brain are narrowed, delivery of contrast to that portion will be delayed. Unless proper care is taken to ensure that the arterial input function is given time to peak and to return to near baseline value, the software may misinterpret delayed flow and present it as diminished perfusion. This is shown in Figure 1-28. Blood flow into the left MCA territory was delayed because of complete occlusion of the proximal left internal carotid artery (ICA) as demonstrated in the CTA. The arterial input function was not given enough time to return to baseline. The resulting perfusion maps show a large perfusion deficit in the left MCA territory even when the patient had no acute stroke. Similar situations may arise in the setting of low ejection fraction, total occlusion of an artery, or transient atrial fibrillation.

■ MDCT IN NEOPLASTIC CONDITIONS

MDCT provides a quick way to detect primary and metastatic disease in the brain. A non–contrast-enhanced CT is relatively insensitive for detection of neoplastic disease, especially when the tumor burden is small. Therefore, a postcontrast CT should always be obtained when evaluating neoplastic conditions using CT. For certain conditions, both precontrast and postcontrast imaging are warranted. For example, if hemorrhage is suspected or the neoplastic condition being ruled out is intrinsically hyperdense (e.g., melanoma, small blue round cell tumors, densely packed lymphomas), then a noncontrast CT in addition to a postcontrast scan should be obtained. Small metastatic foci can be hard to see in a contrast-enhanced CT image (Figure 1-29). Therefore, attention to the scanning protocol is of utmost importance in these cases.

For the scanning protocol, 2.5- to 5-mm thick slices generally are sufficient. Because most institutions now acquire images in a helical mode, thinner overlapping slices can be reconstructed retrospectively if they are required to answer a specific clinical question. Such retrospective reconstruction is feasible as long as the raw projection data still are available in the scanner. Coronal and sagittal images should be reconstructed and reviewed to increase the sensitivity of detection. Bone kernel reconstructions should be obtained in addition to soft tissue kernels to increase sensitivity to bony primary and metastatic disease.

For postcontrast imaging, the contrast agent is slowly infused, and imaging is conducted 2 to 5 minutes after the end of infusion. This timing is different from that used in contrast-enhanced CTA or CTV because the process being imaged has a very different time constant. In CTA or CTV, the arterial or venous phase of the contrast bolus is of interest. These phases commence approximately 20 or 40 seconds after the start of IV contrast injection, depending on the cardiac ejection fraction of the patient. In tumor imaging, the imaging is delayed by several minutes. The rationale for relatively delayed imaging is to give the contrast enough time to "leak out" of the compromised blood–brain barrier in the tumor vasculature. Because different tumors show peak opacification at different times, no single "perfect" time applies to all neoplastic conditions. However, if a patient is known to have a primary tumor and the question is that of ruling out intracranial metastatic disease, the timing of the scan may be appropriately configured. Melanoma, renal cell carcinoma, choriocarcinoma, sarcomas, neuroendocrine tumors, and thyroid cancers typically show early enhancement.

Despite an optimal imaging protocol, MDCT is not as sensitive as MRI for detection of intracranial primary and metastatic disease. Nonetheless, MDCT provides essential information about intracranial neoplasms and should be obtained for more complete characterization. MDCT is essential for postoperative evaluation of tumors and any associated surgical complications. If the patient cannot undergo an MRI scan (e.g., because of a pacemaker), a contrast-enhanced CT scan may be the only alternative for detection and follow-up of intracranial neoplastic conditions.

MDCT contributes to the diagnosis and characterization of intracranial neoplastic disease, either primary or metastatic, in three essential ways:
1. The internal density and composition of the tumor can be readily studied using CT. For example, CT is very sensitive in detecting internal calcifications, necrosis, foci of hemorrhage, and fatty deposits.
2. The presence and extent of calvarial or skull base involvement by tumor are better depicted by CT than MRI.
3. The presence of neovascularity can be evaluated by CT perfusion studies, thus narrowing the differential diagnosis or leading to a diagnosis.

Problem-Solving Tool/Cases in Neoplastic Conditions

The remainder of this section illustrates typical applications of MDCT as a problem-solving tool in neoplastic conditions.

Figure 1-30 shows the case of a 45-year-old woman who presented with a history of slowly progressive spasticity of the upper and lower limbs. CT scan showed an extraaxial mass wrapped around the medulla with considerable mass effect on the brainstem. At MRI, the mass had a cystic component centrally and T2 hypointense component anteriorly. CT feature of uniform hyperdensity in the anterior component suggested a diagnosis of a "white epidermoid." DWI scan confirmed

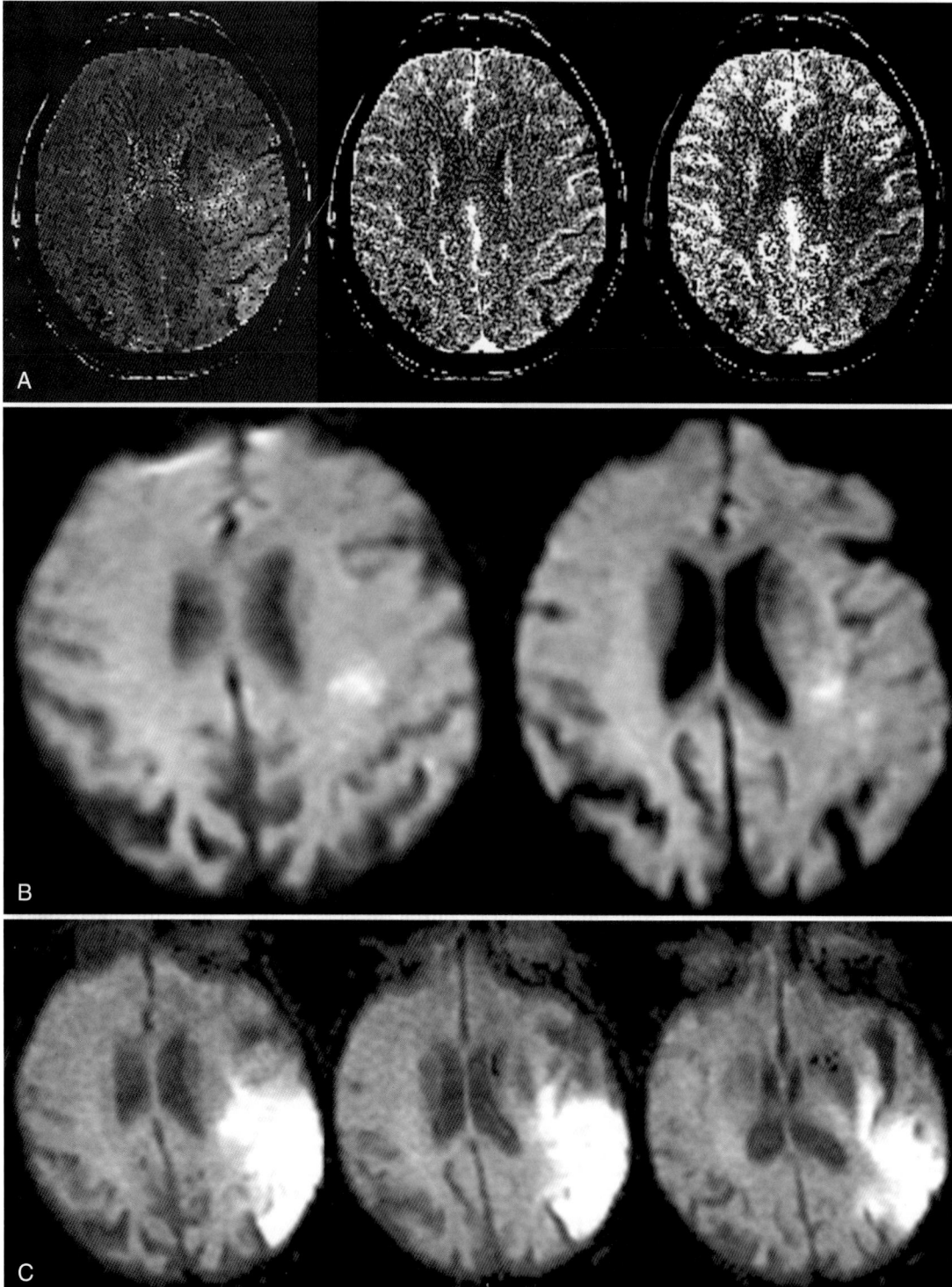

Figure 1-27 A: Admission cerebral blood volume, cerebral blood flow, and mean transit time for a patient who presented with acute stroke. **B:** Diffusion-weighted images at 24 hours showing the core of the infarct. **C:** Diffusion-weighted images 48 hours after presentation. Note that the final infarct size is close to that predicted by the cerebral blood flow map.

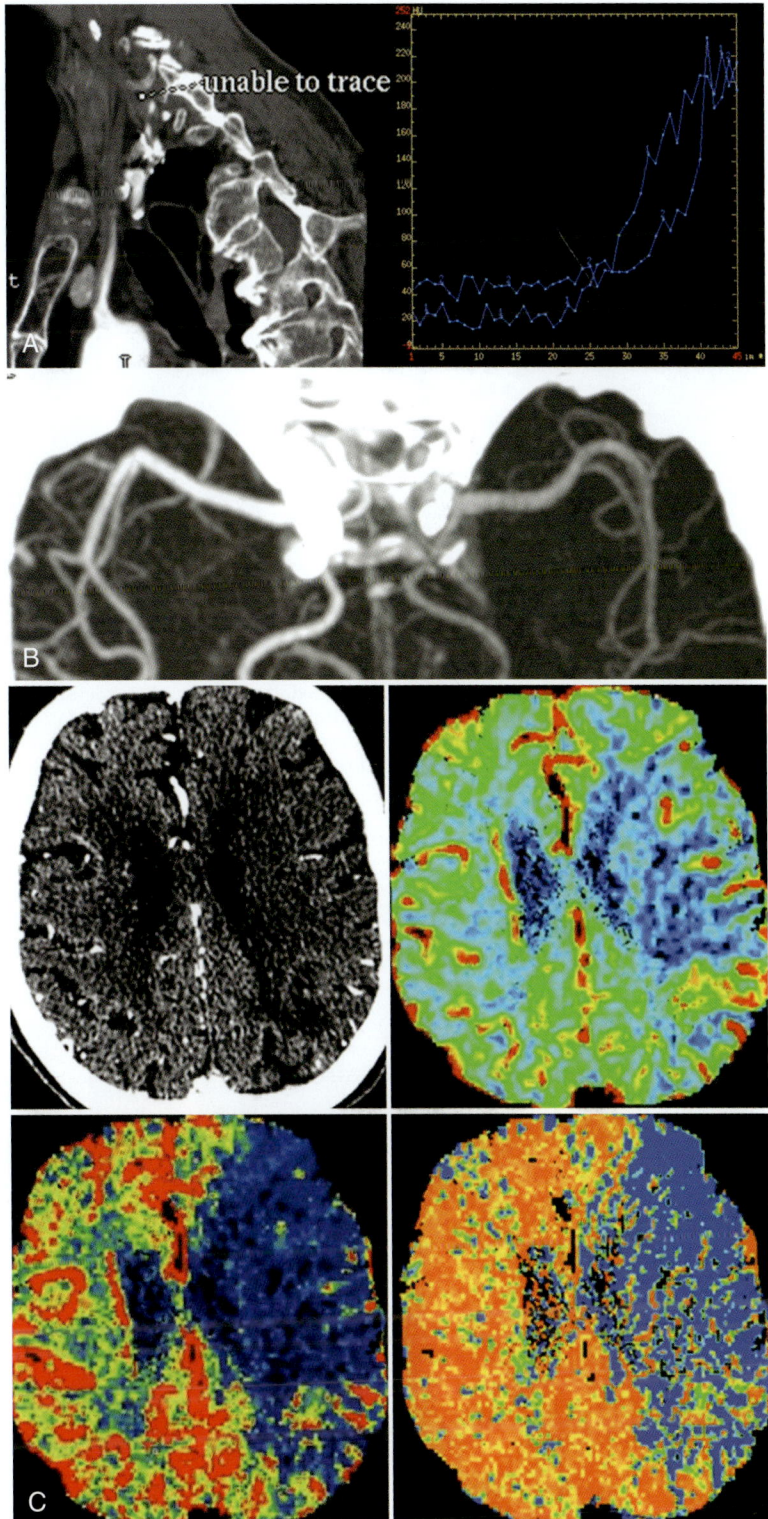

Figure 1-28 A: Contrast-enhanced computed tomography showing inability to trace the internal carotid artery. **B:** Left middle cerebral artery (MCA) is less dense compared to right MCA because of delayed bolus arrival. **C:** Perfusion map showing artificial mean transit time changes in the left hemisphere.

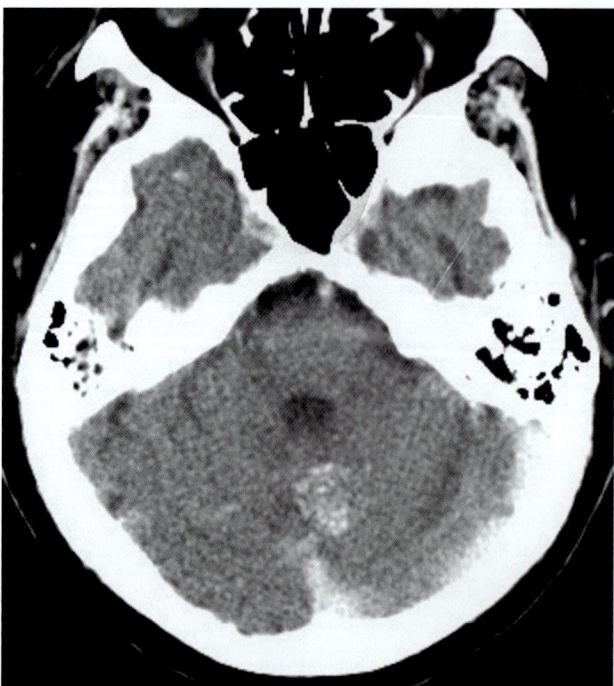

Figure 1-29 Contrast-enhanced computed tomographic slice through the posterior fossa demonstrating an amorphous area of contrast enhancement in a patient known to have colon cancer. This finding confirmed intracranial metastatic disease in the patient, who could not undergo magnetic resonance imaging scan because of a cardiac pacemaker.

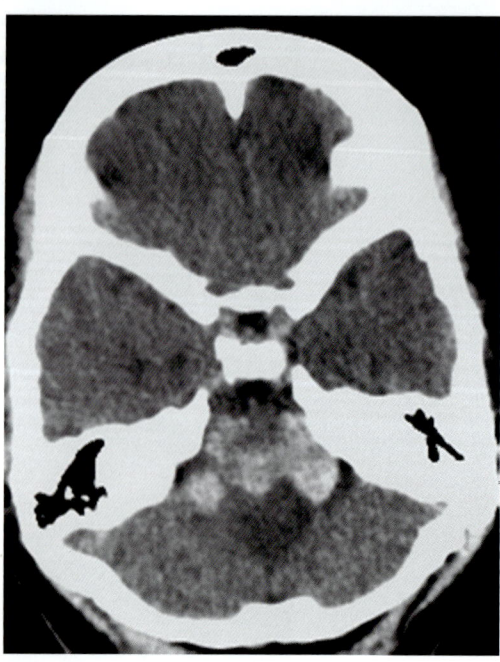

Figure 1-30 Plain computed tomographic section at the level of the medulla showing a hyperdense mass wrapped around the anterior medulla with a cystic component in the region of the fourth ventricle. Magnetic resonance imaging with diffusion imaging (not shown) confirmed an epidermoid tumor in this location.

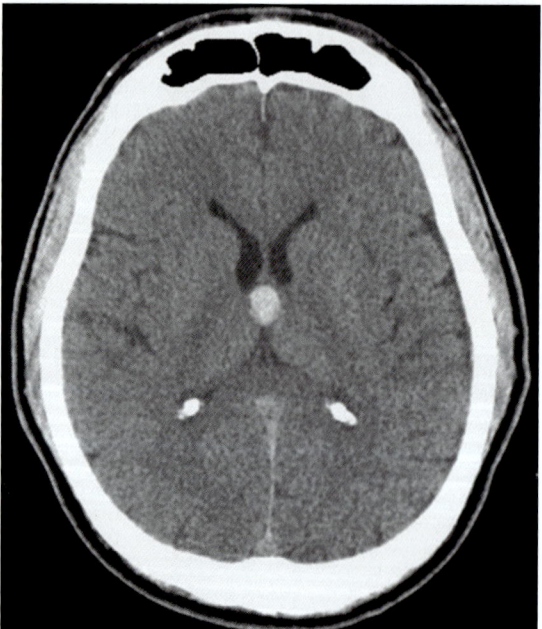

Figure 1-31 Noncontrast computed tomographic slice at the level of the basal ganglia showing a central, well-defined, hyperdense mass along the midline, near the foramen of Monro in the anterior third ventricle, with classic features of a colloid cyst on computed tomography.

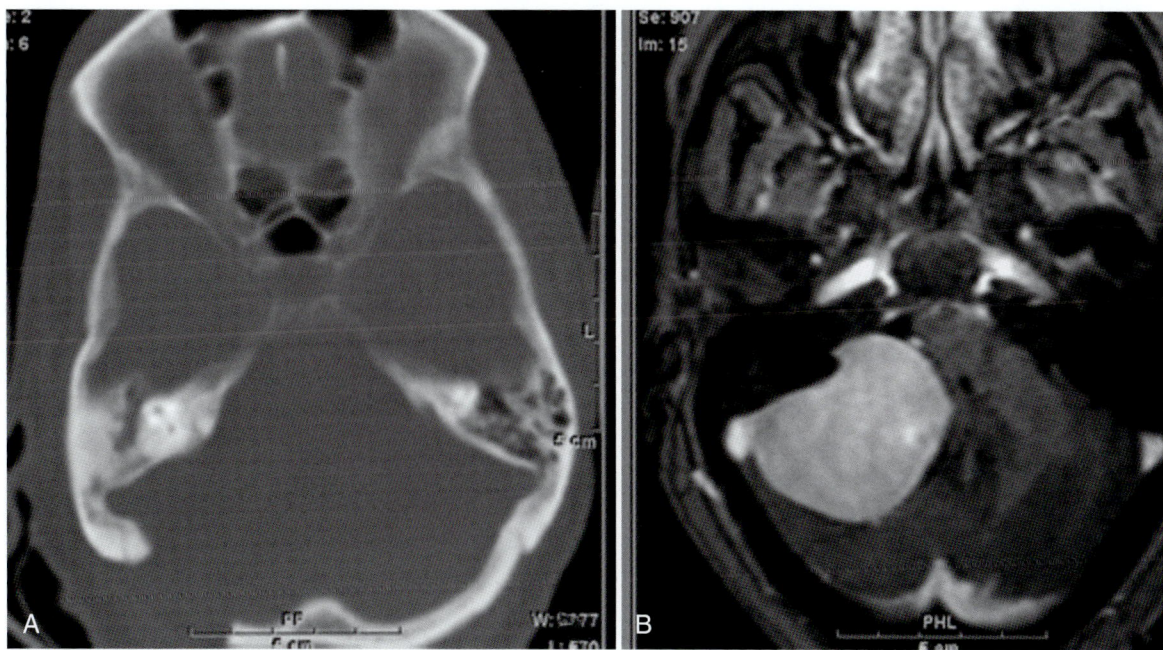

Figure 1-32 A: Postoperative computed tomography (CT) of a patient with a right cerebropontine angle mass, extending into the right internal auditory canal, showing hyperostosis of the petrous ridge and the mastoid air cells on the ipsilateral side. B: Magnetic resonance imaging of the same patient. The hyperostosis demonstrated by CT scan is suggestive of a meningioma.

the diagnosis of an epidermoid. Epidermoid cysts usually are hypodense but infrequently are hyperdense, as illustrated in this case.

Hyperdensity on CT may reflect dense cellularity, diffuse calcification, mineralization (e.g., siderosis), or high protein content in an otherwise cystic structure. Figure 1-31 shows an example of a colloid cyst, which is characteristically seen in this location. The diagnosis of a colloid cyst is virtually confirmed by the CT scan.

Bone remodeling is better illustrated on CT than MRI. Figure 1-32 shows the postoperative scan of a 40-year-old man with a right-sided, peripheral, posterior fossa mass. The CT section confirms hyperostosis of the right petrous ridge, a classic feature of a meningioma.

For a mass adjacent to important vascular structures, a wealth of information can be derived from CTA study. CTA or CTV can be used to study tumor vascularity, mass effect on the adjacent vessels and their dominant blood supply, venous drainage and their patency. Figure 1-33 shows examples of high-convexity meningiomas infiltrating the superior sagittal sinus. MDCT demonstrates complete occlusion of the midsegment of the sinus is case A, with collaterals and incomplete occlusion in case B.

CT can readily show the presence and distribution of calcifications in a mass, narrowing the differential diagnosis. For example, suprasellar masses can have a broad differential that includes pituitary macroadenoma, craniopharyngioma, cavernous ICA aneurysm, germinoma, and metastases. This differential can be considerably narrowed by the extent of the mass, enhancement pattern, calcifications, blood flow, and native CT density. Figure 1-34 shows the case of a young child who presented with increased intracranial pressure and vision loss. The image clearly shows a calcified cystic mass in the suprasellar cistern suggesting the diagnosis of a craniopharyngioma, a diagnosis that is classically made on CT. However, a soft tissue mass confined to the suprasellar region, causing hydrocephalus due to foramen of Monro obstruction, could represent a pilocytic astrocytoma, as illustrated in Figure 1-35.

Interaction of a mass with adjacent bone is well demonstrated by MDCT. Figure 1-36 shows a soft tissue mass that is destroying the lesser wing of the sphenoid. This soft tissue mass projects into the middle cranial fossa, displacing the temporal lobe, and abuts the left cavernous sinus. Small calcific foci are located within the mass. Histopathologic examination revealed the mass to be an eosinophilic granuloma.

Pituitary macroadenoma is typically known to extend into the suprasellar cistern and in up to 40% of cases can invade the cavernous sinus. Cavernous sinus invasion is determined by encasement of the ICA, which can be well identified on CTA (Figure 1-37).

Figure 1-38 illustrates a pitfall of CT and the method for getting around it. The initial CT scan of a 4-year-old child who presented with abdominal pain, vomiting, and recent sinusitis treated with antibiotics was read as normal. A closer look at the skull base in the vicinity of the cavernous sinuses shows an extraaxial hyperdense mass that was misinterpreted as volume averaging and beam hardening artifact. The trick here is to review coronal and/or sagittal reformations, which clearly demonstrate bulging cavernous sinuses, a feature that cannot be attributed to CT artifacts. A repeat scan 1 week later showed that the mass had grown significantly in the interval. Stereotactic biopsy confirmed Burkitt lymphoma, which was hyperdense on CT.

This case illustrates another key point: even soft tissue masses can show differences in CT attenuation that

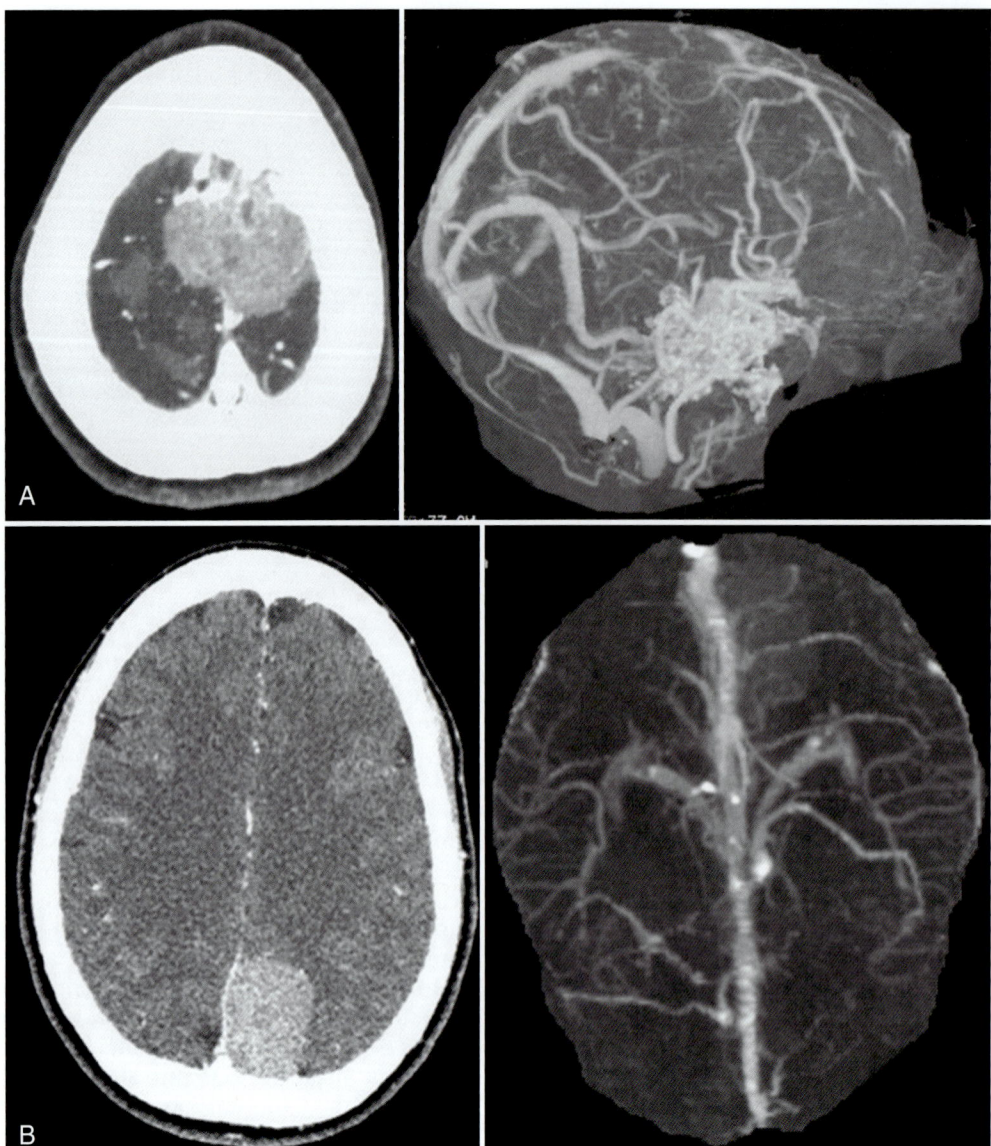

Figure 1-33 **A:** *Case A. Left,* Left high convexity parasagittal meningioma causing complete occlusion of the midsegment of the superior sagittal sinus with formation of collateral venous drainage around it. *Right,* Computed tomographic venogram confirms complete occlusion of the segment of the superior sagittal sinus. **B:** *Case B. Left,* Posterior left parasagittal meningioma abutting and indenting the superior sagittal sinus without occluding it. *Right,* Computed tomographic venogram confirming patency of the superior sagittal sinus at the site of indentation by the mass.

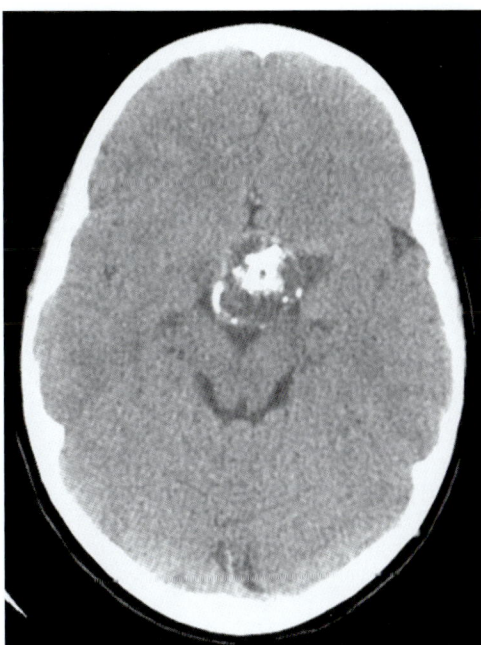

Figure 1-34 Axial section from a non–contrast-enhanced computed tomographic (CT) scan at the suprasellar cistern level showing a well-defined rounded lesion with some cystic components around the central chunky calcification as well as linear calcifications in the rim of the cystic components. The noncontrast CT appearance is highly suggestive of a craniopharyngioma.

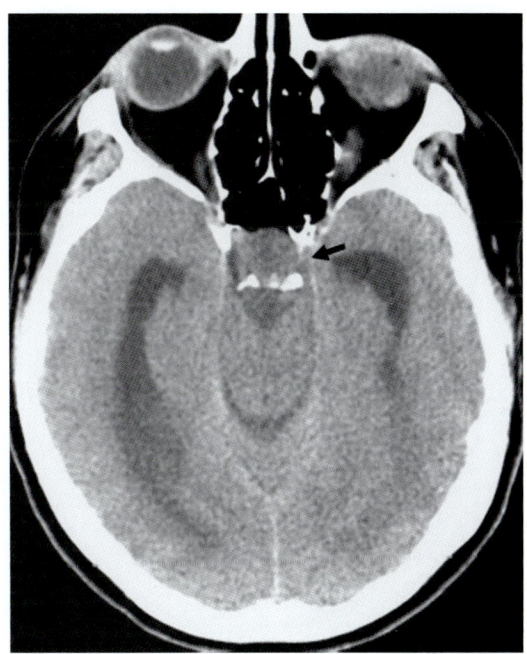

Figure 1-35 Pilocytic astrocytoma in the suprasellar cistern causing dilation of the temporal horns of the lateral ventricles due to compression of the foramen of Monro.

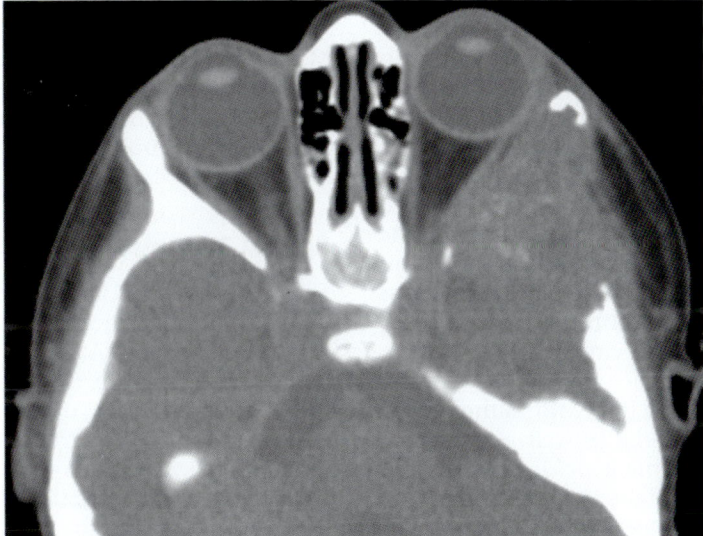

Figure 1-36 Eosinophilic granuloma eroding the left lesser wing of the sphenoid and left squamous temporal bone. This mass also shows punctate calcific foci and a soft tissue component that is indenting on the left temporal lobe and is extending medially to abut the lateral wall of the cavernous sinus.

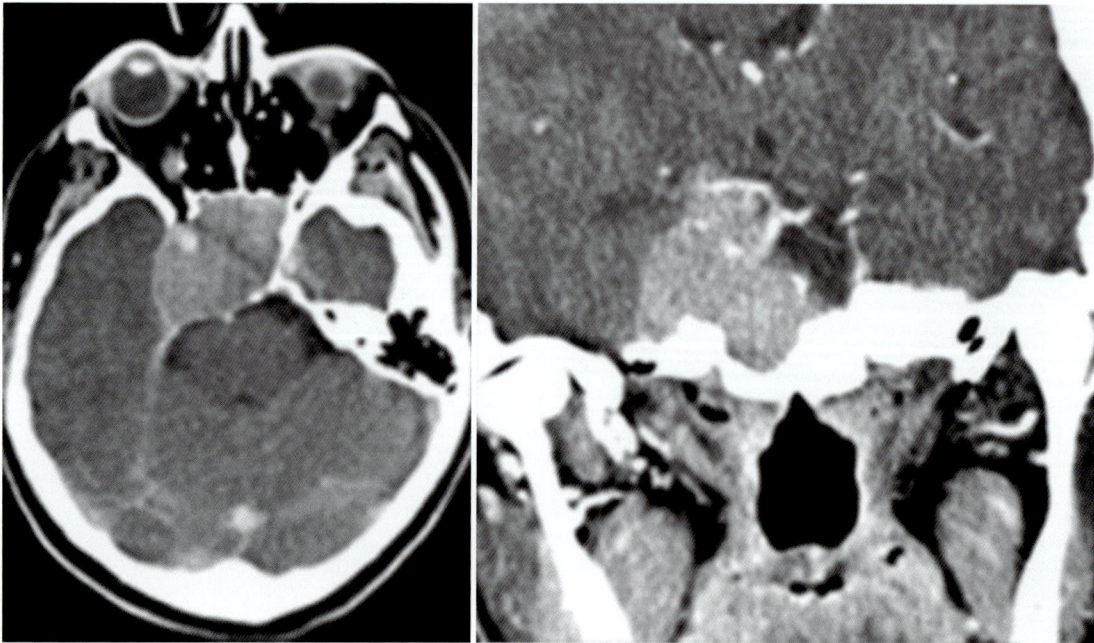

Figure 1-37 Large bilobed, enhancing sellar/suprasellar mass that is expanding the sella and invading the right cavernous sinus representing a typical pituitary macroadenoma. The right cavernous internal carotid artery is completely encased, and there is a convex lateral margin. A lobulated component in the right aspect of the perimesencephalic cistern is seen indenting on the right posterior cerebral artery and proximal right middle cerebral artery without compromising its lumen. The optic chiasm is compressed and displaced, and it cannot be identified separately from the mass.

may be useful in characterizing a mass. For example, densely cellular masses have slightly higher attenuation, a property common to high-grade lymphomas. This is illustrated in Figure 1-39, which shows the case of a 55-year-old man who presented with new-onset seizures. On non–contrast-enhanced CT imaging, he was found to have a large mass in the left cerebral hemisphere. This mass, which is slightly hyperdense compared with normal gray matter and hyperdense compared to normal white matter, crosses the midline and predominantly involves the white matter, with marked edema. MRI with gadolinium showed the mass to be brightly enhancing. MRS showed a high choline peak with an elevated choline-to-creatine ratio and no lipid component. The differential included glioblastoma multiforme and lymphoma. However, the CT finding of a hyperdense mass favors lymphoma. Stereotactic biopsy was performed, and histopathology confirmed a lymphoma.

CT can demonstrate pathologies affecting the calvaria with better sensitivity and detail than MRI. Although CT cannot demonstrate bone edema as well as MRI can, the extent of cortical involvement or destruction can only be demonstrated on CT. Figures 1-40 through 1-42 show some specific conditions in which CT shows characteristic findings pointing to a diagnosis.

MDCT not only shows the primary tumor and it's interrelationship with the adjacent vessels, it often can demonstrate any associated complications. For example, if a mass is compressing an important vascular structure or is eroding the bone to form a fistulous connection between two compartments, CT may be used as a problem-solving tool. Figure 1-43 shows the case of a chordoma that had eroded the skull base, causing extensive pneumocephalus. The same finding would be suboptimally demonstrated on MRI because of susceptibility artifacts from air. CT not only shows the pathology but also the exact place where the fistulous connection is formed. Another case of bone erosion by neuroblastoma is shown in Figure 1-44.

■ MDCT IN EVALUATION OF SPINE

MDCT plays a major role in the diagnosis and management of various conditions involving the spine. The following subsections briefly outline and illustrate the role played by this modality in the management of trauma, infection, neoplastic conditions, and myelography.

Spinal Trauma

The efficacy of CT, along with its high sensitivity and specificity, in detecting traumatic fractures of the spine is well established. Axial CT significantly outperforms plain radiography in the evaluation of trauma to the spine and has largely supplanted it in the management of acute trauma. The excellent structural details of multiplanar reconstructions and 3-D images help in better visualizing spatial relationships. MDCT has become the standard of care for classification and preoperative planning for acute traumatic fractures. CT is much more valuable than MRI in the detection of subtle fractures because of its availability and lack of contraindications. MRI is reserved for evaluation of ligamentous injury.

State-of-the-art MDCT scanners are capable of approximately 0.5-mm isotropic resolution. Thin CT slices, combined with low pitch and overlapping reconstructions, result in marked improvement in the visualization of subtle fractures. It is important to use a sharp kernel, low slice thickness, and appropriate

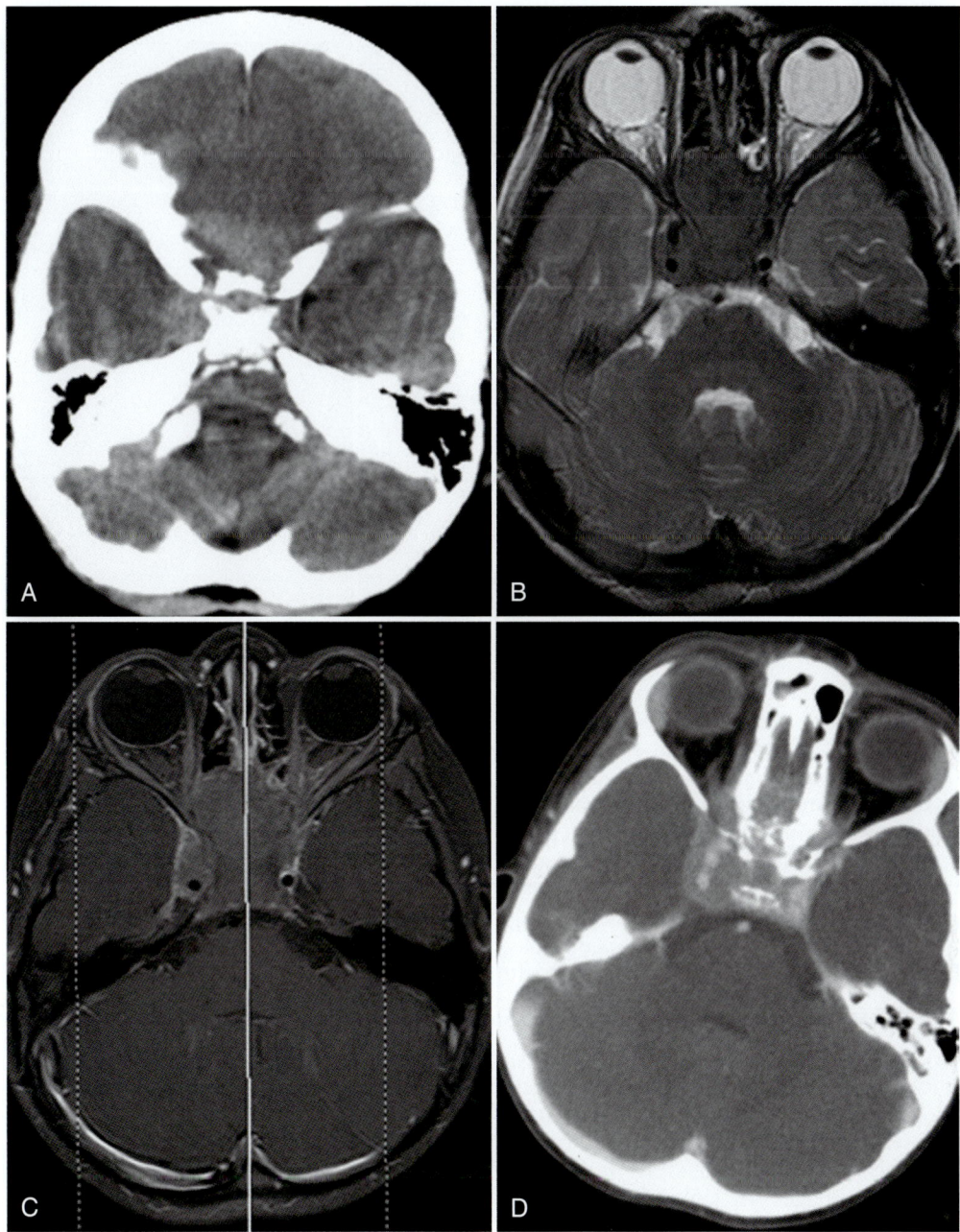

Figure 1-38 A: Axial computed tomographic (CT) image showing a hyperdense mass along the outer margin of the right cavernous sinus. B, C: T2 and postcontrast T1-weighted images confirming midline mass in the posterior ethmoid region, encroaching on the right cavernous sinus. D: CT scan obtained 1 week after the image shown in A showing increased size of the hyperdense, enhancing mass.

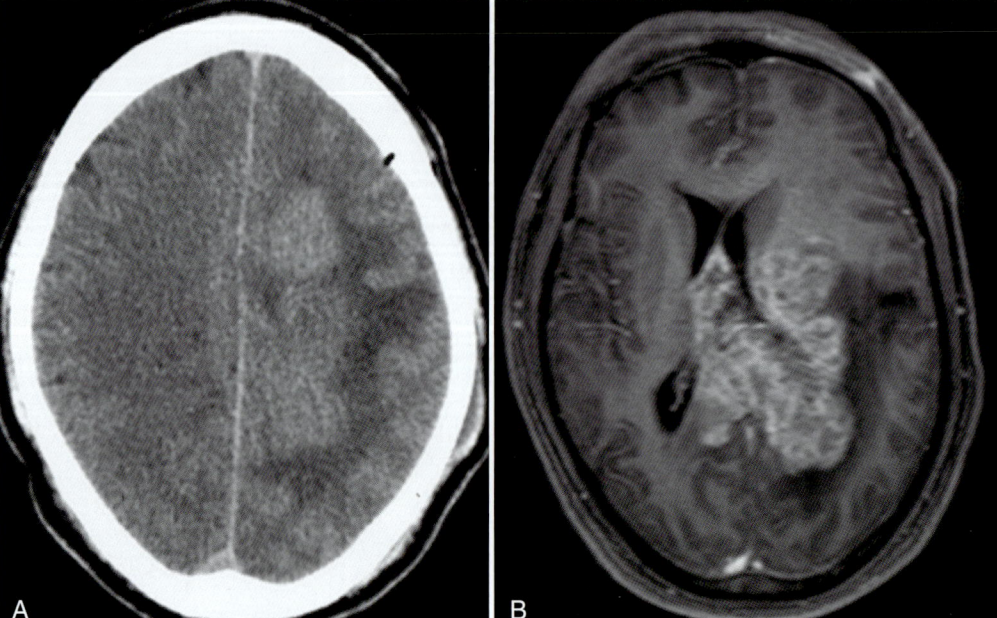

Figure 1-39 A: Computed tomographic scan showing left-sided mass in the white matter that is hyperdense compared with normal white matter and isodense compared to gray matter. B: Post-gadolinium magnetic resonance imaging scan showing a predominantly left-sided mass that is infiltrating and extending across the body and splenium of the corpus callosum to cross the midline.

sagittal and coronal reformations when analyzing spinal CT. Figure 1-45 shows the importance of appropriate choice of scan and reconstruction parameters in a trauma setting. At a slice thickness of 2.5 mm and pitch of 1:1, the fracture in the right posterior arch of C1 was not apparent and initially was missed. However, with a decreased slice thickness of 1.25 mm and pitch of 0.5:1, the fracture became more apparent on CT scan performed after 1 week. In general, decreasing the pitch, along with the decrement in the slice thickness, may allow visualization of an otherwise occult fracture.

With the advent of MDCT, primarily by virtue of oblique reformations and 3-D display technology, fracture classification has become easier and more straightforward. Although extensive literature exists on determining which fractures are unstable based on radiographs, the task is considerably simplified using multiplanar CT images. In simplified terms, a "major" cervical injury includes any of the following: (1) displacement of more than 2 mm in any plane, (2) widening of the vertebral body, (3) widening of the interspinous or interlaminar line, (4) widened facet joints, (5) posterior vertebral body line disruption, (6) widening of the disc space, (7) burst fracture, (8) unilateral or bilateral locked/perched fractures, (9) hangman's fracture, (10) odontoid fracture, and (11) occipital condyle fracture. All other types of fractures may be considered "minor."

Problem-Solving Tool/Cases in the Spine

MDCT is helpful in the detection of the type of fracture, the extent of trauma, and any associated complications. Figures 1-46A and 14-6B show a major injury of the cervical spine seen via sagittal and 3-D surface-rendered views. A unilateral locked/perched inferior articular facet of C5 is easily visualized on these views. Figures 1-46C and 1-46D show the same pathology at the thoracic level.

Neural foraminal compromise or widening after trauma can be well appreciated on MDCT. Posttraumatic pseudomeningoceles occur due to avulsion of nerve roots within the dura. The resulting saccular pockets of cerebrospinal fluid that extend through the neural foramen are best seen on coronal images. Minimum intensity projection images after CT myelography are excellent for demonstrating these dural defects and associated nerve roots (Figure 1-47).

Preoperative and Postoperative Evaluation

CT is an excellent modality for preoperative and postoperative evaluation. With the improved multiplanar and 3-D reconstructions, preoperative assessment of complex spinal deformities has become routine practice. Preoperative CT scan defines the anatomy and avoids any unexpected intraoperative posterior element deficiencies. Because of its high resolution and its ability to obtain oblique views retrospectively, CT provides superior visualization of the bony anatomy. In cases of severe scoliotic deformity, MRI can be limited because only a select number of planes can be specified and obtained. Using CT, curved reformats can be performed and the spine "straightened" out in order to elicit the relationship of the nerves with respect to the neural foramina. One such example is shown in Figure 1-48.

Although CT produces metallic artifacts in the plane of the axial slice, the distribution of the artifacts is very different from that in MRI. In MRI, typically a wide area surrounding the metal is compromised. Using appropriate oblique views, the artifacts can be thrown off the plane of abnormality in order to demonstrate

Chapter 1 Multidetector Computed Tomography as a Problem-Solving Tool in Neuroradiology

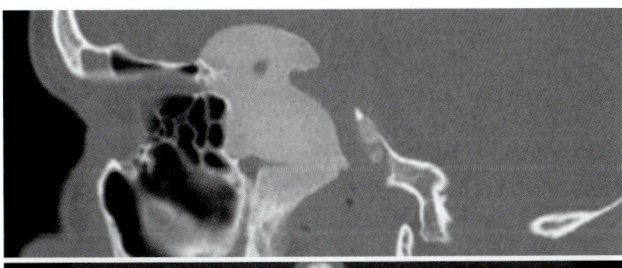
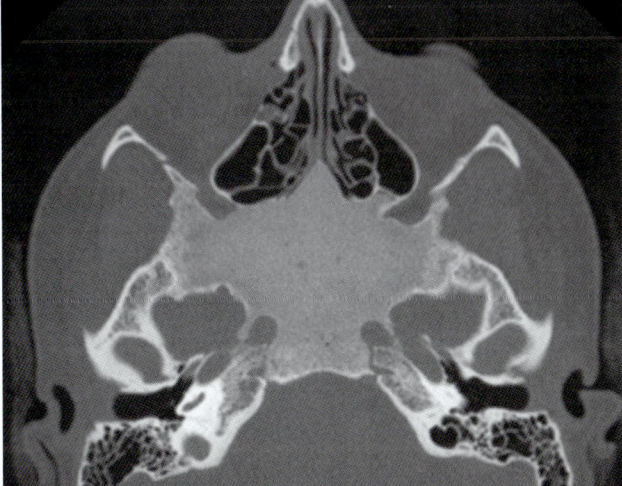
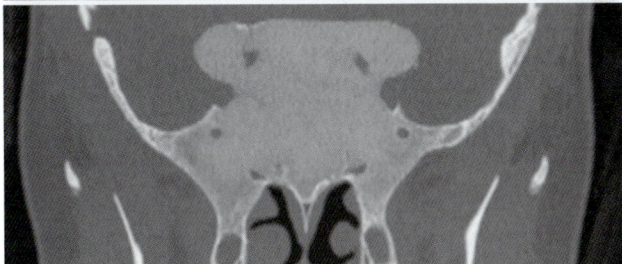

Figure 1-40 Sagittal, axial, and coronal computed tomographic slices showing classic features of fibrous dysplasia of the sphenoid bone, such as expansion of the sphenoid bone with ground-glass appearance with associated distortion of the optic foramina.

certain pathologies. An example is shown in Figure 1-49. Although MRI is better for visualizing nerves and soft tissue abnormalities, the type of nerve impingement shown in this figure would be very difficult to demonstrate using MRI due to the metallic artifacts. However, appropriately angled oblique images clearly demonstrate impingement of the L5 nerve root from malpositioned hardware.

Spinal Infections

Infective spondylodiscitis commonly presents as simple backache. This diagnosis is more effectively made using MRI but also can be made using MDCT. CT scan can show the extent and type of infection causing spondylodiscitis. Assessment of the degree of canal or foraminal compromise and bony destruction is better performed using MDCT than MRI. Signs that differentiate between infection and other conditions, such as neoplasm, have been described. CT can provide maps for intraoperative image-guided biopsy.

In the setting of vertebral body or disc infection, CT is very effective in demonstrating erosion along the end plates. Coronal and sagittal images enable detection of disc involvement and loss of height. Prevertebral and paravertebral components of the infective process are easily identified. Paraspinal abscesses have a characteristic fluid density with peripheral rim enhancement. Any epidural component of an abscess can be identified using CT, although MRI is more sensitive. Use of contrast improves detection of an infected disc, which shows abnormal enhancement.

Although CT is by no means definitive, it can guide in differentiating the causative organism in spinal infections. The features that favor a pyogenic abscess include greater sclerosis and erosions along the end plates, existence of necrotic tissue, and greater involvement of the adjacent disc, which shows abnormal enhancement. However, in tuberculous spondylodiscitis, sclerosis

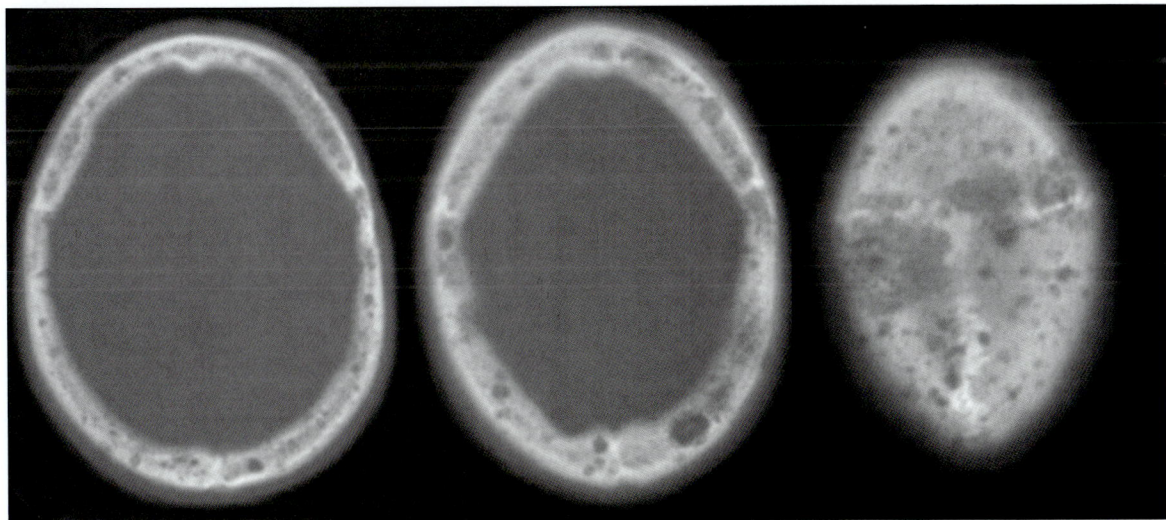

Figure 1-41 Multiple small, similar-sized, teardrop- or raindrop-shaped lytic lesions throughout the skull representing multiple myeloma.

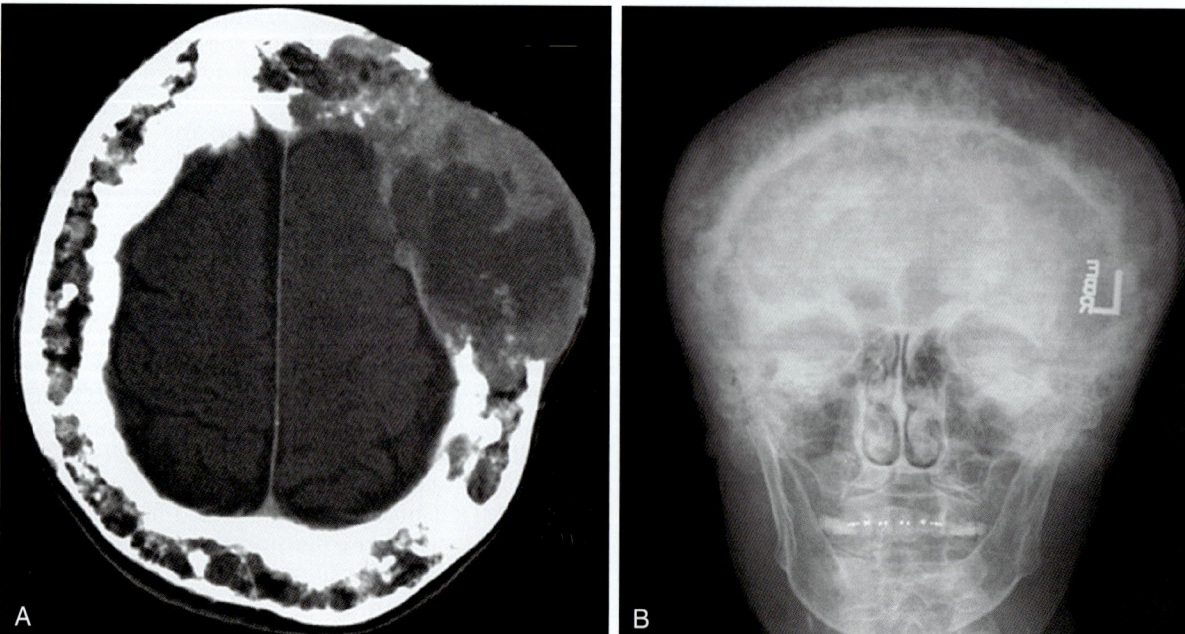

Figure 1-42 A: Computed tomographic section of the brain in the high vertical region showing widened diploic space with cortical thickening, coarse trabeculae, and marked sclerosis of the skull. A large soft tissue mass with a necrotic center is replacing the left frontal bone. These are classic findings of Paget disease with the soft tissue mass representing malignant transformation. B: Skull radiograph showing the cotton-wool appearance with lytic component in the left frontal region representing malignant transformation.

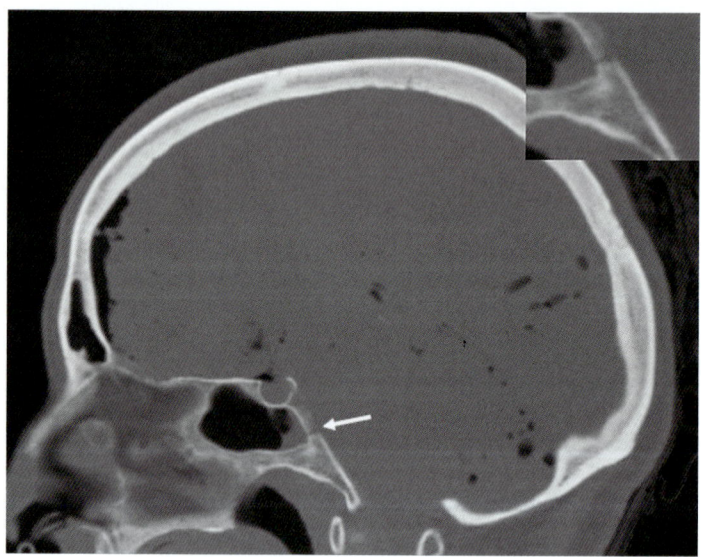

Figure 1-43 Sagittal computed tomographic reformation from multidetector computed tomography of a 65-year-old woman who presented with severe headache. Extensive pneumocephalus due to a defect in the clivus (arrow) is seen. Inset: Magnified view showing the communication between the sphenoid sinus and the posterior fossa responsible for the pneumocephalus.

typically is minimal, and only a thin enhancing rim may be seen around the necrotic components. In Koch spine, CT may identify subligamentous spread of infection and intra-osseous abscesses within the vertebral bodies. Figure 1-50 shows a case of spondylodiscitis. Spinal brucellosis, an uncommon spinal infection, is known to have a "cauliflower" appearance of lytic lesions with sclerosis along the margins of the lesions.

Epidural abscess, a surgical emergency, is rarely encountered in present-day clinical practice. However, a young patient with rapid onset of infective symptoms, or a spinal level quadriparesis should undergo a workup for an epidural abscess. The advantages of CT in the diagnosis of an epidural abscess include (1) possible detection of the source of infection, spondylitis, discitis, or facet joint infection; (2) detection of the extent of epidural abscess; and (3) preoperative planning for image-guided aspiration and biopsy for diagnosis.

Spinal Tumors

Early detection of a spinal tumor is possible on CT if a lytic or sclerotic component is present. In case of diffuse marrow infiltrating tumors, CT may be less valuable.

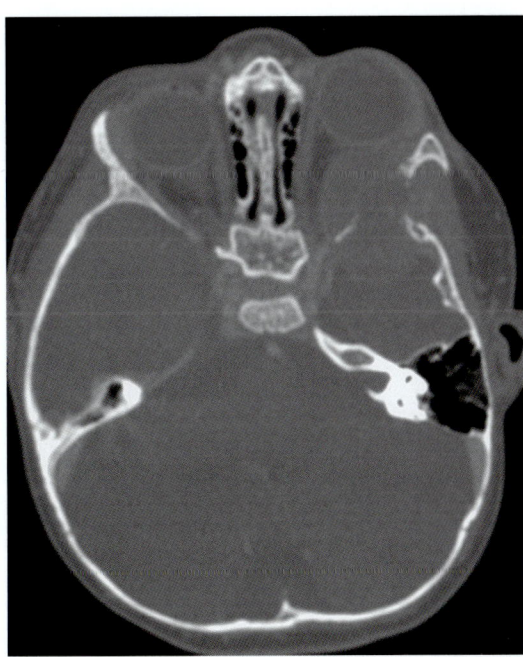

Figure 1-44 Young male who presented with left-sided proptosis. Axial computed tomographic (CT) section showing destruction of the lesser wing of sphenoid on the left side with a large soft tissue component protruding into the left orbit causing proptosis. CT shows the extent of cortical destruction from this biopsy-proven neuroblastoma.

In detecting tumors, CT is more useful than conventional radiography for evaluating lesion location and analyzing bone destruction and condensation.

A "bubbly" lytic lesion that extends across vertebral levels likely is a giant cell tumor or aneurysmal bone cyst. The latter is more common in the younger age group and in the posterior elements. A solitary expansile lytic lesion could also represent a plasmacytoma or a lesion in multiple myeloma. Many solitary lesions, such as bone island, osteoid osteoma, osteochondroma, chondrosarcoma, vertebral hemangioma, and aneurysmal bone cyst, have characteristic features on CT. For example, an isolated bone island is a focal, well-circumscribed osseous density within the marrow. An osteoid osteoma demonstrates extensive sclerosis with a central lytic nidus. A hemangioma shows a typical "corduroy" appearance, and aneurysmal bone cyst is a bubbly lesion.

Mixed lesion with lytic, sclerotic, and soft tissue components could represent a lymphoma or chordoma. The latter is more commonly encountered in the sacrum. Figures 1-51 and 1-52 illustrate some examples of these entities.

■ CT IN HEAD AND NECK IMAGING

Head and neck pathologies and their associated imaging findings are discussed in detail in Chapter 19. This section reviews and highlights areas where MDCT is especially useful in evaluating these pathologies. The role of this modality as a problem-solving tool in this field is illustrated with the help of representative examples. This section is divided into three main subsections: temporal bone, orbital pathologies, and neck tumors/masses.

Temporal Bone

As has been illustrated in other sections, MDCT is an excellent tool for imaging bony pathology. This is especially useful for temporal bone and for structures embedded within it because of their small size and intricate interrelationships. MDCT is the preferred modality for imaging the temporal bone and its associated pathologies. Many congenital abnormalities, such as cochlear aplasia, Mondini malformation, anomalous course of the seventh and eighth cranial nerves, otosclerosis, and tympanosclerosis, are readily demonstrated by MDCT if proper attention is paid to the imaging protocol.

An ideal protocol for temporal bone imaging entails very thin nonoverlapping slices. Typically, slices as thin as 0.5 mm, reconstructed with bone kernel, are required to visualize the small structures of the temporal bone. The anatomy and the structures within the temporal bone are not specifically aligned with the three cardinal planes of the body. For example, the superior semicircular canal (sSCC) is oriented approximately 45 degrees from both the sagittal and coronal planes. The native axial dataset should be reformatted in specially oriented oblique planes to optimize visualization. The two most commonly used planes are the Stenvers plane and the Pöschl plane. The Pöschl plane approximates the plane of the sSCC (Figure 1-53). The Stenvers plane is perpendicular to both the axial plane and the Pöschl plane. The Stenvers plane shows the upper cortex of the sSCC in perfect cross section and is optimal for demonstrating the integrity of the wall of the upper arc of the sSCC.

The Stenvers and Pöschl orientations can be prescribed by the technologist at the scanner and the resulting image data should be archived along with the axial dataset. For prescribing these planes, the plane of the lateral semicircular canal can be used to define the true axial plane. On the true axial dataset, the sSCC can be used to prescribe the Pöschl plane; the Stenvers plane is perpendicular to this plane. In general, the Stenvers plane is approximately parallel to the petrous ridge, and the Pöschl plane is perpendicular to the long axis of the petrous ridge. Visualization of pathologies, such as sSCC dehiscence, cochlear malformations, and vestibular anomalies, is facilitated by these planes.

The sSCC dehiscence syndrome is a typical pathology that shows the power of MDCT. This syndrome, originally described in an article in 1998, requires demonstration of a very small defect in the bony wall of the sSCC. Even a small sliver of bone overlying the SCC excludes the diagnosis of this syndrome. High-resolution imaging and proper attention to protocol are crucial to offset partial volume effect. Figure 1-54 shows CT images from a case demonstrating a defect in the sSCC.

Superior semicircular canal dehiscence is only one of many pathologies that may result in the formation of a "third window" into a semicircular canal causing

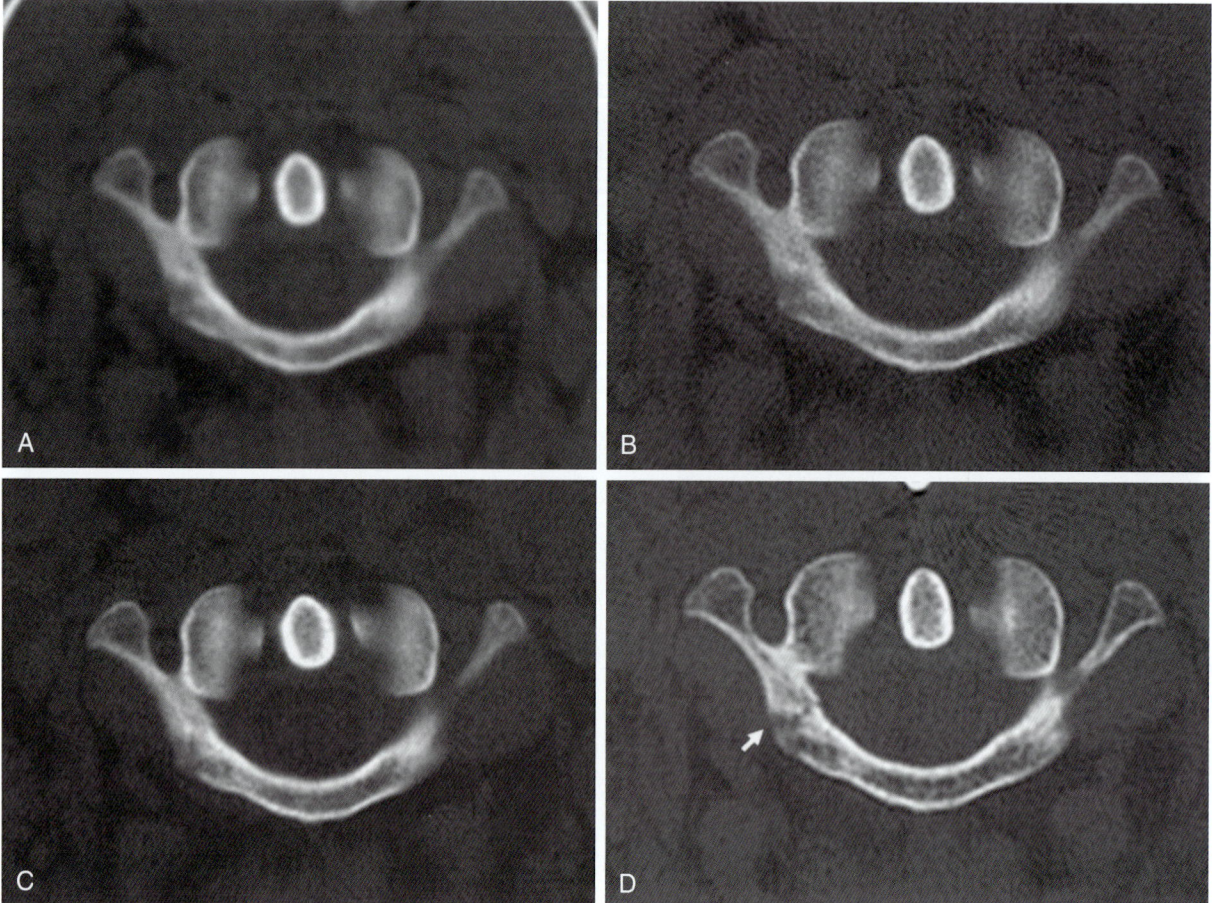

Figure 1-45 Multiple images of a subtle fracture in the right posterior arch of C1. **A:** Standard kernel, slice thickness 2.5 mm, pitch 1:1. **B:** Bone kernel, slice thickness 2.5 mm, pitch 1:1. **C:** Standard kernel, slice thickness 1.25 mm, pitch 0.5:1. **D:** Bone kernel, slice thickness 1.25 mm, pitch 0.5:1. This fracture is not visible at slice thickness 2.5 mm and pitch 1:1 either using the standard kernel (**A**) or the bone kernel (**B**). The fracture becomes more apparent when pitch 0.5:1, slice thickness 1.25 mm, and standard reconstruction kernel are used (**C**). It becomes even more apparent after 1 week (**D**) when a sharper bone kernel with thinner slices and lower pitch is used *(white arrow)*.

Tullio phenomenon. The hallmark of Tullio phenomenon is dizziness in response to loud sound. Tullio phenomenon also results in specific eye movements that depend on the semicircular canal involved. For example, a third window in the lateral SCC results in a horizontal nystagmus, whereas that in the sSCC causes vertical nystagmus with an inward torsion (45-degree tilt of canal) or an opposite direction nystagmus with Valsalva. Entities that can cause a third window into the SCC include cholesteatoma, syphilis, and iatrogenic reasons. All of these entities are well demonstrated using MDCT.

Problem-Solving Tool/Cases in Head and Neck Imaging

Figures 1-55 through 1-57 illustrate other typical applications of MDCT for evaluation of inner ear pathology. Figure 1-55 shows the case of a 10-year-old girl with sensorineural hearing loss. A temporal bone CT scan without contrast illustrates a complex left inner ear dysplasia with aplasia of the left cochlea. Other congenital malformations are equally well illustrated by MDCT (Figures 1-56 and 1-57).

MDCT is the modality of choice for depicting trauma to temporal bone. Traumatic fractures of the temporal bone can be divided into those that are oriented along the long axis of the petrous pyramid and those that are perpendicular to it. These two fracture types result in very different symptoms and can be readily distinguished using MDCT. A transverse temporal bone fracture is shown in Figure 1-58. Such fractures account for about 10% to 30% of all temporal bone fractures and typically are the result of blunt trauma to the occiput. The fracture line commonly extends from the jugular foramen or foramen magnum to the middle cranial fossa. It may pass through bony labyrinth and may destroy both vestibular and cochlear apparatuses. If it is a bit more medial, it may transect the internal auditory meatus and the cochlear nerve within it. A transverse fracture commonly results in sensorineural hearing loss. Over years, an old fracture may result in ossified labyrinth (which can be demonstrated with MDCT), severe vertigo, and nystagmus. It also can cause transection of the vestibule, vestibular nerve, or vestibular aqueduct. These fractures are sometimes hard to detect on axial MDCT images, requiring the Stenvers or Pöschl plane for detection. A perilymph fistula, cerebrospinal

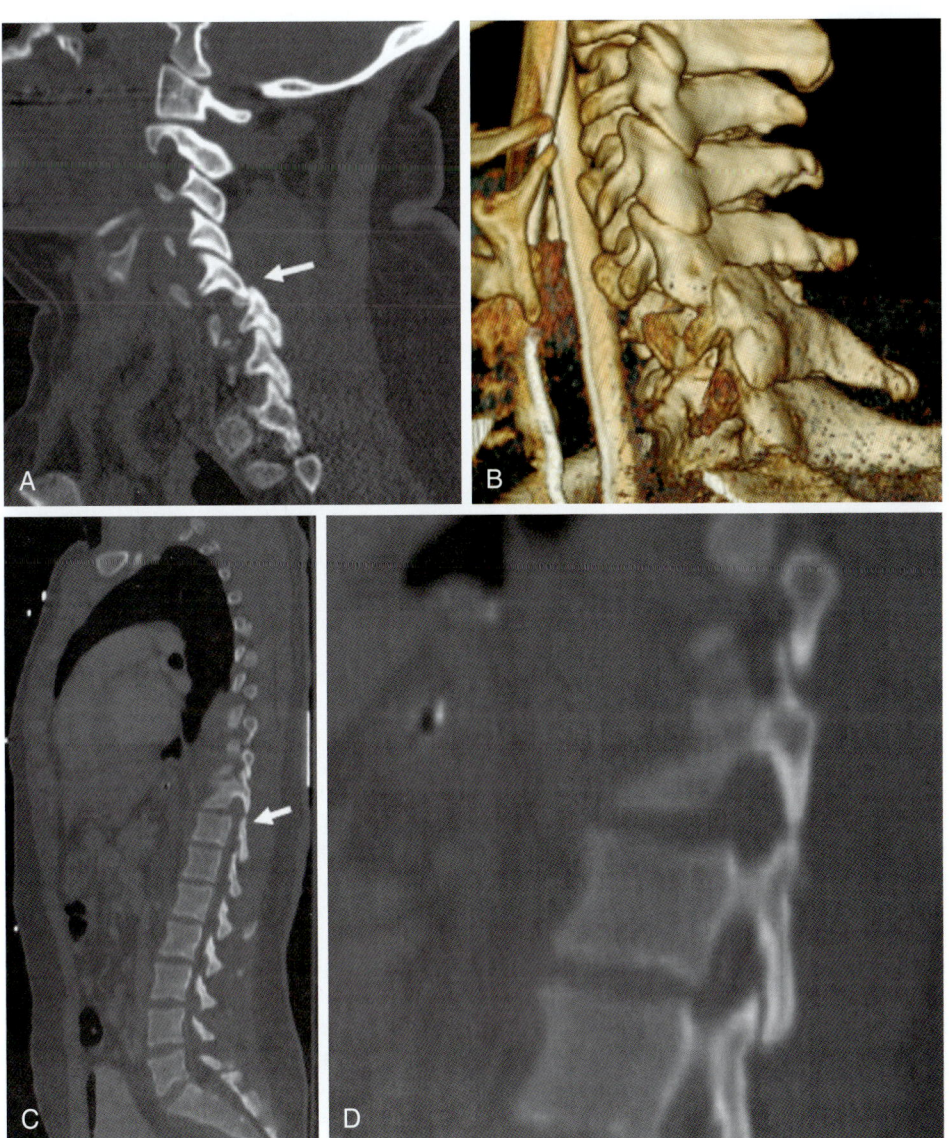

Figure 1-46 A: Sagittal reconstructed multidetector computed tomographic (MDCT) image showing a unilateral locked facet at the C5–6 level *(arrow)*. **B:** Surface-rendered image showing a different view of a perched (locked) facet. Thoracic perched facet at T10–11 shown in sagittal MDCT section **(C)** and focal magnified image at the T10–11 level **(D)**.

fluid level in the middle ear, and fluctuating sensorineural hearing loss are other signs of occult trauma to the inner ear.

The otic capsule is the densest bone in the body. CT is quite sensitive in depicting mineralization (or lack there of) in the otic capsule and ossicles. Figure 1-59 shows a case of tympanosclerosis in a middle-aged man. This pathology may be asymptomatic or may present as conductive hearing loss, often as a sequela of chronic otitis media.

Tympanosclerosis may cause restriction of ossicular movement and may involve the tympanic membrane, suspensory ligaments, and tendon degeneration. Secondary stapes fixation due to oval window annular ligament involvement is not uncommon. Of these changes, only the bony changes are well visualized using CT. Demineralization of the otic capsule from otospongiosis or otosclerosis is also well depicted by MDCT.

Visualization of the temporal bone structures is crucially dependent on spatial resolution. Impressive temporal bone images have been demonstrated using a new type of CT scanner based on flat-panel detector technology. These scanners, called *flat-panel volume CT* (fpVCT) scanners, are characterized by very high spatial resolution and volumetric coverage. They are described in detail later in this chapter. Some example images of temporal bone specimens acquired from one such prototype scanner are shown here.

Figure 1-60 shows a reformatted fpVCT view of the branching of the eighth cranial nerve into its vestibular part (white arrowhead) and the cochlear part (black arrowhead). Its branches (small black arrowhead) can be followed through the modiolus to the bony spiral lamina in the cochlea. The tensor tympani muscle (black arrow) in its canal next to the carotid (cross) and the facial nerve canal (white arrow) next to the middle ear also are visible.

Figure 1-61 shows multiple segments of the facial nerve (small black arrowheads) in another reformatted image obtained from the fpVCT volumetric data. These structures are not as well seen on the MDCT or MRI images due to their limited resolution. The reformation

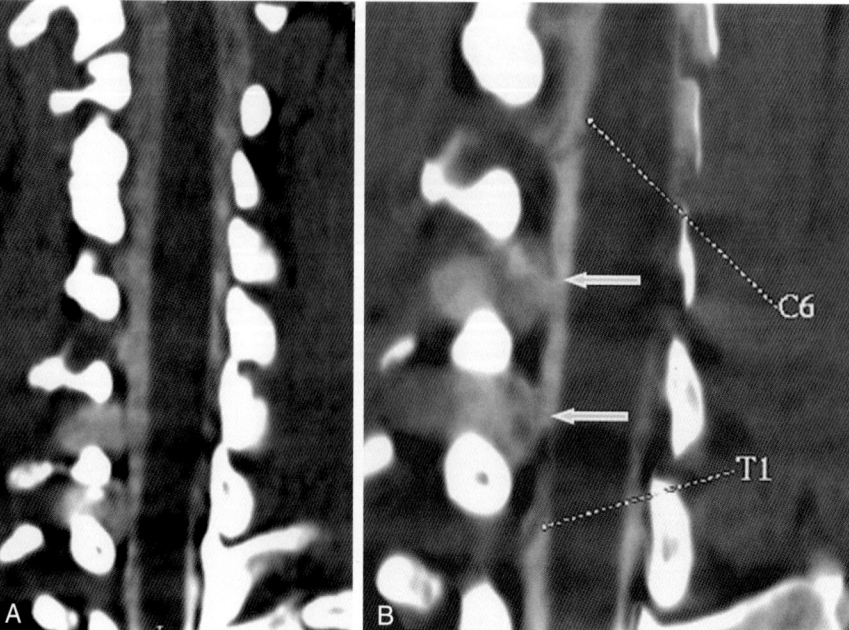

Figure 1-47 Coronal sections from computed tomographic myelogram of cervical spine rendered with minimum intensity projection (MIP) showing posttraumatic saccular outpouching of contrast at the C6–7 and C7–T1 levels *(white arrows)* representing pseudomeningoceles along the right C7 and C8 nerve root sleeves. MIP brings out the nerve roots embedded within the contrast-enhanced cerebrospinal fluid.

plane in Figure 1-61A is close to a horizontal section. It shows the facial nerve leaving the internal auditory canal (black arrow) through its canal (large black arrowhead) into the geniculate ganglion (large white arrowhead). The image plane in Figure 1-61B is situated midway between the sagittal and frontal planes. It shows both the tympanic segment and the descending mastoid segment of the facial nerve. Note that the nerve in the canal is directly imaged in this specimen because air has dissected into this space during specimen preparation. Only a thin bony lamina separates it from the middle ear (white arrow). The canal of the greater petrosal nerve (long white arrow) can also be seen. Due to a high jugular bulb (white star), only a thin bony lamina (small white arrowhead) separates the jugular vein from the middle ear cavity. The tensor tympani muscle (black star) can be found parallel to the eustachian tube. Figure 1-62 shows another high-resolution dataset in which the entire length of the cochlear aqueduct, a structure not normally demonstrated by MDCT, can be seen.

The image quality and resolution of fpVCT are adequate for high-quality segmentation and volume rendering. Figure 1-63 shows a comparison of the volume-rendered views from MDCT and fpVCT. The definition and detail of the high-contrast structures are superior on the fpVCT images. This concept can be taken a step further by making 3-D models of the inner and middle ear structures. Figure 1-64 shows one such 3-D model of the right temporal bone seen from the anterolateral direction. This model was built by individually segmenting out anatomic structures from the fpVCT image stack. In the foreground, the tympanic membrane (yellowish green), malleus (orange), and incus (green) can be seen; the stapes (blue) is partially covered. The facial nerve (purple) can be followed from behind the bony labyrinth (transparent yellow) to its tympanic part. In front of the transparent bony cochlea, in which the spiral osseus lamina (brown) is visible, one branch of the facial nerve (greater petrosal nerve) can be seen. The tensor tympani muscle (pinkish purple) is in the right half of the image; the stapedius muscle (also pinkish purple) can be found in the left half. The stapedius nerve (purple) innervating the stapedius muscle and the vestibulocochlear nerve (dark lilac) are depicted.

The ability to render high-quality surface views opens a unique possibility in the evaluation of temporal bone. "Virtual endoscopy" of the middle and inner ear can be performed by positioning a camera in the temporal bone and prescribing an orientation and motion path. Figure 1-65 shows three snapshots from a virtual endoscopy movie generated using surface-rendered images from fpVCT data. In Figure 1-65A, the virtual endoscope is positioned in the external acoustic meatus, close to the plane of the tympanic membrane, and is facing medially. The tympanic membrane is removed by rendering its opacity level to zero (i.e., making it completely transparent). Its position can be deduced from the handle of the malleus (black star) and the tympanic sulcus (small black arrows) where the circumference of the tympanic membrane is attached. The eustachian tube (white star), long process of the incus (short white arrow), and promontory (black cross) with its round window niche (white long arrowhead) are shown. Behind the tendon of the stapedius muscle (large black arrowhead), the posterior crus of stapes is visible. In the right lower corner of the image can be seen the bulge of a high jugular bulb, which is only partially covered by a thin bony lamina. Spaces that are covered only by soft tissue (small arrowheads) make it a dehiscent high jugular bulb. In Figure 1-65B, the camera is positioned in the distal end of the eustachian tube. It is oriented so that the viewing direction is about 45 degrees laterally and posteriorly. The external auditory canal is visible in the right half of the image. Besides the features described in Figure 1-65A, the anterior crus of stapes can be seen (small black arrowhead). In Figure 1-65C,

Chapter 1 Multidetector Computed Tomography as a Problem-Solving Tool in Neuroradiology

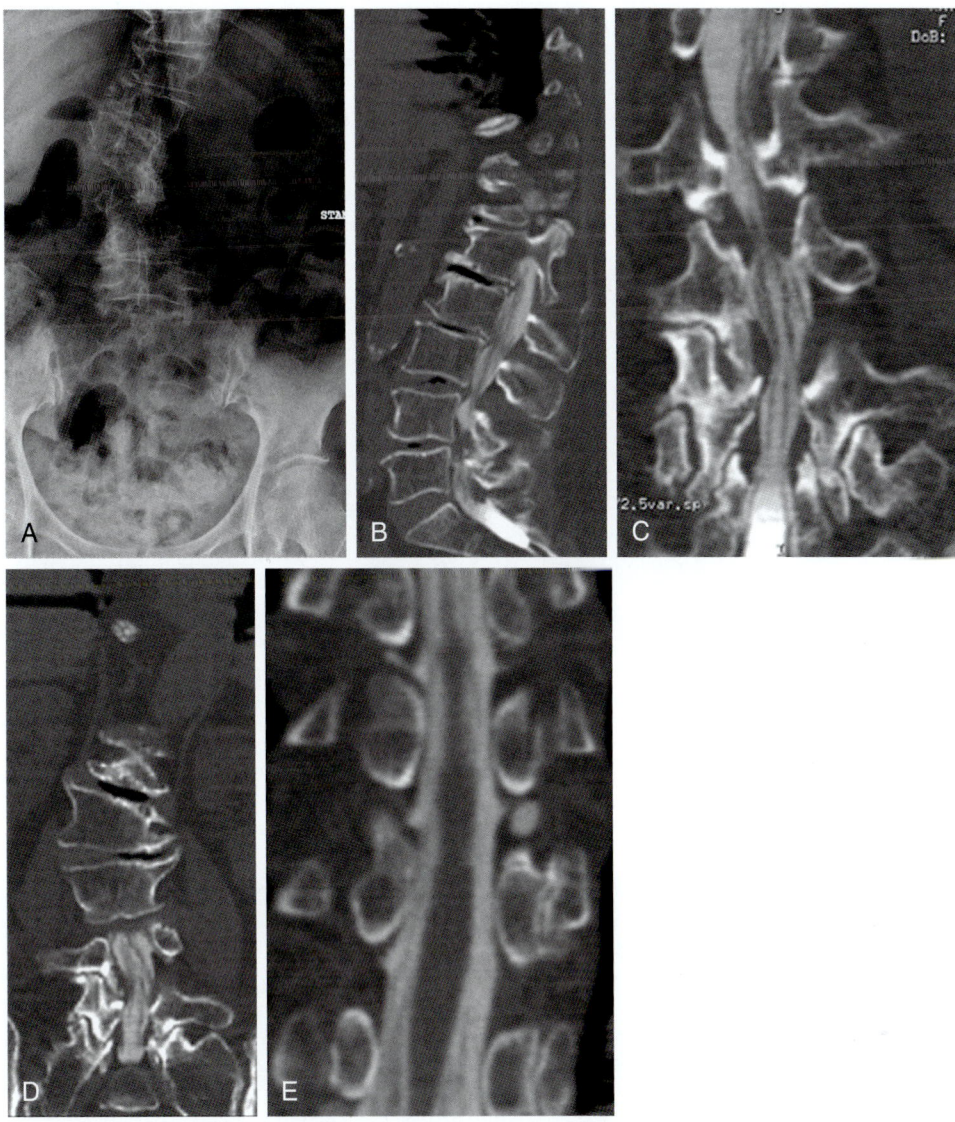

Figure 1-48 A: Plain radiograph of the thoracolumbar spine showing a complex kyphoscoliotic deformity. Straight sagittal and coronal reformations (B, D) and curved sagittal and coronal reformations (C, E) from a computed tomographic myelogram. The curved reformatted images give excellent details regarding multiple levels of thecal sac despite the extensive kyphoscoliotic deformity.

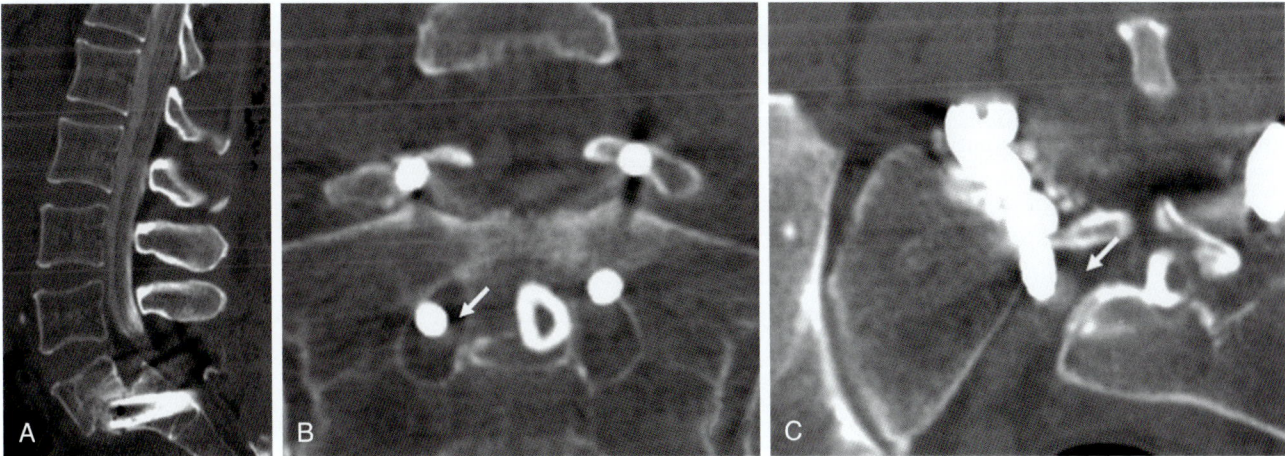

Figure 1-49 Postoperative imaging after laminectomy at L5 with transpedicular fixation at the L5–S1 level. Sagittal (A), coronal reconstruction (B), and axial section (C) at the L5–S1 level demonstrating grade 2 spondylolisthesis of L5 over S1 with impingement of the right S1 nerve root (*white arrow*) between the right-sided screw and the bony margin of the neural foramen.

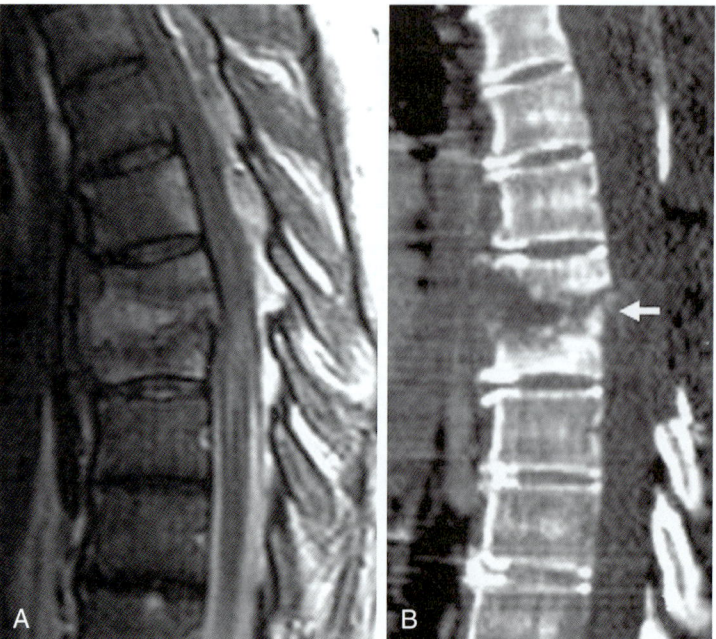

Figure 1-50 Fifty-year-old woman who presented with subacute paraplegia and loss of sensations. **(A)** T2 weighted sagittal section through midthoracic region showing partial collapse of the vertebrae adjoining destroyed disc, no obvious epidural abscess but canal narrowing and cord hyperintensity suggesting cord edema. **(B)** Multidetector computed tomography with sagittal reconstruction showing the extent of vertebral body destruction, disc destruction, and prevertebral necrotic collection in continuity with osseous disease. A minimally sclerotic component *(white arrow)* protruding into the spinal canal indenting on the cord at this midthoracic level is also demonstrated by multidetector computed tomography and likely is responsible for the patient's symptoms.

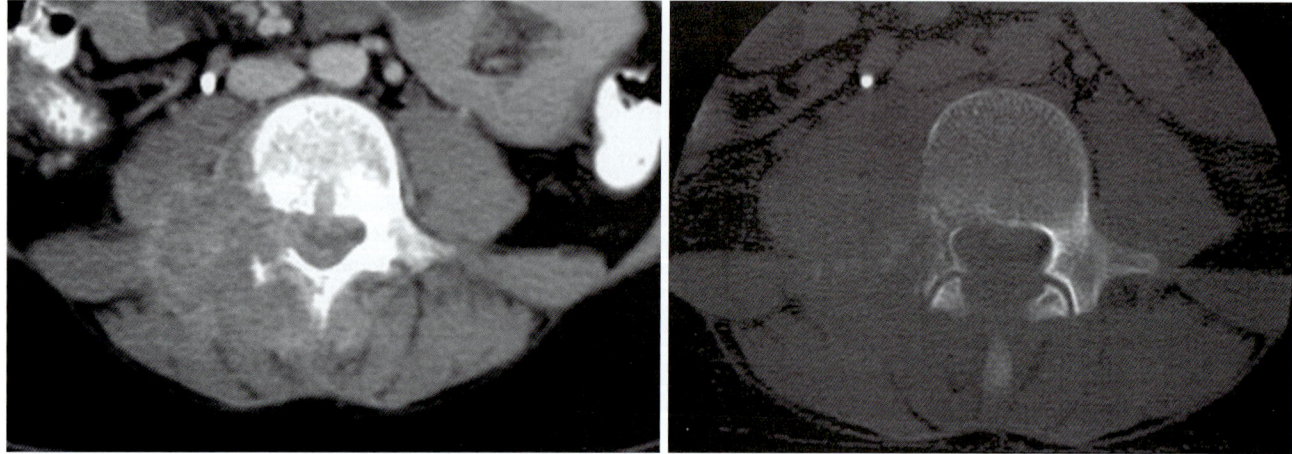

Figure 1-51 Soft tissue and bone kernel axial sections of a 10-year-old boy with back pain and right-sided hip and knee pain. Computed tomography showing permeative necrosis of the right pedicle and transverse process with a soft tissue component extending into the right quadratus lumborum and erector spinae muscles with minimal epidural component. With these imaging characteristics, the differential considerations would include Ewing sarcoma, lymphoma, and eosinophilic granuloma. Histopathology showed this lesion to be an anaplastic lymphoma.

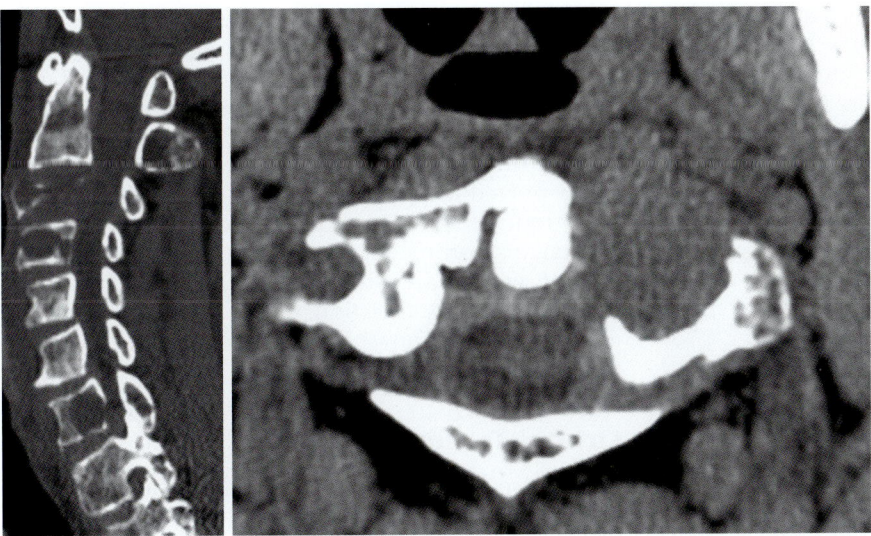

Figure 1-52 Sagittal reformation through the cervical spine and axial section at the C1–2 level showing multiple well-defined lytic lesions in the vertebral bodies with collapse of C3 and a soft tissue component arising from the left anterior arch of C1. The posterior elements are relatively uninvolved. These multidetector computed tomographic features are suggestive of multiple myeloma.

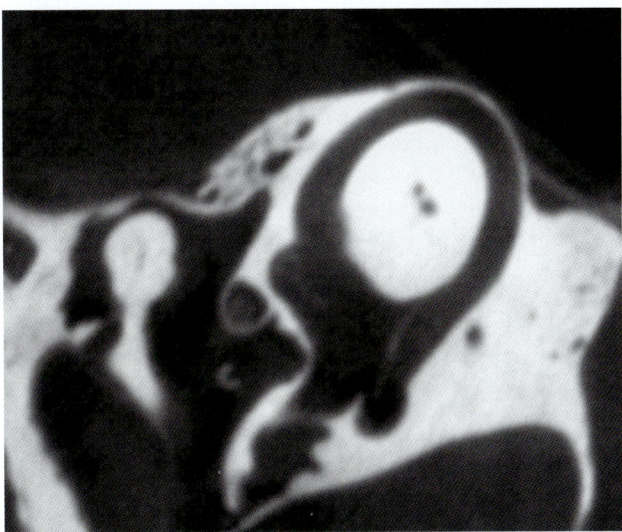

Figure 1-53 Single slice from a stack of images along the Pöschl plane showing a nondehiscent superior semicircular canal.

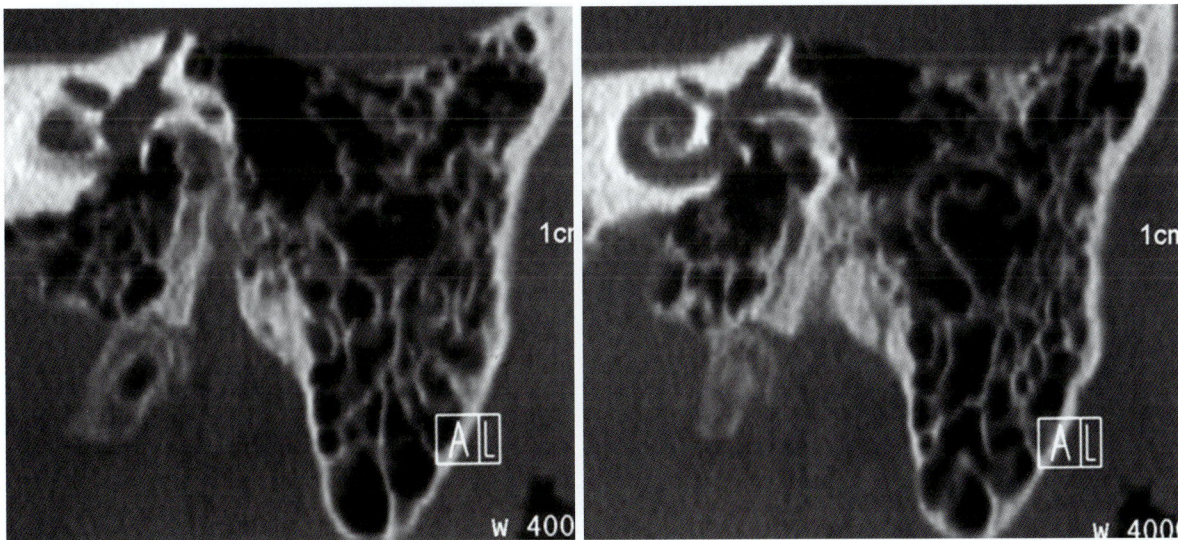

Figure 1-54 Dehiscence of superior semicircular canal.

the camera is positioned beneath the ossicular chain and is facing superiorly. Both crura of the stapes can be clearly assessed. In addition to the features described in Figures 1-65A and 1-65B, the short process of the incus within the tympanic attic is marked (long white arrow). In all of these views, the chorda tympani and the tympanic membrane are not visible because their CT numbers were below the threshold used for surface rendering.

Orbital Pathologies

Orbital pathologies can be broadly divided into traumatic, congenital, vascular/lymphatic, infectious, inflammatory/metabolic, and neoplastic categories. All of these entities are well demonstrated by MDCT, making CT scan the first-line imaging modality for most orbital pathology. CT is most valuable in delineating the shape, size, location, and characteristics of orbital lesions. It also can guide clinicians during surgical interventions because it places a lesion with respect to the various spaces of the orbit. This subsection briefly illustrates some example cases of orbital pathologies that demonstrate the utility of MDCT.

Signs and symptoms of orbital disease that prompt a CT scan include exophthalmos (unilateral or bilateral), displacement of globe, ptosis, diplopia, limitations of extraocular motility, decreased vision, visualization or palpation of an orbital mass, swelling, orbital pain, abnormal vascularity, and trauma. Although the clinician may have a good sense of the state of the superficial aspects of the eye and the globe, evaluation of the retrobulbar areas requires a tomographic modality.

The advantages of MDCT in the evaluation of temporal bone also apply to orbital pathologies. There is natural contrast between the retrobulbar fat, bone, air, and soft tissues of the orbit. CT also detects calcifications easily, a fact that is useful in characterizing an orbital mass. CT scan is quick and generally motion free, and, in most cases, sedation is not required for pediatric patients.

The optimal protocol for MDCT of the orbit must include thin axial slices, approximately 1.5 mm thick, reconstructed using bone and soft tissue kernels. From these routine axial CT slices, it is customary to obtain sagittal and coronal sections. In complex cases, oblique sagittal sections also should be obtained (Figure 1-66). If an orbital mass, infection, or inflammatory condition is suspected, IV contrast must be administered. Noncontrast examination may be sufficient for follow-up cases.

Orbital Trauma

The choice of CT after blunt or penetrating trauma to the orbit, globe, or face is obvious. It can show fractures, hemorrhage, soft tissue swelling, embedded foreign bodies, and other derangements of the orbit in exquisite detail, even in an uncooperative patient. Figure 1-67 shows two cases of trauma resulting in lens dislocation. In the second case, the lens has been displaced from the anterior portion of the globe and has come to rest in the dependent portion of the vitreous humor. Although trauma is the most common cause of lens subluxation, other causes include Marfan syndrome, Ehlers-Danlos syndrome, Weill-Marchesani syndrome, familial ectopia lentis, homocystinuria, cataract surgery, and aniridia.

Inflammatory and Metabolic Conditions

Inflammatory and metabolic conditions form a heterogeneous group that includes idiopathic orbital inflammatory disease (more commonly referred to as *orbital*

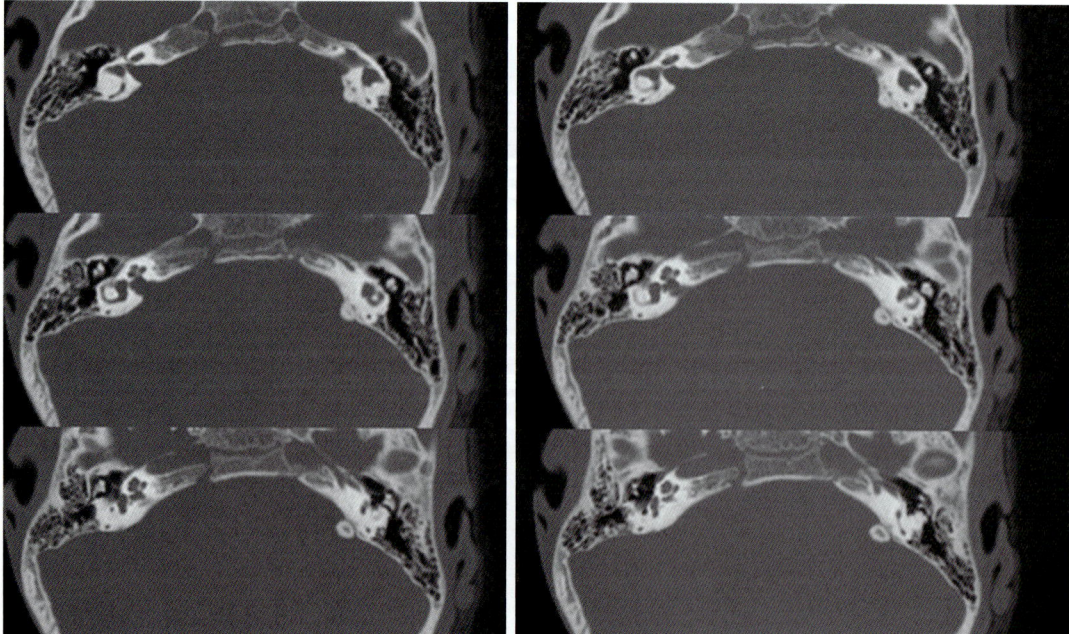

Figure 1-55 Axial sections through the posterior fossa, reconstructed with bone kernel, showing absence of the left internal auditory canal. The semicircular canals protrude into the cerebropontine angle, and the left-sided cochlear turns are aplastic.

pseudotumor), optic neuritis, thyroid-associated orbitopathy, and a variety of granulomatous diseases, such as Wegener granulomatosis, tuberculosis, and sarcoidosis. All of these conditions of the orbit are well demonstrated by MDCT. To illustrate the role of MDCT in the management of these conditions, orbital pseudotumor is examined in detail.

Idiopathic inflammatory orbital pseudotumor is the third most common orbital disease after Graves disease and lymphoproliferative disease. It may involve the orbit, lungs, and other systems. Orbital and periorbital pain is common during acute onset. Other clinical signs and symptoms may include exophthalmos, lid swelling, conjunctival injection and edema, motility restrictions, ptosis, and increased orbital pressure. Orbital pseudotumor may be acute, subacute, or chronic. It may present as a single episode, it may be continuous, or it may be intermittent. The chronic form may evolve from the acute or subacute variety, or it may begin as a chronic process. The chronic form represents the sclerosing type. MDCT is the primary investigative modality; MRI is reserved for evaluation of extraorbital extension.

Orbital pseudotumor is diagnosed using a combination of clinical findings, MDCT findings, and response to steroid therapy. Although MDCT provides useful information, the ultimate diagnosis is clinical. Fine-needle aspiration biopsy with CT guidance can be used when questions arise. For example, CT-guided biopsy may be necessary when the pseudotumor is mass-like, does not respond to steroid therapy, or is a sclerosing type.

Based on its radiologic appearance, pseudotumor can be classified as dacryoadenitis, diffuse orbital infiltration, myositis, orbital mass, sclero-uveitis, perineuritis, or eyelid pseudotumor. Combinations of these pathologic patterns are possible. Although many of these conditions are evaluated during a comprehensive eye examination, MDCT plays a crucial role in the evaluation of retrobulbar disease. For example, CT locates the enlargement of the lacrimal gland in dacryoadenitis. Myositis typically presents as pain during extraocular muscle motion but cannot be directly evaluated clinically. CT scan readily shows tubular, irregular, asymmetric enlargement of the involved extraocular muscles (Figure 1-68). The tendons of the affected muscles also are enlarged and broadened in this condition, a key point that differentiates it from Graves ophthalmopathy. Lateral rectus is most commonly affected; involvement of superior oblique and palpebral muscles is rare.

The appearance of pseudotumor on contrast-enhanced MDCT scan is suggestive but nonspecific. Differential diagnosis of orbital pseudotumor includes

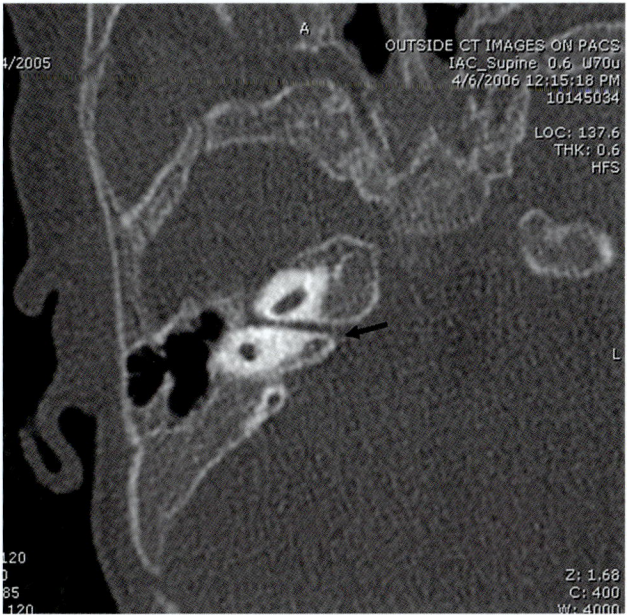

Figure 1-56 Axial section through the right temporal bone using a sharp bone kernel showing a well-defined canal *(black arrow)*, superior and separate from the internal auditory canal, representing an anomalous channel for the seventh cranial nerve.

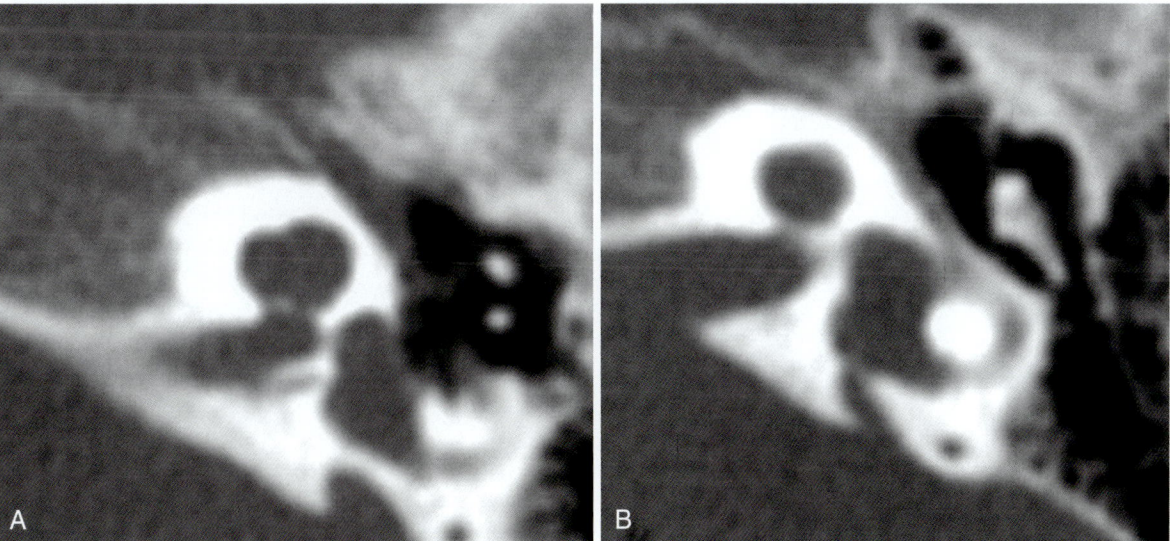

Figure 1-57 Undersegmented left cochlea with poorly formed interscalar septum representing a Mondini malformation.

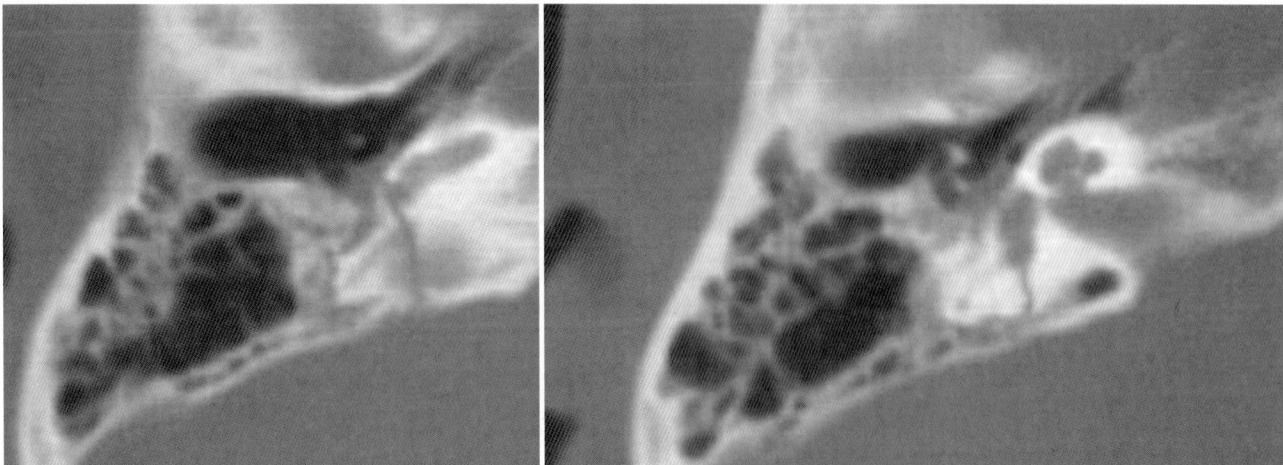

Figure 1-58 Axial sections through the right mastoid of a 31-year-old man who presented with altered mental status after sustaining a head injury from a fall 3 days ago. The bone kernel shows the fracture line perpendicular to the petrous ridge extending through the tympanic portion of the seventh nerve and lateral semicircular canal.

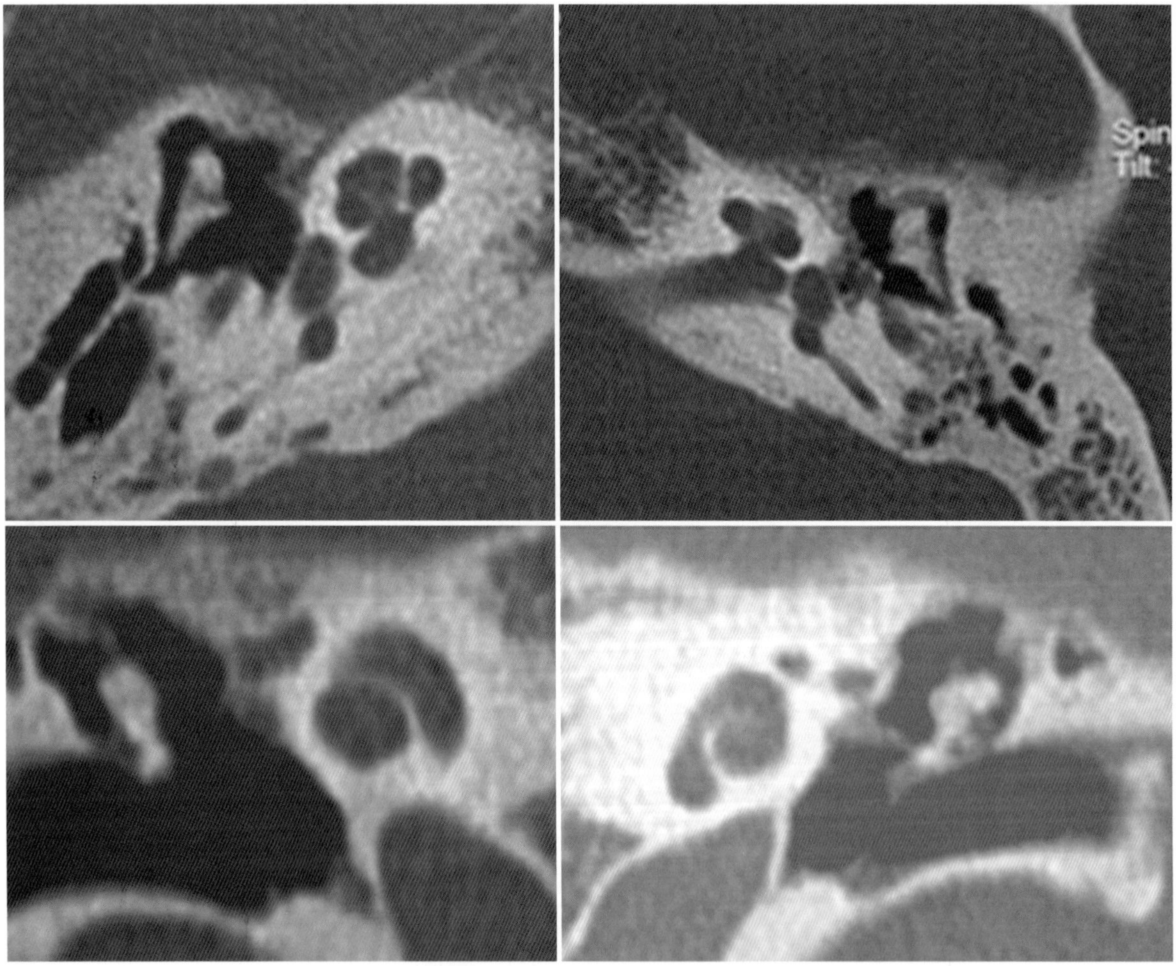

Figure 1-59 Tympanosclerosis involving the ossicles.

Graves ophthalmopathy, infections (bacterial, granulomatous, fungal), other granulomatous conditions (Wegener granulomatosis, sarcoidosis), metastatic disease (typically breast, lung), amyloid infiltration, histiocytosis (primarily in children), and rare entities such as Erdheim-Chester disease.

Thyroid-associated ophthalmopathy or Graves disease presents with eyelid retraction, exophthalmos with bilateral enlargement of the extraocular muscles, and compressive optic neuropathy. Superior, medial, and inferior recti are more preferentially involved, and the involvement is predominantly bilateral (90%) and symmetric (70%). Isolated involvement of a single extraocular muscle is uncommon (~5%). CT scan may show fat expansion and enlargement of the extraocular muscles with more than normal enhancement. Increased orbital fat may secondarily compress nerves. Figure 1-69 shows two cases of thyroid ophthalmopathy.

Periorbital and Orbital Infections

Infections of the obit may result in orbital cellulitis and abscess formation. Orbital infections may be viral, bacterial, or fungal (typically, aspergillus or mucormycosis). Contrast-enhanced MDCT is a reliable modality for assessing orbital infections that require further workup. The rapidity of this test and its wide availability make MDCT the first-line imaging modality for evaluation of infections. The orbital septum is a key landmark in assessment of periorbital/orbital infections. It is a fascia arising from the periosteum of orbital margin and inserts into the aponeurosis and fascia of the upper and lower eyelids at the margins of the superior and inferior tarsal plates. The orbital septum defines the margin between the preseptal and postseptal compartments.

Problem-Solving Tool/Cases in Orbital Lesions

MDCT can readily distinguish preseptal from postseptal cellulitis. This is an important distinction because a preseptal cellulitis can be managed conservatively, whereas a postseptal extension of infection is a potential emergency. CT should be considered in all cases where severe eyelid swelling obstructs the clinician's ability to properly examine the globe. Clinically, preseptal cellulitis presents with erythema and swelling of

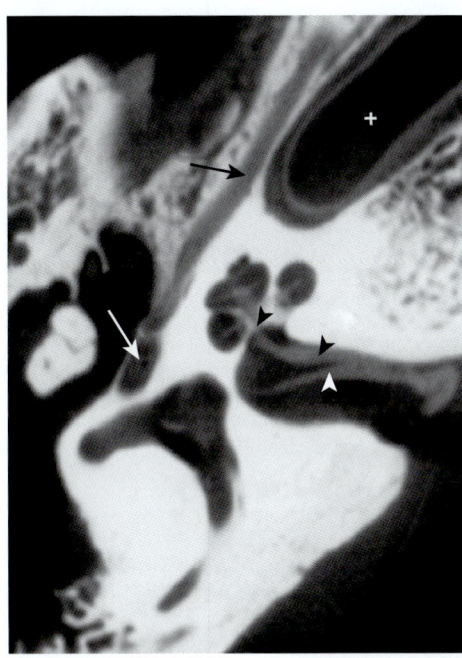

Figure 1-60 Reformatted flat-panel volume computed tomographic view of branching of the eighth cranial nerve into its vestibular part *(white arrowhead)* and cochlear part *(black arrowhead)*. Small black arrowhead, Modiolus; *black arrow*, tensor tympani muscle; *cross*, carotid; *white arrow*, facial nerve canal. (Courtesy of Dr. Soenke Bartling, DKFZ, Heidelberg, Germany)

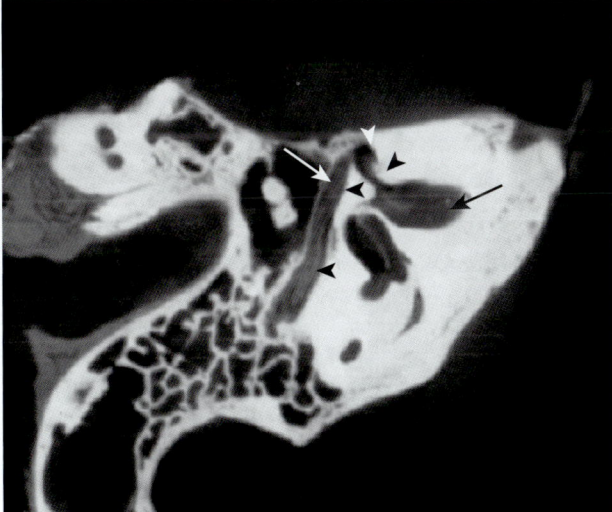 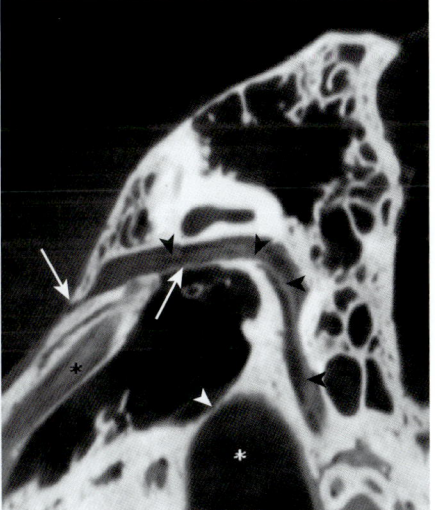

Figure 1-61 Multiple segments of the facial nerve *(small black arrowheads)* in reformatted images from a flat-panel volume computed tomography dataset. **A:** axial reformat and **B:** coronal reformat. Tympanic and descending mastoid segments of the facial nerve *(black arrow heads)*. *Black arrow*, Internal auditory canal; *large white arrowhead*, geniculate ganglion; *white arrow*, thin bony lamina separating tympanic segment from middle ear; *long white arrow*, canal of greater petrosal nerve; *white star*, high jugular bulb; *small white arrowhead*, thin bony lamina separating jugular vein from middle ear cavity; *black star*, tensor tympani muscle. (Courtesy of Dr. Soenke Bartling, DKFZ, Heidelberg, Germany)

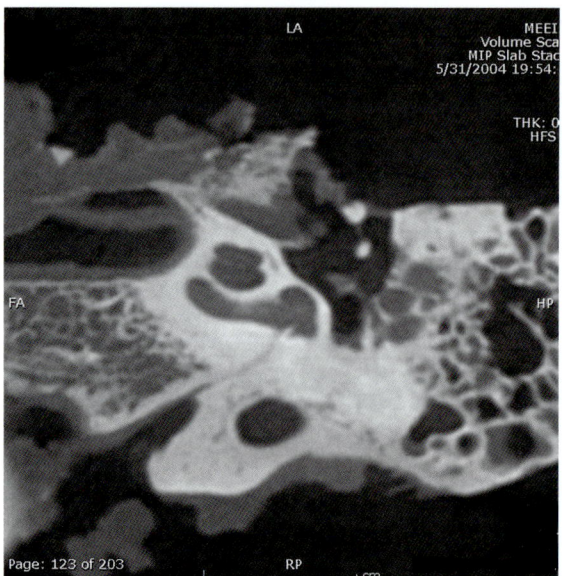

Figure 1-62 Reformatted flat-panel volume computed tomographic image through the base turn of the cochlea showing the entire length of the cochlear aqueduct, a feature that is generally not seen on routine multidetector computed tomographic images. (Courtesy of Dr. Soenke Bartling, DKFZ, Heidelberg, Germany)

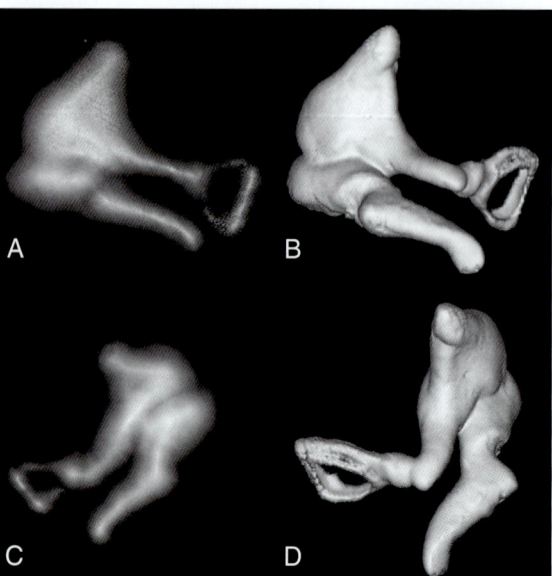

Figure 1-63 Volume-rendered views of the ossicular chain by multidetector computed tomography **(A, C)** and flat-panel volume computed tomography (fpVCT) **(B, D)** from inferior **(A, B)** and posterior **(C, D)** views. The volume-rendering transfer function is separately optimized for both datasets after the ossicular chain was segmented out of the volumes. The structure of the ossicular chain is much better visualized using fpVCT. (Courtesy of Dr. Soenke Bartling, DKFZ, Heidelberg, Germany)

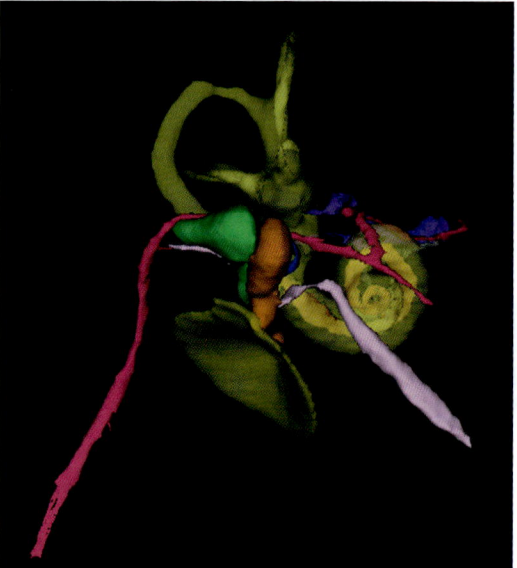

Figure 1-64 Three-dimensional model of the right temporal bone seen from the anterolateral direction. Color code: tympanic membrane—*yellowish green*; malleus—*orange*; incus—*green*; stapes—*blue*; facial nerve—*purple*; bony labyrinth—*transparent yellow*; transparent bony cochlea with osseus lamina spiralis—*brown*; tensor tympani muscle—*pinkish purple structure in right half of image*; stapedius muscle—*pinkish purple in left half of image*; stapedius nerve—*purple structure inserting in stapedius muscle*; vestibulocochlear nerve—*dark lilac*. (Courtesy of Dr. Soenke Bartling, DKFZ, Heidelberg, Germany)

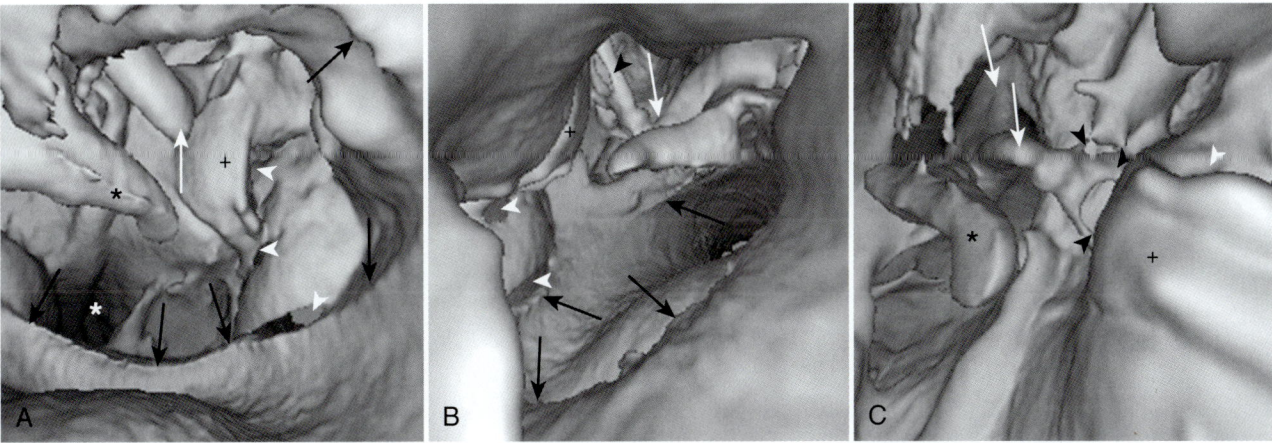

Figure 1-65 Three surface-rendered views from virtual endoscopy movie from flat-panel volume computed tomography dataset. **A:** Camera is positioned in external acoustic meatus and is facing medially through the tympanic membrane, which has been removed. *Black star,* Handle of malleus; *small black arrows,* tympanic sulcus; *white star,* eustachian tube; *short white arrow,* long process of incus; *black cross,* promontory; *long white arrowhead,* round window niche; *large black arrowhead,* tendon of stapedius muscle; *small (white) arrowheads,* dehiscent high jugular bulb. **B:** Camera is positioned in distal end of eustachian tube and is facing the middle ear cavity. *Small black arrowhead,* Anterior crus of stapes. **C:** Virtual endoscope is positioned beneath the ossicular chain and is facing superiorly. *Long white arrow,* Short process of incus within tympanic attic. (Courtesy of Dr. Soenke Bartling, DKFZ, Heidelberg, Germany)

the eyelid without any proptosis, chemosis, or pupillary defect (Figure 1-70). MDCT may show streaky density within the fat anterior to the orbital septum, often secondary to superficial facial infection. Because of a valveless venous plexus, extension posterior to the orbital septum is a dreaded complication. Preseptal cellulitis usually is not sinogenic, and the paranasal sinuses usually are clear.

Clinical findings of postseptal cellulitis, also known as *orbital cellulitis,* include proptosis, chemosis, restriction of ocular motility, and papillary defect. Evaluation of the orbit and sinuses by CT becomes essential in these cases to confirm the diagnosis and to assess the extent of infection. Delayed treatment in such cases may lead to blindness, intracranial abscess, and even death. MDCT in orbital cellulitis demonstrates fat stranding and other inflammatory changes in the retrobulbar orbital fat. These streaky densities within orbital fat may indicate spread of infection through the venous system or periorbita.

Advanced cases of infection may result in a subperiosteal abscess from bacterial infection extending from the retrobulbar fat or, more commonly, from the sinuses through the cortical bone. A subperiosteal abscess, if it is sinogenic, may or may not involve the orbital fat. In all cases, there is central displacement of the adjacent rectus muscle. All complications of orbital infections are well demonstrated by MDCT. They include fat stranding, proptosis, orbital phlegmon, abscess, cavernous sinus thrombosis, and superior orbital vein thrombosis. Figures 1-71 and 1-72 demonstrate two cases of subperiosteal abscess formation. In Figure 1-72, the abscess involves the superior portion of the orbit. Although CT is excellent at demonstrating the orbital extension of the abscess, the intracranial extension may be difficult to elucidate using MDCT.

Besides infection, other conditions involving the sinuses may result in orbital pathology. Figure 1-73 shows an example. MDCT demonstrates orbital asymmetry and spontaneous enophthalmos caused by sinus atelectasis in a condition called *silent sinus syndrome.* This condition is a result of acquired obstruction of the maxillary sinus ostium leading to sinus hypoventilation and accumulation of sinus secretions. Over time, resorption of sinus secretions generates subatmospheric pressure in the maxillary antrum. This causes maxillary sinus collapse, with prolapse of the walls of the sinus. The floor of the orbit formed by the orbital plate of the maxillary bone is relatively thin and gives in easily. This process can be considered the reverse of that occurring in an orbital blowout fracture: the orbital contents are being pulled into the maxillary sinus as opposed to being pushed into it.

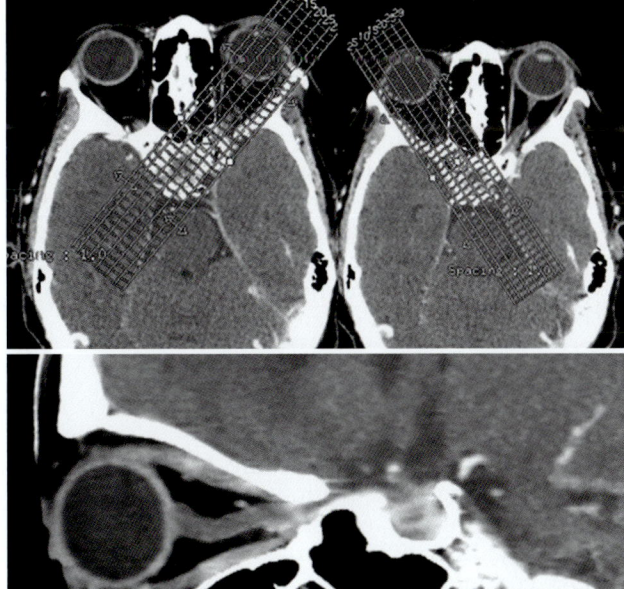

Figure 1-66 Angulation of oblique sagittal sections **(A)** and representative oblique sagittal section through the orbit **(B).**

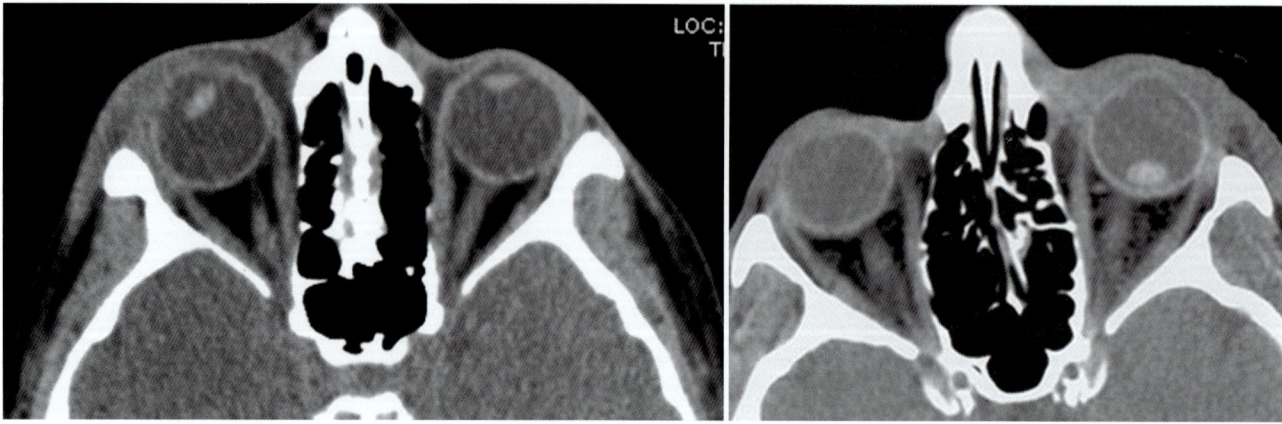

Figure 1-67 Two cases of lens dislocation. A: Thirteen-year-old after trauma to right eye. B: Patient with unilateral trauma to left eye.

Congenital Conditions

Most congenital orbital pathologies are readily demonstrated by MDCT. These conditions include entities such as neurofibromatosis type 1 (NF1), persistent hyperplastic primary vitreous, microphthalmos, coloboma, Coats disease, dermoids, and epidermoids. NF1 is considered here as a representative example.

Figure 1-74 shows a case of NF1 with orbital involvement. A plexiform neurofibroma anywhere within the body is pathognomonic for NF1 and is quite common in the orbit. Typically, the involvement is unilateral, as it is in this case. CT scan shows serpentine masses in the retrobulbar area representing plexiform neurofibromas. These masses may involve intraorbital nerves, muscles, optic nerve sheath, or sclera. Other cranial nerves also may be involved and may result in expansion of the associated foramina at the skull base. Associated sphenoid dysplasia is common. These plexiform neurofibromas in NF1 gradually enlarge until they involve nearly all orbital structures, both internal and external. The differential diagnosis of these lesions includes other infiltrating orbital lesions, such as capillary hemangioma, rhabdomyosarcoma, histiocytosis, lymphoma, leukemia, and metastases.

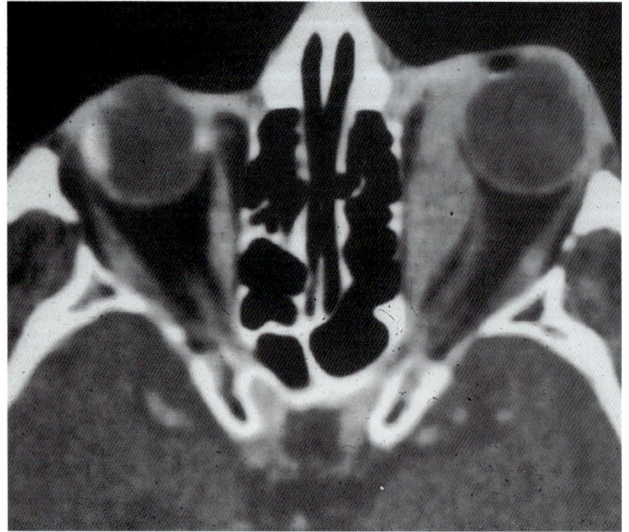

Figure 1-68 Orbital myositis involving the left medial rectus muscle.

Vascular and Lymphatic Malformations

Vascular and lymphatic malformations of the orbit, which form a continuum with varying proportions of arterial, lymphatic, and venous elements, include entities such as capillary and cavernous hemangiomas, lymphangiomas, and venous varices. Pathologically, these malformations have elements of lymphatic, arterial, and venous tissue.

Venous lymphatic malformations arise from a pluripotent venous analogue that develops into both venous and lymphatic structures that do not have any connection to systemic venous or lymphatic structures. They enlarge slowly, producing progressive proptosis. Many manifest abruptly because of hemorrhage after minor trauma or infection. Sometimes, no antecedent cause is identified, and hemorrhage may be spontaneous. Lymphangiomas are associated with intracranial developmental venous anomalies, sinus pericranii, and AVMs. Figure 1-75 shows the CT scan of a 6-year-old with an orbital lymphangioma. Generally, these masses are poorly marginated and lobulated, and show irregular enhancement.

Lymphangiomas show irregular enhancement, but a lobulated, irregular orbital mass that shows intense enhancement in an infant likely is a capillary hemangioma. It may involve any part of the orbit. On noncontrast CT it is slightly hyperdense and turns homogeneously bright on postcontrast images. A rhabdomyosarcoma can have a similar appearance, except that it usually is invasive and shows bone destruction, especially at large sizes. Neuroblastoma and hematopoietic malignancies are other entities in the differential consideration.

Orbital Masses and Neoplastic Conditions

Congenital orbital tumors include hamartomas (e.g., capillary hemangiomas, neurofibromatosis) and choristomas (e.g., dermoids, epidermoids, lipodermoids).

Capillary hemangiomas of the orbit are benign tumors commonly seen in the pediatric age group, whereas cavernous hemangiomas of the orbit are more common in adults. Diagnosis is mostly established

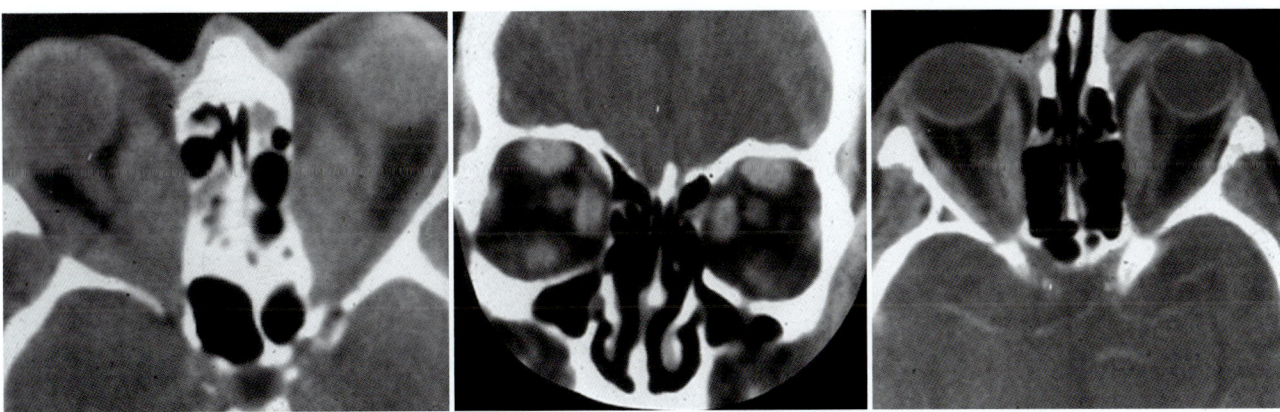

Figure 1-69 Thyroid ophthalmopathy secondary to Graves disease. **A:** Axial section showing extensive involvement of medial rectus muscles resulting in bowing of left optic nerve. **B, C:** Coronal and axial sections from contrast-enhanced computed tomographic scan showing bilaterally symmetric enlargement of superior, medial, and inferior rectus muscles. The lateral rectus muscles are relatively spared.

by CT, but MRI may play a role. Lymphangiomas can occur in the conjunctiva, eyelids, orbit, oropharynx, or sinuses. CT scan with contrast is useful for locating these lesions. Optic nerve sheath meningiomas, optic nerve gliomas, and neurofibromas are the neural tumors for which CT plays a role in detection. Malignant tumors of the orbit include retinoblastoma, ocular melanoma, optic pathway glioma, adenoid cystic carcinoma of the lacrimal gland, and lymphoma. MDCT can be used in both detecting and managing these lesions. CT also is helpful in evaluating the lesions of the lacrimal gland to differentiate between inflammatory and neoplastic conditions.

Contrast-enhanced CT scan can effectively demonstrate these orbital masses and show characteristics that can narrow the differential. Although the soft tissue contrast of MRI is superior in demonstrating these pathologies, CT shows calcifications and the relationship to adjacent bony and vascular structures to better advantage.

For example, consider the two soft tissue masses in the posterior aspect of the left globe shown in Figure 1-76. The mass on the left is hyperdense compared with the normal vitreous humor, occupies a normal-sized globe, and is devoid of any calcifications. A key differentiating feature of the mass on the right is the presence of punctuate and finely speckled calcifications. On postcontrast images, this mass shows moderate enhancement. This pattern of calcifications and enhancement is characteristic of a retinoblastoma. The hyperdense, noncalcified mass on the right represents an exudative retinopathy of Coats disease. As shown in Figure 1-77, MDCT also readily demonstrates the extent of the mass, its bony involvement, and any spread to the adjacent compartments. This case shows a bladder cancer metastasis that has invaded through the superior orbital foramen to involve the intracranial compartment.

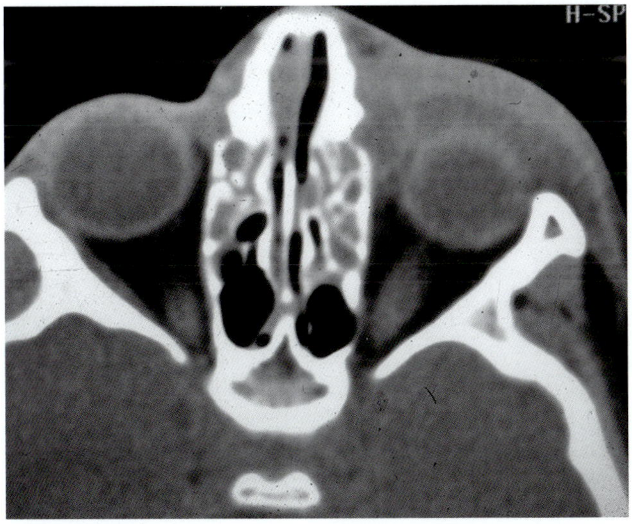

■ MDCT FOR CERVICAL MASSES AND INFECTIONS

MDCT is an indispensible tool in the evaluation of a variety of cervical masses and infectious conditions. This section presents several examples that demonstrate the utility of MDCT for cervical masses and infections.

MDCT shows bone destruction, thinning, and invasion to better advantage than does MRI. These changes can be reliably distinguished from simple remodeling of the bone from a chronic, nonaggressive expansile process. In this case, MRI scan did not really narrow the differential and was not as useful at MDCT scan.

Figure 1-78 shows the case of an 18-year-old man with history of choroid plexus papilloma resected at age 1 year, who presented with increasing nasal congestion. MDCT with contrast demonstrates an aggressive nasal mass that is destroying the adjacent bone. The lamina papyracea and the ethmoid air cells on the right are destroyed, with bowing of the medial rectus. This imaging presentation is consistent with a fast-growing malignancy. Pathology study proved this mass to be an alveolar-type rhabdomyosarcoma.

Figure 1-79 shows axial section and coronal and sagittal reconstructed images from contrast-enhanced MDCT of the face and brain of a young male who presented

Figure 1-70 Case of superficial infection resulting in preseptal cellulitis. The retrobulbar fat is free of any signs of infection.

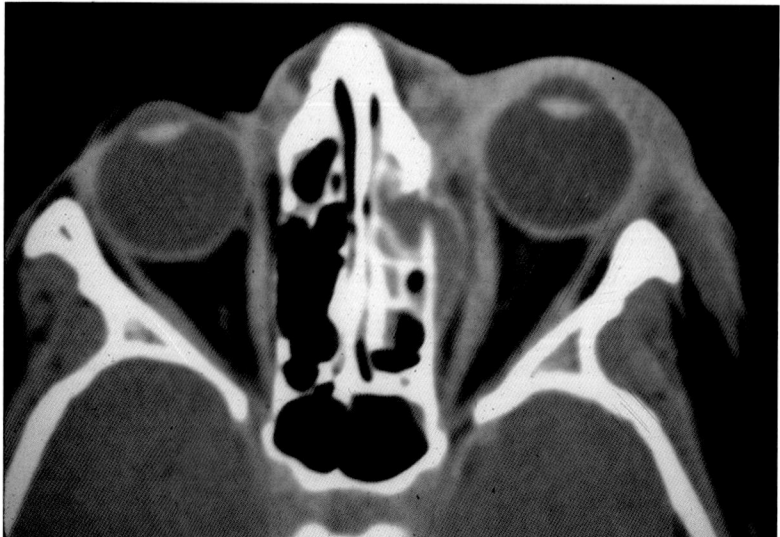

Figure 1-71 Four-year-old girl with 2-day history of fever and acute onset of right eye swelling. A sinogenic subperiosteal abscess that is continuous with an opacified ethmoid air cell through a dehiscence in the lamina papyracea, with resulting central deviation of the medial rectus muscle, can be seen.

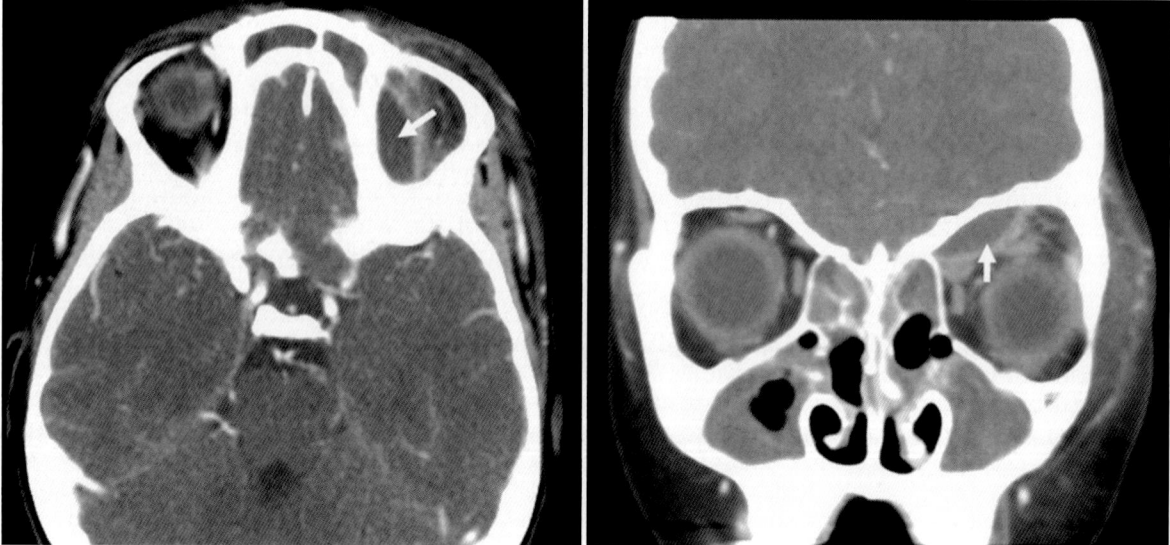

Figure 1-72 Case of orbital cellulitis and subperiosteal abscess formation.

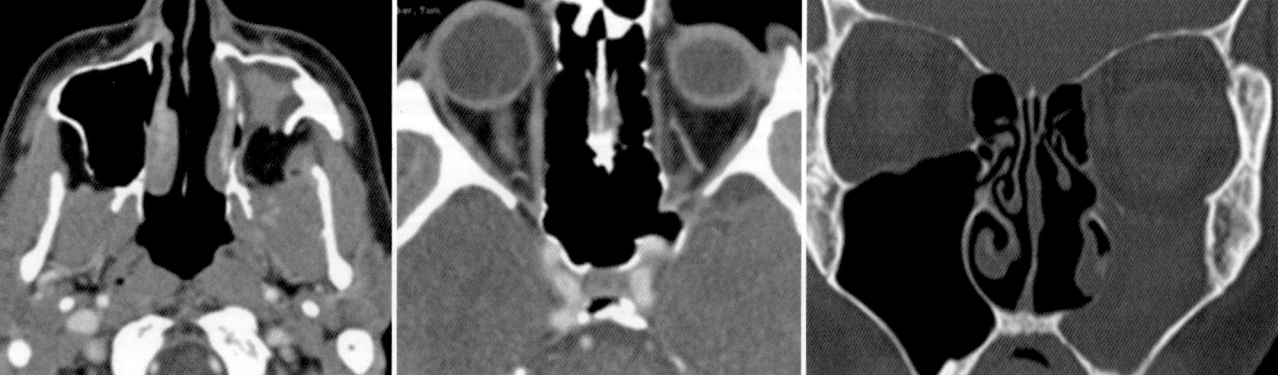

Figure 1-73 Forty-year-old patient with diplopia who presented with a feeling of "sinking of the eye." Atelectasis of left maxillary sinus with resultant enophthalmos can be seen on axial and coronal sections. (Images courtesy Dr. Michelle Rottblatt.)

Chapter 1 Multidetector Computed Tomography as a Problem-Solving Tool in Neuroradiology

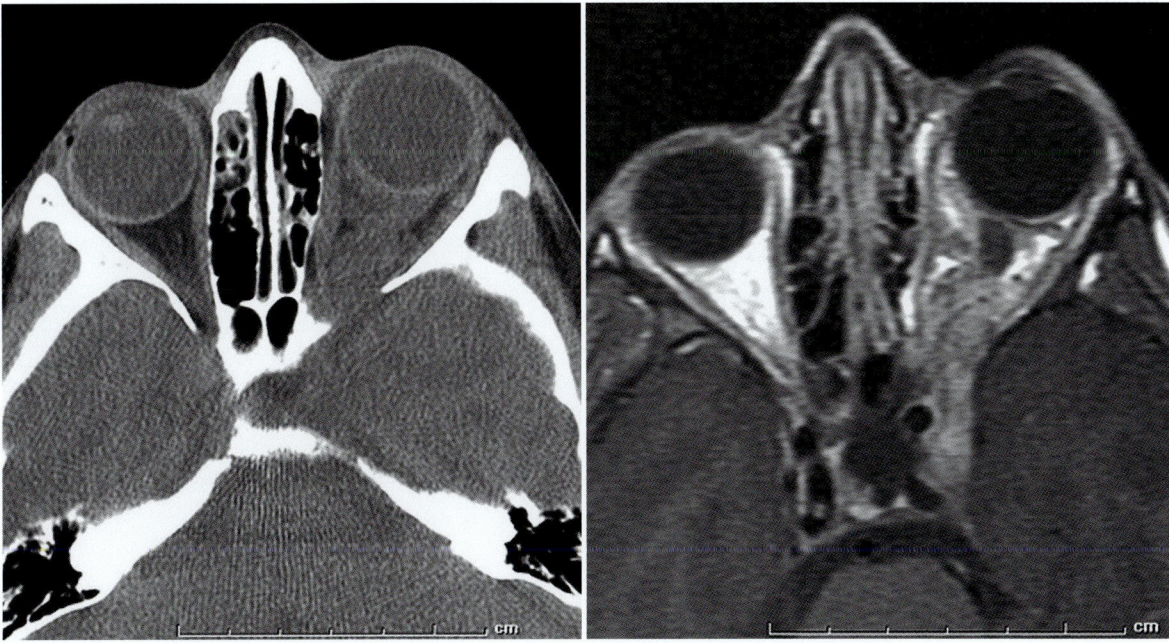

Figure 1-74 Ten-year-old patient with proptosis of the left globe. Noncontrast computed tomography *(left)* demonstrating hypodense infiltrative soft tissue masses representing plexiform neurofibroma that enhance on postcontrast image *(right)*. Bony changes and proptosis are seen. Both the superior orbital fissure and the optic canal are enlarged.

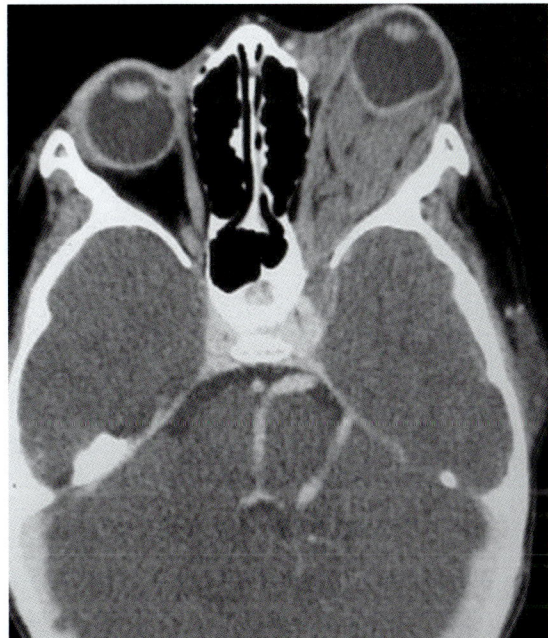

Figure 1-75 Six-year-old patient with orbital proptosis. Noncontrast computed tomographic scan (not shown here) demonstrated multicystic hypodense mass and remodeling of bone. Variable wall enhancement is seen on postcontrast images. Mass effect on the posterior globe can be appreciated.

with epistaxis. The images show an avidly enhancing mass in the right pterygomaxillary fissure extending into the sphenoid sinus, right infratemporal fossa, and posterior nasopharynx with deviation of the nasal septum to the left of midline. Marked neovascularity, characteristic location within the pterygomaxillary fissure, and the overall extent of this mass—features that are well demonstrated by MDCT—characterize it as a juvenile nasopharyngeal angiofibroma.

MDCT is the modality of choice for demonstrating the internal vascularity and relationship of a mass to adjacent vascular structures. A carotid body tumor is a case in point (Figure 1-80). This tumor, also known as *intercarotid paraganglioma, glomus tumor,* or *chemodectoma,* is a neural crest derivative that occurs at the carotid bifurcation. It is a slowly growing, hypervascular, intensely enhancing, compressible mass that is fixed vertically by the carotid bifurcation but can move laterally. It characteristically splays the carotid bifurcation and may encase vessels. Its ovoid shape is best seen with sagittal and coronal MDCT images (Figure 1-80).

MDCT is ideal for demonstrating displacement of the adjacent structures and fascial layers. For example, masses in the carotid sheath displace the fat in the parapharyngeal space anteromedially. Neurogenic tumors, such as those arising from the vagus nerve or the sympathetic chain, cause anterior displacement of the carotid. In general, vagal lesions cause anteromedial displacement of the carotid because the vagus nerve is situated posterior to the carotid. Sympathetic chain schwannomas are located at the posteromedial border of the ICA and typically result in anterior or anterolateral displacement of the carotid. If posterior displacement of the carotid artery is observed, the differential considerations should include lesion arising from the deep lobe of the parotid or from the prestyloid parapharyngeal space.

Several examples of infectious conditions as depicted by MDCT have been shown. The key characteristics of this modality that make it suitable for imaging those sites make it equally applicable for evaluation of head and neck infections. Figure 1-81 shows the case of an

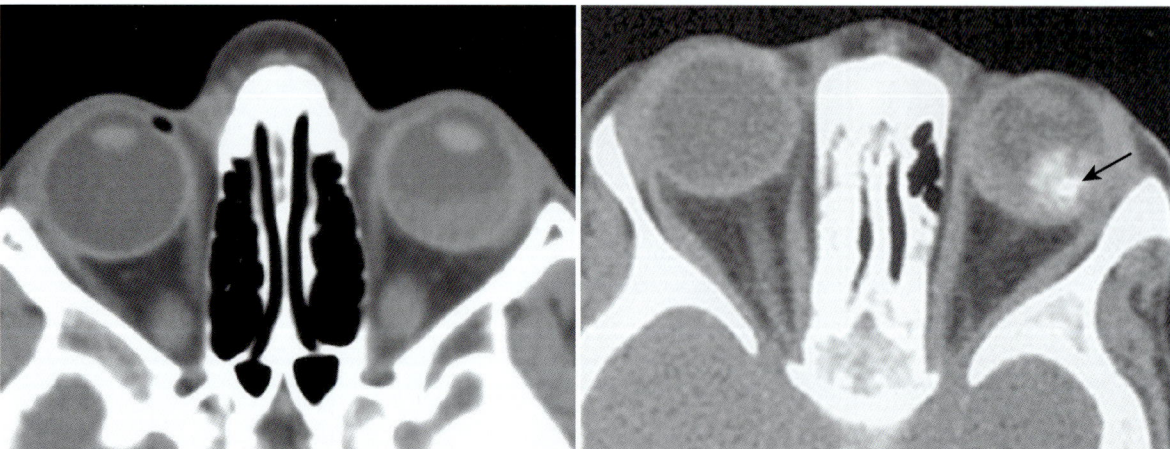

Figure 1-76 Two different soft tissue masses in the posterior aspect of the left globe representing Coats disease *(left)* and retinoblastoma *(right)*.

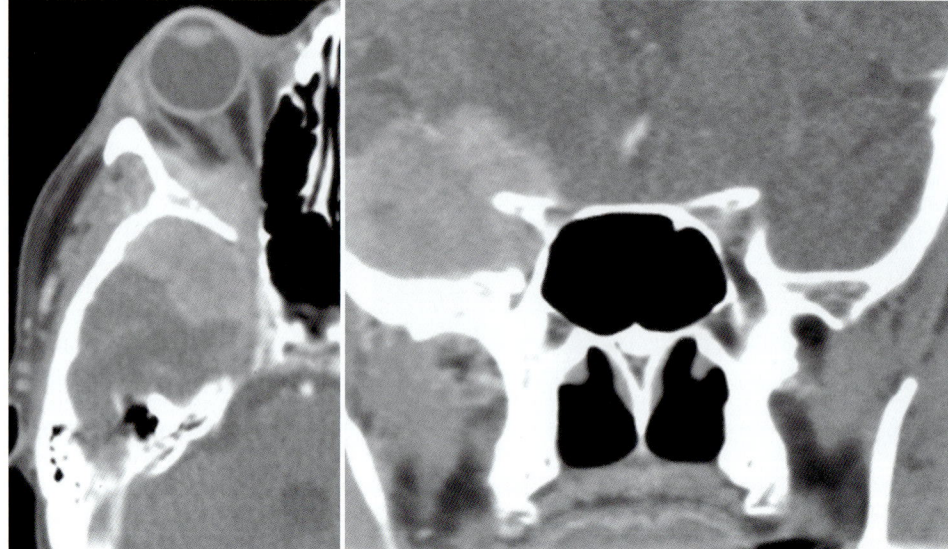

Figure 1-77 Fifty-year-old patient with a history of bladder cancer who presented with right eye pain. Contrast-enhanced multidetector computed tomography showing an enhancing mass in the posterior aspect of the orbit that has spread to the intracranial compartment via the superior orbital foramen.

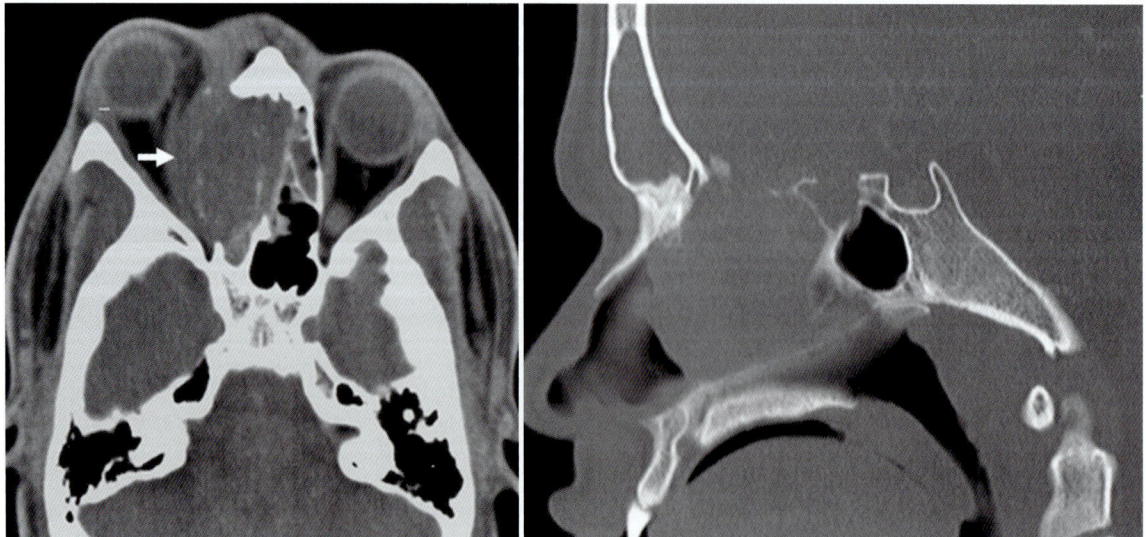

Figure 1-78 Case of rhabdomyosarcoma (alveolar type).

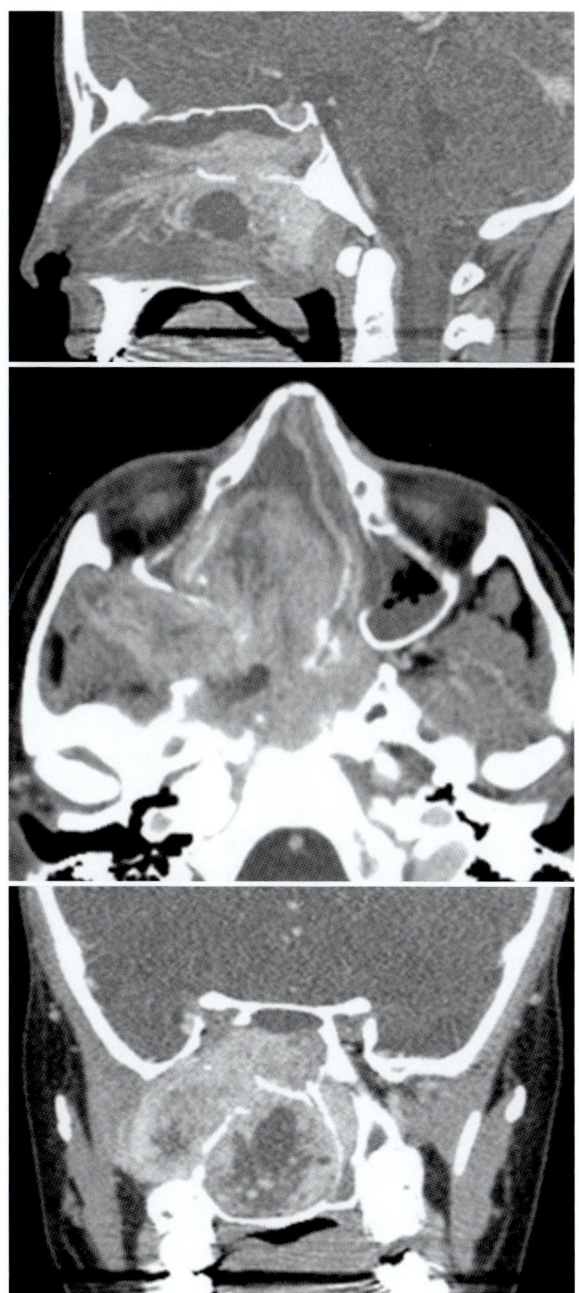

Figure 1-79 Highly vascular mass involving multiple compartments that proved to be juvenile nasopharyngeal angiofibroma at pathology.

11-month-old girl with a retropharyngeal abscess secondary to trauma to the oropharynx from a drum stick. The image clearly shows the abscess with foci of gas within it. Also seen is a hypodense track from the oropharyngeal mucosa down to the abscess cavity, likely representing the traumatic penetration of the foreign body. The relationship of the abscess with the adjacent carotid artery and jugular vein is clearly demonstrated in this image, as is the fact that they are not thrombosed, a dreaded complication of head and neck infections.

A case of cervical infection leading to thrombophlebitis is shown in Figure 1-82. The patient, a 37-year-old man with human immunodeficiency virus and acquired immunodeficiency syndrome, presented with a 12-day history of left neck pain, fever, headaches, nausea, and vomiting. CT scan of the chest, head, and neck with contrast showed a focal, hypoattenuating mass in the left neck, with irregular margins and peripheral enhancement. The sternocleidomastoid muscle is swollen, as are the surrounding subcutaneous soft tissues. The thyroid, trachea, and carotid artery are deviated to the right, and the internal jugular vein (IJV) is thrombosed. Differential considerations for IJV thrombophlebitis include tumor thrombus, lymphoma, otitis media or externa, recent IJV catheterization, and Lemierre syndrome. This case is a classic presentation of Lemierre syndrome. Patients with this syndrome generally are young with pharyngitis or peritonsillar abscess who present with high fever, rigors, cervical adenopathy, and tenderness. Thrombophlebitis of IJV develops, and distant abscess formation from metastasis is common. Distant septic metastases most commonly involve the lungs and cause pulmonary infiltrates, pleural effusions, and cavitations. Joint infections and hepatic or splenic abscesses also may develop. Early treatment with antibiotics is essential.

MDCT is a quick and easy way to show the location and extent of disease by demonstrating the associated inflammatory changes, enhancement, and fluid dissecting in different fascial layers. Rim-enhancing collections, necrotic lymph nodes, and cystic structures (Figure 1-83) are well demonstrated by MDCT.

■ MDCT: STATE OF THE ART AND FUTURE TRENDS

Figure 1-84 illustrates a simplified timeline summarizing the key increments in the capabilities of CT. The evolution of MDCT was made possible by steady improvements in spatial, contrast, and temporal resolution. These, in turn, were the result of continuous engineering advancements in detector design, gantry rotation speed, slip-ring technology, and axial coverage of the detectors. The state of the art of MDCT is summarized here in terms of these key benchmarks, followed by some new and exciting innovations in technology that have recently become available.

State of the Art in MDCT

Spatial Resolution
Detector technology has perhaps seen the most radical changes in CT engineering. The current detectors are solid state and offer a resolution of about 0.4 mm in-plane and 0.5 mm along the Z-direction. The number of detector rows has steadily increased, and 64-slice detectors currently are the norm. Scanners with as many as 320 slices have been introduced recently into clinical practice. The available detectors can be configured in many arrangements, offering a wide variety of settings for collimation, pitch, and slice thickness.

Although traditional MDCT scanners have significantly improved spatial resolution, some of the very fine structures in head and neck radiology are still beyond

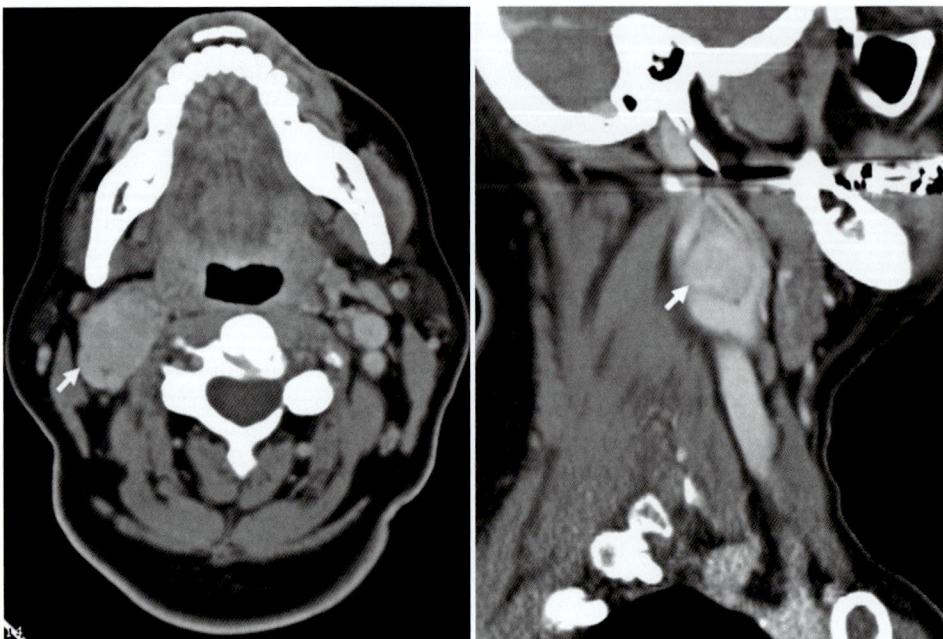

Figure 1-80 Axial and oblique sagittal views of a carotid body tumor.

their reach. For example, the footplate of the stapes, the attachment of the stapedius muscle, the spiral osseous in the cochlea, and many other structures in the temporal bone are more imagined than seen at the clinical resolution available today. Recently, digital flat-panel detector-based CT systems have been developed and shown to provide isotropic spatial resolution of about 130 μm. This innovative design, which provides unprecedented visualization of small intracranial structures, especially those in temporal bone, are briefly described later in this chapter under flat panel volume CT.

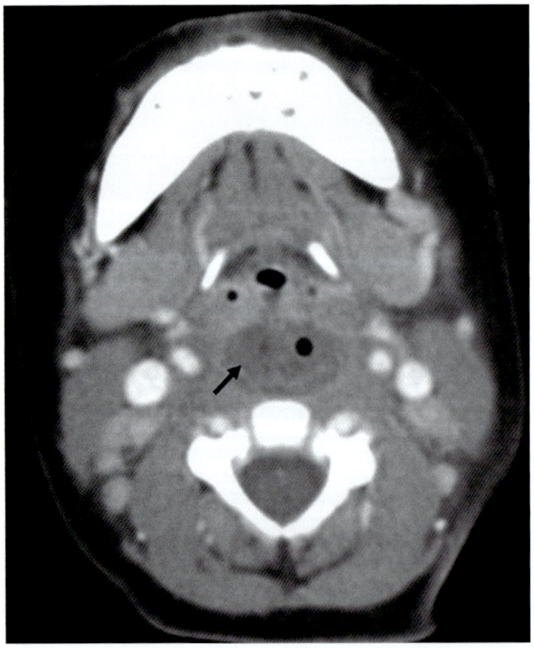

Contrast Resolution

Differentiation between gray matter and white matter, a difference of about 10 HU in CT attenuation, is essential for detection of acute infarctions. Quantification of small changes in parenchymal opacification forms the basis of perfusion imaging. At diagnostic energies (70–150 kVp), such small differences in attenuation can be subtle, and detection of these subtle differences can be challenging in presence of noise, partial volume effects, and motion artifacts. With the advent of highly engineered solid-state detectors using rare earth crystalline materials, the detective quantum efficiency has increased significantly. These advances, coupled with newer acquisition and processing techniques, have resulted in steady improvement in the contrast resolution of the scanners. Currently, single-energy, state-of-the-art MDCT scanners can discriminate differences as subtle as 1 HU. The discriminating power of a scanner can be further augmented using dual-energy scanning, a topic that is further discussed later in this chapter under dual-source and dual-energy CT.

Temporal Resolution

Currently, CT imaging for most neurologic applications, with the exception of perfusion imaging, is static. The need for higher temporal resolution is primarily driven by cardiac imaging. Nonetheless, neuroimaging also benefits from faster scanners. Current MDCT systems provide temporal resolution in the range from 165 to 330 ms depending on gantry speed and the reconstruction algorithm used (i.e., whether projection data from 180 or 360 degrees is used for reconstruction). With the advent of these fast scanners, imaging of a wide swath of anatomy has become possible with one injection of contrast. For example, a head and neck CTA from

Figure 1-81 Eleven-month-old girl who presented with gagging after trauma to the oropharynx from a drum stick. Multidetector computed tomography demonstrating a retropharyngeal abscess with foci of air within it. Adjacent carotid artery and jugular vein are patent.

Chapter 1 Multidetector Computed Tomography as a Problem-Solving Tool in Neuroradiology

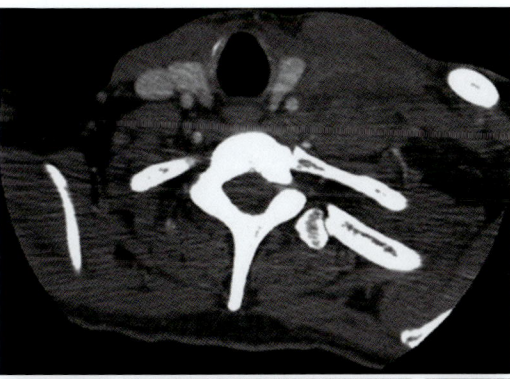

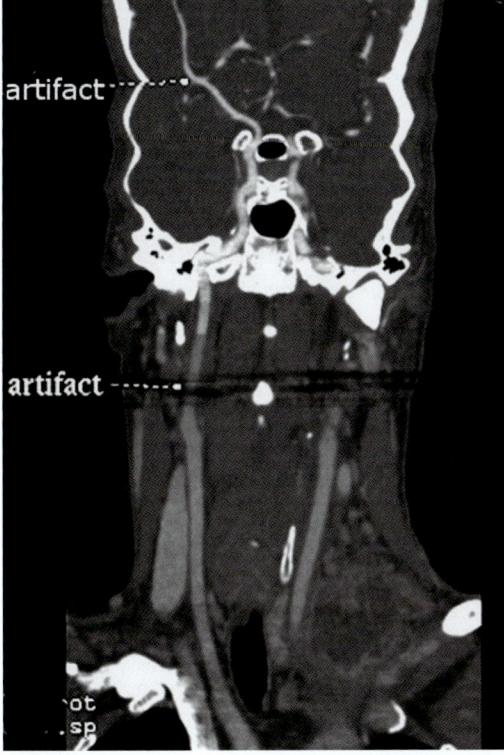

Figure 1-82 Axial and coronal multidetector computed tomography of head and neck demonstrating postanginal sepsis and thrombophlebitis of left internal jugular vein in Lemierre syndrome.

of a gantry rotation is sufficient for reconstructing a single slice. The SOMATOM Definition (Siemens Medical Solutions, Forchheim, Germany), a recently introduced dual-source CT scanner, has a rotation time of 0.33 second. Therefore, a temporal resolution of approximately 0.083 second is feasible. Such high temporal resolution may prove beneficial in studying dynamic phenomena such as neuroperfusion and cardiovascular events. High temporal resolution also may prove useful in visualizing processes such as early venous shunting in an AVM and tumor vascularity.

Of note, with dual-source CT the radiation dose is not increased by a factor of two. Although twice as much power is being delivered per unit time, the scan takes almost half as much time as compared to single source MDCT scanners. Therefore, the overall effective dose is the same as that with a conventional MDCT scanner. In fact, for cardiac examinations that rely on oversampling the projection data to account for ectopic beats, the overall x-ray dose is decreased compared with a single-source CT.

The two x-ray sources of a dual-source CT scanner can be operated at two different tube voltages. This gives rise to dual-energy CT, which is primarily used for tissue characterization. Dual-energy CT is based on the principle that x-ray attenuation is energy dependent. The peak tube voltage (kVp) determines the average energy of the x-ray beam. Therefore, a change in kVp leads to an alteration of average photon energy. Because the beam attenuation caused by different materials is energy dependent, different tissue types can be discriminated by their attenuation characteristics at two different energy levels.

The x-ray absorption depends on the atomic number and the density irrespective of chemical bonding. For example, the high attenuation of iodine at low kVp changes to half at high photon energies. In contrast, the attenuation of bone changes much less when the kVp of the tube is changed. Dual-energy CT uses this key difference to distinguish between different materials. Two x-ray sources perpendicular to each other, running simultaneously at two different energy settings, acquire two datasets using two separate detector arrays. These datasets, at two different energy levels, are perfectly registered with respect to each other as they are acquired very close to each other in time.

The two datasets have different attenuation levels or Hounsfield units for the same tissue. A weighted average image of the two datasets is used to obtain a scan with a cumulative dose from the two tubes. If the energy levels for the two tubes are 80 and 140 kVp, the average scan can be regarded as that obtained at 120 kVp. The real power of dual-energy CT is realized with the help of special software and postprocessing tools that can analyze the two datasets to extract material specific differences in attenuation. These differences, in turn, enable classification of the chemical composition of the scanned tissue.

The overall attenuation of any tissue is primarily determined by two main interactions: photoelectric absorption and Compton scattering. For any material, two unknown parameters weight the contributions of

the aortic arch to the vertex can be completed in less than 10 seconds. Temporal resolution can be further enhanced by using two x-ray sources and two detectors simultaneously. This quantum leap in CT technology is discussed next.

Dual-Source and Dual-Energy CT

Dual-source CT (DSCT) is a new innovation in CT technology. It uses two x-ray sources and two detectors in a single gantry to accelerate image acquisition. Using two imaging chains simultaneously effectively doubles temporal resolution and x-ray tube power. In addition, the two imaging chains can be operated at different tube voltages, enabling dual-energy CT (discussed later in this section). Because projection data from just over half of a rotation is sufficient for image reconstruction, when the scanner is operated in the dual-source mode one quarter

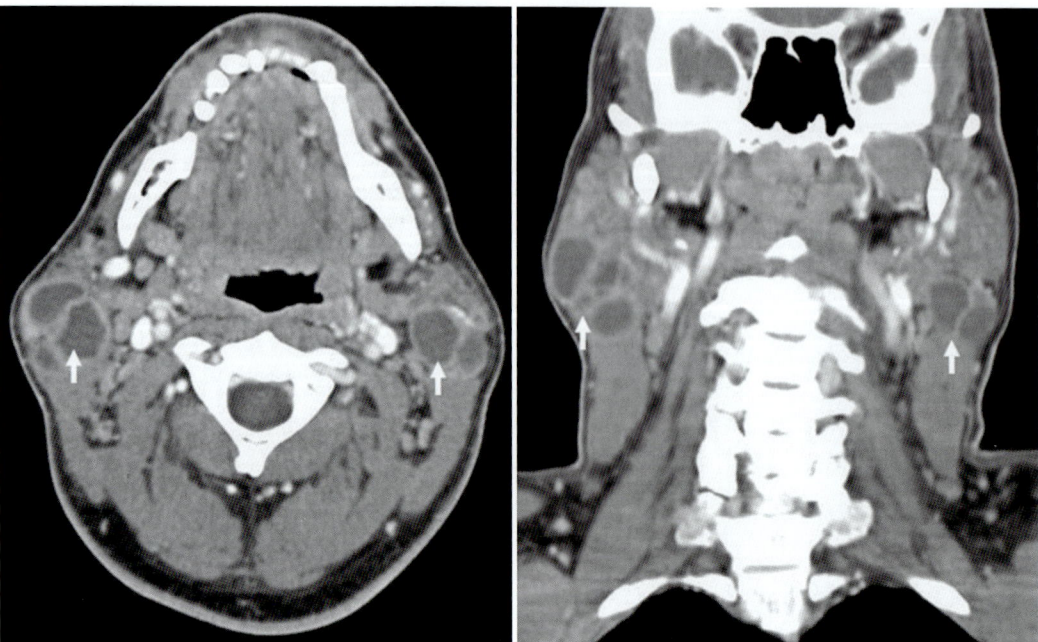

Figure 1-83 Bilateral level 2 well defined, peripherally enhancing cystic lesions (white arrow) representing lymphoepithelial cysts in human immunodeficiency virus lymphadenitis.

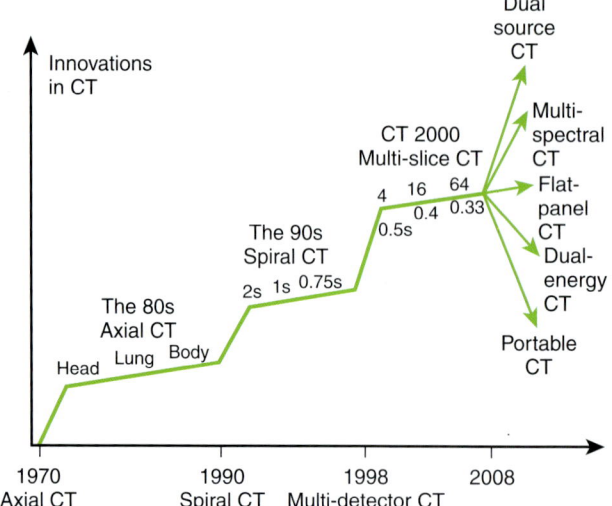

Figure 1-84 Some key milestones in the evolution of multidetector computed tomography.

these two interactions to the overall attenuation coefficient. Therefore, the total attenuation coefficient of a material can be decomposed into two parts that describe the contribution of these two interactions. Each component is energy dependent; however, the energy dependencies can be treated as known functions as they can be calibrated a priori. Dual-energy CT provides two measurements for each voxel from which the two unknown parameters can be estimated.

In a two-component tissue model, each image voxel is assumed to be composed of two known substances (e.g., iodine and calcium). The attenuation coefficients of these substances in their pure form are known at each kVp level. The fraction of these tissue types present within an image voxel can be estimated using dual-energy CT. The contribution to the overall attenuation by these two substances is the desired estimate. For the two-component model, imaging at two energy settings provides a solution because there are two unknowns. The mass fraction of each substance can be derived from the measured weighting factors.

Dual-energy CT may offer clinically useful tissue signatures for different normal and pathologic conditions and currently is an area of active research. For example, dual-energy CT can distinguish between calcium deposits and injected iodine. This property can be used in CTA for automatic bone subtraction (Figure 1-85). Enhancement characteristics of different tissue types

Chapter 1 Multidetector Computed Tomography as a Problem-Solving Tool in Neuroradiology

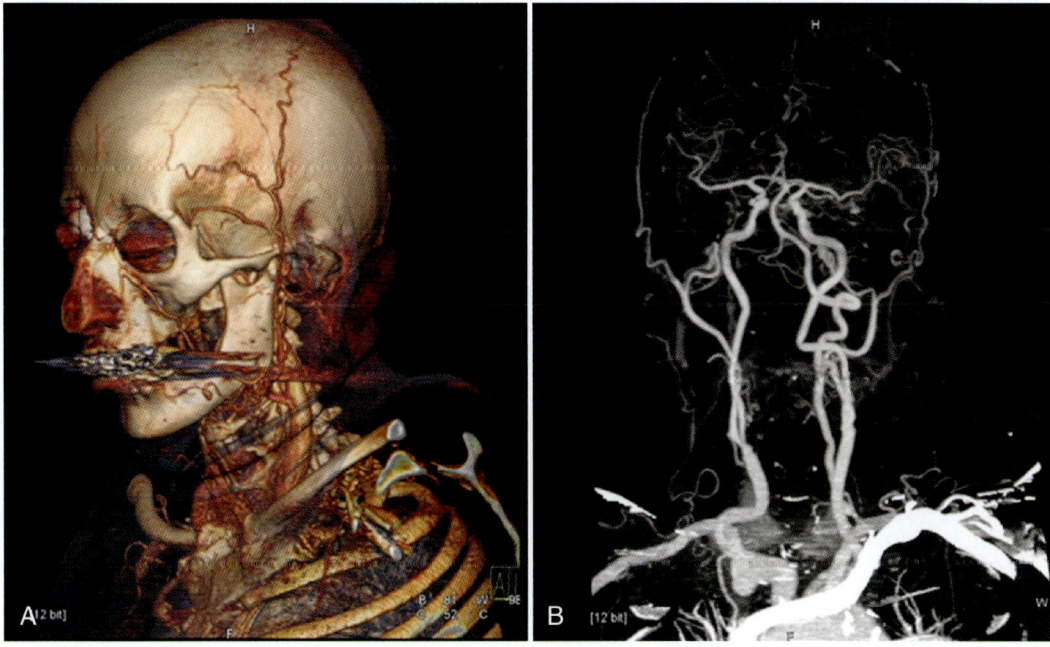

Figure 1-85 Dual-energy computed tomography enables bone subtraction for comprehensive evaluation of complex vascular structures. (Images courtesy University of Munich-Grosshadern Campus, Munich, Germany.)

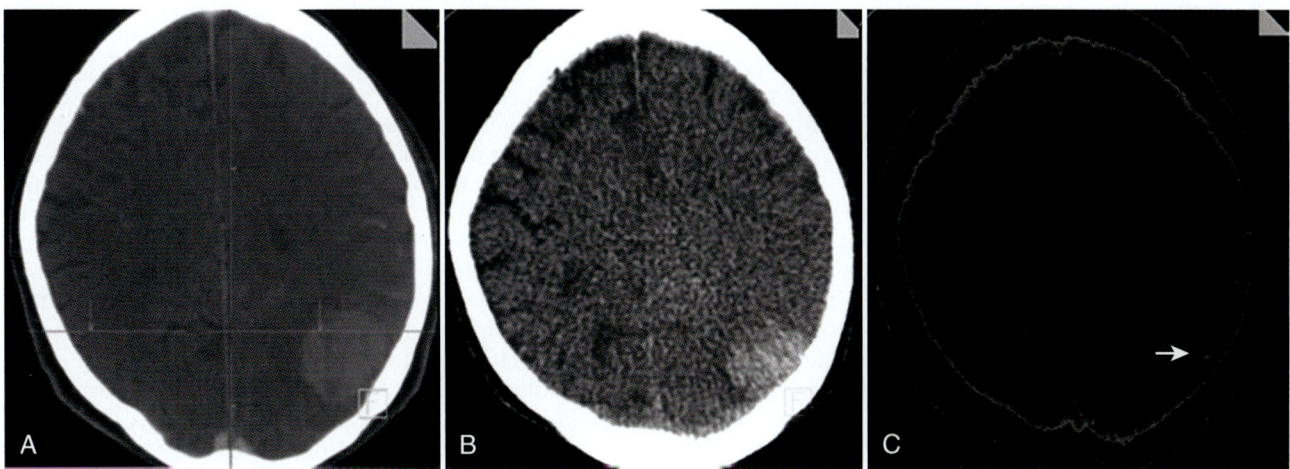

Figure 1-86 Dual-energy computed tomography. **A:** Noncontrast imaging showing a hyperdense intraparenchymal hemorrhage in the left frontoparietal region. **B:** Contrast-enhanced image of the same patient. Any active contrast extravasation into the hematoma is difficult to see. **C:** Iodine-only image obtained by processing the low and the high kVp images showing extravasation of iodine in the hematoma. Such active extravasation may reflect a risk of hematoma expansion with time. (Images courtesy University of Munich-Grosshadern Campus, Munich, Germany.)

also may be better demonstrated using dual-energy subtraction.

On a conventional MDCT scan, acute intracranial hemorrhage and iodine extravasation appear radiodense. It is possible to separate the two using dual-energy CT. Iodine extravasation in a hematoma after IV contrast injection may be a marker of hematoma expansion (Figure 1-86). Analogues of this phenomenon, called the *spot sign*, have been seen on routine MDCT of the brain.

Visualization of soft atherosclerotic plaque is often compromised by the concomitant presence of calcifications. Dual-energy CT can effectively subtract out the calcific portions, making available a pure soft tissue image. Other applications, such as characterization of kidney stones, differentiation of hard plaque from injected contrast, and detection of pulmonary perfusion defect, have been reported in the literature.

Visualization of dual-energy scans poses a unique display challenge because reviewing high-energy and low-energy scans separately is not useful to a human operator. With dual-energy CT, the attenuation caused by iodine can be subtracted out. Therefore, a virtual noncontrast (VNC) image can be made and the contribution from iodine enhancement overlaid on it. The Siemens dual-energy application suite provides a fusion multiplanar reconstruction (multiplanar reformat) tool for postprocessing and visualization. The VNC image can be fused with the iodine image in any proportion. For example, at a setting of 50% VNC and 50% iodine overlay, a fused image is displayed in which each pixel is equally weighted by the VNC and iodine contributions. The visualization tool allows the operator to separate window-level settings for each component.

Wide-Coverage MDCT Scanners

A limitation of current MDCT scanners is their small Z-axis coverage. Clinical scanners with 64 detector rows provide approximately 4 cm of coverage along the Z-dimension. A simple way to increase Z-coverage is to use a greater number of detector rows. Toshiba America Medical Systems Inc. (Tustin, CA, USA) recently introduced the Aquilion 320, which has more than five times the detector coverage of a 64-slice CT scanner. The advantage of such wide coverage is obvious. In 1 second or less a volume as large as 16 cm can be scanned. This is wide enough to capture most organs, including the brain, with one single rotation of the gantry. Phillips Medical Systems (Best, The Netherlands) has announced a system with 128 detector rows.

Wide-volume coverage supported with continuous gantry rotation can produce time-resolved volumetric images of the organ being studied. This is referred to as *dynamic volumetric CT*. Dynamic CT permits visualization of time-evolving processes, such as neuroperfusion, tumor permeability, AVM blood flow patterns, and aneurysm pulsations.

An increased number of detector rows proportionately increases the volumetric coverage if there is a concomitant increase in the number of readout channels and the bandwidth of the slip ring to transfer data from the rotating gantry to the stationary hardware. Larger Z-coverage also leads to a much wider cone angle, with attendant deterioration of the slice selectivity profile further from the isocenter.

In typical scanning, the patient is translated through the gantry bore in one direction during the scan. Effective Z-coverage can be increased by using back-and-forth motion of the patient table. Newer 4-D scanning modes have recently been introduced by different vendors (e.g., Adaptive 4D Spiral, Siemens Medical Solutions, Forchheim, Germany; Shuttle Mode CT, GE Healthcare Inc., Princeton, NJ, USA). These modes allow larger Z-axis coverage up to 27 cm using only 64 detector rows that span only 4 cm. Thus, it is feasible to acquire dynamic scans of a complete organ even on a 64-slice scanner. This technology generates robust, artifact-free neuroperfusion and cardiac imaging at temporal resolution less than 200 ms. It also may be used for 3-D CT-guided interventions.

Flat-Panel Volume CT

The fpVCT is a uniquely designed prototype scanner with enhanced capabilities over conventional MDCT. An fpVCT scanner can be considered a variant of the conventional MDCT scanner in which the individual rows of detectors have been replaced by a 2-D digital flat-panel detector. The detector has an active area of 40 cm × 30 cm. Its digital flat-panel detector makes it capable of ultra-high spatial resolution, and the volumetric coverage of the detector allows studies of whole-organ perfusion, such as perfusion of the liver, kidney, or brain. Furthermore, the gantry can rotate continuously while projection data are being acquired, giving fpVCT the added capability of dynamic CT scanning.

In an fpVCT scanner, Z-direction coverage up to 18 cm around the isocenter by source-side collimation in the Z-direction is possible. This is large enough to scan an entire human head in one rotation. The rotation time of the gantry can be varied from 2 to 20 seconds. Native spatial resolution of the flat panel is a 150-μm cube.

The wide area detector used by the fpVCT prototype enables the operator to scan from a fixed angular position with a high image frame rate as well as scan continuously while the gantry is rotating. This flexibility gives rise to the following scanning modes.

Ultra-high resolution mode: The fpVCT system can be operated in the standard CT scanning mode by acquiring projections during a full rotation and reconstructing them as a volumetric stack. The only difference is that the entire volume is acquired in one rotation, and images have a much higher resolution because of the inherent spatial resolution of the flat-panel detector. For ultra-high spatial resolution scanning the detector is read out in the 1 × 1 binning mode. In this mode every pixel is read out separately, and a spatial resolution of approximately 150 μm is achieved. In order to improve the signal-to-noise ratio and increase the frame readout rate, a 2 × 2 binning mode is used. In this mode, four neighboring pixels are averaged to make one effective pixel with outstanding spatial resolution of approximately 200 μm. Despite this quantum improvement in spatial resolution compared with MDCT, the low contrast resolution is quite reasonable and approaches 5 HU in slices 10 mm thick.

Dynamic CT mode: fpVCT has the ability to monitor a volume of interest continuously over a period of time. The current prototype can rotate continuously for 80 seconds while acquiring projection data. The rotation time can be varied from 2 to 20 seconds. This enables observation of time-evolving processes such as first-pass dynamics of a contrast bolus, aneurysmal pulsations, blood flow pattern through an AVM, and tumor vascularity. This feature is further enhanced by the fact that fpVCT can cover a large volume in each rotation. If the temporal resolution is short enough and the imaging is conducted for an appropriate length of time, depending on the tissue type being studied, the evolution of a contrast bolus can be followed through the arteries, soft tissue, veins, viscera, and even bone marrow. Using such a dataset, a perfusion study of these tissues can be performed, making it possible to combine fpVCT angiography and fpVCT perfusion in one dynamic imaging process.

The temporal resolution of such a dataset will be equal to the rotation time of the gantry. In general, a higher rotation speed improves the temporal resolution at the expense of image noise and spatial resolution because of the fixed frame rate of the detector. By increasing the rotation speed, the number of frames used in reconstruction is proportionately decreased.

Fluoroscopy mode: The imaging chain of the fpVCT can be "parked" in one angular position and real-time projection data acquired. Such a fluoroscopy mode enables visualization and intervention from any user-selectable angular position.

Because of the various application modes that encompass radiography, fluoroscopy, and tomography in a single scanner, fpVCT can be thought of as an omni-scanner that may represent an important tool for neuroimaging in the future. Although this prototype scanner is still in its research phase, the preliminary results look promising. For example, by virtue of its high resolution, fpVCT is very helpful in visualizing small structures such as the ossicles and the pathologies involving the footplate of the stapes and other middle and inner ear structures. Other applications, such as dynamic imaging and real-time fluoroscopy, currently are being developed and explored. It is expected that the fpVCT will play a vital role in diagnosing small emboli, arterial dissections, and other neurovascular pathologies. Animal experiments with dynamic mode have shown that the ultra-high spatial resolution can clearly help in demarcating the narrow vessels of the brain (Figures 1-87 and 1-88). Aneurysm morphology and surface features, such as blebs and perforators, can be well seen using this technology. Animal experiments have demonstrated dynamics of tumor vascularity that may be useful in planning treatment. Together these features offer the promise of improved tomographic imaging in the future, with radiation exposure comparable to that of routine MDCT.

Portable CT Scanners

Compact mobile CT scanners for head and neck imaging recently have become commercially available. Portable CT machines, such as the CereTom (NeuroLogica Corporation, Danvers, MA, USA), provide a new option for critically ill patients. Instead of transporting the patient to a fixed scanner in a radiology suite, the scanner is brought to the patient so that he or she can be scanned in the ICU bed. Besides patient safety, mobile point-of-care imaging allows faster response to imaging requests.

Our experience has shown that use of the CereTom CT scanner is associated with a 58% reduction in request-to-scan times. It also improves personnel utilization because critical care nurses need not leave their premises to bring the patient to the radiology suite.

Because of their ease of use, these scanners are ideal for confirming the position of a shunt catheter, follow-up intracranial hemorrhage, midline shift, or any other neurologic process that may evolve over time and requires tracking by repeat CT scanning. Besides routine follow-up head CTs, the current scanners can perform contrast-enhanced CT, CTA, CT perfusion, and even xenon perfusion without sacrificing image quality.

Mobile scanners are the tool of choice in the neurology ICU setting, where patients often have multiple arterial, venous, and electrical lines, are ventilator dependent, and are too sick to travel to a fixed CT scanner. These scanners also enable deployment of advanced imaging in nontraditional areas, such as outpatient clinics, battlefront and military locations, ships, and sports facilities. Mobile CT scanners have also proven to be a useful tool in operating rooms.

Mobile scanners generally provide a headrest system so that images can be obtained in a sterile environment intraoperatively. Intraoperative scans, which can be obtained in minutes, provide vital data with minimal disruption or delay. For example, they can be used to ascertain the completeness of tumor or AVM resection.

The CereTom (NeuroLogica Corporation) was the first portable CT scanner. It is an eight-slice scanner that can generate images with slice thickness varying from 1.25 to 10 mm. In a 25-cm field of view configured for dedicated head scanning, it offers a resolution comparable to that of clinical MDCT. The tradeoff between the radiation dose delivered to patients and image quality is important for all CT scanners, including mobile CT scanners. Because mobile scanners are designed for bedside imaging of the head and neck, the dose to the personnel is another important consideration.

Mobile scanners typically are designed for multiple operating modes that trade off image quality for faster scan time and reduced dose. For example, in the low-dose mode (2 seconds per rotation), the CereTom delivers a radiation dose that is below or comparable to that of the American College of Radiology's diagnostic reference value. The CereTom can be operated in "standard" or "high-quality" modes that take 4 and 6 seconds per rotation, respectively. With these modes come corresponding increases in image quality, radiation dose, and scan time.

According to the manufacturer's specifications for the CereTom scanner, at 120 kVp and 7 mAs, the $CTDI_{100}$ values for rotation speeds of 2, 4, and 6 seconds are 44.8, 83.5, and 122 mGy, respectively. At 140 kVp and 7mAs, these values increase to 65.3, 126.8, and 176.3 mGy, respectively, and are within expected dose levels for high-quality head CT scans. The choice of imaging mode to be used is dictated by the patient's clinical condition. For example, for a postoperative scan assessing the position of a ventriculostomy catheter, a fast 2-second scan would suffice. However, if the clinical question is to determine if an acute infarction has occurred, a high-quality scan may be warranted to assess gray–white differentiation.

The scanner provides protective lead curtains so that the scatter radiation is well within ALARA (as low as reasonably achievable) standards. The specifications for the CereTom state that "at a distance of 2 meters (6 feet) from the isocenter, an operator can perform over 26 scans per day, for 250 days per year without any additional lead protection." Therefore, the dose to the personnel conducting the scan is well within the acceptable range when proper precautions are taken.

Figure 1-89 illustrates the power of a mobile CT scanner in a neurology ICU setting. The patient, a 43-year-old woman, was found unconscious in her house by Emergency Medical Services (EMS). The patient was in asystole, but EMS achieved a complex perfusing rhythm in the field after administering epinephrine and atropine. In the neurology ICU, the patient, who

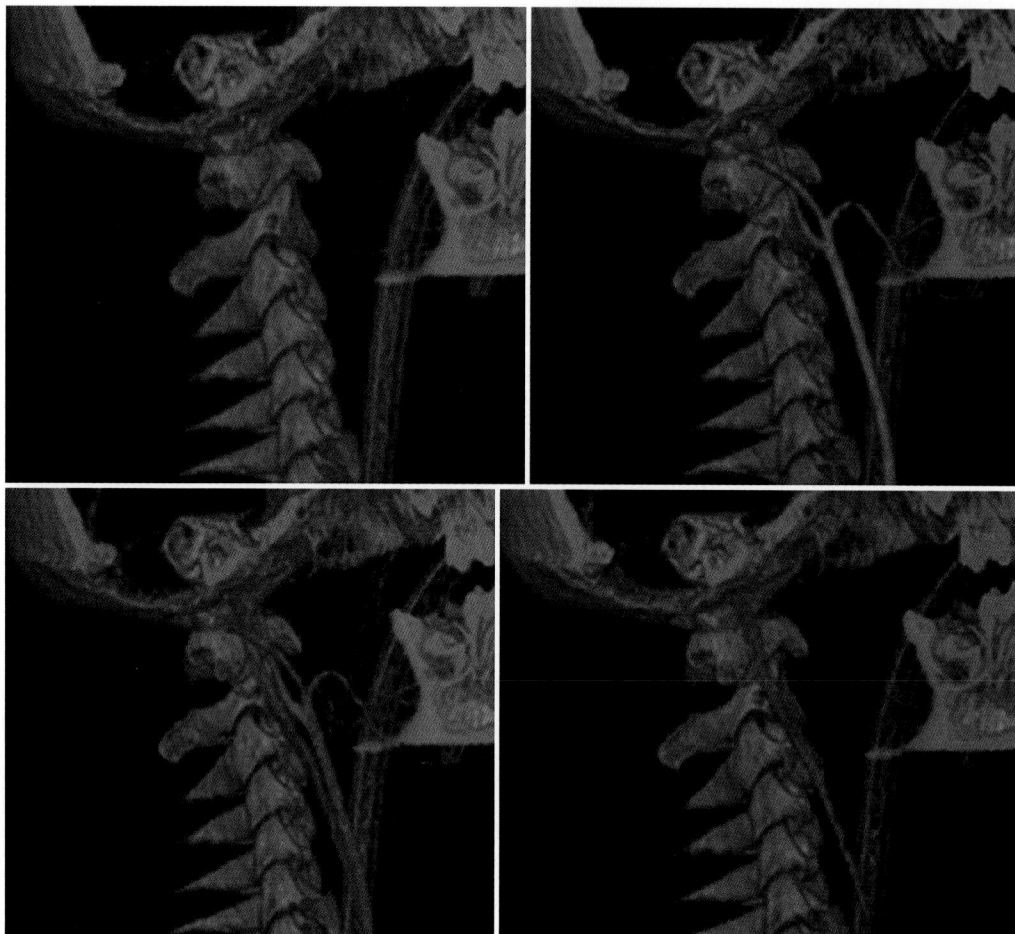

Figure 1-87 Flat-panel volume computed tomographic images of *Macaca sylvanus* showing dynamic filling of the cervical arteries and veins. *Left,* Very early during contrast injection, none of the vessels are visible. *Second from left,* Arterial phase of the bolus shows peak arterial opacification. *Third image from left,* A bit later in time, both arteries and veins are visible. *Right,* Venous phase.

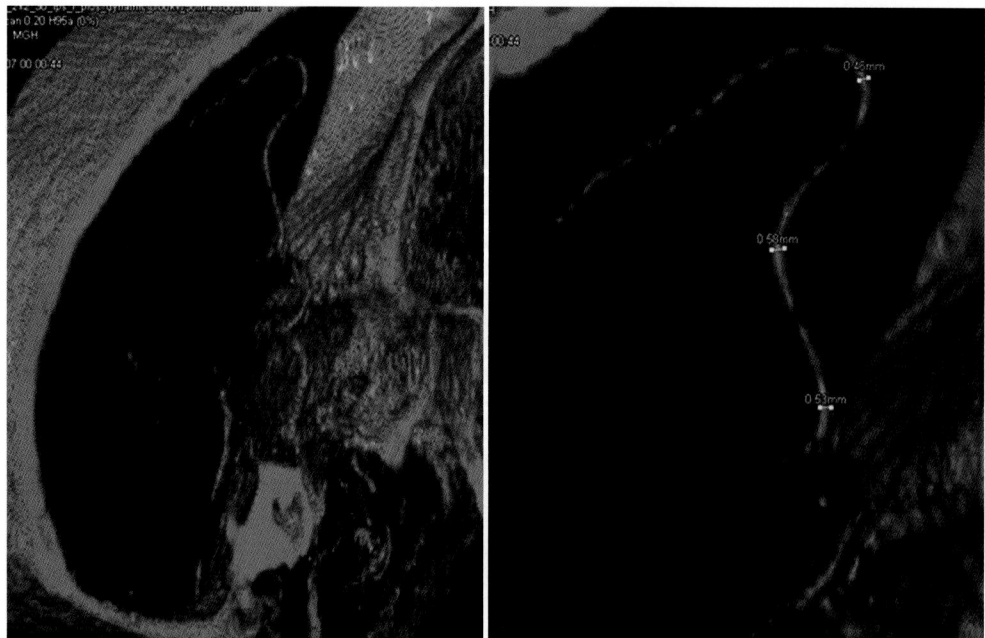

Figure 1-88 Ultra-high spatial resolution of flat-panel volume computed tomography enables visualization of very small vessels of the brain. In this case, the anterior cerebral artery of a *Macaca sylvanus,* measuring approximately 400 μm at the genu, can be visualized.

Chapter 1 Multidetector Computed Tomography as a Problem-Solving Tool in Neuroradiology

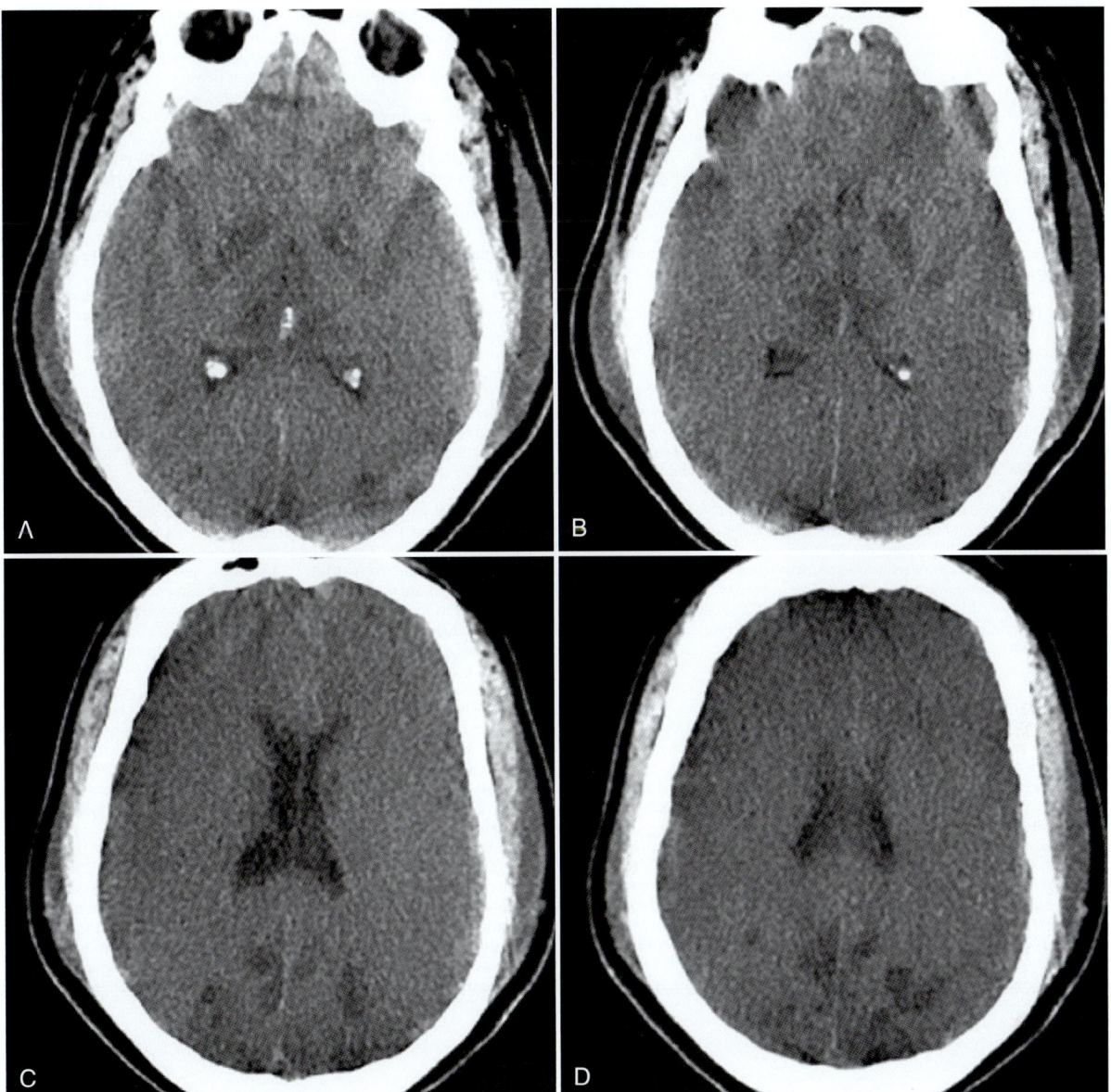

Figure 1-89 Multiple axial computed tomographic slices acquired using a portable scanner (CereTom, NeuroLogica Corporation, Denvers, MA, USA) in a patient with a history of prolonged asystole. Even with a portable device, diffuse loss of gray–white differentiation and sulcal effacement can be appreciated and is compatible with cerebral edema, as is the effacement of perimesencephalic cisterns and uncal herniation. Multiple foci of infarctions suggest widespread hypoxic ischemic injury, which is most severe in the areas of high metabolic activity, such as the basal ganglia.

was hyperkalemic with a blood potassium level in the range from 6.1 to 7.2, was deemed too unstable to undergo a regular head CT or MRI. A portable CT scan using the CereTom was performed. Figure 1-89 shows diffuse loss of gray–white differentiation and sulcal effacement compatible with cerebral edema. There is complete effacement of the third and fourth ventricles, suprasellar cistern, quadrigeminal plate cistern, and ambient cistern. Bilateral uncal herniation has occurred. Hypoattenuation is seen in bilateral caudate bodies, the lentiform nuclei, thalami, bilateral hippocampal formations, and patchy areas in bilateral posterior parietal lobes. These areas of infarctions are consistent with diffuse hypoxemic ischemic injury secondary to prolonged asystole. As demonstrated in this case, portable CT scanners have the requisite contrast resolution and low-contrast detectability to demonstrate subtle differences in attenuation required for neuroimaging.

Suggested Readings

Baleriaux DL, Neugroschl C. Spinal and spinal cord infection. *Eur Radiol.* 2004;14(suppl 3):E72-E83.

Batra S, Ahuja S. Congenital scoliosis: Management and future directions. *Acta Orthop Belg.* 2008;74:147-160.

Braun IF, Naidich TP, Leeds NE, Koslow M, Zimmerman HM, Chase NE. Dense intracranial epidermoid tumors. Computed tomographic observations. *Radiology.* 1977;122:717-719.

Chae EJ, Song JW, Seo JB, Krauss B, Jang YM, Song KS. Clinical utility of dual-energy CT in the evaluation of solitary pulmonary nodules: Initial experience. *Radiology.* 2008;249:671-681.

Chae EJ, Seo JB, Goo HW, et al. Xenon ventilation CT with a dual-energy technique of dual-source CT: Initial experience. *Radiology.* 2008;248:615-624.

Chang MC, Wu HT, Lee CH, Liu CL, Chen TH. Tuberculous spondylitis and pyogenic spondylitis: Comparative magnetic resonance imaging features. *Spine.* 2006;31:782-788.

Chirinos JA, Lichtstein DM, Garcia J, Tamariz LJ. The evolution of Lemierre syndrome: Report of 2 cases and review of the literature. *Medicine (Baltimore)*. 2002;81:458-465.

Coulon A, Lafitte F, Hoang-Xuan K, et al. Radiographic findings in 37 cases of primary CNS lymphoma in immunocompetent patients. *Eur Radiol*. 2002;12:329-340.

Curtin HD. Superior semicircular canal dehiscence syndrome and multi-detector row CT. *Radiology*. 2003;226:312-314.

Daffner RH, Brown RR, Goldberg AL. A new classification for cervical vertebral injuries: Influence of CT. *Skeletal Radiol*. 2000;29:125-132.

Demirci M, Tan E, Durguner M, Zileli T, Eryilmaz M. Spinal brucellosis. A case with "cauliflower" appearance on CT. *Neuroradiology*. 1989;31:282-283.

Frerichs KU, Stieg PE, Friedlander RM. Prediction of aneurysm rupture site by an angiographically identified bleb at the aneurysm neck. *J Neurosurg*. 2000;93:517.

Gallagher CN, Hutchinson PJ, Pickard JD. Neuroimaging in trauma. *Curr Opin Neurol*. 2007;20:403-409.

Geijer M, El-Khoury GY. MDCT in the evaluation of skeletal trauma: Principles, protocols, and clinical applications. *Emerg Radiol*. 2006;13:7-18.

Goldstein JN, Fazen LE, Snider R, et al. Contrast extravasation on CT angiography predicts hematoma expansion in intracerebral hemorrhage. *Neurology*. 2007;68:889-894.

Gupta R, Bartling SH, Basu SK, et al. Experimental flat-panel high-spatial-resolution volume CT of the temporal bone. *AJNR Am J Neuroradiol*. 2004;25:1417-1424.

Gupta R, Grasruck M, Suess C, et al. Ultra-high resolution flat-panel volume CT: Fundamental principles, design architecture, and system characterization. *Eur Radiol*. 2006;16:1191-1205.

Holmes JF, Akkinepalli R. Computed tomography versus plain radiography to screen for cervical spine injury: A meta-analysis. *J Trauma*. 2005;58:902-905.

Imakita S, Onishi Y, Hashimoto T, et al. Subtraction CT angiography with controlled-orbit helical scanning for detection of intracranial aneurysms. *AJNR Am J Neuroradiol*. 1998;19:291-295.

Intracerebral hemorrhage after intravenous t-PA therapy for ischemic stroke. The NINDS t-PA Stroke Study Group. *Stroke*. 1997;28:2109-2118.

Jevtic V. Vertebral infection. *Eur Radiol*. 2004;14(suppl 3):E43-E52.

Kim EY, Heo JH, Lee SK, et al. Prediction of thrombolytic efficacy in acute ischemic stroke using thin-section noncontrast CT. *Neurology*. 2006;67:1846-1848.

Kirchhof K, Welzel T, Mecke C, Zoubaa S, Sartor K. Differentiation of white, mixed, and red thrombi: Value of CT in estimation of the prognosis of thrombolysis phantom study. *Radiology*. 2003;228:126-130.

Klein GR, Vaccaro AR, Albert TJ, et al. Efficacy of magnetic resonance imaging in the evaluation of posterior cervical spine fractures. *Spine*. 1999;24:771-774.

Koroshetz WJ, Lev MH. Contrast computed tomography scan in acute stroke: "You can't always get what you want but...you get what you need." *Ann Neurol*. 2002;51:415-416.

Lee BK, Lopez F, Genovese M, Loutit JS. Lemierre's syndrome. *South Med J*. 1997;90:640-643.

Leugers CM, Clover R. Lemierre syndrome: Postanginal sepsis. *J Am Board Fam Pract*. 1995;8:384-391.

Lev MH, Farkas J, Gemmete JJ, et al. Acute stroke: Improved nonenhanced CT detection—Benefits of soft-copy interpretation by using variable window width and center level settings. *Radiology*. 1999;213:150-155.

Lev MH, Segal AZ, Farkas J, et al. Utility of perfusion-weighted CT imaging in acute middle cerebral artery stroke treated with intra-arterial thrombolysis: Prediction of final infarct volume and clinical outcome. *Stroke*. 2001;32:2021-2028.

Li F, Zhu S, Liu Y, Chen G, Chi L, Qu F. Hyperdense intracranial epidermoid cysts: A study of 15 cases. *Acta Neurochir (Wien)*. 2007;149:31-39.

Miller JD, Murray LS, Teasdale GM. Development of a traumatic intracranial hematoma after a "minor" head injury. *Neurosurgery*. 1990;27:669-673.

Minor LB, Solomon D, Zinreich JS, Zee DS. Sound- and/or pressure-induced vertigo due to bone dehiscence of the superior semicircular canal. *Arch Otolaryngol Head Neck Surg*. 1998;124:249-258.

Pieper DR, Al-Mefty O, Hanada Y, Buechner D. Hyperostosis associated with meningioma of the cranial base: Secondary changes or tumor invasion. *Neurosurgery*. 1999;44:742-746.

Rodallec MH, Feydy A, Larousserie F, et al. Diagnostic imaging of solitary tumors of the spine: What to do and say. *Radiographics*. 2008;28:1019-1041.

Saver JL. Time is brain—Quantified. *Stroke*. 2006;37:263-266.

Schaefer PW, Roccatagliata L, Ledezma C, et al. First-pass quantitative CT perfusion identifies thresholds for salvageable penumbra in acute stroke patients treated with intra-arterial therapy. *AJNR Am J Neuroradiol*. 2006;27:20-25.

Schramm P, Schellinger PD, Fiebach JB, et al. Comparison of CT and CT angiography source images with diffusion-weighted imaging in patients with acute stroke within 6 hours after onset. *Stroke*. 2002;33:2426-2432.

Sekhar LN, Heros RC. Origin, growth, and rupture of saccular aneurysms: A review. *Neurosurgery*. 1981;8:248-260.

Servadei F, Vergoni G, Staffa G, et al. Extradural haematomas: How many deaths can be avoided? Protocol for early detection of haematoma in minor head injuries. *Acta Neurochir (Wien)*. 1995;133:50-55.

Shapiro MD, Neilan TG, Jassal DS, et al. Multidetector computed tomography for the detection of left atrial appendage thrombus: A comparative study with transesophageal echocardiography. *J Comput Assist Tomogr*. 2007;31:905-909.

Tissue plasminogen activator for acute ischemic stroke. The National Institute of Neurological Disorders and Stroke rt-PA Stroke Study Group. *N Engl J Med*. 1995;333:1581-1587.

Toyama Y, Kobayashi T, Nishiyama Y, Satoh K, Ohkawa M, Seki K. CT for acute stage of closed head injury. *Radiat Med*. 2005;23:309-316.

Velez MR, Dorsett Jr C, Ferguson HW, Hansen K. Lemierre's syndrome: A case report. *J Oral Maxillofac Surg*. 2003;61:968-971.

Wada R, Aviv RI, Fox AJ, et al. CT angiography "spot sign" predicts hematoma expansion in acute intracerebral hemorrhage. *Stroke*. 2007;38:1257-1262.

Wintermark M, Flanders AE, Velthuis B, et al. Perfusion-CT assessment of infarct core and penumbra: Receiver operating characteristic curve analysis in 130 patients suspected of acute hemispheric stroke. *Stroke*. 2006;37:979-985.

Wintermark M, Reichhart M, Thiran JP, et al. Prognostic accuracy of cerebral blood flow measurement by perfusion computed tomography, at the time of emergency room admission, in acute stroke patients. *Ann Neurol*. 2002;51:417-432.

CHAPTER 2
Magnetic Resonance Imaging as a Problem-Solving Tool

Jane J. Kim and Pratik Mukherjee

■ INTRODUCTION

Computed tomography (CT) and magnetic resonance imaging (MRI) have been the mainstays of diagnostic neuroradiology into the first decade of the twenty-first century. CT has shown particular utility in the evaluation of bone, blood, calcium, and metal in the brain and spine. Contrast-enhanced CT angiography also affords exquisite detail of the cerebrovascular system. However, MRI has become the dominant technique for problem solving in neuroradiology due to its inherent multiplanar and three-dimensional (3D) capability, sensitivity, and versatility and its multitude of available contrast mechanisms for evaluating the diverse tissues of the neuraxis. Using appropriate procedures and widely accepted precautions, MRI is very safe, with no exposure to ionizing radiation or iodinated contrast media.

■ PHYSICAL BASIS OF MRI

The MR signal from biologic tissues arises when an external magnetic field (B_0) is applied and the hydrogen nuclei, primarily from water protons, begin to rotate ("precess") at the resonance frequency, known as the *Larmor frequency*, and align along the direction of the B_0 field, designated the z-axis or the longitudinal direction. The precession of the aligned hydrogen nuclei at the Larmor frequency creates a net magnetization, but this cannot be detected along the z-axis; it can only be detected when its magnetization lies in the transverse (x/y) plane orthogonal to the z-axis. To measure the MR signal, a radiofrequency (RF) pulse is applied to tip the net magnetization by a certain angle (the flip angle) toward the transverse plane. Immediately after the RF pulse, protons in the transverse plane precess together at the same frequency and coherently at the same phase, creating a signal. However, the signal is rapidly lost as inhomogeneities in the magnetic field cause the nuclei to lose their phase coherence ("dephase") and spin at different frequencies, a process known as *free induction decay* (FID). FID cannot be measured directly for imaging purposes. Instead, an echo of the FID, either a spin echo or gradient echo, must be produced by rephasing the nuclei. These two basic rephasing methods are the basis for many RF pulse sequence designs that result in the diverse forms of contrast available from MRI.

■ MR IMAGE GENERATION

To form images, magnetic field gradients are applied that steadily increase in strength along a particular direction. Because of the gradients, a proton in one location will be at a different magnetic field strength and therefore will precess at a different Larmor frequency than a proton in another location along the gradient direction. To localize protons within the body in all three orthogonal axes $(x, y,$ and $z)$, three mutually perpendicular gradients are applied, designated the *frequency-encoding, phase-encoding,* and *slice-select gradients.*

Two-dimensional MRI uses a specific RF pulse to excite a slice of tissue. The slice-select gradient is turned on while the excitatory RF pulse is given so that the only nuclei to respond are those in the slice whose Larmor frequency matches that of the exciting RF pulse. The stronger the slice-select gradient, the thinner the excited slice. The frequency-encoding gradient is used during detection or "readout" of the MR signal. The phase-encoding step, which is performed between slice selection and frequency-encoded readout, must be performed many times at different gradient strengths, making this one of the key determinants of the length of a scan. Two-dimensional imaging typically produces a series of slices that are greater than 1 mm each in thickness and may be contiguous and consecutive, contiguous and interleaved, or noncontiguous with small gaps between the 2D slices.

In 3D imaging, the RF pulse and slice-select gradient excite an entire volume of tissue along the z-axis, rather than a single thin slice. Phase encoding is performed in the two directions mutually orthogonal to the frequency-encode direction, not just in one direction as in 2D imaging, and is followed by the frequency-encoded readout. Three-dimensional imaging can generate very thin slices (each <1 mm) that are contiguous with each other, permitting excellent multiplanar reconstructions. However, 3D imaging is slower than 2D imaging because it performs the relatively time-consuming process of phase encoding in two directions, not just one.

Generation of an actual image from an MR signal usually requires multiple excitations with an RF pulse to produce enough data for the image. The period between excitations is the *time to repetition* (TR); the period from RF excitation to echo readout is the *time to echo* (TE). The measured echoes from a particular slice are sampled and

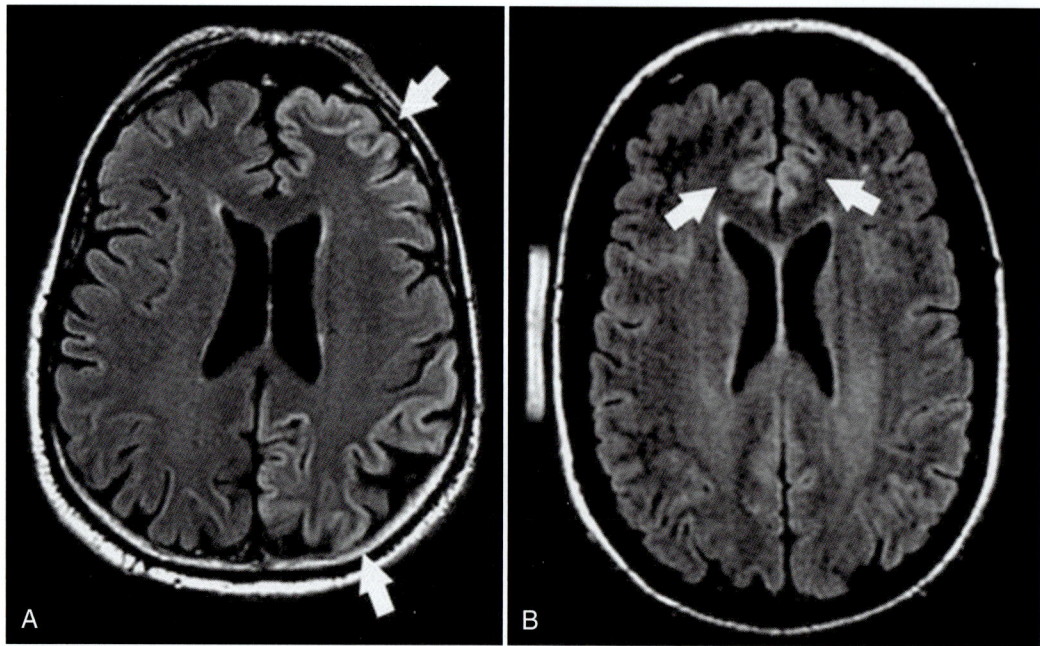

Figure 2-1 Importance of proper coil selection. Patients with prion disorders, such as Creutzfeldt-Jakob disease (CJD), may have high signal in the cerebral cortex, as was the case for a patient **(A)** who had bright cortical signal particularly in the left cerebral hemisphere *(arrows)*. A different patient **(B)**, who did not have CJD, was imaged in a surface coil and showed high signal in the paramedian frontal cortex bilaterally *(arrows)*. This is an artifact from the closer proximity of superficial tissues to the surface coil. Because of the potential for confusion with artifactually inhomogeneous signal, diagnosis of CJD may be easier with a volume coil, which encircles the entire head and provides better signal uniformity.

then encoded within k-space. The k-space is a mathematical construct consisting of a blank grid or matrix onto which frequency and phase data can be mapped prior to their transformation into an MR image. In k-space, frequency information typically is mapped along the x-axis and phase information along the y-axis. In a conventional spin-echo sequence, one echo generates the data for a single line in k-space and corresponds to a single phase-encoding step. The center of k-space contains information about general form (low spatial resolution) at high image contrast. The periphery of k-space holds information about fine detail (high spatial resolution) at low image contrast. The data within k-space are rendered into an image by Fourier transformation, a computerized mathematical process of MR signal decoding that converts frequency information into the pixels of an image.

RF COILS

RF antennas called *coils* are used to transmit the RF pulse and receive the MR signal. Separate coils can be used for transmission and reception, or the same coil can be used for both functions. MR coils may be constructed to have different regions of coverage. A *volume coil* is a circumferential structure that surrounds the body part completely, whereas a *surface coil* is typically flat or curved and placed on the skin surface overlying a specific region of interest. Volume coils both transmit and receive the MR signal. They encircle the body part completely, so they provide very uniform signal throughout the entire MR image. A typical volume coil used for neuroimaging is the birdcage head coil. Surface coils are generally receive-only coils, so a separate volume head or body coil is needed to transmit the RF pulse. Surface coils have very high signal-to-noise ratio, especially for superficial structures close to the coil. However, they have a reduced field of view (FOV) and are more prone to inhomogeneity of signal across an MR image, with signal loss for deeper tissues. Phased-array coils are composite coils composed of multiple small surface coils arranged to form an array. These have been developed to try to increase the FOV while maintaining the high signal-to-noise ratio of surface coils. Imaging for Creutzfeldt-Jakob disease illustrates the importance of proper coil selection (Figure 2-1).

TISSUE CONTRAST IN MRI

T1, T2, and proton density are the fundamental parameters of MRI and determine the contrast between tissues. Following the excitatory RF pulse and tilting of the net magnetization into the transverse or x/y-plane, the transverse magnetization is lost at a rate determined by a particular tissue's T2 relaxation time. Simultaneously, longitudinal magnetization along the z-axis is regained at a rate set by the tissue's T1 relaxation time.

Fat has a shorter T1 than cerebrospinal fluid (CSF) and recovers its longitudinal magnetization quickly following an RF pulse. If TR is short, fat recovers more of its longitudinal magnetization than CSF and produces a stronger MR signal. More longitudinal magnetization leads to more transverse magnetization and stronger signal with the next RF pulse. Making TR short emphasizes the differences in T1 relaxation times of tissues, so tissues with short T1, such as fat, melanin, and protein, produce high signal. MR sequences that emphasize tissue differences in T1 relaxation are designated *T1 weighted*.

Fat has a shorter T2 relaxation time than CSF and loses its transverse magnetization (T2 signal) more rapidly. Making TE long provides greater time for transverse magnetization to decay and emphasizes differences in T2 relaxation times of tissues. When TE is long, tissues with short T2 relaxation times (fat) show greater loss of T2 signal and appear dark, whereas tissues with long T2 relaxation times (CSF) retain a larger portion of their T2 signal and appear bright. MR sequences that use long TE to emphasize tissue differences in T2 relaxation times are designated *T2 weighted*.

If TR is long and TE is short, neither the T1 nor T2 difference between fat and CSF is emphasized. Any difference in contrast observed between the two tissues is then due to differences in the proton densities of the tissues. Tissues with higher proton density supply greater signal than tissues with lower proton density. MR sequences that use long TR and short TE to capture differences in tissue proton density are designated *proton-density (PD) weighted sequences*.

Image Quality

In MR, image quality depends on spatial resolution and the signal-to-noise ratio. Like CT, spatial resolution reflects voxel size. Pixel size influences in-plane or x/y-axis spatial resolution, whereas slice thickness determines z-axis spatial resolution. Therefore, spatial resolution can be improved by reducing voxel size through decreasing FOV, increasing matrix size, or obtaining thinner slices. However, reducing voxel size to improve spatial resolution tends to increase the relative noise in an image. Spatial resolution and signal-to-noise ratio are competing considerations.

The sampling bandwidth refers to the rate at which an echo is sampled. A high bandwidth samples an echo quickly but requires a stronger frequency-encoding gradient and results in a greater range of frequencies. A low bandwidth takes longer to sample an echo but has a smaller range of frequencies and includes less sampling of noise. High bandwidths reduce acquisition time, so there is less opportunity for image degradation from signal decay. Low bandwidths prolong acquisition time but improve the signal-to-noise ratio.

Basic MR Sequences

Spin echo and gradient echo are the only two basic sequences in MRI; all other sequences are variations of one of these two sequences. To create either a spin echo or gradient echo following the FID, a specific pulse sequence must be designed. A pulse sequence diagram illustrates the series and timing of requisite events, including application of the RF pulse and various gradients, to produce the sampled echo.

Spin Echo

The spin echo (SE) sequence is created by following the 90-degree excitatory pulse with a 180-degree refocusing pulse at time TE/2. Following the 90-degree RF pulse, transverse magnetization (FID) is quickly lost because of (1) macroscopic magnetic field inhomogeneities due to factors such as adjacent ferromagnetic objects, non-uniformities in the B_0 magnetic field, and tissue interfaces, and (2) microscopic magnetic interactions among spinning nuclei. The loss of magnetization due to both microscopic and macroscopic factors is termed *T2* relaxation*. Signal loss due only to microscopic nuclear interactions is "true" T2 decay and occurs more slowly than $T2^*$ decay.

The 180-degree refocusing pulse is able to rephase nuclei that have begun precessing at different frequencies and can prevent the signal loss that is due to macroscopic factors. However, it cannot prevent the signal loss that is due to random, microscopic nuclear interactions (i.e., T2 decay). The spin echo that results from the rephasing effects of the 180-degree pulse is still susceptible to T2 decay; therefore, SE sequences with long TE are said to be T2 weighted (not $T2^*$ weighted).

Figure 2-2, *A* illustrates the pulse sequence diagram for the spin-echo technique.

Gradient Refocused Echo

If the 180-degree refocusing pulse is not given, an echo of the FID can still be produced by using gradients of opposite polarity (equal strength, opposite direction) to first dephase and then rephase the spins. Opposite-polarity lobes of the frequency-encoding gradient are used to bring spins together in phase and produce a gradient echo at time TE. Because they do not use a 180-degree refocusing pulse, gradient-recalled echo (GRE) images are prone to signal loss from both macroscopic and microscopic factors ($T2^*$ decay). Depending on various sequence parameters, GRE sequences can be T1 or $T2^*$ weighted, but typically not T2 weighted (exceptions are discussed later). Figure 2-2, *B* illustrates the components of a GRE sequence.

Unlike SE, GRE sequences use small flip angles less than 90 degrees. Flip angles less than 90 degrees do not completely eliminate longitudinal magnetization. Some longitudinal magnetization remains, so it recovers more completely before the next pulse. This permits use of a shorter TR and helps achieve faster scan time. In GRE sequences, the tissue weighting depends on TR, TE, and the value of the flip angle. Larger flip angles accentuate differences in T1 relaxation time because more longitudinal magnetization must recover to produce the image. Therefore, larger flip angles produce T1-weighted images.

"Spoiling" or "refocusing" transverse magnetization provides another means of tissue weighting. To reduce scan times, GRE sequences frequently use very short TR (shorter than the T2 relaxation times of many tissues) so that transverse magnetization does not have time to decay completely before the next excitatory pulse. In this situation, there is both residual transverse magnetization and recovered longitudinal magnetization just before the next RF pulse. If the residual transverse magnetization is "spoiled" or destroyed, only the longitudinal magnetization is left for the next RF pulse, resulting in T1-weighted images. Spoiling of transverse magnetization is achieved by use of spoiler gradients or

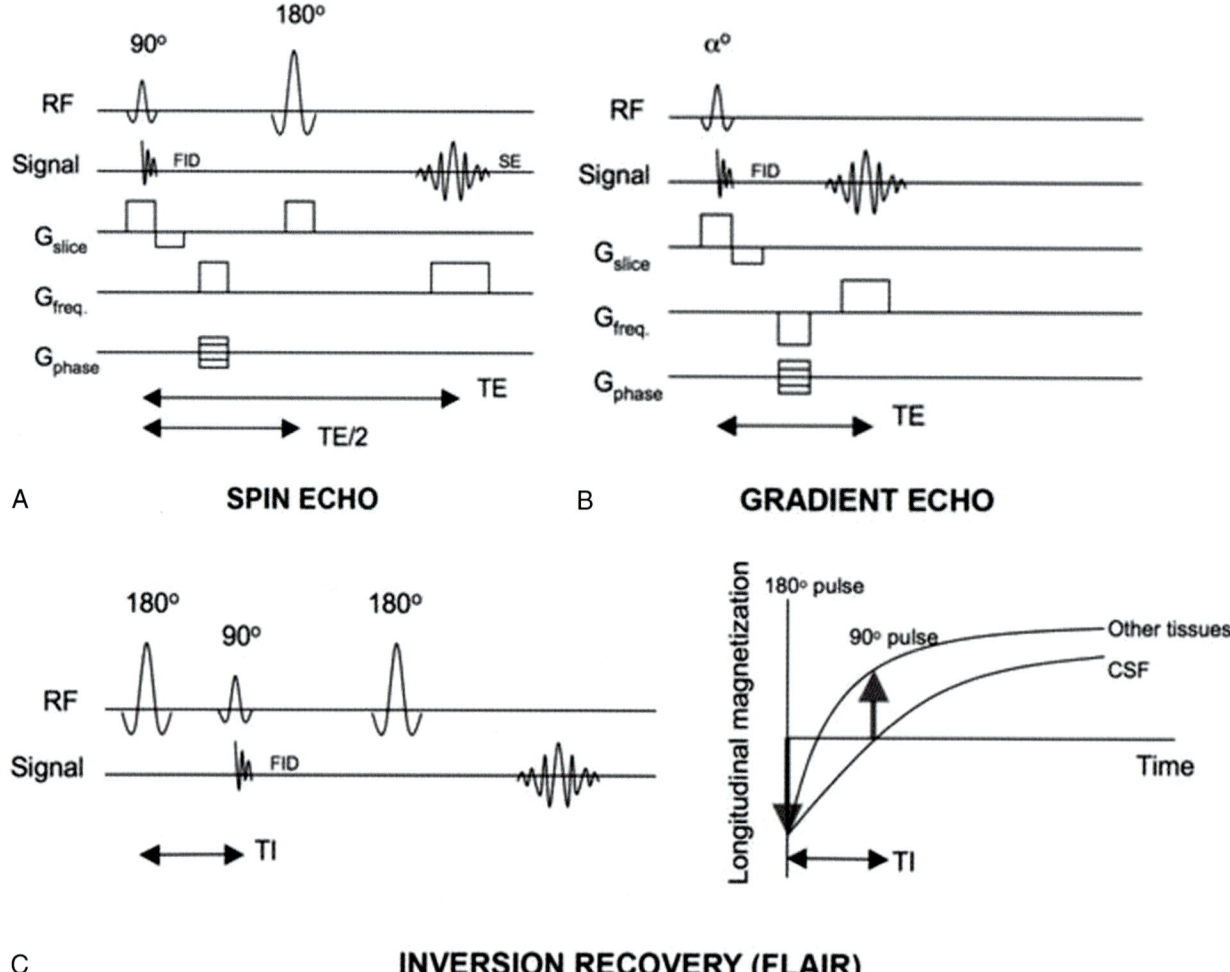

Figure 2-2 Pulse sequence diagrams. **A:** Spin echo. Following the 90° excitation pulse, which occurs at the same time as the slice-selection gradient, free induction decay quickly disappears. The 180-degree refocusing pulse given at time TE/2 rephases the spins to create the spin echo that is read out at time TE with application of the frequency-encoding gradient. The phase-encoding step must be performed many times at different gradient strengths, so it is pictured with multiple lines denoting different gradient amplitudes. **B:** Gradient echo. Following the radiofrequency pulse (with flip angle α <90 degrees), free induction decay is rapidly lost. No 180-degree refocusing pulse is given; instead, opposing lobes of the frequency-encoding gradient are used to first dephase then rephase the spins, creating an echo at time TE. The negative (dephasing) lobe of the frequency-encoding gradient is shown below baseline, and the positive (rephasing) lobe is shown above baseline. **C:** Inversion recovery and fluid-attenuated inversion recovery (FLAIR). A 180-degree pulse is given at the beginning of the sequence, which flips the net magnetization vector into the −z-axis. Tissues recover longitudinal magnetization according to their T1 properties, and cerebrospinal fluid (CSF), with long T1, regains magnetization more slowly than other tissues. The 90-degree excitatory pulse at time TI is given at the null point for CSF, when there is no longitudinal magnetization for CSF. However, other tissues have recovered longitudinal magnetization, which is flipped into the transverse plane with the excitatory pulse to generate the magnetic resonance signal. FLAIR is performed on a spin-echo sequence.

RF spoiling, a discussion of which is beyond the scope of this chapter. These T1-weighted GRE sequences are known as *spoiled* or *incoherent GRE sequences*.

Alternatively, *unspoiled* or *coherent GRE imaging* preserves the transverse magnetization that accumulates between RF pulses in short TR sequences. The subsequent RF pulse rotates residual transverse magnetization into the longitudinal plane while flipping recovered longitudinal magnetization into the transverse plane. Over time and with successive RF pulses, there is an intricate mixing of transverse and longitudinal components known as steady-state free precession. Unlike spoiled GRE sequences, signal intensity in unspoiled sequences depends not only on the amount of longitudinal magnetization that has recovered but on the amount of transverse magnetization that remains. Because recovery of longitudinal magnetization is determined by T1 and decay of transverse magnetization by T2, these sequences reflect a mixture of T1 and T2 weighting. Note that if TR is sufficiently long to allow complete decay of transverse magnetization and leave only longitudinal magnetization, the unspoiled/coherent sequence becomes T1 weighted, much like a spoiled/incoherent GRE.

Another consequence of preserving residual transverse magnetization in unspoiled GRE imaging is the generation of a spin echo with the next excitatory RF pulse. The excitatory pulse behaves like a refocusing pulse on residual transverse magnetization and is conceptually similar to (though less effective than) the

180-degree refocusing pulse used in SE imaging. The residual transverse magnetization that was becoming dephased is suddenly refocused and generates a spin echo in addition to the usual FID that is created immediately after an RF pulse. Depending on sequence design, either the FID or spin echo can be favored to achieve more T2* or T2 weighting, respectively. Balanced GRE sequences are constructed so that all gradients are balanced and the FID and spin echo signals coincide, achieving a complex mix of T1 and T2 weighting.

Inversion Recovery Imaging

Inversion recovery imaging applies a preparatory pulse just before an SE or GRE sequence to emphasize T1 contrast or to eliminate signal from undesired tissues such as CSF or fat. A 180-degree inversion pulse is first given to flip the initial net magnetization vector from the +z axis to the −z axis. Nuclei recover longitudinal magnetization from −z to +z according to their T1 properties. If an excitatory 90-degree pulse is given during relaxation (at inversion time TI), nuclei with shorter T1 will have recovered more longitudinal magnetization and thus produce greater transverse magnetization and MR signal. This creates T1 weighting.

As nuclei recover longitudinal magnetization from −z to +z following the 180-degree inversion pulse, they pass through a null point at which the net magnetization vector is zero. A 90-degree excitatory pulse given at this time for CSF (or fat) would have very little effect on and generate no MR signal from CSF (or fat). In this manner, specific tissues can be made dark on imaging. *Short tau inversion recovery* (STIR) is the name of the sequence used for fat elimination. Because fat has a relatively short T1, STIR sequences typically use inversion times of approximately 150 to 175 ms at 1.5 T. *Fluid-attenuated inversion recovery* (FLAIR) is the name of the sequence used for CSF suppression. Because water has a long T1, FLAIR sequences typically use inversion times ranging from 1,800 to 2,400 ms at 1.5 T. Figure 2-2, *C* illustrates a typical inversion recovery sequence.

The concept of tissue contrast is more complex than simple T1 or T2 weighting for FLAIR. Whereas FLAIR sequences have long TE and are T2 weighted so that fluid other than CSF is bright, an element of T1 weighting is also present. The 180-degree inversion pulse introduces T1 weighting, because the degree to which tissues recover longitudinal magnetization before the excitation pulse is given depends on their T1 properties.

Fast Imaging Techniques

The main drawback of conventional SE imaging is its long imaging time. Long imaging time results because each excitatory RF pulse generates a single echo that fills only a single line of *k*-space, corresponding to a single phase-encoding step. The SE technique does not considerably lengthen the time required for obtaining T1-weighted images because T1-weighted sequences use short TR and short TE. However, the SE technique significantly lengthens the time required for obtaining T2-weighted images because T2-weighted sequences use long TR and long TE. *Rapid acquisition with refocused echo* (RARE) sequences were developed to reduce imaging time. Commercially, these are known as *fast spin-echo* (FSE) or *turbo spin-echo* (TSE) sequences. In this approach, each 90-degree RF pulse is followed by multiple 180-degree refocusing pulses (not just one) in order to generate more spin echoes and fill multiple lines of *k*-space per excitation pulse. The number of echoes generated after each excitatory pulse is termed the *echo train length* (ETL) and corresponds to the number of phase-encoding steps acquired in a single TR. Therefore, FSE or TSE reduces the scan time to 1/ETL of the time required for standard SE imaging.

The *k*-space demonstrates a certain symmetry and redundancy of information that allows an image to be derived from a portion of the complete dataset. If enough echoes are collected to fill one-half of *k*-space after a single 90-degree excitatory pulse (designated a *shot*), the data in the other half of *k*-space can be inferred based on the known symmetry of *k*-space. The technique used to produce images from a half set of data is known as *single-shot RARE* (or commercially as half-Fourier acquisition single-shot turbo spin echo [HASTE] or single-shot fast spin echo [SSFSE]).

A similar rapid imaging technique using gradient echoes is designated *echo planar imaging* (EPI). In EPI, the single excitatory pulse or shot is followed by a long stream of gradient echoes generated by rapidly switching gradients. The multiple gradient echoes fill all of *k*-space after a single shot. EPI is one of the fastest MR sequences available, so it is used for diffusion-weighted imaging (DWI). Because DWI characterizes the microscopic movement or diffusion of water molecules through tissue, corruption by bulk macroscopic motion due to long scan time cannot be permitted.

Figure 2-3 summarizes the differences between single and multiple echo techniques. Note that all multiple echo techniques are subject to image contrast blurring because transverse magnetization decays over the course of the long echo train. This T1, T2, or T2* blurring increases with ETL and reaches its extreme in the single-shot techniques (HASTE, SSFSE, and EPI).

■ NORMAL APPEARANCE OF IMAGES WITH MRI

On T1-weighted images of the normal adult brain, white matter is of slightly higher signal intensity than gray matter. However, the unmyelinated or partially myelinated white matter of infants younger than 2 years is hypointense to gray matter. Fat is bright and CSF is dark on T1-weighted images, as previously discussed.

On T2-weighted images of the normal adult brain, white matter is hypointense to gray matter. The unmyelinated or partially myelinated white matter of infants younger than 2 years is hyperintense to gray matter on T2-weighted images. Fat is dark and CSF is bright on spin-echo T2-weighted images. However, fat may appear bright on FSE or TSE T2-weighted images due to a decrease in a phenomenon known as *J-coupling*. Any pathologic process that increases tissue water content

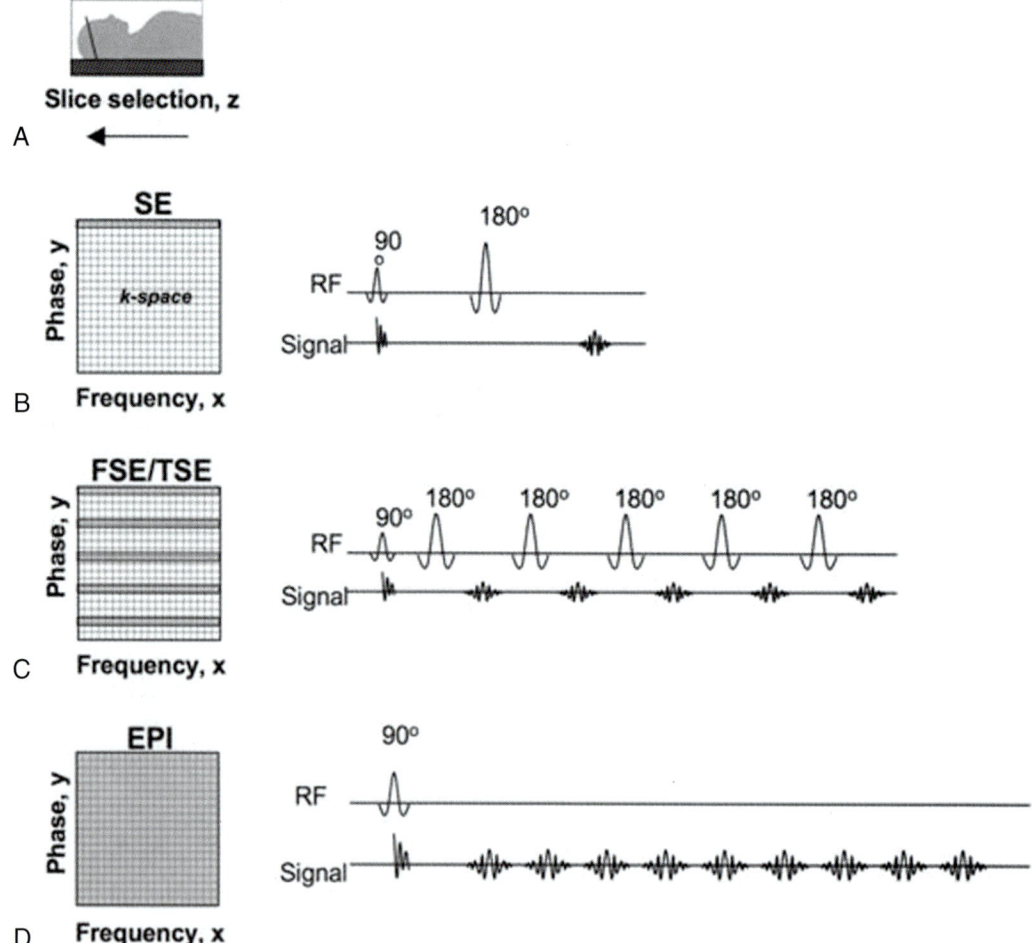

Figure 2-3 Comparison of single and multiple echo techniques, following a single excitatory pulse. **A:** An axial level in the brain is determined by the slice-selection gradient at the time of radiofrequency excitation. **B:** In conventional spin echo, a single 180-degree refocusing pulse after the excitatory pulse produces a spin echo that fills a single line of k-space (shaded in *gray*). The sequence must be repeated, with phase encoding performed at a different amplitude, to generate another spin echo that fills a different line of k-space. **C:** In fast or turbo spin echo, each excitatory pulse is followed by n number of 180-degree refocusing pulses (five in our case) that generate n echoes to fill n lines of k-space. The echo train length (ETL) is 5 and scan time is 1/5 (1/ETL) of the conventional spin-echo sequence. Phase encoding is performed at a different amplitude for each echo, to fill a different line of k-space. **D:** In single-shot echo planar imaging, the excitatory pulse is followed by rapid gradient switching that generates a long stream of gradient echoes enough to fill all of k-space after a single pulse.

will be readily seen as bright signal on T2-weighted sequences.

Artifacts Associated with MRI, Including False Positive/False Negative

Some of the common MR artifacts are discussed here. Artifacts associated with specific MR sequences are explained later in the chapter.

Wraparound/aliasing occurs when the body part imaged is larger than the FOV, causing "wraparound" of the data outside the FOV. This occurs along the phase-encoding direction(s) and can be eliminated by enlarging the FOV or by increasing the number of phase-encoding steps. Truncation or Gibbs ringing artifact occurs because of undersampling or truncation of high-frequency data. It appears as alternating light and dark bands at high–low signal tissue interfaces, characteristically at the brain–skull interface and in the spine on sagittal images, where it can simulate a syrinx. Truncation artifact can be reduced by decreasing interface contrast (e.g., by using fat suppression) or by increasing matrix size. Motion/ghost artifacts typically occur in the phase-encoding direction because time-consuming phase-encoding steps allow more time for motion to disrupt the MR signal and create artifact. Both patient and physiologic motion (e.g., CSF or blood pulsation) can cause artifact, which may appear as blurred areas or as "ghosts" (discrete lines or objects). Motion artifact can be reduced by using fast imaging techniques or applying presaturation pulses to minimize signal from moving or pulsating structures. If the artifact obscures a structure of interest, swapping the phase-encoding and frequency-encoding directions can redirect the artifact away from that specific structure.

Chemical shift artifact occurs in the frequency-encoding direction. Frequency encoding spatially localizes the MR signal on the basis of frequency, and differences in frequency are automatically equated to differences in signal origin. The magnetic field experienced by a proton is influenced by the precise chemical environment in which it resides. Electron clouds of adjacent chemical groups may partially "shield" a proton from the applied gradient field so that the proton experiences a slightly different magnetic field than its neighbor and responds by precessing at a slightly different frequency from its neighbor. The difference in precessional frequency caused by the different chemical environment is designated *chemical shift*. Within the same voxel, the protons in fat and water precess at slightly different Larmor frequencies (chemical shift) because they experience different magnetic fields due to differential shielding by their electron clouds. Bright and dark signal at the fat–water interface results from mismapping of fat and water protons in the same voxel during frequency encoding and is known as *chemical shift artifact*. Chemical shift artifact can be reduced by suppressing signal from fat, by switching frequency-encoding and phase-encoding directions to minimize disruption to a specific area, or by increasing the sampling bandwidth. Increasing the bandwidth increases the range of sampled frequencies and decreases the relative importance or conspicuity of the chemical shift difference. However, increasing the bandwidth will reduce the signal-to-noise ratio.

Susceptibility is a property of different materials that describes their interaction with a magnetic field. Certain materials, such as iron-containing hemorrhage or gadolinium-based contrast, weakly increase the local magnetic field and are known as *paramagnetic*. Superparamagnetic or ferromagnetic materials such as iron and various metal alloys more strongly increase and distort the local magnetic field, causing signal dropout and a warped appearance of nearby tissues. GRE sequences are more prone to susceptibility artifact because they do not use a 180-degree refocusing pulse and signal dephases rapidly due to field inhomogeneities. Susceptibility artifact can be decreased by using SE rather than GRE technique (especially FSE or TSE with long ETLs), by using short TE (decreasing the time for dephasing to occur), and by increasing the sampling bandwidth (faster acquisition, decreasing the time for dephasing to occur). Alternatively, susceptibility artifact may be used to advantage to identify very small and otherwise easily overlooked foci of hemorrhage, such as those found with trauma, amyloid angiopathy, and cavernous malformations. These effects form the basis of susceptibility imaging and are especially prominent at higher field strengths.

Figure 2-4 illustrates several commonly encountered artifacts.

SPECIFIC USES FOR THE TECHNIQUE

MR is the workhorse of neuroimaging for the adult brain. It can be used to evaluate intracranial tumors, infection or inflammation, demyelinating processes, degenerative disease, ischemic injury, and developmental anomalies. Very small anatomic structures, such as the sella turcica and cranial nerves, can be depicted more precisely with MR than CT. The following section highlights specific uses of common MR techniques for clinical neuroimaging.

SYSTEMS FOR ANALYZING IMAGES USING MRI

Illustrated Approach

1. Spin Echo and Fast/Turbo Spin Echo
SE has traditionally been considered the mainstay of neuroimaging. T2-weighted SE or FSE/TSE highlights pathologic processes because of its sensitivity to fluid and changes in tissue cellularity and often is superior to CT in depicting pathologic lesions (Figure 2-5). Appearance on T1 imaging can be helpful for identifying substances such as fat, melanin, and proteinaceous material because they all appear bright on T1. Hemorrhage has variable appearance on T1-weighted and T2-weighted images depending on the age of the hematoma.

Gadolinium-based contrast material can be administered intravenously to highlight pathology. Gadolinium is a paramagnetic metal that, by itself, is toxic to the human body, so it must be tightly chelated to another substance such as diethylenetriamine-pentaacetic acid (DTPA) before it is used. Gadolinium shortens T1 relaxation times, causing increased signal on T1-weighted images wherever the blood–brain barrier has been breached and contrast material is able to enter (e.g., in tumor).

2. Gradient Echo
The lack of a 180-degree refocusing pulse and the specific vulnerability to $T2^*$ decay can be exploited to detect intracranial hemorrhage. Paramagnetic blood products create local magnetic field inhomogeneities, cause adjacent spinning nuclei to dephase, and induce a striking, characteristic signal loss on GRE sequences (Figure 2-6). In contrast, blood can be more difficult to detect on SE sequences, which are less sensitive to susceptibility effects due to the 180-degree refocusing pulse. FSE and TSE sequences are even less sensitive to hemorrhage than SE because they use multiple refocusing pulses. GRE MRI, especially at high magnetic field strength such as 3 T, is even superior to CT for detecting microhemorrhages (e.g., due to traumatic brain injury) (Figure 2-7). This is because susceptibility effects increase dramatically with field strength, rendering high-field $T2^*$-weighted GRE very sensitive to small amounts of blood breakdown products.

The faster imaging time of GRE is particularly useful in scanning uncooperative patients or in 3D imaging, which requires longer scan times than 2D imaging. In particular, 3D spoiled GRE sequences are T1 weighted and provide excellent anatomic detail. Three-dimensional GRE T1-weighted sequences are useful for evaluating subtle cortical abnormalities in seizure patients or for characterizing tumor extension in conjunction with gadolinium-based contrast.

3. Fluid-Attenuated Inversion Recovery
FLAIR is typically a T2-weighted FSE/TSE sequence that uses an inversion pulse to eliminate the signal from CSF. It is useful for highlighting lesions that lie close to ventricles or sulci and are not as conspicuous on

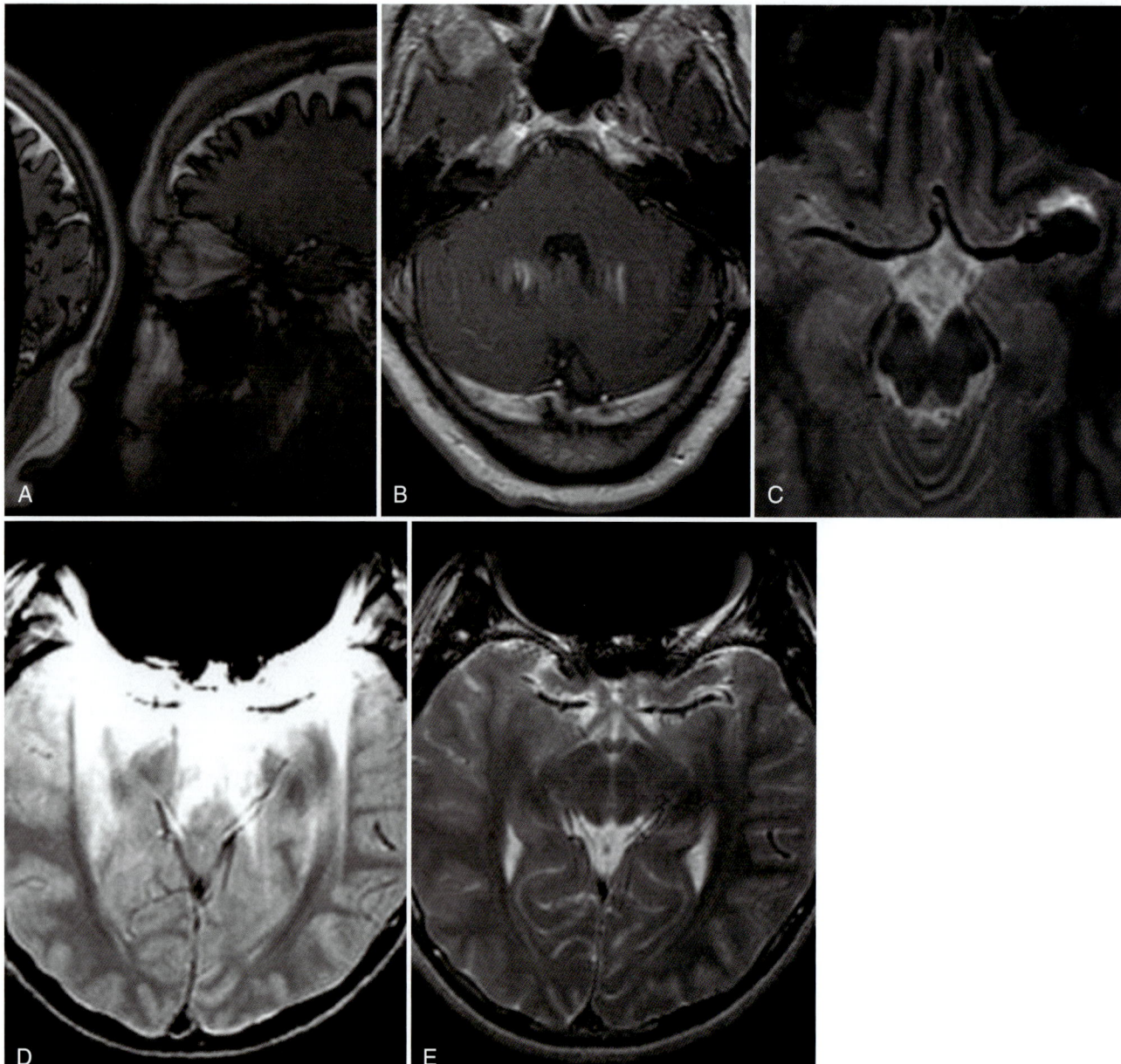

Figure 2-4 Magnetic resonance artifacts. **A:** Wraparound or aliasing caused by small field of view. **B:** Typical location of pulsation artifact from the dural venous sinuses in the phase-encoding direction (left/right). **C:** Lipoma in the left sylvian fissure causes chemical shift artifact in the frequency-encoding direction (anterior/posterior). **D:** Susceptibility from patient's dental braces causes marked signal loss and distortion on this conventional spin-echo sequence. **E:** Fast/turbo spin-echo sequence in the same patient as in D shows dramatic reduction of artifact. The multiple 180-degree refocusing pulses used for fast/turbo spin echo make it less vulnerable to magnetic field inhomogeneities than conventional spin echo.

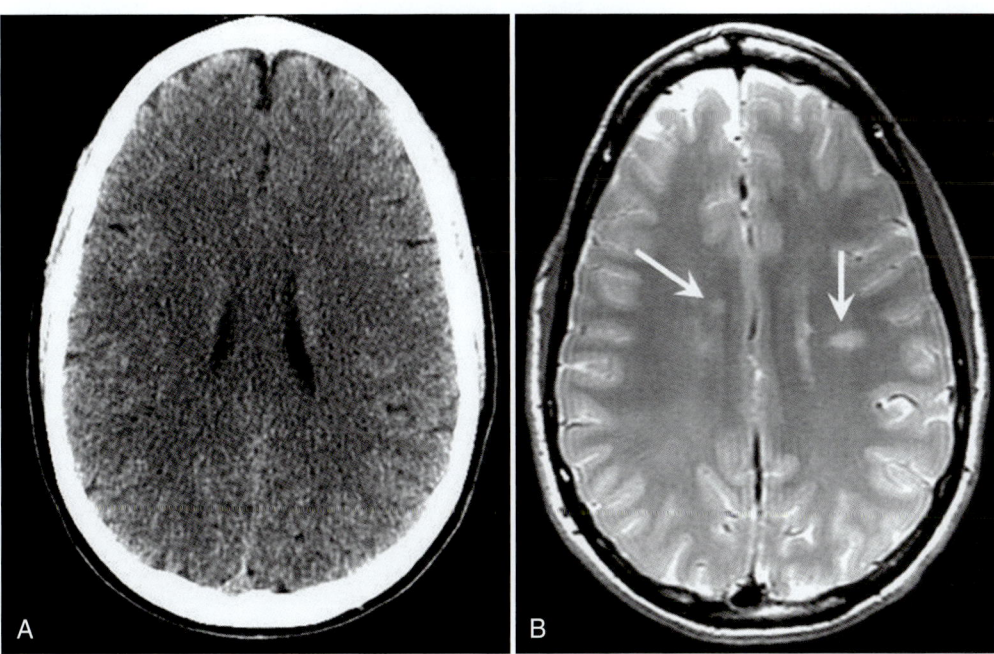

Figure 2-5 T2-weighted magnetic resonance imaging is superior to computed tomography (CT) for detection of primary demyelinating diseases, such as multiple sclerosis. **A:** Axial slice from a normal head CT in a 30-year-old woman with multiple sclerosis. **B:** Axial slice at approximately the same level as the CT image from a two-dimensional T2-weighted fast spin-echo sequence shows hyperintense periventricular and subcortical white matter lesions *(arrows)* in a characteristic distribution for multiple sclerosis. The ovoid shape and orientation orthogonal to the margin of the lateral ventricle displayed by the largest lesion in the left hemisphere are also characteristic of demyelinating plaques.

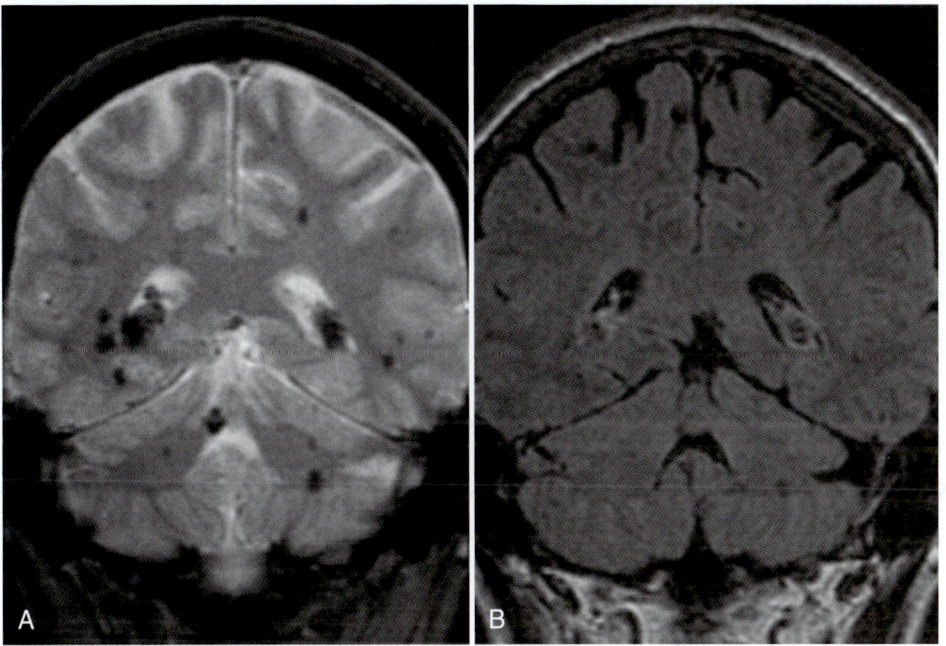

Figure 2-6 Detecting hemorrhage with gradient-recalled echo (GRE) sequences. **A:** Coronal refocused or coherent GRE (T2*-weighted) image shows numerous foci of susceptibility in a patient with familial multiple cavernous malformations. **B:** These lesions are much more difficult to appreciate on coronal fluid-attenuated inversion recovery, which is typically performed on a fast/turbo spin-echo sequence and is less sensitive to hemorrhage because of multiple refocusing pulses.

T2-weighted sequences (e.g., plaques of multiple sclerosis or small infarcts abutting the cortex). Suppression of CSF signal allows for distinction between epidermoid cysts (bright) and arachnoid cysts (dark). Because FLAIR sequences normally suppress the signal of CSF within the sulci, failure of suppression of sulcal signal on FLAIR sequences suggests leptomeningeal disease with replacement of normal CSF by blood (subarachnoid hemorrhage), pus (meningitis), or tumor (leptomeningeal carcinomatosis). Because supplemental oxygen,

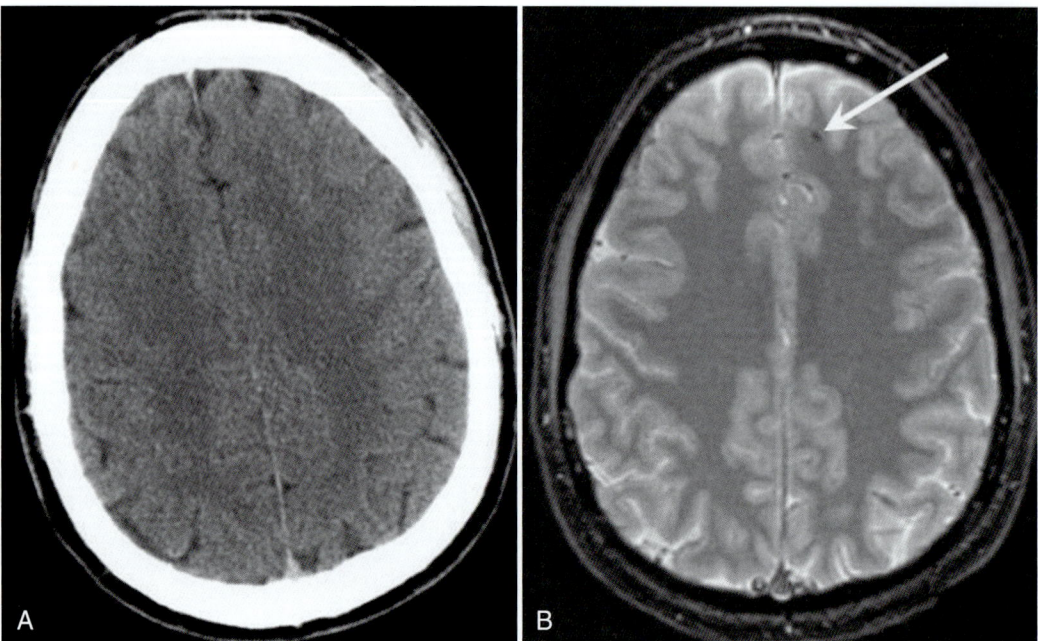

Figure 2-7 Magnetic resonance imaging with gradient-recalled echo (GRE) sequences is superior to computed tomography (CT) for detection of traumatic microhemorrhage due to axonal shearing injury. **A:** Axial slice from a normal head CT in a patient who presented with head trauma. **B:** Axial slice at the same level as the CT image from a two-dimensional T2*-weighted GRE sequence acquired at 3 T shows a microhemorrhage in the subcortical white matter of the left superior frontal gyrus (arrow), indicating traumatic axonal injury.

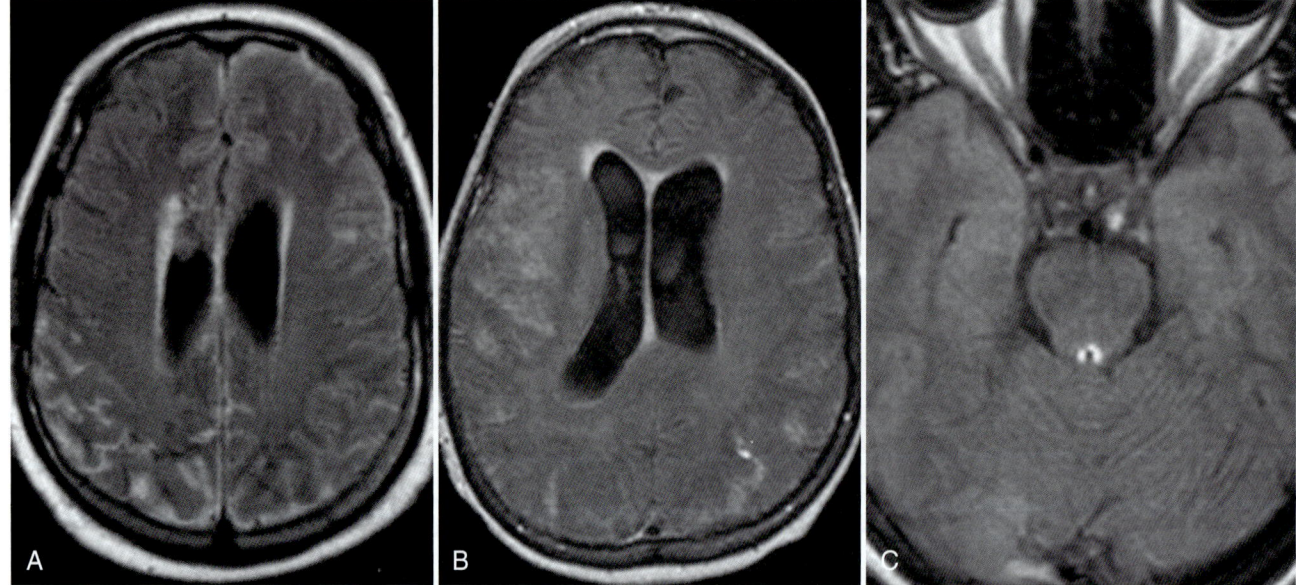

Figure 2-8 Uses and artifacts of fluid-attenuated inversion recovery (FLAIR). **A:** Axial FLAIR image in a patient with tuberculous meningitis shows high T2 signal within the subarachnoid space, particularly in the right parietal lobe, consistent with pus. **B:** Similar high T2 signal within the subarachnoid space is observed on axial FLAIR in a patient requiring general anesthesia for sedation, consistent with high-flow oxygen artifact. This high FLAIR signal in the subarachnoid space will disappear within minutes after cessation of oxygen supplementation. **C:** High T2 signal around the cerebral aqueduct is typical of FLAIR artifact caused by incomplete cerebrospinal suppression.

especially at high concentrations, can artifactually create bright signal within the cisterns and sulci by reducing the T1 relaxation time of CSF, no diagnosis of cisternal abnormality on FLAIR images should be made before determining whether the patient was receiving oxygen during the MR scan.

FLAIR imaging is also limited in evaluation of the posterior fossa because of CSF flow artifacts in the basilar cisterns and third/fourth ventricles. Unsuppressed CSF can flow very rapidly into these narrow areas, after the 180-degree inversion pulse but before signal sampling, creating bright FLAIR signal. Three-dimensional FLAIR is not as susceptible to CSF flow artifact as 2D FLAIR because the inversion pulse is applied to the entire volume imaged and not just a single slice. Figure 2-8 illustrates some important features of FLAIR.

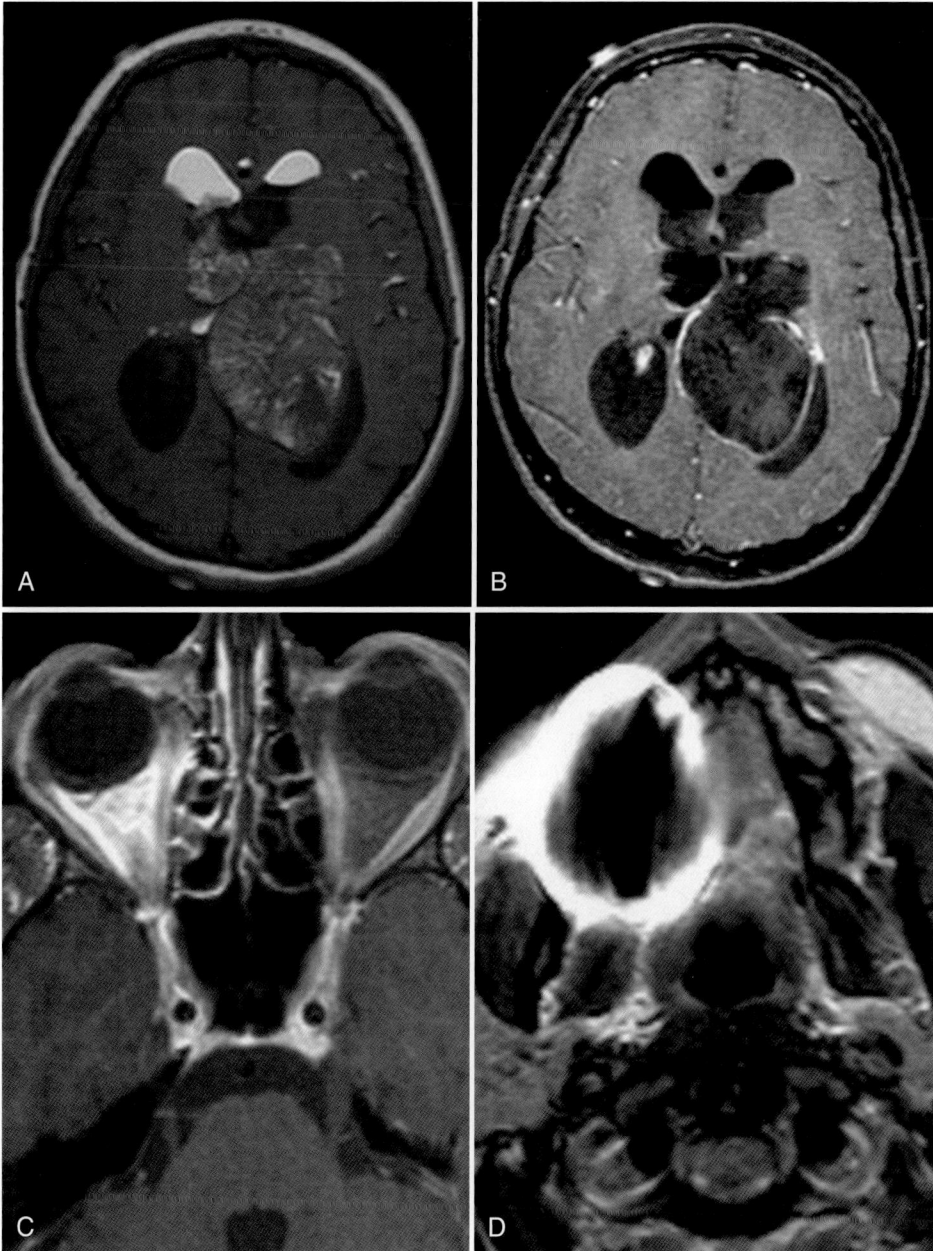

Figure 2-9 Uses and pitfalls of fat saturation. **A:** Axial unenhanced T1-weighted image demonstrates a large lesion mostly in the region of the left lateral ventricle, with high signal layering nondependently in the frontal horns of both lateral ventricles as well as within the sulci bilaterally. The intrinsic T1 shortening is suspicious for fat-containing dermoid with rupture into the ventricular system and subarachnoid space. **B:** Loss of signal within the lesion, ventricles, and sulci following fat saturation confirms this diagnosis. **C:** Axial T1-weighted postgadolinium image with fat saturation demonstrates abnormal high signal within the right retrobulbar fat, concerning for enhancement. **D:** Inspection of more caudal images shows extensive susceptibility from dental hardware. This creates magnetic field inhomogeneities, leading to failure of fat saturation in the right orbit, which should not be mistaken for enhancement.

4. Fat Saturation

Frequency-selective fat saturation (FS) is an alternative technique to STIR for eliminating signal from fat. FS exploits the chemical shift between protons in fat and those in water to reduce or remove the signal from the fat. In FS, a 90-degree saturation pulse specifically tuned to the Larmor frequency of fat is given to flip only the magnetization of fat into the transverse plane. This signal is then eliminated by a spoiler gradient. FS is clinically useful for diagnosing lipomas or dermoid cysts. Good FS requires that the main magnetic field be exactly uniform throughout. Field inconsistencies can make fat or water protons precess at slightly different frequencies from their Larmor frequency, making the saturation pulse less effective (Figure 2-9). Field inhomogeneities are especially pronounced along the periphery of the patient (farther from the isocenter of the magnet) and at air–tissue and bone–tissue interfaces, including the skull base and sinuses.

5. Diffusion-Weighted Imaging

DWI is a way to display the molecular motion or diffusion of water protons within tissue. To achieve diffusion weighting, paired diffusion gradients of equal magnitude are added to a spin-echo (T2-weighted) echo

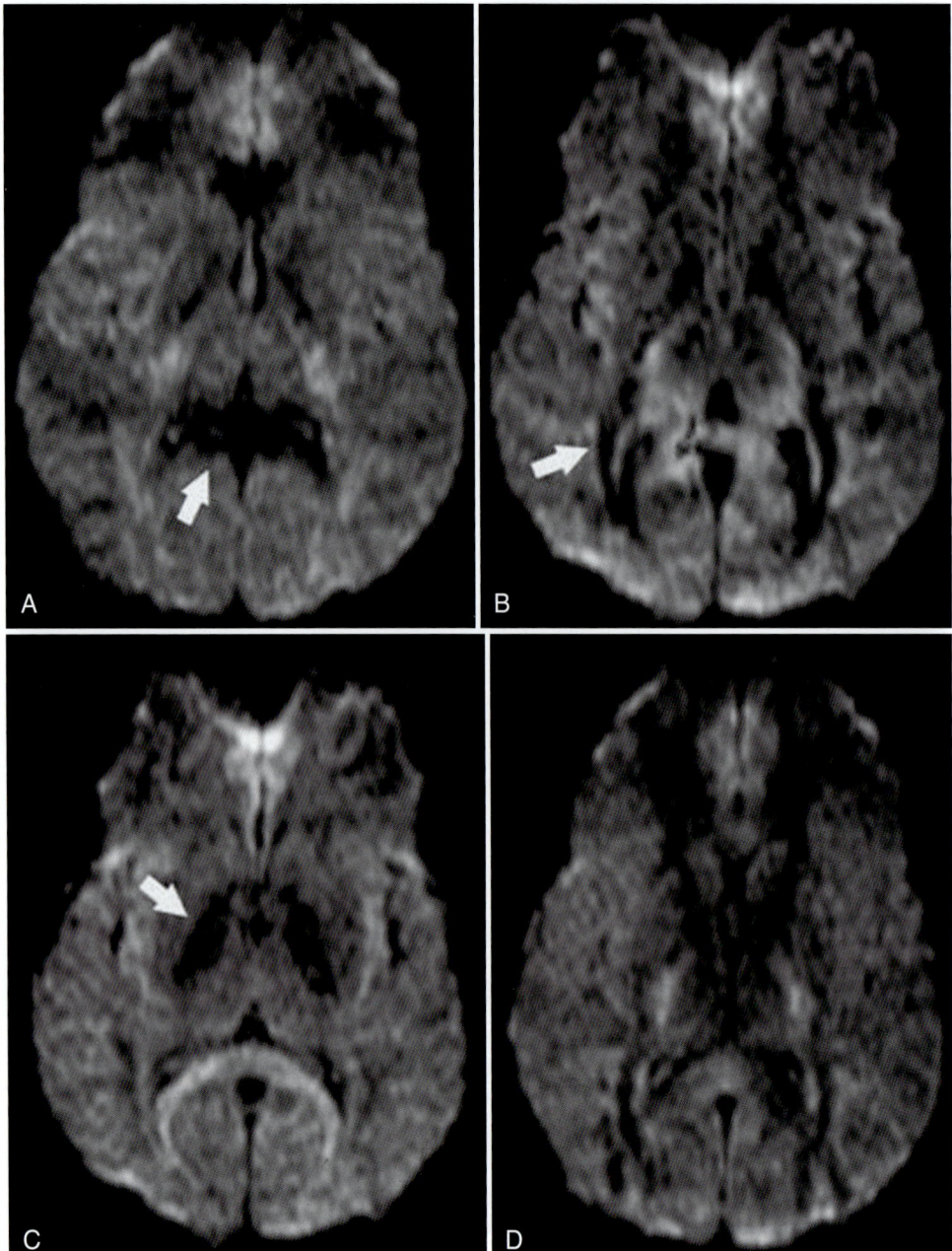

Figure 2-10 The anisotropic nature of diffusion requires that diffusion be assessed in multiple directions (A–C), then the images combined to yield an isotropic map (D). Signal loss is appreciated when diffusion occurs along the direction of the gradient. Diffusion gradients were applied along the transverse (A–x), anterior/posterior (B–y), and craniocaudad (C–z) directions, as diffusion occurs along fibers of the splenium of the corpus callosum (A–x), frontoparietal white matter (B–y), and corticospinal tract (C–z).

planar sequence. The first diffusion gradient is applied before the refocusing pulse, and the second gradient is applied after the refocusing pulse. If there is motion of water protons (diffusion is not restricted), the diffusion gradients cause dynamic dephasing of the moving nuclei that cannot be rephased, resulting in loss of MR signal that is proportional to the rate of water motion. This phenomenon is distinct from the static dephasing that can be rephased by the 180-degree refocusing pulse.

In the brain, especially the white matter, diffusion of water varies in all directions (anisotropic) rather than occurring to the same degree in all directions (isotropic) because diffusion occurs more easily parallel rather than perpendicular to axon bundles. Because of anisotropy, diffusion is measured in multiple different orientations (e.g., x, y, and z gradient directions), and the results are combined into one "isotropic" image (Figure 2-10).

MR signal intensity on DWI depends in part on the strength of the diffusion weighting (i.e., b value). When $b = 0$ s/mm^2, there is no diffusion weighting, so the image displays only the effects of T2 weighting. As b is raised to 1,000 s/mm^2, diffusion weighting increases, and signal from CSF (which has unrestricted diffusion) decreases. However, T2 weighting does not disappear entirely, even at high b values, so the T2 signal may still appear within the image (T2 shine-through artifact) and

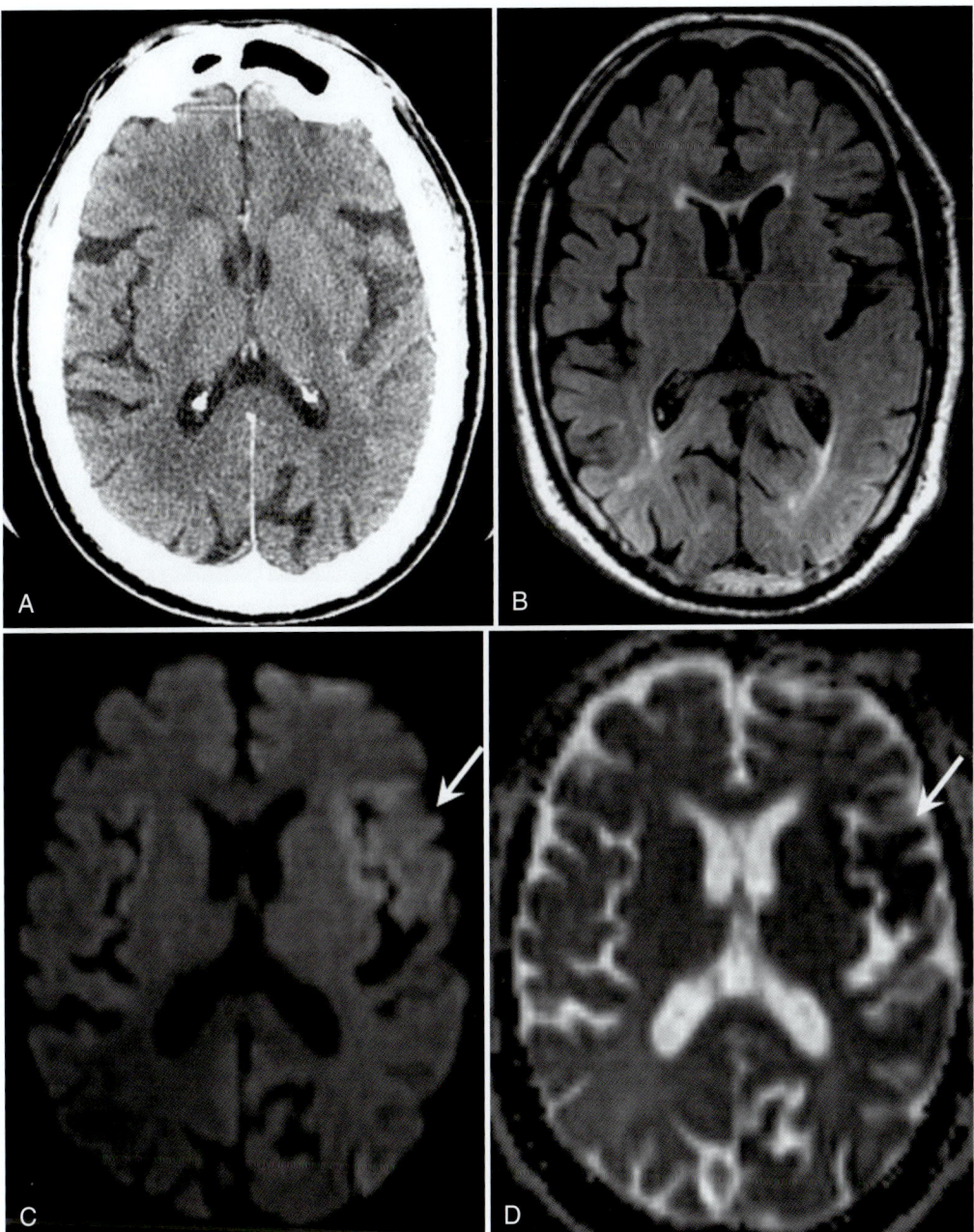

Figure 2-11 Diffusion-weighted imaging is more sensitive than noncontrast computed tomography (CT) or other magnetic resonance (MR) imaging modalities for hyperacute ischemic stroke. **A:** Axial CT performed 30 minutes after the patient experienced ischemic symptoms during a coronary angiogram shows no definite abnormality. **B:** Axial T2-weighted fluid-attenuated inversion recovery image from an MR scan initiated 15 minutes after the CT shows no acute abnormality. **C:** Axial diffusion-weighted imaging from the same MR scan reveals abnormal cortical hyperintensity in the anterior left perisylvian region (*arrow*). **D:** Corresponding apparent diffusion coefficient map confirms reduced diffusion in the anterior left perisylvian cortex, consistent with a hyperacute left middle cerebral artery infarct (*arrow*).

make it difficult to determine whether the bright signal seen on DWI represents restricted diffusion, T2 prolongation (T2 shine-through), or both in some proportion.

This difficulty is resolved by use of an apparent diffusion coefficient (ADC) map, which the computer derives mathematically by comparing the diffusion-weighted images obtained at two different b values (e.g., $b = 0$ s/mm^2 and $b = 1,000$ s/mm^2). ADC is a measure of the rate of diffusion, and the ADC map is a "pure diffusion map" free of T2 shine-through effects. On the ADC map, pixel intensity corresponds directly to the ADC value itself, so areas with high ADC (rapid diffusion), such as CSF, will be bright, whereas areas with low ADC (slow diffusion) will be dark. Note that the signal intensities displayed on an ADC map are the inverse of what is seen on a diffusion-weighted image: areas of restricted diffusion will appear bright on DWI but dark on the ADC map.

Acute cerebral infarction is the most commonly encountered pathologic process to reduce diffusion (bright on DWI and dark on ADC), with MR findings seen as early as 30 minutes after ischemia onset, when it is not detectable by CT or by other types of MR sequences (Figure 2-11). Because the high DWI signal decreases over the course of days to weeks, diffusion imaging is

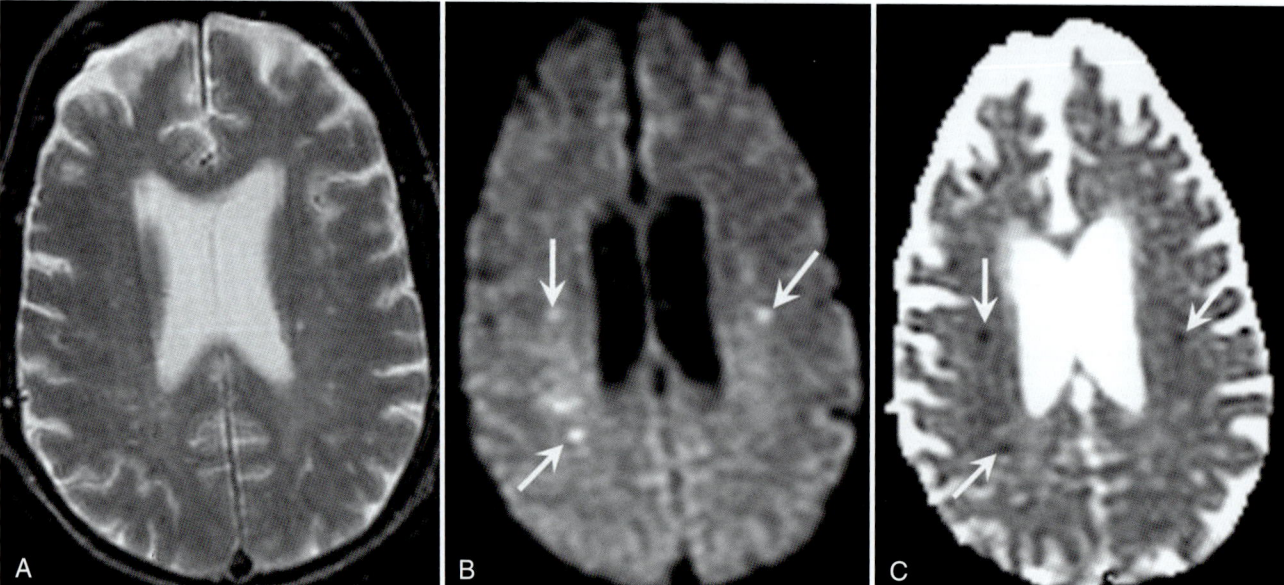

Figure 2-12 Diffusion-weighted imaging can differentiate acute from chronic ischemia. **A:** Axial T2-weighted spin-echo image in a patient with endocarditis and new neurologic deficits shows numerous periventricular and subcortical white matter lesions of indeterminate acuity. **B:** Axial diffusion-weighted imaging demonstrates hyperintensity in several of the subcortical lesions *(arrows)*. **C:** Corresponding apparent diffusion coefficient map confirms reduced diffusion in these lesions *(arrows)*, consistent with acute embolic infarcts and not T2 shine-through on the diffusion-weighted imaging from subacute or chronic ischemia.

also very helpful in distinguishing acute from chronic ischemia (Figure 2-12). Reduced diffusion can also be seen in pyogenic abscesses, epidermoid masses, herpes encephalitis, Creutzfeldt-Jakob disease, and tumors with high cellular density (e.g., lymphoma). Limitations of DWI include susceptibility to field inhomogeneities, particularly at tissue–air interfaces of the skull base, adjacent to postsurgical metallic hardware, and at large collections of blood breakdown products (Figure 2-13), leading to signal dropout and image distortion.

An interesting application of DWI is diffusion tensor imaging (DTI), which assesses diffusion in at least six different directions. This yields a more complete set of diffusivity information that can be used to deduce axonal fiber orientation and thereby create 3D maps of white matter tracts in the brain.

6. Time-of-Flight MR Angiography

To visualize the intracranial vasculature, time-of-flight (TOF) imaging is most commonly used. TOF imaging provides an "MR angiogram" (MRA) of the circle of Willis by (1) minimizing signal from stationary background tissues and (2) maximizing signal from flowing blood.

GRE sequences with a rapid succession of RF pulses and very short TR are used. If the TR is shorter than the T1 of background tissue, the rapid RF pulses prevent the tissue spins from regaining their normal full longitudinal magnetization. Because longitudinal magnetization is reduced to a minimum, the next RF pulse produces less transverse magnetization, and the background tissue appears dark. In this state, the background tissue is described as saturated. Blood situated outside the imaging slice, however, is relatively unaffected by the successive RF pulses, retains its longitudinal magnetization, and remains unsaturated. When the unsaturated spins of the blood flow into the imaging plane with intact longitudinal magnetization, they generate a bright MR signal known as *flow-related enhancement*.

TOF MRA can be performed by both 2D and 3D techniques. Two-dimensional TOF MRA has higher sensitivity to slow blood flow than does 3D because 2D TOF imaging excites individual thin slices whereas 3D excites entire slabs of tissue simultaneously. Because blood must travel a longer distance through a thicker slab with 3D imaging than with 2D imaging, the blood experiences some saturation effects from successive RF pulses and loses some signal. The signal loss is particularly pronounced for 3D imaging of slowly moving blood. For that reason, 3D TOF MRA may fail to display vessels with slow flow. However, 3D TOF MRA achieves thinner, contiguous imaging sections and much higher spatial resolution than does 2D TOF. Three-dimensional TOF is also less prone to signal loss from turbulent blood flow within an area of stenosis, so 3D TOF MRA is less likely to overestimate the severity of a stenosis. Cervical MRA for the carotid and vertebral arteries in the neck is typically performed with 2D TOF because 2D TOF is more sensitive for detecting slow flow within an area of stenosis. Intracranial MRA of the circle of Willis is typically performed with 3D TOF imaging because 3D TOF MRA provides better spatial resolution and depiction of small distal cerebral arteries (Figure 2-14, *A*).

7. Contrast-Enhanced MRA

Contrast-enhanced MRA is often used for evaluation of cervical vessels (Figure 2-14, *B* and *C*). A large coronal FOV can be used to image the vessels from their origins at the aorta to their vascular territories within the brain in a fraction of the time required for conventional axial plane TOF MRA. Contrast-enhanced MRA also suffers less signal loss secondary to slow or turbulent flow.

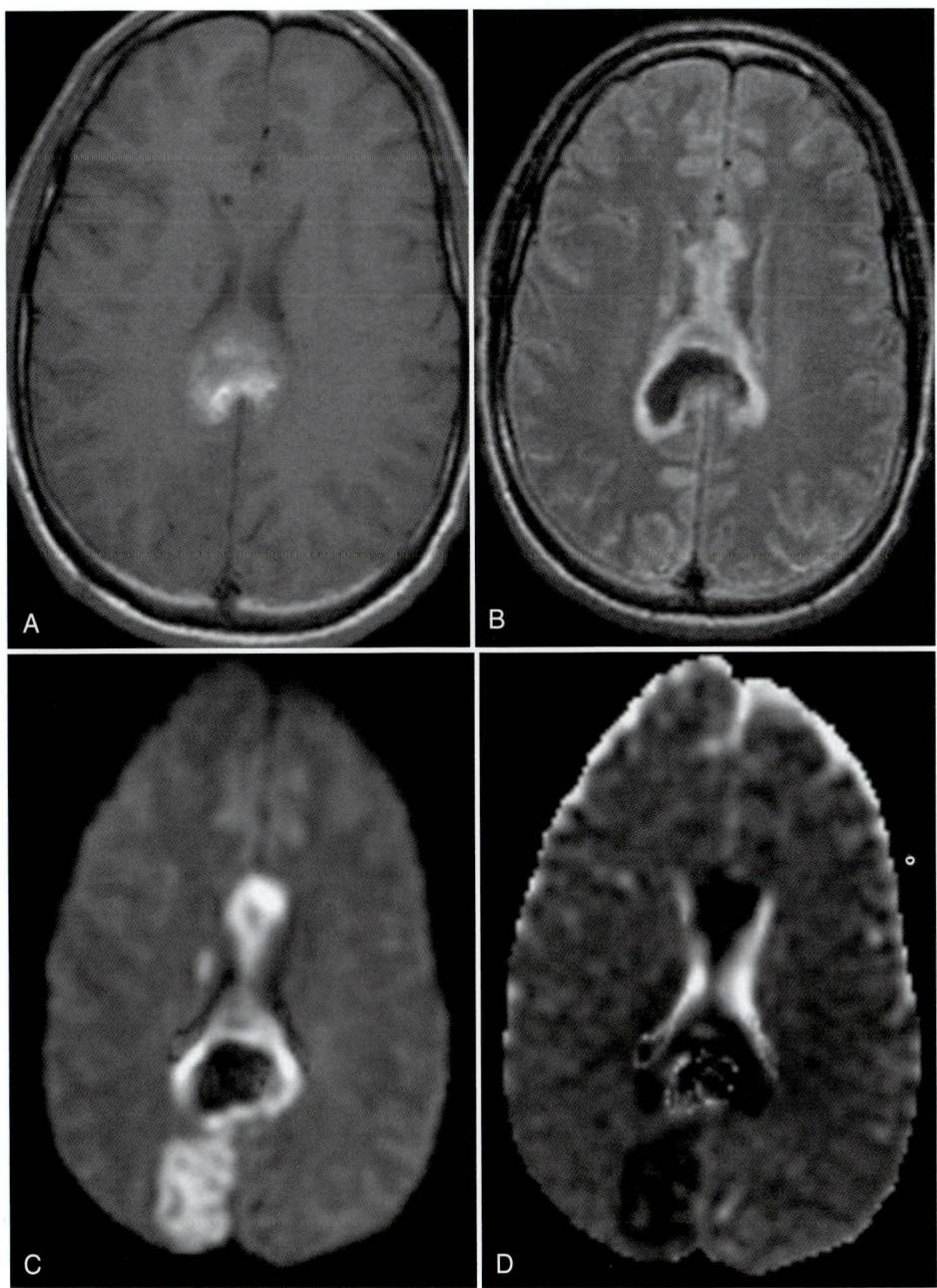

Figure 2-13 A: Axial T1-weighted spin echo shows hyperintensity in the splenium of the corpus callosum, compatible with hemorrhage. **B:** Axial fluid-attenuated inversion recovery shows signal loss within the hemorrhage as well as bright signal in the sulci posteriorly suspicious for subarachnoid hemorrhage. Increased signal is seen in the caudate body and along the body of the corpus callosum, with subtly increased signal in the right posteromedial parietal and occipital lobes. **C:** Axial diffusion-weighted imaging more dramatically demonstrates high signal in the right posterior parietal lobe, caudate body, and corpus callosum. This may reflects reduced diffusion due to acute infarction. Diffusion-weighted imaging is prone to susceptibility effects, seen as signal loss within the hemorrhage. **D:** Apparent diffusion coefficient map shows reduced diffusion in the right posterior cerebral artery territory and corpus callosum, consistent with acute infarction.

■ PITFALLS AND LIMITATIONS OF MRI

Use of MRI is limited in several important situations. The magnetic field can induce voltages or currents in electrically conductive materials (wires, leads, implants), which may result in heating. Patients with medical implants or devices made of ferromagnetic materials (e.g., certain aneurysm clips) may be at risk for object displacement or heating. MR should not be performed unless the specific type of implant or device is documented to be MR compatible. Information regarding MR compatibility and safety testing of thousands of specific objects can be found online at www.MRIsafety.com. Cardiac pacemakers and defibrillators are considered a contraindication to MR. Patients with these implanted devices should be studied by MR only after specific evaluation of risks and benefits and after consideration of alternative means for obtaining the data needed for care. Such studies should

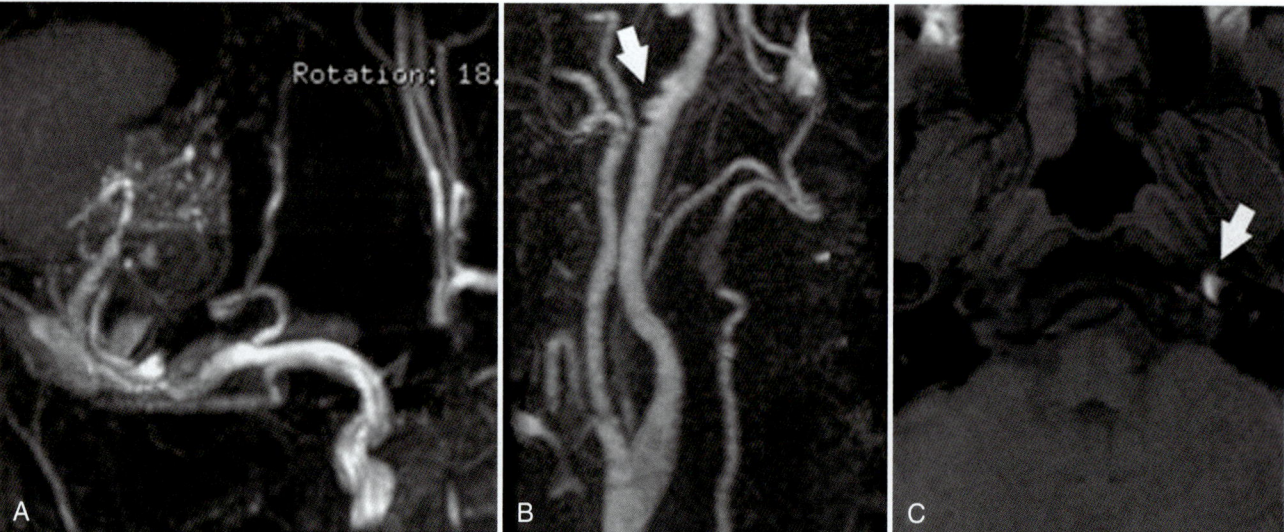

Figure 2-14 Intracranial and cervical magnetic resonance angiography (MRA). **A:** Three-dimensional time-of-flight MRA of the circle of Willis shows a tangle of vessels with enlarged right middle cerebral and lenticulostriate artery branches, consistent with arteriovenous malformation and hemorrhage. **B:** Gadolinium-enhanced cervical MRA shows focal lobular irregularity *(arrow)* of the left internal carotid artery (cervico–petrous junction), concerning for injury such as dissection with pseudoaneurysm. **C:** Given the concern for dissection, axial unenhanced T1-weighted fat-saturated sequence was obtained, which shows crescentic high signal in the left internal carotid artery *(arrow)* consistent with methemoglobin in an intramural hematoma due to acute arterial dissection.

be performed on a case-by-base basis and only if sufficient radiology and cardiology expertise is available.

MR can be performed at any stage of pregnancy, following thoughtful consideration of risks and benefits by appropriate attending radiologists, obstetricians, and perinatologists. Gadolinium-based contrast agents may be administered on a case-by-case basis but should not be given routinely during pregnancy because their risks to the fetus are not known. (Because gadolinium-based contrast agents can enter the amniotic fluid, there is theoretical potential for dissociation of the toxic gadolinium from its chelating compound and concern for theoretical risk of fetal injury.) Again, any decision to administer gadolinium-based contrast should be preceded by careful analysis of the risks and benefits by the team of attending physicians.

Much has been recently written about nephrogenic systemic fibrosis and its association with gadolinium-based contrast agents in patients with severe renal disease. Nephrogenic systemic fibrosis refers to tissue fibrosis with skin thickening and hardening as well as fibrosis of other body parts, including the heart, lung, and skeletal muscles. It occurs following gadolinium-based contrast administration in approximately 3% to 5% of patients with severe renal disease. Although most published cases have been reported in patients who received gadodiamide (Omniscan, GE Healthcare), nephrogenic systemic fibrosis has been associated with other gadolinium chelates, such as gadopentetate dimeglumine (Magnevist, Bayer Schering) and gadoversetamide (OptiMARK, Mallinckrodt). The most recent 2007 MR safety guidelines released by the American College of Radiology recommend that patients with chronic renal disease and glomerular filtration rates (GFR) less than 60 ml/min/1.73 m^2 not receive gadolinium-based contrast unless the benefits of contrast clearly exceed the risks. In those cases, the lowest possible dose necessary should be used, and hemodialysis should be performed immediately following the scan (if the patient is already on dialysis). Patients with GFR greater than 60 ml/min/1.73 m^2 need no special treatment, although gadodiamide should not be given in patients with any level of renal disease.

■ CURRENT RESEARCH AND FUTURE DIRECTION

MRI at 1.5 T is the current clinical standard, although there has been an increasing shift to 3-T imaging for clinical use in the past few years. Systems at field strengths of 7 T and higher are now under investigation but currently used only for research. The primary appeal of 3-T over 1.5-T imaging is its better signal-to-noise ratio. Field strength and MR signal are linearly related, with twice the MR signal at 3 T than at 1.5 T for the same scan time. Figure 2-15 illustrates the utility of imaging at higher field strength.

Higher field strengths prolong T1 recovery times but leave T2 relatively unaffected. This allows for higher-quality TOF MRA images at 3 T compared to 1.5 T because the background is better suppressed at 3 T (less recovery of longitudinal magnetization), whereas inflowing, unsaturated blood has higher signal at 3 T (double the signal of 1.5 T). Longer T1 recovery times do result in poor tissue contrast between gray and white matter on T1-weighted SE or FSE/TSE sequences performed at 3 T if the same TR is used, but this can be avoided by using inversion-prepared sequences for T1 weighting. Higher field strengths also have greater chemical shift effects, allowing for more effective fat suppression but suffering from more chemical shift artifacts if a greater bandwidth is not used. Susceptibility effects increase with field strength, so sequence parameters must be optimized to decrease artifact.

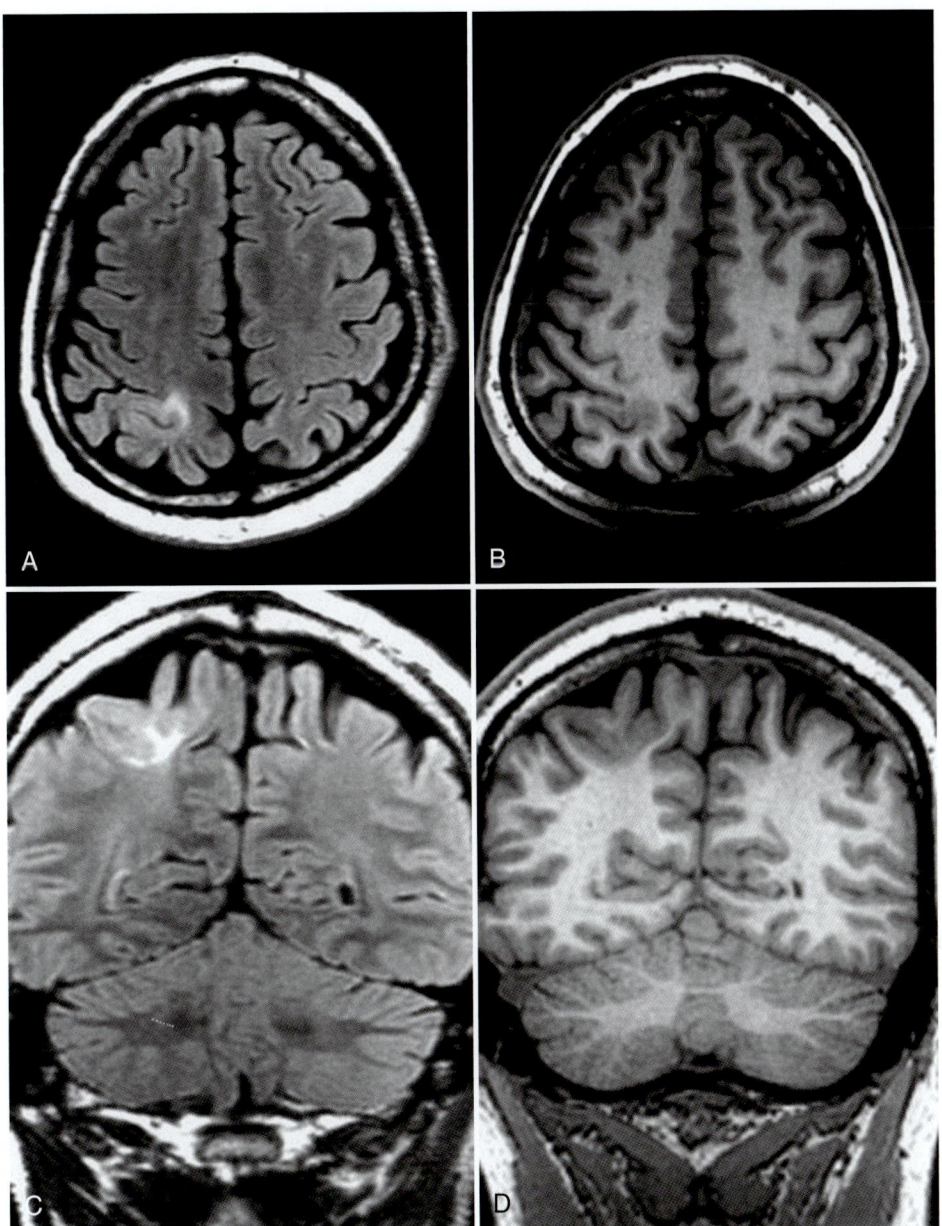

Figure 2-15 Imaging at 3 T. A 29-year-old man with epilepsy reported to have "abnormal fluid-attenuated inversion recovery (FLAIR) signal in the right parietal lobe" on prior outside magnetic resonance imaging presented for further workup. Imaging at 3 T demonstrates T2 prolongation in the right parietal lobe on axial (**A**) and coronal (**C**) FLAIR. T1-weighted spoiled gradient recalled-echo (GRE) sequences, axial (**B**) and coronal (**D**) planes, show that the abnormal T2 signal corresponds to a focal area of cortical thickening and blurring. This is suggestive of a cortical dysplasia that, although subtle, can be better delineated at 3 T due to its superior signal-to-noise ratio. The FLAIR and spoiled GRE sequences were three-dimensional acquisitions to ensure thin, contiguous slices for detection of subtle abnormalities in this seizure patient.

One of the chief concerns with high-field imaging is the greater *specific absorption rate* (SAR), which is the energy absorbed by tissue following an RF pulse, potentially leading to tissue heating. SAR quadruples when field strength is doubled from 3 to 1.5 T. SAR also increases with greater flip angles and more RF pulses during a given TR, so SAR is particularly high for FSE/TSE sequences where multiple 180-degree pulses are given. Modifications to limit SAR include decreasing the flip angle or refocusing pulse (although this also decreases MR signal). The synergistic and tandem development of parallel imaging techniques, which reduce scan time and limit energy exposure, has greatly facilitated imaging at 3 T.

In parallel imaging, k-space is undersampled by decreasing the number of phase-encoding steps. This reduces scan time. However, the resultant loss of spatial information is recovered by taking advantage of the redundant spatial information provided by the phased-array coils used for parallel imaging. Because signal strength varies according to distance from the receiver coil, spatial information afforded by differences in signal strength at the receiver coil can be used to complete the dataset for the MR image. Undersampling k-space reduces FOV, which produces severe aliasing in the MR image. However, mathematical models have been developed to correct for aliasing and produce a proper image;

the two most commonly used techniques are sensitivity encoding (SENSE) and variants of the original simultaneous acquisition of spatial harmonics (SMASH) parallel imaging technique, such as generalized autocalibrating partially parallel acquisitions (GRAPPA).

With these techniques and with newer developments (e.g., compressed sensing) that will enable even faster scanning, MR should remain the primary tool for neuroimaging for the foreseeable future.

Suggested Readings

Brant-Zawadzki M, Atkinson D, Detrick M, Bradley WG, Scidmore G. Fluid-attenuated inversion recovery (FLAIR) for assessment of cerebral infarction. Initial clinical experience in 50 patients. *Stroke.* 1996;27(7):1187-1191.

De Coene B, Hajnal JV, Gatehouse P, et al. MR of the brain using fluid-attenuated inversion recovery (FLAIR) pulse sequences. *AJNR Am J Neuroradiol.* 1992;13(6):1555-1564.

Feinberg DA, Hale JD, Watts JC, Kaufman L, Mark A. Halving MR imaging time by conjugation: demonstration at 3.5 kG. *Radiology.* 1986;161(2):527-531.

Hashemi RH, Bradley Jr WG, Chen DY, et al. Suspected multiple sclerosis: MR imaging with a thin-section fast FLAIR pulse sequence. *Radiology.* 1995;196(2):505-510.

Kanal E, Barkovich AJ, Bell C, et al. ACR guidance document for safe MR practices: 2007. *AJR Am J Roentgenol.* 2007;188(6):1447-1474.

Kuo PH, Kanal E, Abu-Alfa AK, Cowper SE. Gadolinium-based MR contrast agents and nephrogenic systemic fibrosis. *Radiology.* 2007;242(3):647-649.

Le Bihan D, Breton E, Lallemand D, Grenier P, Cabanis E, Laval-Jeantet M. MR imaging of intravoxel incoherent motions: application to diffusion and perfusion in neurologic disorders. *Radiology.* 1986;161(2):401-407.

Lee H, Wintermark M, Gean AD, Ghajar J, Manley GT, Mukherjee P. Focal lesions in acute mild traumatic brain injury and neurocognitive outcome: CT versus 3T MRI. *J Neurotrauma.* 2008;25(9):1049-1056.

Lustig M, Donoho D, Pauly JM. Sparse MRI: The application of compressed sensing for rapid MR imaging. *Magn Reson Med.* 2007;58(6):1182-1195.

Mukherjee P, Berman JI, Chung SW, Hess CP, Henry RG. Diffusion tensor MR imaging and fiber tractography: theoretic underpinnings. *AJNR Am J Neuroradiol.* 2008;29(4):632-641.

Mukherjee P, Chung SW, Berman JI, Hess CP, Henry RG. Diffusion tensor MR imaging and fiber tractography: technical considerations. *AJNR Am J Neuroradiol.* 2008;29(5):843-852.

Pierpaoli C, Jezzard P, Basser PJ, Barnett A, Di Chiro G. Diffusion tensor MR imaging of the human brain. *Radiology.* 1996;201(3):637-648.

Pruessmann KP, Weiger M, Scheidegger MB, Boesiger P. SENSE: sensitivity encoding for fast MRI. *Magn Reson Med.* 1999;42(5):952-962.

Sadowski EA, Bennett LK, Chan MR, et al. Nephrogenic systemic fibrosis: risk factors and incidence estimation. *Radiology.* 2007;243(1):148-157.

Sodickson DK, Manning WJ. Simultaneous acquisition of spatial harmonics (SMASH): fast imaging with radiofrequency coil arrays. *Magn Reson Med.* 1997;38(4):591-603.

Stehling MK, Turner R, Mansfield P. Echo-planar imaging: magnetic resonance imaging in a fraction of a second. *Science.* 1991;254(5028):43-50.

Thomsen HS. European Society of Urogenital Radiology guidelines on contrast media application. *Curr Opin Urol.* 2007;17(1):70-76.

Warach S, Gaa J, Siewert B, Wielopolski P, Edelman RR. Acute human stroke studied by whole brain echo planar diffusion-weighted magnetic resonance imaging. *Ann Neurol.* 1995;37(2):231-241.

Webb JA, Thomsen HS, Morcos SK. The use of iodinated and gadolinium contrast media during pregnancy and lactation. *Eur Radiol.* 2005;15(6):1234-1240.

CHAPTER 3

Advanced MR (MR Spectroscopy, Diffusion Imaging, Diffusion Tensor Imaging, and Perfusion Imaging): A Multiparametric Algorithmic Approach to Problem Solving in Neuroradiology

Meng Law, Saulo Lacerda, and Pascal Bou-Haidar

■ INTRODUCTION

Neuroradiology has progressed rapidly in recent times to be in the forefront of imaging technology. Advanced magnetic resonance imaging (MRI) techniques, such as magnetic resonance spectroscopy (MRS), diffusion-weighted imaging (DWI), diffusion tensor imaging, and perfusion MRI techniques can give important in vivo physiologic and metabolic information, complementing morphologic findings from conventional MRI in the clinical setting. Combining these new tools can help in solving difficult cases and increase diagnostic specificity and confidence.

■ IMAGING TECHNIQUES

Magnetic Resonance Spectroscopy

The basic metabolite changes common to brain pathology include elevations in choline (Cho), lactate, and lipids, and decreases in N-acetylaspartate (NAA) and creatine (Cr) (Figure 3-1). As clinical spectroscopy becomes more sophisticated, metabolites identified by short echo time (TE) MRS are becoming important in increasing the specificity of MRS in brain tumor diagnosis. The increase in Cho in simple terms is attributed to cell membrane turnover and proliferation. To determine whether elevation in Cho is pathologic and, more importantly, to increase specificity, the more optimal approach involves comparing Cho in the pathologic voxels with Cho in the contralateral normal brain tissue, the so-called normalized Cho levels. This method may be useful in the clinical setting of focally enhancing lesions for characterizing inflammatory, ischemic, demyelinating, and tumoral lesions.

As mentioned, most of these lesions can present with "apparent" elevation of Cho (relative to NAA or Cr), decrease in NAA, and elevation of lipids and lactate. When Cho in the pathologic voxels is compared with Cho in the contralateral normal brain tissue [Cho(n)], in some of cases total Cho is, in fact, reduced compared to the normal side.

Diffusion-Weighted and Diffusion Tensor Imaging

Water molecules undergo random brownian *diffusion* over time due to differences in concentration according to Fick's law. Although diffusion is a random process, directional preference may result from local barriers; for example, barriers to diffusion in white matter tracts include axonal proteins and myelin. DWI has been instrumental in the early diagnosis of acute ischemic stroke. More recently, restricted diffusion has been demonstrated in very cellular gliomas and lymphomas. We will apply these diffusion changes in the characterization of brain and spinal cord lesions.

Several reports have shown that glioma grade correlates inversely with minimum apparent diffusion coefficient (ADC), likely the result of increasing tumor cellularity with grade. Although the initial reports on correlation between minimum ADC and glioma grade have shown promise, the role of DWI in preoperative assessment of glioma grade is controversial and remains investigational because of substantial overlap in ADC values among different grades of glioma. The finding of abnormally reduced diffusion in, around, and remote from the resection bed immediately after surgery for brain tumor resection is not uncommon. The important

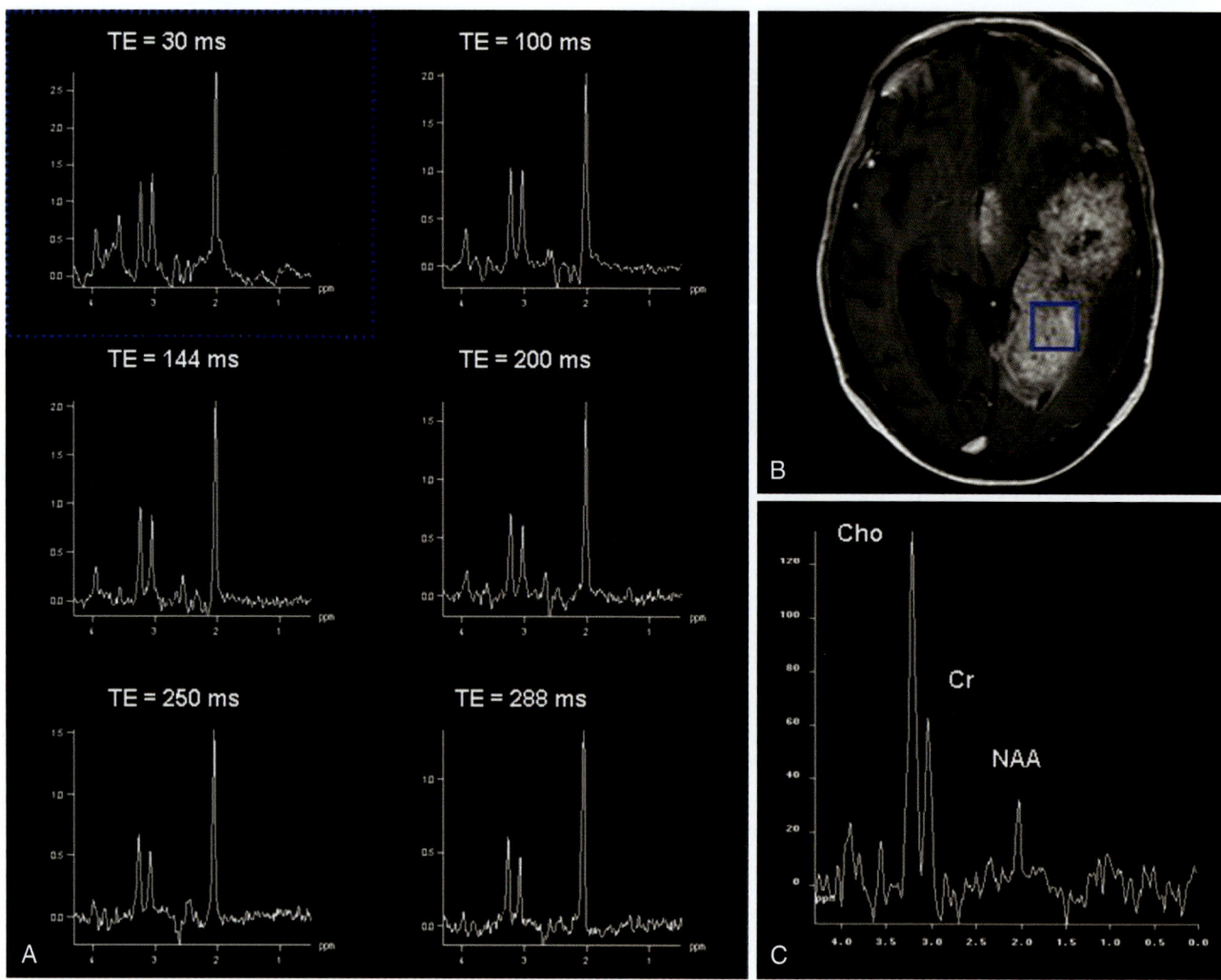

Figure 3-1 **A:** Normal spectra acquired at different echo times demonstrating normal concentrations of choline (Cho), creatine (Cr), and N-acetylaspartate (NAA). The relative concentration (e.g., Cho/Cr or Cho/NAA) of each of the metabolites is different at different echo times because of the differences in T2 relaxation time for different metabolites. This is a pitfall when comparing metabolite ratios at different echo times. **B:** Localizing postcontrast T1-weighted image demonstrating a mass with the location of the blue voxel. **C:** Abnormal spectrum within a recurrent glioma demonstrating marked elevation in Cho relative to Cr and NAA. (Courtesy Nouha Salibi, Siemens Medical Solutions.)

clinical implication is that these areas of immediate postoperative diffusion abnormality invariably undergo a phase of contrast enhancement on routine anatomic images that easily can be misinterpreted as tumor recurrence and as early treatment failure, prompting aggressive therapy with high potential for toxicity. These areas of enhancement invariably evolve into encephalomalacia or gliotic cavity on long-term follow-up studies (Figure 3-2), indicating the occurrence of some immediate postoperative ischemia from either surgical retraction or venous insufficiency.

Diffusion tensor imaging is the application of DWI in six or more directions. This allows the calculation of fractional anisotropy, relative anisotropy, mean diffusivity, and the major and minor eigenvalues, which can be color coded. Colors are assigned as blue = superoinferior orientation; green = anteroposterior; and red = laterolateral (Figure 3-3).

In white matter, the direction of the major eigenvector tends to be parallel with the orientation of axonal fibers. Using this observation, algorithms have been developed that may generate three-dimensional representations of axonal fibers, or *three-dimensional fiber tractography*. These algorithms in effect attempt to "string together" adjacent voxels based on similarity in the direction of their major eigenvectors (Figure 3-3).

Although useful in tract visualization, white matter fiber tractography represents a more postprocessed representation of diffusion tensor imaging data compared to visualization of tensor maps and maps of fractional anisotropy and mean diffusivity metrics; therefore, it is prone to the addition of error. In voxels that contain crossing fiber tracts from two or more directions, the association between diffusion tensor measurement and axonal fiber direction is less direct. Algorithms have been developed to mitigate this problem, which arises commonly in central nervous system (CNS) structures such as the brainstem and in areas with complex crossing association fibers. High angular resolution diffusion tensor imaging techniques have been developed in an effort to resolve the crossing fibers in the brain and brainstem. Various data smoothing and interpolation

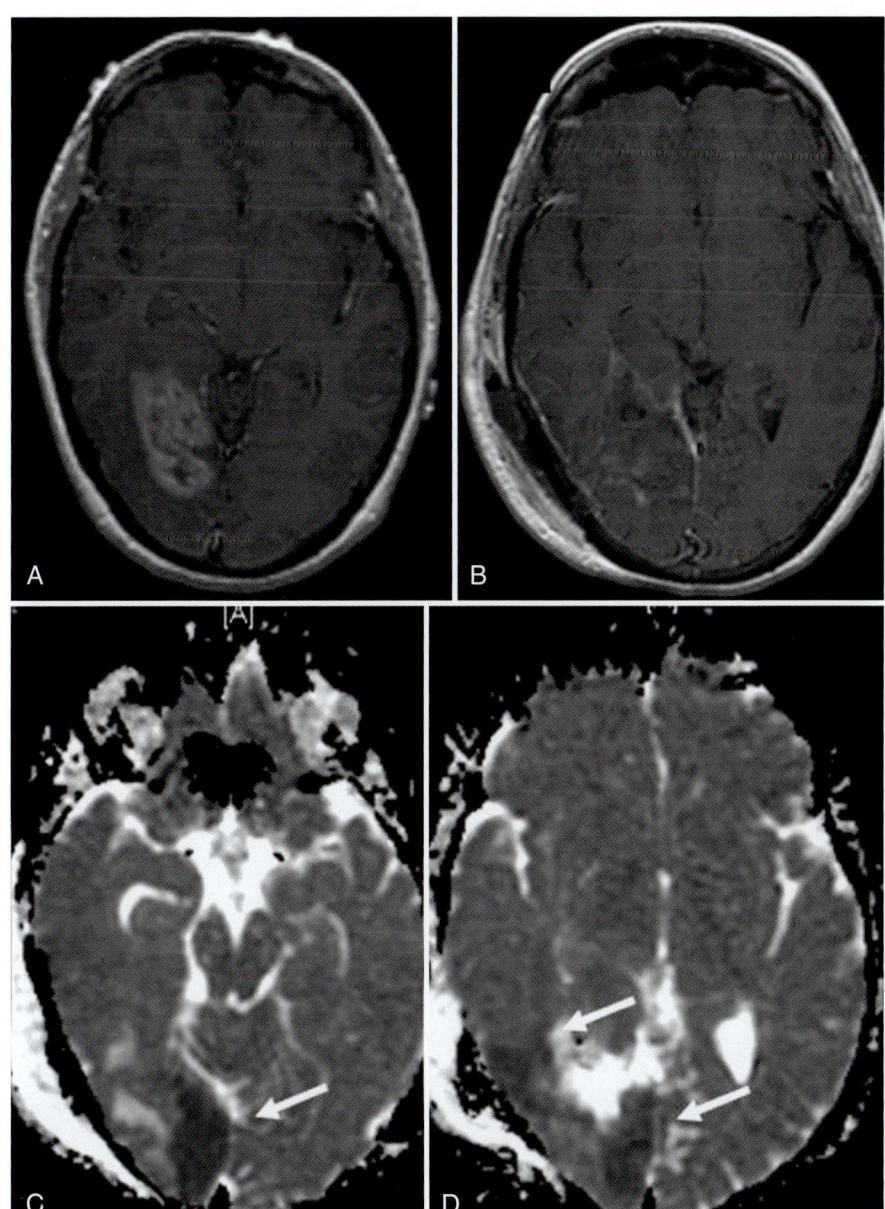

Figure 3-2 A 52-year-old-man with glioblastoma multiforme in the right occipital lobe. **A:** Axial T1-weighted image postcontrast showing a mass with heterogeneous enhancement in the occipital lobe. **B:** Axial T1-weighted image postcontrast on the first postoperative day demonstrating radical resection of the tumor. **C, D:** Diffusion apparent diffusion coefficient maps showing diffusion restriction areas along the margin of the surgical cavity *(arrows).*

Continued

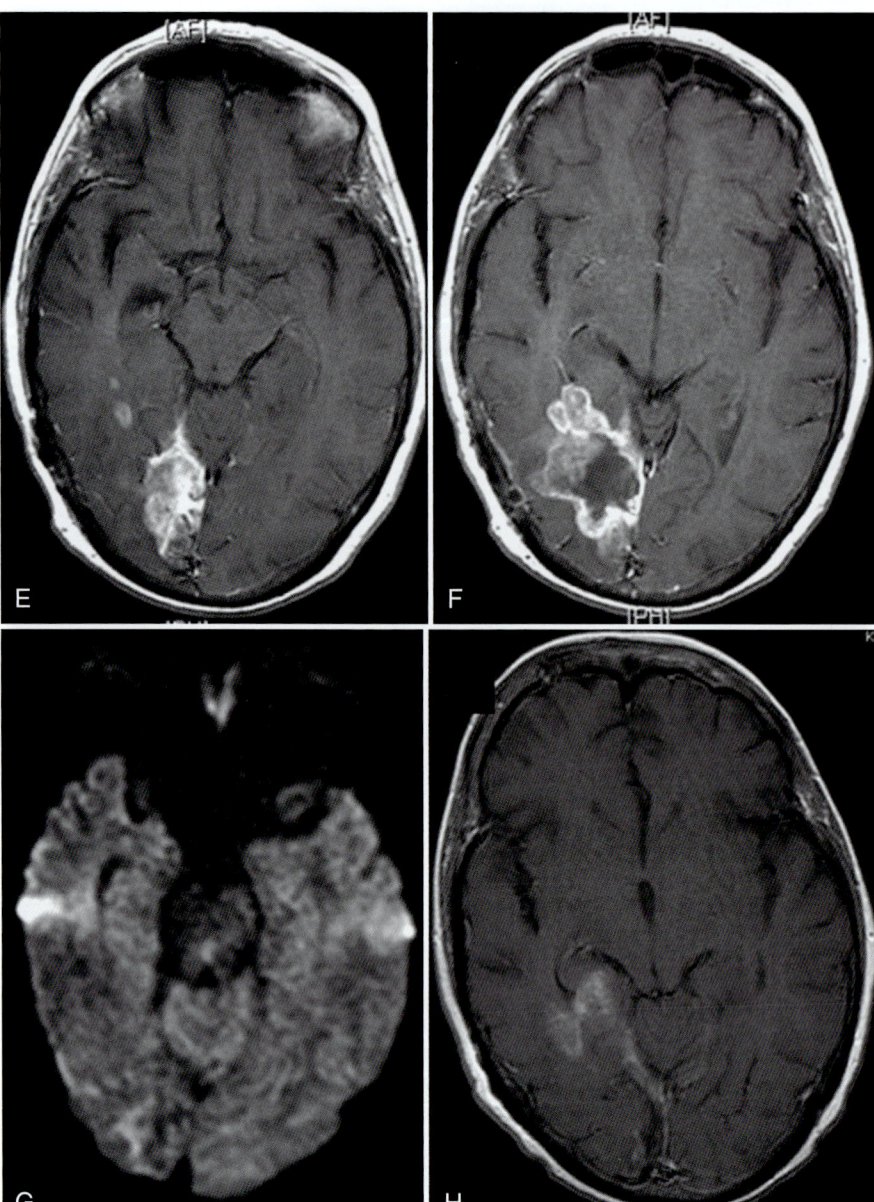

Figure 3-2—cont'd E, F: Postcontrast T1-weighted image demonstrating enhancement 1 month after initial surgery. The enhancement relates to transient operative ischemia rather than recurrent tumor. G: Diffusion-weighted image demonstrating resolution of the ischemic findings. H: Almost complete resolution of the enhancing regions at a later time interval.

techniques also have been used to minimize the propagation of noise error.

Perfusion Imaging Dynamic Susceptibility Contrast Perfusion MRI and Dynamic Contrast-Enhanced MRI

Perfusion MRI (with diffusible contrast) can be performed using two major techniques. Dynamic susceptibility contrast perfusion magnetic resonance imaging (DSC MRI), which utilizes a first-pass $T2^*$-weighted technique, is most commonly distributed by the major MRI vendors and is used more frequently. Dynamic contrast-enhanced magnetic resonance imaging (DCE MRI) is a steady-state T1-weighted technique that is not commonly used because the T1 technique yields a slightly lower signal-to-noise ratio, and the kinetic modeling algorithms for the estimation of blood volume and vascular permeability are more complex. Here we discuss both techniques and show how characterization of signal intensity curves using both DSC MRI and DCE MRI techniques can be useful in problem solving, particularly in addressing difficult questions such as differentiating recurrent tumoral disease from therapy-related necrosis.

Technical Pitfalls and Limitations in DSC MRI

Even though DSC MRI is the most commonly used and easily applied technique for studying brain tumor perfusion, use of a gradient echo sequence is associated with a number of important limitations. First, because the technique is weighted to measure susceptibility, it is extremely sensitive to lesions that cause

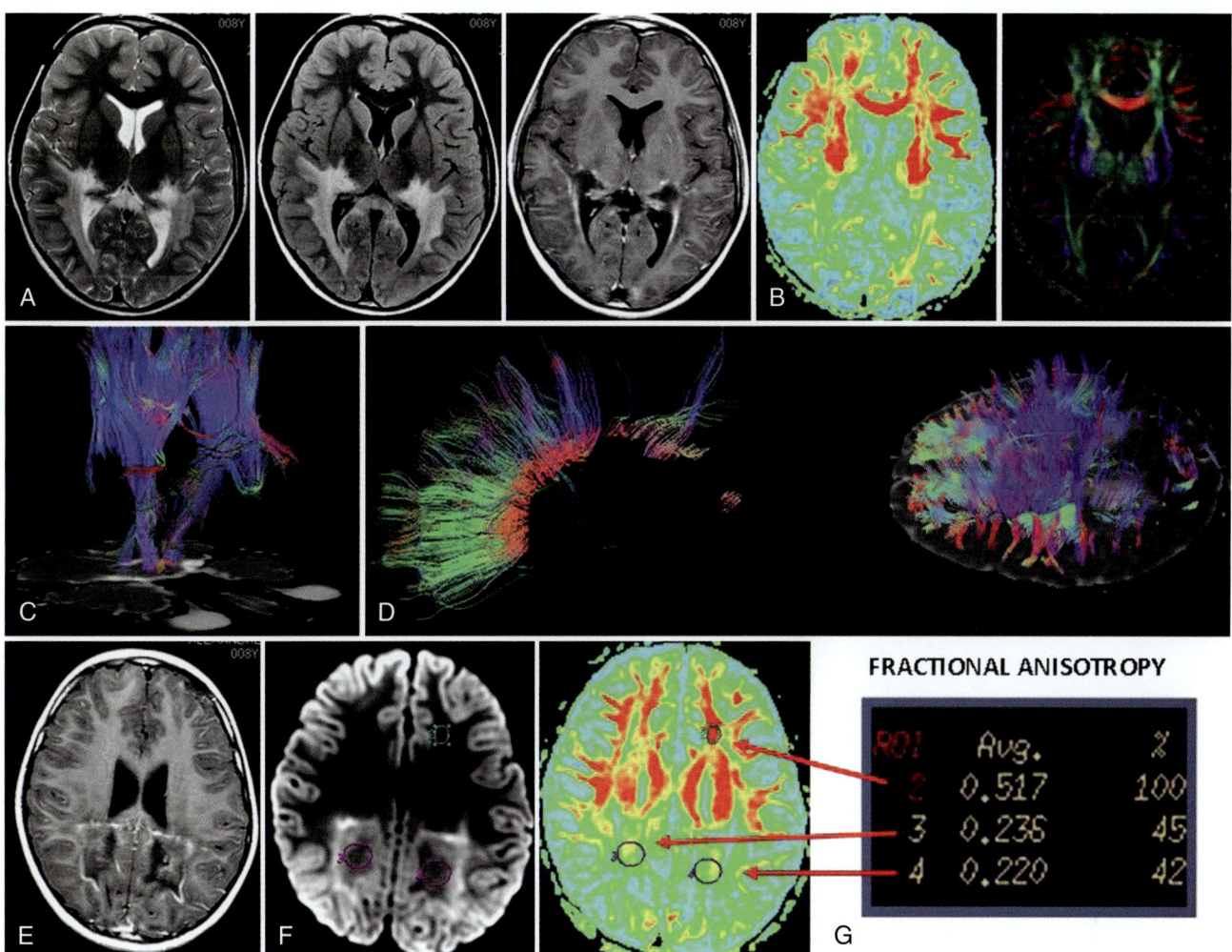

Figure 3-3 Patient with adrenoleukodystrophy. **A–C:** Axial T2-weighted, FLAIR, and postcontrast T1-weighted images demonstrating the typical regions of demyelination involving the posterior periventricular white matter. **B:** Magnitude and directional color-coded fractional anisotropy (FA) maps from diffusion tensor imaging (DTI) demonstrating a marked decrease in FA in the posterior periventricular white matter. **C, D:** Color-coded fiber tractography demonstrating a decrease in the projected fiber tracts in the posterior white matter. **E, F:** Postcontrast T1-weighted, gray scale and color FA maps demonstrating regions of interest for quantitation of FA show a marked decrease in FA in the posterior white matter compared with the anterior white matter. This case illustrates how DTI data can be presented.

magnetic field inhomogeneity, such as blood products, calcium, bone, melanin, metals, and lesions near the brain–bone–air interface, such as the skull base. This factor becomes important when characterizing both high-grade gliomas, which may contain blood products, and low-grade gliomas, which may contain some calcification. Solutions for reducing inhomogeneity and susceptibility include decreasing slice thickness, which also reduces the signal-to-noise ratio and slice coverage. Parallel imaging methods also can reduce both susceptibility and scan time, thus allowing more brain coverage and a higher signal-to-noise ratio. If a larger lesion requires increased brain coverage, then the interslice gap can be increased while maintaining thinner slices to reduce susceptibility. Second, quantification of perfusion metrics, such as cerebral blood volume (CBV) and vascular permeability (K^{trans}), can be inaccurate in lesions having a very leaky blood–brain barrier, such as glioblastoma multiforme (GBM), choroids plexus tumors, and meningiomas. Therefore, extremely low or high perfusion values must be considered with caution. Correction algorithms can be applied to compensate for leakiness. When T1 effects are exaggerated, relative cerebral blood volume (rCBV) will be underestimated, which may affect tumor grade prediction. Preloading with a small dose of contrast (which can also serve to produce T1 steady-state permeability maps) along with gamma variate and linear fitting to correct for the leakage will improve the accuracy of rCBV estimations. Where T2* effects are exaggerated in the setting of a very leaky lesion, rCBV will be overestimated. Hence, correction algorithms can result in either an increase or a decrease in rCBV (Figure 3-4). Finally, some controversy still exists regarding the effect of corticosteroid/dexamethasone administration on perfusion and permeability estimations in the brain. Anecdotally and physiologically, it appears that steroid significantly reduces vascular permeability; however, in

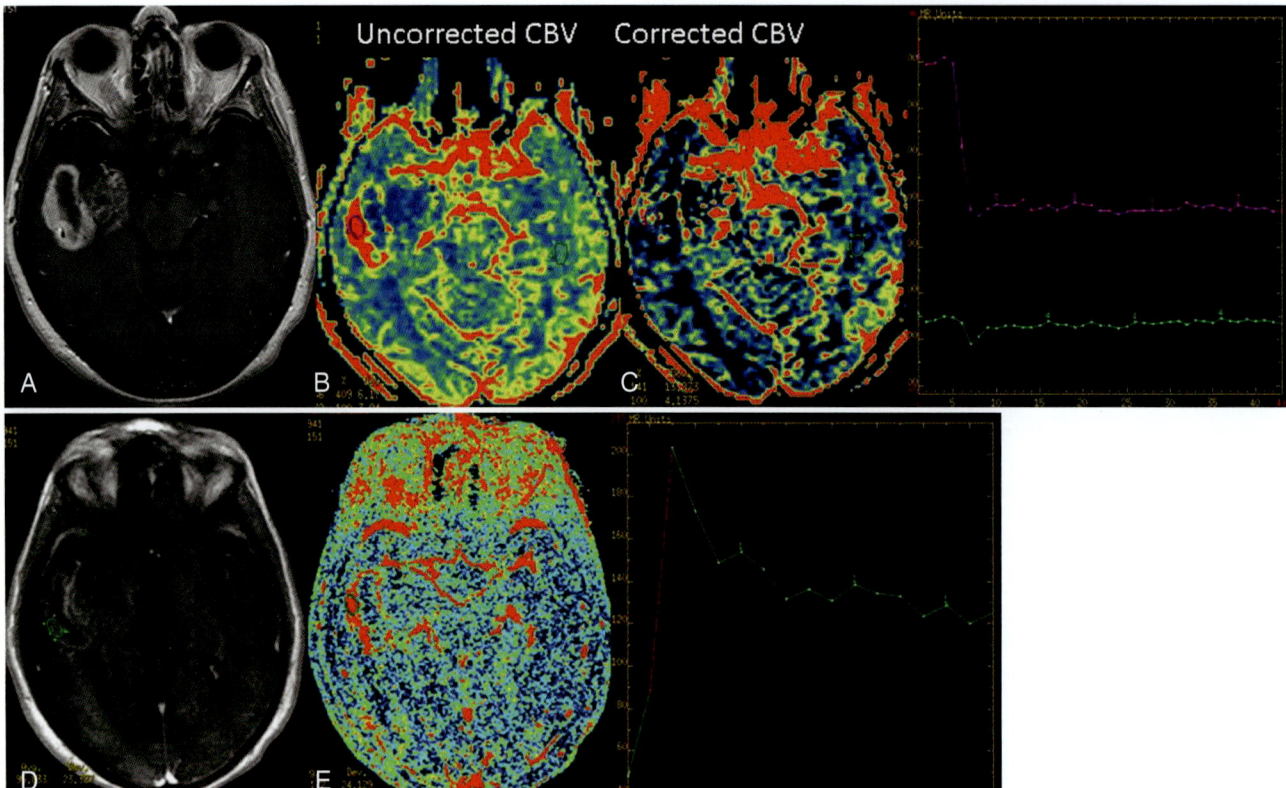

Figure 3-4 Heterogeneously enhancing right temporal high-grade glioma in a 50-year-old man. **A:** Axial T1-weighted image showing an enhancing mass in the right temporal region. **B:** Dynamic susceptibility contrast perfusion magnetic resonance imaging (DSC MRI) uncorrected relative cerebral blood volume (rCBV) color overlay demonstrating elevated rCBV. **C:** DSC MRI corrected rCBV color overlay demonstrating decrease in rCBV. DSC MRI T2* signal intensity curves demonstrating increased leakiness as well as exaggerated T2* effect of gadolinium resulting in overestimation of rCBV. **D, E:** Overestimation and underestimation can be corrected by preloading with contrast as well as applying a linear or gamma variate fit that will produce corrected rCBV maps that provide a more accurate estimation of rCBV. **Bottom row:** Dynamic contrast-enhanced magnetic resonance imaging permeability map demonstrating increased vascular permeability.

terms of perfusion metrics, a recent paper seems to suggest that dexamethasone does not significantly affect tumor blood flow, blood volume, or transit time but may, by reducing peritumoral water content and local tissue pressure, subtly increase perfusion in the edematous brain.

PROBLEM SOLVING IN BRAIN TUMORS

Multiparametric Algorithmic Approach

The ring-enhancing mass lesion in the brain can have a number of differential diagnoses. They include high-grade glioma, metastasis, infarct, radiation necrosis, abscess, or tumefactive demyelinating lesion. An algorithmic multiparametric approach combining findings from each of the advanced MRI techniques can be used to differentiate these pathologies (Figure 3-5). A potential approach to a mass lesion would initially be evaluation to determine whether the lesion enhanced. If enhancement is seen, then review the DWI. If ADC is low, then consider CNS lymphoma. If ADC is higher, then review the perfusion imaging. If rCBV (perfusion) is less than 1.75, then consider an abscess or tumefactive demyelinating lesion. If rCBV is greater than 1.75, then consider either a high-grade glioma or metastasis. Review of the rCBV in the perienhancement T2 signal abnormality will help differentiate between an infiltrating high-grade glioma and a well-circumscribed metastasis.

Figures 3-6 to 3-16 show 10 illustrative cases of how these imaging techniques are applied to problem solving. In clinical practice, this is done on an ad hoc basis for each case. The algorithm provides a more structured approach that can benefit both the novice and the more experienced neuroradiologist in problem solving. We review a number of problematic cases and, based on the algorithm, demonstrate how a multiparametric algorithmic technique can be used in the clinical setting. We also highlight some important teaching points that will help to increase accuracy when using this algorithm.

Perfusion and Tumor Vascularity

This case illustrates an important pitfall in terms of perfusion of low-grade oligodendrogliomas. The typical signs found on conventional images are characterized by heterogeneous cortically based tumors, with variable enhancement. Foci of calcifications may be seen on MRI or computed tomography. However, perfusion imaging often is elevated in low-grade oligodendrogliomas (Figure 3-7). Law et al. reviewed 160 glioma patients and found sensitivity of 95% and specificity of 57.5% for differentiating high-grade from low-grade gliomas. In Figure 3-8, all of the conventional imaging findings and the spectroscopic ratios favor a high-grade glioma; the perfusion study demonstrates high capillary density compatible with a high-grade tumor. This situation illustrates a pitfall of this algorithm and seems to undermine the role of DSC MRI in glioma grading.

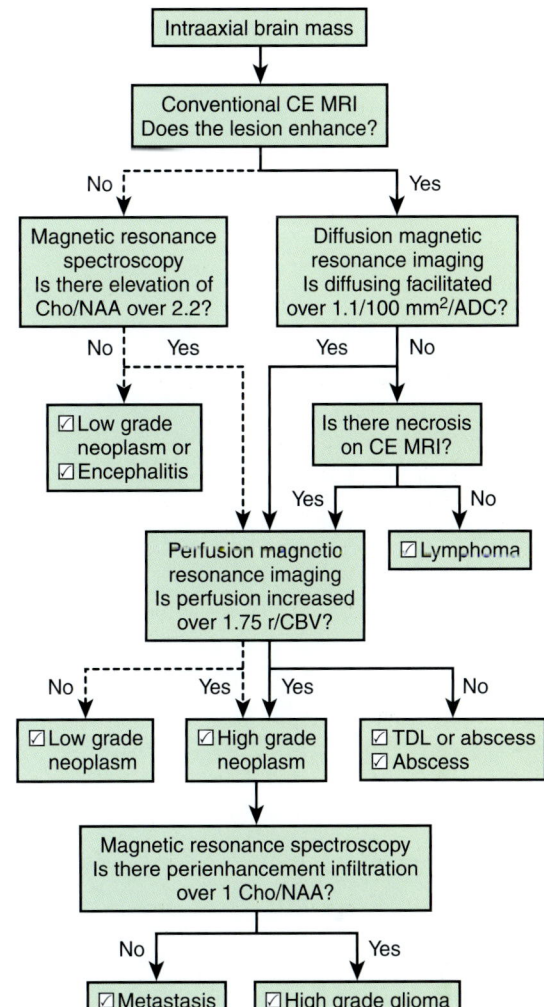

Figure 3-5 Flowchart illustrating order of methods used to diagnose and differentiate intraaxial masses. Each method provides an answer to a specific question, which is used as a discriminator to distinguish lesions. $1.1/100\ mm2/ADC$, $1.1 \times 10^{-3}\ mm^2/s$; *ADC*, apparent diffusion coefficient; *CE*, contrast material enhanced; *Cho*, choline; *NAA*, N-acetylaspartate; *r/CBV*, relative cerebral blood volume; *TDL*, tumefactive demyelinating lesion. (From Al-Okaili RN, Krejza J, Woo JH, et al. Intraaxial brain masses: MR imaging-based diagnostic strategy—Initial experience. Radiology 2007;243(2):539-550.)

DWI and Tumor Cellularity

DWI can demonstrate areas of high cellularity indicated by low ADC values. Figure 3-10 shows a typical example of a high-grade glioma, which not uncommonly can present with areas of very low ADC levels, probably related to its high cellularity. In these cases, following the algorithm, other findings such as high capillary density within areas of T2 hyperintensity suggest a primary high-grade glioma over lesions such as a lymphoma, which may have decreased ADC because of cellularity but does not tend to have very high perfusion.

Typically, infective or inflammatory lesions are known as "cold lesions," although investigators have demonstrated increased rCBV and vascular endothelial growth factor (VEGF) expression in the capsule of bacterial abscesses, which probably are responsible for the high perfusion along the edge of the lesion. Thus,

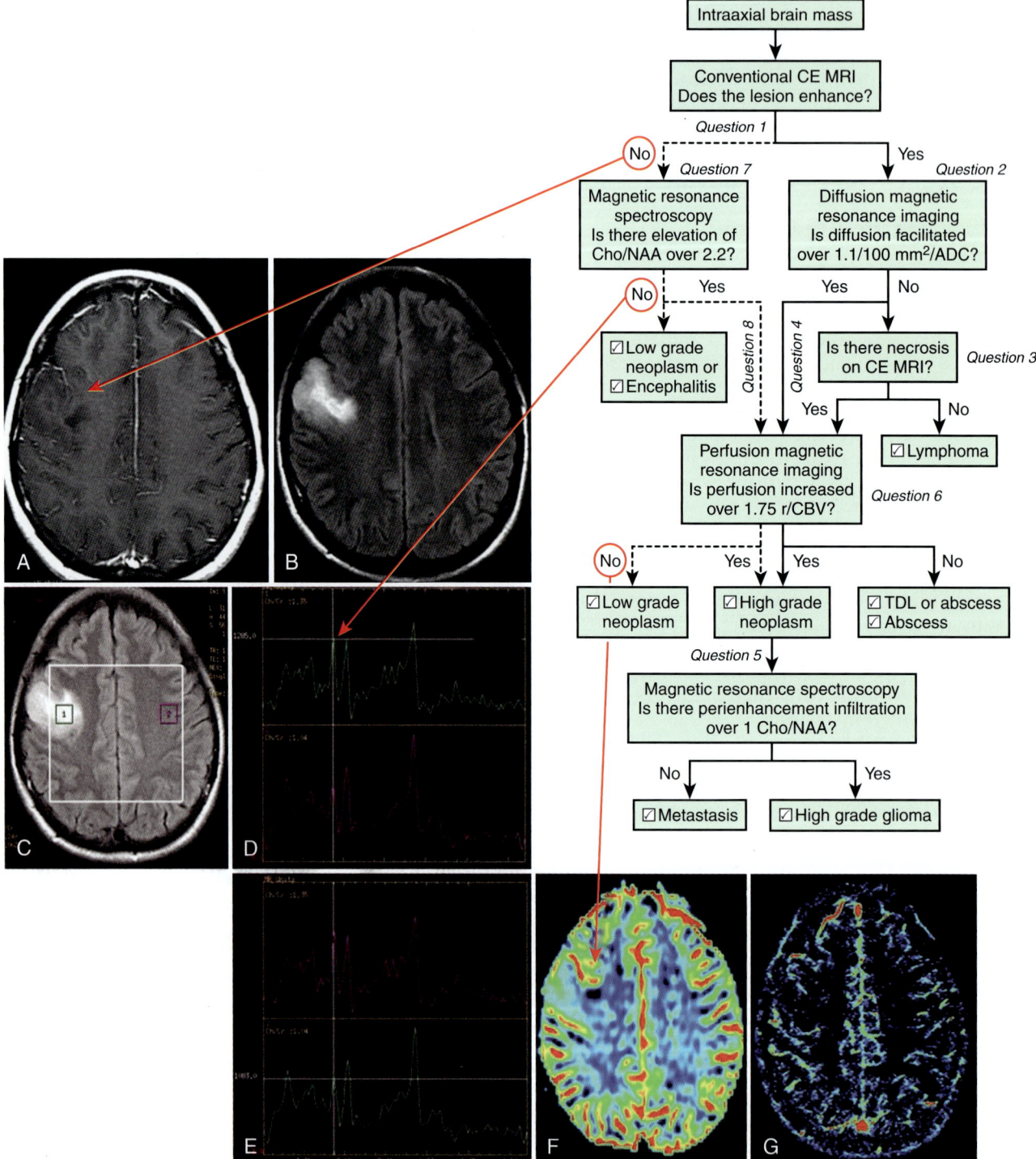

Figure 3-6 A 41-year-old woman with a history of headaches demonstrating a low grade-glioma (LGG) that follows all the magnetic resonance findings for an LGG. **A:** Axial T1-weighted image showing a mass within the right perirolandic region with no enhancement. **B:** Axial FLAIR image demonstrating the right perirolandic region mass with hyperintensity but minimal edema. **C–E:** Magnetic resonance spectroscopy demonstrating no increase in choline, even compared to choline in contralateral normal brain (purple spectra), in keeping with LGG. **F:** Gradient-echo axial dynamic susceptibility contrast T2* magnetic resonance imaging with relative cerebral blood volume color overlay demonstrating reduced relative cerebral blood volume within the lesion. **G:** Spin-echo dynamic contrast-enhanced T1 magnetic resonance image showing a decrease in vascular permeability.

Chapter 3 Advanced MR (MR Spectroscopy, Diffusion Imaging, and Perfusion Imaging)

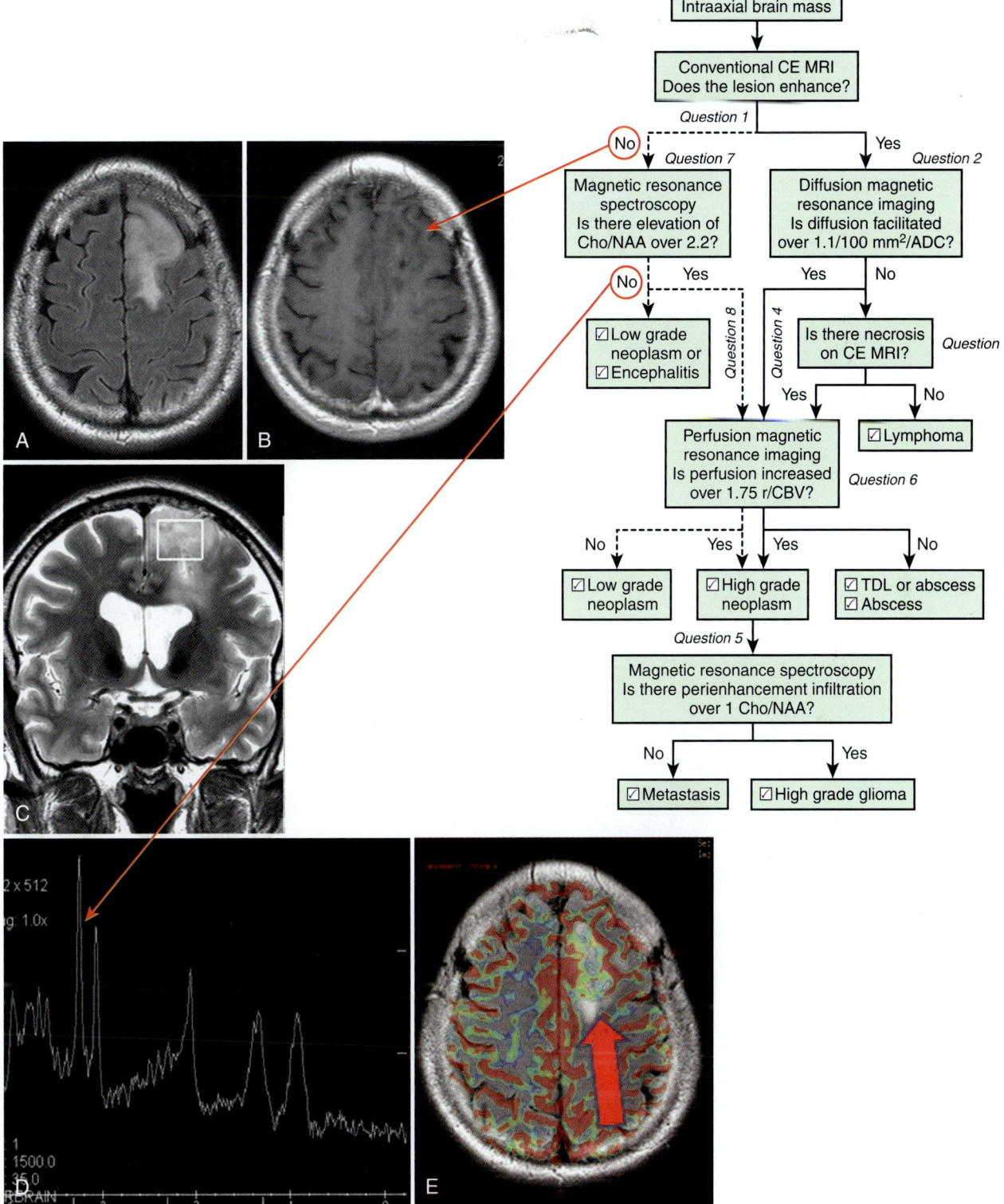

Figure 3-7 A 45-year-old woman with a history of headaches. Example of nonenhancing low-grade oligodendroglioma with high perfusion. **A:** Axial FLAIR image showing a mass in the left frontal lobe. **B:** Contrast-enhanced axial T1-weighted image demonstrating no contrast enhancement. **C, D:** Magnetic resonance spectroscopy demonstrating minimal increase in choline, in keeping with a low-grade glioma. **E:** Gradient-echo axial dynamic susceptibility contrast perfusion magnetic resonance imaging with relative cerebral blood volume color overlay demonstrating slightly elevated cerebral blood volume within the lesion. As a pitfall this was found to be an oligodendroglioma, a tumor known to have high cerebral blood volume levels even when low grade.

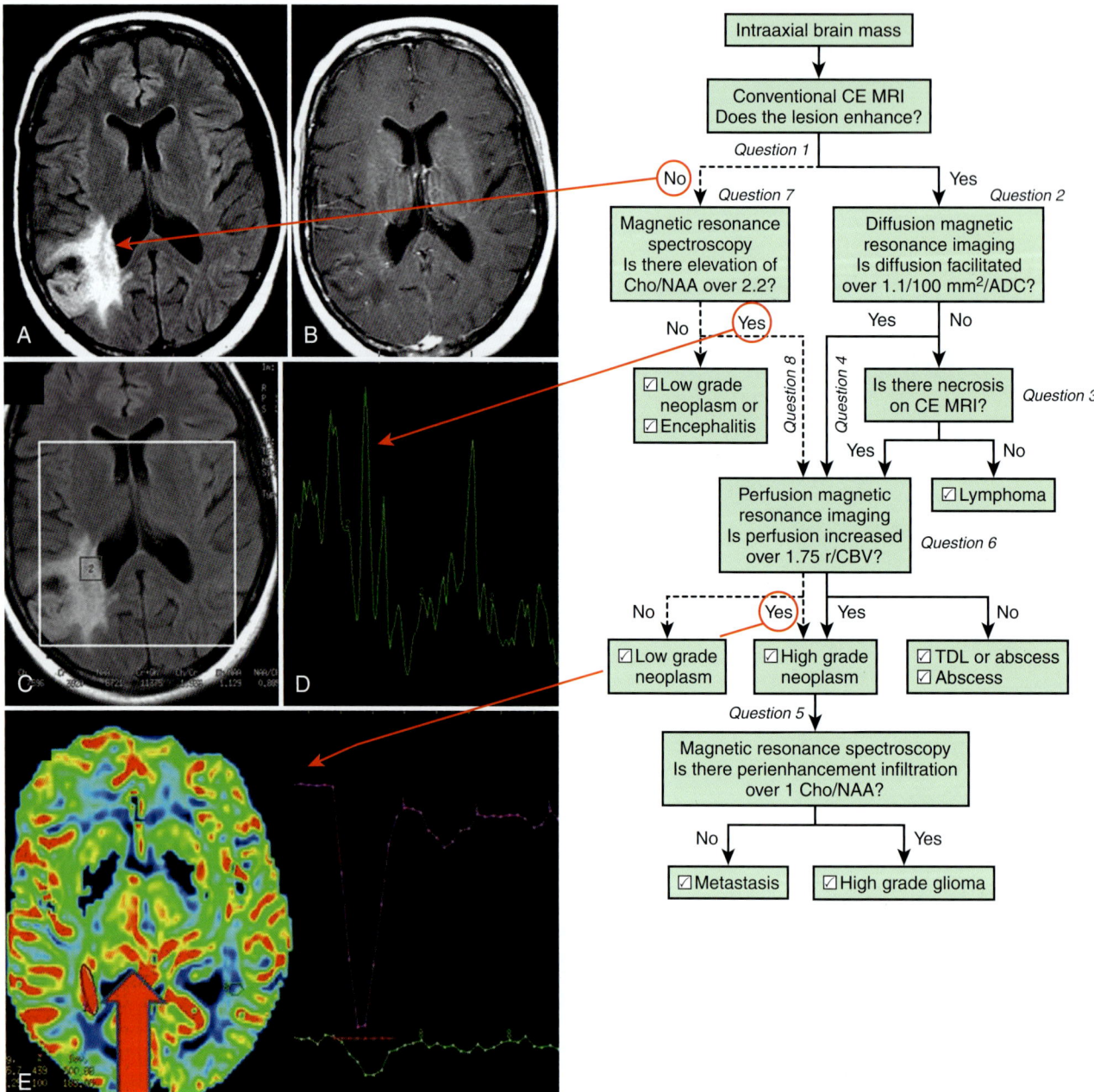

Figure 3-8 Nonenhancing high-grade glioma with low choline but high relative cerebral blood volume (rCBV) in a 59-year-old man with pathology-proven anaplastic astrocytoma. **A:** Axial FLAIR image demonstrating a hyperintense right parietal tumor. **B:** Axial T1-weighted image showing no contrast enhancement. **C, D:** Magnetic resonance spectroscopy demonstrating a moderate increase in choline levels. **E:** Gradient-echo axial dynamic susceptibility contrast perfusion magnetic resonance imaging with rCBV color overlay demonstrating increased relative cerebral blood volume within the lesion, in keeping with the diagnosis of anaplastic astrocytoma (World Health Organization grade III).

Chapter 3 Advanced MR (MR Spectroscopy, Diffusion Imaging, and Perfusion Imaging)

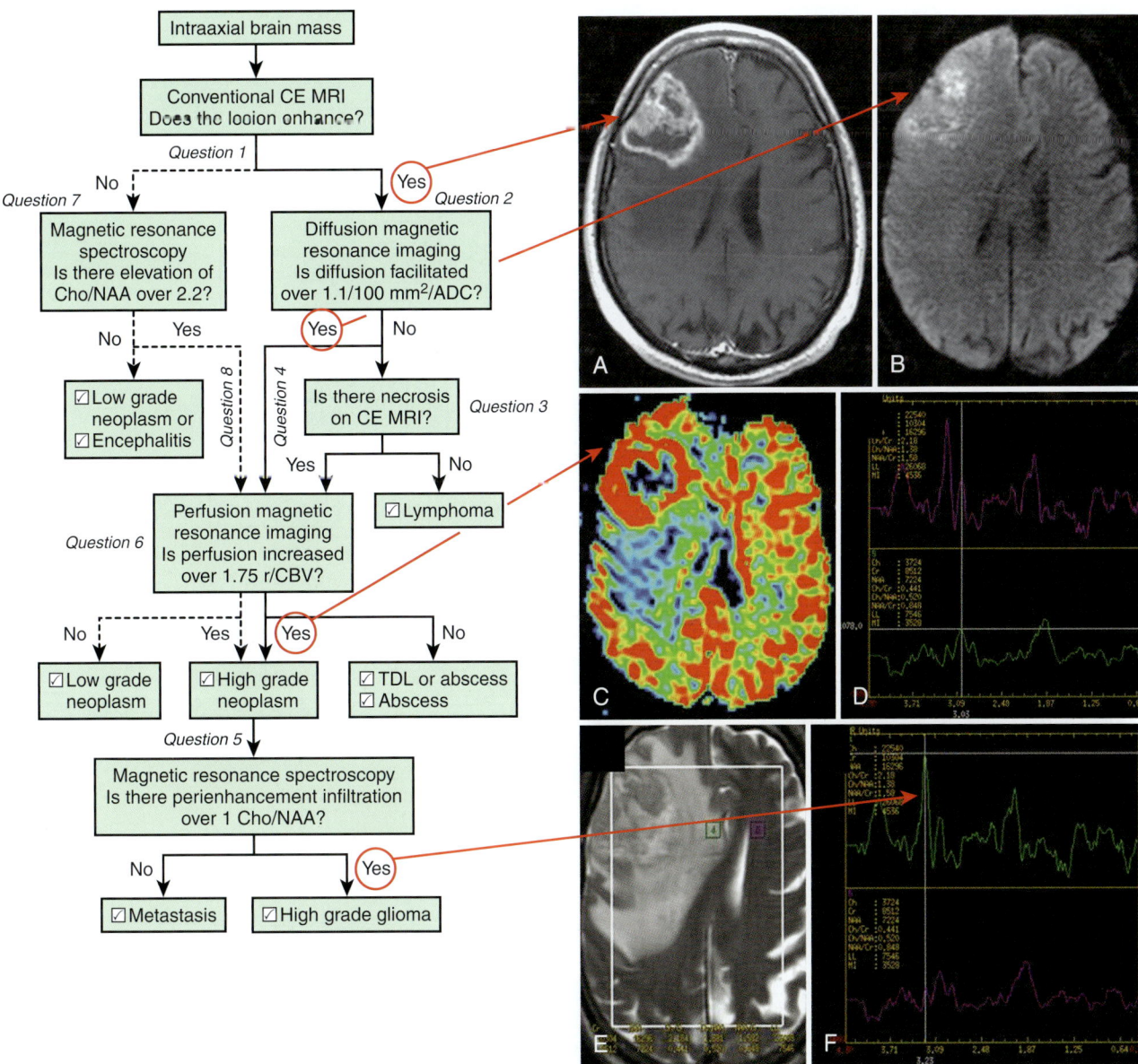

Figure 3-9 Typical advanced magnetic resonance findings for a high-grade glioma in a 62-year old man with a history of behavioral changes. **A:** Axial T1-weighted image showing a mass with central necrosis and predominantly peripheral enhancement. **B:** Diffusion-weighted image demonstrating no diffusion restriction, unlikely to be lymphoma. **C:** Gradient-echo axial dynamic susceptibility contrast perfusion magnetic resonance imaging with relative cerebral blood volume (rCBV) color overlay demonstrating marked increase in rCBV within the lesion. **D–F:** Magnetic resonance spectroscopy of the peritumoral region showing increased choline, compatible with an infiltrating high-grade tumor (World Health Organization grade IV).

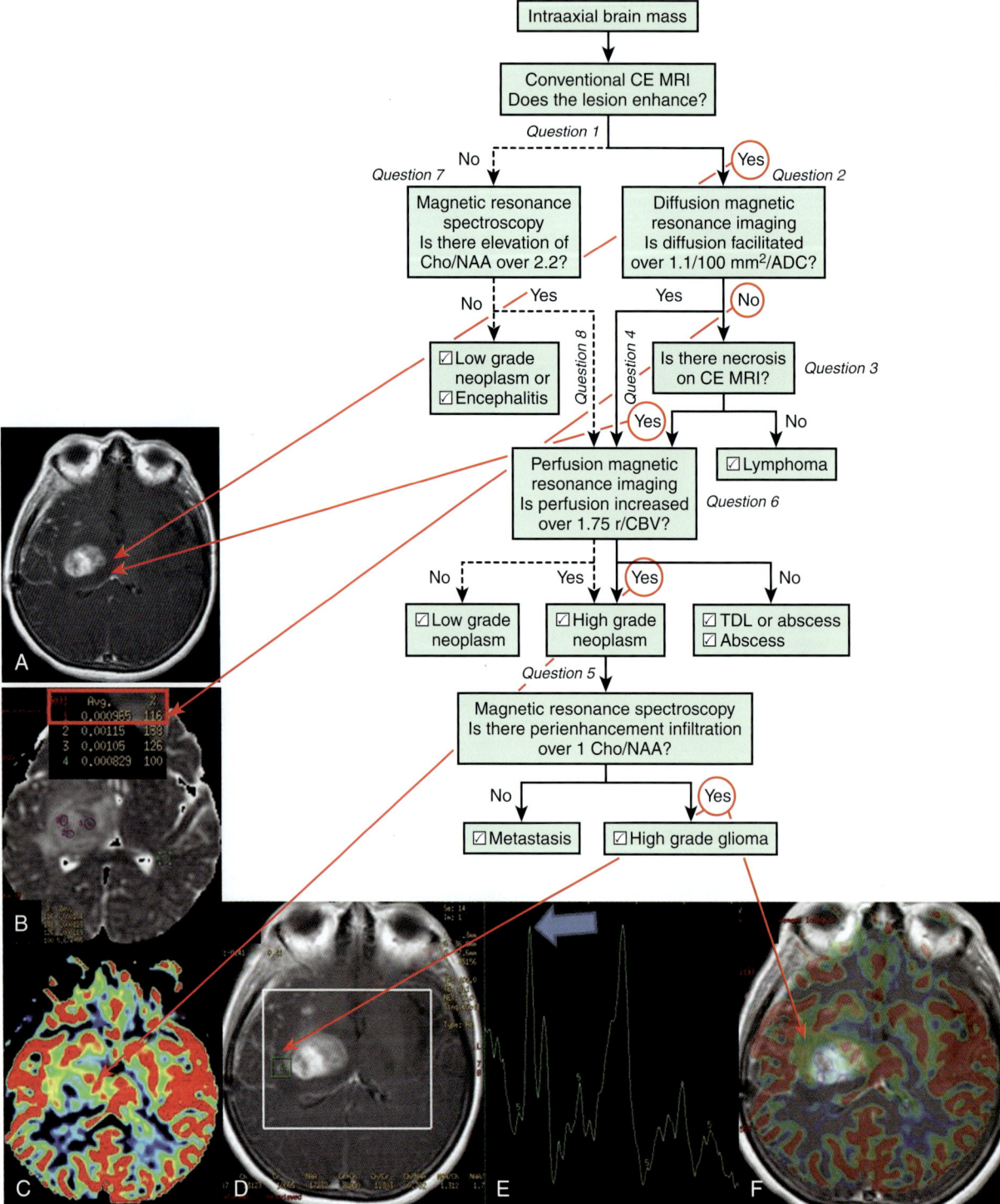

Figure 3-10 A high-grade glioma in a 62-year-old man with a history of behavioral changes. The remainder of the advanced magnetic resonance imaging was able to problem solve and make an accurate diagnosis. **A:** Axial T1-weighted image showing a mass in the right thalamus with heterogeneous enhancement and minimal central necrosis. **B:** Apparent diffusion coefficient (ADC) map demonstrating some areas with low ADC values, suggesting central nervous system lymphoma or a glioma with high cellularity. **C:** Gradient-echo axial dynamic susceptibility contrast perfusion magnetic resonance imaging (DSC MRI) with relative cerebral blood volume (rCBV) color overlay demonstrating increased rCBV within the lesion. **D, E:** Magnetic resonance spectroscopy of the peritumoral region showing increased choline, compatible with an infiltrating high-grade tumor (World Health Organization grade IV). **F:** Gradient-echo axial DSC MRI with rCBV color overlay demonstrating increased rCBV within the peritumoral region, again suggesting infiltration by the tumor.

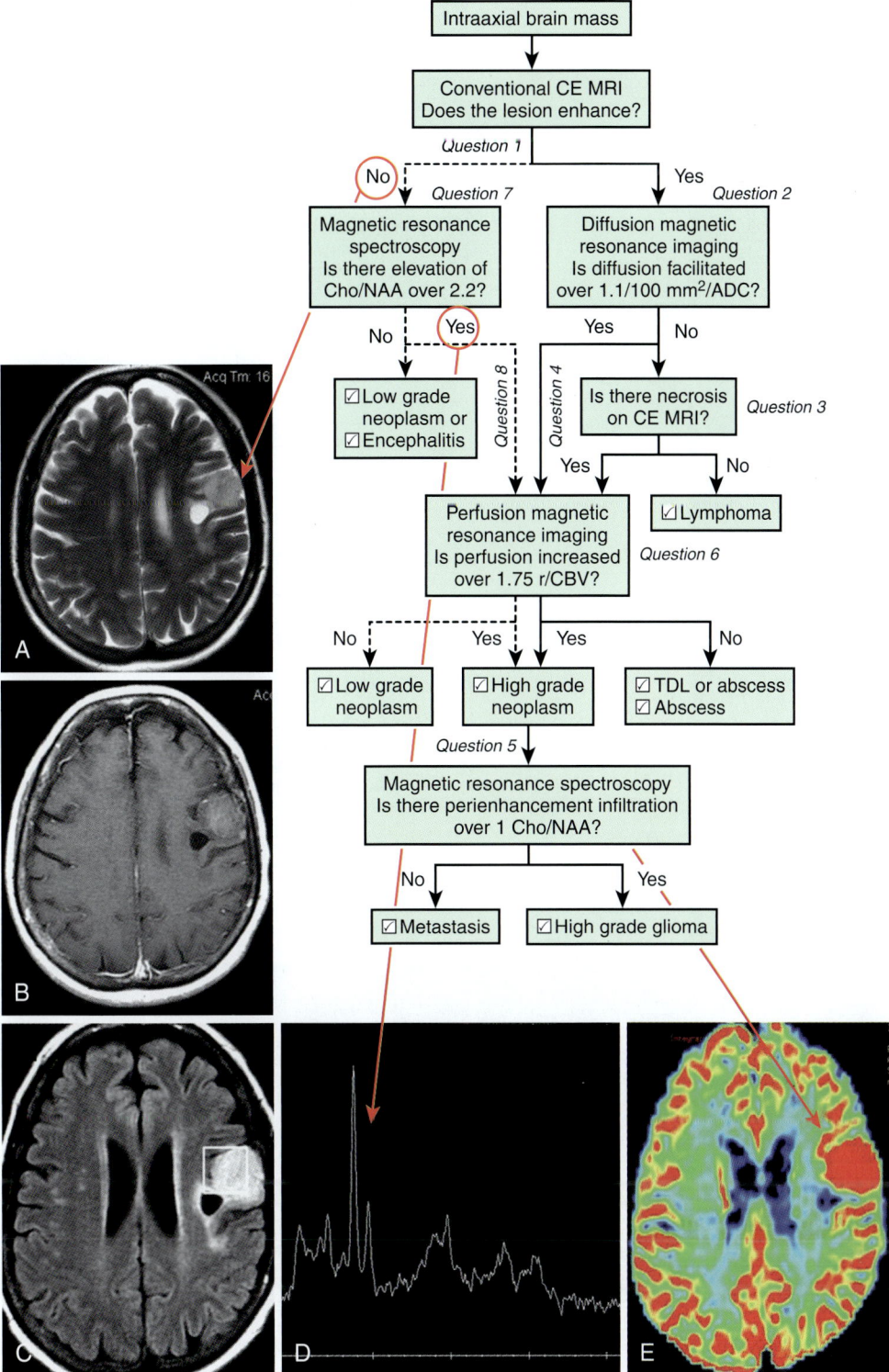

Figure 3-11 A 48-year-old man with a history of right hemiparesis. **A:** Axial T2-weighted showing a lesion in the left perirolandic region. **B:** Postcontrast axial T1-weighted image demonstrating minimal, if any, contrast enhancement. **C, D:** Magnetic resonance spectroscopy demonstrating increase in choline levels (Cho/N-acetylaspartate >2.2) within the lesion. **E:** Gradient-echo axial dynamic susceptibility contrast perfusion magnetic resonance imaging with relative cerebral blood volume (rCBV) color overlay demonstrating significant elevation in rCBV (>1.75) within the lesion, compatible with the diagnosis of fibrillary astrocytoma (World Health Organization grade III).

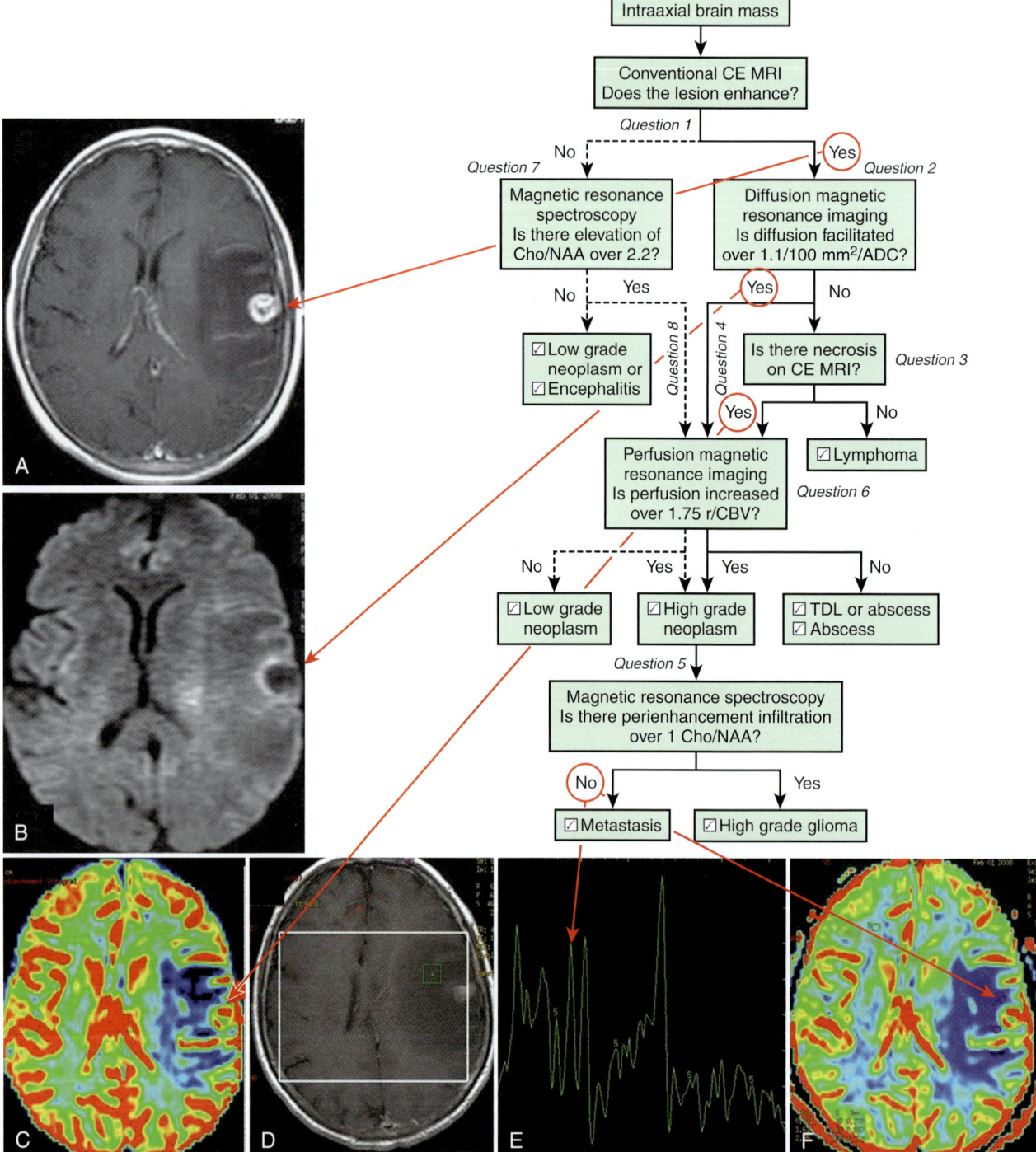

Figure 3-12 Advanced magnetic resonance findings of a metastasis in a 48-year-old man with a history of breast cancer and right hemiparesis. **A:** Axial T1-weighted image showing a mass in the left frontoparietal operculum with ring enhancement and minimal central necrosis. **B:** Diffusion-weighted image demonstrating no restriction diffusion within the lesion. **C:** Gradient-echo axial dynamic susceptibility contrast perfusion magnetic resonance imaging (DSC MRI) with relative cerebral blood volume (rCBV) color overlay demonstrating increased rCBV within the lesion. **D, E:** Magnetic resonance spectroscopy of the peritumoral region showing no increased choline, in keeping with the pathophysiology of the peritumoral region in metastatic lesions. The region contains no infiltrating tumor cells and shows almost purely vasogenic edema. **F:** Gradient-echo axial DSC MRI with rCBV color overlay demonstrating decreased rCBV within the peritumoral region, again compatible with vasogenic edema.

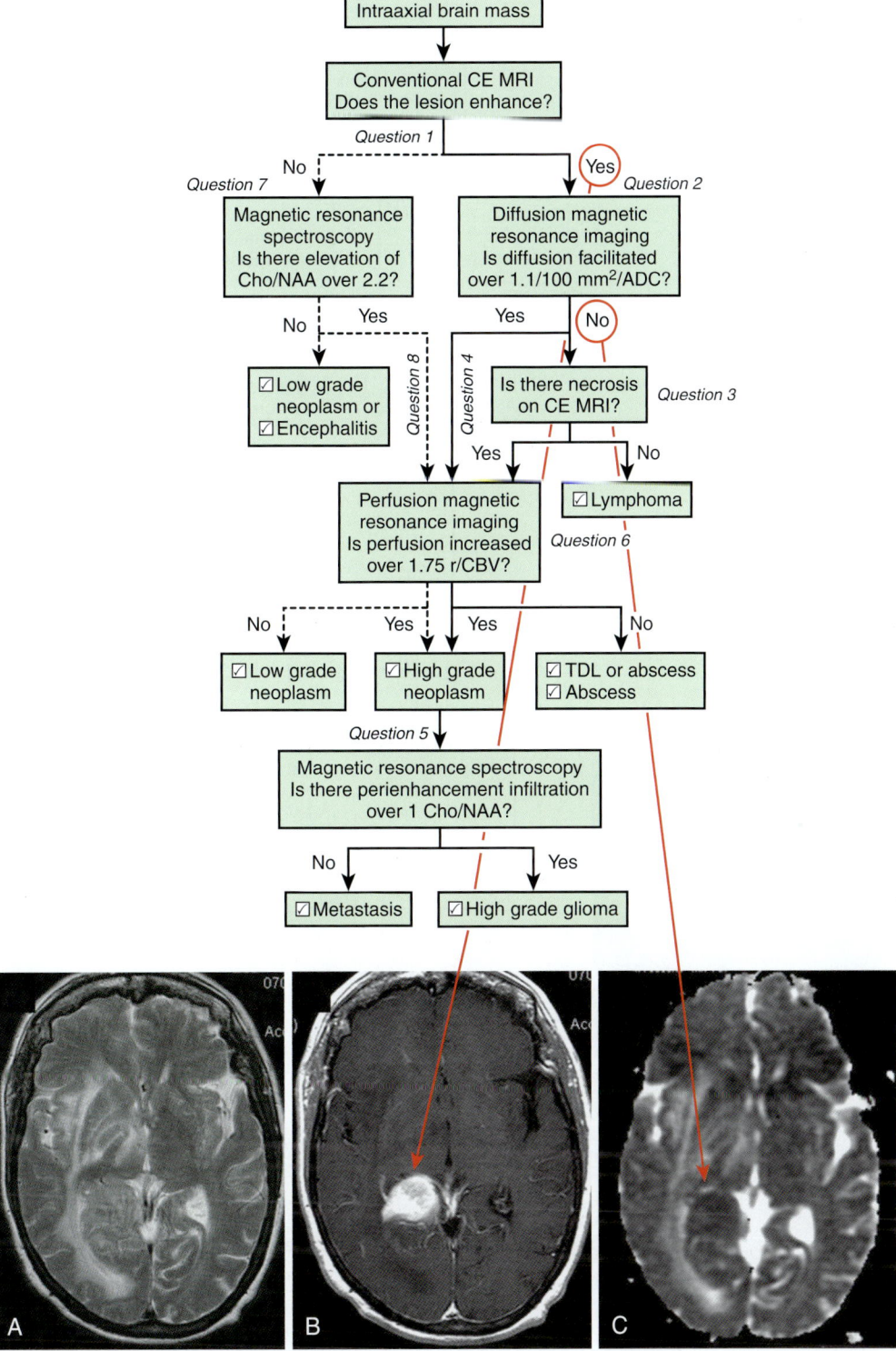

Figure 3-13 Periventricular lesion compatible with central nervous system lymphoma in an immunocompetent 74-year-old woman with a history of headaches. **A:** Axial T2-weighted image showing a mildly hyperintense mass in the isthmus of the cingulum on the right, surrounded by significant edema. **B:** Axial T1-weighted image showing homogeneous enhancement of the mass suggestive of either a glioma or lymphoma. **C:** Apparent diffusion coefficient (ADC) map demonstrating significantly low ADC values, suggesting an lesion with high cellularity. Based on the algorithm, the absence of necrosis suggests lymphoma as the most probable diagnosis, which was confirmed by biopsy. Lymphoma can be necrotic in an immunosuppressed patient.

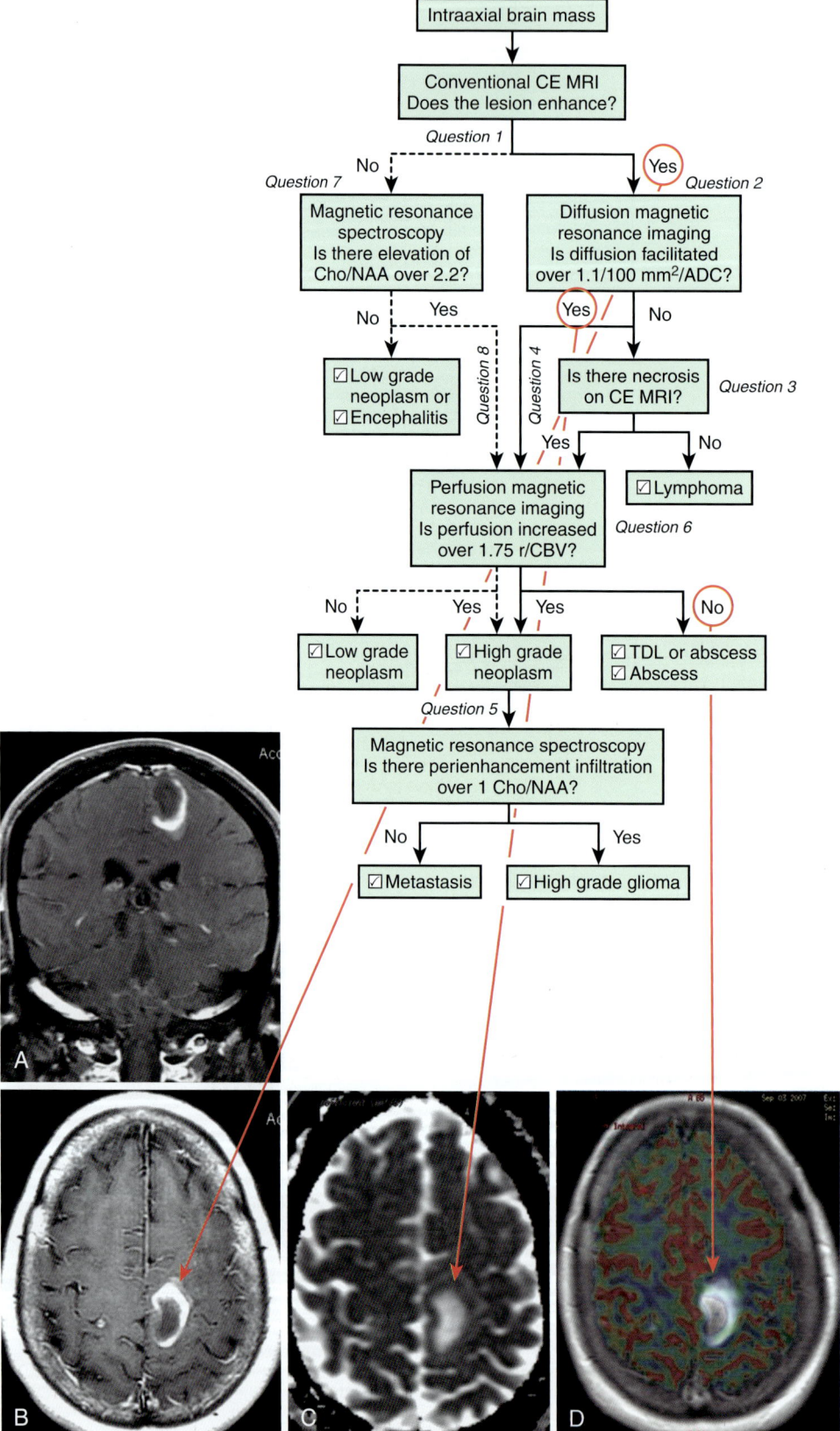

Figure 3-14 A 55-year-old-man with a tumefactive demyelinating lesion (TDL). **A, B:** Postcontrast T1-weighted images (coronal and axial) demonstrating an incomplete ring of enhancement that is often seen in TDLs. **C:** Apparent diffusion coefficient map demonstrating no evidence of diffusion restriction within the lesion, although some diffusion restriction is seen, possibly from acute demyelination, on the leading edge of the lesion. **D:** Gradient-echo axial dynamic susceptibility contrast perfusion magnetic resonance imaging with relative cerebral blood volume color overlay demonstrating reduced perfusion/vascularity within the lesion, even at the enhancing so-called leading edge.

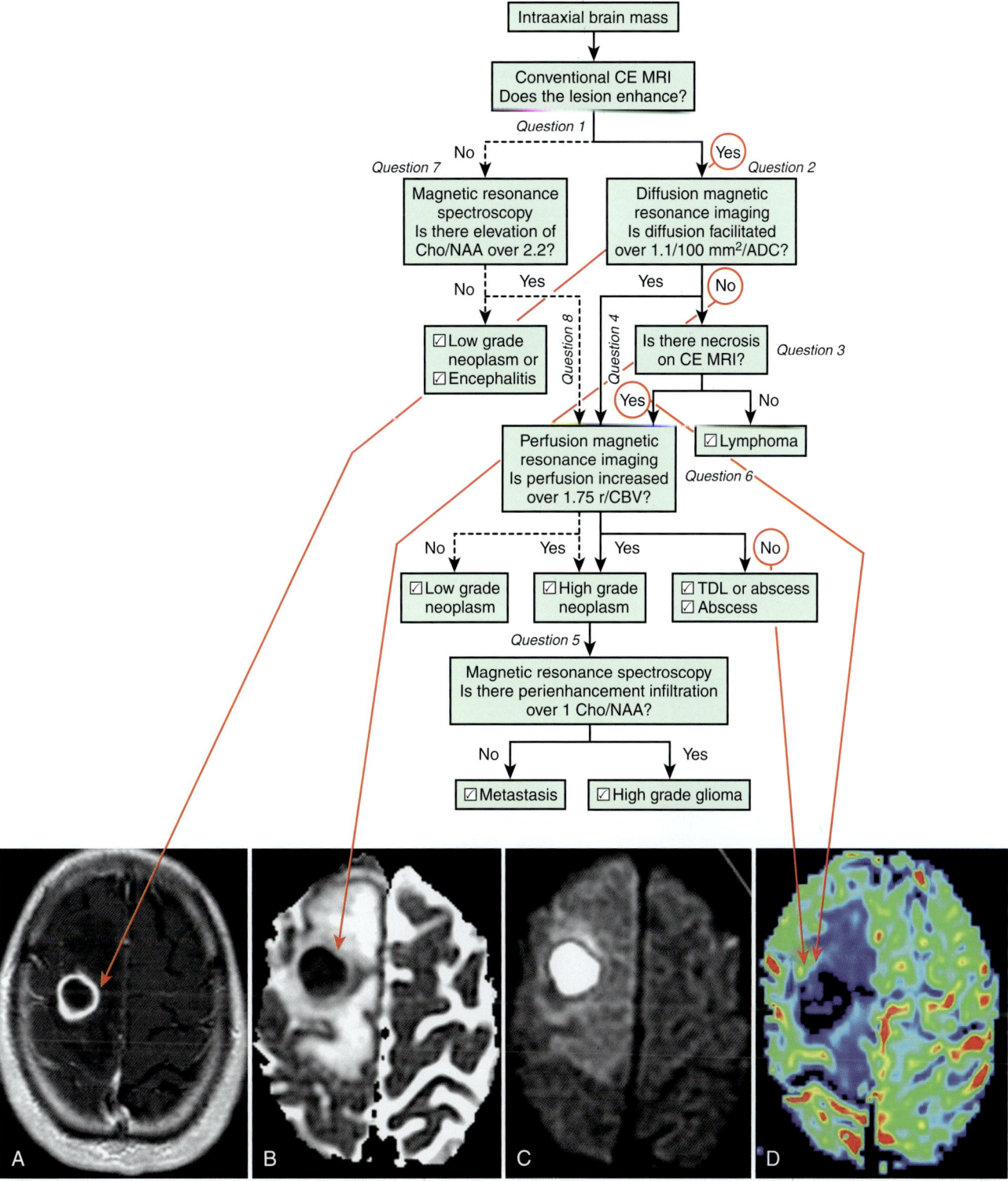

Figure 3-15 A 47-year-old man with a history of tooth extraction, who presented with fever and left hemiparesis. **A:** Mass with central necrosis and ring enhancement in the right frontal region. **B, C:** Diffusion-weighted imaging with apparent diffusion coefficient map demonstrating diffusion restriction in the center of the lesion. Considerable vasogenic edema is seen. **D:** Gradient-echo axial dynamic susceptibility contrast perfusion magnetic resonance imaging with relative cerebral blood volume (rCBV) color overlay demonstrating reduced rCBV within the lesion. Advanced magnetic resonance imaging findings are in keeping with a bacterial abscess.

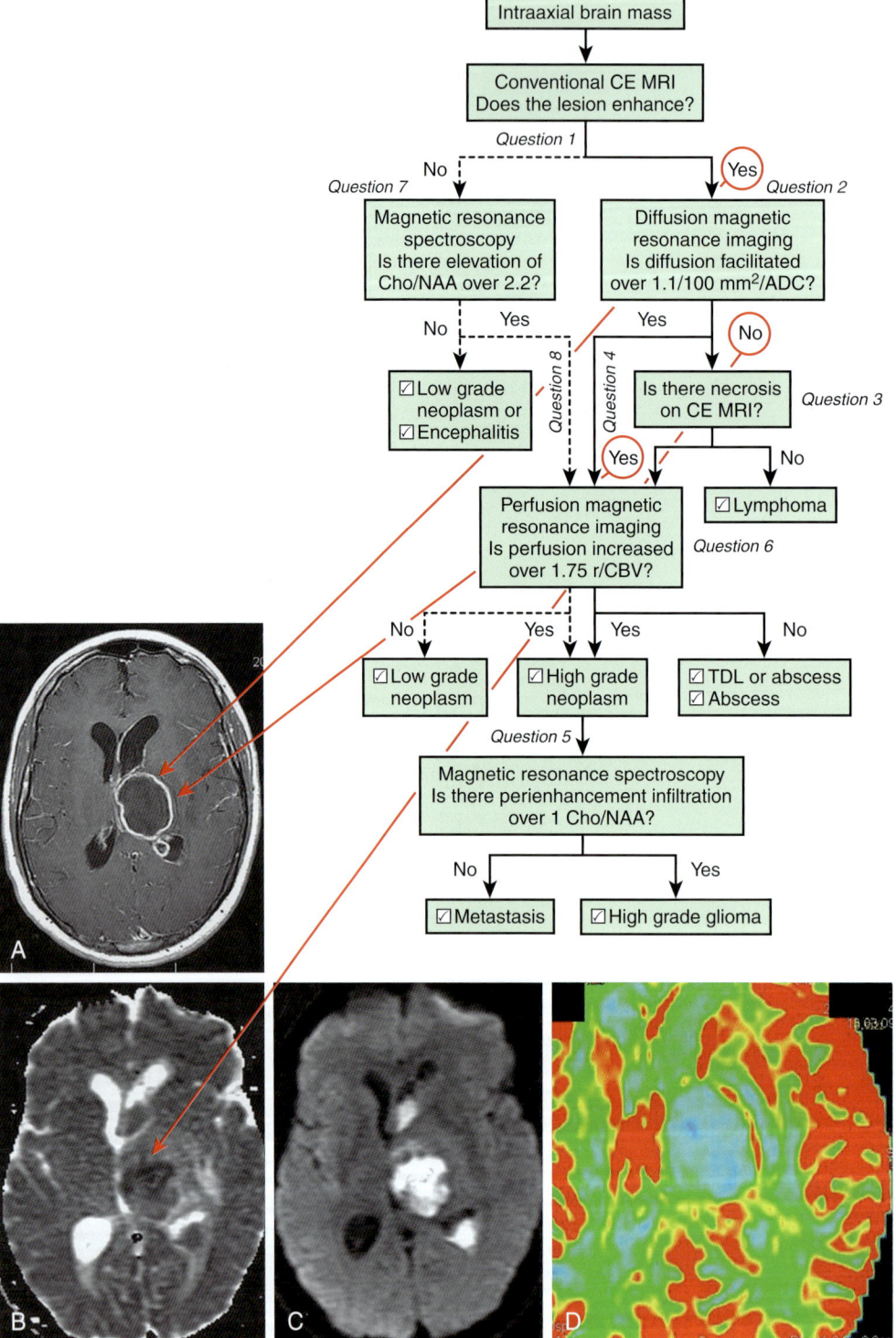

Figure 3-16 A 52-year-old man with a history of colon cancer, who presented with altered conscious state. **A:** Postcontrast T1-weighted image demonstrating a left thalamic mass with central necrosis and ring enhancement. **B, C:** Diffusion-weighted imaging and apparent diffusion coefficient map demonstrating diffusion restriction in the center of the lesion suggesting a bacterial abscess. **D:** Gradient-echo axial dynamic susceptibility contrast perfusion magnetic resonance imaging with relative cerebral blood volume (rCBV) color overlay demonstrating increased rCBV within the edge of the lesion.

ALGORITHMIC-MULTIPARAMETRIC APPROACH

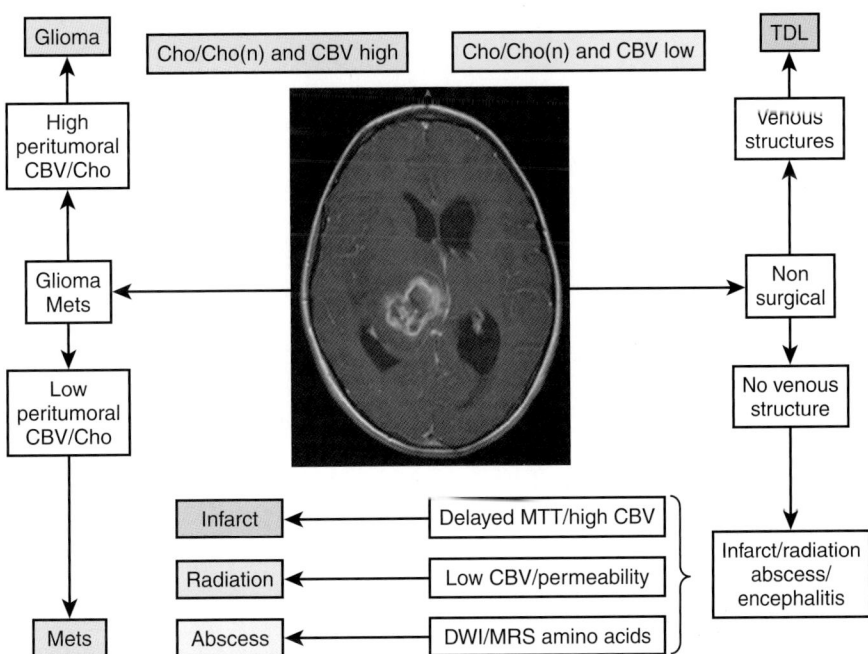

Figure 3-17 An alternate algorithm that incorporates normalized Cho/Cho(n) and relative cerebral blood volume levels as well as perfusion metrics such as mean transit time and vascular permeability. *CBV*, Cerebral blood volume; *Cho*, choline; *DWI/MRS*, diffusion-weighted imaging/magnetic resonance imaging; *MTT*, mean transit time; *TDL*, tumefactive demyelinating lesion.

care should be taken when dealing with a focal lesion having restricted diffusion and high rCBV levels. Using the algorithm, this lesion would be classified as a high-grade neoplasm. Figure 3-16 shows another pitfall in this algorithm in that some infective bacterial abscesses may demonstrate increased perfusion.

Alternate Multiparametric Algorithmic Approach

An alternate multiparametric algorithmic approach that differs slightly from the algorithm shown in Figure 3-5 uses normalized metabolite ratios and perfusion metrics such as mean transit time and time to peak. The algorithm also incorporates vascular permeability for differentiating radiation/therapeutic necrosis from recurrent tumoral disease (Figure 3-17). Although the two approaches have some overlap, normalizing metabolite ratios to the contralateral normal brain tissue likely will increase diagnostic specificity. Figures 3-18 to 3-27 are illustrative cases showing how this algorithm can be used in problem solving.

Normalizing Cho – Cho/Cho(n) and Normalizing rCBV, Glioma and Metastases

The first step in this algorithm is to determine what the pathologic Cho and CBV levels are relative to either contralateral or adjacent normal tissue (Figure 3-18). If considerable elevation in Cho/Cho(n) or rCBV is seen, then the two major pathologies to be considered are high-grade primary glioma or metastasis. If rCBV and Cho are high upon review of the peritumoral or perienhancement region, then there is infiltrating tumor found in an infiltrating high-grade glioma. If rCBV and Cho are low, then consider a circumscribed metastasis (Figure 3-12).

Infiltrating and Well-Circumscribed Gliomas

Pathologically, some high-grade gliomas are well circumscribed lesions with minimal tumor infiltration in the peritumoral edema (Figure 3-19). These so-called circumscribed gliomas are uncommon but represent a potential pitfall in investigating peritumoral edema when differentiating a primary glioma from a metastasis using perfusion and MRS.

Tumefactive Demyelinating Lesions

When reviewing the perfusion images or using new techniques such as susceptibility weighted imaging, tumefactive demyelinating lesions have a predilection for periventricular white matter and demonstrate venous structures running through the lesion. These periventricular veins maintain their normal architecture and are not disrupted or destroyed as would be expected in a glioma (Figure 3-20).

Elevation of the Cho level is consistently found in acute multiple sclerosis (MS) lesions. Explanations for this finding have included reactive astrogliosis, demyelination, and inflammation. Law et al. showed that the mean Cho/Cr ratio in all regions of tumefactive demyelinating lesions was not significantly different from that of normal-appearing contralateral brain. In some patients, however, the Cho/Cr ratio demonstrated prominent elevation in Cho/Cr, which suggests that different degrees of inflammation or membrane proliferation in reactive astrocytes may occur in different lesions. Typically,

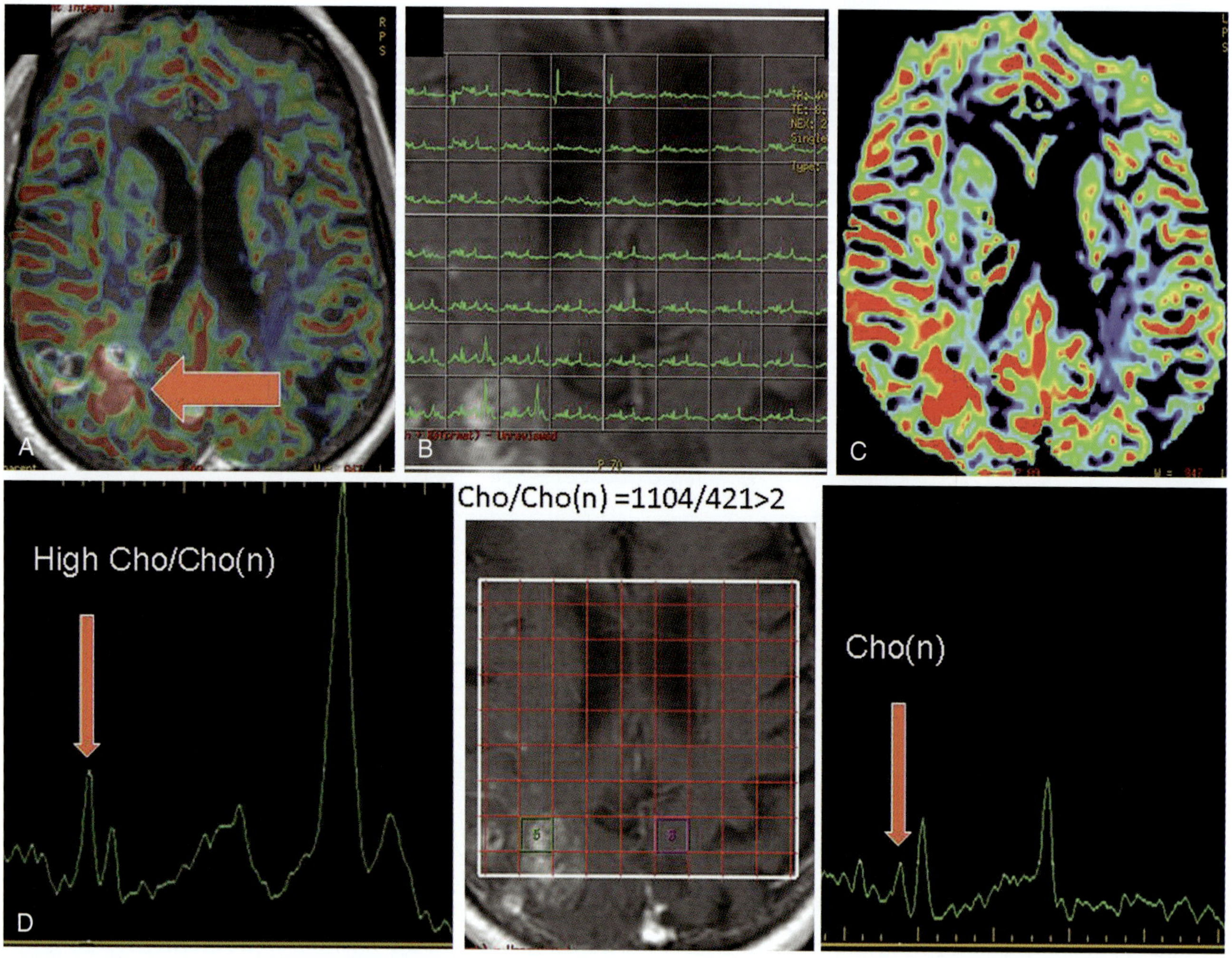

Figure 3-18 Patient with a primary high-grade glioma. **A:** Dynamic susceptibility contrast perfusion magnetic resonance imaging T2* perfusion color overlay map demonstrating an increase in relative cerebral blood volume (rCBV). Cerebral blood volume relative to the contralateral brain is markedly elevated. **B:** Magnetic resonance spectroscopy two-dimensional spectral map demonstrating marked elevation in choline (Cho) compared with normalized Cho(n) in the adjacent and contralateral brain. **C:** rCBV color map confirming elevated rCBV. **D:** Elevation in Cho. Tumoral Cho is at least twice as high as normalized Cho.

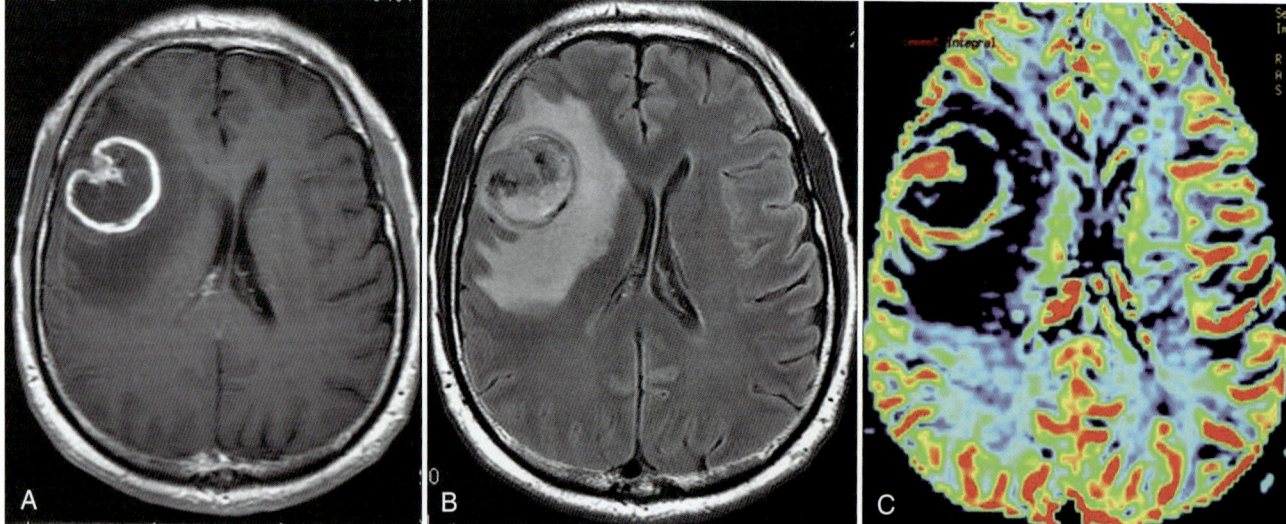

Figure 3-19 Patient with biopsy-proven primary high-grade glioma. **A:** Axial T1-weighted image postgadolinium showing a peripherally enhancing mass in the right frontal region with mass effect. **B:** Axial FLAIR weighted image demonstrating edema surrounding the enhanced component of the lesion. **C:** Gradient-echo axial dynamic susceptibility contrast perfusion magnetic resonance imaging with relative cerebral blood volume color overlay map demonstrating increase in perfusion at the rim of enhancement. However, hypovascularity in the peritumoral region suggests vasogenic edema without infiltrating tumor. This finding suggests a metastasis as a first option, but in this case it was proven to be glioblastoma multiforme.

Chapter 3 Advanced MR (MR Spectroscopy, Diffusion Imaging, and Perfusion Imaging)

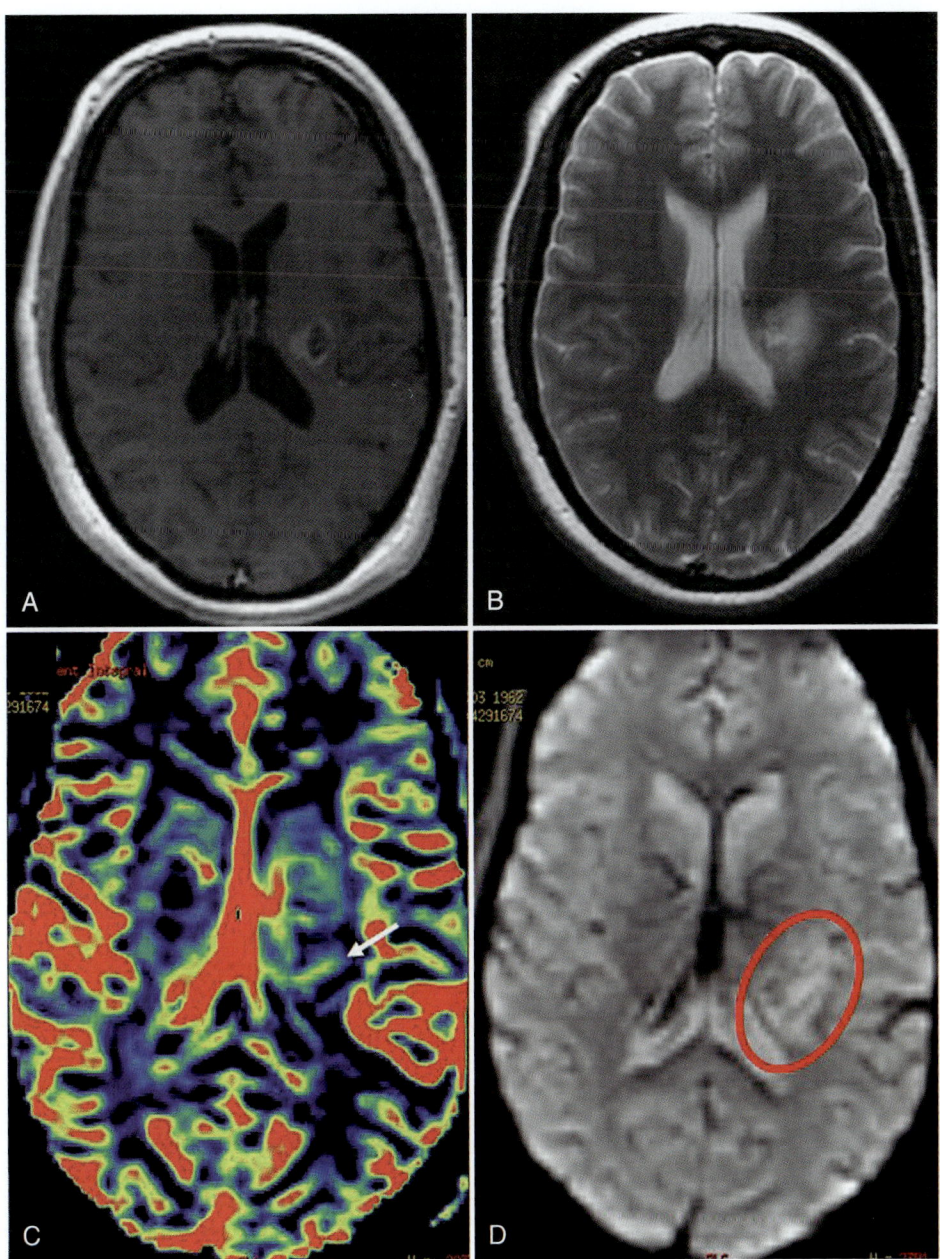

Figure 3-20 A 26-year-old-woman with a tumefactive demyelinating lesion **A, B:** Axial postcontrast T1-weighted and axial FLAIR images showing a lesion in the left corona radiata with minimal edema and ring enhancement. **C:** Gradient-echo axial dynamic susceptibility contrast perfusion magnetic resonance imaging (DSC MRI) with relative cerebral blood volume color overlay demonstrating reduced vascularity within the lesion *(arrow)*. However, venules within the lesion are inflamed and prominent and not destroyed or distorted, as would be seen in a high-grade glioma. **D:** These venous structures are seen best on gradient-echo DSC MRI raw images at the time of contrast bolus peak. Area outlined by red oval indicates periventricular venules.

tumefactive demyelinating lesions have relatively lower Cho/Cho(n) or rCBV than gliomas or metastases (Figure 3-14). A more variable finding in tumefactive demyelinating lesions is the presence of lactate. Local ischemia, neuronal mitochondrial dysfunction, and inflammation all have been proposed as possible mechanisms for lactate and lipid elevation. Another common finding is reduced NAA levels, related to neuronal damage.

Acute Ischemic Stroke

If an acute ischemic stroke is considered a likely differential and the findings are not conclusive on DWI, again review Cho/Cho(n) or rCBV. Importantly, the normalized Cho/Cho(n) is lower in ischemia than glioma, so it is critical to compare the relative concentrations of the abnormal Cho to the normal side. The perfusion maps should also demonstrate abnormal perfusion involving gray and white matter (Figure 3-21). Review of the signal intensity curves from perfusion MRI should demonstrate prolongation in the mean transit time or time to peak.

Therapeutic Monitoring

Therapy-Induced Necrosis and Recurrent Tumor

Treatment options for brain tumors include surgical resection, chemotherapy, and radiation therapy,

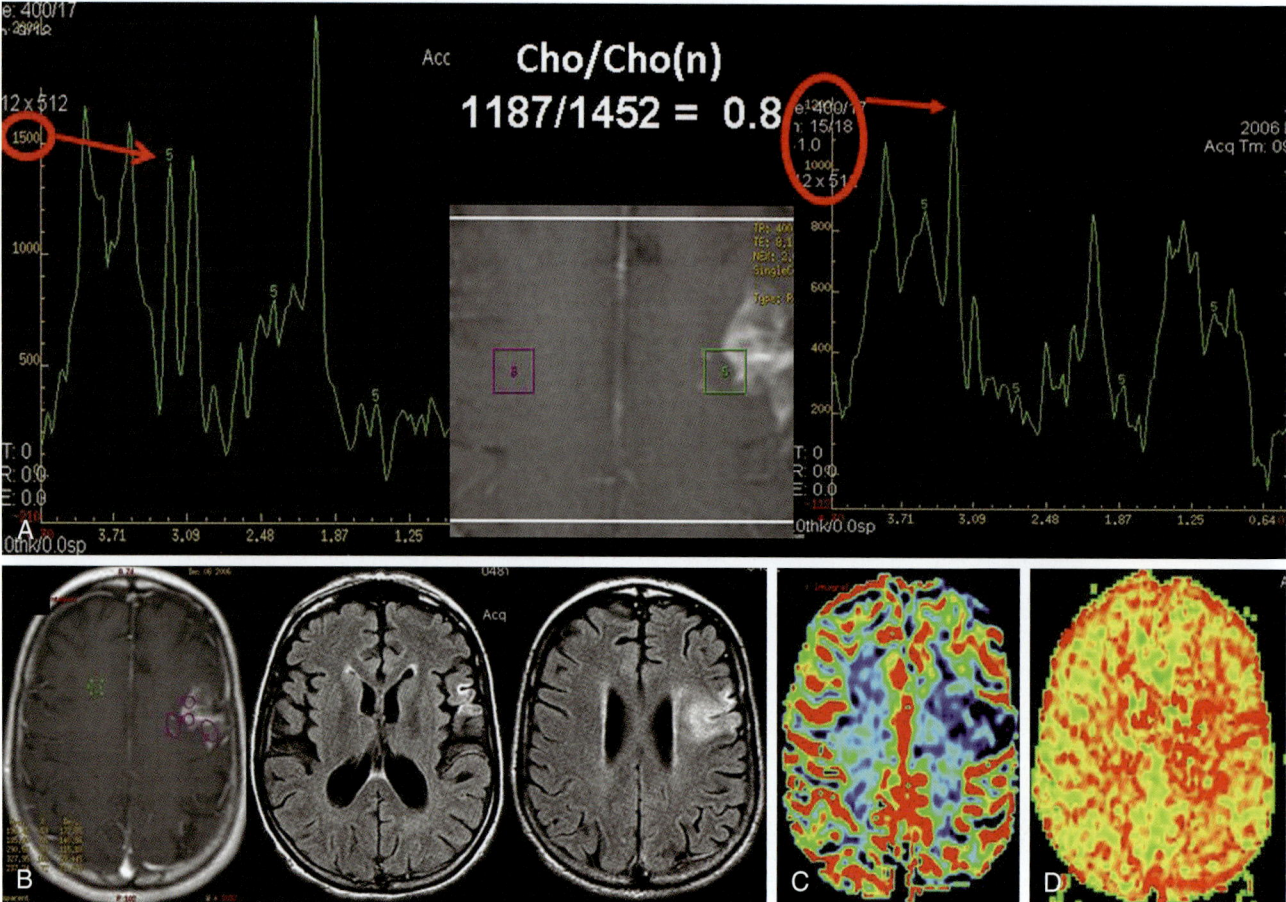

Figure 3-21 Patient with a left insular ischemia stroke that, in the subacute stage, could demonstrate contrast enhancement simulating a glioma. **A:** Normalized choline (Cho)/Cho(n) demonstrating a decrease in relative Cho levels within the enhancing lesion. Cho/Cho(n) levels are approximately 0.8, indicating that this is unlikely to be tumoral disease despite very high Cho/creatine ratio within the lesion. **B:** Postcontrast axial T1-weighted and FLAIR images demonstrating some contrast enhancement and edema. Involvement of the gray and white matter suggests that this may be ischemic. **C:** Dynamic susceptibility contrast perfusion magnetic resonance imaging T2* perfusion color overlay map for relative cerebral blood volume and mean transit time (MTT) demonstrating decrease in perfusion and prolongation in MTT compatible with an ischemic stroke.

which includes gamma-knife radiosurgery, brachytherapy, and intensity-modulated radiation therapy. The differentiation of therapy-induced necrosis (radiation or chemotherapy) from recurrent or residual tumor is challenging. In the clinical setting it is best to simplify these two entities into two diagnoses that are potentially separable with DSC MRI, namely, delayed radiation necrosis (DRN)/chemotherapy-induced necrosis versus recurrent tumor. Unfortunately, most times in clinical practice and at histopathology these two entities coexist, as it is primarily in the setting of residual tumor that the patient receives adjuvant radiation or chemotherapy.

Some investigators have suggested that, particularly in the first 6 months after initiation of treatment, a combination of residual tumor *and treatment effects* or *radiation leukoencephalopathy* must coexist in the same patient. By clinical definition, residual disease must be within the surgical cavity for the patient to receive postoperative radiation therapy. DRN is an entity very distinct from radiation leukoencephalopathy and diffuse radiation injury. DRN results in vascular and myelin damage, and it occurs from a few months to several years and even decades after the end of therapy.

Posttherapeutic conventional MRI often depends on enhancement patterns, edema patterns, and interval change in dimensions to discriminate among gliosis, DRN, and recurrent tumor. These variables often are nonspecific and confusing. Six months after initiation of therapy, DSC MRI can help in determining a good or a poor response to treatment. If substantial elevation in rCBV occurs at any point in time, recurrent tumoral disease is present. DSC MRI is proving to be a sensitive technique in differentiating DRN, and perhaps even radiation leukoencephalopathy, from recurrent tumor. Histopathologically, DRN is an occlusive vasculopathy that results in "stroke-like episodes." Endothelial proliferation can be seen in the early phase of DRN and may result in obliteration of the vessel lumen. Endothelial injury from radiation leads to fibrinoid necrosis of small vessels, endothelial thickening, hyalinization, and vascular thrombosis. If radiation necrosis is a consideration, then CBV and cerebral blood flow typically are low because of vascular narrowing. K^{trans} may be reduced because even

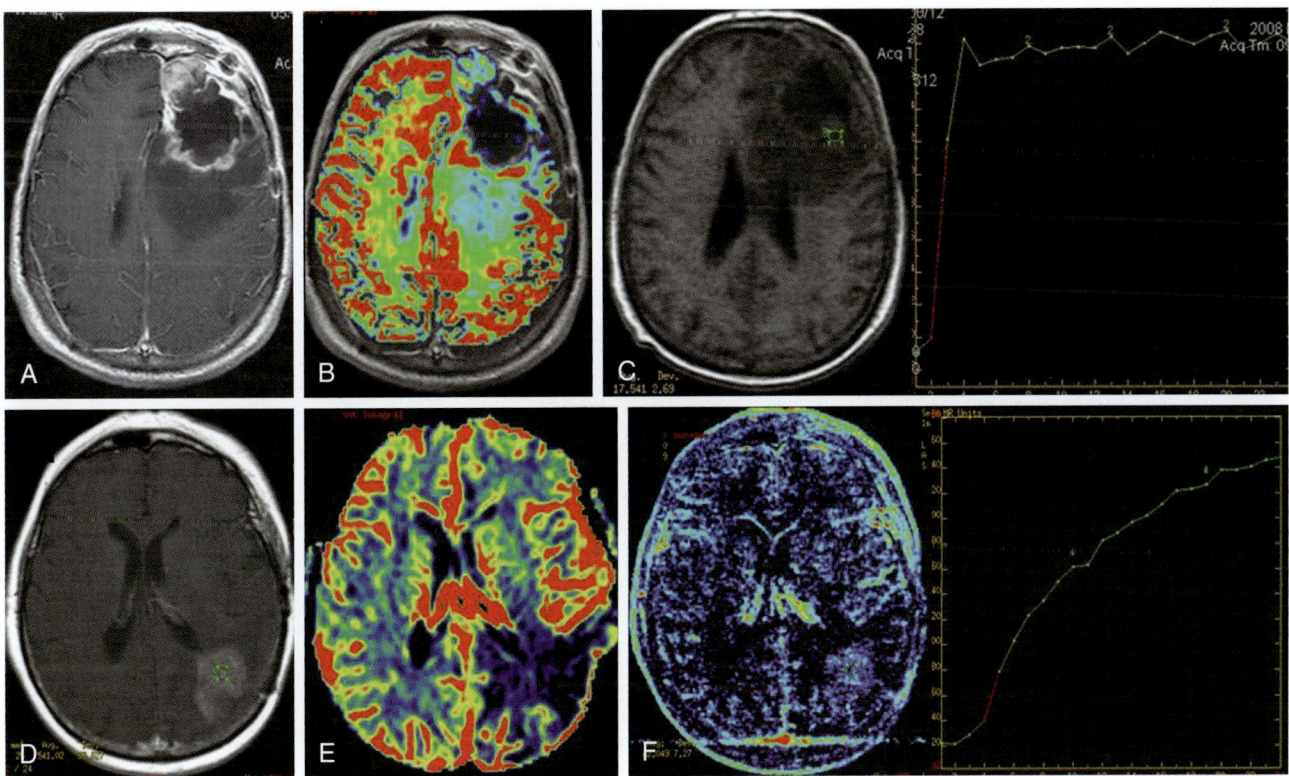

Figure 3-22 Two different patients with recurrent tumor and radiation necrosis, respectively. **A:** Axial postcontrast T1-weighted image demonstrating prior left frontal craniotomy with a ring-enhancing lesion and marked edema. **B:** Dynamic susceptibility contrast perfusion magnetic resonance imaging (DSC MRI) T2* perfusion color overlay demonstrating elevation in relative cerebral blood volume (rCBV) in the enhancing component of the lesion. **C:** Dynamic contrast-enhanced magnetic resonance imaging (DCE MRI) T1 steady-state permeability curve demonstrating a very rapid initial increase in permeability compatible with a vascular phase, then a more steady leakage typical for a highly vascular, highly permeable recurrent tumor. **D:** Slightly less avidly enhancing left parietooccipital lesion. **E:** DSC MRI T2* perfusion color overlay demonstrating a decrease in rCBV throughout the enhancing lesion. **F:** DCE MRI T1 steady-state permeability color overlay and curve demonstrating a much slower rise in signal compatible with a leaky blood–brain barrier from fibrinoid necrosis but no vascular phase.

though enhancement is seen, the rate of enhancement typically is very slow (Figures 3-22 and 3-23). As in the algorithm shown in Figure 3-17, normalized Cho/Cho(n) will be decreased compared to the contralateral Cho (Figure 3-24). Perfusion (rCBV) and vascular permeability appear to be measuring different pathophysiologic changes in the brain. As a result, in some instances not only are spatial differences seen in the distribution of rCBV versus permeability changes, but one metric may be better than the other in characterizing radiation necrosis versus recurrent tumor (Figure 3-25).

DWI in Therapeutic Follow-up

Another application of DWI is in the follow-up of tumors with very high cellularity. A classic example is the use of DWI in demonstrating recurrent tumor in the follow-up of medulloblastoma, which is known to be a very cellular tumor (Figure 3-26). Despite promising results reported in the recent literature, the role of DWI in the quantification of treatment response of brain tumors remains investigational because of the heterogeneous and dynamic reorganization of tumor structure leading to varying changes in tumor ADC values.

Chemoradiation-Induced Pseudoprogression

Data recently reported in the randomized EORTC 22981/26981–NCIC CE.3 (European Organization for Research and Treatment of Cancer/National Cancer Institute of Canada) phase III trial of newly diagnosed patients with GBM given temozolomide plus radiotherapy have provided a new standard of care. With the introduction of chemoradiotherapy with temozolomide as the new standard of care for patients with GBM has come an increasing awareness of posttherapeutic progressive and enhancing lesions on MRI noted immediately after the end of treatment. These lesions are not related to tumor progression but are a treatment effect. This so-called therapy-induced necrosis or pseudoprogression, which can occur in up to 20% of patients who have been treated with temozolomide chemoradiotherapy, can explain about half of all cases of increasing lesions and enhancement after the end of treatment. The lesions decrease in size or stabilize without additional treatments and often remain clinically asymptomatic (Figure 3-27). The mechanisms behind these events have not yet been fully elucidated, but chemoradiotherapy likely causes a higher degree of (desired) tumor cell and endothelial cell killing. The increased cell kill might lead to secondary reactions,

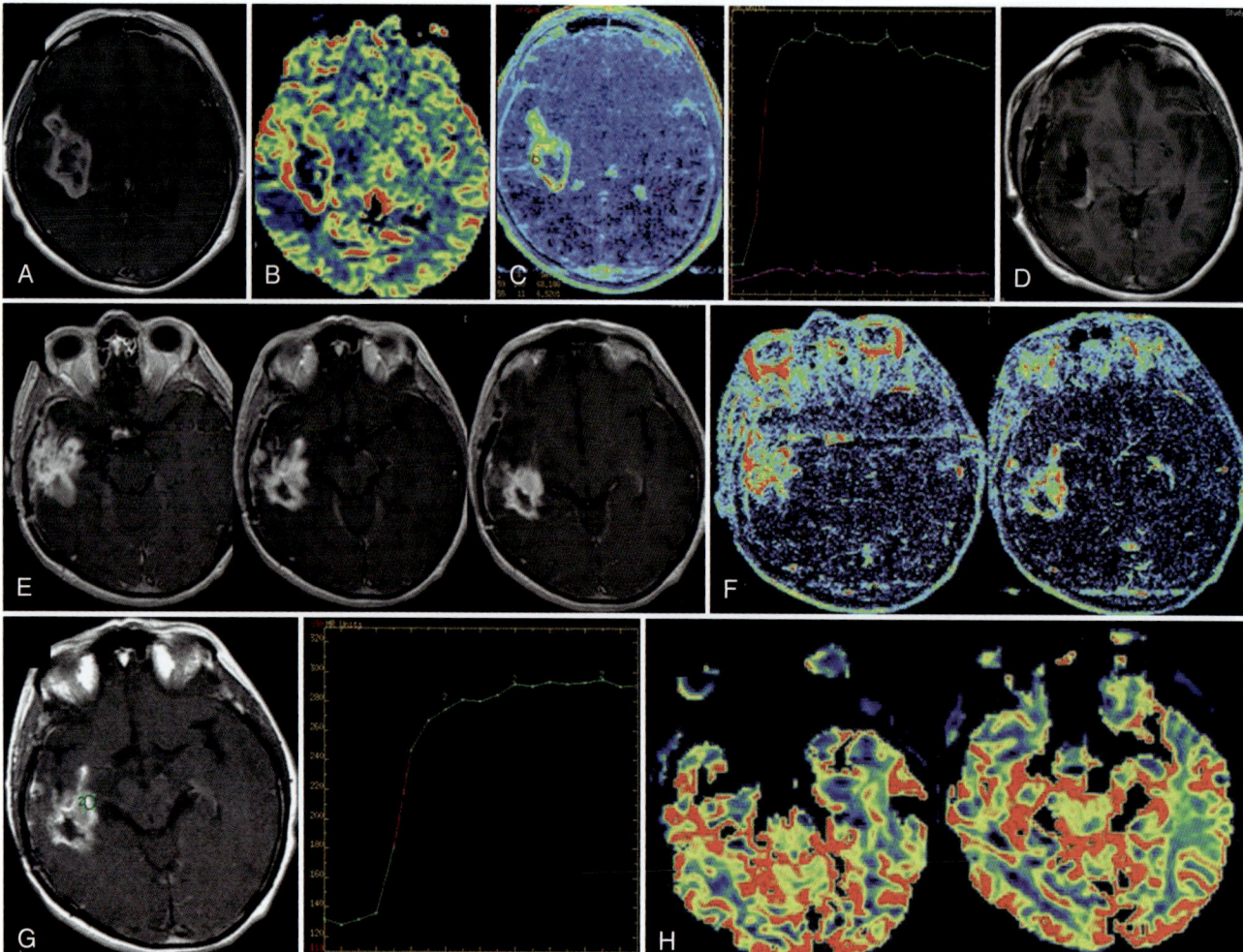

Figure 3-23 Patient with recurrent tumor over a 6-month period. **A:** Axial postcontrast T1-weighted image presurgery demonstrating a right temporal high-grade glioma. **B:** Dynamic susceptibility contrast perfusion magnetic resonance imaging (DSC MRI) T2* perfusion relative cerebral blood volume (rCBV) color overlay demonstrating increased perfusion. **C:** Dynamic contrast-enhanced magnetic resonance imaging (DCE MRI) T1 permeability color overlay with signal intensity curve demonstrating increase in vascular permeability with marked vascular phase. **D:** Immediate postoperative scan demonstrating surgical cavity with a small amount of residual enhancement in the medial aspect of the surgical cavity. **E:** MRI 6 months from the initial surgery demonstrating recurrent tumoral disease. **F:** DCE MRI T1 steady-state permeability maps and curve **(G)** demonstrating a very rapid initial increase in permeability compatible with a vascular phase, then a more steady leakage typical for a highly vascular, highly permeable recurrent tumor. **H:** DSC MRI T2* perfusion color overlay demonstrating a decrease in rCBV throughout the enhancing lesion compatible with a recurrent tumor.

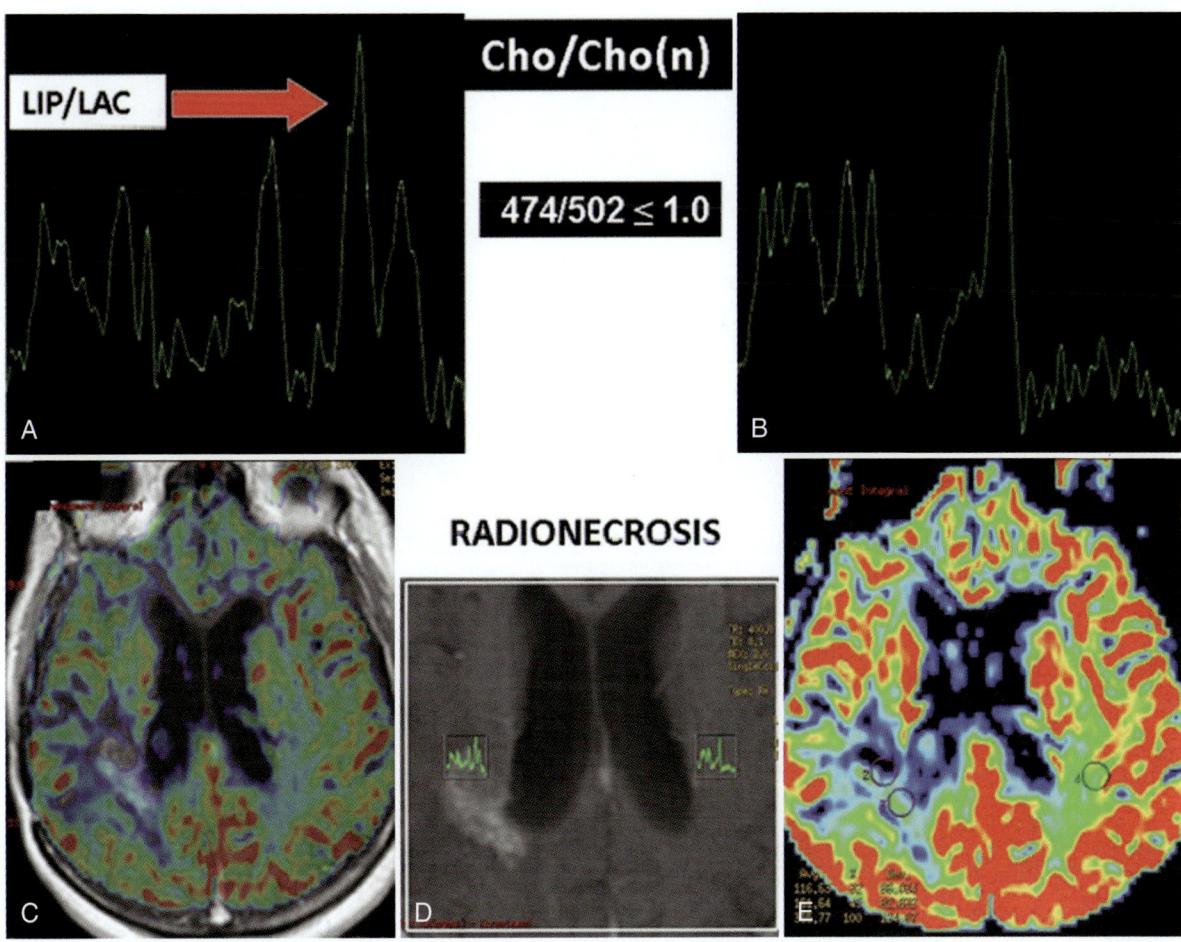

Figure 3-24 Patient with radiation necrosis. **A:** Magnetic resonance spectrum from the enhancing lesion demonstrating lower choline (Cho) levels than the contralateral normal Cho(n) in **B**. Elevation in lipid and lactate is in keeping with radiation necrosis. **B:** Normal contralateral spectrum. Cho/Cho(n) is <1.0. **C:** Dynamic susceptibility contrast perfusion magnetic resonance imaging T2* perfusion color overlay demonstrating decrease in relative cerebral blood volume (rCBV) in the enhancing component of the lesion. **D:** Localizing image demonstrating the location of the abnormal spectrum in **A** and the normal spectrum in **B**. **E:** Color overlay demonstrating the location of the region of interest placed to demonstrate low rCBV in the lesion.

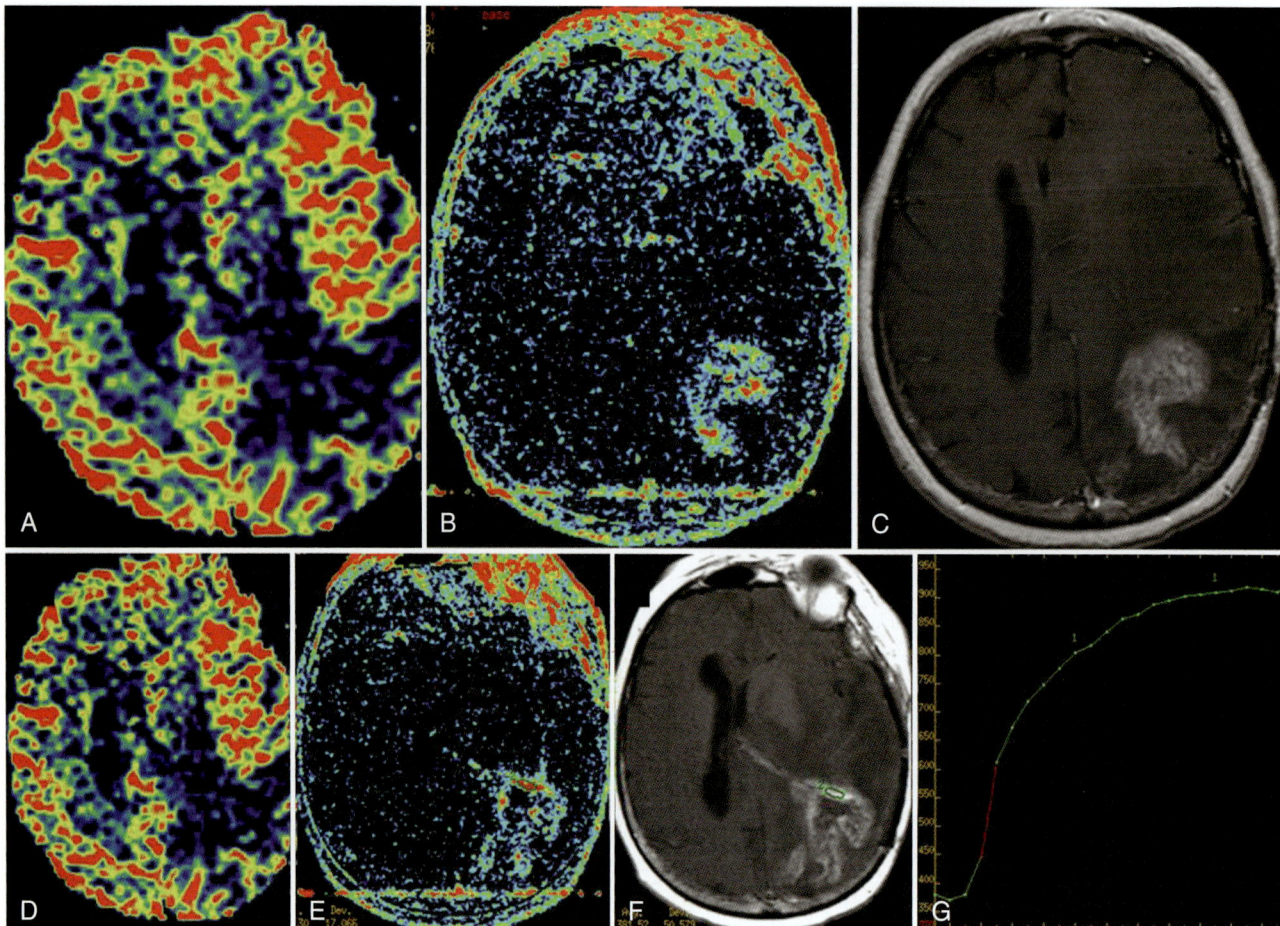

Figure 3-25 Follow-up of glioblastoma multiforme after chemoradiotherapy in a 50-year-old patient. Mismatch between relative cerebral blood volume (rCBV) and permeability. **A:** Gradient-echo T2* axial dynamic susceptibility contrast perfusion magnetic resonance imaging (DSC MRI) with rCBV color overlay demonstrating reduced rCBV within the lesion. **B:** T1 dynamic contrast-enhanced magnetic resonance imaging (DCE MRI) showing some foci of high vascular permeability within the lesion. **C:** Axial T1-weighted postcontrast image showing heterogeneously enhancing lesion in the left parietal lobe in the region of the previously resected tumor. **D:** Gradient-echo axial DSC MRI with rCBV color overlay just above the previous slice again demonstrating reduced rCBV within the lesion. **E–G:** Spin-echo DCE MRI showing some focus of high vascular permeability within the lesion. DCE MRI T1 steady-state permeability curve shows a very rapid initial increase in permeability compatible with recurrent tumor. This case demonstrates a situation where permeability shows recurrent tumor in a lesion with relatively low perfusion, indicating that perfusion and permeability correlate with different pathophysiology. In many lesions there is also often a combination of necrosis and tumor.

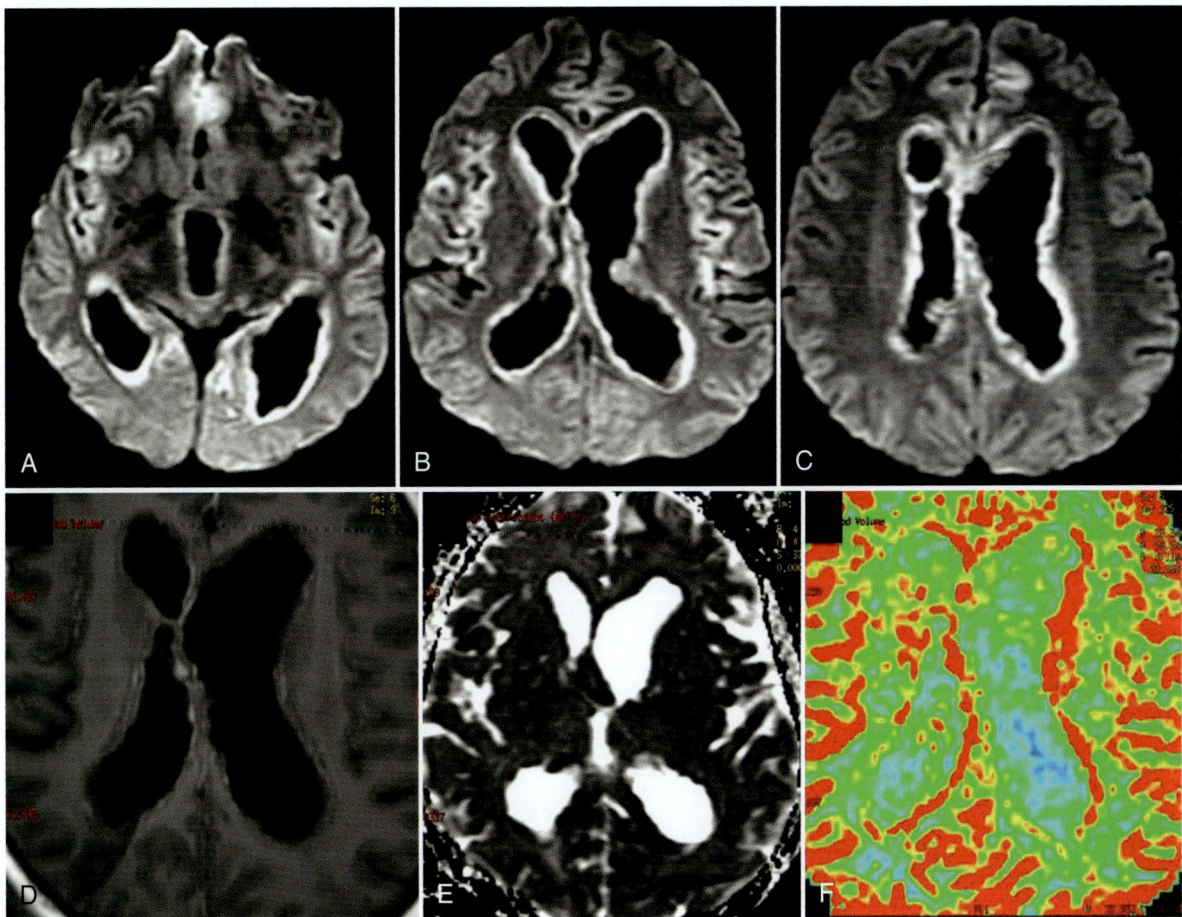

Figure 3-26 Follow-up of medulloblastoma in the posterior fossa. **A–C:** Diffusion-weighted images showing diffusion restriction along the ependymal surface of the ventricular wall, with some nodularity. **D:** Axial T1-weighted image postcontrast demonstrating minimal contrast enhancement. **E:** Apparent diffusion coefficient map confirming restriction of diffusion. **F:** Dynamic susceptibility contrast perfusion magnetic resonance imaging with color overlay demonstrating increased cerebral blood volume along the ependymal surface of the ventricular wall, all in keeping with recurrent medulloblastoma.

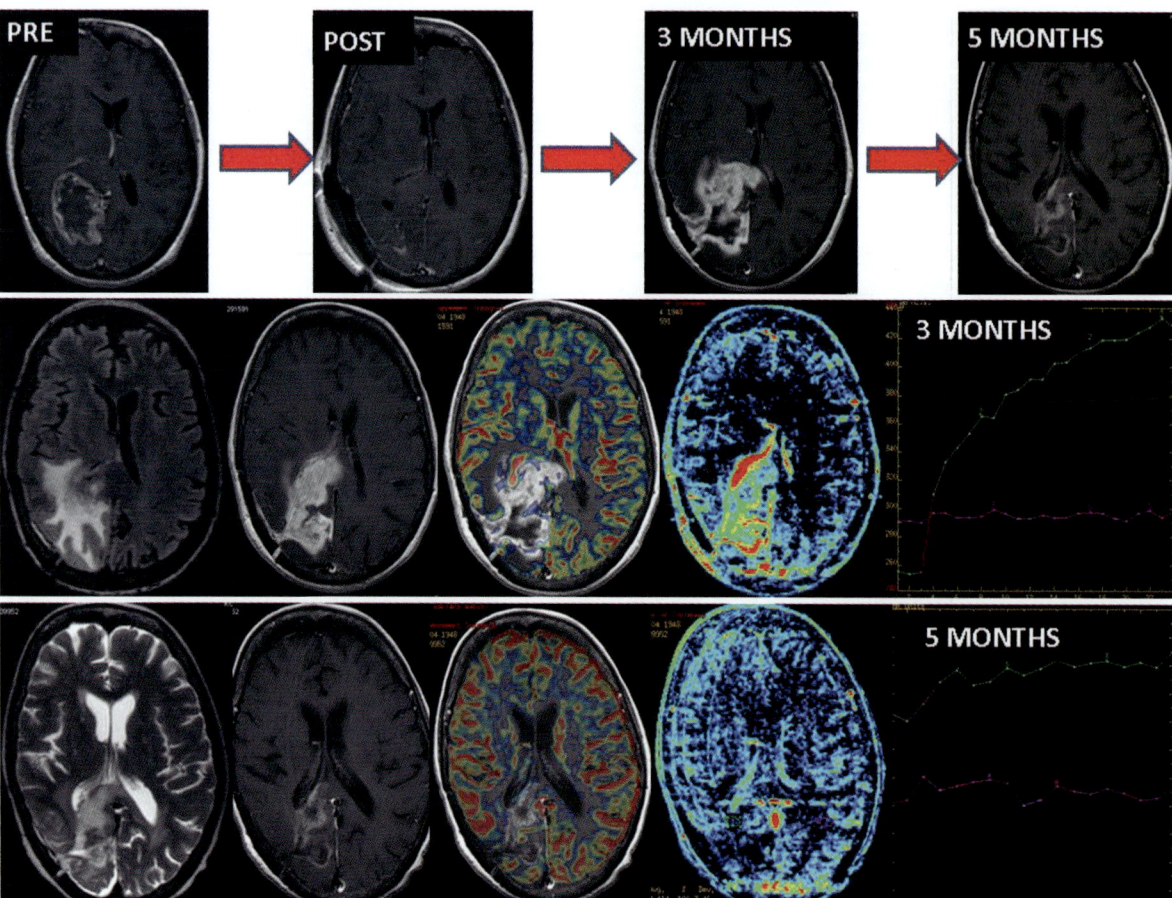

Figure 3-27 Right parietooccipital glioblastoma multiforme in a 54-year-old man. **Top row:** Axial T1-weighted images with contrast demonstrating preoperative enhancing lesion with central necrosis. Immediately postsurgery, there appears to have a gross total resection. The patient received radiation therapy as well as chemotherapy with temozolomide. Three months after chemoradiotherapy, increased nodular contrast enhancement may represent pseudoprogression. Five months after therapy, the lesion demonstrates substantially decreased contrast enhancement. **Middle row:** Axial FLAIR, T1-weighted image postgadolinium demonstrating increased enhancement at the surgical site. Dynamic susceptibility contrast perfusion magnetic resonance imaging (DSC MRI) demonstrates decreased perfusion and dynamic contrast-enhanced magnetic resonance imaging (DCE MRI) T1-weighted permeability color overlay map with corresponding signal intensity curve demonstrates increased permeability, which could indicate recurrent tumor or pseudoprogression. **Bottom row:** Axial FLAIR, T1-weighted image postgadolinium demonstrating decreased edema, mass effect, and enhancement at the surgical site. DSC MRI demonstrates decreased perfusion and DCE MRI T1-weighted permeability color overlay map with corresponding signal intensity curve demonstrates decreased permeability, which could indicate pseudoprogression. (Reproduced from Law M, Lacerda S. Magnetic resonance perfusion and permeability imaging in brain tumors. *Neuroimaging Clin N Am* 2009;19(4):527-557.)

such as edema and abnormal vessel permeability in the tumor area, that mimic tumor progression, in addition to subsequent early treatment-related necrosis in some patients and milder subacute radiotherapy reactions in others. Advanced neuroimaging findings in pseudoprogression suggest a decrease in CBV values and a slight decrease in vascular permeability (as well as an increase in Cho levels), which are in keeping with the proposed pathophysiology previously described. These findings (along with the contrast enhancement) usually regress 6 to 9 months after the initial commencement of temozolomide and radiation therapy and possibly other chemoradiation regimens. Further research is needed to establish reliable imaging parameters that distinguish between true tumor progression and pseudoprogression or treatment-related necrosis.

Radiation injury to the CNS may, in fact, depend on increased capillary permeability induced by radiotherapy, leading to fluid transudation into the interstitial space and consequent brain edema. Furthermore, if capillary permeability is altered, damage from chemotherapy may occur earlier and be more severe. Radiotherapy may enhance the efficacy of chemotherapy by maximizing drug uptake at the cell membrane, disrupting the blood–brain barrier, and/or altering cell metabolism. This can lead to the observation of early radiologic increase in contrast enhancement on MRI consequent to alterations in the blood–brain barrier, thus falsely suggesting tumor progression. This phenomenon may be the expression of treatment-induced necrosis leading to disruption of the blood–brain barrier and passage of contrast material. The potential impact of O^6-methylguanine–DNA methyltransferase (MGMT) promoter methylation status has been described in this group of patients. A retrospective analysis of newly diagnosed GBM patients with assessable MGMT methylation status found that MGMT promoter methylation status can predict the incidence and outcome of pseudoprogression.

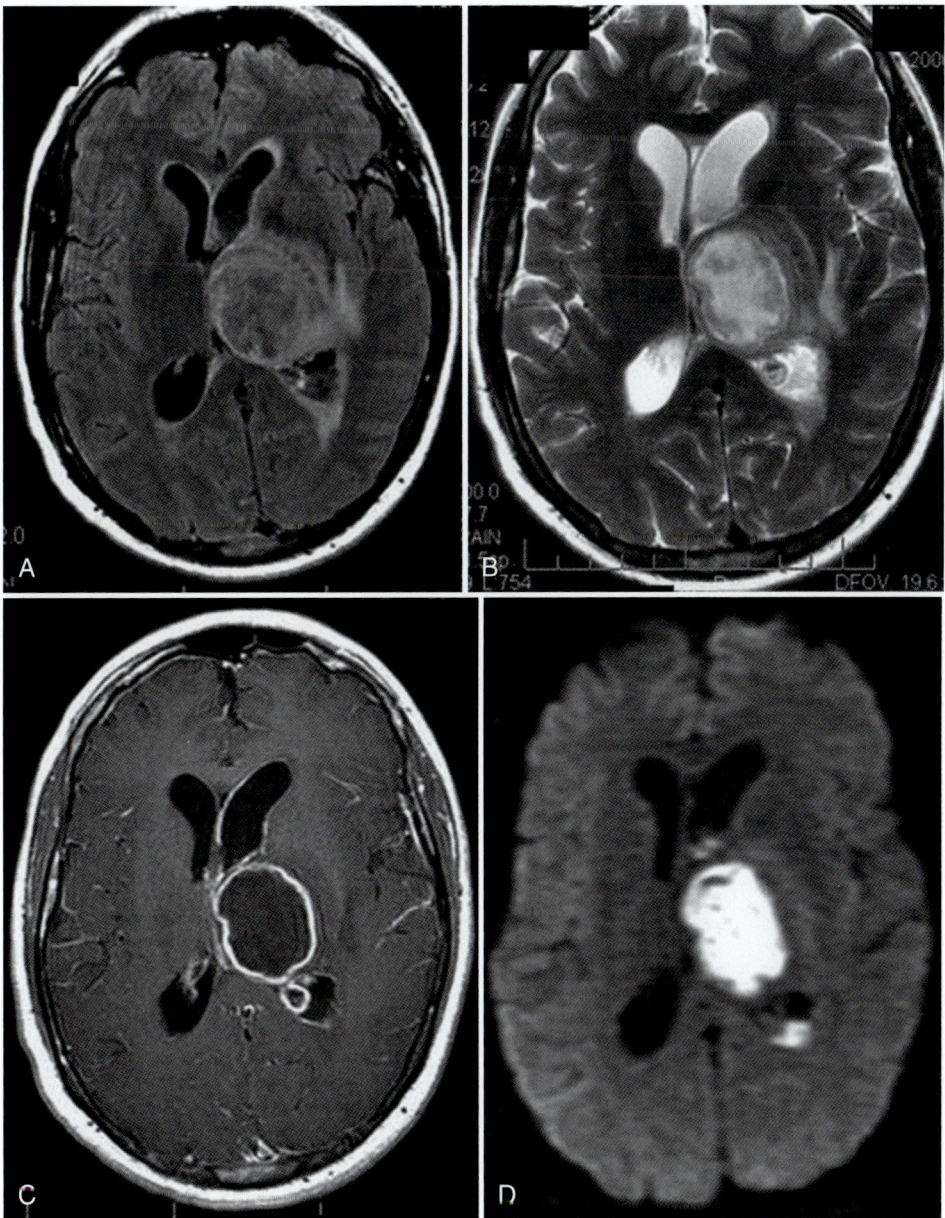

Figure 3-28 A 52-year-old man with a history of colon cancer, who presented with altered conscious state. **A, B:** Axial FLAIR and T2-weighted images demonstrating a bacterial abscess in the left thalamus. **C:** Postcontrast axial T1-weighted image demonstrating ring enhancement with a likely "daughter" component in the left ventricle. **D:** Axial diffusion-weighted images demonstrating diffusion restriction and hyperintensity in keeping with a pus-filled cavity rather than tumor necrosis.

Continued

■ CNS INFECTIONS: BACTERIAL AND TUBERCULOUS INFECTIONS

A major differential diagnosis for ring-enhancing lesions are intracranial abscesses, which may be bacterial, tuberculous, or parasitic. The diagnosis of a brain abscess usually is made by reviewing the clinical, hematologic, and conventional imaging findings. In some instances where the diagnosis is not straightforward, combining MRSI and DSC MRI may increase the specificity of neurodiagnosis. There is decreased perfusion within the central portion of an abscess and in the regions of surrounding edema compared with a neoplasm. There may be a very thin rim of increased perfusion between the enhancing capsule and the region of surrounding edema. Typically bacterial abscesses demonstrate some restriction of diffusion on DWI (Figure 3-28). Bacterial abscesses also have demonstrated the by-products of bacterial metabolism, amino acid levels of 0.9 ppm with or without the presence of succinate, acetate, alanine, and glycine (Figure 3-29). Although ring-enhancing lesions with diffusion restriction are believed to likely represent bacterial abscesses, other pathologies, such as gliomas, metastases, and lymphomas, can demonstrate diffusion restriction (Figures 3-30 and 3-31). This is a well-recognized pitfall.

Typically tuberculous granulomas do not show diffusion restriction, as well as toxoplasmosis, whereas

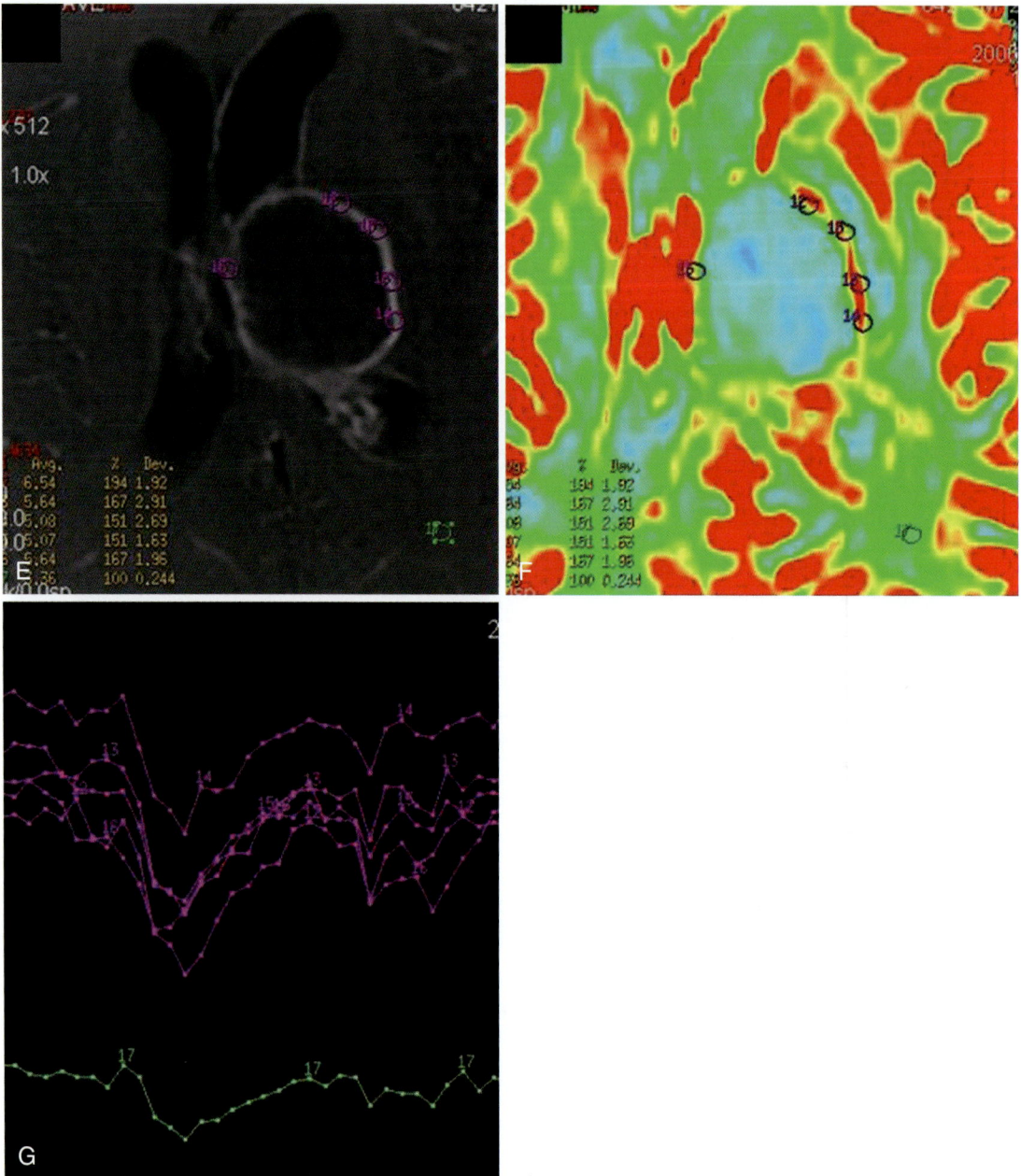

Figure 3-28—cont'd E, F: Gradient-echo axial dynamic susceptibility contrast perfusion magnetic resonance imaging with relative cerebral blood volume (rCBV) color overlay demonstrating multiple regions of interest within the capsule of the lesion show a thin rim of increased rCBV on the lateral cortical side of the lesion. **G:** rCBV signal intensity curve again confirms some increased perfusion in the capsule of the lesion. Haris et al. have demonstrated that the inflammatory cells in the wall of the abscess are positive for vascular endothelial growth factor expression.

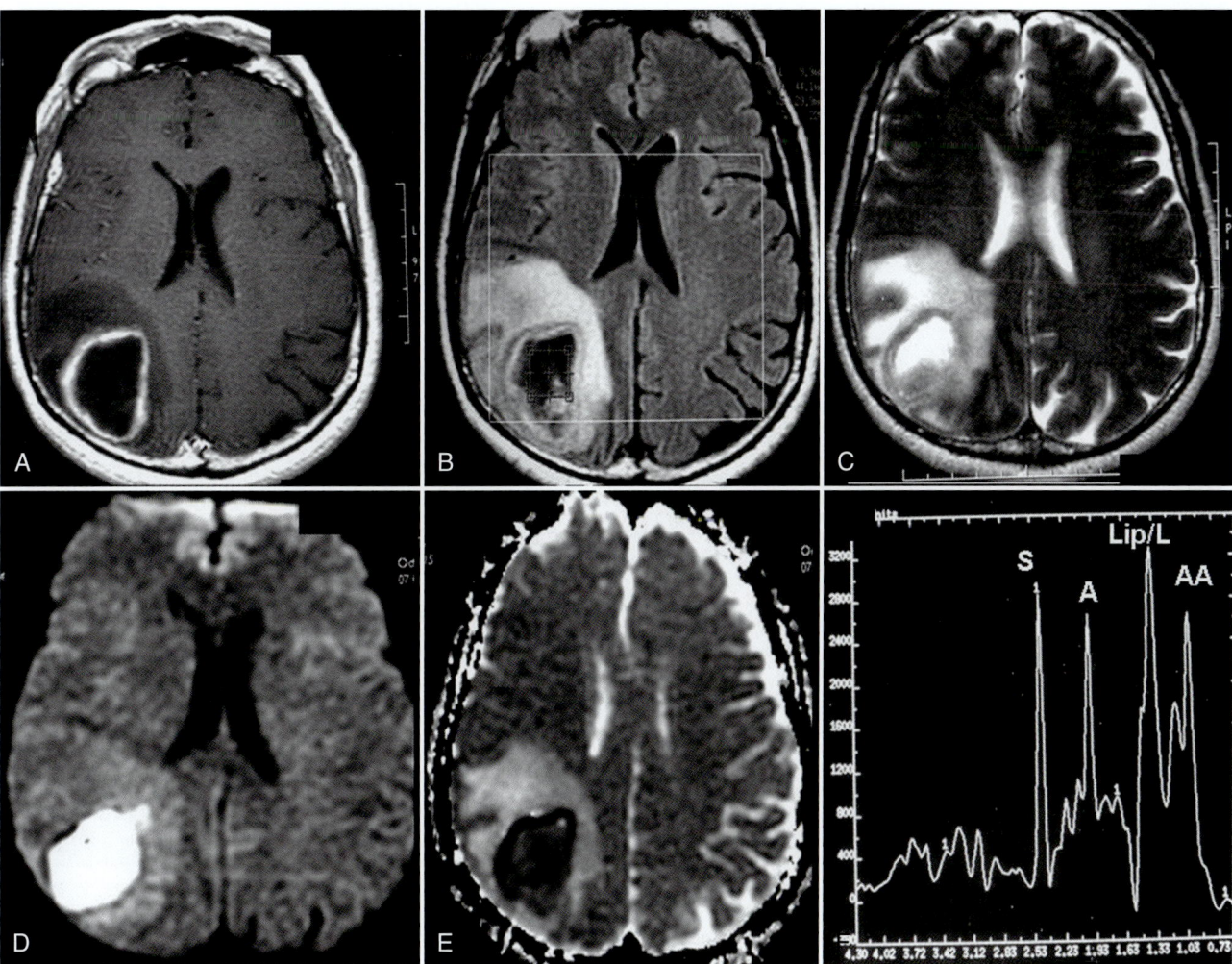

Figure 3-29 A 61-year-old man with a bacterial abscess. **A:** Postcontrast axial T1-weighted image demonstrating a ring-enhancing lesion in the right parietooccipital regions. **B, C:** Axial FLAIR and T2-weighted images demonstrating a moderate degree of vasogenic edema seen in bacterial abscesses. **D, E:** Diffusion-weighted imaging with apparent diffusion coefficient map demonstrating diffusion restriction with hyperintensity in keeping with bacterial pus. **F:** Magnetic resonance spectroscopy showing the presence of succinate (S) at 2.4 ppm; acetate (A) at 1.92 ppm; lipid/lactate (Lip/L) at 1.3 ppm; and leucine, isoleucine, and valine (AA) at 0.9 ppm. Glycine (Gly) at 3.56 ppm and alanine (Al) at 1.5 ppm can sometimes also be seen but are not clearly seen in this patient.

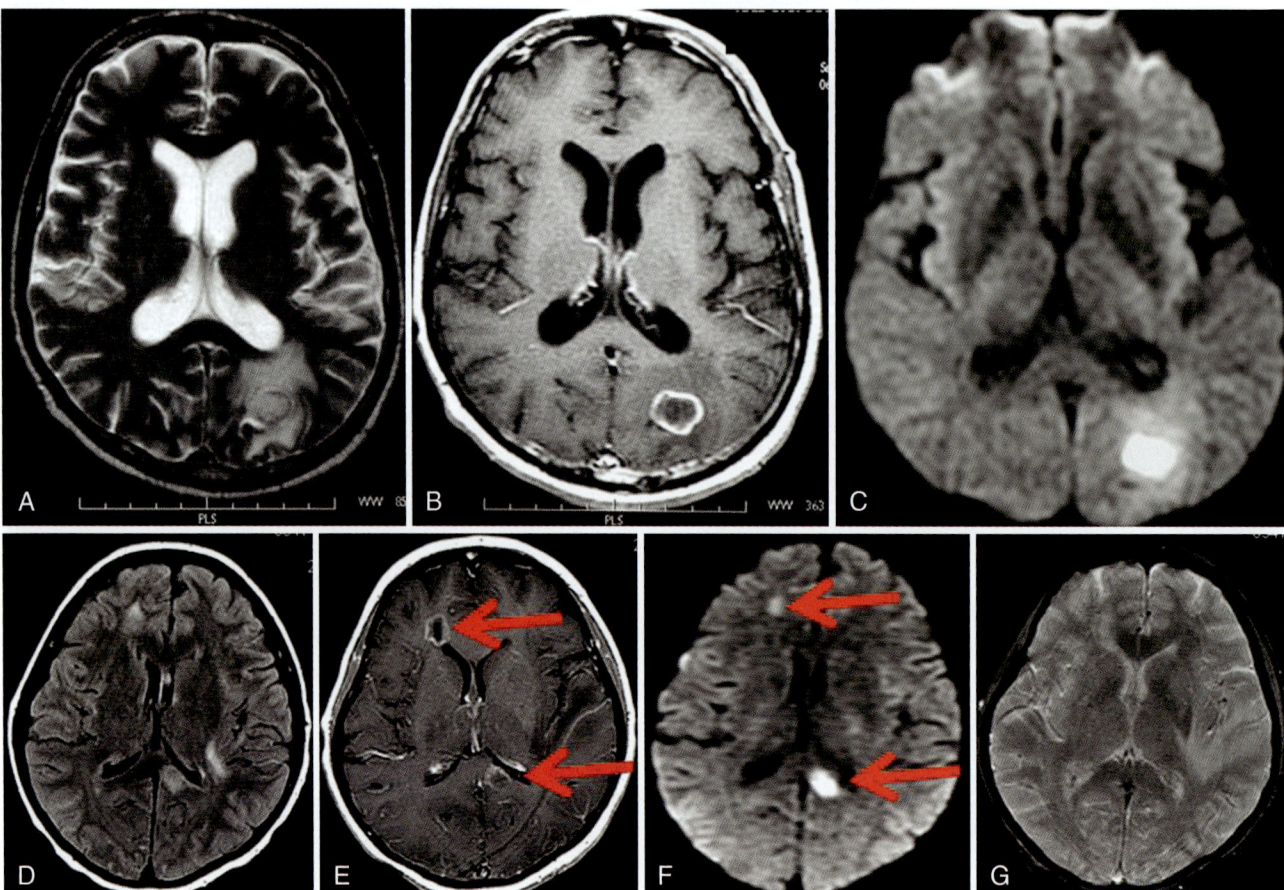

Figure 3-30 A 50-year-old patient with a history of lung cancer and biopsy-proven metastasis to the central nervous system (CNS). **A, B:** Axial T2- and postcontrast T1-weighted images demonstrating a mass with central necrosis and ring enhancement located in the occipital lobe. **C:** Diffusion-weighted image demonstrating diffusion restriction in the center of the lesion. **D:** A 68-year-old patient with a history of breast cancer and biopsy-proven metastasis to the CNS. **D:** Axial FLAIR image showing at least three lesions: one in the white matter of the right frontal lobe, one in the splenium of the corpus callosum, and one in the posterior aspect of the left insula. **E:** Axial T1-weighted image showing peripherally enhancing lesions *(red arrows)*. **F:** Diffusion-weighted image demonstrating restricted diffusion within these lesions *(red arrows)*. **G:** Gradient-echo axial image demonstrating no blood products within the lesions. These two cases illustrate that some metastases can, at least in the early stages, show some diffusion restriction and in this regard must be recognized as a pitfall not to be confused with a bacterial abscess. (Courtesy Dr. Nelson Fortes, Med Imagem, Brazil.)

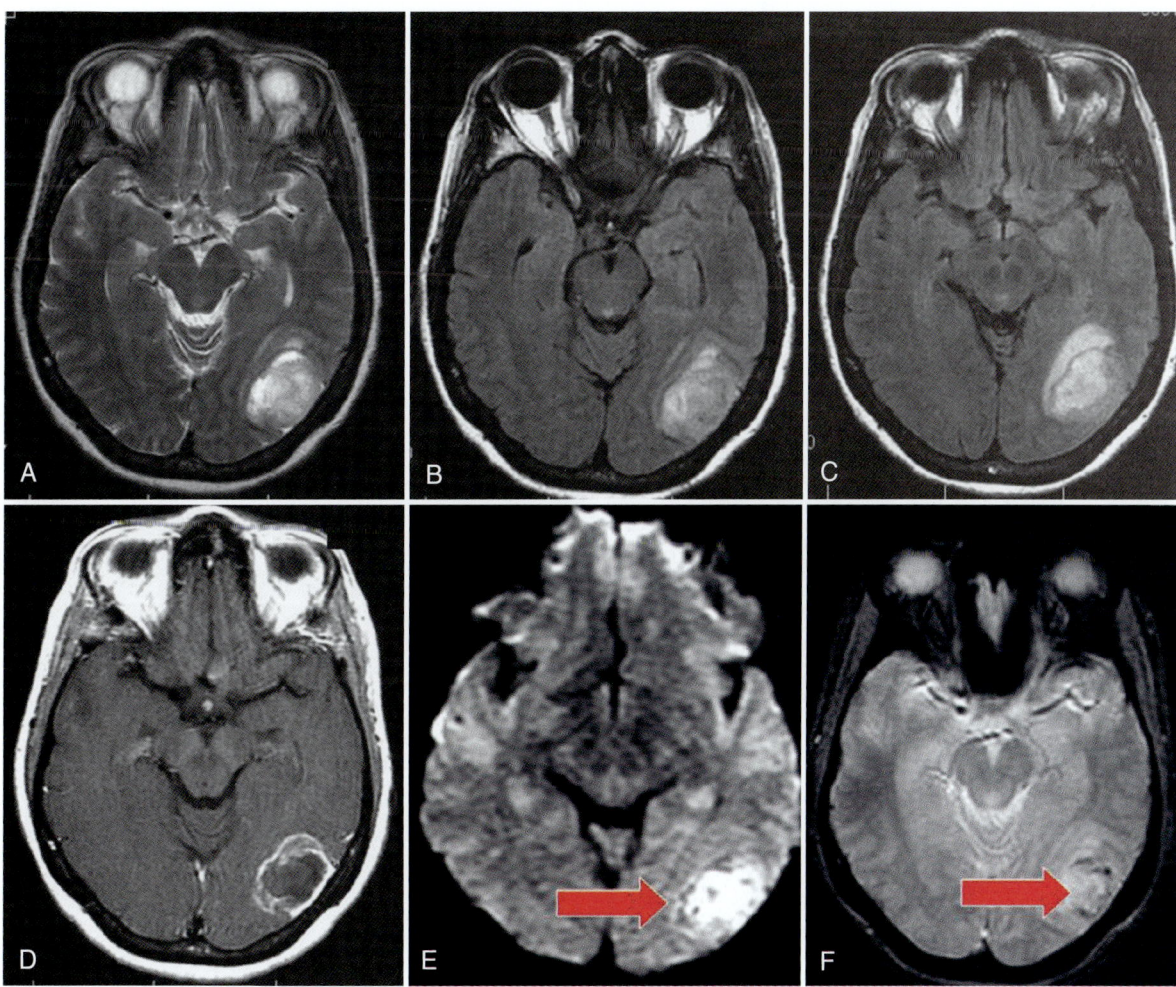

Figure 3-31 A 62-year-old man with biopsy-proven glioblastoma multiforme (GBM). **A–C:** Axial T2-weighted and axial FLAIR images showing a mass in the left occipital region. **D:** Axial postcontrast T1-weighted image showing a mass with central necrosis and predominantly peripheral enhancement. **E:** Diffusion-weighted image demonstrating high signal in the central portion of the lesion. **F:** Gradient-echo axial image demonstrating some blood products within the lesion, which may explain the high signal intensity observed in diffusion-weighted imaging. This is another pitfall in that GBMs can present with blood products centrally, which can be misinterpreted as a bacterial abscess.

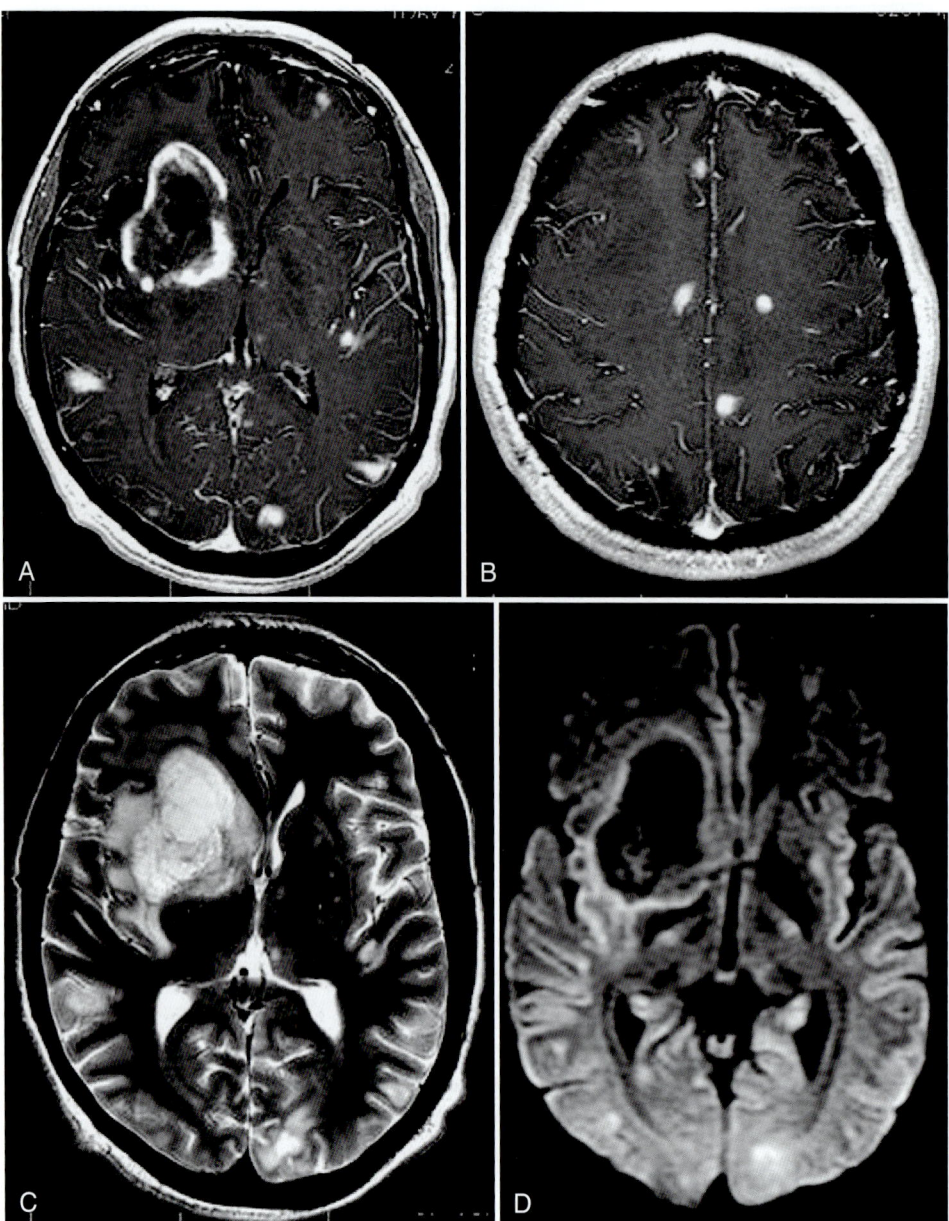

Figure 3-32 A 26-year-old woman with toxoplasmosis (perfusion, diffusion, and spectroscopic findings often similar to those seen in tuberculous abscesses). **A, B:** Axial T1-weighted images demonstrating a dominant mass in the right frontal region with a moderate degree of edema. There are multiple other enhancing lesions close to the corticomedullary junction sometimes seen in toxoplasmosis. **C:** Axial T2-weighted image demonstrating edema as well as mass effect on the left frontal horn. **D:** Diffusion-weighted image demonstrating low signal in the abscess cavity indicating free diffusion.

Continued

tuberculous abscesses can present with diffusion restriction. However, different from bacterial abscesses, tuberculous abscesses demonstrate only lactate and lipid peaks (Figure 3-32) without the presence of glycine, succinate, acetate, and alanine. In vivo studies have demonstrated these metabolites (including lipids) at 0.9, 1.3, 2.0, and 2.8 ppm and phosphoserine at 3.7 ppm. Haris et al. also recently demonstrated that physiologic perfusion indices such as rCBV, cerebral blood flow, and K^{trans} appear to be useful in differentiating infective from neoplastic brain lesions. Their study of 103 patients demonstrated that infective lesions showed the highest permeability, followed by high-grade gliomas and low-grade gliomas. CBV measurements also correlated with microvascular density and the expression of VEGF in excised tuberculomas. There was also a significant decrease in rCBV in response to antituberculous therapy.

■ OTHER INFLAMMATORY MIMICS/ ENCEPHALITIS/ENCEPHALOPATHY

Inflammatory lesions of the CNS, such as cerebritis, encephalitis, and encephalopathy, can mimic tumor. Typically brain inflammation is associated with an element of vasculitis. A full discussion of all of the etiologies of vasculitis is beyond the scope of this chapter. Noninfectious vasculitides are characterized

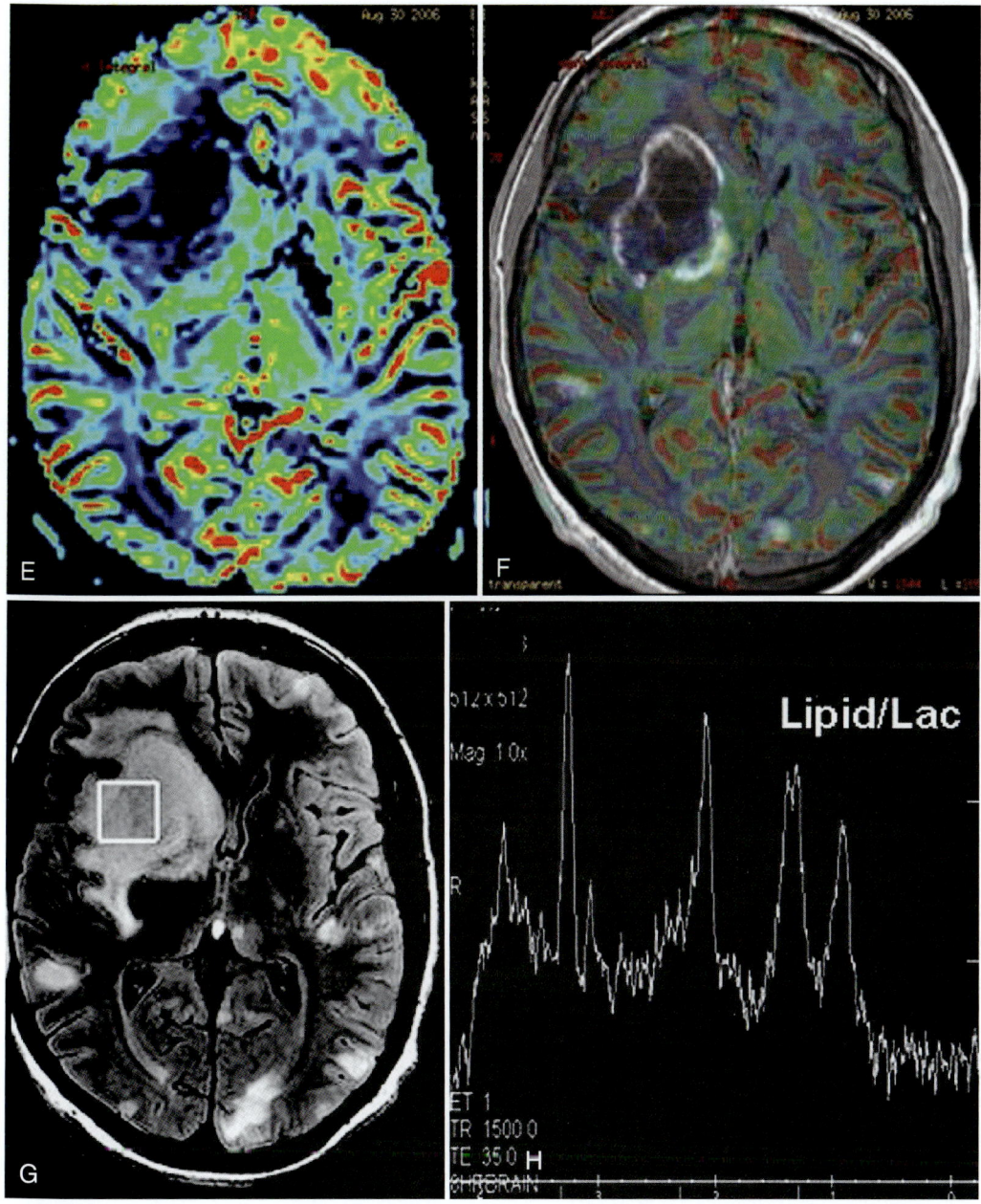

Figure 3-32—cont'd E, F: Gradient-echo axial perfusion MRI with relative cerebral blood volume (rCBV) color overlay maps demonstrating some decrease in rCBV. G, H: Axial FLAIR localizing image showing the location of a voxel placed for magnetic resonance spectroscopy, which demonstrates elevation in lipid and lactate. The finding of the combination of lipid, lactate, decreased rCBV, and diffusion is consistent with either toxoplasmosis or a tuberculous abscess.

by inflammatory cell infiltrates, with varying degrees of multinucleated giant cells, granuloma formation, and fibrinoid necrosis. Several of these vasculitides result in vessel wall fibrosis if the disease state becomes chronic. There is variation within the vasculitides in terms of the part of the vessel wall (intima, media, adventitia) and the type of vessel (large-vessel, medium-vessel, small-vessel, or vein) involved. Systemic vasculitides can cause neurologic symptoms either primarily by affecting cranial vessels or secondarily by causing vascular occlusion or embolism. Consequently, inflammatory lesions of the brain usually result in reduced rCBV use of perivascular infiltrate causing some vascular wing (Figures 3-33). The caveat is the occurrence of substantial blood–brain barrier breakdown, which may artifactually cause an elevation in rCBV. CBV correction should demonstrate a more accurate estimation of true CBV.

■ PITFALL CASES WITH ADVANCED IMAGING

Low-Grade Oligodendrogliomas Usually Have Elevated Perfusion

Numerous investigators have characterized DSC MRI findings in oligodendroglial tumors. Oligodendrogliomas are slowly growing, typically low-grade

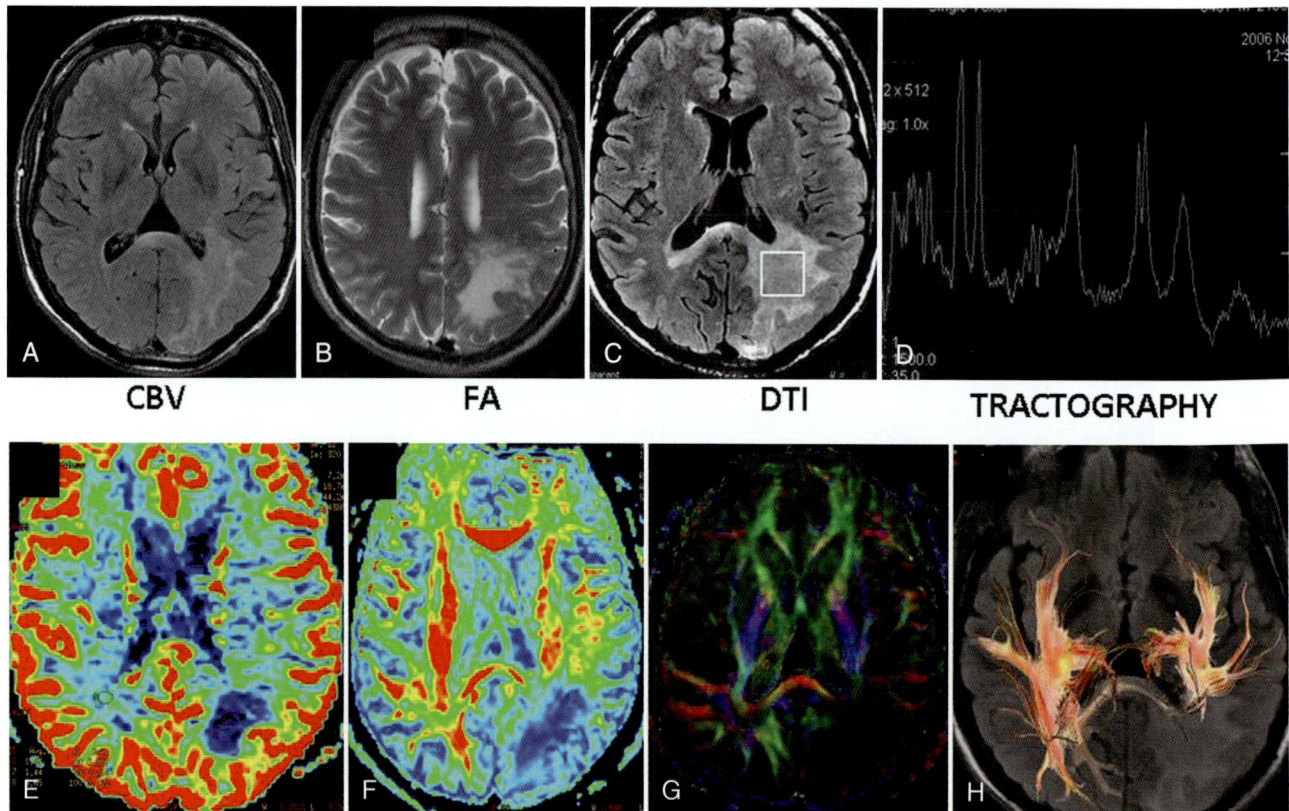

Figure 3-33 A 46-year-old-man with human immunodeficiency virus and progressive multifocal leukoencephalopathy (PML) (perfusion, diffusion, and spectroscopic findings often similar to those seen in encephalitis). **A, B:** Axial FLAIR and T2-weighted images demonstrating abnormal increase in signal in the left parietooccipital white matter. **C:** Axial FLAIR image demonstrating the position of the voxel for magnetic resonance spectroscopy. **D:** Magnetic resonance spectroscopy demonstrating decrease in N-acetylaspartate as well as increased lipid and lactate. The normalized Cho/Cho(n) should be low. **E:** Gradient-echo axial perfusion MRI with relative cerebral blood volume (rCBV) color overlay map demonstrating decrease in rCBV. **F, G:** Axial diffusion tensor imaging (DTI) color overlay fractional anisotropy (FA) and directional color image demonstrating decrease in white matter integrity. **H:** Fiber tractography generated from DTI confirms loss of white matter integrity in the left parietooccipital white matter.

tumors. Oligodendrogliomas have been shown to demonstrate high CBV even in lower-grade tumors. The histologic appearance of oligodendrogliomas consist of a dense network of branching capillaries that produce a vascular pattern resembling chicken wire in addition to the "fried-egg" appearance of the tumor cells, which in part accounts for the increase in rCBV.

Recently, there has been promise in the treatment of oligodendrogliomas with the discovery of the association between 1p 19q chromosomal arm deletions and improved responsiveness to chemotherapy. Given the histopathologic and molecular evidence supporting increased neovascularity in gliomas with oligodendroglial components, the association between 1p 19q deletions and increased perfusion seems to warrant further investigation. Investigators found that elevated rCBV raises the possibility of a 1p 19q chromosomal deletion in human gliomas. Thus, rCBV may serve as an important physiologic imaging biomarker for identifying gliomas with 1p 19q chromosomal deletions conferring higher chemosensitivity (Figure 3-34). Furthermore, DSC MRI may provide noninvasive physiologic imaging markers of potential molecular signatures that identify microvascular proliferation, malignant transformation, patient outcome, and response to therapy.

Extraaxial Neoplasms (Meningioma, Schwannoma) Also Have High Perfusion

Relative CBV may not be as reliable in differentiating extraaxial from intraaxial lesions in the brain because substantial contrast leakage from the lack of a blood–brain barrier in extraaxial lesions can give erroneously low or high uncorrected CBV values. However, evaluating the signal intensity–time curve and determining the degree of permeability may be helpful in the clinical setting. In extraaxial lesions, the signal intensity–time curve demonstrates immediate and continued leakage of contrast compared with intraaxial lesions. Meningiomas are the most common extraaxial tumors and usually are a straightforward diagnosis on conventional MRI, obviating the need for DSC MRI or biopsy. rCBV and K^{trans} usually are elevated in meningiomas.

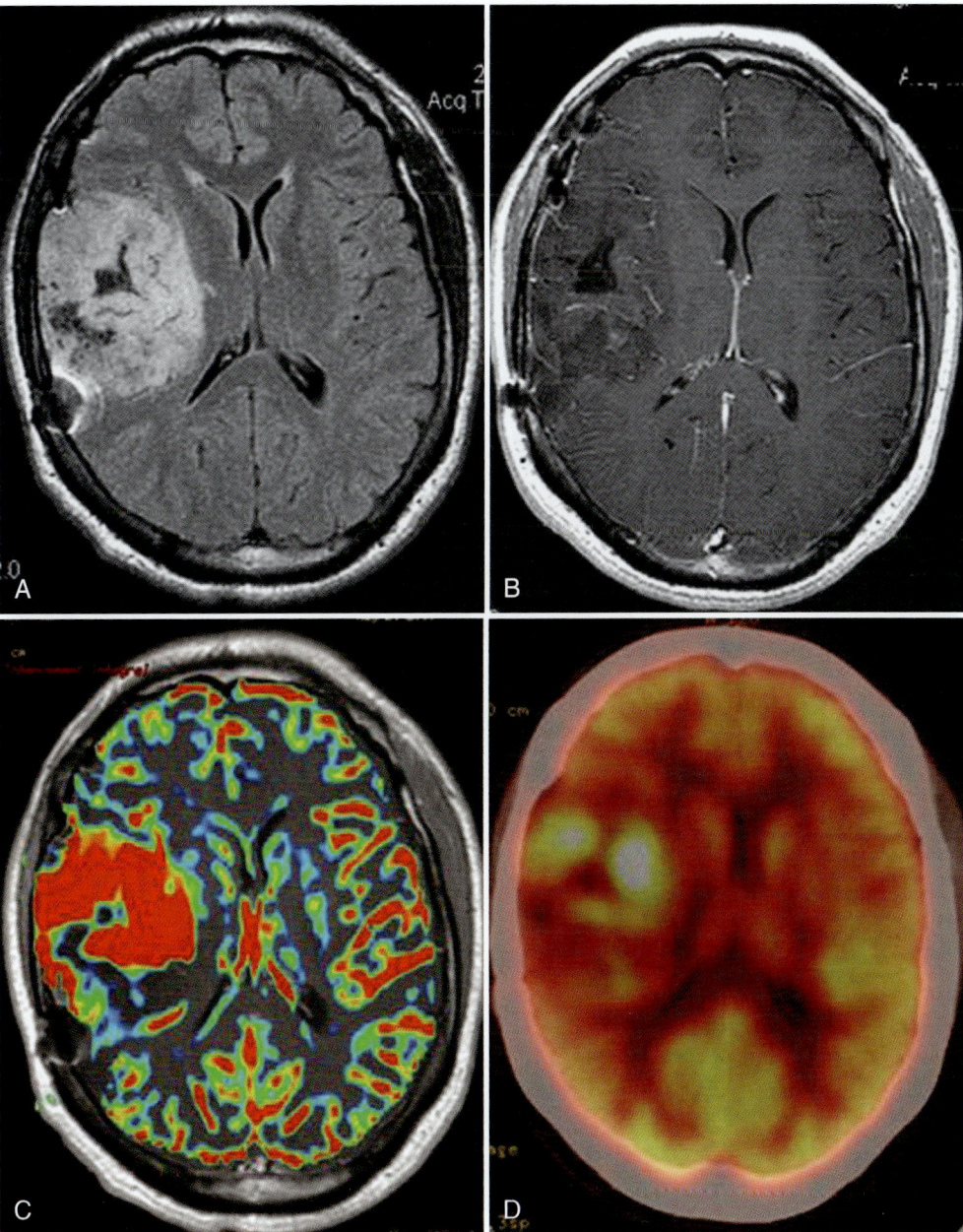

Figure 3-34 A 63-year-old man with pathology-proven oligodendroglioma and high perfusion relative cerebral blood volume (rCBV) of 6 and 1p19q allelic deletions. **A:** Axial FLAIR image demonstrating a cortically based right frontal lesion with mass effect. **B:** Contrast-enhanced axial T1-weighted image demonstrating a minimally enhancing mass in the right frontotemporal region. **C:** Axial dynamic susceptibility contrast perfusion magnetic resonance imaging with rCBV color overlay map showing a lesion with very high perfusion and rCBV of 6. Low-grade oligodendrogliomas have been described to have elevated perfusion. This is a pitfall when using perfusion to determine tumor grade. **D:** Fluorodeoxyglucose positron emission tomographic (FDG PET) image demonstrating increased FDG uptake in the lesion.

Continued

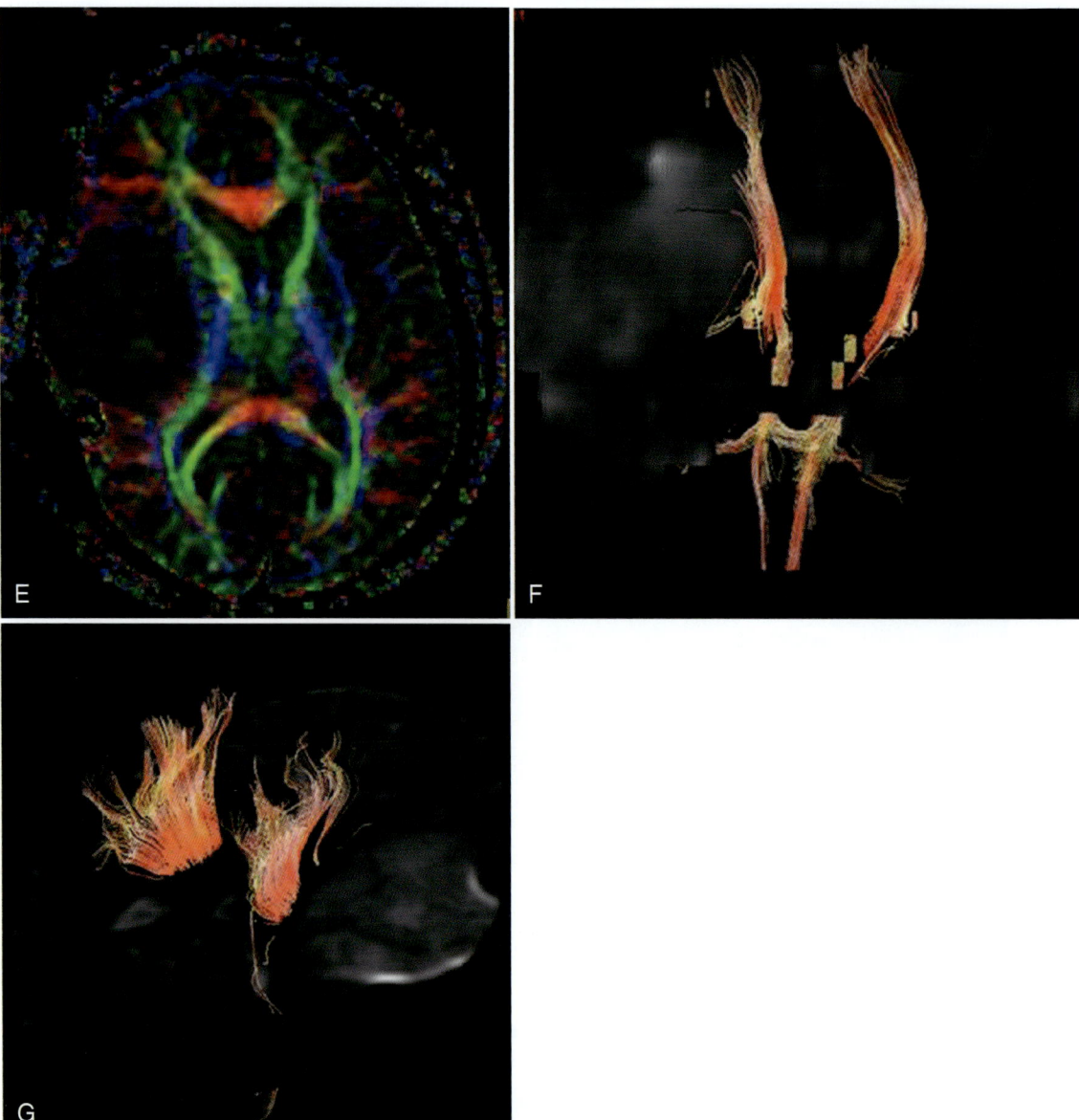

Figure 3-34—cont'd E: Color-coded directional fractional anisotropy map demonstrating the circumscribed oligodendroglioma likely is displacing rather than destroying the adjacent corticospinal tracts in the posterior *(blue)* and anterior *(green)* limbs of the internal capsule. **F, G:** Fiber tractography confirms the integrity of the corticospinal tracts.

Meningiomas are known pathologically and at angiography to be vascular tumors. There also appears to be good correlation between K^{trans} and the histologic grade of meningiomas (Figure 3-35). Pathologically, higher K^{trans} measurements may be related to the degree of micronecrosis found in atypical meningiomas. Because the atypical and typical variants of meningioma have different recurrence rates, measurement of K^{trans} provides a prospective measure of tumor behavior, and this information could help avoid surprises, such as brain invasion, that could be planned for successfully if the information were available to the neurosurgeon preoperatively.

DSC MRI can increase the sensitivity of diagnosis in extraaxial masses. Differentiating between meningioma and acoustic neuroma at the cerebellopontine angle can be a challenge. Lower vascular permeability has been found in typical meningiomas compared to acoustic neuromas.

Advanced MRI as Biomarkers for Therapeutic Response in Novel Antiangiogenic Agents

Malignant gliomas, particularly recurrent anaplastic gliomas and GBM, are highly refractory to therapy. A key feature of malignant gliomas, such as GBM, is their tendency to infiltrate surrounding tissues. This invasive property often precludes total surgical resection and makes it difficult to treat with radiation without damaging normal brain parenchyma. Because of the difficulty in obtaining total resection, patients with GBM have a

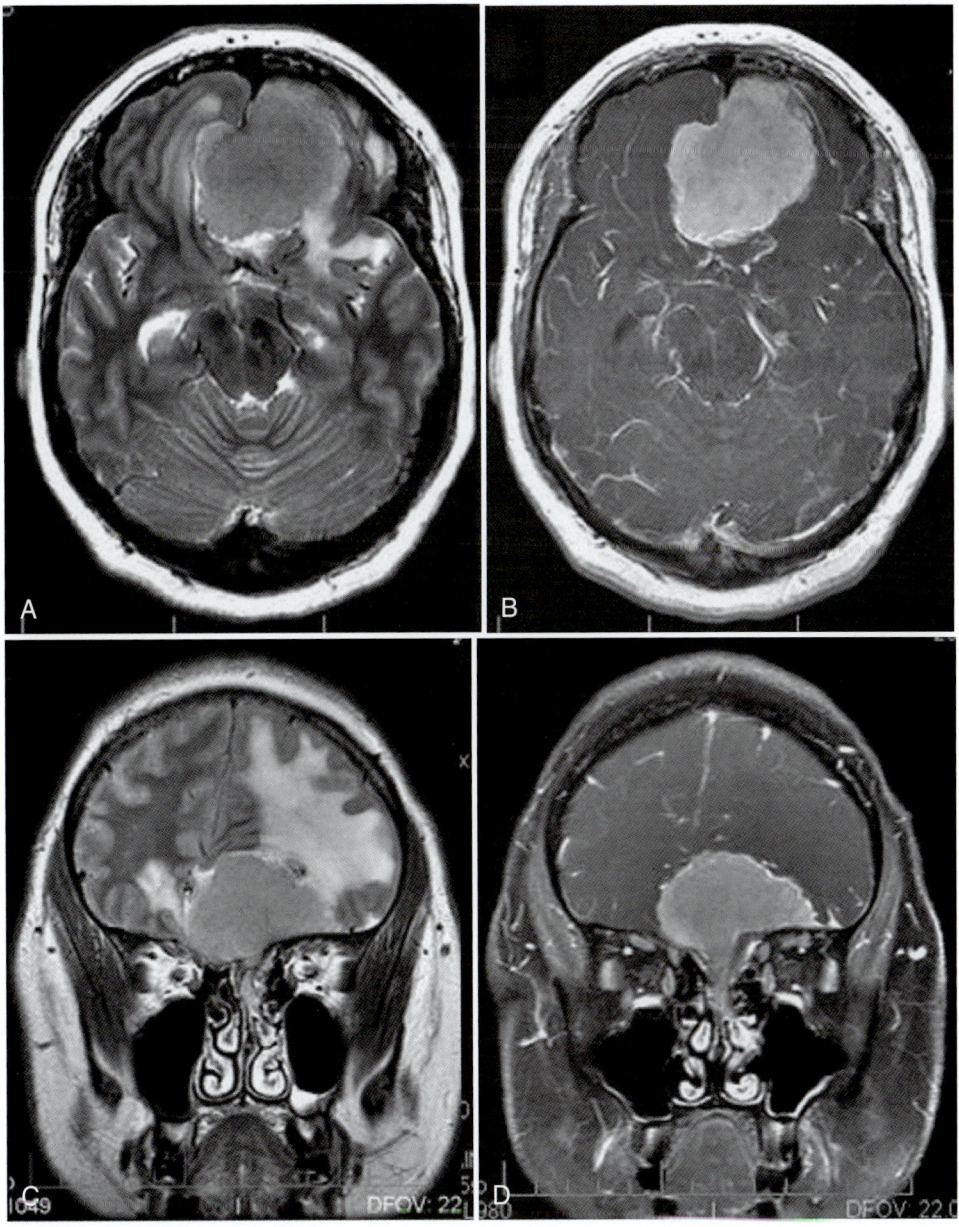

Figure 3-35 Pathologically confirmed atypical meningioma (World Health Organization grade II). **A, B:** Axial T2- and T1-weighted postgadolinium images. **C, D:** Coronal T2- and T1-weighted images demonstrating a falcine meningioma with moderate edema.

Continued

median survival of less than 1 year, despite aggressive treatment. Of the approximately 35,000 Americans diagnosed with primary brain cancer each year, almost half with high-grade (World Health Organization class III– IV) gliomas will die of their disease within 2 years if treated and in less than 6 months if untreated. These gliomas are highly vascular and likely are the result of tumoral up-regulation of angiogenic growth factors, such as VEGF. Angiogenesis appears to play a major role in the recurrent and refractory nature of these high-grade tumors. As a result, pharmaceutical companies have invested heavily into researching and developing effective antiangiogenesis agents. One of the few agents currently approved by the United States Food and Drug Administration (FDA) is bevacizumab (Avastin).

Bevacizumab (Avastin) is a humanized murine monoclonal antibody against the VEGF receptor. Published data on the role of Avastin in primary brain tumors are much more limited. One study demonstrated a 50% conventional MRI response rate in 14 patients with recurrent high-grade gliomas. Of these patients, four died (mean survival after treatment: 116 days). Two had what the authors described as "mixed progressive disease," and the other two had "partial response," suggesting that radiographic improvement does not correlate well with clinical outcome.

Initial studies with antiangiogenic agents such as thalidomide demonstrated that perfusion imaging was able to more accurately predict overall survival and progressive disease than conventional MRI. More recently,

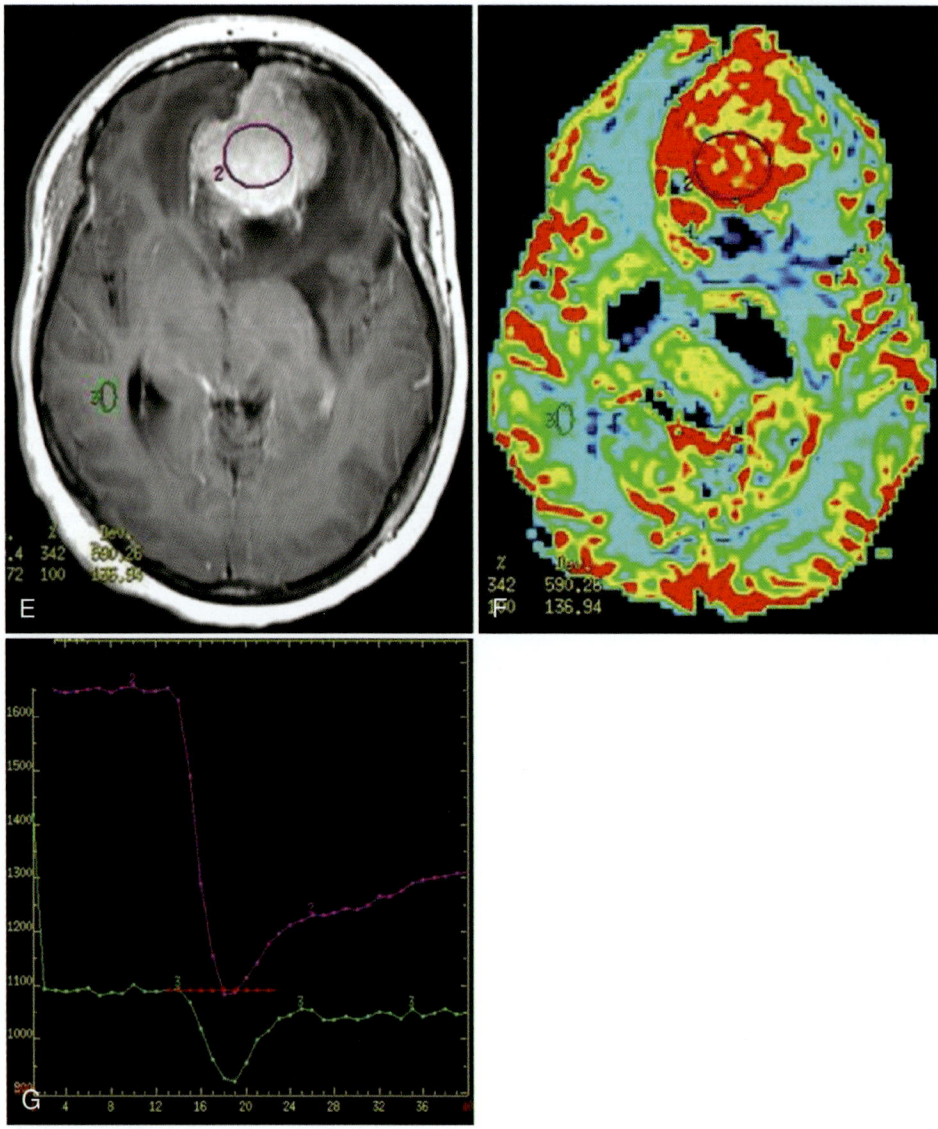

Figure 3-35—cont'd **E:** T1 localizing image with gradient-echo axial dynamic susceptibility contrast perfusion magnetic resonance imaging (DSC MRI) and relative cerebral blood volume color overlay demonstrating high rCBV throughout the lesion. **F:** Gradient-echo axial DSC MRI signal intensity curve depicting signal intensity drop with the curve not returning to the preinjection baseline, indicating increased leakage/vascular permeability. **G:** T2* signal intensity curve demonstrating increased vascular permeability in atypical meningiomas compared with typical meningiomas.

we have used CBV and permeability measurements to follow patients taking Avastin. To date, it appears that radiographically on conventional MRI, CBV, and permeability measurements, most patients demonstrate a response to treatment with a decrease in enhancing volume, CBV, and vascular permeability. However, many of these patients do not demonstrate significant improvement in time to progression or overall survival (Figures 3-36 and 3-37). Pathologically, treatment with antiangiogenic agents may alter glioma biology such that the tumor becomes more invasive and cellular in response to the deprivation of angiogenesis. DWI and/or diffusion tensor imaging are beginning to demonstrate the increased cellularity in some of the treated gliomas.

As with many other disease processes such as human immunodeficiency virus and tuberculous infection, it is likely that, in the future, a combination of drugs will target different components of glioma biology that will be most effective. Regardless of therapy, it will be evident that quantitative MR measures of perfusion, diffusion, and other pathophysiologic parameters will become early surrogate biomarkers of therapeutic response.

■ PROBLEM SOLVING IN NEURODEGENERATIVE DISEASES

Neurodegenerative diseases include the dementias, which comprise various pathologic entities such as primary demyelinating disease, Parkinson disease, amyotrophic lateral sclerosis, Alzheimer disease, frontotemporal dementia, corticobasal degeneration, progressive supranuclear palsy, and dementia with Lewy bodies.

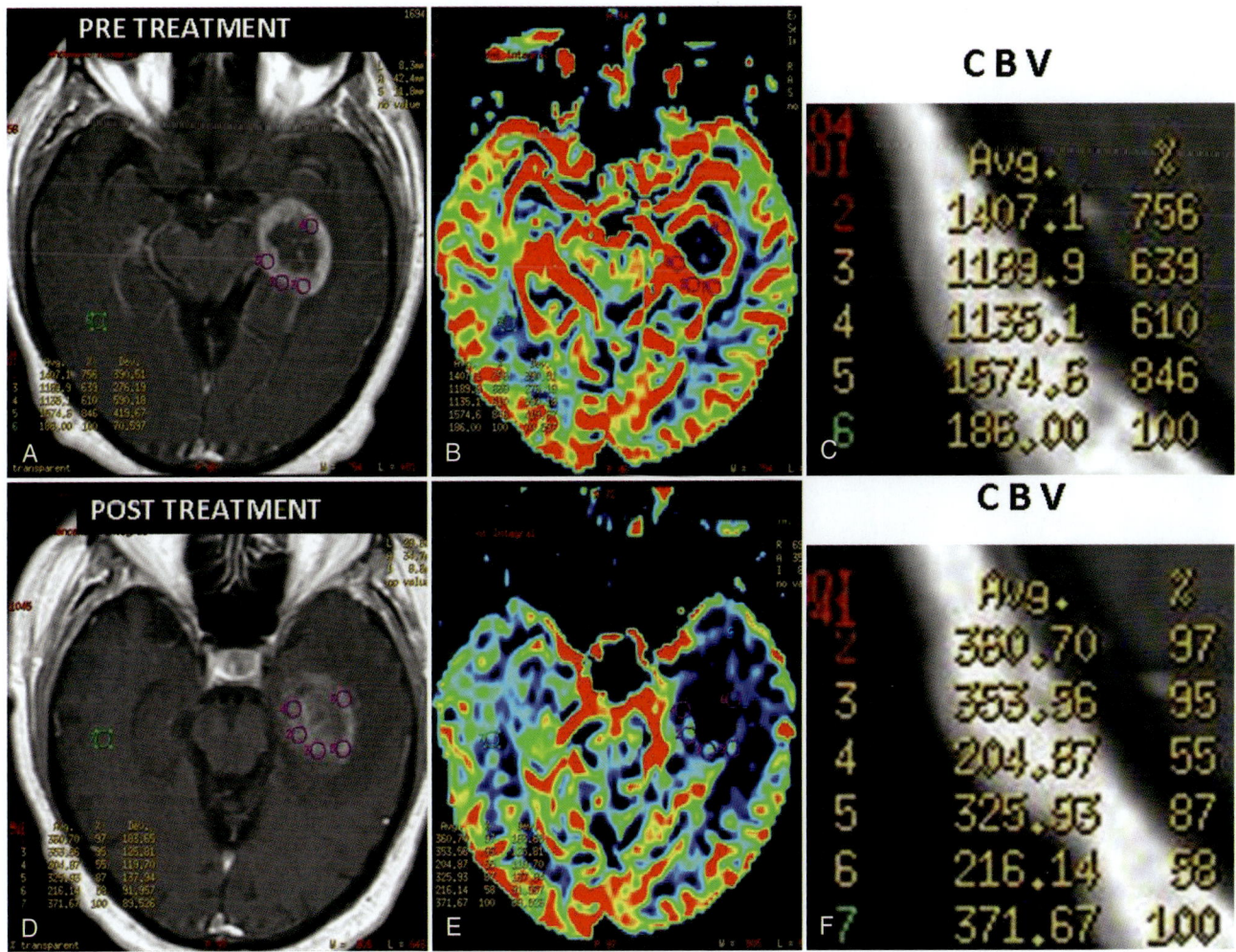

Figure 3-36 Pathologically proven recurrent glioblastoma multiforme (World Health Organization grade IV). **A:** Axial T1-weighted postgadolinium image. **B:** Gradient-echo axial dynamic susceptibility contrast perfusion magnetic resonance imaging (DSC MRI) with relative cerebral blood volume (rCBV) color overlay demonstrating high rCBV within the lesion. **C:** rCBV values within the lesion demonstrating high rCBV values. **D:** Follow-up T1-weighted image demonstrating a good response to therapy. **E:** Gradient-echo axial DSC MRI with rCBV color overlay demonstrating reduced rCBV within the lesion. **F:** rCBV values following treatment demonstrate marked decrease in rCBV values.

Advanced imaging techniques have been used to help in problem solving some of these neurodegenerative disorders.

The clinical diagnosis of these dementia subtypes is based on proposed consensus clinical criteria for each disease. However, distinguishing among the dementia subtypes by clinical examination alone, particularly during the early stages, continues to be difficult. The diagnosis of Alzheimer disease has benefited from the utility of fluorodeoxyglucose positron emission tomographic imaging. MRS has also demonstrated its utility in demonstrating elevation in myoinositol and decrease in glutamine/glutamate complexes during the early stages of the disease. Usually a decrease in NAA also is seen. These metabolite changes are believed to occur globally. In addition, early during the course of the disease, particularly in patients with mild cognitive impairment, metabolite changes are seen in the posterior cingulate gyrus and temporal lobes (Figure 3-38).

Frontotemporal dementia is a clinical syndrome associated with volume loss of the frontal and anterior temporal lobes of the brain. Originally known as Pick disease, the name and classification of frontotemporal dementia has been a topic of discussion for more than a century. Although pharmacologic treatment of dementia patients has not been satisfactory, recent meta-analyses have shown that early treatment with cholinesterase inhibitors could be beneficial for patients with Alzheimer disease. Thus, early discrimination of patients with Alzheimer disease from those with frontotemporal dementia/Pick complex has become more important than the precise differentiation of dementia subtypes. Patients with frontotemporal dementia/Pick complex have been shown to demonstrate a frontal predominant decrease in NAA/Cr ratios, whereas patients with Alzheimer disease showed a posterior dominant decrease. These different distributions of metabolic changes may represent the underlying pathologic processes in each disease (Figure 3-39).

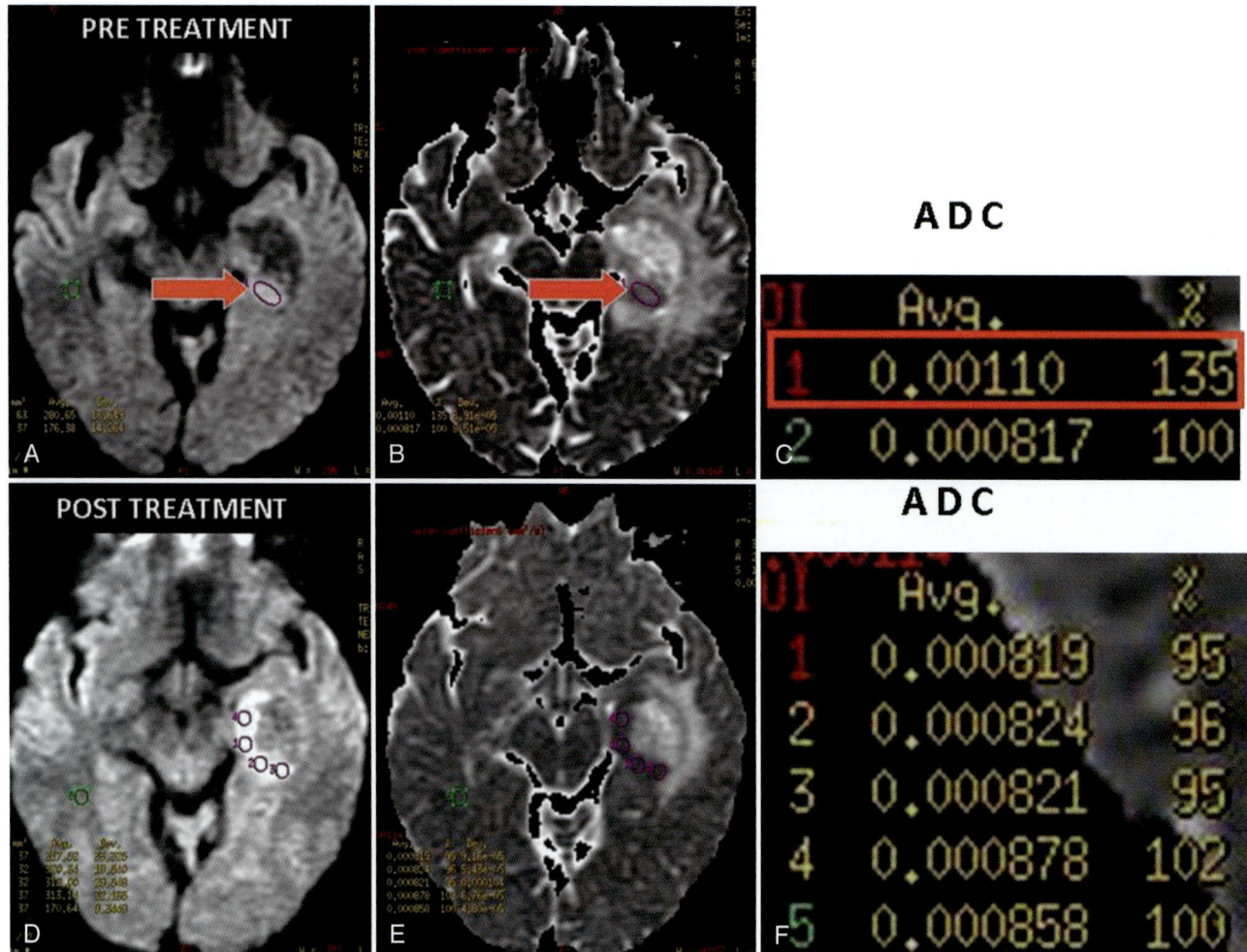

Figure 3-37 Pathologically proven recurrent glioblastoma multiforme after 2 months of therapy with Avastin. Same patient as shown in Figure 3-36. **A, B:** Axial diffusion-weighted imaging (DWI) with apparent diffusion coefficient (ADC) map demonstrating diffusion restriction within the lesion. **C:** Region of interest demonstrating diffusion values. **D:** DWI and ADC image demonstrating a marked decrease in signal suggesting possible increase in tumor cellularity, decrease in edema, and possible increase in invasiveness within the recurrent glioma. This may be a biologic response to removal of the angiogenic component as well as decrease in edema from lower vascular permeability.

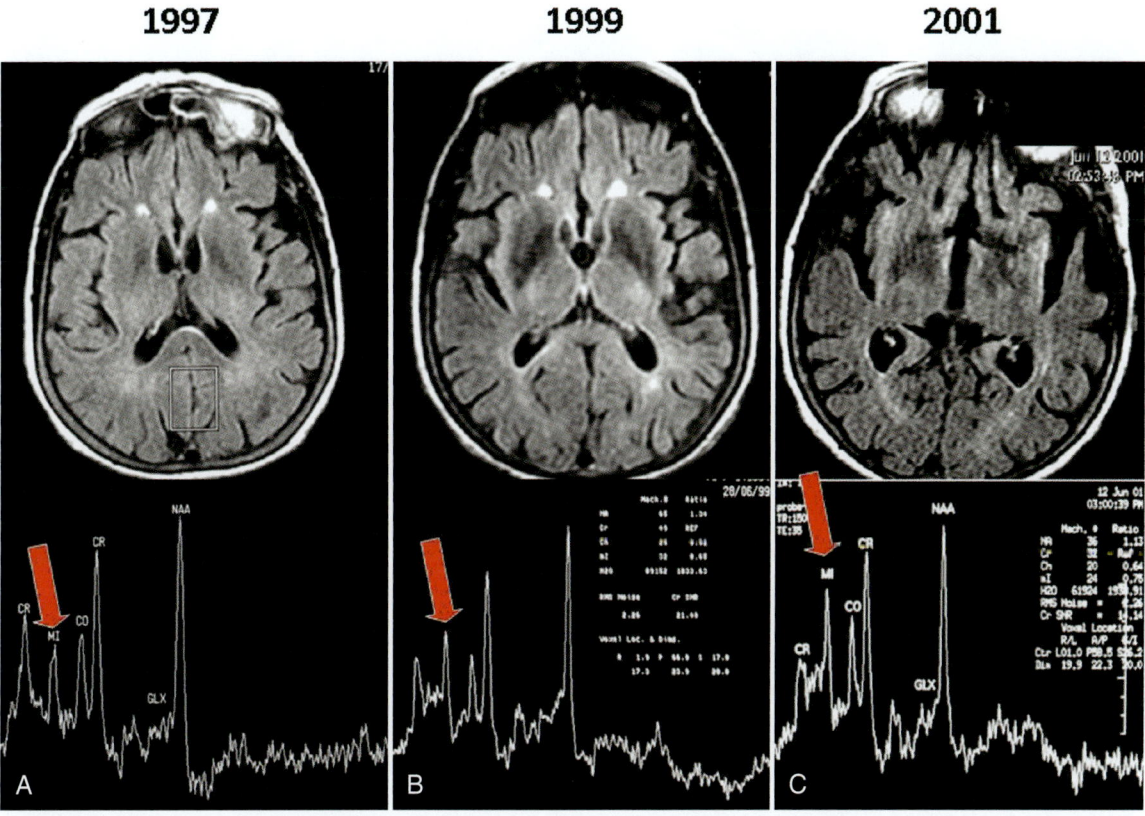

Figure 3-38 Patient who initially presented with mild cognitive impairment progressing to Alzheimer disease (AD). **A:** Initial magnetic resonance scan (MRS) in 1997 demonstrating minimal volume loss and location of the MRS voxel within the posterior cingulate gyrus. MRS shows mild elevation in myoinositol (MI), decrease in glutamine/glutamate (Glx), and decrease in N-acetylaspartate (NAA). **B:** Follow-up scan in 1999 demonstrating similar findings to those seen in 1997. **C:** MRI and MRS in 2001 in the same patient demonstrating increasing volume loss, particularly involving the temporal lobes. MRS demonstrates progressively increasing MI and decreasing NAA in AD. (Courtesy Dr. Nelson Fortes, Med Imagem, Brazil.)

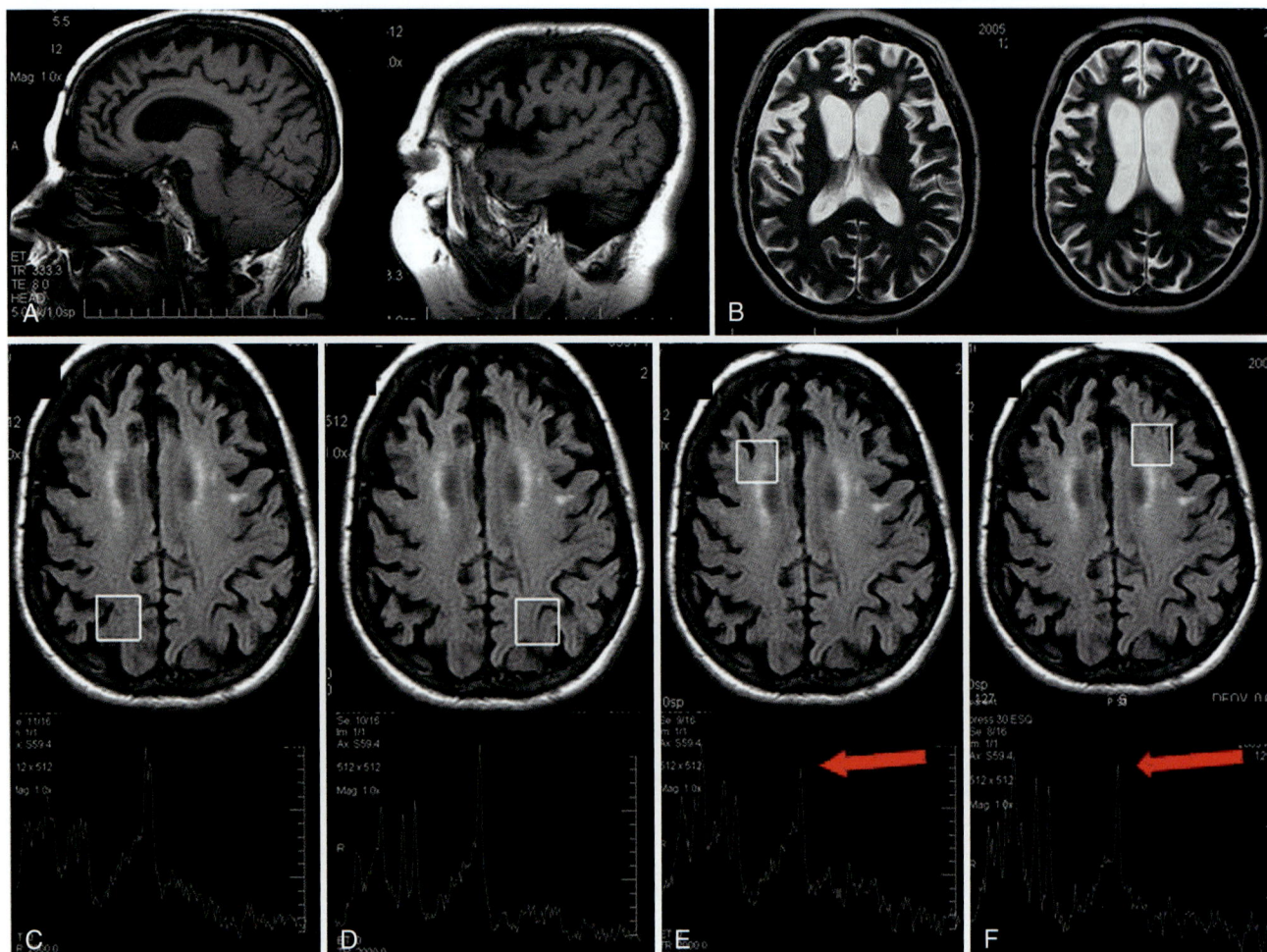

Figure 3-39 Patient who presented with frontotemporal dementia (FTD). **A, B:** Sagittal T1- and axial T2-weighted images demonstrating some volume loss in the frontotemporal regions. Typically with marked volume loss, the sulci are described as having a "knife-like" appearance. **C, D:** Magnetic resonance spectroscopy(MRS) in the posterior gray and white matter demonstrating fairly normal metabolite concentrations. **E, F:** MRS in the frontal regions demonstrating a marked decrease in N-acetylaspartate (NAA) in FTD. The predilection from the frontal regions helps to differentiate it from Alzheimer disease, which has a more posterior predilection (see Figure 3-38). (Courtesy Dr. Nelson Fortes, Med Imagem, Brazil.)

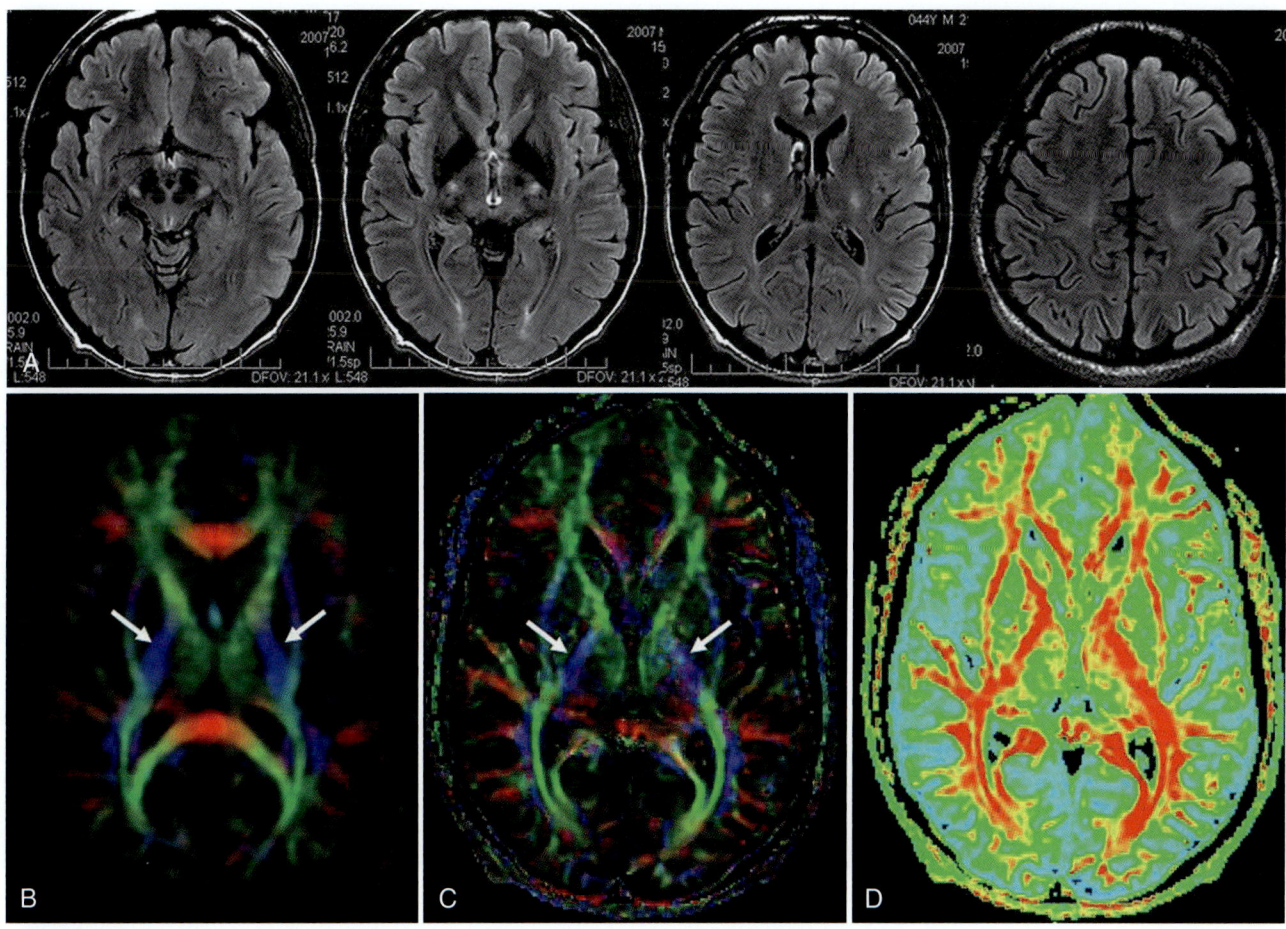

Figure 3-40 Patient with amyotrophic lateral sclerosis (ALS). **A:** Axial FLAIR image demonstrating increase in signal along the corticospinal tracts (CST) extending from the precentral sulcus through the posterior limb of the internal capsule down into the brainstem. **B:** Axial directional color-coded fractional anisotropy (FA) maps in a normal patient demonstrating the superior to inferior direction of the CST *(white arrows)*. **C, D:** Patient with ALS demonstrating decrease in FA along the CST *(white arrows in C)* seen on both the directional and magnitude color-coded maps.

Amyotrophic lateral sclerosis (ALS), or motor neuron disease, is a neurodegenerative disorder of unknown origin. It occurs in sporadic (90%–95% of cases) and familial (5%–10%) forms. It is characterized pathologically by selective degeneration of somatic motor neurons of the brainstem and spinal cord (lower motor neurons) and of large pyramidal neurons of the motor cortex (upper motor neurons), with eventual loss of fibers in the corticospinal tracts. MRI studies using T2-weighted and fluid-attenuated inversion recovery (FLAIR) or fast spin-echo (FSE) sequences have shown that qualitatively increased signal intensity in the corticospinal tracts (Figure 3-40), decreased signal intensity in the precentral gyrus gray matter (motor cortex), or both occur in some patients with ALS. Metabolic changes also have been demonstrated in the subset of ALS patients with precentral gyrus signal changes on imaging, and significantly increased Ins was associated with cortical hypointensity on FSE images have been shown in the precentral sulcus. Diffusion tensor imaging demonstrates a decrease in fractional anisotropy within the corticospinal tracts seen on color-coded fractional anisotropy maps (Figure 3-40). These findings can be important for differentiating ALS from other neurodegenerative diseases.

PROBLEM SOLVING IN WHITE MATTER, METABOLIC DISEASES, AND DEVELOPMENTAL DISEASES

For a more complete review of how to problem solve with MRS in metabolic and pediatric white matter disease, see the review by Cecil and Kos entitled "Magnetic resonance spectroscopy and metabolic imaging in white matter diseases and pediatric disorders." Numerous metabolite disease have a metabolic signature on MRS, and a discussion of this topic is beyond the scope of this text. An example of how MRS can be useful in problem solving is Canavan disease, which has a fairly specific metabolite finding. Canavan disease is an inherited disorder (autosomal recessive) caused by a deficiency in aspartoacylase, which results in progressive white matter vacuolization. This disorder has been localized to chromosome 17p. Patients present with early psychomotor retardation, megalencephaly, blindness, and spasticity. Aspartoacylase aids in the metabolism of NAA into acetate and aspartate, and NAA buildup ensues in patients with aspartoacylase deficiency. Prominent NAA peaks have been reported in all published cases of MRS and Canavan disease (Figure 3-41). Decreased choline has been noted, as has lactate elevation and Cr decrease in a few cases.

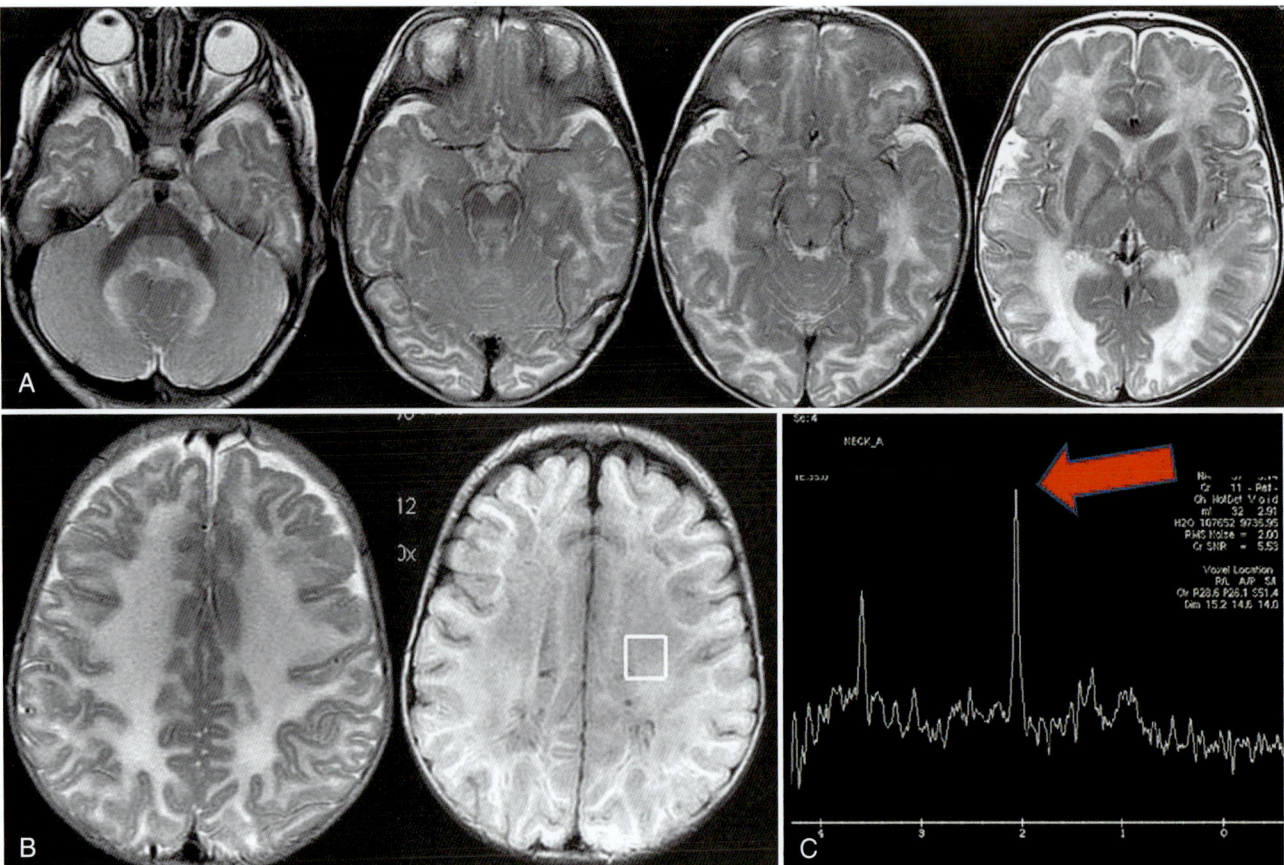

Figure 3-41 Patient with Canavan disease. **A:** Axial T2-weighted images demonstrating diffuse increase in signal intensity throughout the visualized white matter. There is also increased signal within the globus pallidus and anterior thalami bilateral, sometimes seen in Canavan disease. **B:** Localizing T2-weighted image showing the location of the voxel for magnetic resonance spectroscopy (MRS). **C:** MRS showing the very characteristic elevation in *N*-acetylaspartate *(red arrow)*. There is also a pronounced decrease in creatine. (Courtesy Dr. Ronnie Peterson, Santa Casa, Porto Alegre, Brazil.)

Suggested Readings

Alger JR, Frank JA, Bizzi A, et al. Metabolism of human gliomas: Assessment with H-1 MR spectroscopy and F-18 fluorodeoxyglucose PET. *Radiology.* 1990;177(3):633-641.

Al-Okaili RN, Krejza J, Wang S, Woo JH, Melhem ER. Advanced MR imaging techniques in the diagnosis of intraaxial brain tumors in adults. *Radiographics.* 2006;26(Suppl 1):S173-S189.

Al-Okaili RN, Krejza J, Woo JH, et al. Intraaxial brain masses: MR imaging-based diagnostic strategy—Initial experience. *Radiology.* 2007;243(2):539-550.

Bastin ME, Carpenter TK, Armitage PA, Sinha S, Wardlaw JM, Whittle IR. Effects of dexamethasone on cerebral perfusion and water diffusion in patients with high-grade glioma. *AJNR Am J Neuroradiol.* 2006;27(2):402-408.

Bauman GS, Ino Y, Ueki K, et al. Allelic loss of chromosome 1p and radiotherapy plus chemotherapy in patients with oligodendrogliomas. *Int J Radiat Oncol Biol Phys.* 2000;48(3):825-830.

Bowen BC, Pattany PM, Bradley WG, et al. MR imaging and localized proton spectroscopy of the precentral gyrus in amyotrophic lateral sclerosis. *AJNR Am J Neuroradiol.* 2000;21(4):647-658.

Boxerman JL, Schmainda KM, Weisskoff RM. Relative cerebral blood volume maps corrected for contrast agent extravasation significantly correlate with glioma tumor grade, whereas uncorrected maps do not. *AJNR Am J Neuroradiol.* 2006;27(4):859-867.

Brandes AA, Franceschi E, Tosoni A, et al. MGMT promoter methylation status can predict the incidence and outcome of pseudoprogression after concomitant radiochemotherapy in newly diagnosed glioblastoma patients. *J Clin Oncol.* 2008;26(13):2192-2197.

Brandsma D, Stalpers L, Taal W, Sminia P, van den Bent MJ. Clinical features, mechanisms, and management of pseudoprogression in malignant gliomas. *Lancet Oncol.* 2008;9(5):453-461.

Buckner JC. Factors influencing survival in high-grade gliomas. *Semin Oncol.* 2003;30(6 Suppl 19):10-14.

Cairncross J, Ueki K, Zlatescu M, et al. Specific genetic predictors of chemotherapeutic response and survival in patients with anaplastic oligodendrogliomas. *J Natl Cancer Inst.* 1998;90(19):1473-1479.

Cecil KM, Kos RS. Magnetic resonance spectroscopy and metabolic imaging in white matter diseases and pediatric disorders. *Top Magn Reson Imaging.* 2006;17(4):275-293.

Cha S. Dynamic susceptibility-weighted contrast-enhanced perfusion MR imaging in pediatric patients. *Neuroimaging Clin N Am.* 2006;16(1):137-147:ix.

Cha S. Update on brain tumor imaging: From anatomy to physiology. *AJNR Am J Neuroradiol.* 2006;27(3):475-487.

Cha S, Johnson G, Yuz M. The role of contrast-enhanced perfusion MR imaging in differentiating between recurrent tumor and radiation necrosis (abstr). *Radiology.* 1999;213:188.

Cha S, Knopp EA, Johnson G, Wetzel SG, Litt AW, Zagzag D. Intracranial mass lesions: Dynamic contrast-enhanced susceptibility-weighted echo-planar perfusion MR imaging. *Radiology.* 2002;223(1):11-29.

Cha S, Knopp EA, Johnson G, et al. Dynamic, contrast-enhanced T2*-weighted MR imaging of recurrent malignant gliomas treated with thalidomide and carboplatin. *Am J Neuroradiol.* 2000;21(5):881-890.

Cha S, Tihan T, Crawford F, et al. Differentiation of low-grade oligodendrogliomas from low-grade astrocytomas by using quantitative blood-volume measurements derived from dynamic susceptibility contrast-enhanced MR imaging. *AJNR Am J Neuroradiol.* 2005;26(2):266-273.

Chamberlain MC. Pseudoprogression in glioblastoma. *J Clin Oncol.* 2008;26(26):4359.

Engelhard HH, Stelea A, Cochran EJ. Oligodendroglioma: Pathology and molecular biology. *Surg Neurol.* 2002;58(2):111-117.

Essig M, Waschkies M, Wenz F, Debus J, Hentrich HR, Knopp MV. Assessment of brain metastases with dynamic susceptibility-weighted contrast-enhanced MR imaging: Initial results. *Radiology.* 2003;228(1):193-199.

Fuss M, Wenz F, Scholdei R, et al. Radiation-induced regional cerebral blood volume (rCBV) changes in normal brain and low-grade astrocytomas: Quantification and time and dose-dependent occurrence. *Int J Radiat Oncol Biol Phys.* 2000;48(1):53-58.

Graham ML, Herndon 2nd JE, Casey JR, et al. High-dose chemotherapy with autologous stem-cell rescue in patients with recurrent and high-risk pediatric brain tumors. *J Clin Oncol.* 1997;15(5):1814-1823.

Gupta RK, Haris M, Husain N, et al. Relative cerebral blood volume is a measure of angiogenesis in brain tuberculoma and its therapeutic implications. *Proceedings of ISMRM.* 2006:181.

Gupta RK, Roy R, Dev R, et al. Finger printing of mycobacterium tuberculosis in patients with intracranial tuberculomas by using in vivo, ex vivo, and in vitro magnetic resonance spectroscopy. *Magn Res Med.* 1996;36(6):829-833.

Gupta RK, Vatsal DK, Husain N, et al. Differentiation of tuberculous from pyogenic brain abscesses with in vivo proton MR spectroscopy and magnetization transfer MR imaging. *AJNR Am J Neuroradiol.* 2001;22(8):1503-1509.

Haque S, Law M, Abrey LE, Young RJ. Imaging of lymphoma of the central nervous system, spine, and orbit. *Radiol Clin North Am.* 2008;46(2):339-361:ix.

Haris M, Gupta RK, Husain M, et al. Assessment of therapeutic response in brain tuberculomas using serial dynamic contrast-enhanced MRI. *Clin Radiol.* 2008;63(5):562-574.

Haris M, Gupta RK, Singh A, et al. Differentiation of infective from neoplastic brain lesions by dynamic contrast-enhanced MRI. *Neuroradiology.* 2008;50(6):531-540.

Hess C, Mukerjee P, Han ET, et al. High angular resolution diffusion tensor imaging (HARDI). *Magn Reson Med.* 2006;56:104-117.

Hourani R, Brant LJ, Rizk T, Weingart JD, Barker PB, Horska A. Can proton MR spectroscopic and perfusion imaging differentiate between neoplastic and nonneoplastic brain lesions in adults? *AJNR Am J Neuroradiol.* 2008;29(2):366-372.

Jenkinson MD, Smith TS, Joyce KA, et al. Cerebral blood volume, genotype and chemosensitivity in oligodendroglial tumours. *Neuroradiology.* 2006;48(10):703-713.

Kantarci K, Jack Jr CR, Xu YC, et al. Regional metabolic patterns in mild cognitive impairment and Alzheimer's disease: A 1H MRS study. *Neurology.* 2000;55(2):210-217.

Kantarci K, Reynolds G, Petersen RC, et al. Proton MR spectroscopy in mild cognitive impairment and Alzheimer disease: Comparison of 1.5 and 3 T. *AJNR Am J Neuroradiol.* 2003;24(5):843-849.

Kono K, Inoue Y, Nakayama K, et al. The role of diffusion-weighted imaging in patients with brain tumors. *AJNR Am J Neuroradiol.* 2001;22(6):1081-1088.

Law M, Cha S, Knopp EA, Johnson G, Arnett J, Litt AW. High-grade gliomas and solitary metastases: Differentiation by using perfusion and proton spectroscopic MR imaging. *Radiology.* 2002;222(3):715-721.

Law M, Brodsky JE, Babb J, et al. High cerebral blood volume in human gliomas predicts deletion of chromosome 1p: Preliminary results of molecular studies in gliomas with elevated perfusion. *J Magn Reson Imaging.* 2007;25(6):1113-1119.

Law M, Yang S, Wang H, et al. Glioma grading: Sensitivity, specificity, and predictive values of perfusion MR imaging and proton MR spectroscopic imaging compared with conventional MR imaging. *AJNR Am J Neuroradiol.* 2003;24(10):1989-1998.

Lev MH, Ozsunar Y, Henson JW, et al. Glial tumor grading and outcome prediction using dynamic spin-echo MR susceptibility mapping compared with conventional contrast-enhanced MR: Confounding effect of elevated rCBV of oligodendrogliomas [corrected]. *AJNR Am J Neuroradiol.* 2004;25(2):214-221.

Matalon R, Michals-Matalon K. Biochemistry and molecular biology of Canavan disease. *Neurochem Res.* 1999;24:507-513.

Mihara M, Hattori N, Abe K, Sakoda S, Sawada T. Magnetic resonance spectroscopic study of Alzheimer's disease and frontotemporal dementia/Pick complex. *Neuroreport.* 2006;17(4):413-416.

Moffat BA, Chenevert TL, Lawrence TS, et al. Functional diffusion map: A noninvasive MRI biomarker for early stratification of clinical brain tumor response. *Proc Natl Acad Sci USA.* 2005;102(15):5524-5529.

Moseley ME, Kucharczyk J, Mintorovitch J, et al. Diffusion-weighted MR imaging of acute stroke: Correlation with T2-weighted and magnetic susceptibility-enhanced MR imaging in cats. *Am J Neuroradiol.* 1990;11:423-429.

Pope WB, Lai A, Nghiemphu P, Mischel P, Cloughesy TF. MRI in patients with high-grade gliomas treated with bevacizumab and chemotherapy. *Neurology.* 2006;66(8):1258-1260.

Ross BD, Bluml S, Cowan R, Danielsen E, Farrow N, Gruetter R. In vivo magnetic resonance spectroscopy of human brain: The biophysical basis of dementia. *Biophys Chem.* 1997;68(1-3):161-172.

Saindane AM, Cha S, Law M, Xue X, Knopp EA, Zagzag D. Proton MR spectroscopy of tumefactive demyelinating lesions. *AJNR Am J Neuroradiol.* 2002;23(8):1378-1386.

Schaefer PW, Hunter GJ, He J, et al. Predicting cerebral ischemic infarct volume with diffusion and perfusion MR imaging. *AJNR Am J Neuroradiol.* 2002;23(10):1785-1794.

Uematsu H, Maeda M, Sadato N, et al. Vascular permeability: Quantitative measurement with double-echo dynamic MR imaging—Theory and clinical application. *Radiology.* 2000;214(3):912-917.

Watanabe T, Nakamura M, Kros JM, et al. Phenotype versus genotype correlation in oligodendrogliomas and low-grade diffuse astrocytomas. *Acta Neuropathol (Berl).* 2002;103(3):267-275.

Wenz F, Rempp K, Hess T, et al. Effect of radiation on blood volume in low-grade astrocytomas and normal brain tissue: Quantification with dynamic susceptibility contrast MR imaging. *Am J Roentgenol.* 1996;166(1):187-193.

Whitmore RG, Krejza J, Kapoor GS, et al. Prediction of oligodendroglial tumor subtype and grade using perfusion weighted magnetic resonance imaging. *J Neurosurg.* 2007;107(3):600-609.

Yang S, Law M, Zagzag D, et al. Dynamic contrast-enhanced perfusion MR imaging measurements of endothelial permeability: Differentiation between atypical and typical meningiomas. *AJNR Am J Neuroradiol.* 2003;24(8):1554-1559.

CHAPTER **4**

PET/CT Imaging in Squamous Cell Carcinoma of the Head and Neck

Lale Kostakoglu

■ INTRODUCTION

Squamous cell carcinoma (SCC) of the head and neck (HNSCC) constitutes more than 90% of head and neck cancers, and salivary gland tumors, lymphoma, melanoma, and sarcoma account for the remaining 10%. The majority of HNSCC patients present with locally advanced disease; less than 50% of newly diagnosed patients have early-stage disease. Management depends primarily on a combination of T and N staging. The TNM (tumor node metastasis) system is used for staging HNSCC, with the T stages being specific to each anatomic subdivision but the N and M staging being shared (Table 4-1). Usually, the presence of subclinical nodal and distant metastases determines whether the patient can be treated with function-sparing therapy. Contrast-enhanced computed tomography (ceCT) or magnetic resonance imaging (MRI) has been the primary imaging modality for evaluating HNSCC at both staging and restaging. Nonetheless, this approach has been shifting toward the use of positron emission tomography integrated with computed tomography using fluorodeoxyglucose (FDG PET/CT) in the past several years. Although rare at initial presentation, the presence of distant metastasis as well as second primary cancers of the upper aerodigestive tract should be evaluated by whole body imaging, preferably by FDG PET/CT as a metabolic imaging modality. If concern exists regarding the invasion of muscle, nerves, or bone, an MRI study may be appropriate for better evaluation of the extent of tumor involvement. This chapter reviews FDG PET/CT imaging in oral cavity, oropharyngeal, and laryngeal SCCs, which constitute the majority of HNSCC. Other malignancies of the head and neck do not fall in the scope of this review. In addition, this chapter reviews the subsites of HNSCC with respect to regional anatomy and nonmalignant causes of FDG uptake, because proper interpretation of PET/CT images requires a thorough understanding of these subjects.

■ ORAL AND OROPHARYNGEAL CANCERS

What Are the Anatomic Subsites to Evaluate in Oral Cavity and Oropharyngeal Cancers?

Oral cancers are anatomically divided into the oral cavity and oropharynx, which in turn are divided into several anatomic subsites. The SCCs of these two regions have distinct biologic behavior such that regional lymph node and distant metastases occur more frequently in oropharyngeal SCCs due to a rich lymphatic network that is not as abundantly present in the oral cavity.

The borders for oral cavity consist of the lips, floor of the mouth, gingivobuccal mucosa, hard palate, oral tongue (anterior two thirds of tongue), floor of mouth, and retromolar trigone. The most common tumors of the oral cavity involve the oral tongue and the floor of the mouth. The oropharynx contains the base of the tongue (posterior third of the tongue) and the tonsils and extends from the palate to the epiglottic valleculae, including the posterior and lateral pharyngeal walls. The most common cancers in this location arise from the tonsils and base of the tongue.

Patients who present with early-stage SCCs often can be successfully treated with either surgery or radiotherapy alone. The treatment strategy for more advanced disease depends on the involved subsite and may involve chemoradiation followed by resection and/or neck dissection if necessary, followed by adjuvant chemoradiation.

Does FDG PET/CT Have a Primary Role in Evaluation of Primary Tumor in Oral Cavity and Oropharyngeal Cancers?

Accurate determination of the T stage requires knowledge of the size of the primary tumor, depth of invasion, and infiltration of adjacent structures. ceCT or MRI has been widely used when assessing the T stage at initial presentation. MRI is the preferred modality for evaluation of perineural spread or invasion of the bone. FDG PET/CT is highly sensitive for detection of primary HNSCCs; however, it has not been proven to be superior to standard anatomic imaging modalities in T staging. Understandably, the metabolic information alone is not sufficient to provide T-stage information without the association of a high-resolution ceCT study or MRI. The best approach is the combination of both FDG PET and ceCT data into one study, particularly when the objective is to improve diagnostic specificity (Figures 4-1 through 4-3). The other goal is accurate determination of bone invasion to avoid unnecessary morbid results with surgical intervention (see Is FDG PET Useful in Evaluation of Bone Invasion for further discussion with case examples).

Chapter 4 PET/CT Imaging In Squamous Cell Carcinoma of the Head and Neck

Table 4-1 N and M Staging for Squamous Cell Carcinomas of the Head and Neck

N STAGING	
NX	Regional lymph nodes cannot be assessed
N0	There is no regional nodes metastasis
N1	Metastasis in a single ipsilateral lymph node, <3 cm*
N2	Metastasis in a single ipsilateral lymph node, > 3 cm and ≤ 6 cm; or metastasis in multiple ipsilateral lymph nodes, none > 6 cm; or metastasis in bilateral or contralateral lymph nodes, none >6 cm
	N2a Metastasis in a single ipsilateral lymph node, > 3cm but < 6 cm
	N2b Metastasis in multiple ipsilateral lymph nodes, none > 6 cm
	N2c Metastasis in bilateral or contralateral lymph nodes, none > 6 cm
	N3 Metastasis in a lymph node > 6 cm
M STAGING	
MX	distant metastasis cannot be evaluated
M0	no distant metastasis
M1	distant metastasis

*All measurements are in greatest dimension
"U" and "L" are designations that may be given in addition to indicate the level of metastasis above the lower border of the cricoid cartilage (U) or below the lower border of the cricoid cartilage (L).
Adapted from the American Joint Committee on Cancer (AJCC), Chicago, Illinois. The original source for this material is the AJCC Cancer Staging Manual, Seventh Edition (2010) published by Springer-Verlag New York, www.cancerstaging.net.

What Are the Oral Cavity Cancer Subtypes?

SCC of Oral Tongue

The majority of oral tongue SCC involves the lateral border or ventral surface of the tongue (Figure 4-4, *A*). The tongue contains intrinsic and extrinsic musculature in which the genioglossus muscle forms the main bulk of the extrinsic tongue. Owing to the anatomic characteristic of the genioglossus muscle, tumors can easily extend toward the anterior floor of the mouth (Figures 4-4, *B*, and 4-5, *A* and *B*). The prognosis mainly depends on the depth of invasion. Involvement of the extrinsic muscles of the tongue and extension into the floor of mouth are relatively easy to detect on PET/CT imaging (Figure 4-5, *B*). Extensive local tumor spread may involve the soft palate via the palatoglossus muscle and from the soft palate to the nasopharynx (Figures 4-5, *A* and *C*). The management changes if the tumor crosses the midline of the tongue and/or extends, posteriorly into the base of tongue (Figure 4-5, *B*). Treatment of the tongue and floor of the mouth SCC is performed based on a compromise between therapeutic necessity and functional and esthetic preservation. Surgery and postoperative radiation are mainstays of therapy. Most tongue SCCs involving the tongue base are confined to one side of the tongue, allowing for a partial glossectomy. However, medial extension crossing the midline necessitates a total glossectomy in surgically resectable cases (Figure 4-4). In large excisions, a myocutaneous flap is used to cover the defect. Mandibular extension of tongue base carcinoma can dramatically change the operative

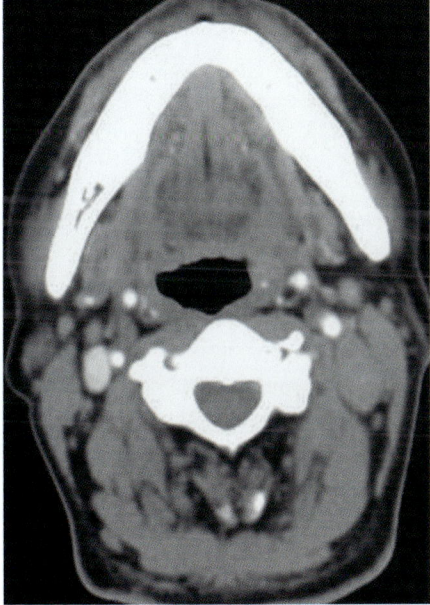
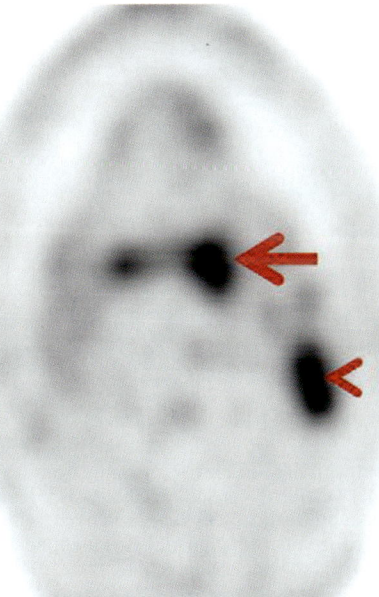
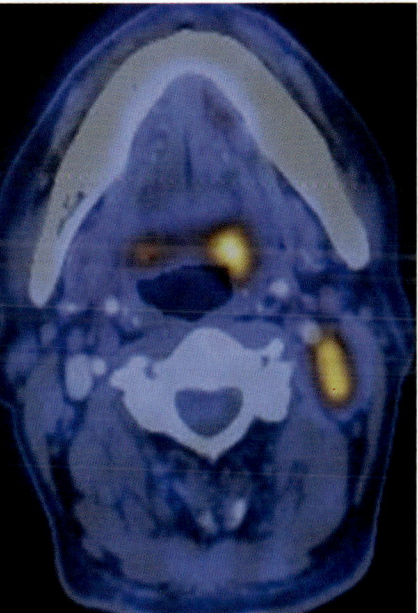

Figure 4-1 A 49-year-old man recently diagnosed with tonsillar squamous cell carcinoma (SCC), referred for staging with FDG PET/CT performed with contrast-enhanced high-resolution CT. PET/CT axial images demonstrate increased FDG uptake (SUV_{max} 12.0) in the left tonsillar fossa corresponding to a soft tissue fullness with ill-defined margins, with enhancement equal to that of muscles and measuring approximately 2.0 cm (T1), consistent with tonsillar SCC *(arrow)*. Additionally, an enlarged level IIB lymph node measuring 2.3 cm (N1) shows heterogeneous attenuation with increased FDG uptake (SUV_{max} 6.6), consistent with ipsilateral lymph node metastasis *(arrowhead)*. AJCC staging: T1N1MX, stage III disease.

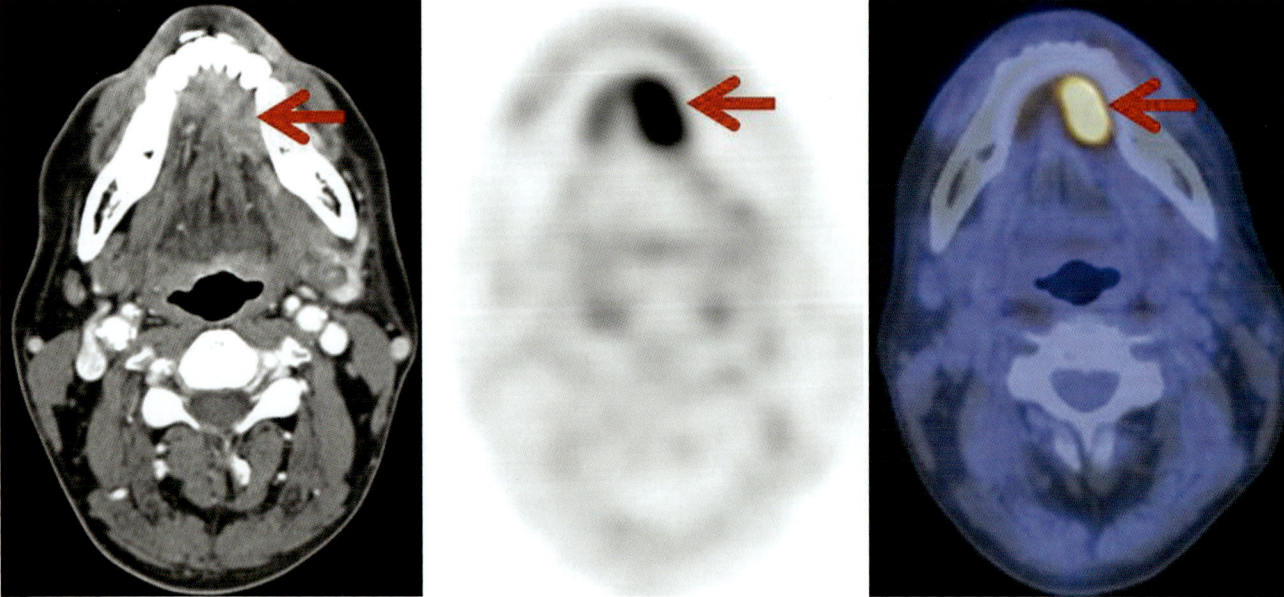

Figure 4-2 A 62-year-old patient recently diagnosed with floor of the mouth squamous cell carcinoma, referred for staging with FDG PET/CT performed with contrast-enhanced high-resolution CT. FDG PET/CT axial images reveal increased FDG uptake (SUV_{max} 8.5) in the left floor of the mouth, anteriorly, corresponding to an enhancing mass abutting the mandible and measuring 2.8 cm (T2), consistent with the patient's primary malignancy *(arrows)*. There is no evidence of bone invasion (bone windows not shown) or lymph node metastasis (N0). AJCC staging: T2N0MX, stage II disease.

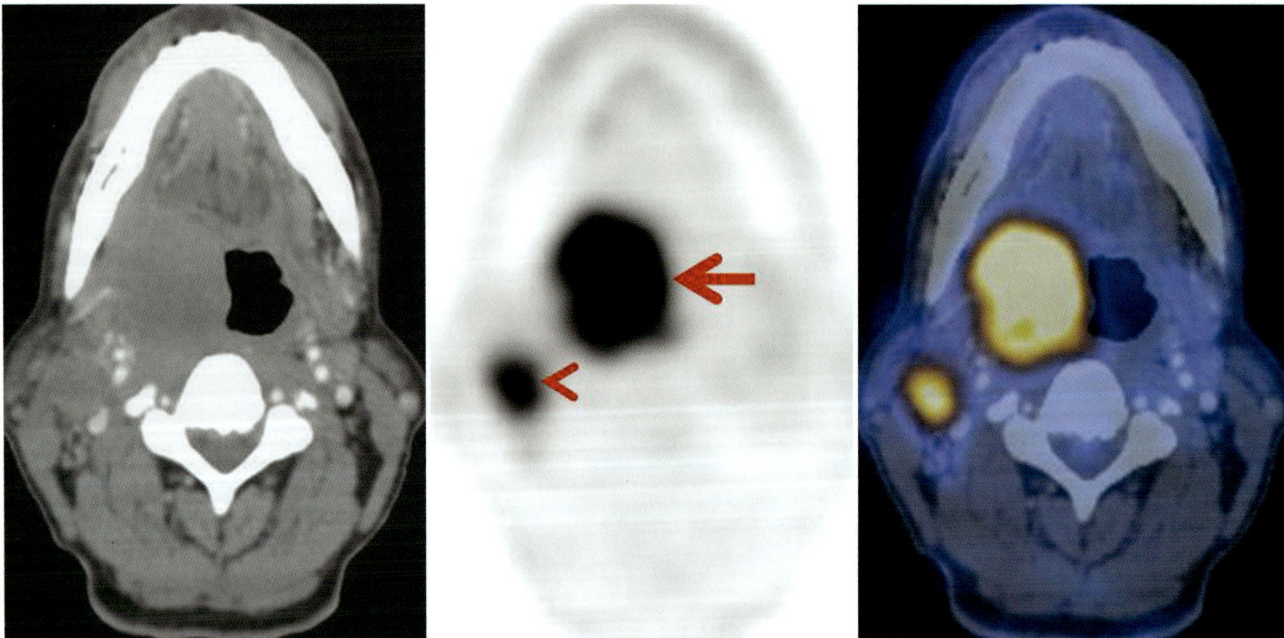

Figure 4-3 A 50-year-old man recently diagnosed with base of tongue squamous cell carcinoma, referred for staging with FDG PET/CT performed with contrast-enhanced high-resolution CT. FDG PET/CT axial images reveal increased FDG uptake (SUV_{max} 13.5) corresponding to a bulging mass situated in the right base of tongue extending caudally to the oropharynx, with narrowing of the pharyngeal lumen and measuring 4.1 cm (T3), consistent with the patient's known oropharyngeal malignancy. A nonenhancing enlarged right level II lymph node with increased FDG uptake (SUV_{max} 10) is consistent with ipsilateral regional metastatic disease (N1). AJCC staging: T3N1MX, stage III disease.

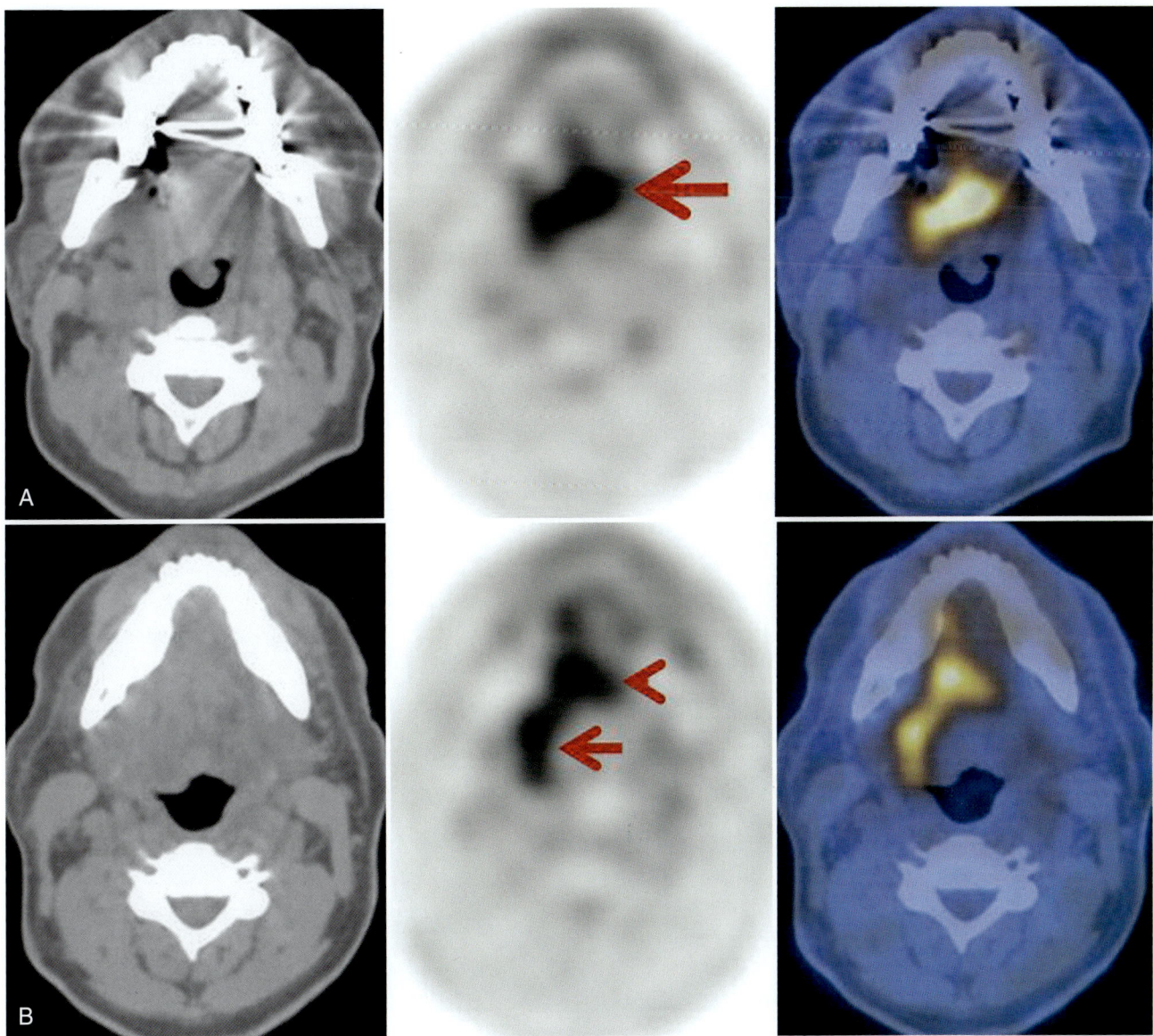

Figure 4-4 A 42-year-old man recently diagnosed with tongue cancer, referred for staging with FDG PET/CT performed with noncontrast-enhanced low-dose CT. **A:** FDG PET/CT axial images reveal an irregular area of increased FDG uptake (SUV_{max} 8.4) in the ventral surface of the mobile tongue, measuring between 2 and 4 cm (T2), mainly on the right but crossing the midline *(arrow)*. **B:** The tongue mass extends into the base of tongue and spreads caudally into the floor of mouth involving the right-sided genioglossus muscle *(arrowhead)* and probably hyoglossus muscle *(small arrow)*. Squamous cell carcinoma of the tongue often involves genioglossus muscle. There is no evidence of lymph node metastasis. AJCC staging: T2N0MX, stage II disease.

approach for therapy (see Is FDG PET Useful in Evaluation of Bone Invasion for further discussion).

SCC of the Floor of the Mouth

The floor of the mouth is a crescent-shaped area between the lower gingiva and the ventral surface of the tongue consisting of neurovascular structures and the sublingual glands. The majority of the SCC of the floor of the mouth originate within 2 cm of the anterior midline floor of the mouth (Figures 4-2 and 4-6, A). These tumors can invade the adjacent osseous structures and underlying soft tissues early during the course of disease (Figure 4-6, B). Because the genioglossus muscle is an essential part of both the floor of the mouth and the tongue, inferior tumor extension into this muscle raises suspicion for involvement of the tongue (Figure 4-2).

SCC of the Buccal Mucosa

Buccal SCC comprises less than 10% of oral cavity cancers. Similar to other subsites within the oral cavity, advanced tumors involving the adjacent muscles lymph nodes have poor prognostic features. Buccal SCC can deeply invade the neighboring structures along the parotid duct, masseter muscle, or palate, or may break

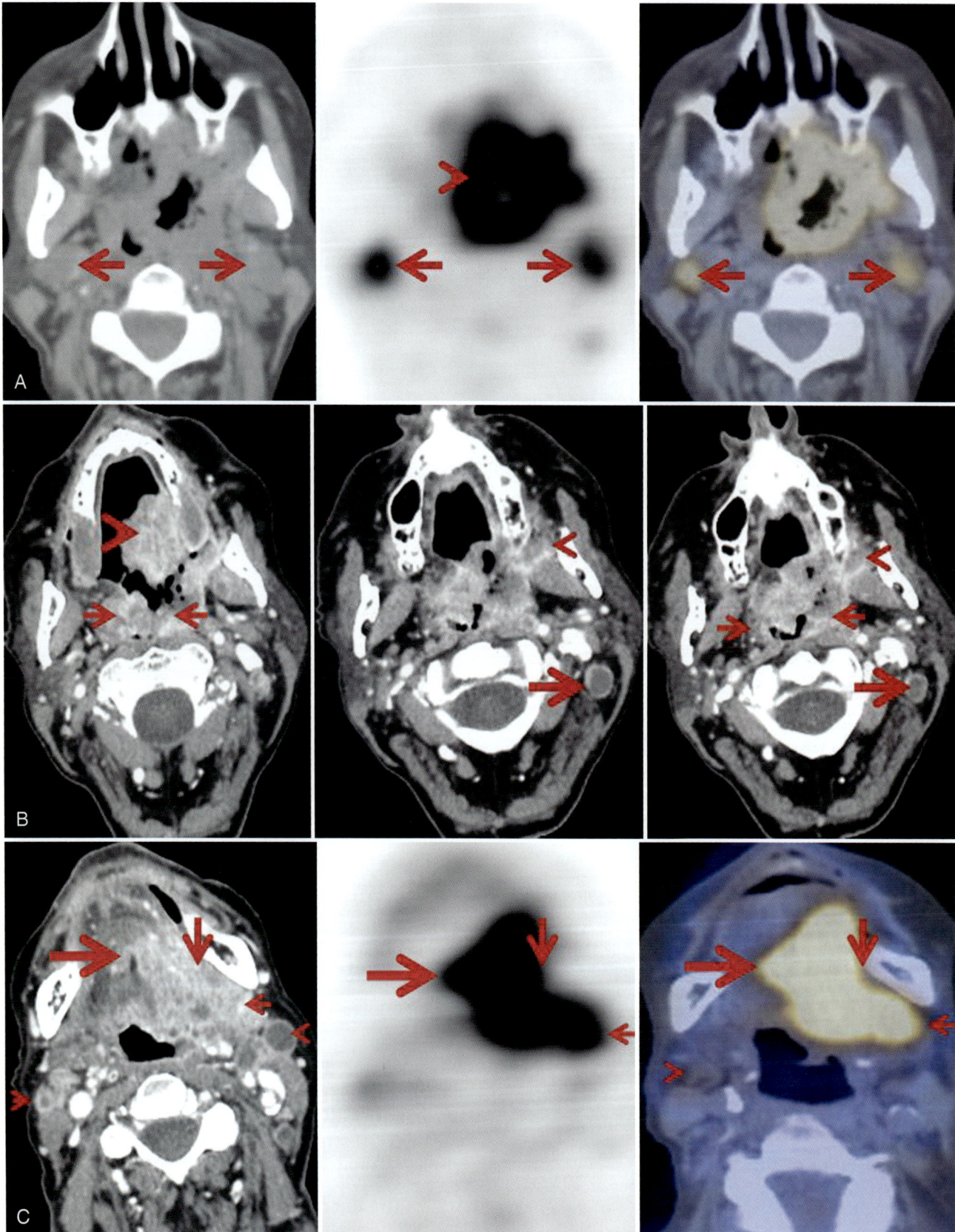

Figure 4-5.

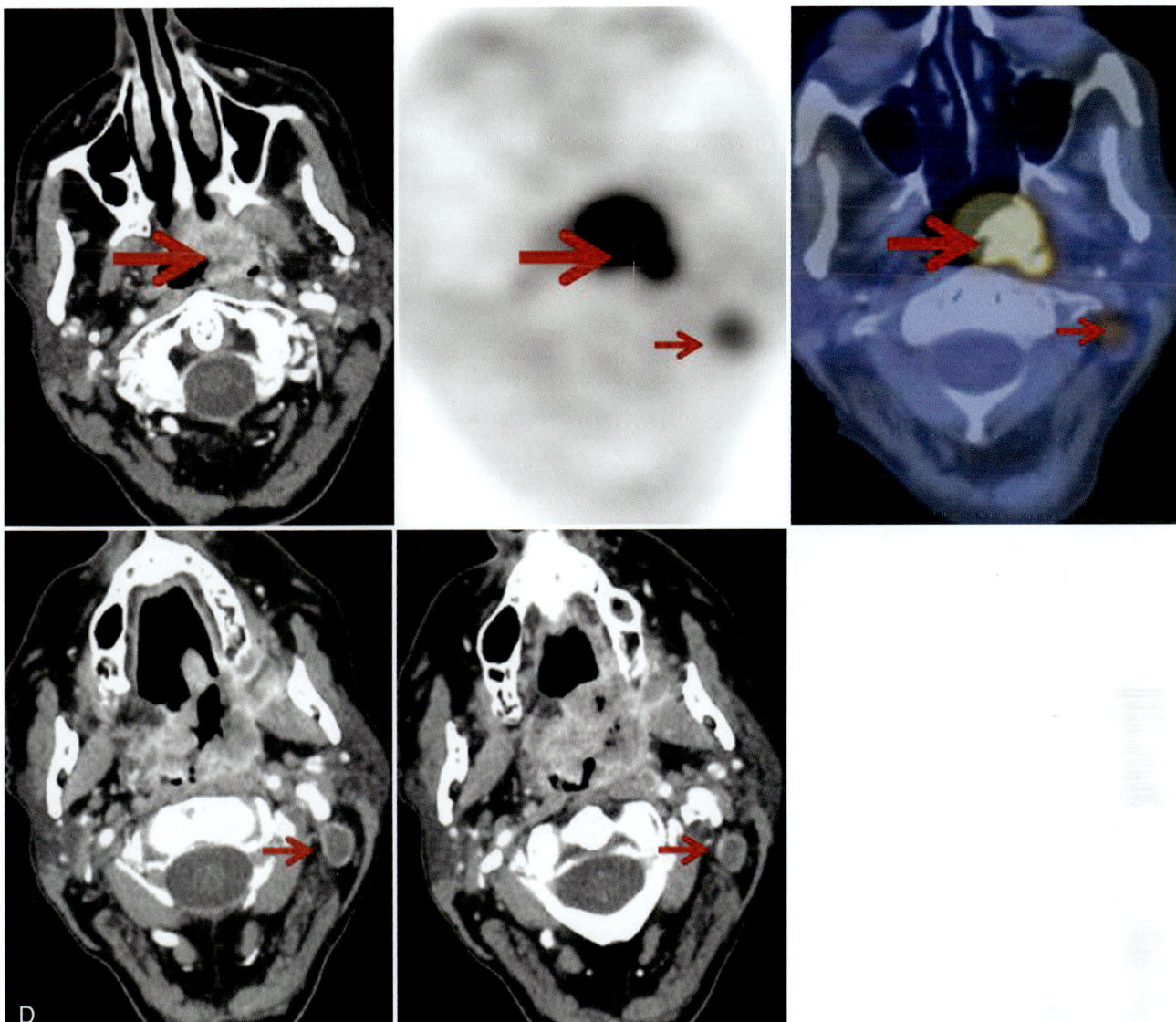

Figure 4-5, cont'd A 65-year-old woman recently diagnosed with tongue cancer, referred for staging with FDG PET/CT performed with low-dose CT (**upper panel**), and a separately acquired contrast-enhanced high-resolution CT (**lower panel**). **A:** FDG PET/CT axial images reveal increased FDG uptake (SUV_{max} 18) corresponding to a large enhancing mass involving the entirety of the mobile tongue, measuring >4 cm (T3), and showing multiple necrotic areas on the CT portion of the study (right *arrowheads*; **upper and lower panels**). **B:** On the CT portion, the tumor is noted to extend caudally to the oropharyngeal wall (small right and left arrows) and spreads to both sides of the base of tongue, oropharynx. Tumor extension is also seen into the pterygoid muscles and in the retromolar trigone (*left arrowheads*). There are multiple necrotic nodes bilaterally in the left level II nodal regions (N2c) (*large arrows*). Note that the contrast-enhanced CT and PET slices do not align well due to separate acquisition sessions (see panel B for better orientation). **C:** Corresponding slices of contrast-enhanced high-resolution CT and FDG PET slices show tumor spread in the left genioglossus (*large right arrows*), and left myelohyoid muscles (*vertical arrows*). Note mildly hypermetabolic necrotic, metastatic level II lymph nodes (left small *arrows*) that again do not align well with the PET slices. **D:** Hypermetabolic tongue mass extends cranially to the left side of the nasopharynx and involves the pharyngeal recess (fossa of Rosenmüller) and palate (*arrows*). Note the mildly hypermetabolic, necrotic left level IIB lymph node (SUV_{max} 3.6) (*small arrows*), consistent with metastatic disease. The low-grade uptake is attributable to central necrosis. Note the value of contrast-enhanced CT for accurate staging of the primary tumor as well as necrotic lymph nodes. AJCC staging: T3N2cMX, stage IV disease.

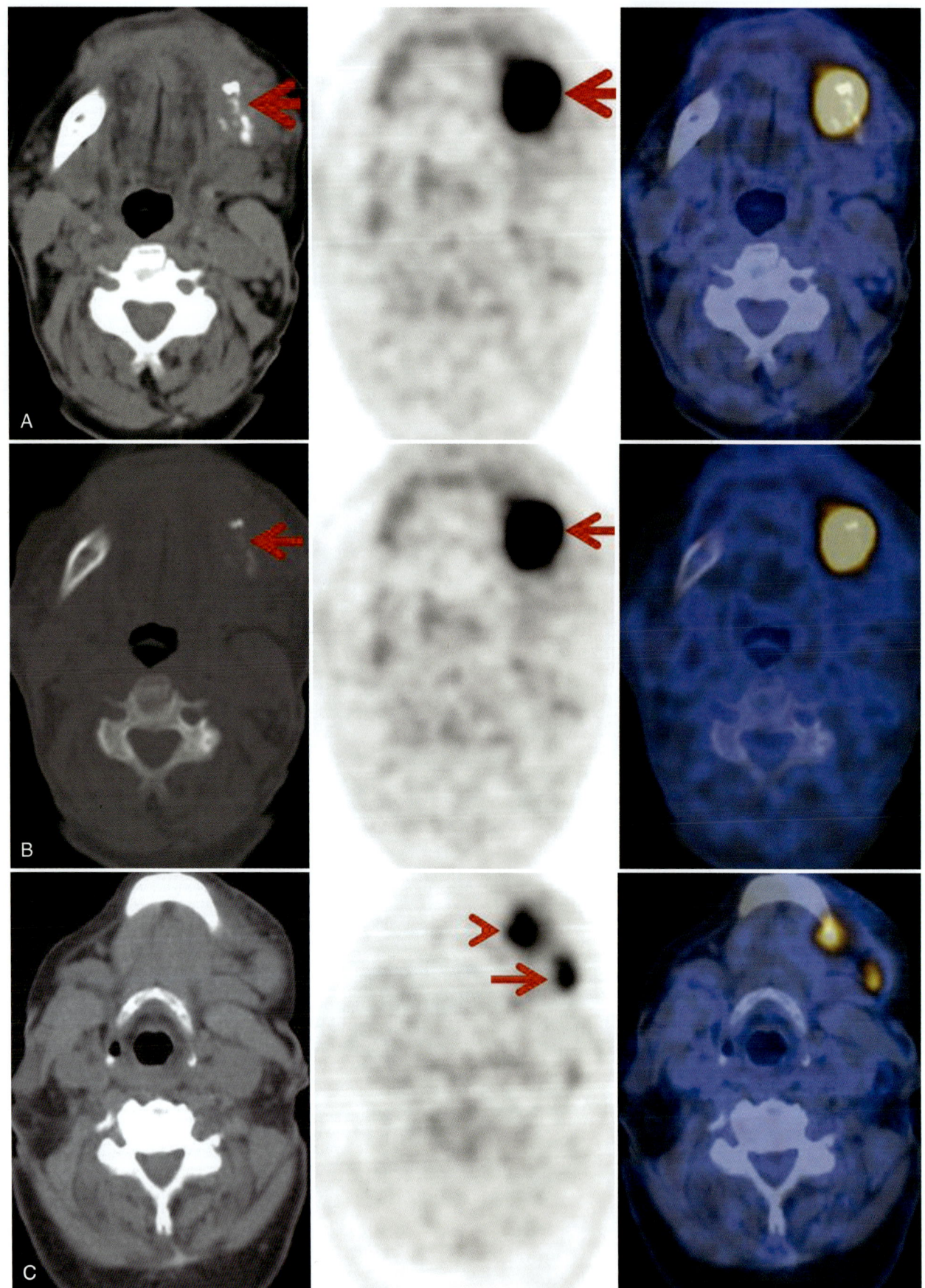

Figure 4-6 A 62-year-old woman recently diagnosed with floor of the mouth squamous cell carcinoma, referred for staging with FDG PET/CT performed with noncontrast-enhanced low-dose CT. FDG PET/CT axial images reveal increased FDG uptake (SUV_{max} 18.7) corresponding to an infiltrating tumor in the left floor of the mouth with destruction of the left symphysis and body of the mandible (T4) noted in both soft tissue **(A)** and bone **(B)** windows. **C:** An enlarged hypermetabolic (SUV_{max} 7.9) left level IB lymph node (N1) consistent with locoregional metastatic disease node (*arrow*). Note inferior border of the tumor abutting the rim of the left mandibular body (*arrowhead*). AJCC staging: T4N1MX, stage IV disease.

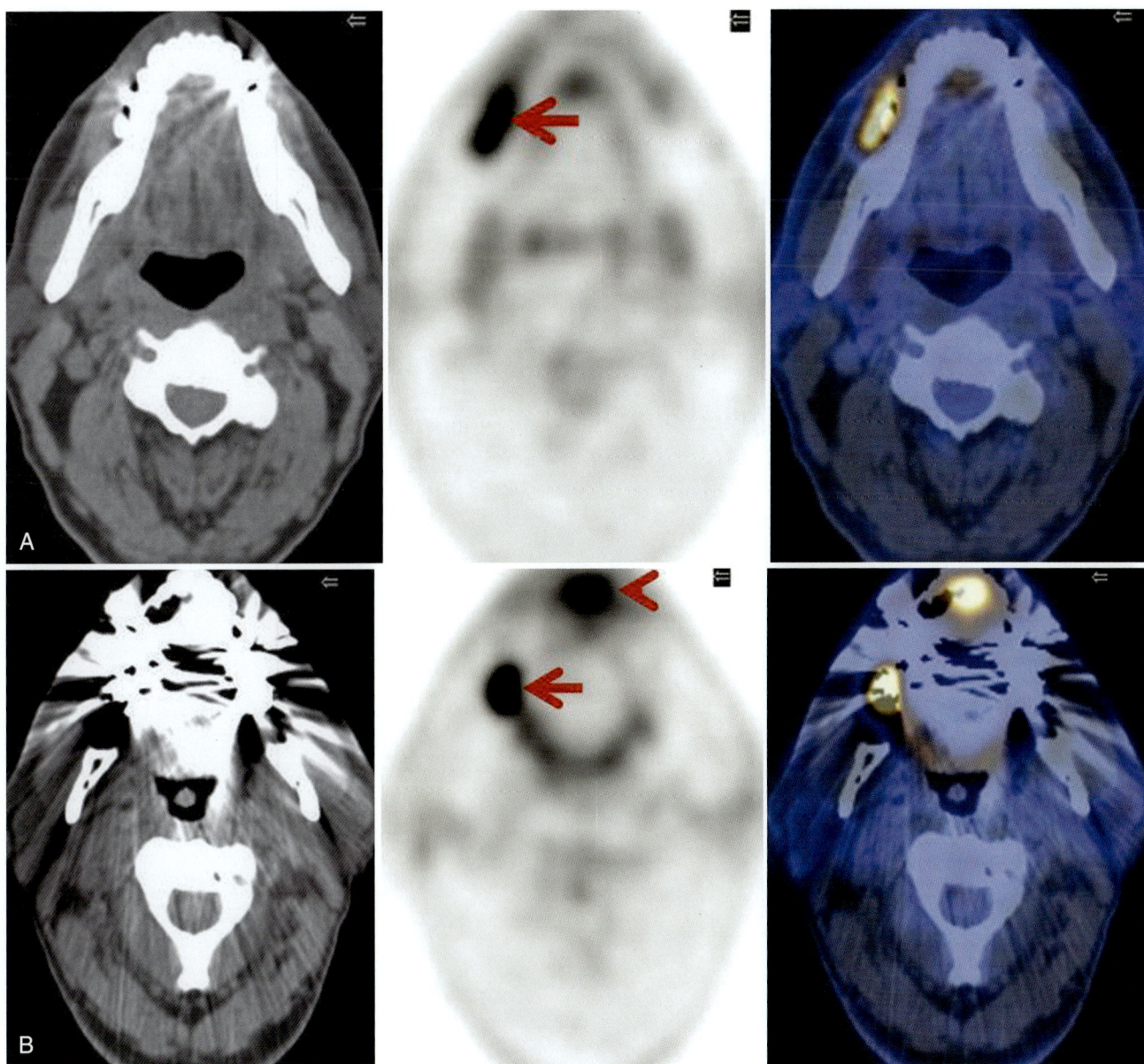

Figure 4-7 A: A 48-year-old woman recently diagnosed with buccal squamous cell carcinoma (SCC), referred for staging with FDG PET/CT performed with noncontrast-enhanced low-dose CT. FDG PET/CT axial images reveal a fusiform area of increased FDG uptake (SUV$_{max}$ 9.5) corresponding to a soft tissue mass, situated in the inferior margin of the masseter muscle along the right alveolar ridge, and measuring 1.9 cm (T1), consistent with buccal carcinoma that has infiltrated the muscle (*arrow*). AJCC staging: T1N0MX, stage I disease. **B:** A 54-year-old man recently diagnosed with buccal SCC. FDG PET/CT performed with noncontrast-enhanced low-dose CT reveals intensely increased FDG accumulation corresponding to the alveolar ridge at the right mandibular angle in close proximity to the mandible (*arrow*) (SUV$_{max}$ 14.3). Mandibular bone may be involved; however, streak artifacts emanating from the dental implants preclude appropriate evaluation of both CT and PET images. The patient underwent composite resection with right selective neck dissection which revealed no evidence of mandibular invasion. AJCC staging: T1N0MX, stage I disease. Note physiologic uptake in anterior midline of oral cavity, which is usually seen at the confluence of sublingual glands and insertion of the genioglossus muscle (*arrowhead*).

into the buccal fat pad (Figure 4-7, *A*). Accurate identification of these areas of involvement change surgical approach. Although MRI is ideal for imaging of the buccal mucosa and the masticator space, PET/CT may complement anatomic imaging with useful metabolic information, particularly for lesions whose evaluation is hampered by artifacts (Figure 4-7, *B*). Nonetheless, streak artifacts can hinder the evaluation of FDG PET and CT images alike despite appreciable FDG uptake. Without the delineation of an obvious mass on the corresponding CT images, FDG findings can be of equivocal value to both interpreting and referring physicians.

Cancers of the Hard Palate

Dissimilar to other subsites of the oral cavity, SCC does not constitute the overwhelming majority of malignant processes of the hard palate, which is rich in minor salivary glands. The adenoid cystic carcinoma and mucoepidermoid carcinoma originate from the minor salivary glands, which can be found everywhere

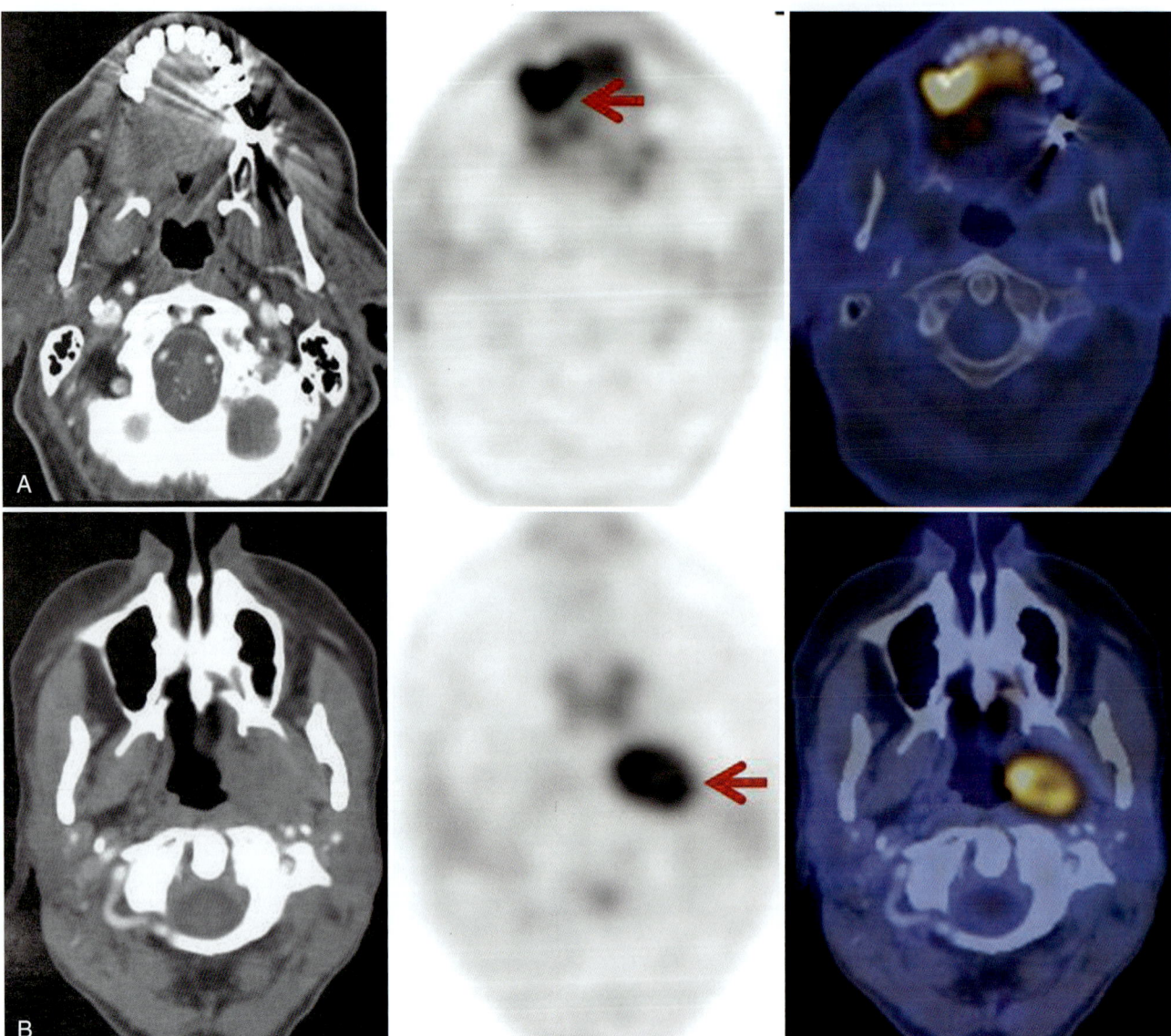

Figure 4-8 A: A 74-year-old man with recently diagnosed palate squamous cell carcinoma (SCC), referred for staging with FDG PET/CT performed with low-dose CT and a separately acquired contrast-enhanced high-resolution CT (low-dose CT not shown). FDG PET axial image reveals increased FDG uptake (SUV_{max} 17.4) in a soft tissue density situated in the left anterior hard palate abutting the maxilla (*arrow*), consistent with hard palate SCC. Nonetheless, diagnostic CT does not demonstrate a well-defined discrete focal mass in this location. The patient subsequently underwent hemimaxillectomy, which revealed well-differentiated SCC of the palate. Bone and bone margins were free of carcinoma. **B:** 55-year-old male presented with a mass in his left nasopharynx. FDG PET/CT performed with a contrast-enhanced high-resolution CT demonstrates a moderately hypermetabolic (SUV_{max} 5.5, measured in hottest slice) well-delineated mass, measuring 3.0 cm in the left side of the nasopharynx (*arrow*), extending into the palatine tonsil, consistent with the patient's known adenocystic carcinoma. There is obliteration of the left fossa of Rosenmüller. There is lateral displacement but no gross invasion of the adjacent pterygoid musculature. Note the difference in FDG uptake (SUV_{max}) between the tumors presented in **A** and **B** reflecting the differences in metabolic activity between SCC and adenocytic carcinoma despite the smaller size of the palatine SCC.

in the oral cavity including the palate. Although these tumors cannot be distinguished from SCC (Figure 4-8, A and B) by cross-sectional imaging, FDG PET metabolic features display may differentiate high-grade tumors from those of lower grade (Figures 4-8, A, and 4-9). In low-grade malignancies, FDG uptake with standard uptake value (SUVs) less than 4.0 may be obscured by the normal physiologic FDG uptake, particularly in organs with high background uptake (Figure 4-9, A).

What Are the Oropharyngeal Cancer Subtypes?

SCC of the Base of Tongue

The tongue base is the second most common site within the oropharynx for SCC after the tonsillar SCC. Patients with SCC of the base of the tongue often present with advanced disease with regional lymph node metastases (Figures 4-10 and 4-11). The base of the tongue parallels the oropharyngeal posterior wall and extends to

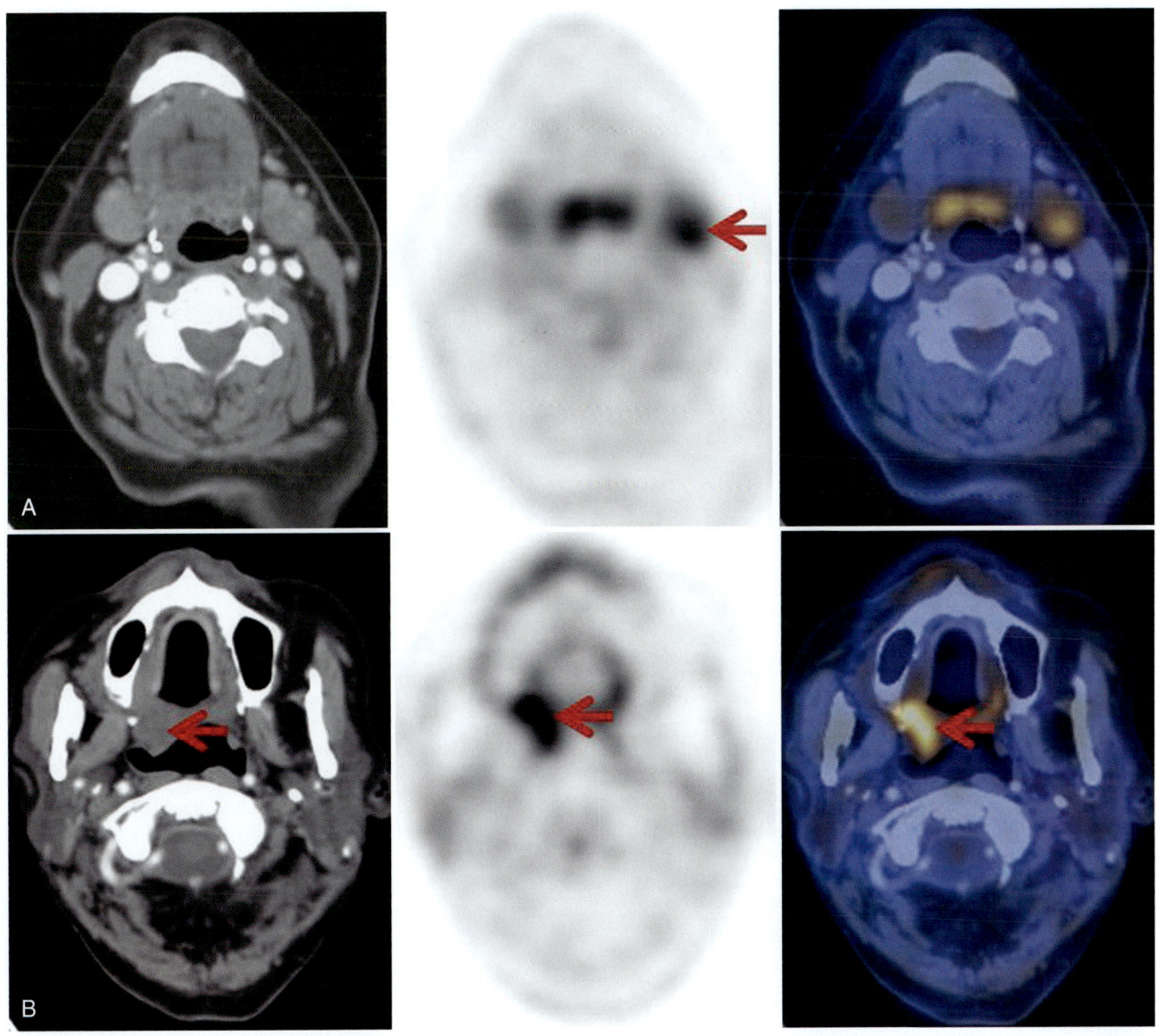

Figure 4-9 A: 59-year-old man recently diagnosed with adenocystic carcinoma of the left submandibular gland. FDG PET/CT performed with a contrast-enhanced high resolution CT demonstrates mild-to-moderately increased FDG uptake in the left mandibular gland (SUV_{max} 5.6; *arrow*). Note marginal difference in FDG metabolism between the two submandibular glands suggesting a low grade tumor involving the left side. **B:** A 66-year-old man recently diagnosed with palate squamous cell carcinoma (SCC). FDG PET/CT performed with a contrast-enhanced high resolution CT demonstrates significantly increased FDG uptake (SUV_{max} 9.8) in the posterior aspect of the right palate, consistent with high-grade SCC (*arrows*). The significant difference in FDG metabolism between the two tumor types represents the difference in tumor grades.

the pharyngoepiglottic folds and vallecula. The anterior spread of base of the tongue SCC can involve the floor of the mouth (Figure 4-10, *A*). Tumor can also spread posterolaterally to the lingual and faucial tonsils or inferiorly to the preepiglottic fat, vallecula, epiglottis, or supraglottic larynx (Figure 4-10, *B*). Inferior extension of a tumor from the tongue base into the preepiglottic fat space implies supraglottic larynx involvement and often requires partial supraglottic laryngectomy. The accuracy of CT or MRI for determining preepiglottic fat infiltration is high at approximately 90%. Thus, FDG PET does not play an essential role in evaluating this region but may still be a complement in special circumstances where anatomic imaging is not definitive (Figure 4-11).

One caveat is that small lesions are difficult to detect on FDG PET imaging due to physiologic uptake within the lymphoid tissue at the base of the tongue. Although asymmetry at the base of the tongue can be a sign of pathologic process, not all asymmetries can account for malignancy. Conservation therapy with chemoradiation is the standard definitive treatment of oropharyngeal cancers. Small-volume tumors can be treated with surgery or radiation therapy. Larger T-staged lesions are

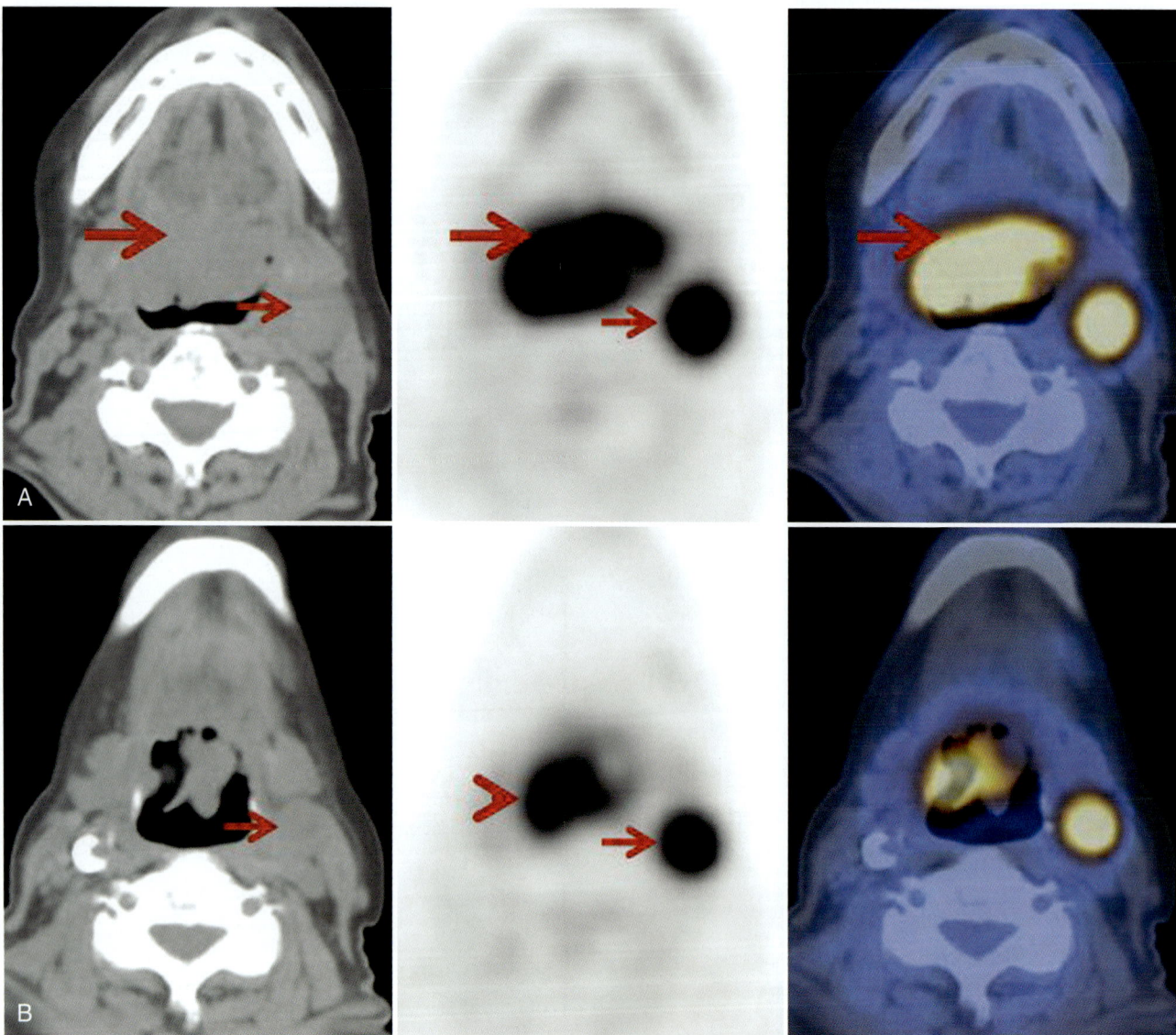

Figure 4-10 A 57-year-old woman recently diagnosed with base of tongue squamous cell carcinoma, referred for staging with FDG PET/CT performed with noncontrast-enhanced low-dose CT. **A:** Large area of increased FDG uptake (SUV_{max} 14.8) involving the base of tongue encompasses both the right and left sides of the midline, measures 4.2 cm and apparently involves the extrinsic tongue muscles (T4?) in the posterior floor of the mouth (*arrows*). Increased FDG uptake (SUV_{max} 12.8) in an enlarged left level IIA lymph node which measures 2.9 cm (N1) (*small arrows*). These findings represent T4?N1MX disease, stage IV (see Figure 4-43 for further evaluation). However, the association of a contrast-enhanced CT study would increase the accuracy and reader confidence, particularly with respect to T staging. **B:** The tumor extends inferiorly to the right oropharyngeal wall, vallecula, and the epiglottis (*arrowhead*). This finding suggests supraglottic laryngeal involvement and prompts consideration of a partial laryngectomy. The patient subsequently underwent neoadjuvant therapy with chemoradiation followed by surgical resection with partial laryngectomy and lymph node dissection.

generally treated with concurrent chemotherapy and radiation therapy in an attempt to preserve function.

SCC of the Tonsils

Carcinomas that arise from the tonsillar fossa are the most common oral cavity cancers. The anterior and posterior tonsillar pillars are mucosal folds over the palatoglossus and palatopharyngeal muscles, respectively. There may be inferior involvement of the tongue base or posterior extension along the lateral oropharyngeal wall (Figure 4-12). Anteriorly, the lesions may extend into the oral cavity (Figures 4-13 and 4-14). Laterally, tumors may invade the parapharyngeal space or mandible. Superior spread of the tumor involves the soft and hard palate (Figure 4-14, A). In cases with advanced tumors, invasion of the masticator and parapharyngeal space is readily detected on FDG PET imaging.

Similar to base of tongue lesions, small lesions located within a tonsillar crypt can be undetectable on PET/CT imaging. As the tumor grows, asymmetry becomes more evident. However, subtle tonsillar asymmetry can be present as a normal anatomic variant in normal individuals. Tonsillar asymmetry should raise suspicion for tumor. However, without the presence of clinical symptoms (e.g., painful swallowing, ipsilateral otalgia, adenopathy), the incidence of an asymmetric tonsil harboring cancer is approximately 5% (Figure 4-15, *A* and *B*). If intravenous contrast is administered,

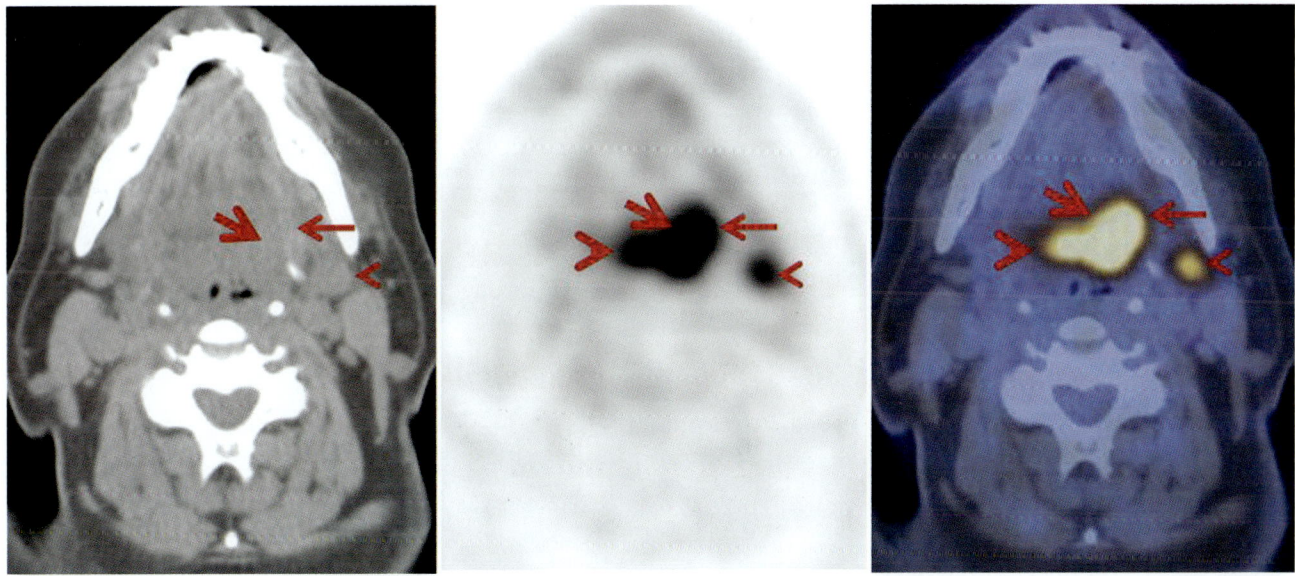

Figure 4-11 A 67-year-old man recently diagnosed with base of tongue squamous cell carcinoma, referred for staging with FDG PET/CT performed with noncontrast-enhanced low-dose CT and a separately acquired contrast-enhanced CT study (not shown). There is increased FDG uptake (SUV_{max} 9.4) in the left base of tongue (*right diagonal arrows*), with extension into the midline as evidenced by FDG uptake in this region (*arrowheads*), tumor extent could not be assessed well on the separately acquired contrast-enhanced dedicated CT (not shown). In this case, FDG PET complemented the findings of CT imaging, suggestive of more extensive local involvement that might lead to a change in the surgical plan. There is also suggestion of involvement of the extrinsic tongue muscles (mylohyoid) in the posterior floor of the mouth (*left small arrows*). An unenlarged hypermetabolic (SUV_{max} 5.4) left level IIA lymph node is suggestive of metastatic disease (*arrowheads*). PET findings upstaged disease to from T1N0M0 to T1N1M0, with migration from stage I to stage III disease per clinical and CT evaluation. Lymph node metastasis was confirmed after subsequent neck dissection.

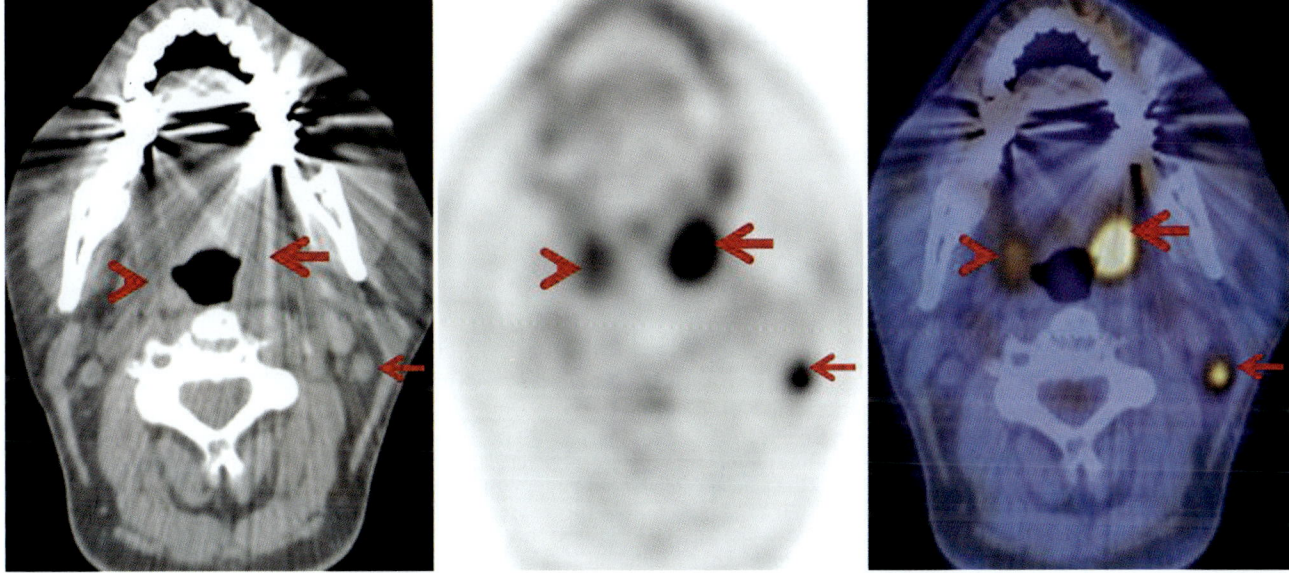

Figure 4-12 A 57-year-old man recently diagnosed with moderately differentiated tonsil squamous cell carcinoma, referred for staging with FDG PET/CT performed with noncontrast-enhanced low-dose CT and a separately acquired contrast-enhanced CT study (not shown). There is increased FDG uptake (SUV_{max} 10.2) in the left tonsillar fossa demonstrating fullness in the oropharyngeal wall (*arrows*), consistent with the patient's known primary tumor. Note the physiologic uptake (SUV_{max} 2.7) in the contralateral tonsil (*arrowhead*). There is a subcentimeter hypermetabolic left level IIB lymph node (*small arrows*) suggestive of metastatic disease (N1) despite its small size (N0 disease by CT criteria). This finding upstaged disease to T1N1M0, representing stage III disease rather than stage I per clinical and CT evaluation. Lymph node metastasis was confirmed on subsequent histopathologic examination.

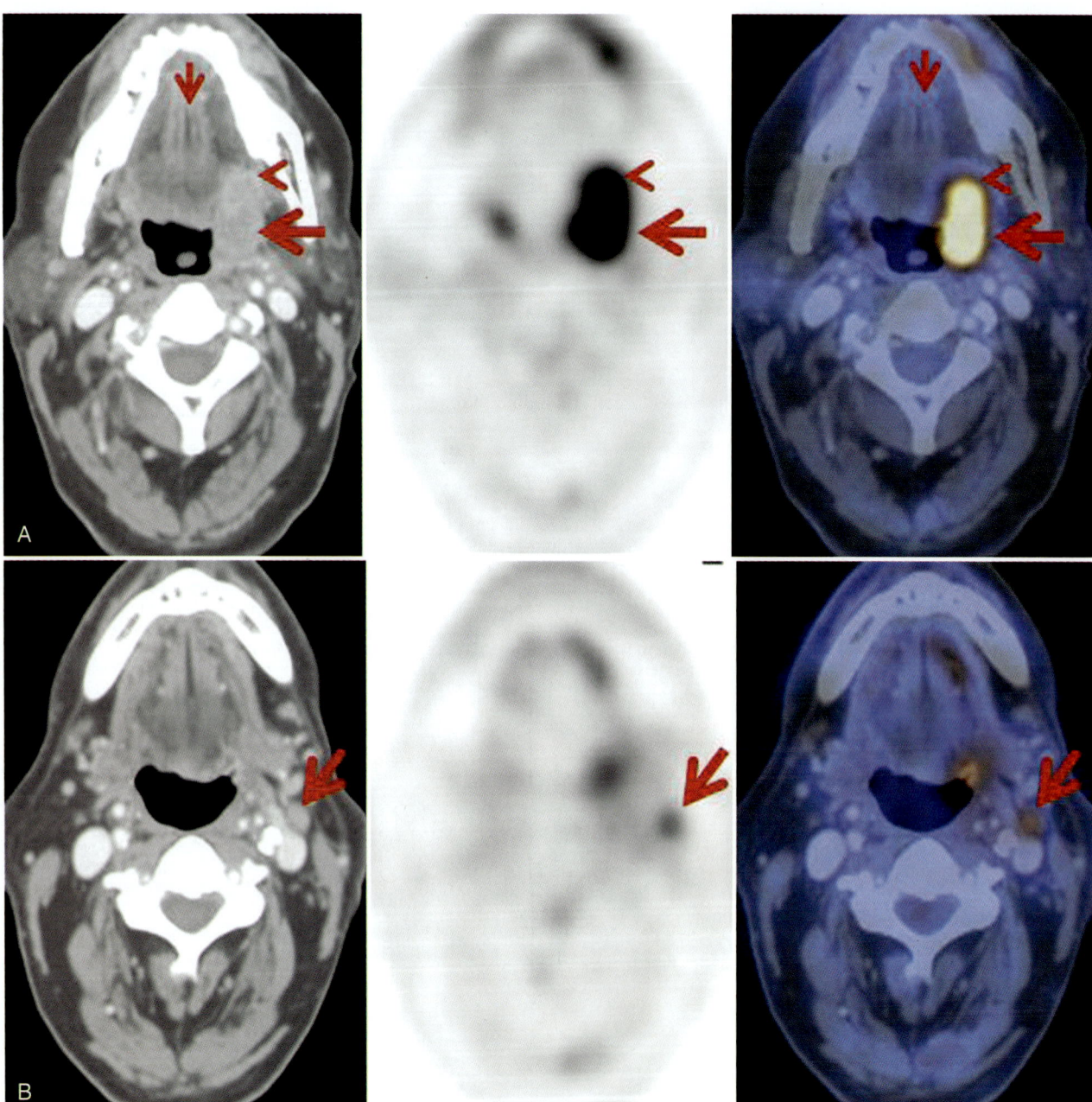

Figure 4-13 A 66-year-old woman recently diagnosed with well-differentiated tonsil squamous cell carcinoma, referred for staging with FDG PET/CT performed with contrast-enhanced high-resolution CT. **A:** There is increased FDG uptake (SUV_{max} 12.8) corresponding to a heterogeneously enhancing mass in the left tonsillar fossa causing prominence of the oropharyngeal wall, measuring 3.2 cm (T2) on the accompanying contrast-enhanced CT study (*arrows*), consistent with the patient's known primary tumor. This mass extends anteriorly to invade the base of tongue (*arrowhead*) but spares the genioglossus muscle (*vertical arrows*). **B:** A subcentimeter mildly hypermetabolic (SUV_{max} 2.7) left level IIA lymph node (*diagonal arrows*) raises suspicion for metastatic disease (N1?). However, histopathologic evaluation of the neck dissection specimen revealed no evidence of lymph node metastasis, proving the FDG PET finding as false positive. Note that inflammatory or reactive changes in lymph nodes, particularly in those that are draining the primary tumor can cause false positive findings. AJCC staging: T2N0M0, stage II disease.

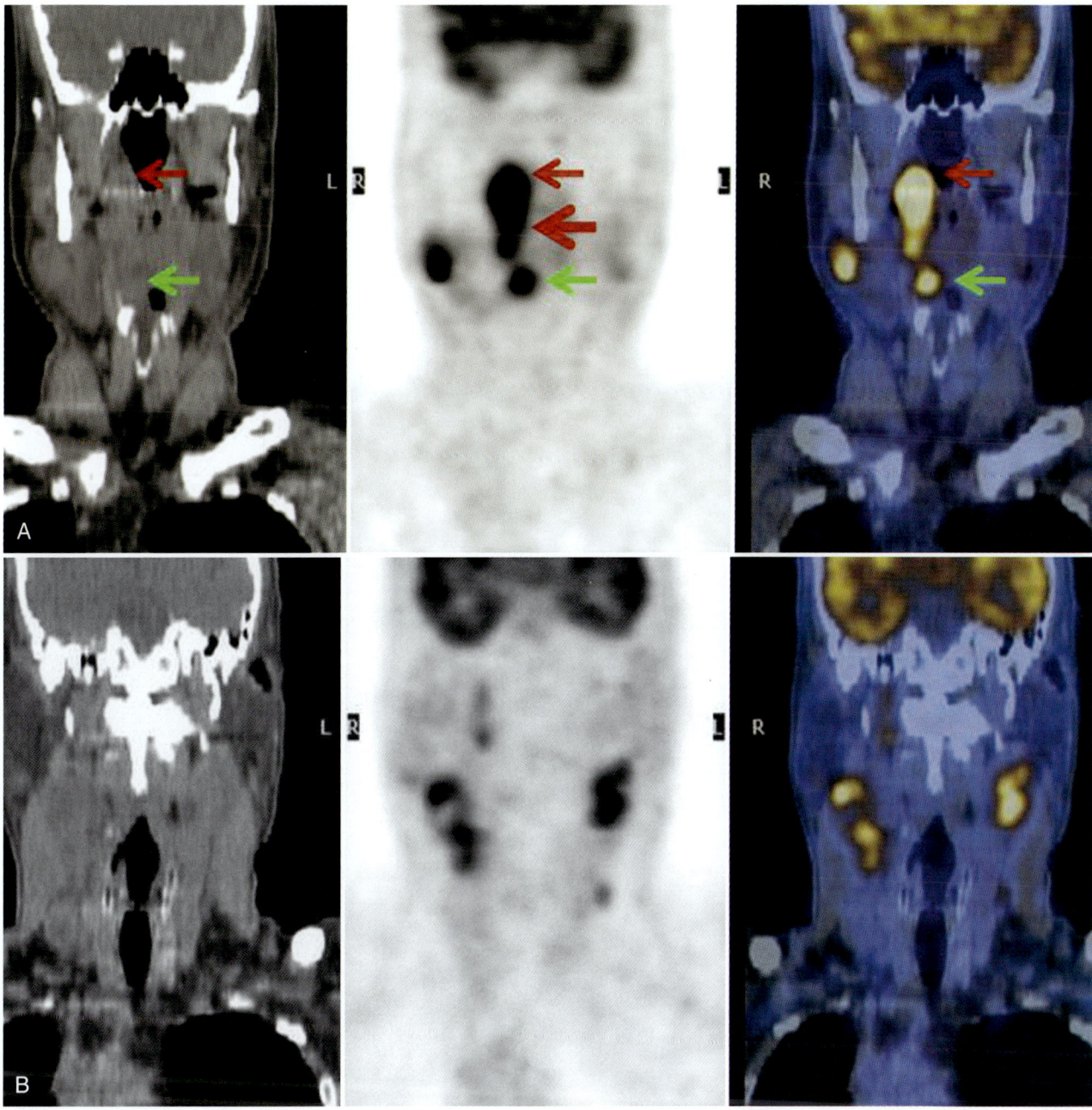

Figure 4-14 A 59-year-old man recently diagnosed with squamous cell carcinoma (SCC) of the right tonsil, referred for staging with FDG PET/CT performed with noncontrast-enhanced low-dose CT. **A:** Coronal images of the FDG PET/CT study demonstrates a large area of hypermetabolic (SUV_{max} 20) conglomerate mass involves the right oropharyngeal wall and extends from the region of the right tonsil and epiglottis, consistent with the primary tumor (4.2 cm, T3). There are multiple, enlarged, confluent lymph nodes at the levels of right IB (SUV_{max} 9.5, size 1.8 cm), right IIA (SUV_{max} 11, size 2.2 cm), right IIB (SUV_{max} 6.7, size 1.47 cm), left IIA (SUV_{max} 13, size 2.3 cm), and left IIB (SUV_{max} 9.5, size 1.45 cm) with extension into level III on the right side. **B:** There are lymph nodes with increased FDG uptake at the right level III (SUV_{max} 4.5, size 10 mm) and left level III stations (SUV_{max} 6, size 7.3 mm). Subsequent lymph node biopsy revealed moderately to poorly differentiated SCC. In advanced T-stage tumors, the likelihood of bilateral neck involvement (stage IV disease) is high.

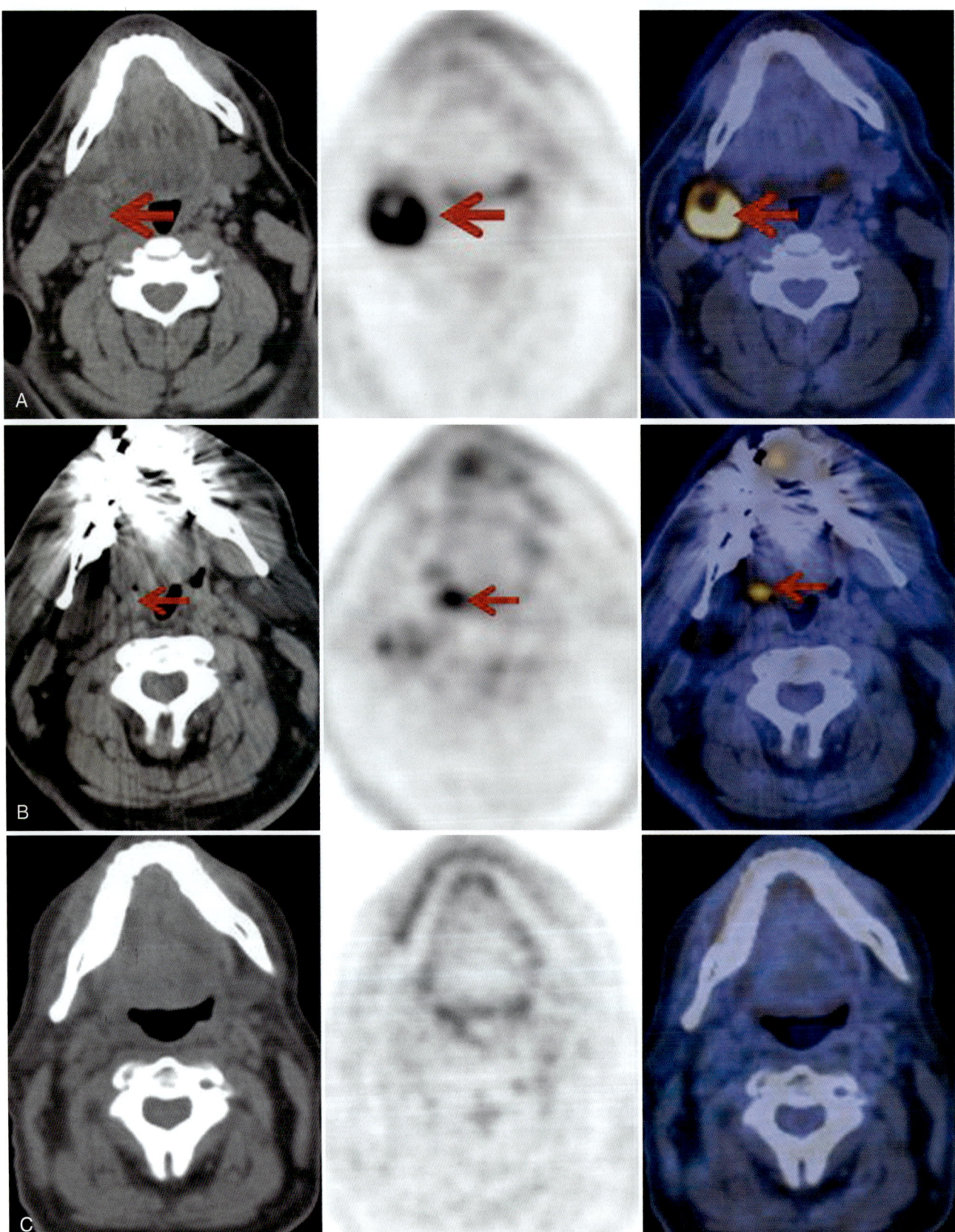

Figure 4-15 **A:** A 47-year-old patient who presented with metastatic SCC of unknown origin in the right neck, referred for evaluation of extent of disease and identification of the primary malignancy. PET/CT scan performed with noncontrast enhanced low-dose CT demonstrates increased FDG uptake in a large level IIA mass showing central necrosis and only peripherally prominent FDG uptake (SUV_{max} 23; *arrows*), consistent with metastatic disease of unknown primary. **B:** Asymmetric uptake in the right tonsillar fossa (SUV_{max} 5.6; *small arrow*). This finding originally was interpreted as "consistent with the tonsillar primary SCC"; however, subsequent surgery confirmed acute tonsillitis, proving the FDG PET finding as false positive for malignancy. **C:** The patient subsequently underwent chemoradiation therapy and follow-up study 3 months after completion of definitive therapy. FDG PET study demonstrates complete resolution of the level II mass, suggestive of favorable response to therapy. Importantly, the planned lymph node dissection was deferred based on resolution of neck disease.

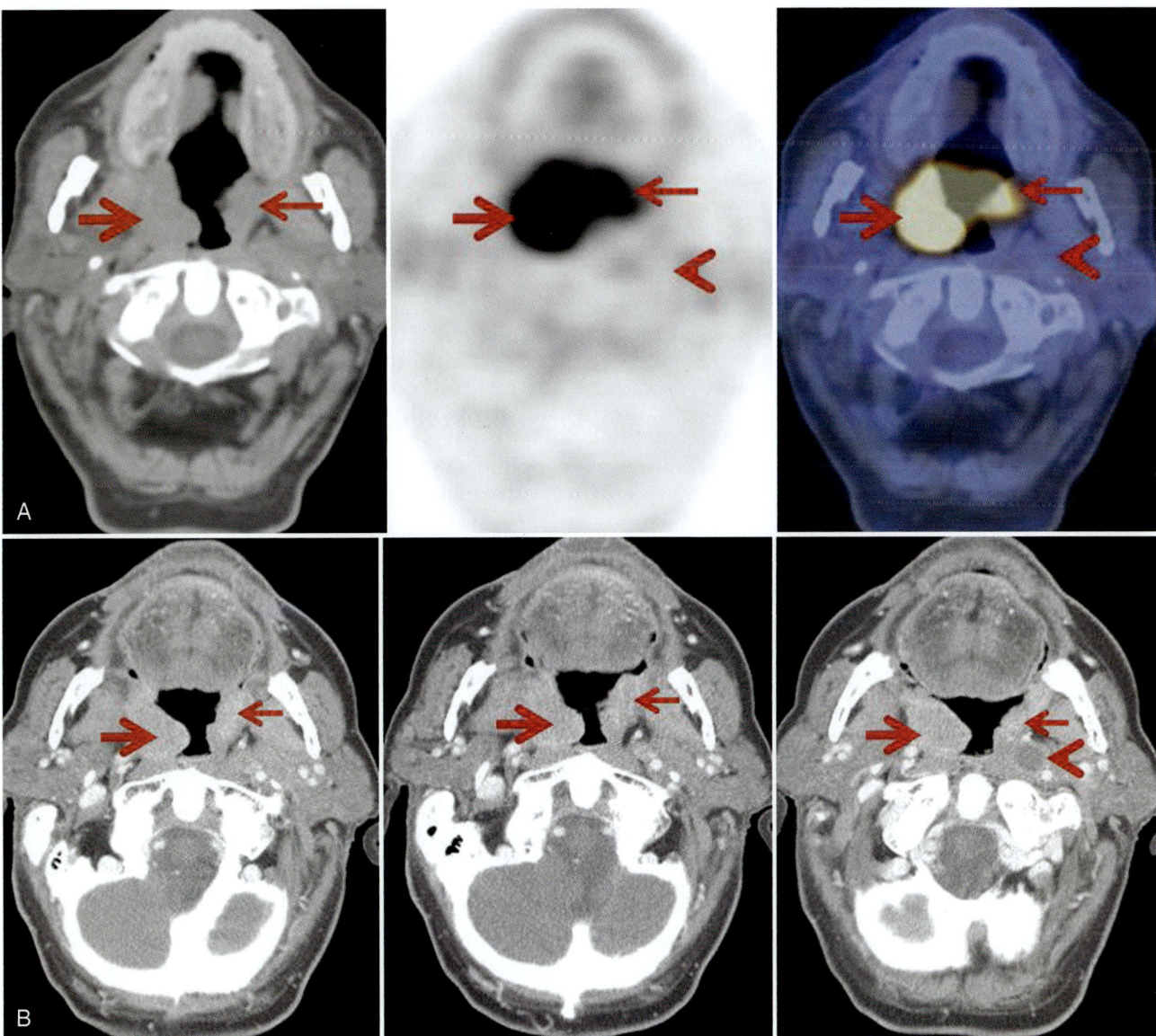

Figure 4-16 A 71-year-old patient recently diagnosed with soft palate squamous cell carcinoma, referred for evaluation of extent of disease with PET/CT study performed with noncontrast enhanced low-dose CT (**A**) and a separately acquired contrast-enhanced CT study (**B**). PET/CT axial slices (**A**) and contrast-enhanced CT (**B**) demonstrate a large hypermetabolic (SUV_{max} 16) soft tissue mass involving the right palatine tonsil extending to the soft palate (*right arrows*). The tumor extends across the midline and thickens the left aspect of the soft palate (*small arrows*). The left tonsillar region is slightly less full, but whether tumor extends into this region is uncertain based on the CT study. However, based on the distribution of FDG uptake, both tonsils appear involved. There is a 1.4-cm necrotic left retropharyngeal lymph node with no FDG uptake (*arrowheads*). The necrotic lymph nodes can be completely false negative on FDG PET imaging. In this case, both dedicated CT and PET complemented each other by showing more findings together than with each test alone.

the CT portion of PET imaging demonstrates enhancement similar to that of the tonsils.

Given the equal performance, primary radiation therapy is the preferred treatment of choice for early tonsillar carcinoma due to the morbidity of surgery. The role of salvage surgery after radiation for early tonsillar carcinomas is well established. As with tumors in other oropharyngeal subsites, multimodality therapy has become the standard of care for advanced tumors of the tonsillar complex for superior local control.

SCC of the Soft Palate

The soft palate is a much less frequent subsite for SCC than are the faucial tonsils or the base of the tongue. As expected, SCC is the most common tumor of the soft palate, but minor salivary gland cancers are not infrequent. Carcinomas of the soft palate most commonly involve the oral aspect of the palate. These lesions have the potential to involve the tonsillar pillars and the hard palate (Figure 4-16) or the skull base. Minor salivary gland tumors (e.g., mucoepidermoid and adenoid cystic carcinomas) can be encountered in this area, although much less so than SCCs.

Either primary surgical resection or radiation therapy is the treatment of choice for early (T1–T2) soft palate SCCs. Locally advanced (T3–T4) soft palate SCCs currently are treated by multimodality therapy involving chemoradiation and surgery. Laser surgery, prostheses, and microvascular free flaps have recently gained more momentum in designing surgical approaches.

II. WHAT ARE THE ANATOMIC SUBSITES TO EVALUATE IN LARYNGEAL CANCERS?

There are three anatomic levels to larynx, supraglottis, glottis and subglottis. The cartilaginous frame of the larynx consists of the thyroid, cricoid, and arytenoid cartilages. Superiorly, the epiglottis forms the border with the pharynx. Inferiorly, it extends to the lower margin of the cricoid. The cricoarytenoid joint demarcates glottic from supraglottic and subglottic structures. The distinction between supraglottic structures; epiglottis, aryepiglottic folds, false vocal cords, laryngeal ventricle, and superior superficial mucosa of the arytenoids and glottic larynx; true vocal cords; and anterior and posterior commissures is crucial for proper management. The subglottis starts below the level of the true vocal cords and extends to the first tracheal ring.

Does FDG PET/CT Have a Primary Role in the Evaluation of Primary Tumor in Laryngeal Cancers?

Similar to oral and oropharyngeal SCCs, the determination of T staging is based on the assessment of depth of tumor invasion. Although endoscopic assessment is the mainstay of T staging, imaging correlates are important for management. ceCT is the imaging modality of choice, with sensitivity and specificity of approximately 95% and 85%, respectively. FDG PET performed with noncontrast CT does not provide additional clinically relevant information due to its inability to differentiate among various depths of invasion in soft tissues. However, a baseline FDG PET/CT acquired with intravenous contrast on board considerably increases the interpretation accuracy of subsequent follow-up studies (Figures 4-17 through 4-19).

Does FDG PET Have a Role in Evaluation of Cartilage Involvement?

Cartilage invasion by laryngeal and hypopharyngeal SCCs leads to upstaging of the tumor to T4 status. Cricoid or thyroid cartilage invasion is associated with a higher recurrence risk and precludes organ-sparing laryngectomy. The presence of tumor may cause new bone formation and osteolysis in the adjacent cartilage. However, variable ossification and chondrification of the laryngeal cartilages render the evaluation for tumoral involvement difficult. Thus, the patterns of ossification caused by neoplastic growth cannot easily be distinguished from benign sclerotic variants. Extrathyroidal extension, erosion, and lysis of the cartilage occur in overt invasion of the cartilage with specificity greater than 90%. However, sensitivity usually is low for these findings unless all coexist. FDG PET/CT imaging can increase the sensitivity of detection of cartilage involvement in cases with unequivocally increased glucose metabolism corresponding to the cartilaginous structures also associated with morphologic abnormalities, particularly for the thyroid cartilage (Figures 4-19, 4-20 and 4-21). Overall sensitivity and specificity of approximately 80% were reported for the combination of these findings. However, it is conceivable that inflammatory changes associated with the adjacent neoplasm may cause findings similar to those of direct tumor invasion leading to false-positive results, particularly on FDG PET/CT imaging (Figure 4-22). Hypopharyngeal tumors involving the piriform sinus often invade the cornua and superior border of the thyroid cartilage (at the transition site with the thyrohyoid membrane).

Other areas that affect management with respect to the extent of primary tumor include the preepiglottic and paraglottic fat planes (Figure 4-23). Invasion of these contiguous spaces not only increases the likelihood of nodal metastases but also portends potential involvement of the base of the tongue and the hyoid bone.

What Are the Laryngeal Cancer Subtypes?

Supraglottic SCC

Supraglottic SCC accounts for 30% of laryngeal cancers and often are diagnosed at advanced T stages because of its insidious onset. Critical sites for assessment include the laryngeal ventricles, arytenoids, and anterior commissure, the involvement of any of which precludes supraglottic laryngectomy. These tumors primarily invade the preepiglottic space, which may lead to involvement of the anterior commissure (Figures 4-23 and 4-24), glottis, or subglottis, and thus eventually become transglottic tumors. Supraglottic tumors originating from the false cord, laryngeal ventricle, or aryepiglottic fold primarily infiltrate the paraglottic space (Figure 4-23), the vallecula anteriorly, or the pharyngeal wall laterally, or can extend into the tongue base through the glossoepiglottic fold by submucosal spread. Destruction of thyroid cartilage can be seen with more advanced tumors. Infiltration of the hypopharynx is common with posteriorly situated supraglottic SCCs.

Despite the high sensitivity of CT and MRI, the specificity of anatomic imaging is limited due to peritumoral inflammatory changes that may lead to overestimation of tumor extent. In these situations, FDG PET/CT may be helpful in increasing diagnostic certainty by demonstrating increased metabolism in the involved regions. Nonetheless, caution still should be exercised because FDG is not specific to malignant processes. Severe inflammation may also cause false-positive findings.

Glottic SCC

Greater than 50% of laryngeal SCCs originate from the glottic larynx. Patients present in early phases of disease due to abrupt development of hoarseness. Glottic SCC typically arises from the anterior half of the vocal cord and spreads via the anterior commissure to invade the contralateral cord or thyroid cartilage (Figure 4-25).

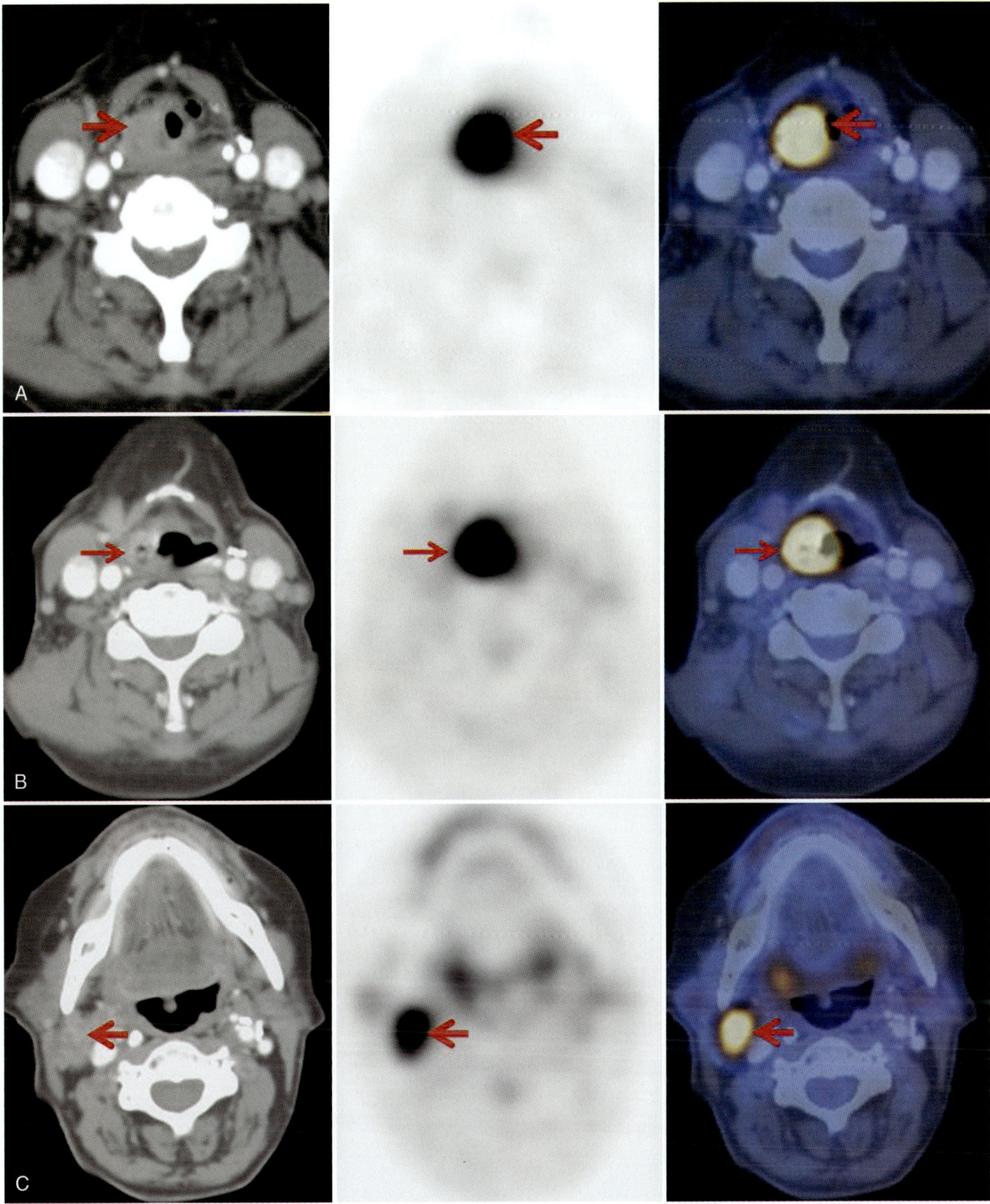

Figure 4-17 A 57-year-old woman recently diagnosed with a supraglottic squamous cell carcinoma (SCC), referred for staging with FDG PET/CT performed with contrast-enhanced high-resolution CT. **A, B:** Increased FDG uptake (SUV_{max} 11.0) corresponds to a mildly enhancing mass in the right supraglottic larynx involving the paraglottic fat planes (*arrows*) with extension into the right piriform sinus (T3) (*small arrows*). **C:** Increased FDG uptake (SUV_{max} 10) in a heterogeneously enhancing right level II lymph node represents metastatic disease (N1) with suggestion of a necrotic component. The patient underwent supraglottic laryngectomy and right selective neck dissection, which revealed invasive moderately differentiated SCC as well as replacement of the level II lymph node by metastatic tumor causing necrotic changes but without extranodal invasion. AJCC stage: T3N1MX, stage III disease.

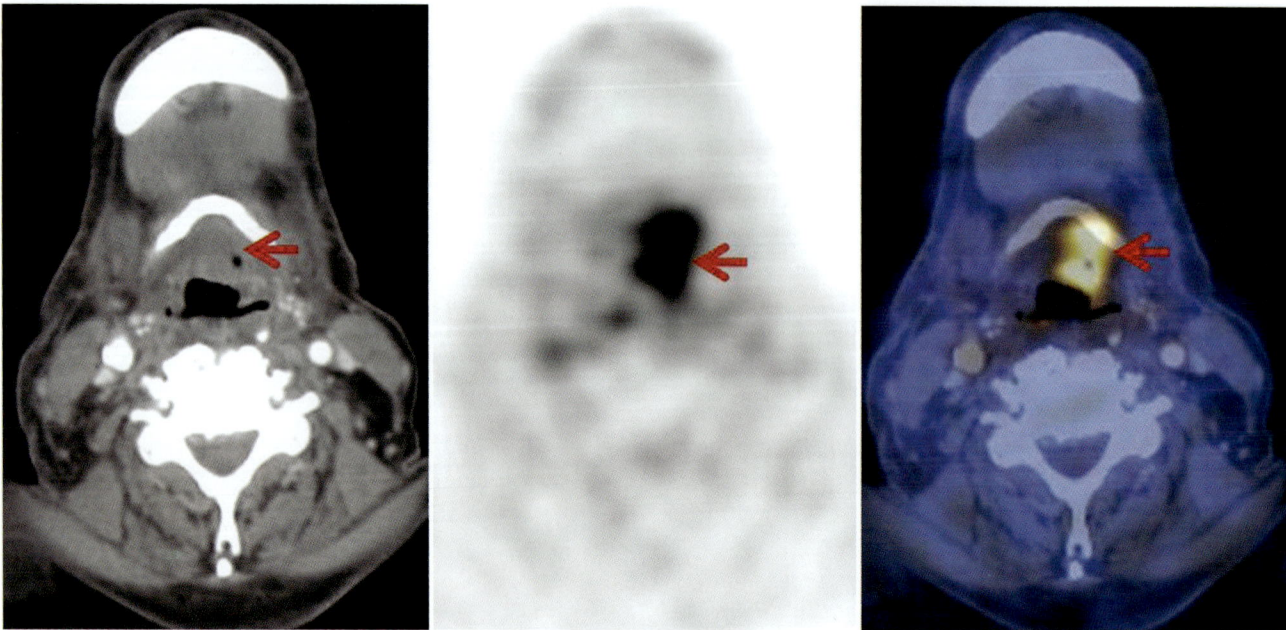

Figure 4-18 A 65-year-old man recently diagnosed with a supraglottic squamous cell carcinoma, referred for staging with FDG PET/CT performed with contrast-enhanced high-resolution CT. Axial images of a PET/CT study show increased FDG uptake (SUV_{max} 12.5) corresponding to nodular thickening of the left supraglottic region (*arrows*) involving the preepiglottic space and the vallecula extending from the median glossoepiglottic fold toward the left side without fixation of the vocal cords (determined by laryngoscopy) (T3). There is no evidence of lymph node involvement (N0). AJCC stage: T3N0MX, stage III disease.

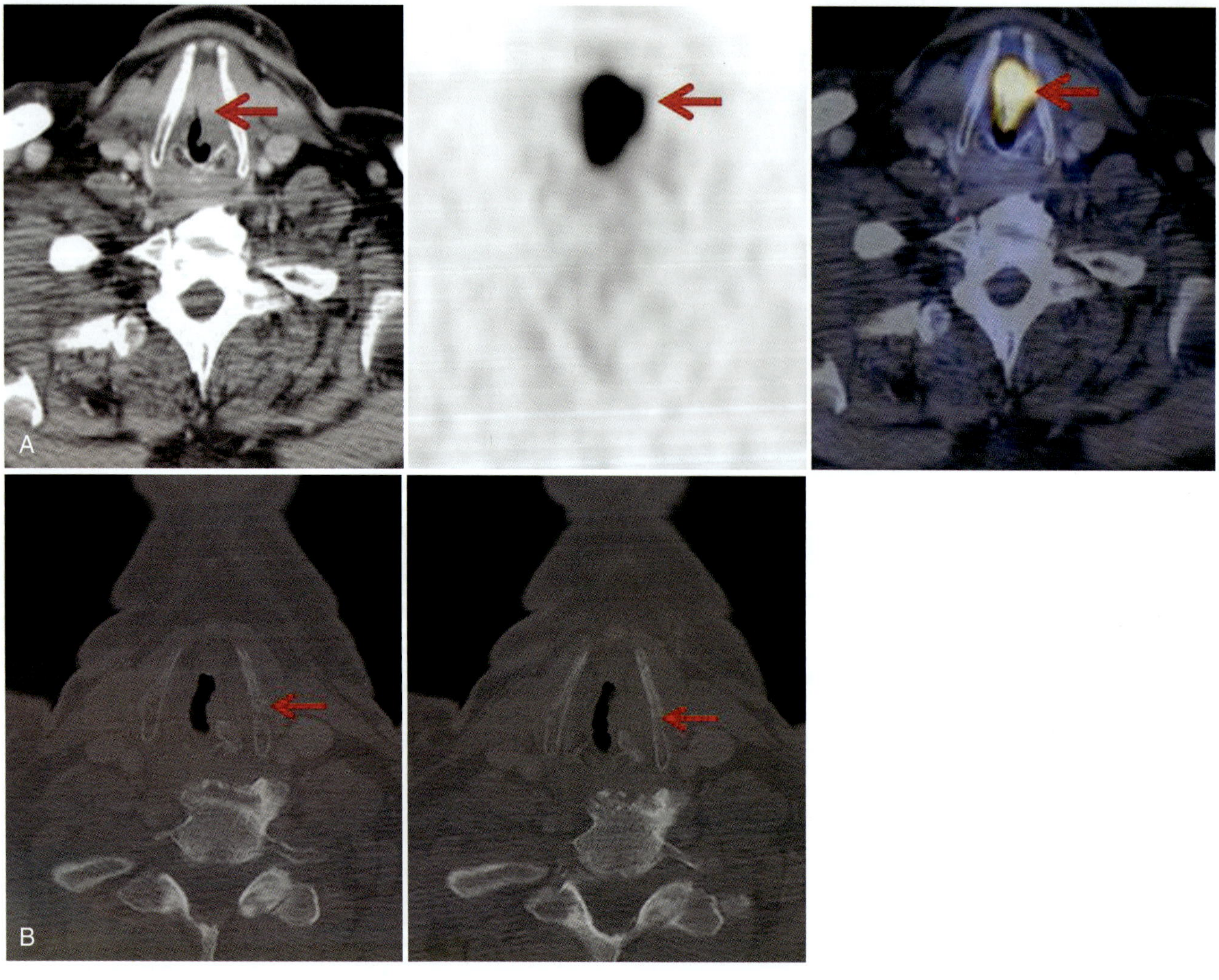

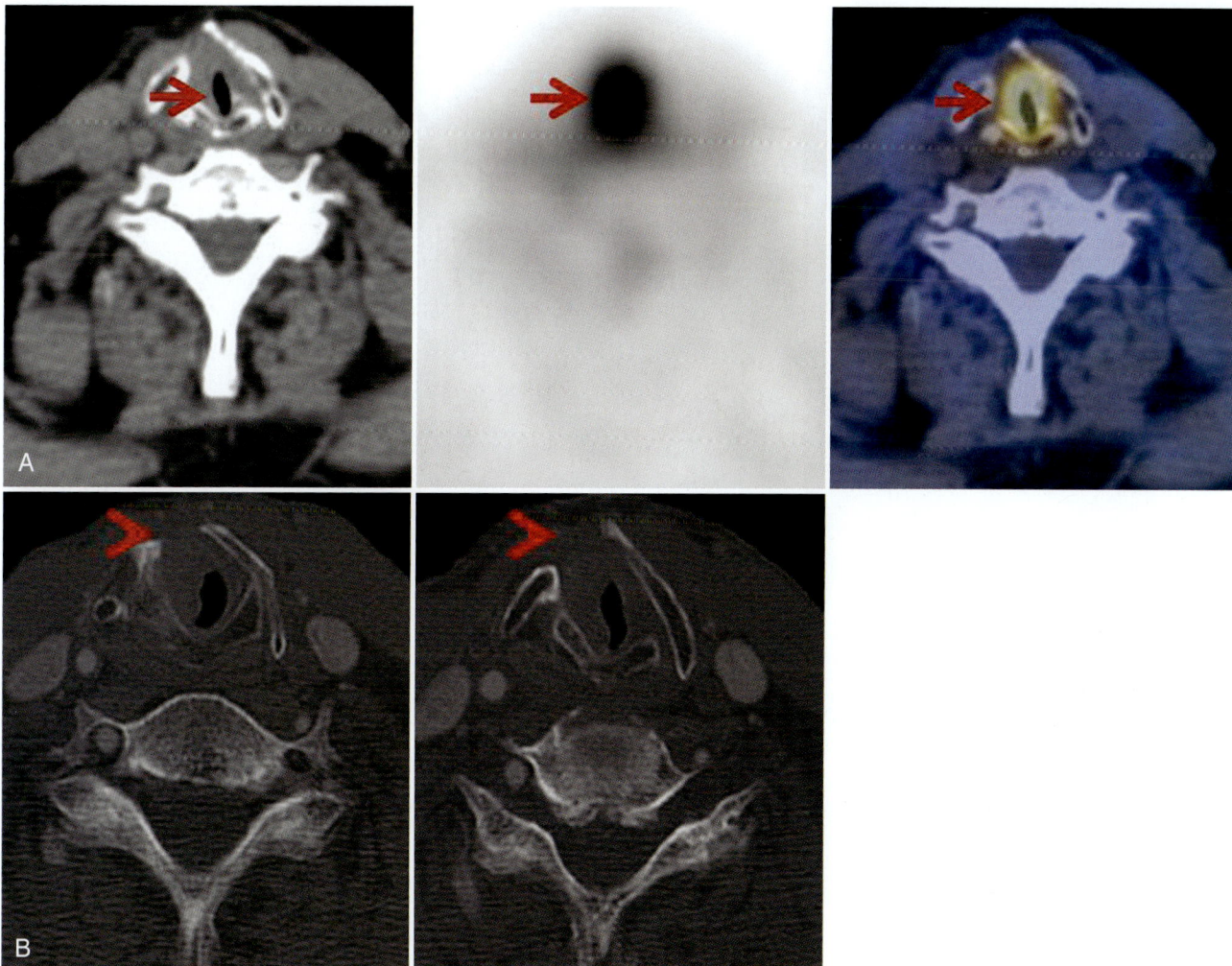

Figure 4-20 A 74-year-old man recently diagnosed with glottic squamous cell carcinoma, referred for staging with FDG PET/CT performed with a noncontrast-enhanced low-dose CT and separately acquired dedicated CT. **A:** Axial images of PET/CT study demonstrate a hypermetabolic (SUV_{max} 9.5) enhancing mass mainly involving the right vocal cord (*arrows*) extending across the anterior commissure to involve the anterior half of the left vocal cord. **B:** Bone windows of the dedicated CT study demonstrate complete destruction/lysis of the right anterior aspect of the thyroid cartilage (T4) (*arrowheads*). There is no evidence of metastatic cervical lymph nodes. AJCC stage: T4N0MX, stage IV disease.

Figure 4-19 A 63-year-old man recently diagnosed with glottic squamous cell carcinoma, referred for staging with FDG PET/CT performed with contrast-enhanced high-resolution CT. **A:** Axial images of PET/CT study demonstrate an intensely hypermetabolic (SUV_{max} 22) enhancing mass centered on the left true vocal cord, involving the anterior commissure and apparent extension into the anterior third of the right true vocal cord with fixation of the vocal cord (determined by laryngoscopy) (T3) (*arrow*). **B:** Bone windows demonstrate that FDG uptake also extends into the left thyroid cartilage, which shows subtle erosion with sclerotic and lytic changes on the accompanying CT (*small arrows*), consistent with cartilage involvement. There is no evidence of metastatic cervical lymph nodes. AJCC stage: T4N0MX, stage IV disease.

146 SECTION I ADVANCED MODALITIES: PROTOCOLS AND OPTIMIZATION

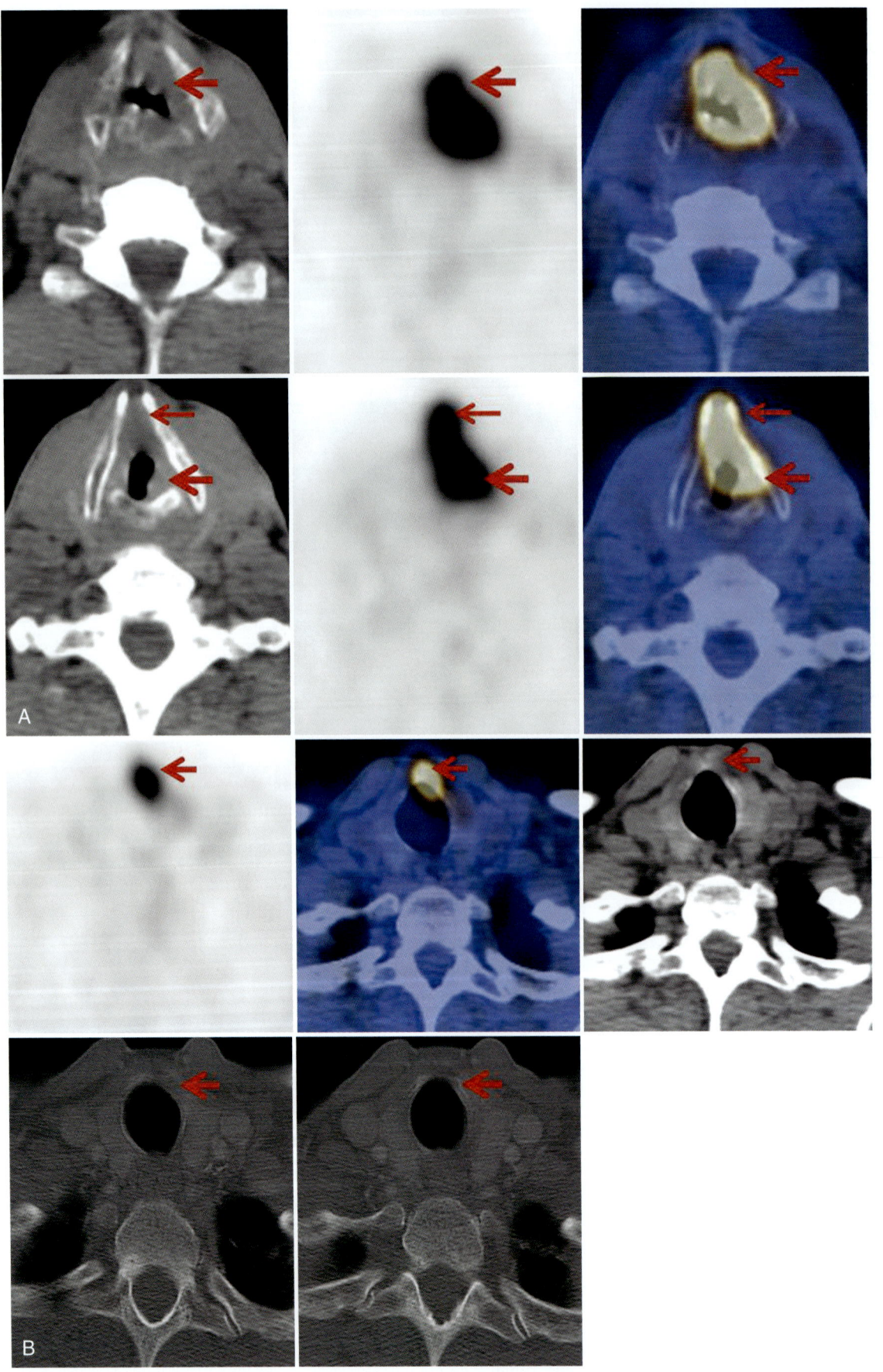

Figure 4-21 A 52-year-old man recently diagnosed with glottic squamous cell carcinoma, referred for staging with FDG PET/CT performed with a noncontrast-enhanced low-dose CT and a separately acquired contrast-enhanced CT study. **A:** Axial images of PET/CT study demonstrate a bulky hypermetabolic (SUV$_{max}$ 26) mass extending from the left supraglottic region (**upper panel,** *arrows*). At the level of the true cords, it appears to extend across the anterior commissure to involve the anterior right true vocal cord (**lower panel,** *arrows*). **B:** The tumor extends through the level of vocal cords and involves the subglottic larynx, and the thyroid cartilage anteriorly (*arrows*). FDG PET image shows definite evidence of involvement by tumor, although the findings on the accompanying CT are subtle with no frank cartilage destruction (**lower panel,** bone windows). Histopathology revealed cartilage invasion proving the CT to be false negative. AJCC stage: T4N0MX, stage IV disease.

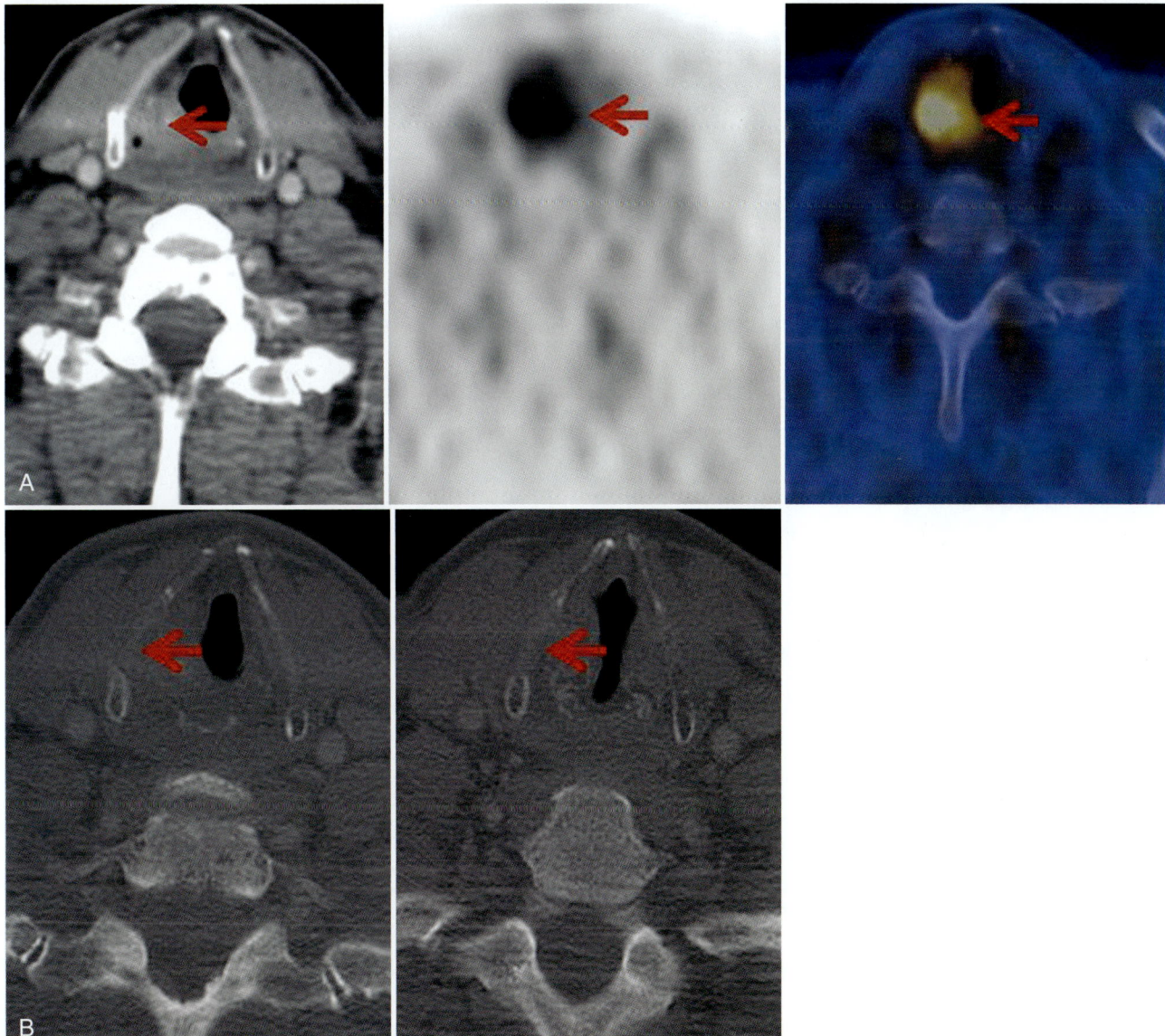

Figure 4-22 A 61-year-old man recently diagnosed with supraglottic squamous cell carcinoma, referred for staging with FDG PET/CT performed with contrast-enhanced high-resolution CT. **A:** Axial images of PET/CT study demonstrate a hypermetabolic mass (SUV$_{max}$ 11.3) involving the right side of the supraglottic larynx effacing the paraglottic fat plane, posteriorly. The tumor involves the right arytenoid and appears to extend through the apex of the piriform sinus (*arrows*) with cord fixation (determined by laryngoscopy) (T3). **B:** Although the tumor appears to be close to the right thyroid cartilage on FDG PET imaging, the bone windows of the diagnostic CT study reveal no evidence of thyroid cartilage involvement (*arrows*). There is no evidence of metastatic cervical lymph nodes. AJCC stage: T3N0MX, stage III disease.

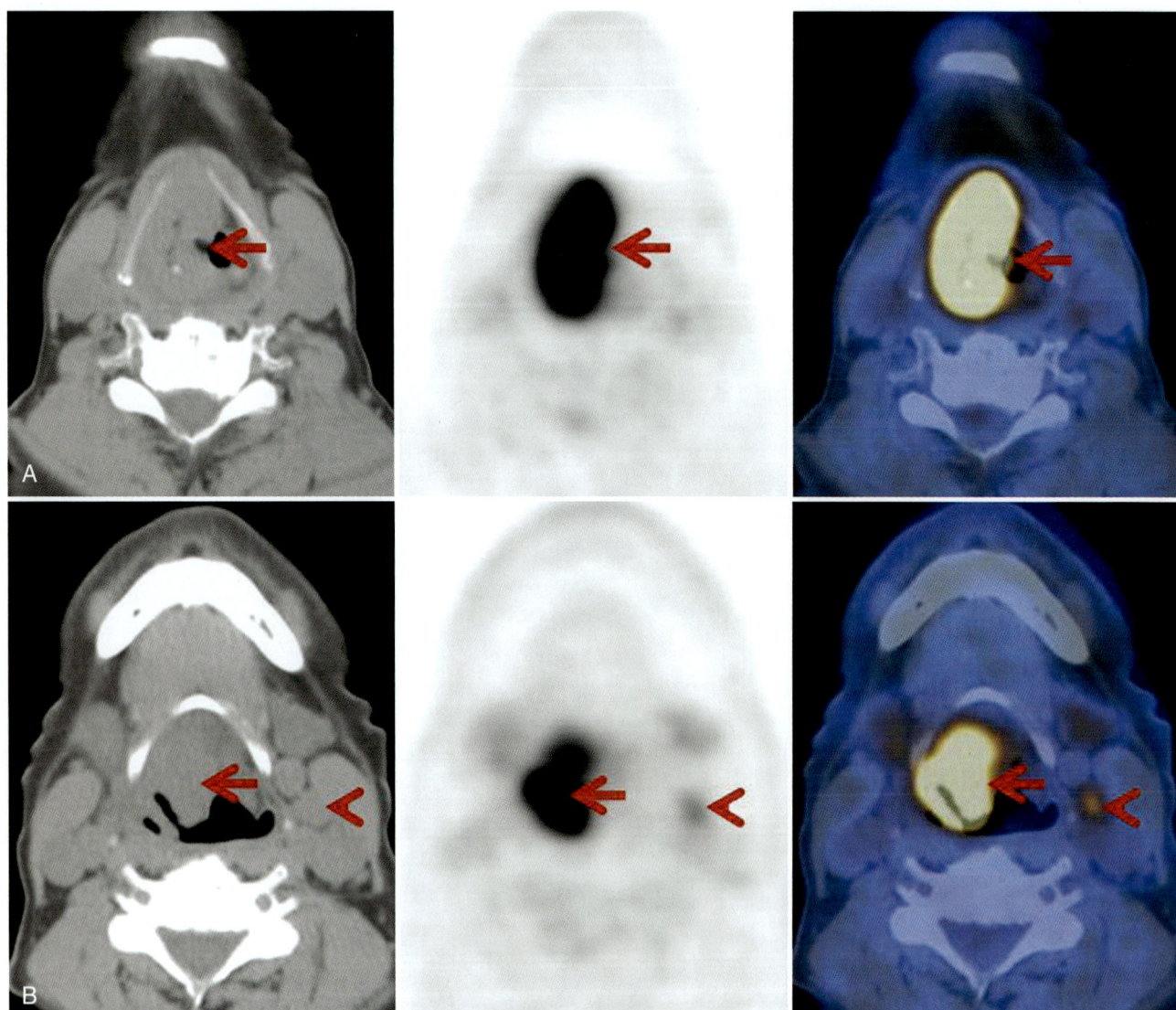

Figure 4-23 An 88-year-old man recently diagnosed with transglottic squamous cell carcinoma involving both supraglottic and glottis larynx, referred for staging with FDG PET/CT performed with noncontrast-enhanced low-dose CT. **A:** Axial images of PET/CT study demonstrate a large hypermetabolic (SUV_{max} 17.8) predominantly supraglottic tumor involving the right vallecula, aryepiglottic folds, and paralaryngeal fat. **B:** Tumor extends to involve the right glottis with vocal cord fixation as well as the surrounding right arytenoid cartilage (T3) (*arrows*). A nodular component in the anterior commissure extends slightly to the anterior left glottis. Tumor abuts a large portion of the right thyroid cartilage but does not involve it (bone windows not shown). There is a 1.0-cm left level III lymph node with mild FDG uptake (SUV_{max} 2.6) (*arrowheads*) that may be either metastatic or reactive in nature (N1 vs N0). AJCC stage: T3N0 or N1MX, either setting stage III disease. The patient underwent neoadjuvant therapy with chemoradiation followed by resection and elective lymph node dissection. The level III lymph node was negative for tumor but there was suggestion of treated tumor on histology (see Figure 4-45 for M staging).

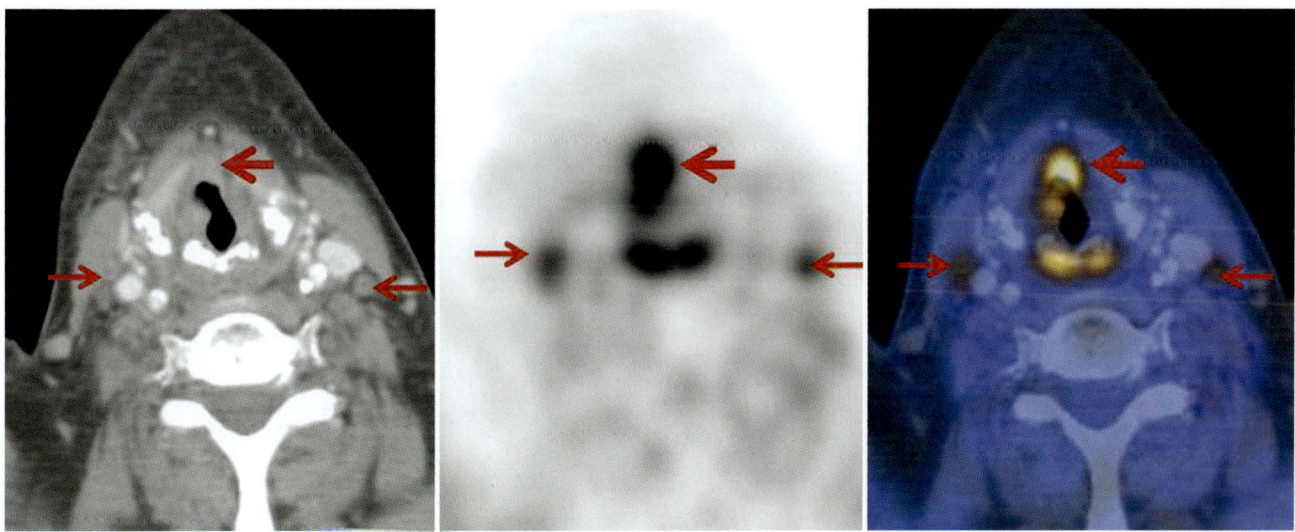

Figure 4-24 A 60-year-old man recently diagnosed with supraglottic squamous cell carcinoma (SCC), referred for staging with FDG PET/CT performed with contrast-enhanced high-resolution CT. Axial images of PET/CT study demonstrate a hypermetabolic (SUV_{max} 12.7) soft tissue mass involving the right vocal cord invading the anterior commissure (*arrow*) suggestive of involvement of the contralateral site. Subcentimeter lymph nodes in level III stations, bilaterally, demonstrate increased FDG uptake (*small arrows*) (SUV_{max} 3.7) and are suspicious for metastatic foci regardless of their small size. The patient underwent neoadjuvant therapy followed by total laryngectomy and lymph node dissection, which revealed poorly differentiated SCC. On histopathology, the level III lymph nodes revealed metastatic disease. AJCC stage: T3N2cMX, stage IV disease.

Once the tumor reaches the anterior commissure, it may easily spread into the supraglottis or subglottis and become transglottic. Of note, the term *transglottic carcinoma* generally refers to tumors that involve both the glottis and supraglottis. Transglottic extension is critical for the surgical approach as transglottic involvement implies advanced disease and an unfavorable prognosis. Transglottic tumors, particularly those that spread vertically in the anterior midline, have a tendency to invade the laryngeal framework and cricothyroid membrane. Vocal cord fixation usually is determined by endoscopic examination and indicates at least T3 tumor, which requires T3 combination chemoradiotherapy in an effort to prevent the morbidity associated with total laryngectomy.

At initial staging, in an untreated patient, the anterior commissure should have no FDG uptake and no soft tissue present in the interthyroidal notch on the accompanying CT study. Even a small degree of FDG uptake in the opposite cord should raise suspicion for tumor spread to the contralateral site. If the FDG PET is accompanied by ceCT, soft tissue thickening of the anterior commissure should increase the confidence of interpretation (Figure 4-25). Glottic tumors can invade the thyroid cartilage superiorly into the paraglottic space (Figures 4-19 through 4-21), inferiorly into the subglottic space, and posteriorly into the posterior commissure, arytenoid cartilage, cricoid cartilage, or cricoarytenoid joint. Subglottic involvement and cricoid cartilage invasion necessitate total laryngectomy. Posterior glottic tumors are rare. These tumors may invade the cricoarytenoid cartilage and piriform sinus, thereby gaining access to its lymphatic drainage. Subglottic spread is commonly seen. The sensitivity of CT and MRI to detect subglottic involvement is higher than endoscopic biopsy, but peritumoral inflammatory changes make it difficult to accurately determine the exact tumor extent for both anatomic and FDG PET imaging.

Subglottic SCC

Involvement of the subglottis by laryngeal cancer usually represents inferior spread of a glottis or supraglottic tumor rather than a primary tumor originating in the subglottis. True subglottic SCCs account for only 5% of laryngeal SCCs and are highly aggressive with a poor prognosis. These tumors subclinically advance to late stages with invasion of the surrounding structures, notwithstanding the relative paucity of lymphatic drainage in this region. Subglottic SCC can spread into the true cords, supraglottis, and trachea, or through the cricothyroid membrane into the thyroid gland or posteriorly into the esophagus.

■ HYPOPHARYNGEAL CARCINOMA

Hypopharynx is defined as is the region between the oropharynx at the level of the hyoid bone and the esophagus at the lower end of the cricoid cartilage. Most hypopharyngeal SCCs (~70%) arise from the piriform sinus (Figure 4-26), but they can also involve the lateral pharyngeal wall (25%), posterior pharyngeal wall, or postcricoid pharynx (5%). Most patients present with large T3 or T4 tumors. Tumors originating from the lateral wall of the piriform sinus infiltrate toward the common carotid artery. Tumors involving primarily the medial wall of the pyriform sinus usually infiltrate the aryepiglottic folds and can invade the laryngeal framework by involving the paraglottic space. Tumors of the lateral wall and apex commonly invade the thyroid cartilage.

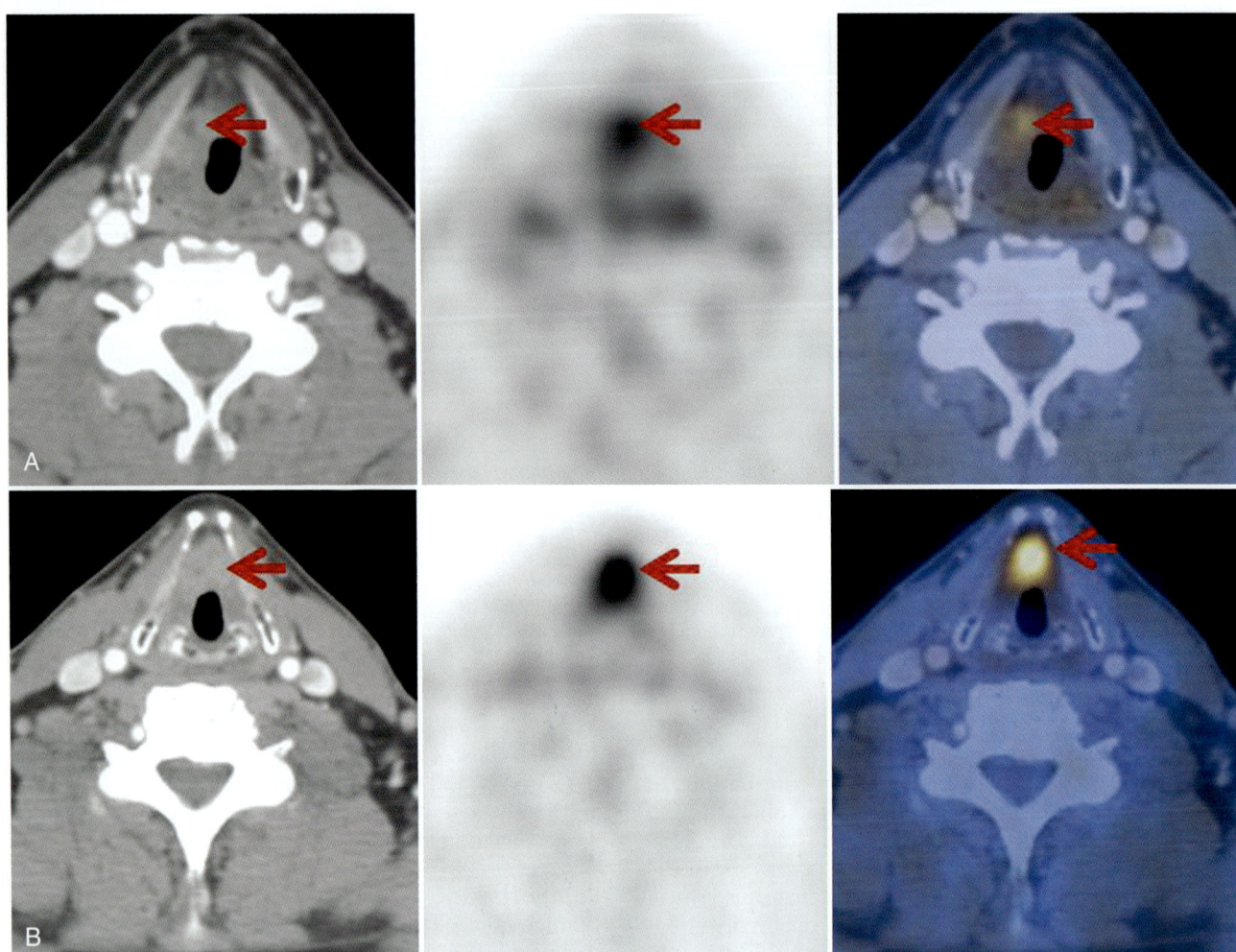

Figure 4-25 A 58-year-old man recently diagnosed with transglottic squamous cell carcinoma involving both the supraglottic and glottis larynx, referred for staging with FDG PET/CT performed with contrast-enhanced high-resolution CT. **A:** Axial images of PET/CT study demonstrate a hypermetabolic (SUV_{max} 9.4) mass in the supraglottic larynx extending from the preepiglottic space to the right paraglottic space (*arrows*). **B:** Caudally, the mass appears to extend into the anterior commissure (*arrows*) and possibly involves the anterior aspect of both true vocal cords without fixation of the cords (determined by laryngoscopy) (T2). There is no erosion of the laryngeal cartilages, no extension of the tumor outside of the laryngeal superstructure, and no evidence of lymph node involvement. AJCC stage: T2N0cMX, stage II disease.

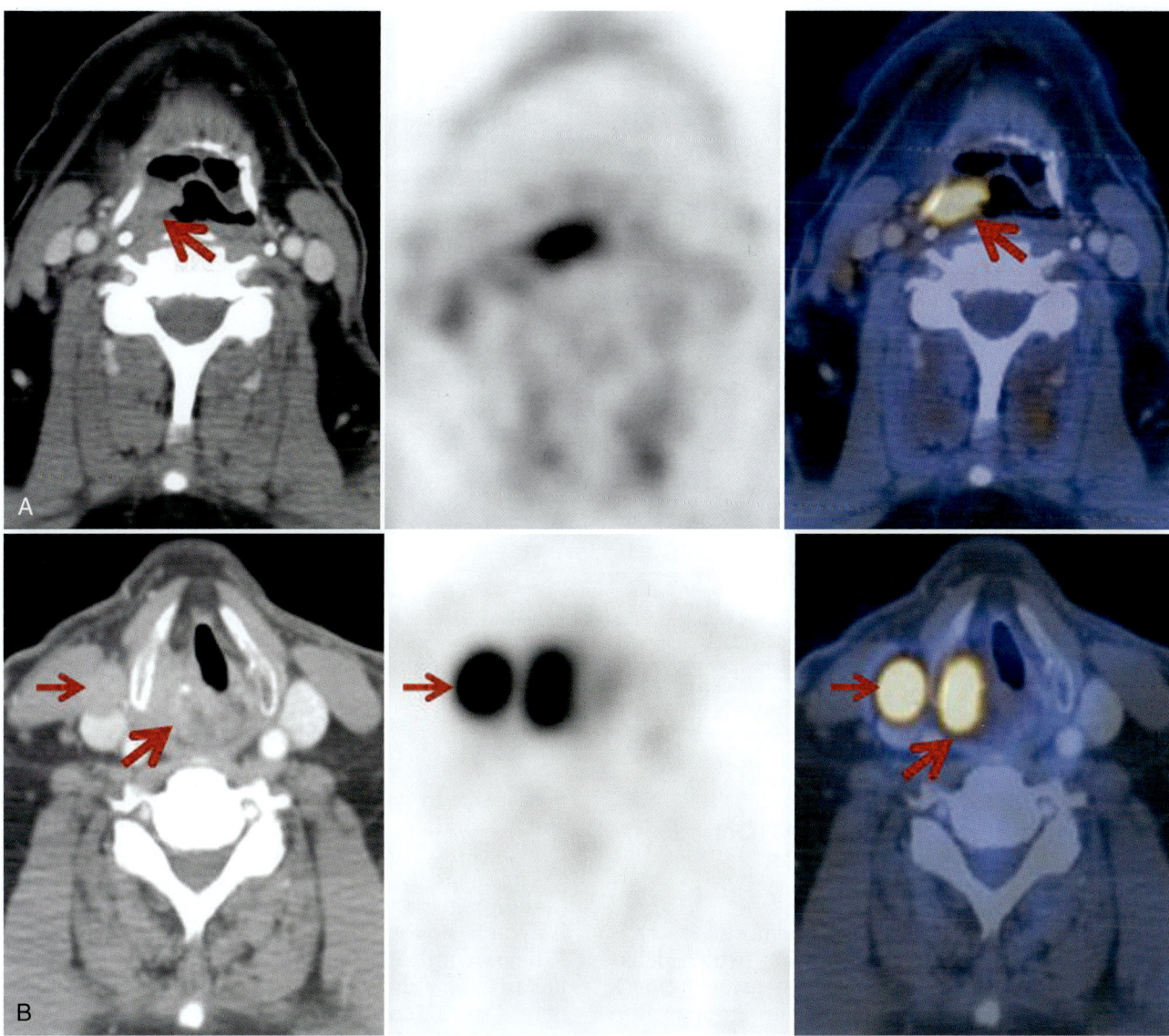

Figure 4-26 A 61-year-old man recently diagnosed with hypopharyngeal squamous cell carcinoma (SCC), referred for staging with FDG PET/CT performed with contrast-enhanced high-resolution CT. **A:** Axial images of PET/CT study show a mass involving the right side of the hypopharynx extending toward the midline, measuring 2.1 cm. The tumor invades the supraglottic larynx, extends around the right arytenoid, and appears to extend through the apex of the piriform sinus (T2) (*arrows*). There is no evidence of lymph node involvement (N0). **B:** A 70-year-old man with a recent diagnosis of hypopharyngeal SCC, referred for staging with FDG PET/CT performed with contrast-enhanced high-resolution CT. Axial images of PET/CT study demonstrate a large hypopharyngeal soft tissue mass with heterogeneous enhancement and intense FDG uptake (SUV$_{max}$ 22) measuring 3.1 cm (T2) (*arrows*). Additionally, there is an enlarged hypermetabolic (SUV$_{max}$ 15) right level III lymph node measuring 2.7 cm (N1) (*small arrows*), consistent with metastatic disease. The patient subsequently underwent chemotherapy and hyperfractionated radiation therapy, followed by selective neck dissection. The patient responded well to therapy with no evidence of residual disease at 8-month follow-up, which included repeat PET/CT and diagnostic CT studies.

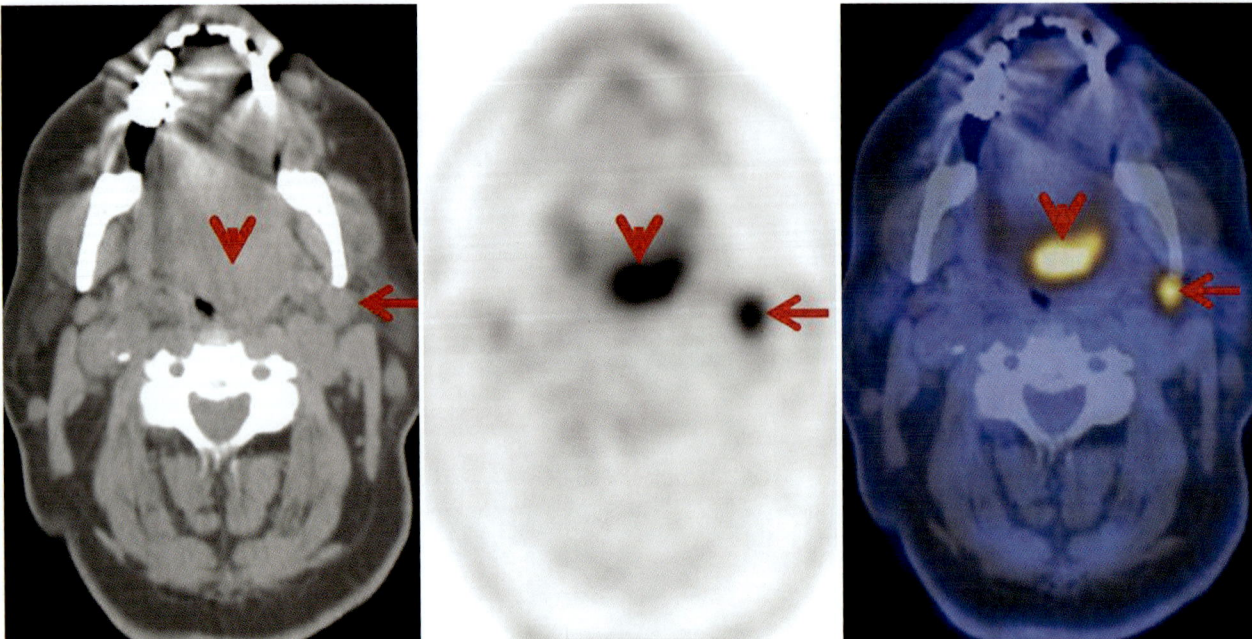

Figure 4-27 A 58-year-old man recently diagnosed with base of tongue squamous cell carcinoma, referred for staging with FDG PET/CT performed with noncontrast-enhanced high resolution CT. Axial images of PET/CT study demonstrate a hypermetabolic (SUV_{max} 13.4) mass, measuring 2.0 cm (T1) in the left base of tongue extending to the midline, consistent with the patient's known primary tumor (*arrowheads*). There is a 1.0-cm hypermetabolic (SUV_{max} 7.0) left level IIA lymph node (*arrows*), consistent with metastatic disease regardless of its small size based on the intense FDG uptake. This PET finding upstaged disease from T1N0M0 to T1N1M0, with migration from stage I to stage III disease per clinical and CT evaluation. Subsequent histopathology confirmed lymph node metastasis.

■ DOES FDG PET/CT HAVE A PRIMARY ROLE IN EVALUATION OF REGIONAL LYMPH NODE METASTASES?

In HNSCC, the most important prognostic factor is locoregional lymph node involvement, which determines the subsequent elective treatment of the neck (Table 4-1). Cervical lymph nodes are grouped into levels I through VI. CT and MRI interpretation depends on size criteria, whereas FDG PET reading is dictated by metabolic characteristics of the lymph nodes. Generally, for level I to II lymph nodes, a measurement ≥1.5 cm in the greatest dimension and ≥0.8 mm for retropharyngeal lymph nodes and >1.0 cm for all other neck nodes is the established definition for lymphadenopathy. However, FDG PET can demonstrate uptake in normal-sized lymph nodes, implying metastatic disease and thereby increasing the detection sensitivity by 10% to 30% compared to ceCT (Figures 4-11, 4-13, *B*, 4-24, and 4-27). More specifically, the sensitivity and specificity of FDG PET in detecting cervical nodal disease ranges from 74% to 94% and 82% to 100%, respectively, compared to CT, which ranges from 65% to 81% and 47% to 81%, respectively. Of note, FDG PET/CT has been shown to be useful in detecting nodal metastases in patients with more advanced T stages when nodal disease is more likely (Figure 4-5).

Oral Cavity SCC
Cervical lymph node metastases are common and occur in nearly half of patients who present with oral cavity SCCs. This group of cancers has a high propensity to metastasize to lymph node levels I to III (Figures 4-5 and 4-28); thus, selective neck dissection is the procedure of choice for management of the neck.

The major lymphatic drainage of the oral tongue (anterior two thirds of the tongue) is to level I to II lymph nodes, often with bilateral involvement. Patients with tongue SCC can present with level IIB metastases, although this sublevel of involvement is rare in oral cavity SCCs (Figure 4-5, *C*). Isolated metastases to level IV, known as "skip metastases," can also occur in tongue SCC. In large tumors (Figure 4-14) and those crossing the midline, the chance for bilateral lymph node involvement is significantly high.

The floor of the mouth SCC frequently metastasizes to the lymph nodes due to the absence of a fascial barrier with free communication between the submandibular space, sublingual space, and inferior parapharyngeal fatty space. Commonly, metastasis occurs to level I and II lymph node basins (Figure 4-6, *C*). As many as 20% of patients with greater than T1 lesions have occult lymph node metastasis, and elective neck dissection with adjuvant radiotherapy may be necessary for increased regional control.

The rich lymphatic network of the buccal region results in lymph node metastasis in a high number of patients, essentially involving levels I to III. In contrast, minor salivary gland tumors of the hard palate usually do not metastasize to the neck, obviating the need for neck dissection in clinically negative cases. In the case of metastatic disease, SCCs of the hard palate metastasize to level I cervical lymph nodes, particularly in patients with stage T2 or higher tumors.

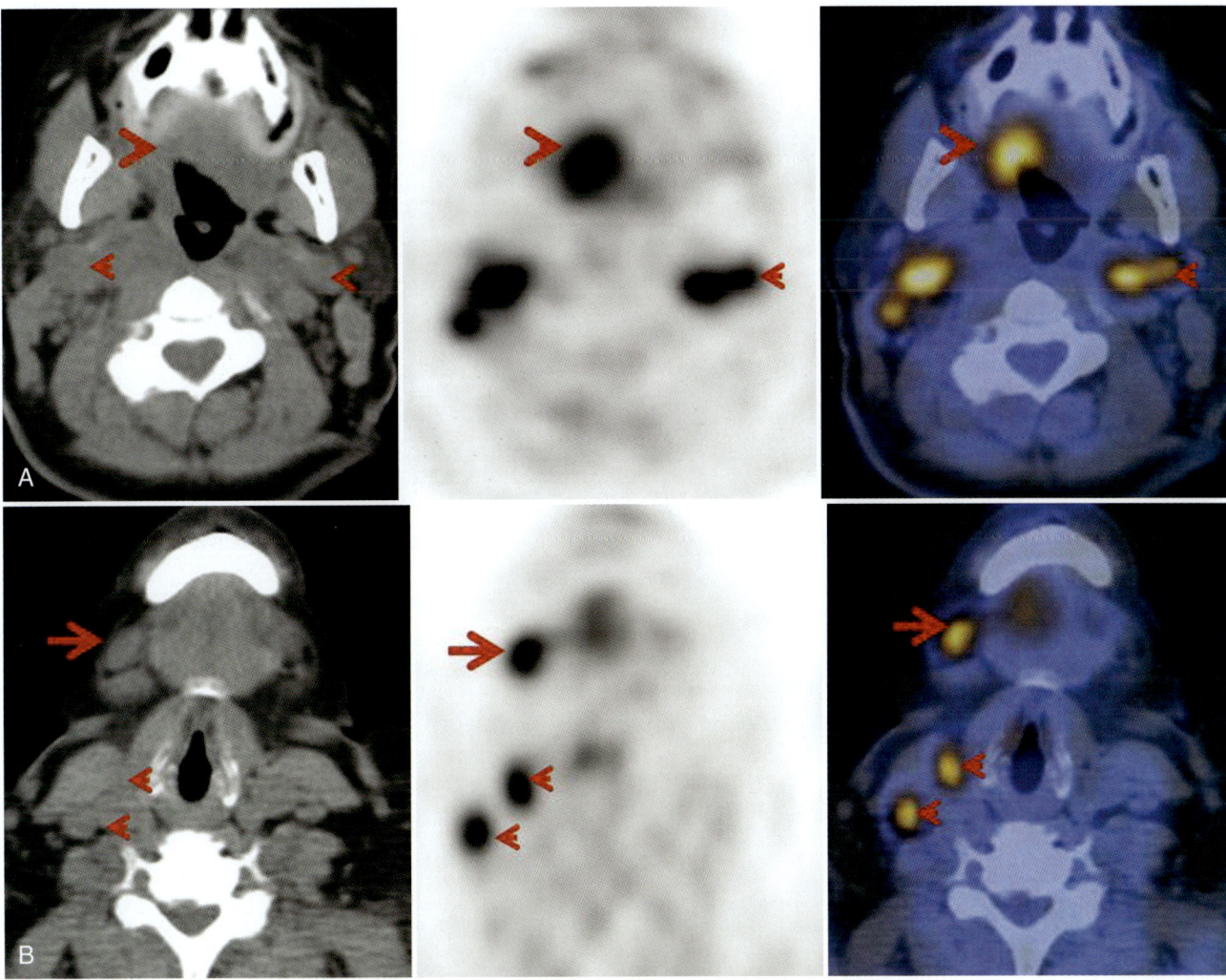

Figure 4-28 A: A 65-year-old woman recently diagnosed with squamous cell carcinoma of the tongue, referred for staging with FDG PET/CT performed with noncontrast-enhanced low-dose CT. **A:** Axial images of PET/CT study demonstrate a hypermetabolic mass (SUV$_{max}$ 18) on the lateral aspect of the left tongue (*arrowheads*), consistent with the patient's primary disease. There are bilateral, multiple, prominent, hypermetabolic (SUV$_{max}$ 10.2) lymph nodes involving the level IIA (*small arrowheads*), consistent with bilateral lymph node metastases (N2c) **B:** Additional hypermetabolic lymph nodes are noted in levels IB (*arrows*) and III (*small arrowheads*) (SUV$_{max}$ 8.0), consistent with additional metastatic disease (N2c). The major lymphatic drainage of the oral tongue is to levels I and II lymph nodes, often with bilateral involvement. Level III lymph nodes may also be involved in advanced cases.

Oropharyngeal SCC

Regional lymph node metastases are seen even more frequently in oropharyngeal SCC patients at the time of diagnosis, with rates exceeding 50%. Bilateral neck involvement occurs in 15% of patients with cervical metastases. Lymphatic drainage from the oropharynx is often directed to level II to III cervical nodes and may also involve level I cervical and retropharyngeal lymph nodes, with level II being the most commonly involved subsite (Figures 4-1, 4-3, 4-11, and 4-12). In the previously untreated neck, metastases to level IV or V are rare in the absence of obvious lymphadenopathy at levels I to III. Systematic reviews have shown that sublevel IIB metastases are rare in oral cavity SCC (Figures 4-1 and 4-12).

The base of tongue has rich lymphatic drainage with significant cross-drainage, resulting in up to 40% of patients presenting with contralateral cervical lymph node metastases, primarily to levels II through IV lymph nodes (Figures 4-3, 4-10, and 4-11). Even early T-stage lesions typically present with cervical metastasis in close to one fourth of patients who present with bilateral neck involvement. Tongue base carcinoma may also extend laterally to encase the internal carotid artery, upstaging the tumor to stage IVB and making the tumor unresectable.

In tonsillar SCCs, clinically positive nodal metastases are common at the time of diagnosis in nearly three fourths of patients (Figures 4-1 and 4-12). These metastases usually are ipsilateral, although contralateral nodal disease has been reported in 20% of patients. The most frequently involved site is the level II lymph node basin, which may extend to the level III region. Predominantly cystic SCC metastasis in the neck can be seen with palatine and lingual tonsil tumors. Such cystic metastases may not be differentiated from liquefaction

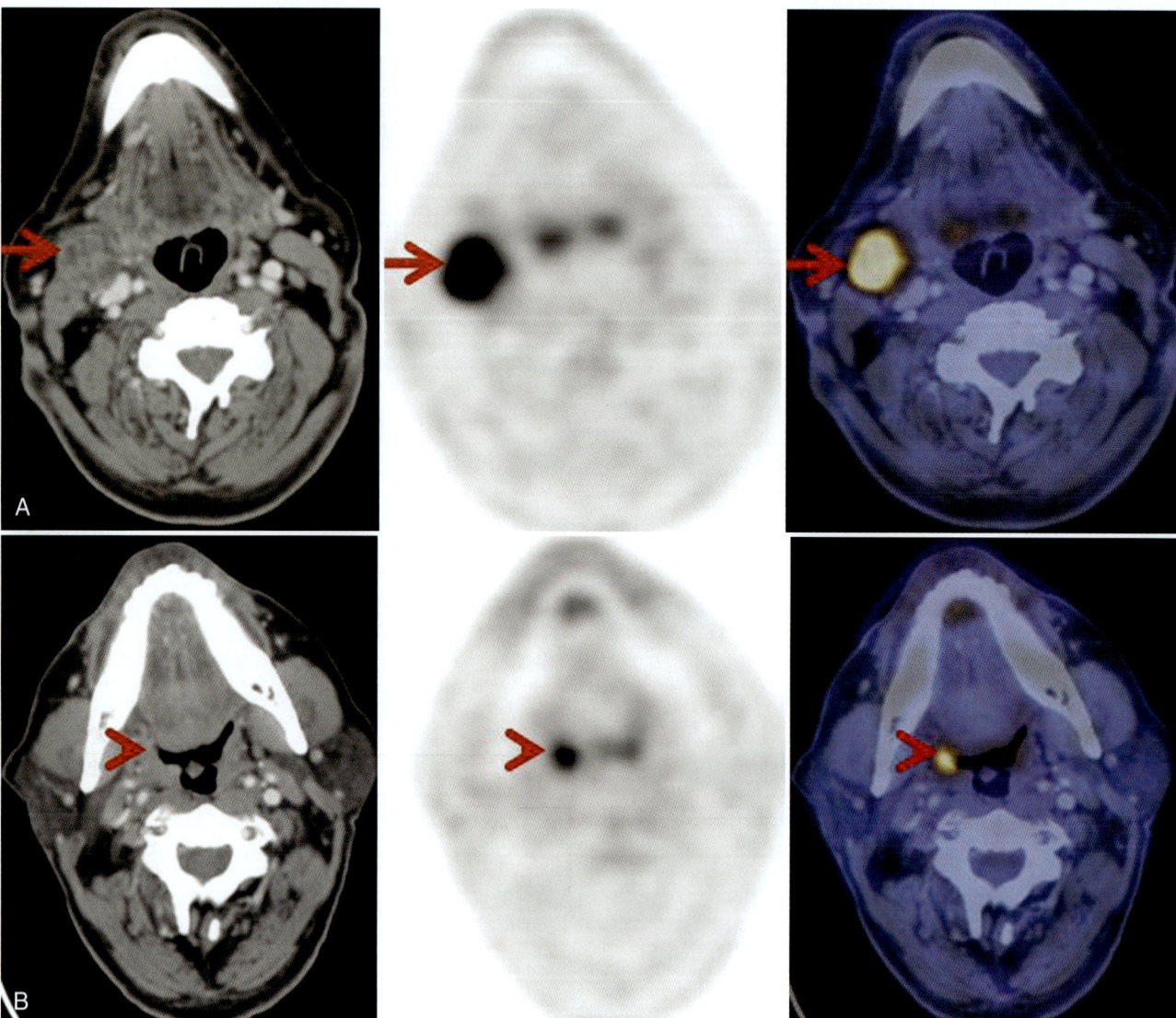

Figure 4-29 A 66-year-old woman recently diagnosed with carcinoma of unknown primary (CUP) of the right neck, referred for determination of the primary and evaluation of extent of disease with FDG PET/CT performed with contrast-enhanced high-resolution CT. **A:** Axial images of PET/CT study demonstrate a heterogeneously enhancing hypermetabolic (SUV_{max} 11) mass in the right level IIA region (*arrows*), consistent with the patient's known metastatic disease of unknown origin. **B:** There is asymmetric uptake in the right tonsil compared to the left (SUV_{max} 5.8 vs 2.0), suggestive of the primary disease site (*arrowheads*). The subsequent biopsy proved this interpretation accurate. Note that no definite mass is demonstrated on the accompanying contrast-enhanced CT scan in the right tonsillar fossa. In patients with CUP, meticulous investigation of the ipsilateral tonsil should be pursued due to the characteristic lymphatic drainage network.

necrosis, which can occur in solid adenopathy by imaging modalities. These primary tumors arise in the tonsillar crypts and are of the transitional type rather than the usual SCC. In a patient with cystic level II nodal metastasis, the ipsilateral tonsil should be targeted for further investigation to diagnose the occult tumor. A caveat associated with tonsillar carcinoma is metastatic SCC of unknown origin involving level I through III cervical lymph nodes. In these cases, meticulous investigation of the ipsilateral tonsils should be pursued due to the typical lymphatic drainage network (Figures 4-15, 4-29, and 4-30). The differential diagnosis includes lymphomas of the tonsils, whose imaging features are similar to those of SCC (Figure 4-31).

Soft palatal carcinomas have a high incidence of nodal metastasis involving levels II, III and retropharyngeal lymph node stations (Figure 4-16, *B*). Approximately 60% of patients have nodal disease at the time of diagnosis. Prognoses of soft palate carcinomas are related to the extent of nodal disease, which is in return related to T stage.

Laryngeal SCC
Primary lymphatic spread of supraglottic carcinomas is directed toward level II to III lymph nodes. Lymph node metastases are common and often bilateral (Figures 4-17, *C*, 4-24, and 4-32). The glottis has sparse lymphatic drainage; thus, nodal metastases

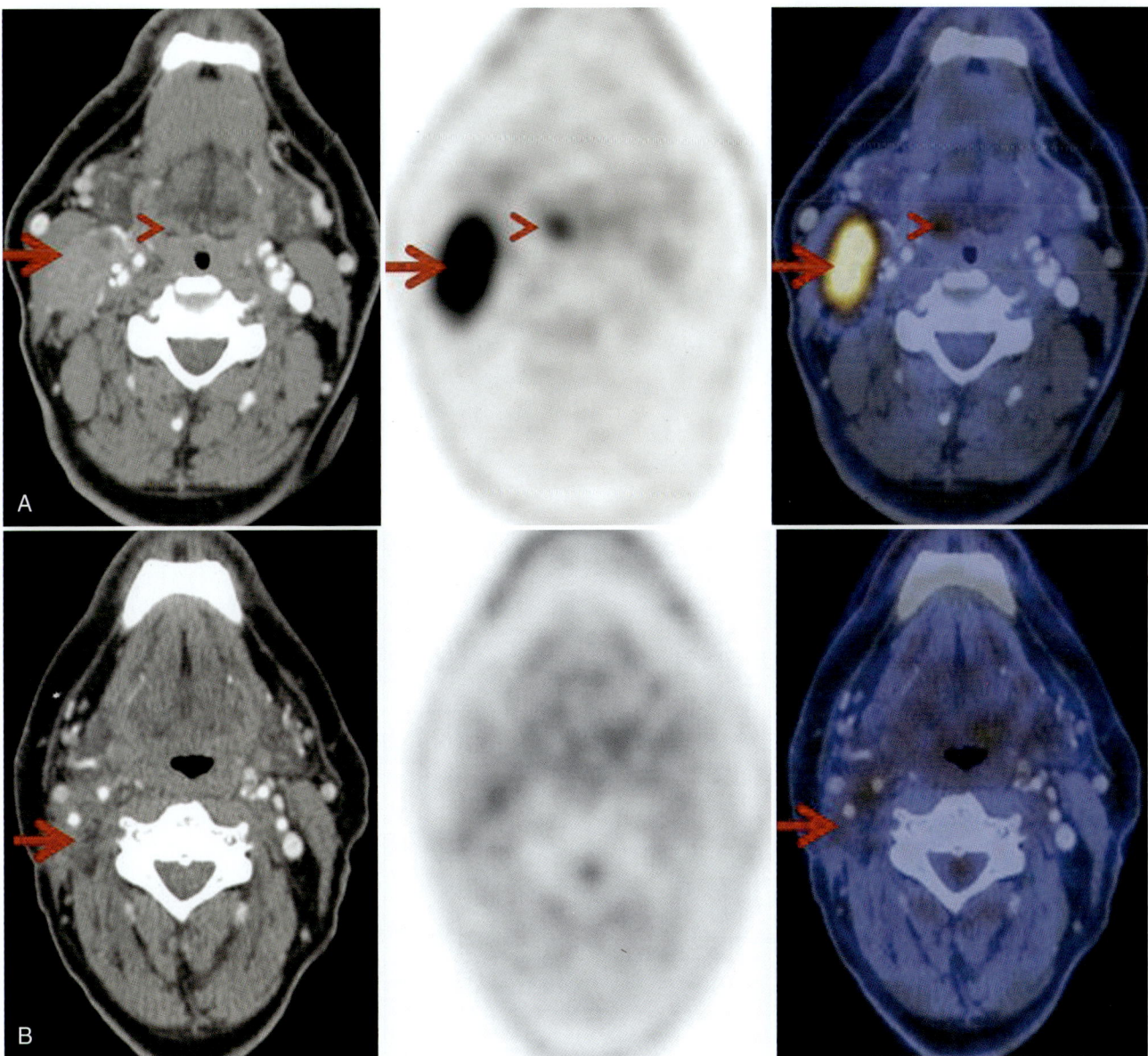

Figure 4-30 A 69-year-old man recently diagnosed with carcinoma of unknown primary in the right neck, referred for determination of the primary and evaluation of extent of disease with FDG PET/CT performed with contrast-enhanced high-resolution CT. **A:** Axial images of PET/CT study demonstrate a heterogeneously enhancing hypermetabolic (SUV$_{max}$ 15) mass in the right level IIB region (*arrows*), consistent with the patient's known metastatic disease of unknown primary. Asymmetric uptake in the right base of tongue/tonsillar fossa is suggestive of primary disease (*small arrowheads*). The patient underwent panendoscopy and right neck dissection, which proved the right tonsil to be the primary site of disease. **B:** The patient underwent chemoradiotherapy. PET/CT study 2.5 months after completion of therapy reveals complete resolution of disease. Note residual soft tissue fullness on the CT study (*arrows*) consistent with fibrotic changes.

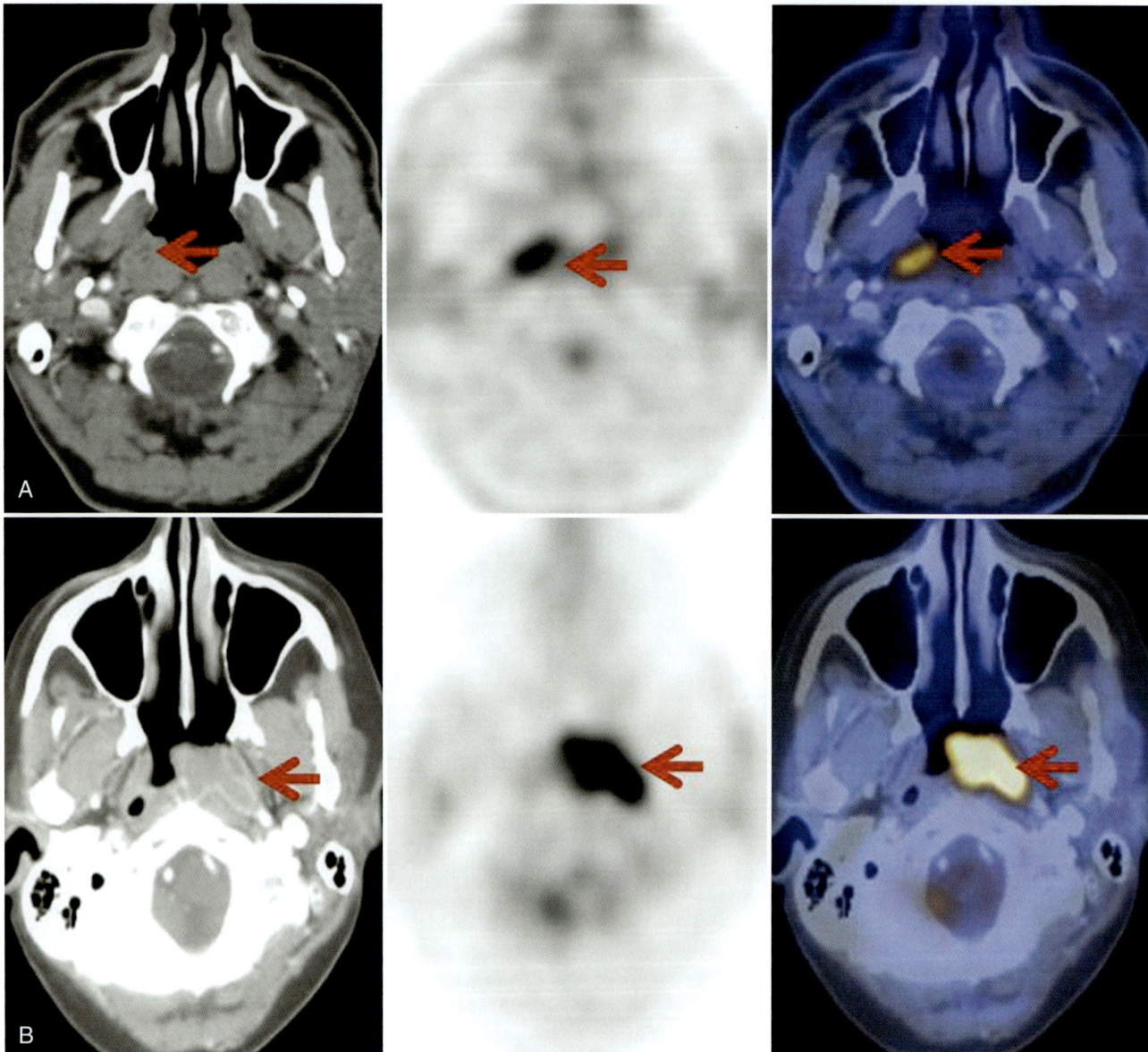

Figure 4-31 **A:** A 49-year-old man recently diagnosed with oropharyngeal squamous cell carcinoma, referred for evaluation of extent of disease with FDG PET/CT performed with contrast-enhanced high-resolution CT. Axial images of PET/CT study demonstrate asymmetric fullness in the right Rosenmüller fossa corresponding to a heterogeneously enhancing hypermetabolic mass (SUV_{max} 9.4) (*arrows*), consistent with a oropharyngeal tumor. **B:** A 43-year-old man recently diagnosed with Burkitt lymphoma of the left tonsil. Axial images of PET/CT study demonstrate asymmetric fullness in the left Rosenmüller fossa corresponding to a heterogeneously enhancing hypermetabolic (SUV_{max} 11.9) (*arrows*) mass, consistent with lymphoma.

occur in less than 10% of patients with truly confined glottic tumors. Once the tumor has traversed the cricothyroid membrane, however, the frequency of lymph node metastases increases significantly. Transglottic carcinoma is often accompanied by lymph node metastases (Figure 4-23). Subglottic SCC or subglottic extensions of a glottic cancer are associated with a high incidence of cervical lymph node metastases. The primary drainage is directed toward levels III and IV and less commonly to the delphian node. Subsequently, pretracheal and paratracheal lymph nodes can be involved.

Hypopharyngeal SCC has a high propensity for lymphatic invasion because of the abundant lymphatics in the region and the extent of primary tumor, with 50% to 75% of patients presenting with nodal metastases at the time of diagnosis, mainly involving level II, III, IV, retropharyngeal, and less frequently level V basins (Figures 4-26, *B*, and 4-33). Occult cervical lymph node metastases are also common, with the overall incidence of cervical lymph node metastases at presentation of approximately 75%. SCC can harbor malignancy in small lymph nodes, making FDG PET valuable in tumor staging.

Chapter 4 PET/CT Imaging In Squamous Cell Carcinoma of the Head and Neck

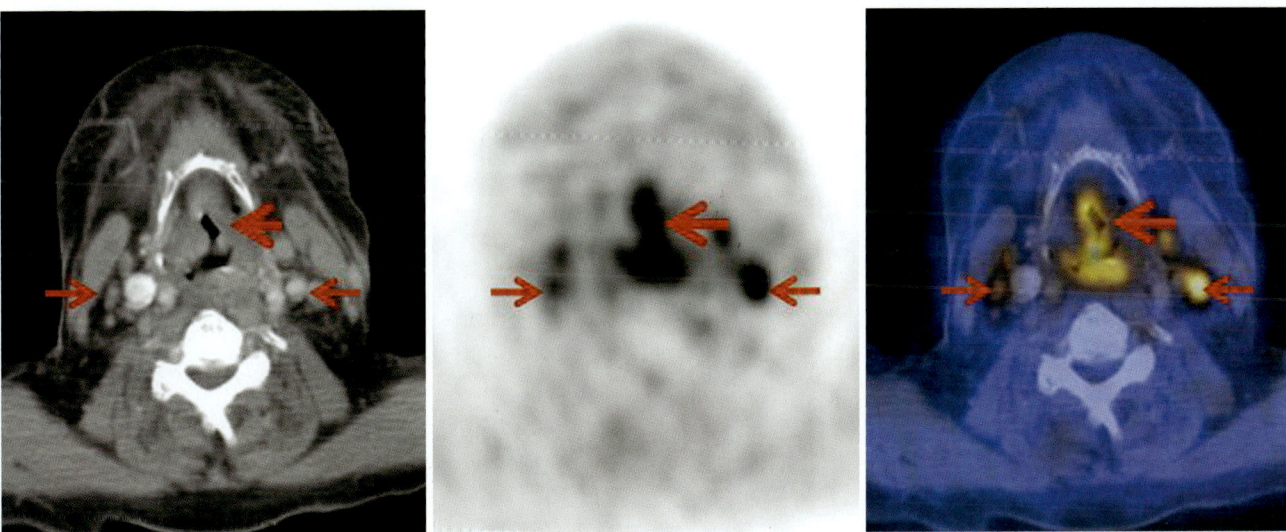

Figure 4-32 A 53-year-old man recently diagnosed with supraglottic squamous cell carcinoma, referred for determination of extent of disease with FDG PET/CT performed with contrast-enhanced high-resolution CT. Axial images of PET/CT shows intense FDG uptake (SUV_{max} 7.3), corresponding to a soft tissue fullness that is centrally located in the supraglottic larynx involving the pre-epiglottic fat, anteriorly as well as the aryepiglottic folds and piriform sinuses, posteriorly (*arrows*). This finding is consistent with the patient's known primary tumor. Bilateral hypermetabolic (SUV_{max} right 4.4, left 6.3) lymph nodes involve the right and left level III regions (*small arrows*) consistent with metastatic disease (N2c), which was proven by a subsequent neck dissection.

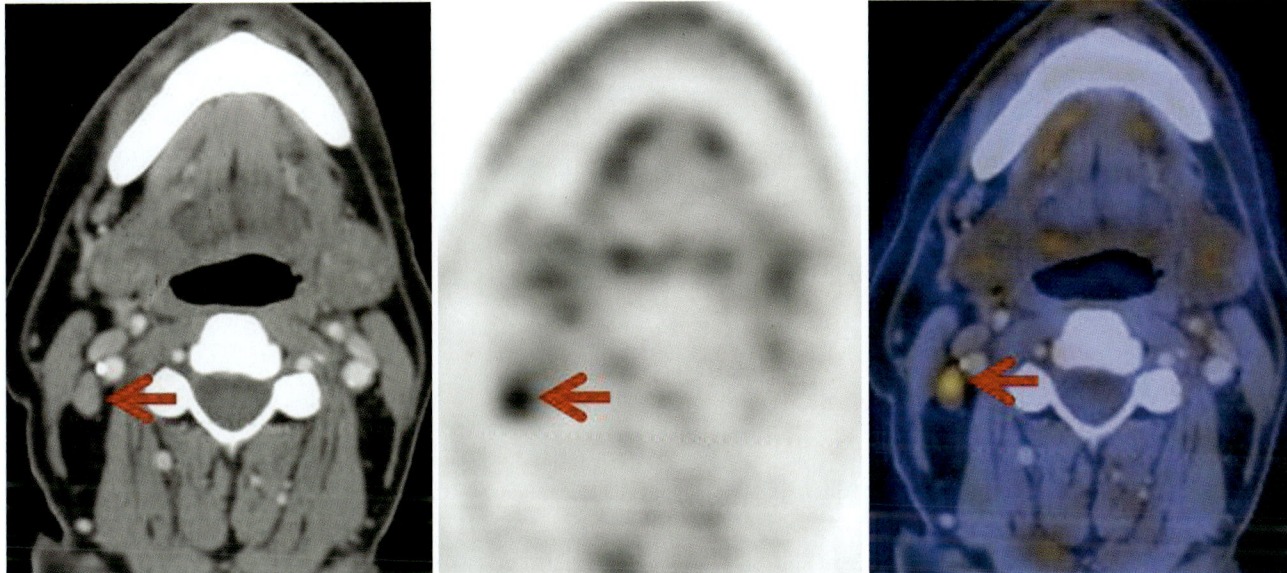

Figure 4-33 A 61-year-old man recently diagnosed with hypopharyngeal squamous cell carcinoma (same patient as shown in Figure 4-26, *A*). Axial images of PET/CT study demonstrate increased uptake in a right level IIB lymph node (SUV_{max} 4.7) (*arrows*). Although this lymph node appears to be benign based on its morphology (smooth margins, no infiltration of the fat, and longer than wider) on the accompanying contrast-enhanced high-resolution CT, subsequent biopsy revealed metastatic disease.

Do FDG PET and ceCT Complement Each Other in Evaluating Nodal Status?

The overall accuracy of PET/CT can be significantly higher than that of CT or MRI for the neck on a level-by-level basis due to enhanced sensitivity rather than specificity. For example, in oral cancer SCC, on a level-by-level basis, the sensitivity of FDG PET for nodal metastases is about twofold higher than that of CT or MRI (Figures 4-11, 4-12, 4-24, 4-27, 4-32, and 4-33). Ideally, both PET and ceCT data should contribute equally to the interpretation of PET/CT. For example, a node that has increased in width but still is smaller than predefined size limits or with evidence of central necrosis despite low levels of FDG uptake should be considered as harboring metastatic disease (Figures 4-5, *C*, 4-16, *B*, and 4-34). Regardless of FDG PET findings, extracapsular spread is suggested by stranding at the nodal margins.

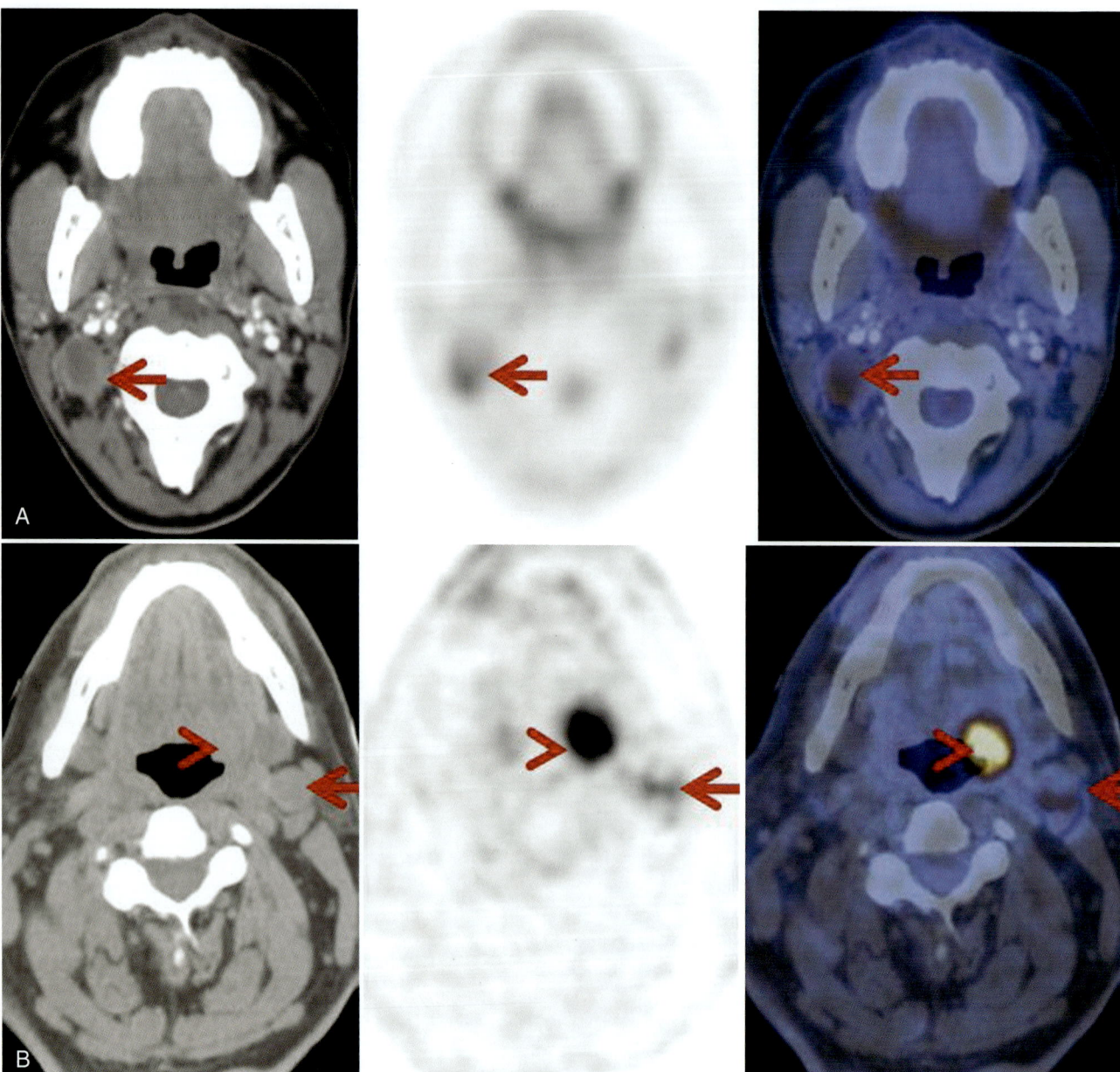

Figure 4-34 Two patients recently diagnosed with tonsillar squamous cell carcinoma. **A:** Axial slice of PET/CT study with contrast-enhanced high-resolution CT. A centrally hypodense right level IIB lymph node demonstrates mild peripheral enhancement on contrast-enhanced study and only mildly increased FDG uptake (SUV_{max} 2.1) on the FDG PET portion of the study (*arrows*). This finding is consistent with a necrotic lymph node with metastatic disease. Note that the primary tumor is not included in the presented PET/CT slice. **B:** Axial slice of PET/CT study performed with non-contrast enhanced low-dose CT. The primary tumor in the left tonsillar fossa (*arrowheads*) demonstrates increased FDG uptake (SUV_{max} 10) corresponding to a soft tissue density. Note the difficulty in delineating the soft tissue mass due to lack of intravenous contrast. There is a heterogeneously attenuating enlarged left level IIA lymph node (*arrows*) with negligible FDG uptake (SUV_{max} 1.4). This finding is consistent with a necrotic metastatic lymph node, which was confirmed by a separately acquired contrast-enhanced CT study (not shown). For both cases, without the help of contrast-enhanced CT study, determination of a metastatic lymph node would prove challenging on the FDG PET portion of the study and sometimes can be completely false negative.

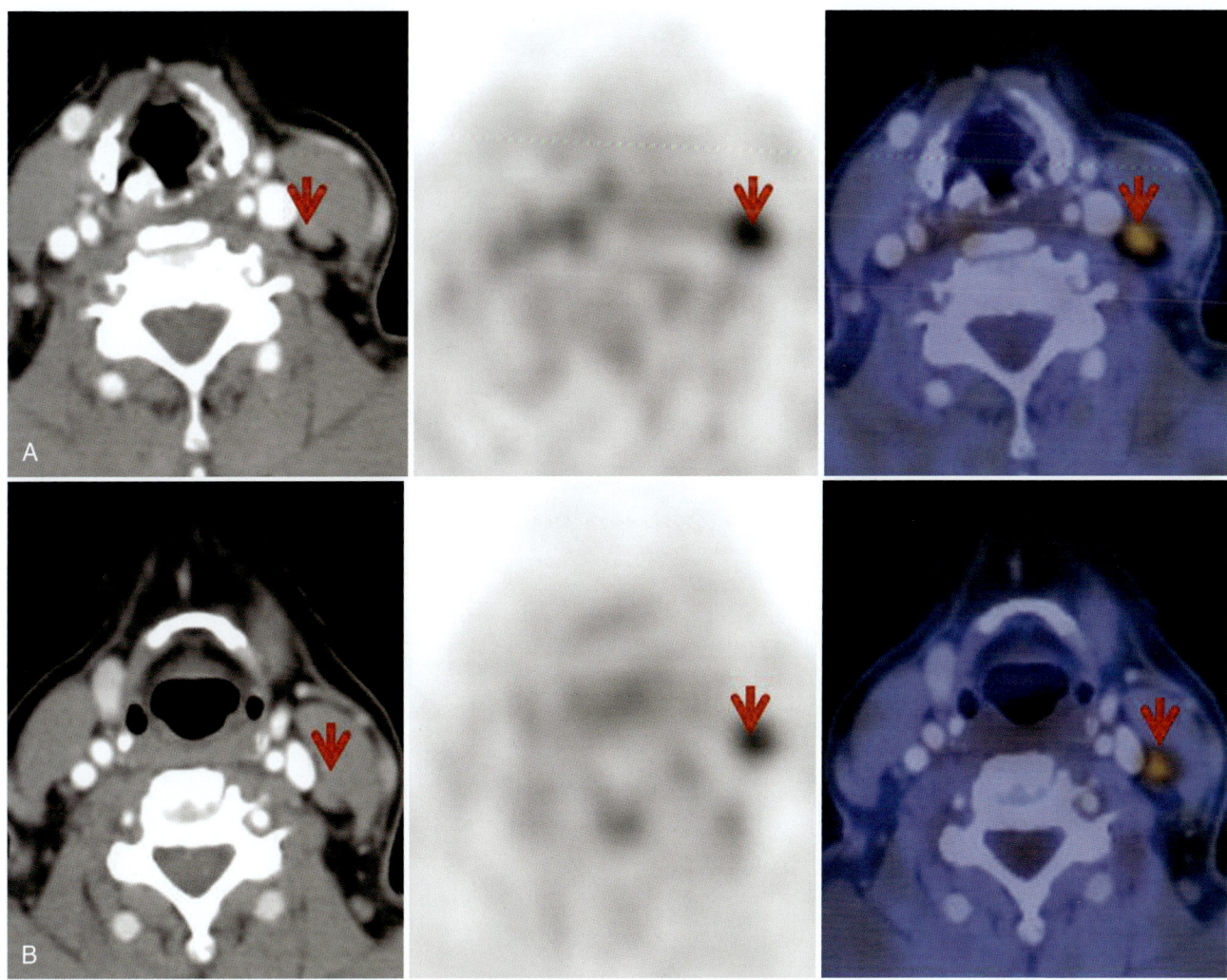

Figure 4-35 A 73-year-old man with a history of tonsillar squamous cell carcinoma, status post primary therapy, referred for determination of extent of disease with FDG PET/CT performed with contrast-enhanced high-resolution CT. **A:** Six-month follow-up PET/CT study demonstrates increased FDG uptake (SUV_{max} 4.9) corresponding to a left level III lymph node that shows benign morphologic features (smooth margins, no infiltration of the fat, and longer than wider) (*vertical arrows*). This finding may represent metastatic disease, although a reactive lymph node cannot be excluded. **B:** Nine-month follow-up PET/CT study demonstrates slightly decreased FDG uptake (SUV_{max} 3.8) and slight decrease in size of the lymph node (*vertical arrows*). Provided the patient had not received any interim therapy, these findings are consistent with reactive changes within this lymph node. When evaluating FDG PET studies, false-positive results seen in reactive lymph nodes must be considered.

Encasement of the carotid artery with more than 270 degrees of circumference is an ineligibility criterion for surgery and significantly increases the risk of recurrence. When evaluating FDG PET studies, false-positive results seen in reactive lymph nodes must be considered (Figures 4-13, *B*, 4-35, and 4-36, *B*).

Does Reactive Lymphoid Hyperplasia Pose Challenges to Classification of Lymph Node Status?

PET/CT fusion may increase specificity of FDG/PET (Figures 4-11, 4-12, 4-24, and 4-27) but cannot prevent misclassification of lymph node status when reactive lymphoid hyperplasia is present (Figures 4-13, *B*, 4-35, and 4-36). Overexpression of the glucose transporter protein GLUT1 in the lymph nodes can be held accountable for preferential FDG uptake in reactive lymph nodes (see the section How Do the Cervical Lymph Nodes Cause False-Positive Readings? for further discussion).

Does Use of Semiquantitative PET Methods Help in Defining a Pathologically Positive Lymph Node?

SUVs have been helpful to a certain extent (Figures 4-11 through 4-13, 4-24, 4-27, 4-35, and 4-36) in differentiating benign from malignant tumors but have not definitively solved the problem. In one study, according to receiver operating characteristic analysis, the size-based SUV_{max} cutoff values of 1.9, 2.5, and 3.0 for lymph nodes measuring <1.0 cm, 1.0 to 1.5 cm, and >1.5 cm, respectively, yielded 79% sensitivity and 99% specificity for nodal level staging. In another study, the sensitivity and specificity for neck nodal staging were 75% and 94%, respectively, with a cutoff value of 3.5. However,

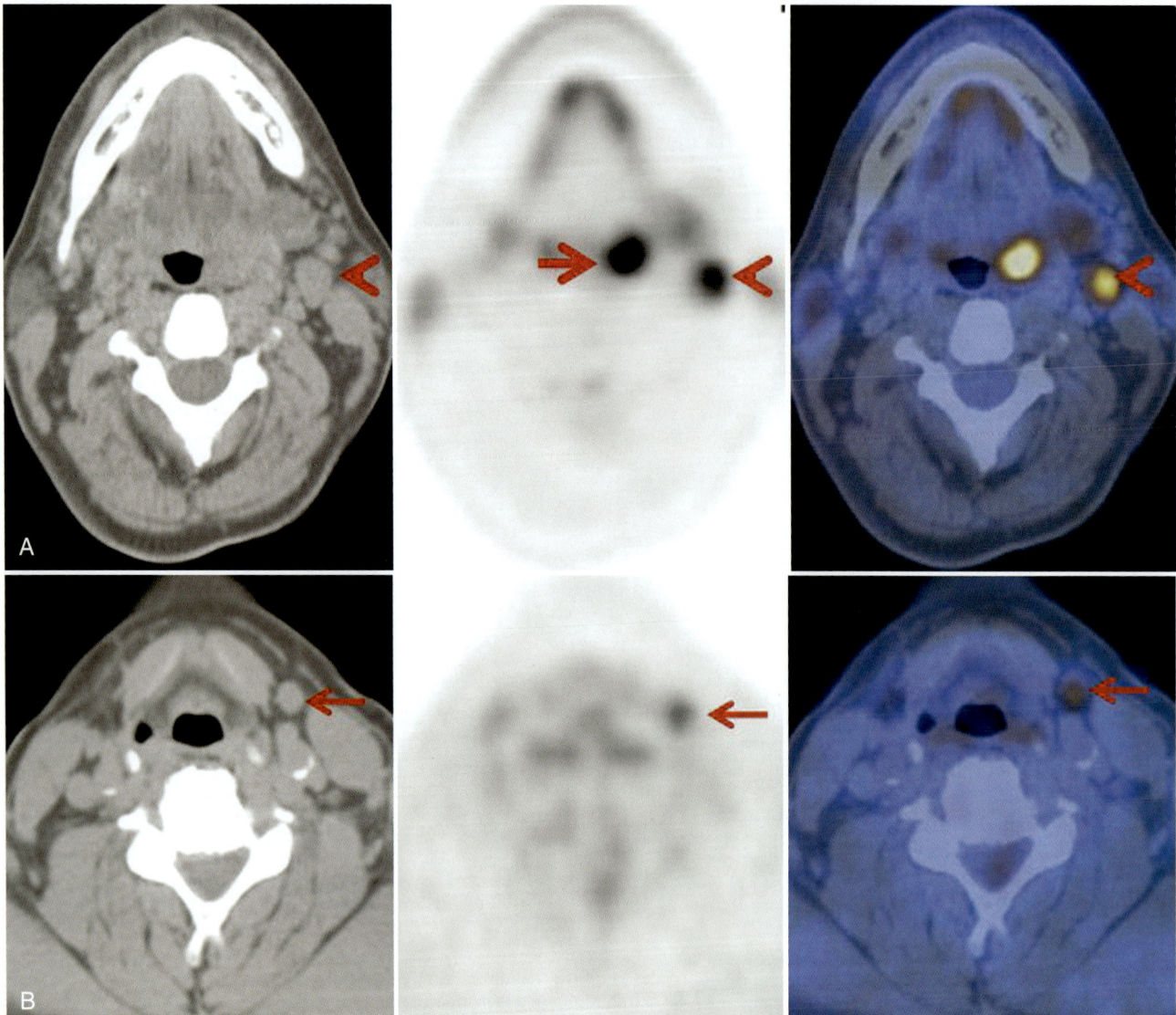

Figure 4-36 A 53-year-old man recently diagnosed with base of tongue squamous cell carcinoma, referred for determination of extent of disease with FDG PET/CT performed with noncontrast enhanced low-dose CT. **A:** Axial images of PET/CT study shows intense FDG uptake (SUV_{max} 16.3), corresponding to a soft tissue mass in the left base of tongue, consistent with primary tumor (*arrows*). There is increased FDG uptake (SUV_{max} 10.4) in an enlarged left level IIA lymph node (*arrowheads*), measuring 1.8 cm in long axis, most consistent with locoregional metastatic disease. **B:** There is also increased FDG uptake in a left level III lymph node (SUV_{max} 1.8), measuring 1.0 cm in long axis and showing benign morphology (smooth margins, no infiltration of the fat) (*small arrows*), which may represent a reactive lymph node considering both the low-grade FDG accumulation and CT features. However, these characteristics may be misleading in many other cases with metastatic disease. False-positive results may be unavoidable in many circumstances because of lack of clear-cut definition of lymph node metastasis by PET criteria and the relatively nonspecific nature of FDG uptake.

SUVs are highly variable in uncontrolled conditions because they depend on a host of variables, such as body fat, insulin and glucose levels, wait time, reconstruction algorithms, and lesion size (partial volume averaging). The pervasiveness of false-positive results associated with FDG PET imaging can be alleviated to a great extent by integration of PET and CT, which improves the positive predictive value (PPV) with the help of precise anatomic definition. It should be emphasized that for both oral and laryngeal SCCs, no validated SUV threshold has been determined to differentiate benign from malignant nodal disease. Hence, SUVs should not be used in routine clinical management until sufficient data accumulate to establish it as a diagnostic criterion.

What Is Clinically N0 Neck?

Across all subsites and T stages, occult cervical metastasis occurs in 10% to 50% of HNSCC patients, particularly in those with oral cavity cancers. Because most of N0 neck metastases harbor microscopic tumor foci, they may go undetected in up to 70% of cases using currently available anatomic and metabolic imaging modalities alike due to resolution limits. Therefore, all patients with oral and oropharyngeal SCC should

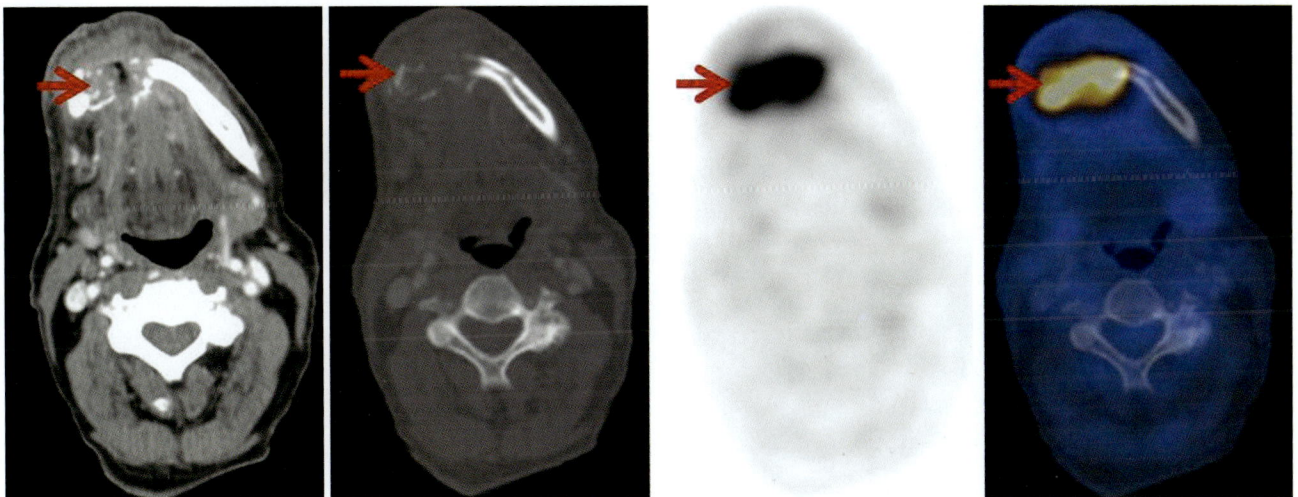

Figure 4-37 A 68-year-old man with floor of mouth squamous cell carcinoma (SCC), referred for determination of extent of disease with FDG PET/CT performed with contrast-enhanced high-resolution CT. Axial images of PET/CT study demonstrate increased FDG uptake (SUV$_{max}$ 17.5) corresponding to a soft tissue mass in the anterior floor of mouth, invading the anterior mandible, displaying destructive changes on the companion contrast-enhanced CT slice in both the soft tissue (A) and bone (B) windows (*arrows*). If sufficiently large, floor of mouth SCC often involves the mandible.

be considered candidates for regional nodal therapy, such as radiotherapy or elective neck dissection. The management approach to N0 disease is not universal. Some groups support observation only, and whereas others advocate a more aggressive surgical approach.

Does FDG PET Guide the Surgeon in N0 Neck?

One consequence of the innate limitations of image resolution associated with PET/CT imaging (at ~6–7 mm) is its suboptimal capability to detect N0 disease. This limitation is heightened even more given that nearly 50% of metastatic cervical lymph nodes measure less than 7 mm in diameter. In a meta-analysis, Kyzas et al found an overall FDG PET sensitivity of 79% in detecting cervical nodal metastases; however, the sensitivity decreased to 50% for clinically N0 patients. Yamazaki et al reported that metastatic nodes measuring 1 cm or greater in the short axis can be detected at a high rate close to 100%, whereas nodes smaller than 5 mm go undetected. Despite its better performance compared to conventional imaging modalities (Figures 4-12, 4-24, 4-27, 4-32, and 4-33) and some promising reports with sensitivities of greater than 75%, FDG PET still is not sufficiently sensitive to allow the surgeon to determine which patients will benefit from neck dissection. Furthermore, false-positive results can occur due to reactive changes that occur in the draining lymph nodes (Figures 4-13, *B*, and 4-36, *B*).

■ IS FDG PET USEFUL IN EVALUATION OF BONE INVASION?

An important clinical concern is the possibility of bone invasion, especially mandibular and maxillary invasion. In patients with oral cavity and oropharyngeal SCCs involving the floor of the mouth, retromolar trigone, or lower alveolus, tumors with mandibular involvement (Figure 4-37), and those with palate cancers, invasion of the maxilla, palatal bone, and nasal vault should be ruled out (Figures 4-38 and 4-39). Although the periosteum serves as an early and effective barrier against bone invasion in edentulous patients, tumor cells gain entrance to the mandible through dental pits or mental or mandibular canals. Tumors of the palate can vertically invade the nasal vault or maxillary sinus, thus requiring resection of underlying bone and deeper structures as necessary.

The poor sensitivity associated with preoperative imaging (both FDG PET and anatomic imaging) has decreased reliance on imaging as the primary method for determining mandibular invasion. Currently, even with an effective preoperative imaging strategy, the decision for segmental mandibulectomy is clinically made based on tumor depth and proximity to the mandible. In general, tumor invasion of the cortex or periosteum can be managed with marginal resection, whereas involvement of the medullary bone requires segmental resection. Diagnosis of unequivocal invasion of the bone requires segmental resection (Figure 4-37), whereas close proximity to the mandible or maxilla even without invasion usually is treated with marginal resection of the bone (Figures 4-2, 4-39, and 4-40). CT with contrast enhancement is the most widely used imaging technique, with a higher specificity than sensitivity of 80% to 95%. MRI apparently is superior for evaluating invasion of the medullary cavity of the mandible, but its specificity is approximately 50% due to false-positive findings. PET/CT imaging in conjunction with ceCT can be helpful in delineating mandibular involvement by increasing the sensitivity and certainty in equivocal cases. One study reported a superior sensitivity for FDG PET compared to CT (100% vs 33%) but an inferior specificity at 85% versus 100% in identifying mandibular invasion. The suboptimal specificity of FDG PET imaging can be attributed to false-positive findings in inflammatory processes (Figure 4-41, *A*) as well as a scattering of photons from the avidly positive primary tumor into the adjacent structures (Figure 4-42).

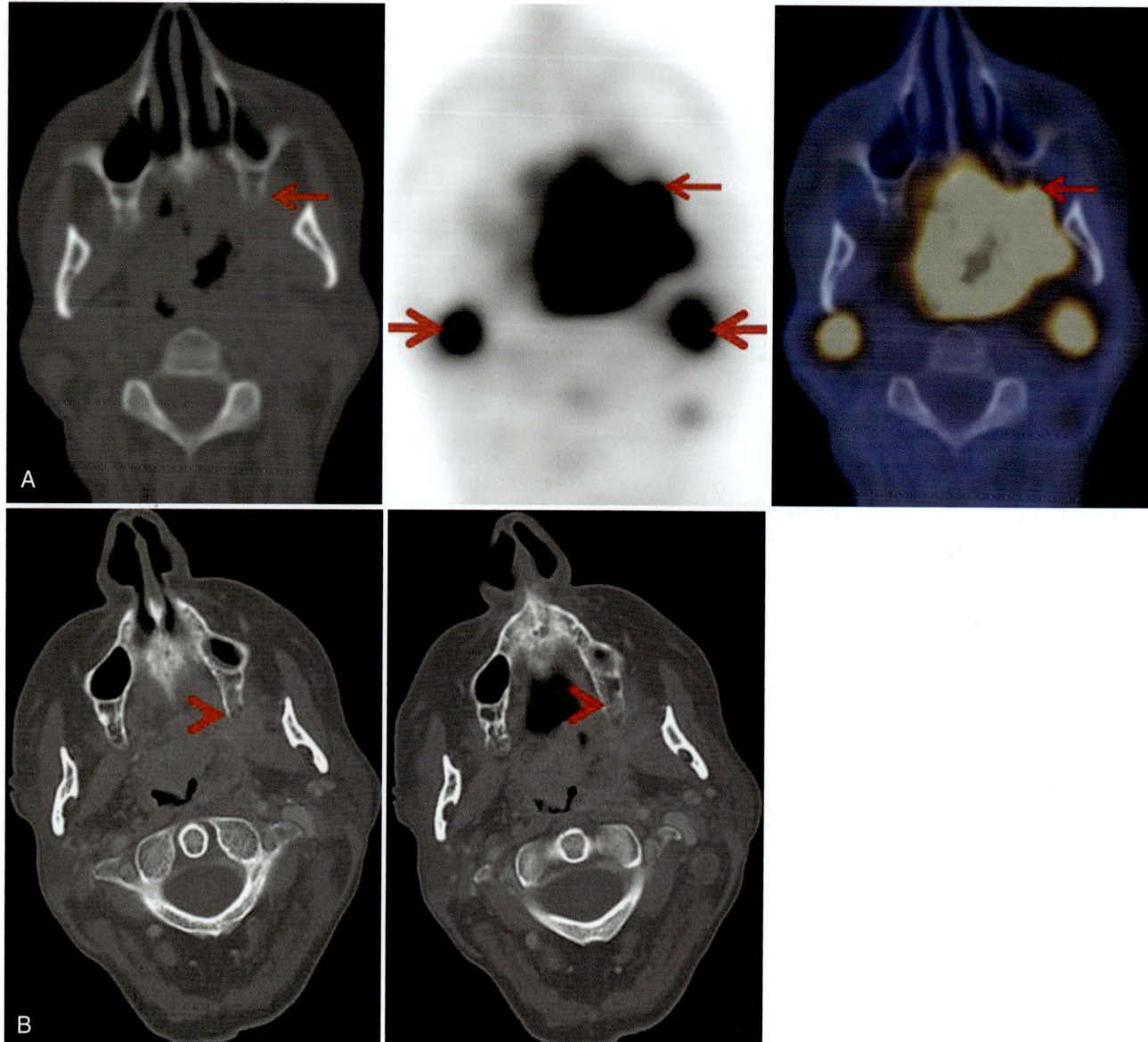

Figure 4-38 A 65-year-old woman recently diagnosed with tongue cancer (same patient as shown in Figure 4-5), referred for determination of extent of disease with FDG PET/CT performed with low-dose CT study **(A)**. In addition, contrast-enhanced high-resolution CT was separately obtained **(B)**. Axial images of PET/CT study demonstrate increased FDG uptake (SUV_{max} 18) corresponding to a soft tissue mass involving the tongue with extension to the oropharyngeal wall and left retromolar trigone. The tumor abuts the left maxillary tuberosity, which shows erosion on bone windows of the contrast-enhanced CT study (*arrowheads*). The uptake extending into this region on the PET/CT images increases the confidence of CT interpretation of bone involvement or vice versa. On CT, the left mandibular ramus is in close proximity to the tumor but shows no evidence of erosion, consistent with sparing of the mandible. There are bilateral level II lymph nodes with increased FDG uptake consistent with metastatic disease (N2c) (*arrows*). The patient underwent chemoradiation therapy followed by glossectomy and bilateral lymph node dissection of partial maxillectomy, which confirmed maxillary bone invasion.

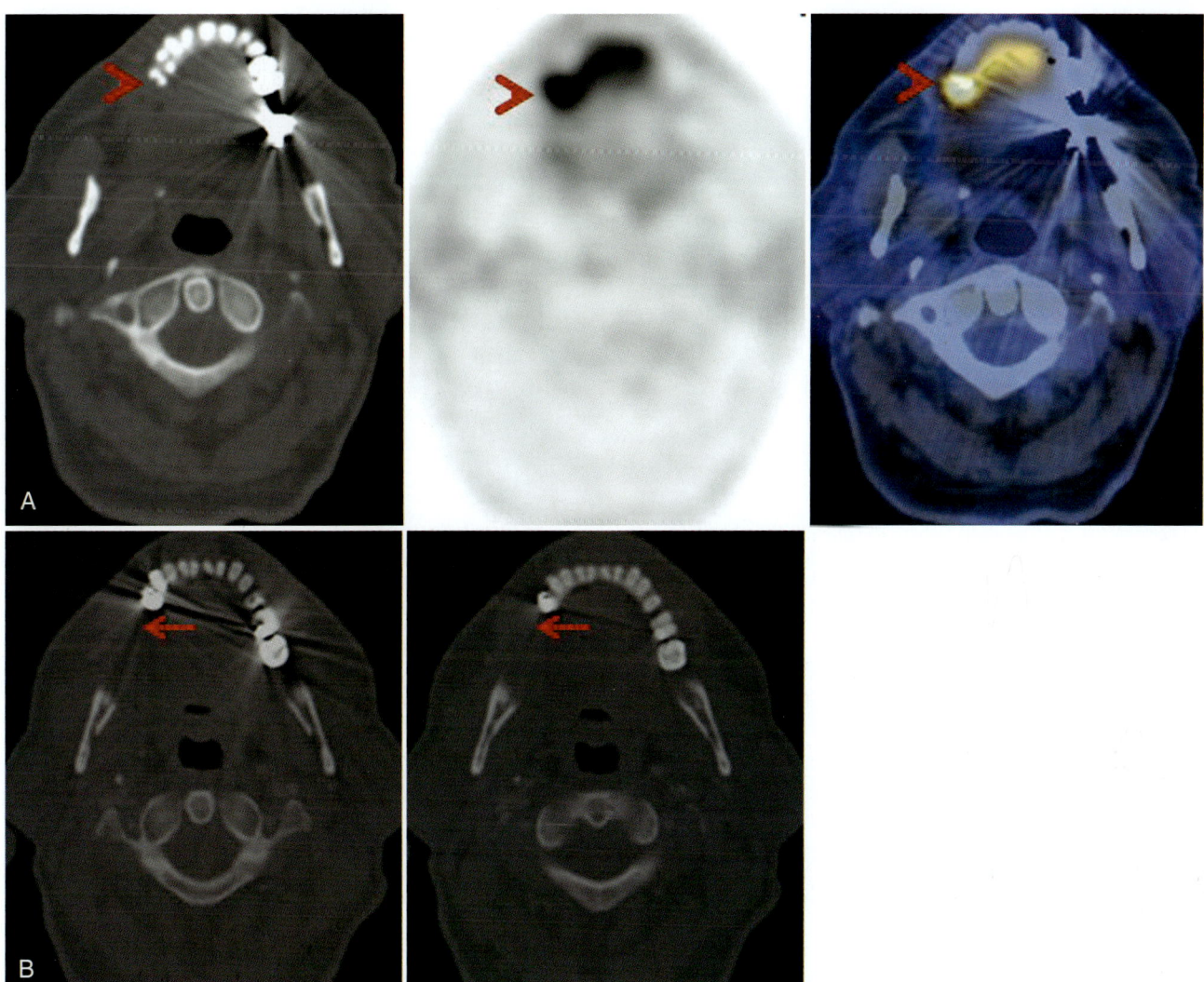

Figure 4-39 A 74-year-old man with recently diagnosed palate squamous cell carcinoma (same patient as shown in Figure 4-8, *A*). **A:** Hypermetabolic mass (SUV$_{max}$ 17.4) in the left anterior hard palate abuts the maxilla (*arrowheads*). **B:** On separately acquired diagnostic CT (bone windows), there is no clear evidence of osseous involvement (*small arrows*). Evaluation of the CT study is limited due to artifacts emanating from dental fillings. The patient subsequently underwent hemimaxillectomy, which revealed no evidence of the bone involvement. The diagnosis of unequivocal invasion of the bone requires segmental resection. The close proximity to the mandible or maxilla even without invasion usually is treated with marginal resection of the bone.

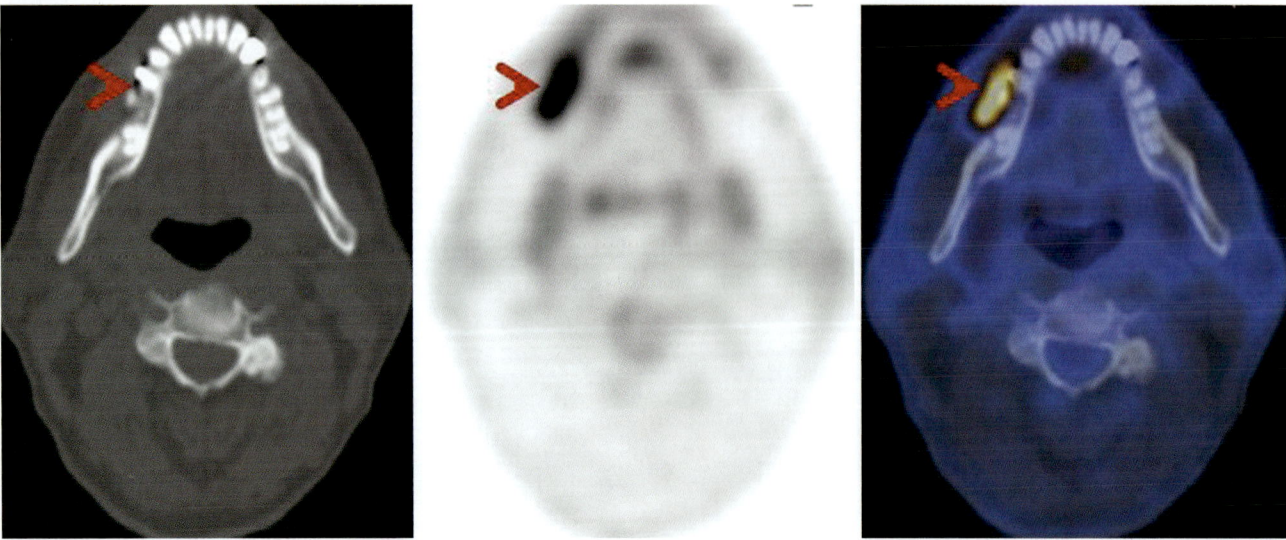

Figure 4-40 A 48-year-old woman recently diagnosed with buccal squamous cell carcinoma (same patient as shown in Figure 4-7, *A*). Hypermetabolic mass (SUV$_{max}$ 9.5) in the right alveolar ridge abuts the mandible, although with no clear evidence of osseous involvement on the bone windows of the accompanying CT study (*arrowheads*). The patient underwent a partial mandibular resection, which revealed no bone involvement on the tumor specimen.

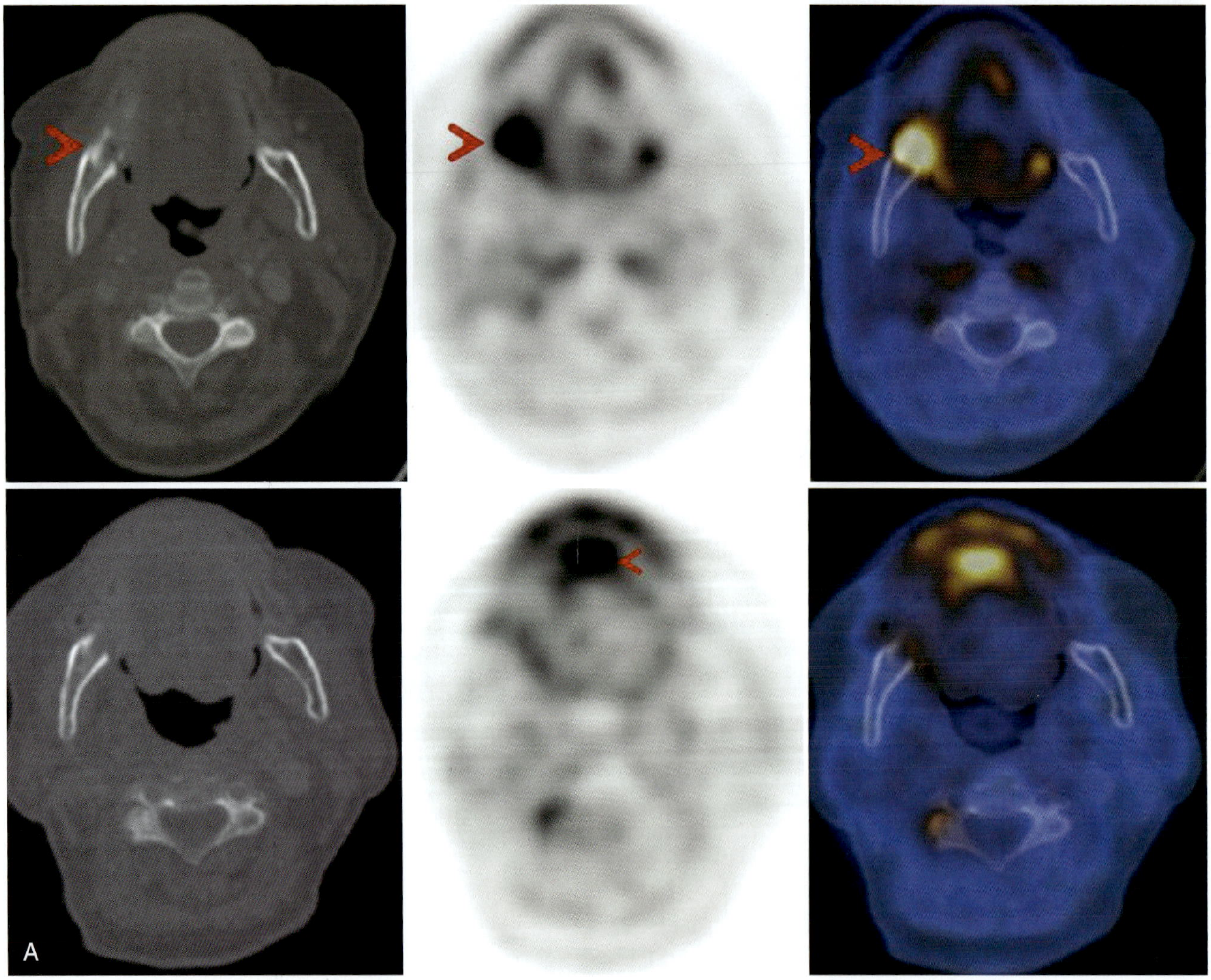

Figure 4-41 A 77-year-old man with a diagnosis of right base of tongue squamous cell carcinoma, referred for FDG PET/CT study performed with noncontrast enhanced low-dose CT study for evaluation of the disease status 3 months after completion of chemoradiation. **A:** Axial images of PET/CT study demonstrate increased FDG uptake (SUV$_{max}$ 9.5) corresponding to the right angle of the mandible (*arrowheads*), raising suspicion for disease recurrence, although there is no pathologic finding on the accompanying CT study. Subsequent biopsy revealed acute inflammation of the gum line with no evidence of malignancy.

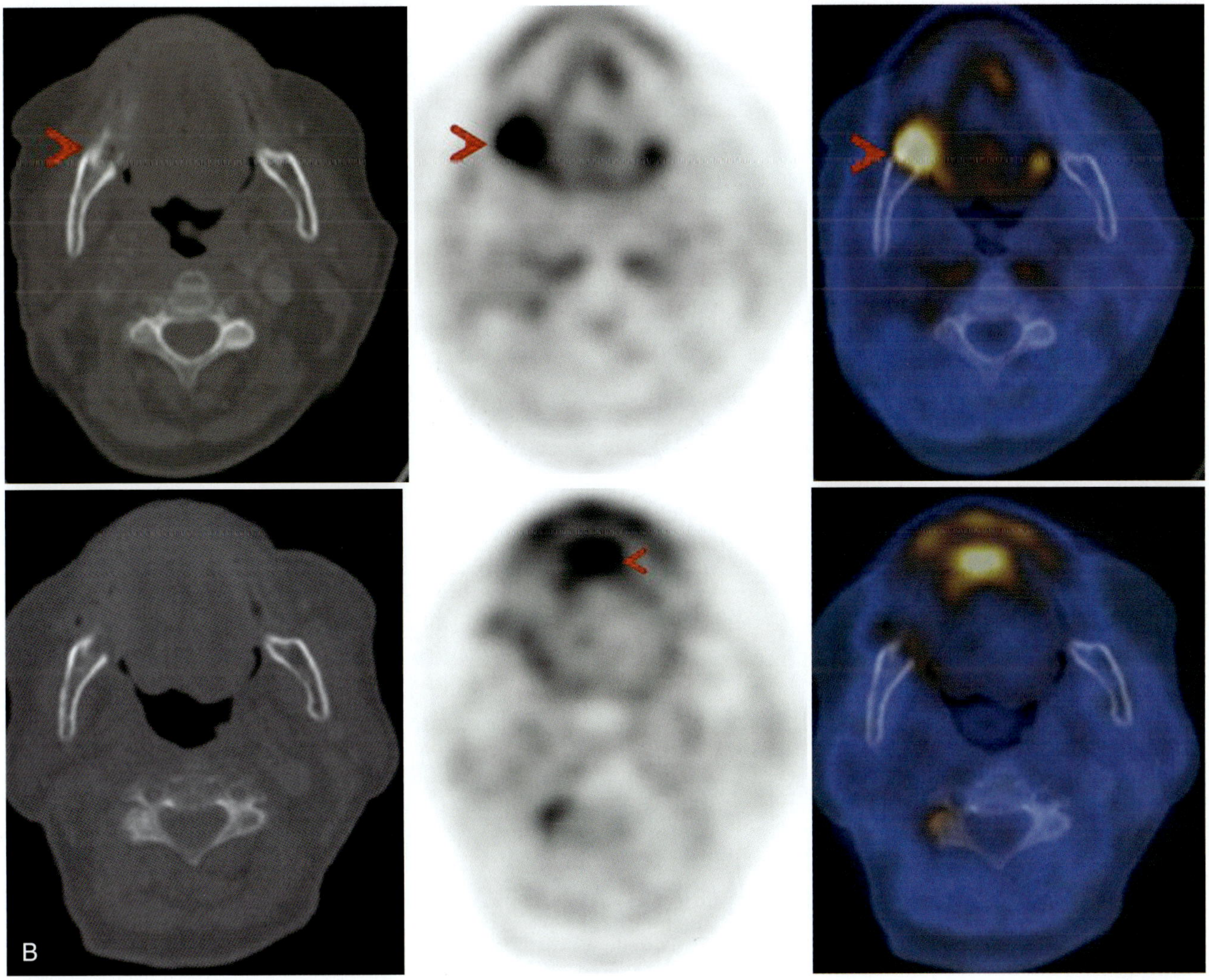

Figure 4-41, cont'd B: Three-month follow-up PET/CT study revealed resolution of the previously increased FDG uptake. This finding may represent radiation-related inflammatory epithelial changes. Note the physiologic uptake in the anterior midline of the oral cavity, which usually is seen at the confluence of sublingual glands and the insertion of the genioglossus muscle (*small arrowhead*).

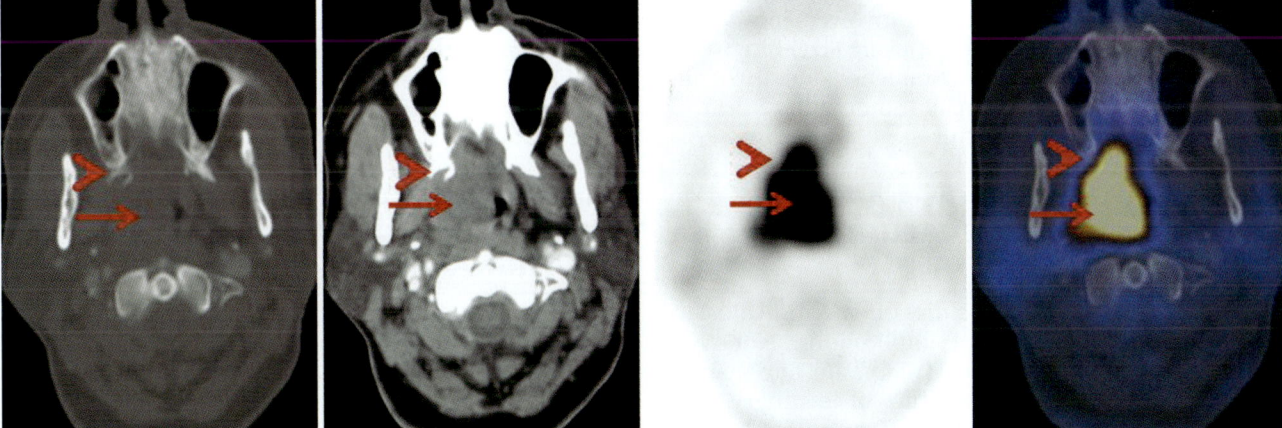

Figure 4-42 A 67-year-old man with a diagnosis of oropharyngeal squamous cell carcinoma, referred for FDG PET/CT study performed with contrast-enhanced high-resolution CT study for evaluation of extent of disease. Axial images of PET/CT study performed with contrast-enhanced CT demonstrate increased FDG uptake (SUV_{max} 16.5) mainly in the right tongue with extension cranially to the palate, evident on the soft tissue windows (**second image from the left**; *small arrows*). On the bone windows, the tumor abuts the right maxillary tuberosity, although there is no definite evidence of bone destruction or erosion (**first image from the left**; *arrowheads*). Subsequent partial maxillectomy specimen revealed no evidence of bone invasion. This finding probably is due to scattered photons from a highly FDG avid primary tumor that is situated in close proximity to the maxillary bone.

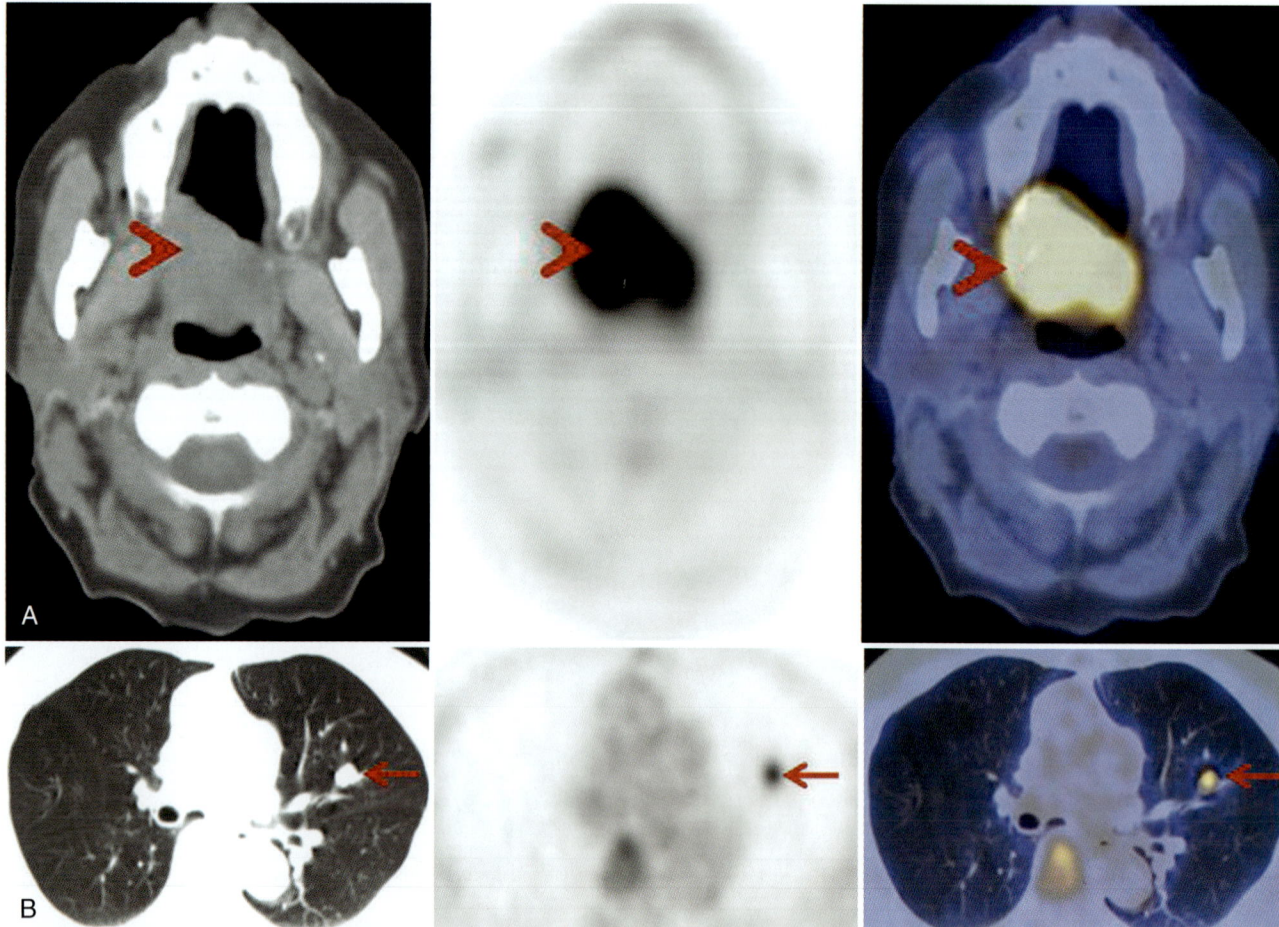

Figure 4-43 A 57-year-old woman recently diagnosed with base of tongue squamous cell carcinoma (same patient as shown in Figure 4-10). **A:** There is a large area of increased FDG uptake (SUV_{max} 14.8) involving the base of tongue extending into the supraglottic larynx (*arrowheads*) (T2N1). **B:** On axial images of the chest of the whole-body PET/CT study, there is increased FDG uptake (SUV_{max} 6.5) in a left upper lobe pulmonary nodule (*small arrows*), consistent with distant metastasis (T2N1M1).

Appropriate preoperative assessment using a combination of clinical and imaging studies may enhance the accuracy in detection of bone involvement. It may be sensible to adopt a strategy of using FDG PET when there is a need to increase confidence and to better define the extent of the primary tumor with respect to involvement of osseous structures.

■ DOES FDG PET/CT HAVE A PRIMARY ROLE IN EVALUATION OF DISTANT METASTASES?

Early detection of metastatic disease is critical due to prognostic and management implications. Nonetheless, distant metastases from HNSCC are rare at presentation, with an overall incidence of less than 15%, whereas patients with locoregionally advanced tumors may be at higher risk for distant metastasis. The lungs are the most common site of distant metastases (Figure 4-43), followed by bone (Figure 4-44) and abdomen. Mediastinal lymph node metastases are considered distant metastatic disease (Figure 4-45). Patients with oropharyngeal and laryngeal SCC are at higher risk than are those with oral cavity SCC for the development of distant metastases. Although more research is necessary to establish the superiority of PET over CT, currently FDG PET appears to be a better imaging modality in identifying distant metastasis, with sensitivity and specificity of 80% to 95% and 85% to 95%, respectively, in advanced stage HNSCC.

■ WHAT ARE THE COMMON SITES FOR SYNCHRONOUS MALIGNANCIES?

Synchronous tumors can occur in the head and neck itself, lung, or upper aerodigestive tract, likely due to shared risk factors. The reported prevalence of synchronous or metastatic chest malignancy in patients with HNSCC varies from 2% to 37.5%, with a significantly higher prevalence in patients with recurrent disease compared to those at initial staging. In general, patients with HNSCC have a 10% risk of developing a second aerodigestive tract primary malignancy. This number is slightly higher at 15% for tonsillar and base of the tongue cancers. Patients with N2 or N3 neck disease

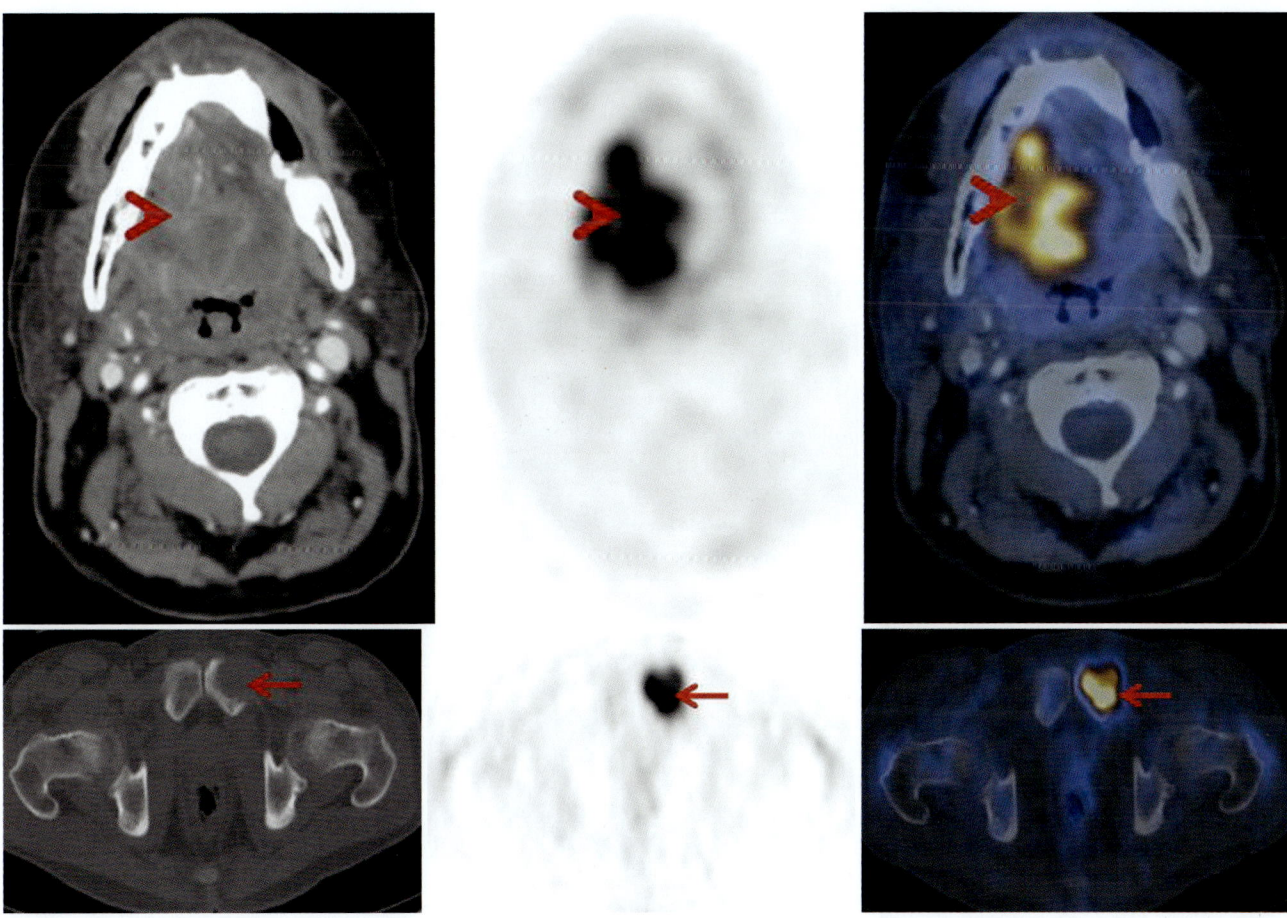

Figure 4-44 A 79-year-old man with a diagnosis of tongue squamous cell carcinoma, referred for FDG PET/CT study performed with contrast-enhanced high-resolution CT study for evaluation of extent of disease. **A:** Axial images of the head and neck portion of the PET/CT study demonstrate increased FDG uptake (SUV$_{max}$ 15.3) corresponding to a heterogeneously enhancing tongue mass crossing the midline, measuring 4.5 cm (T3) (*arrowheads*). There is no evidence of lymph node metastasis (T3N0). **B:** On axial images of the pelvis of the whole-body PET/CT study, there is increased FDG uptake (SUV$_{max}$ 8.6) corresponding to the left pubic symphysis displaying a lytic lesion with a soft tissue component (*small arrows*), consistent with distant metastatic disease (M1), confirming stage IV disease.

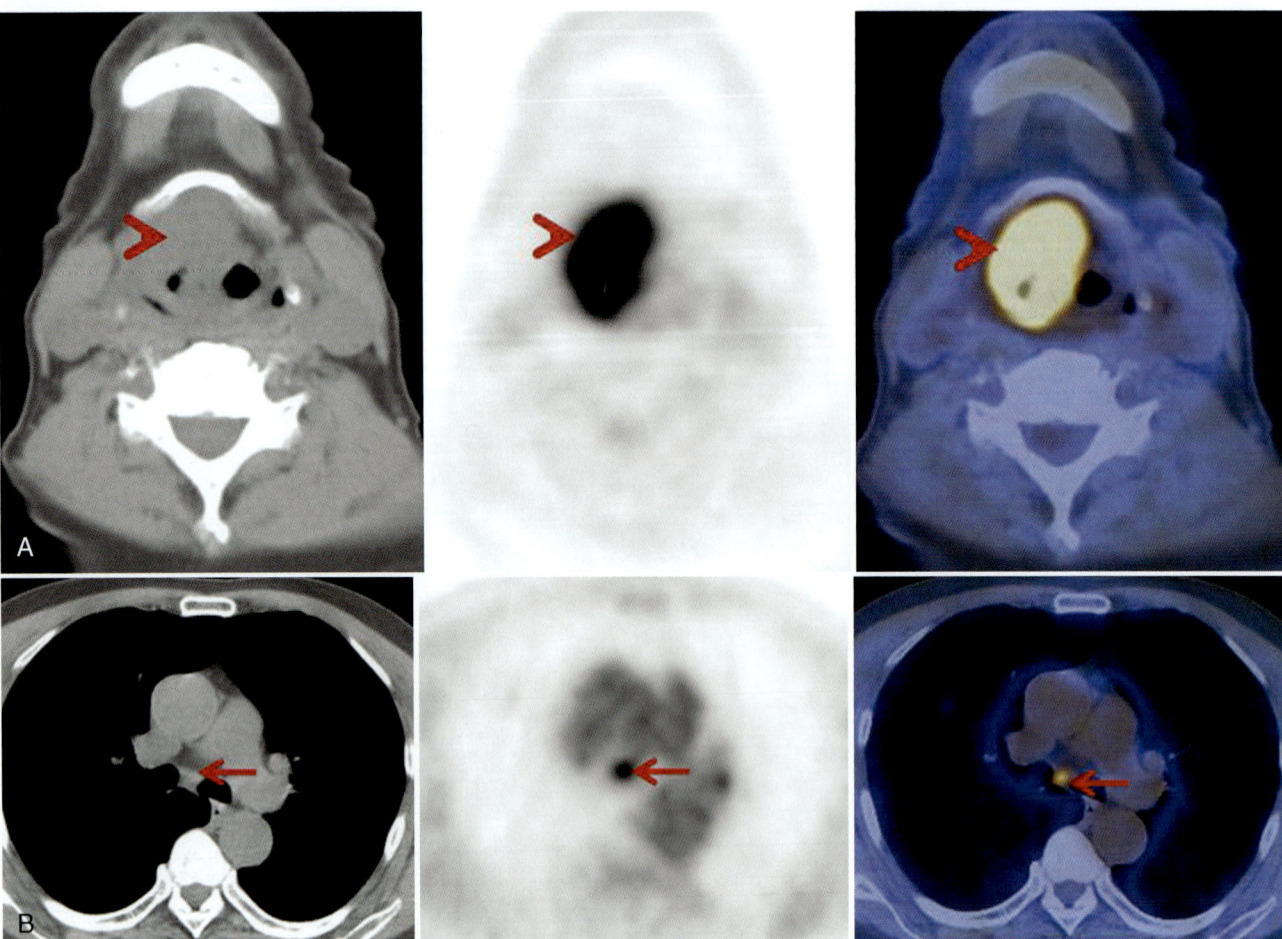

Figure 4-45 A 88-year-old man recently diagnosed with transglottic squamous cell carcinoma (same patient as shown in Figure 4-23), referred for staging with FDG PET/CT performed with noncontrast-enhanced low-dose CT. **A:** Axial images of PET/CT study demonstrate a large hypermetabolic (SUV_{max} 14.8) predominantly supraglottic tumor with vocal cord fixation (determined by laryngoscopy) (T3) (*arrowheads*). **B:** On axial images of the chest of the whole-body PET/CT study, there is increased FDG uptake (SUV_{max} 5.6) corresponding to a subcarinal lymph node (*small arrows*). Subsequent biopsy revealed metastatic disease (M1), stage IV disease. The 1.0-cm mildly hypermetabolic right level III lymph node shown in Figure 4-23 was not biopsied (NX). However, following chemoradiation, uptake has resolved (not shown). Thus, the presence of metastatic disease in this lymph node could not be proven but in a stage IV setting would not change clinical management.

are more likely to have synchronous or metastatic chest malignancy that are those with stage III or stage IV disease, and these indices could be used to select high-risk patients.

Is FDG PET Useful in Detecting Synchronous or Metachronous Malignancies?

The sensitivity of PET/CT is higher (96%–100%) than chest CT in identifying chest malignancy, but its specificity does not exceed 80%. The risk for development of metachronous cancers increases with time after completion of primary treatment of oral cavity and laryngeal cancers (Figure 4-46). The role FDG PET in detecting synchronous malignancies has not been fully investigated due to the relatively low risk for developing subsequent second malignancies in this group of patients. Nonetheless, it may be appropriate to use FDG PET in a surveillance setting for selected high-risk groups (see the section, Does FDG PET/CT Have a Role in Surveillance of HNSCC After Therapy? for further discussion).

■ DOES FDG PET CHANGE MANAGEMENT AT INITIAL STAGING?

FDG PET/CT yields additional information leading to upstaging in 30% to 40% (Figures 4-11, 4-12, 4-24, 4-27, 4-32, 4-43, and 4-45) and thereby can alter management in approximately 30% of patients. According to a physician survey study, FDG PET changed primary surgical plans to neoadjuvant therapy followed by surgery in approximately 20% and eliminated neoadjuvant therapy in approximately 10% of patients. In addition, surgical plans were modified in greater than 50% of patients based on FDG PET findings. The better definition of N staging using FDG PET/CT versus anatomic imaging led to modification of radiotherapy volume and dose in at least 30% of cases.

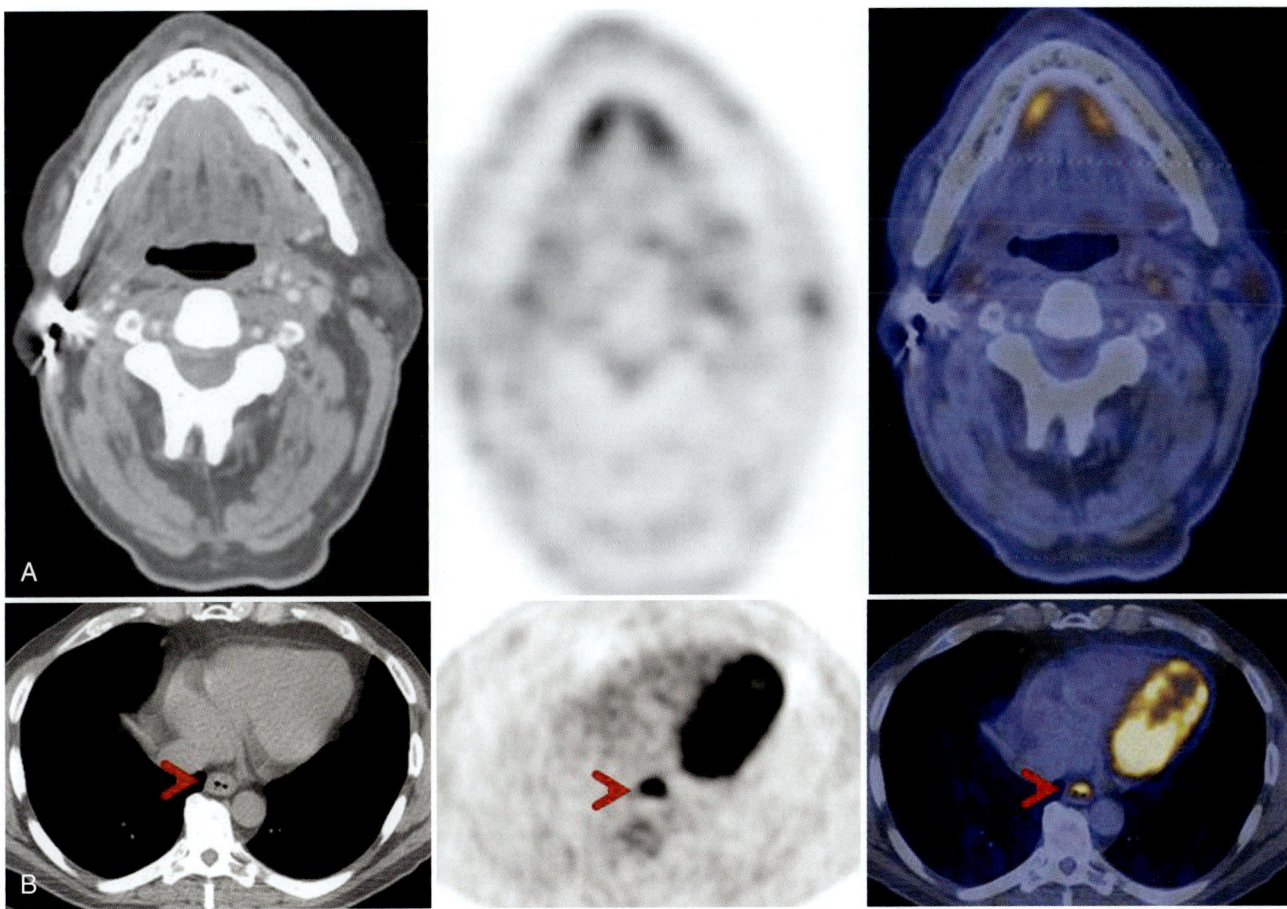

Figure 4-46 A 57-year-old man with a history of base of tongue squamous cell carcinoma, status post primary therapy and right neck dissection, referred for evaluation of disease status 12 months after therapy performed with FDG PET/CT performed with contrast-enhanced high-resolution CT study. **A:** Axial images of the head and neck portion of the PET/CT study demonstrate no evidence of recurrence. **B:** On axial images of the chest of the whole-body PET/CT study, there is increased uptake (SUV_{max} 9.5) corresponding to the mid to distal esophagus (*arrowheads*), which was subsequently proven to be a metachronous cancer in the esophagus of squamous cell origin.

■ DOES FDG PET HAVE A ROLE IN IDENTIFYING PRIMARY DISEASE IN PATIENTS WITH CARCINOMA OF UNKNOWN PRIMARY?

Cervical metastases from an occult primary (carcinoma of unknown primary [CUP]) constitute 5% to 10% of all HNSCC patients. Histologic categorization of the CUP is important to allow for site-specific therapy, which offers better survival than a generic therapeutic approach. The majority of these cases are unresolved with respect to the primary pathology despite vigorous workup and multiple directed biopsies. Generally, lymph node metastases from CUP in the levels I to III and V are associated with primary HNSCC, particularly of tonsil origin (Figures 4-29 and 4-30), whereas level IV involvement is linked to primaries of the chest and less frequently the abdomen or pelvis.

Compared with conventional imaging, FDG PET provides a twofold higher sensitivity, with absolute values usually ranging between 22% and 87% depending on the patient population. However, the specificity is similar to that of CT at approximately 85%. In a meta-analysis, the pooled sensitivity and specificity of FDG PET/CT were 37% and 84%, respectively. Lung and oropharyngeal carcinomas were the most frequently detected primary tumors by FDG PET/CT (33% and 16%, respectively). The most common locations of false-positive PET/CT findings are the lung and the oropharynx due to nonspecific uptake in granulomatous lung nodules and oropharyngeal and nasopharyngeal lymphoid tissues. The asymmetric nature of FDG uptake noted in the tonsillar fossa in some patients does not seem to increase test sensitivity because it can be seen as a normal variant or due to tonsillitis (Figure 4-15).

Despite its marginally better results in detecting the primary site (usually in 30%–40% of cases), FDG PET imaging still is associated with a higher number of false-negative results in the detection of CUP. Because a normal FDG PET result does not eliminate the need for panendoscopy with multiple biopsies and tonsillectomy in the case of CUP, it should be considered a supplemental test to conventional methods for achieving the best possible yield.

IS THERE A ROLE FOR FDG PET/CT IN ASSESSMENT OF TREATMENT RESPONSE?

Sufficient evidence now indicates that FDG PET imaging is valuable in the assessment of response to therapy if timed properly. Significantly decreased FDG accumulation after chemoradiotherapy is associated with favorable tumor response, survival, and local control. Conversely, persistent FDG uptake indicates incomplete response and poor outcomes. This topic is discussed for the primary tumor and nodal disease separately in the following sections.

What Is the Best Timing for Evaluation of Response to Therapy?

The optimal timing of FDG PET/CT after radiation and chemotherapy is subject to ongoing debate due to the long-term persistence of posttreatment inflammatory changes. Radiation-induced inflammation can be considerable within the first 2 months after treatment and can last up to 18 months (Figure 4-47). If imaged very early after treatment, however, both false-positive and false-negative results equally challenge proper management. The majority of studies found that FDG PET/CT yields the highest negative predictive value (NPV) when performed 8 to 12 weeks after completion of radiation therapy (~95%). Imaging performed more than 1 month after completion of radiation therapy was found to have a significantly higher sensitivity compared with PET scans performed within 1 month (95% vs 55%).

Does FDG PET/CT Predict Response in Cervical Lymph Nodes? Does It Have a Primary Role in Deferring Planned Neck Dissection of HNSCC in the Posttherapy Setting?

Following neoadjuvant therapy, identification of posttherapy residual disease in cervical lymph nodes poses a clinical challenge in patients with N2 to N3 disease. In this group of patients, planned posttreatment neck dissection is advocated; however, this aggressive approach may not be indicated in all patients.

After neoadjuvant chemoradiotherapy, the median sensitivity, specificity, and NPV for FDG PET imaging were reported to be 73%, 83%, and 92%, respectively (Figures 4-15, C, 4-30, and 4-48 through 4-50). Negative PET results are highly reliable in excluding the possibility of residual nodal disease with negligible false–negative results. However, FDG PET results can be false positive in at least one third of these patients. In addition, several studies have reported unfavorable results for FDG PET imaging, revealing a false-negative rate as high as 20%. Nonetheless, PET-based assessment changes the response category in approximately 30% of patients, mostly by upgrading partial response based on conventional assessment alone to a complete response (Figures 4-15, C, 4-30, B, and 4-48).

In summary, FDG PET currently has not been fully validated to have the capability to guide the surgeon in deciding whether or not to perform or withhold neck dissection. However, it is conceivable that a combinatorial approach including clinical assessment, CT, and FDG PET imaging may yield the highest predictive value. For example, in one study, combining PET and CT results increased the specificity to 91%, which was approximately 10% higher than that of each test alone, at no cost to the NPV of 94%.

Does FDG PET Predict Response in Primary Tumor?

In the detection of persistent disease at the primary site, similar to nodal response evaluation, the timing of posttreatment FDG PET is particularly critical after radiation therapy. The most optimal timing for FDG PET is suggested to be 2 to 3 months after completion of chemoradiotherapy, yielding mean sensitivity, specificity, PPV, and NPV of 90%, 70%, 30%, and 90%, respectively (Figures 4-48 through 4-50). In addition to the false-positive results, management is challenged by false-negative results. This is attributable to the fact that radiation therapy (RT) may hamper the FDG uptake mechanism early after therapy, leading to inability of the tumor to accumulate FDG.

Although the accuracy of PET/CT is superior to that of ceCT in the neck, it appears to be equivalent at the primary site in predicting persistent disease due to false-positive results associated with PET readings (82% vs 86%).

DOES FDG PET/CT HAVE A PRIMARY ROLE IN DETECTION OF RECURRENT HNSCC DURING FOLLOW-UP AFTER THERAPY?

The high risk of recurrence or the development of second primary malignancies warrants close follow-up of HNSCC patients after definitive therapy. Two thirds of locoregional and metastatic recurrences occur in the initial 2-year time period. Once the absence of residual disease is established, continued surveillance with clinical examination and imaging is pursued, especially in the first 2 years of completion of treatment. Persistent or increased radiotracer uptake in the region of the treated tumor may indicate residual or recurrent disease, especially if a mass is also detected on the corresponding CT section (Figure 4-51). Nonetheless, appreciation of an accompanying mass on CT can be hampered by posttherapy changes (Figure 4-52). For the detection of locoregional recurrence, FDG PET has a higher specificity (~90%) and NPV (>95%) than sensitivity (~80%) and PPV (64%) owing to false-positive findings (Figures 4-53 and 4-54). For detection of distant metastases during follow-up, PET has a higher sensitivity (~90%) and PPV (85%) and equal specificity (>95%) and NPV (>95%) compared to detection of locoregional recurrence.

What Are the Characteristics of Recurrent Disease in Oral and Oropharyngeal Cancers?

The pattern of recurrence in oral cavity SCC differs from that of oropharyngeal SCC in the higher rate of nodal and distant metastases seen in the latter disease entity.

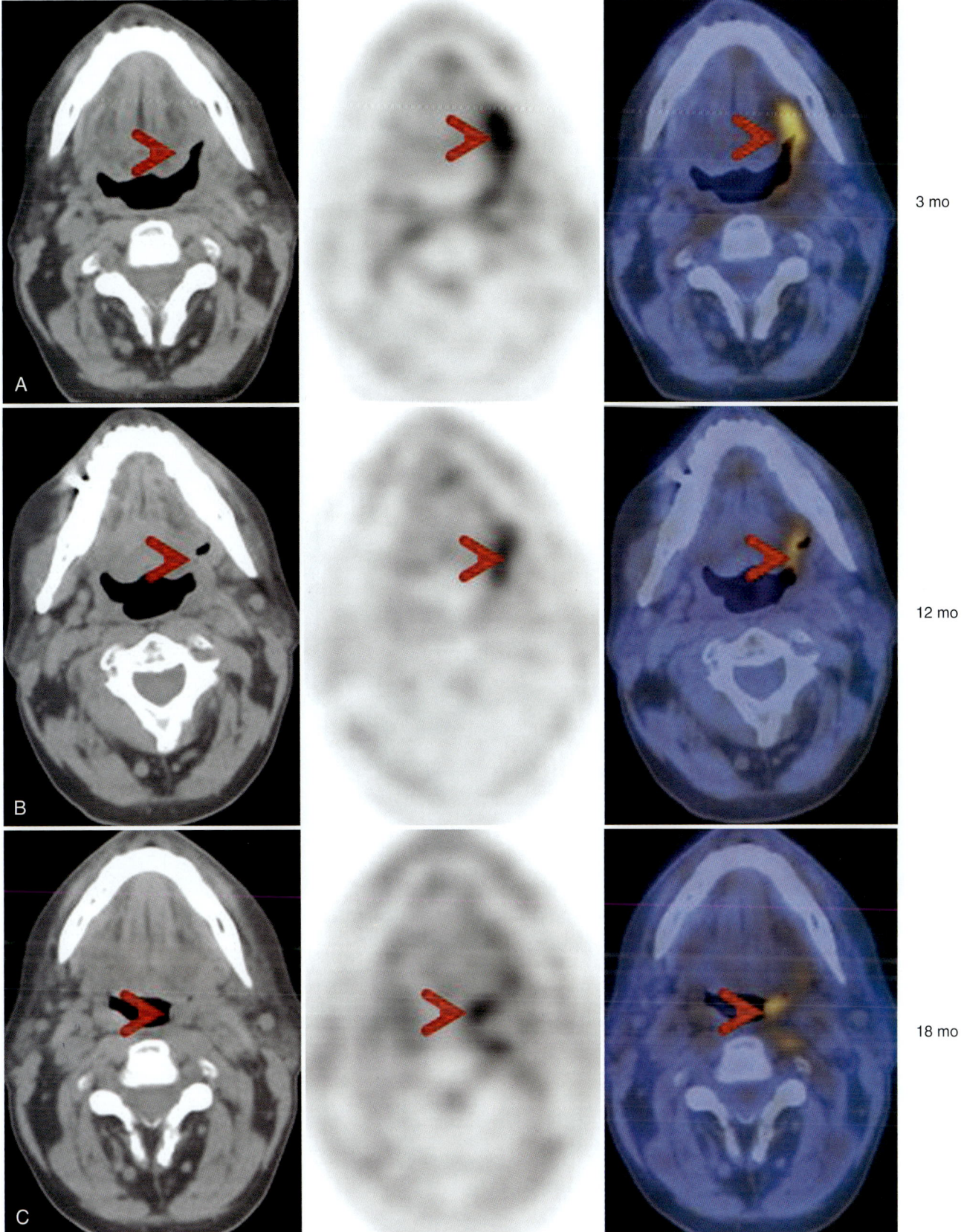

Figure 4-47 A 68-year-old man with a history of left base of tongue squamous cell carcinoma, status post primary therapy with chemoradiation, referred for evaluation of disease status with FDG PET/CT with low-dose CT, 3, 12, and 18 months after completion of therapy. A: Three-month PET/CT study demonstrated increased uptake in the left base of tongue (*arrowheads*), most consistent with postradiation changes. However, residual tumor cannot be definitively excluded. Uptake gradually decreased over time at 12-month **(B)** and 18-month **(C)** PET/CT studies (*arrowheads*), consistent with gradual regression of inflammation induced by radiation therapy.

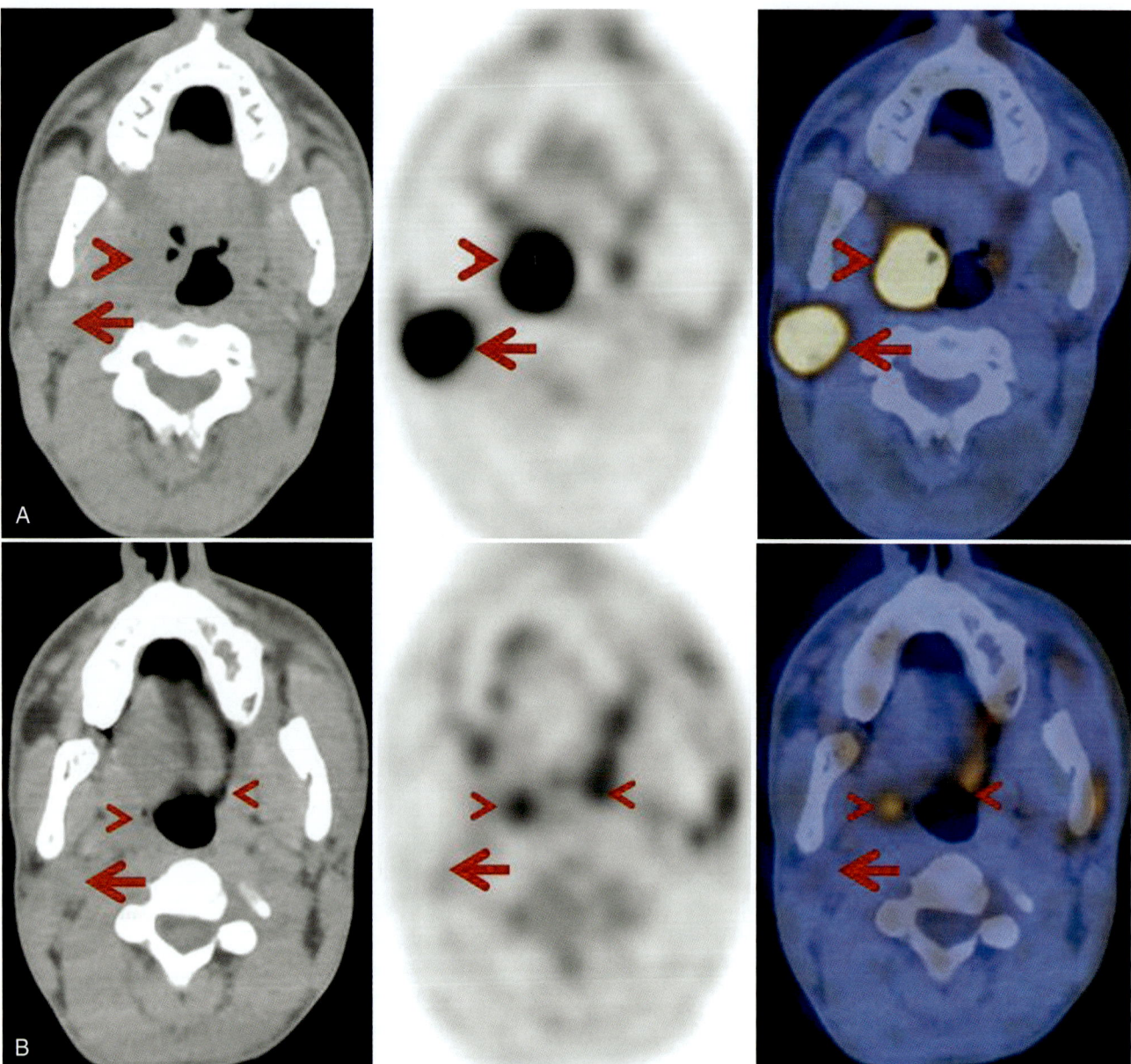

Figure 4-48 A 59-year-old man with recent diagnosis of right base of tongue squamous cell carcinoma. **A:** Pretherapy PET/CT study performed with noncontrast-enhanced low-dose CT demonstrates increased FDG uptake (SUV$_{max}$ 19) in the right base of tongue (*arrowheads*), consistent with the patient's known primary tumor. There is increased uptake (SUV$_{max}$ 14.5) in an enlarged right level II lymph node (*arrows*), consistent with metastatic disease. **B:** The patient subsequently underwent neoadjuvant therapy with chemoradiation and was referred for evaluation of therapy response 11 weeks after completion of therapy. There is complete resolution of uptake in the right base of tongue and in the right level II lymph node station despite the presence of a residual soft tissue density in the neck (*arrows*), consistent with complete response to therapy. The mild uptake noted in the oropharyngeal wall bilaterally probably represents normal lymphoid tissue (*small arrowheads*).

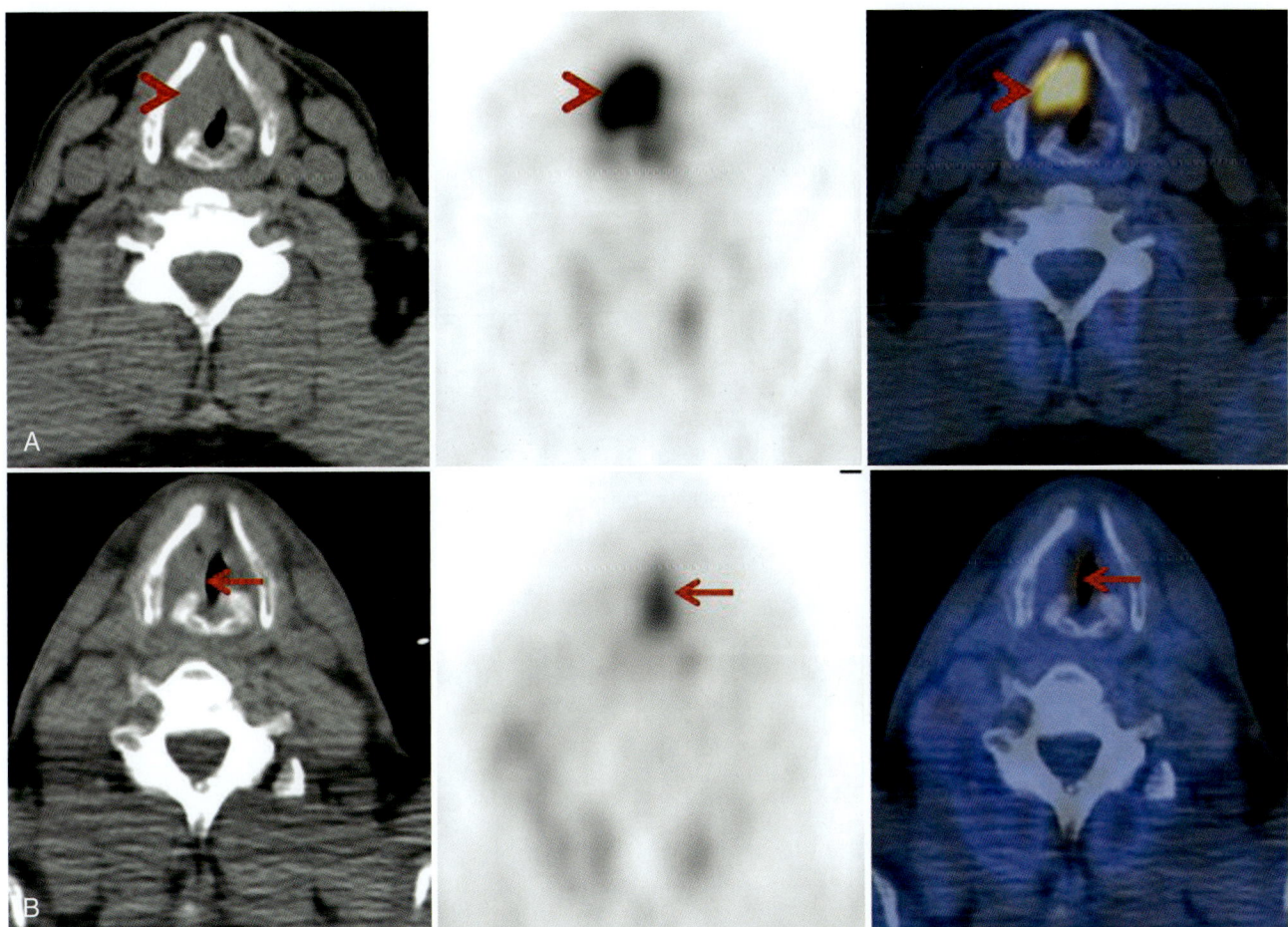

Figure 4-49 A 49-year-old man with recent diagnosis of right supraglottic squamous cell carcinoma. **A:** Pretherapy PET/CT study performed with low-dose CT demonstrates increased FDG uptake (SUV_{max} 11) in a large right supraglottic soft tissue mass, consistent with the primary tumor (*arrowheads*). The right preglottic space is obliterated. **B:** The patient underwent neoadjuvant therapy with chemoradiation and was referred for evaluation of therapy response 11 weeks after completion of therapy. There is resolution of uptake in the supraglottic region with mild residual uptake (SUV_{max} 1.8) (*arrows*). Although minimal residual disease cannot be ruled out, the pattern of uptake is diffuse and also is confined to the luminal/mucosal aspect of the larynx. Thus, this finding is most consistent with postradiation inflammatory changes in the epithelial surfaces. This finding persisted on the following 3-month PET/CT study, warranting a biopsy that revealed squamous cell proliferation with no evidence of malignancy.

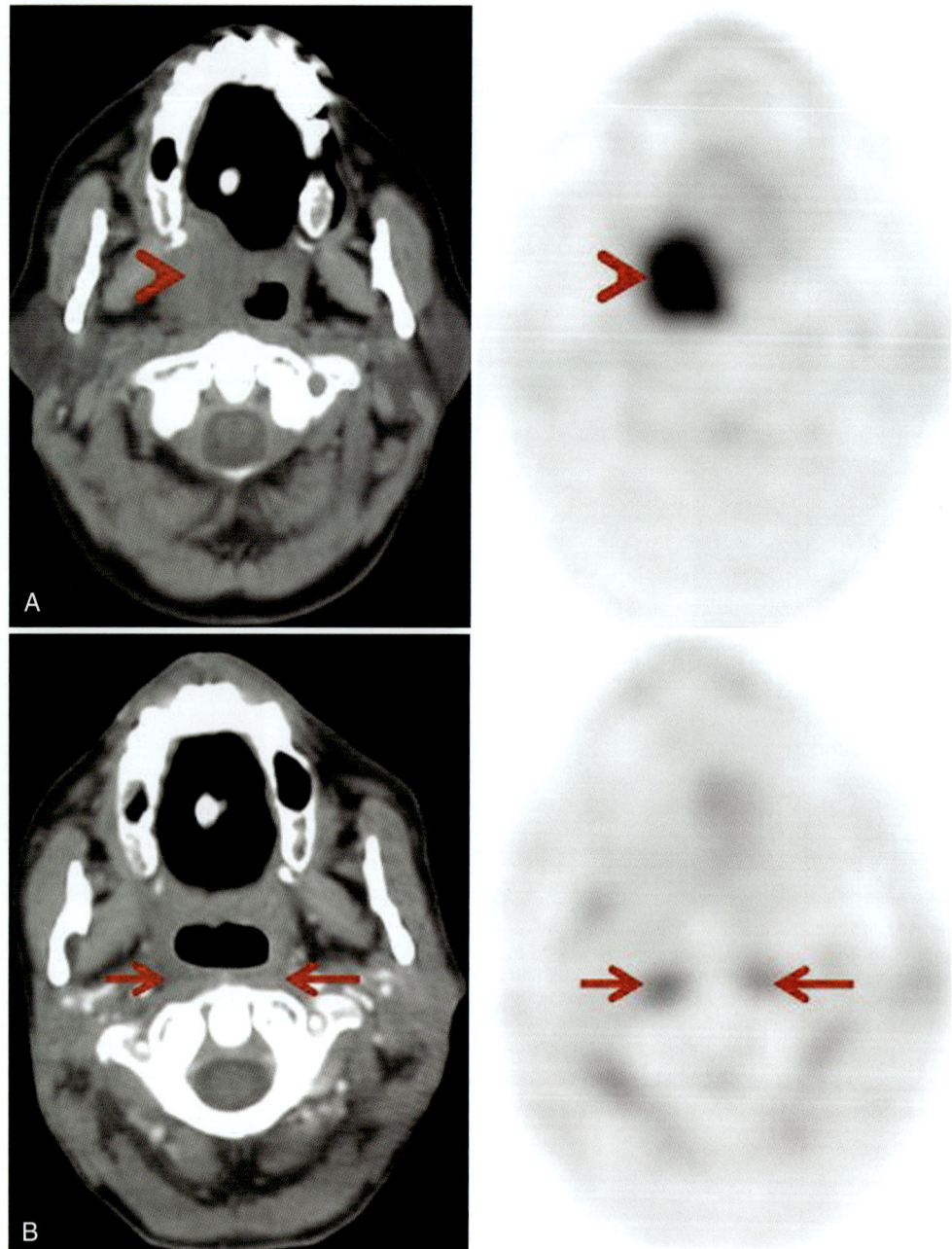

Figure 4-50 A 59-year-old woman who presented with a tonsillar squamous cell carcinoma. **A:** Pretherapy PET/CT study performed with low-dose CT demonstrates increased FDG uptake (SUV$_{max}$ 13.6) corresponding to a soft tissue mass involving the right palatine tonsil (*arrowheads*), consistent with the patient's primary tumor. The patient subsequently underwent neoadjuvant therapy with chemoradiation. **B:** Posttherapy FDG PET study performed 4 months after completion of chemoradiation therapy demonstrates no area of abnormal FDG uptake in the corresponding region, consistent with complete response to therapy. Note minimal uptake in the prevertebral (longus colli) muscles (*small arrows*) probably as a result of tension.

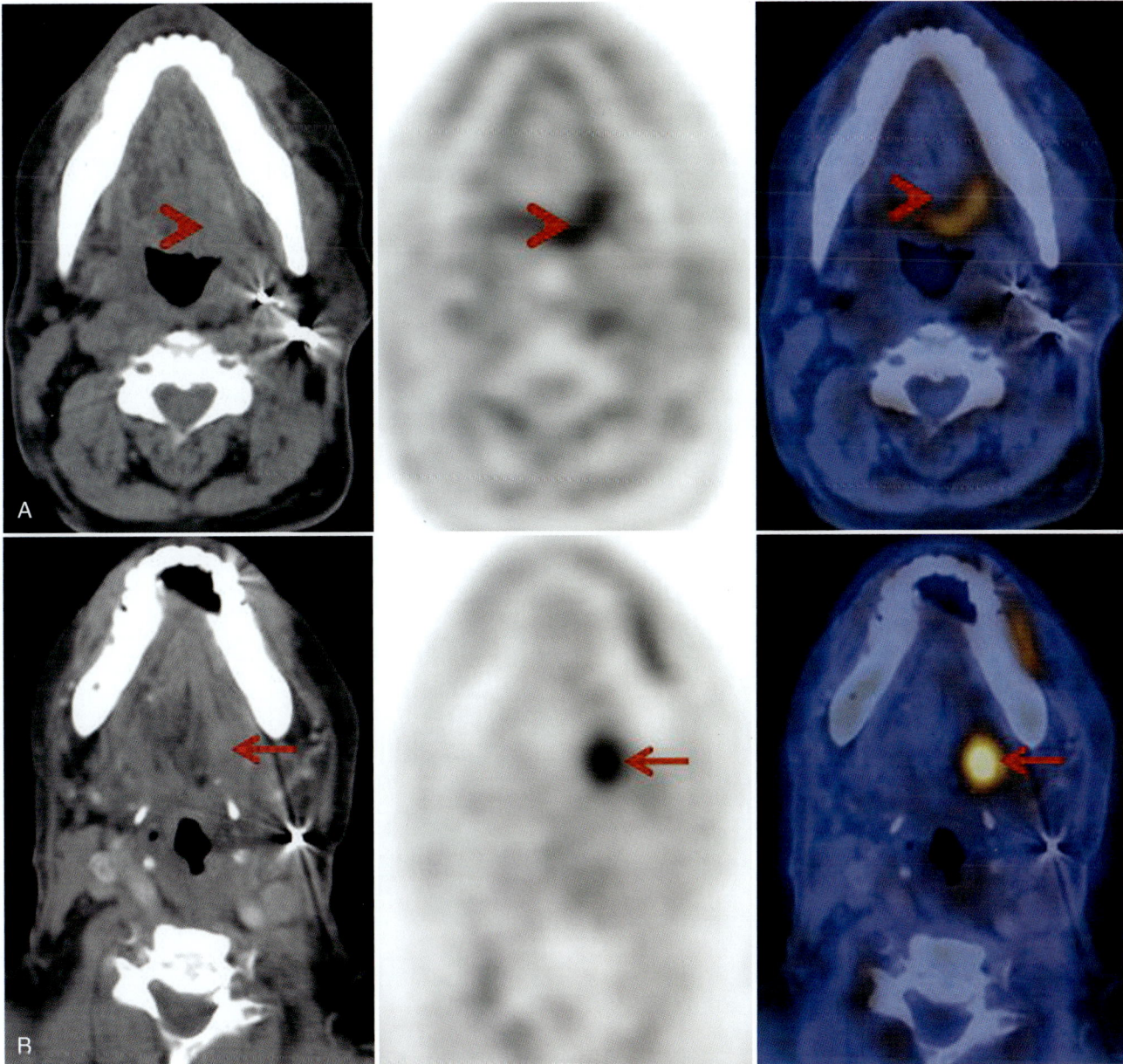

Figure 4-51 A 66-year-old man with a history of stage III left base of tongue squamous cell carcinoma. **A:** Posttherapy PET/CT study performed with low-dose CT 4 months following primary therapy demonstrates postsurgical changes, including architectural distortion in the left neck but no area of abnormal FDG uptake except for mild uptake (SUV_{max} 4.1) in the left base of tongue (*arrowheads*) with minimal extension to the midline, which can be attributable to lymphoid tissue. Subsequent biopsy of this region revealed hyperplastic squamous mucosa with no evidence of tumor recurrence. Because the patient's primary tumor was in the left base of tongue, close follow-up was indicated. **B:** Three-month follow-up PET/CT study performed with contrast-enhanced CT demonstrates a distinct focus of increased FDG uptake (SUV_{max} 6.9) in the left base of tongue, medial to the mylohyoid muscle in the posterior aspect of the genioglossus muscle, where an ill-defined mildly enhancing mass is noted (*arrows*) on the accompanying CT study, most consistent with recurrent tumor. Subsequent biopsy revealed malignant squamous cells. If FDG PET was not performed, contrast-enhanced CT alone would prove equivocal, and the diagnosis of recurrence would have been delayed. The patient subsequently underwent salvage surgery after biopsy confirmation of the recurrence.

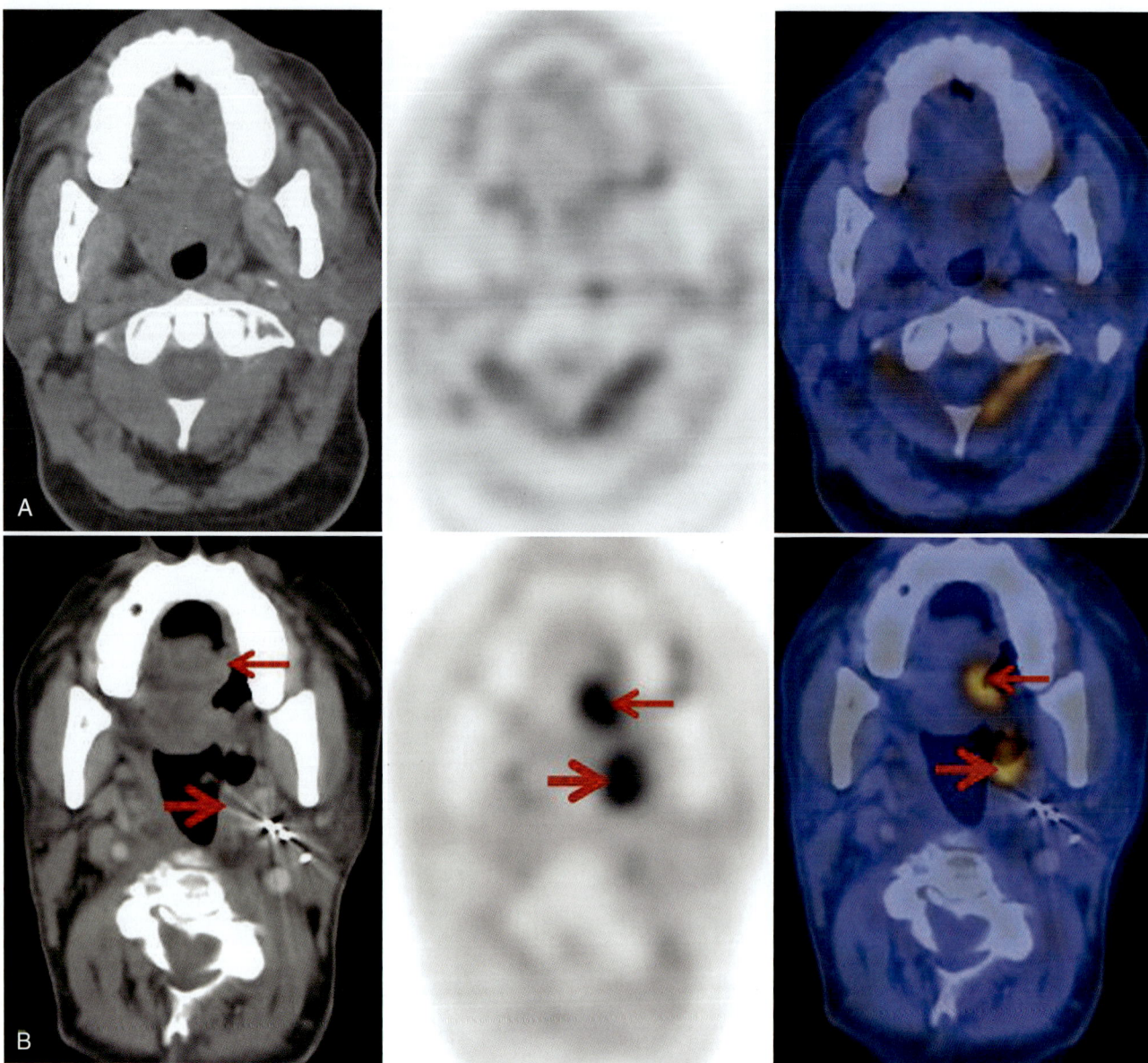

Figure 4-52 A 59-year-old man with a history of tongue squamous cell carcinoma. **A:** Posttherapy PET/CT study performed with low-dose CT 6 months after primary therapy demonstrates no area of abnormal FDG uptake. **B:** Three-month follow-up PET/CT study performed with contrast-enhanced high-resolution CT demonstrates distinct foci of increased FDG uptake (SUV_{max} 7.6) in the left lateral surface of the tongue (*small arrows*) and oropharyngeal wall (*right arrows*) associated with a nonenhancing mass on the accompanying CT study, consistent with recurrent tumor. Subsequent biopsy confirmed recurrence. In this case, both PET and CT complement each other, increasing the certainty of diagnosis of recurrent disease. The patient underwent salvage surgery and has been alive until the last follow-up visit in 2010.

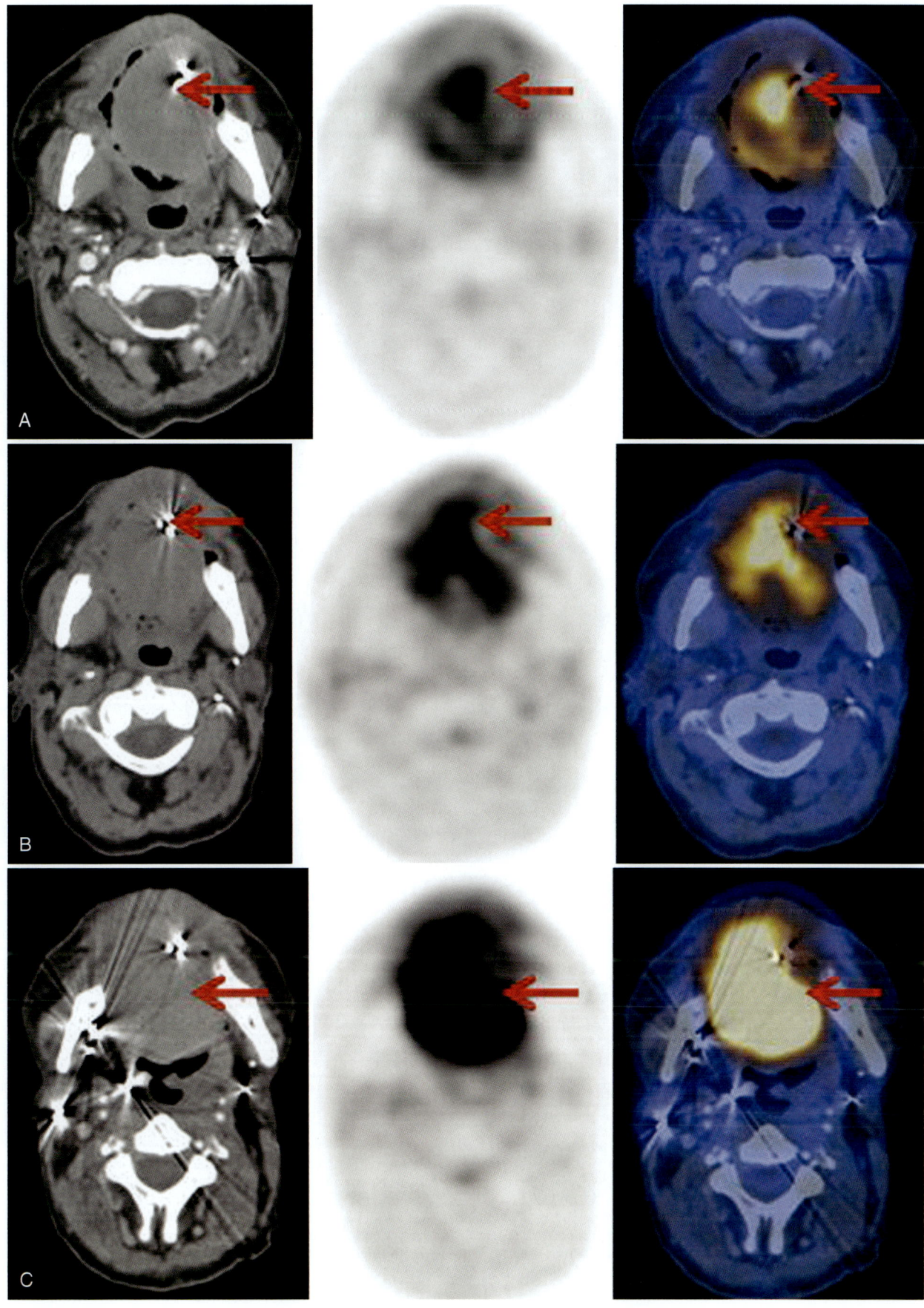

Figure 4-53 A 78-year-old man with a history of tongue squamous cell carcinoma, status post primary treatment with chemoradiation followed by partial glossectomy involving bilateral neck dissection. PET/CT studies performed, 6 months (**A**), with contrast-enhanced high-resolution CT, 12 months with low-dose CT (**B**), and 18 months with contrast-enhanced high-resolution CT (**C**) after completion of primary therapy demonstrate significantly increased uptake [SUV_{max} range 9 (**A**) to 26 (**C**)] corresponding to the tongue with either partial (**A** and **B**) or diffuse involvement of the tongue (**C**; *arrows*). Although these findings can be easily interpreted in favor of recurrent disease, in the absence of a dominant mass noted on the accompanying contrast-enhanced CT, this is rather unlikely. In this patient, subsequent biopsy at the central tongue revealed only skeletal muscles and fibroadipose tissue. Note that this pattern of uptake is frequently seen in patients with partial glossectomy and can be attributable to constant use of unusual muscle groups activated after surgery leading to significant physiologic uptake by these otherwise unused muscle groups.

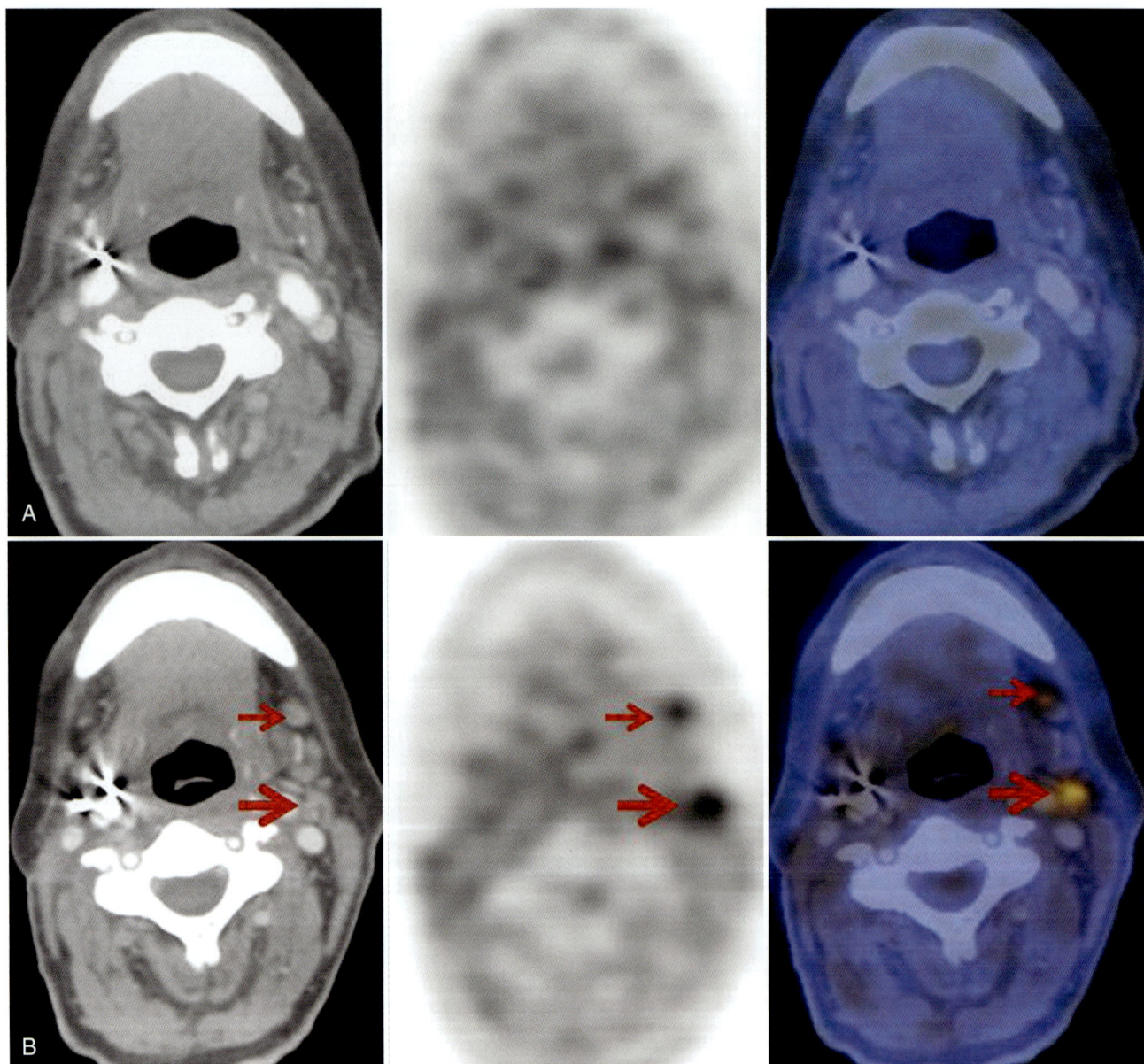

Figure 4-54 A 62-year-old man with a history of right neck carcinoma of unknown origin, status post right selective neck dissection and diagnostic laryngoscopy. **A:** Six-month posttherapy PET/CT study performed with contrast-enhanced high-resolution CT shows surgical clips in the right neck with no evidence of recurrence. **B:** Nine-month follow-up PET/CT study performed with contrast-enhanced CT demonstrates interval appearance of increased uptake (SUV_{max} 3.6) in left-sided level IB (*small arrows*) and level IIA lymph nodes (*large arrows*) measuring up to 1.3 mm (previously measured 6 mm). Note that these lymph nodes demonstrate a fatty hilum, smooth margins, and no pathologic enlargement. Although recurrence cannot be excluded, in the absence of obvious pathologic findings on the accompanying CT, reactive changes should be considered first. Subsequent fine needle aspiration (FNA) biopsy of one of these lymph nodes revealed no evidence of malignancy.

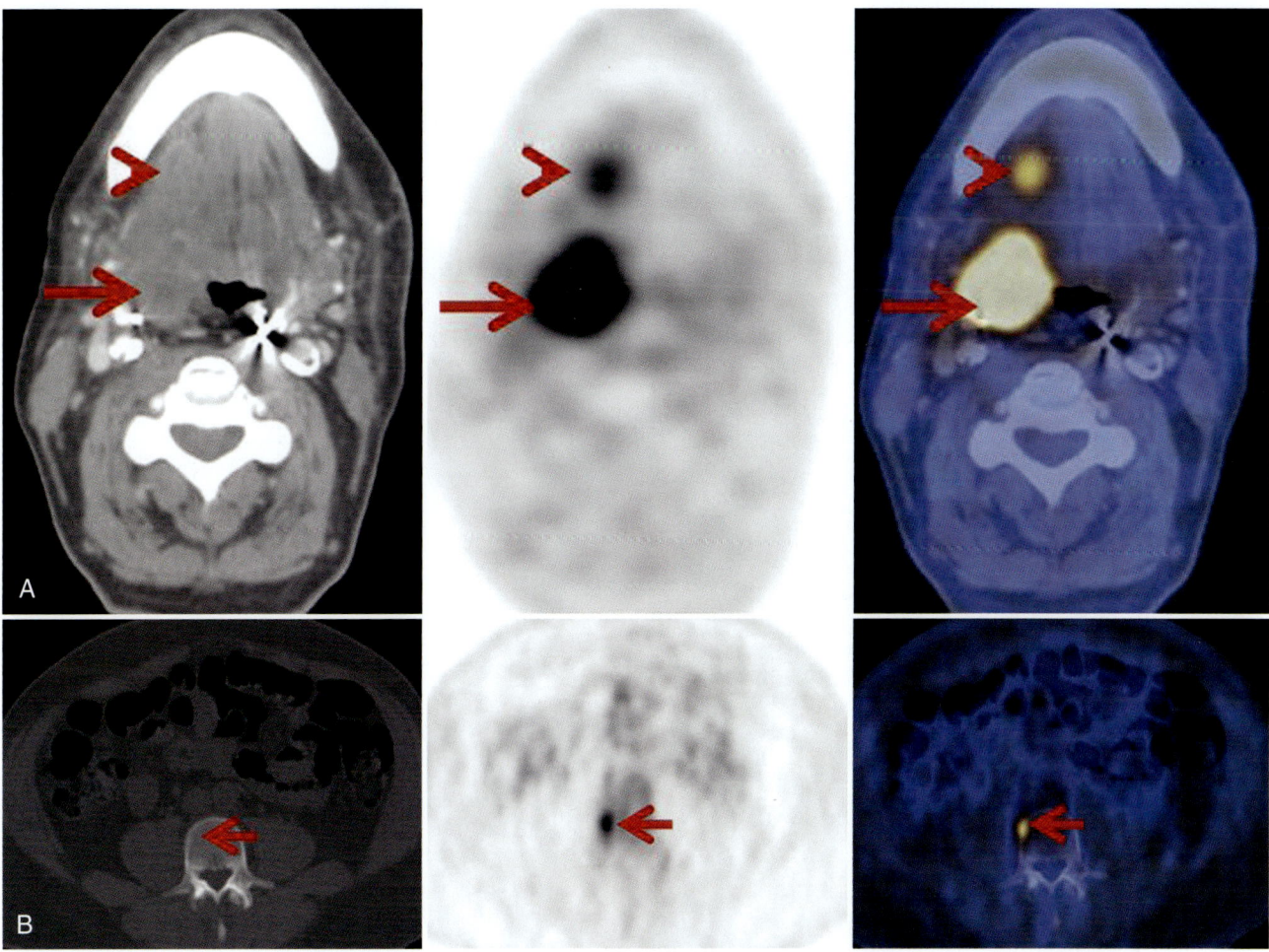

Figure 4-55 A 57-year-old man with right base of tongue squamous cell carcinoma, status post pharyngectomy, base of tongue resection, and radiation therapy. **A:** Eighteen-month follow-up PET/CT study performed with contrast-enhanced high-resolution CT demonstrates an area of increased FDG uptake (SUV_{max} 12) in the right base of tongue corresponding to a hypodense lesion (*arrows*). There is also increased FDG uptake in the anterior right floor of mouth, corresponding to an ill-defined soft tissue density (*arrowheads*), consistent with a second focus of recurrent tumor. **B:** On axial images of the abdomen/pelvis of the whole-body PET/CT study, there is increased FDG uptake (SUV_{max} 11.5) in the right aspect of the L4 vertebral body (*arrows*), associated with no obvious pathology seen on CT study. These findings are consistent with distant metastasis, which is common in patients who have precipitous disease course and high disease burden at recurrence.

Posttreatment follow-up usually focuses on detection of locoregional recurrences, which dominate the clinical presentations following primary therapy (Figures 4-51 and 4-52). Distant metastatic disease is not commonly observed except in patients who have not responded to multiple therapies or have high disease burden at recurrence (Figure 4-55). FDG PET/CT features that indicate locally recurrent disease include increased uptake associated with masses with or without enhancement (Figure 4-56). Abnormalities at the margin of a previous resection or reconstruction are difficult to detect without a FDG PET study due to altered anatomic planes and the presence of metallic artifacts (Figure 4-57). One special concern following radiation therapy is the increased risk for developing osteoradionecrosis or cartilage necrosis which accumulate significant amounts of FDG.

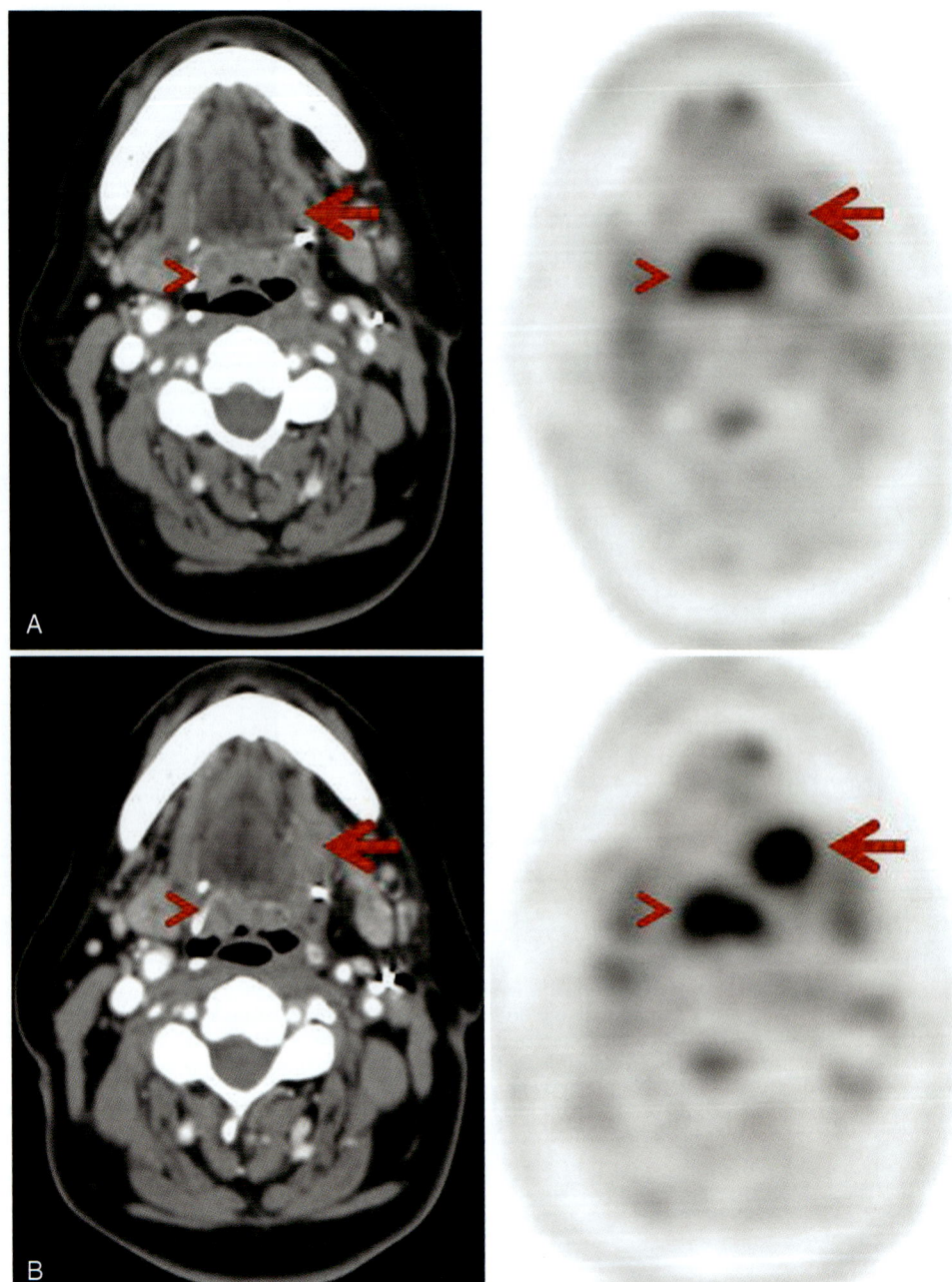

Figure 4-56 A 76-year-old man with left base of tongue squamous cell carcinoma, status post base of tongue resection, left neck dissection, and radiation therapy four months ago. **A:** PET/CT study performed with contrast-enhanced high-resolution CT demonstrates a vague area of increased FDG uptake (SUV$_{max}$ 3.8) in the left base of tongue (*arrows*) in the vicinity of a surgical clip with no association of a mass noted on the accompanying CT study. **B:** Four months later, repeat PET/CT with contrast-enhanced CT shows significant interval increase in FDG uptake in the corresponding region (SUV$_{max}$ 14.5), now associated with an enhancing mass (*arrows*), consistent with recurrent tumor, which was proven by a subsequent biopsy. Note the stable FDG uptake at the midline base of tongue near the vallecula seen in both **A** and **B** (*small arrowheads*), consistent with lymphoid tissue.

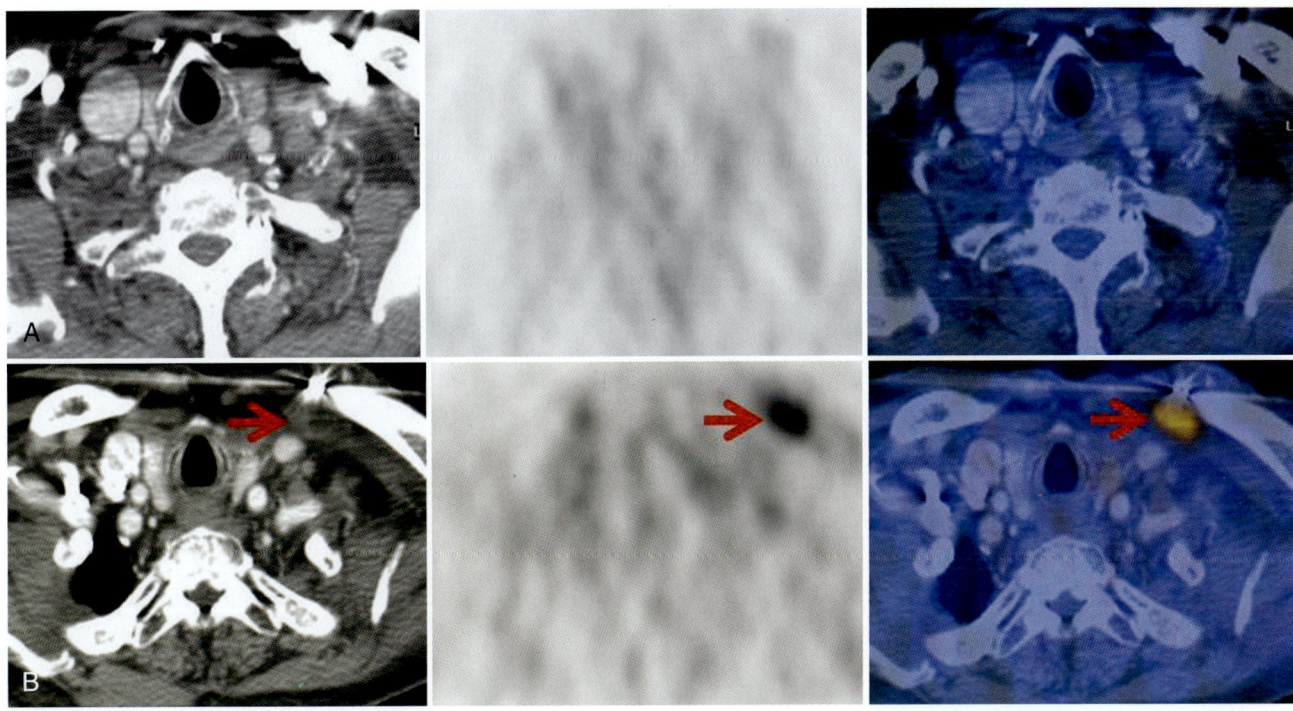

Figure 4-57 A 90-year-old man with a history of tongue squamous cell carcinoma (SCC), status post glossectomy and left neck dissection. **A:** Nine-month follow-up PET/CT study with contrast-enhanced high-resolution CT demonstrates multiple surgical clips in the left supraclavicular region with no definite evidence of pathologically increased FDG uptake. There was no abnormal FDG uptake in the tongue and adjacent structures at this time (not shown) in the tongue or the neck. **B:** Twelve-month follow-up PET/CT with contrast-enhanced CT shows interval appearance of an area of increased uptake in the left supraclavicular region near the surgical clips (*arrows*). Although evaluation with CT is limited due to metallic artifacts, a vaguely enhancing soft tissue mass can be seen on the corresponding CT study (*arrows*). These findings are consistent with recurrent tumor. Subsequent biopsy of this lesion revealed poorly differentiated SCC.

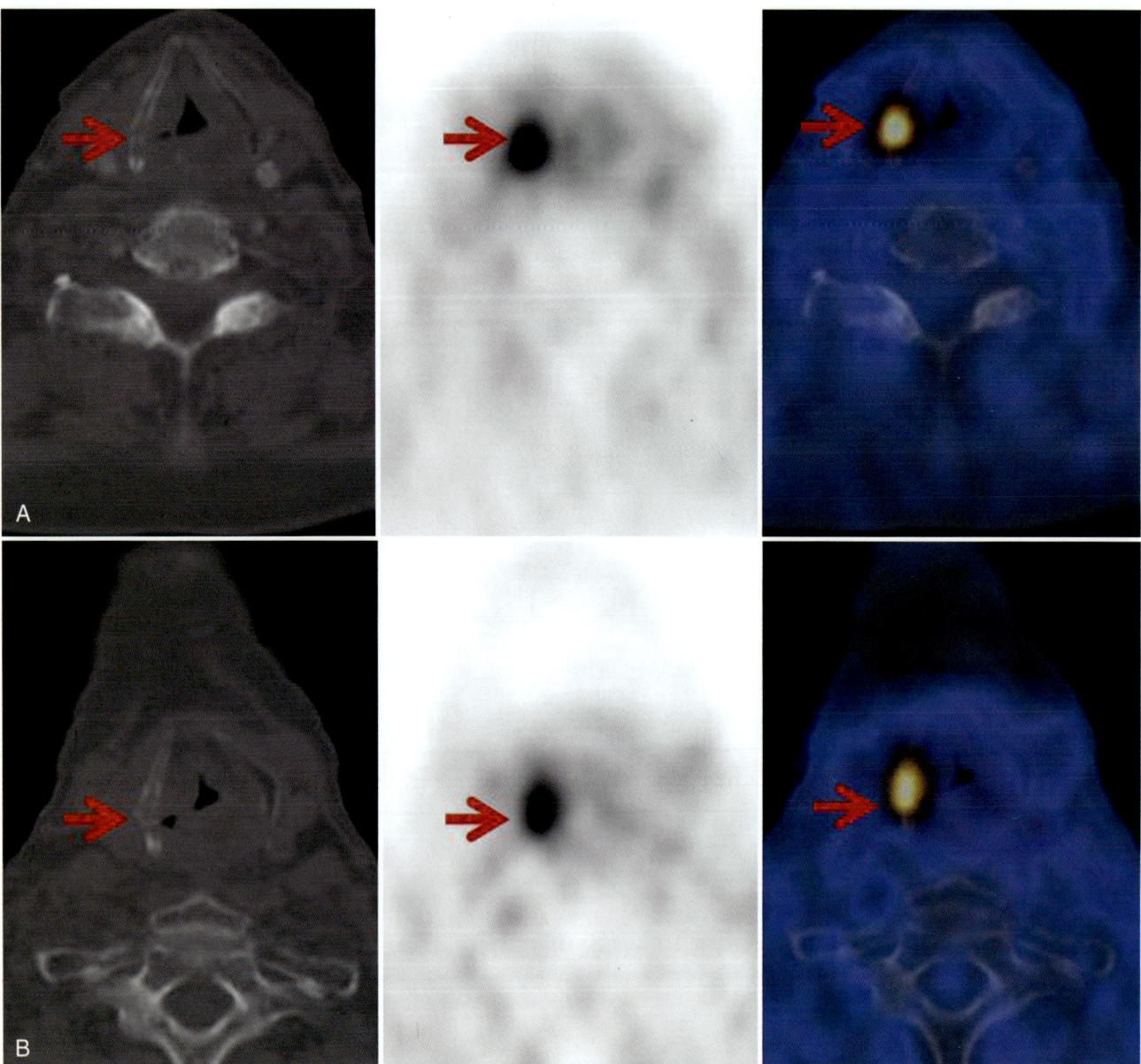

Figure 4-58 A 77-year-old man with laryngeal squamous cell carcinoma, status post radiation therapy. **A:** Six-month follow-up PET/CT study with high-resolution CT but no contrast administration demonstrates increased FDG uptake (SUV_{max} 9.2) in the posterior aspect of the right thyroid cartilage, adjacent to the piriform sinus (*arrows*). The cartilage displays sclerotic changes. Although a malignant process cannot be ruled out, the location of this finding is more consistent with chondronecrosis. **B:** Nine-month follow-up PET/CT with contrast-enhanced CT shows slight progressive sclerosis of the posterior edge of the right thyroid cartilage with focal increased FDG uptake (SUV_{max} 7.0). Areas of lack of ossification have progressed compared to the earlier area of increased uptake (*arrows*). Biopsy revealed benign portion of larynx with ossified thyroid cartilage showing degenerative changes. The patient gradually developed a nonfunctional larynx with aspiration and weight loss and ultimately underwent total laryngectomy. The surgical specimen revealed chondronecrosis with acute and chronic inflammation.

Thus, differentiation from recurrent tumor usually is difficult with all imaging modalities including FDG PET/CT (Figures 4-58 and 4-59) (see the section, What Are the Pitfalls in Evaluation of HNSCC? For further discussion).

What Are the Characteristics of Recurrent Disease in Laryngeal Cancers?

The sensitivity of FDG PET in the detection of recurrence is significantly high, but its specificity can be as low as 65% due to varying degrees of inflammatory processes. Patients whose primary tumors manifest deep invasion have positive margins after surgical resection and extracapsular extension of disease in cervical lymph nodes, or have multiplicity of involved lymph nodes that constitute high-risk categories for tumor recurrence. Laryngoscopy with general anesthesia is routinely performed in patients suspected of having residual or recurrent disease; however, laryngeal edema negatively affects the performance of this test. In this circumstance, FDG PET/CT performs better than ceCT in identifying the presence of residual disease (Figures 4-60 and 4-61). However, in the postsurgical period, particularly in the vicinity of the tracheostomy site, the specificity of FDG findings can be marred by FDG uptake due to the chronic

Chapter 4 PET/CT Imaging In Squamous Cell Carcinoma of the Head and Neck

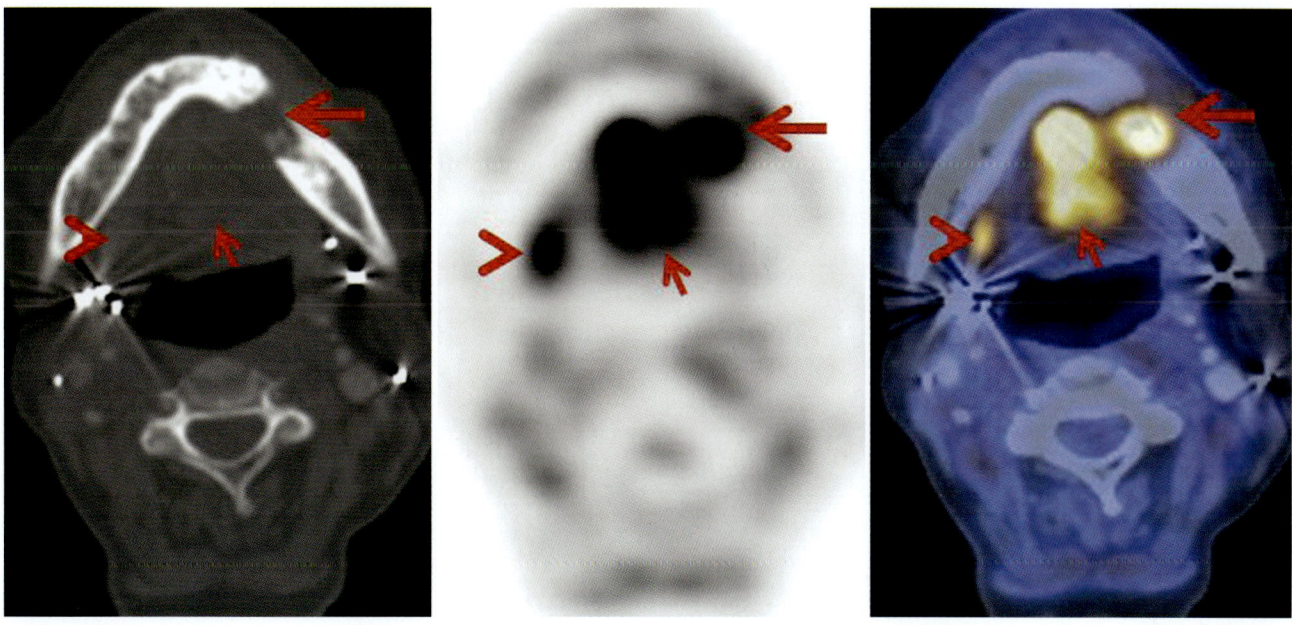

Figure 4-59 A 79-year-old woman with a history of tongue squamous cell carcinoma, status post radiation therapy, partial glossectomy, and bilateral neck dissection. Nine-month follow-up PET/CT study performed with contrast-enhanced high-resolution CT demonstrates significantly increased uptake (SUV_{max} e 9.5) corresponding to the left mandible, displaying destructive changes (*arrows*). Although these findings can be interpreted as favoring recurrent disease with involvement of the bone, osteoradionecrosis should be a strong consideration, particularly in the absence of a soft tissue density (soft tissue windows not shown). Subsequent partial mandibular resection revealed osteonecrosis with no evidence of tumor. Note diffuse uptake in the residual viable tongue (*diagonal arrows*) and right mylohyoid muscle, not well shown without the soft tissue windows (*arrowheads*). Subsequent biopsy at the central tongue revealed no evidence of a malignant process. This pattern of uptake can be attributable to constant use of unusual muscle groups activated after surgery.

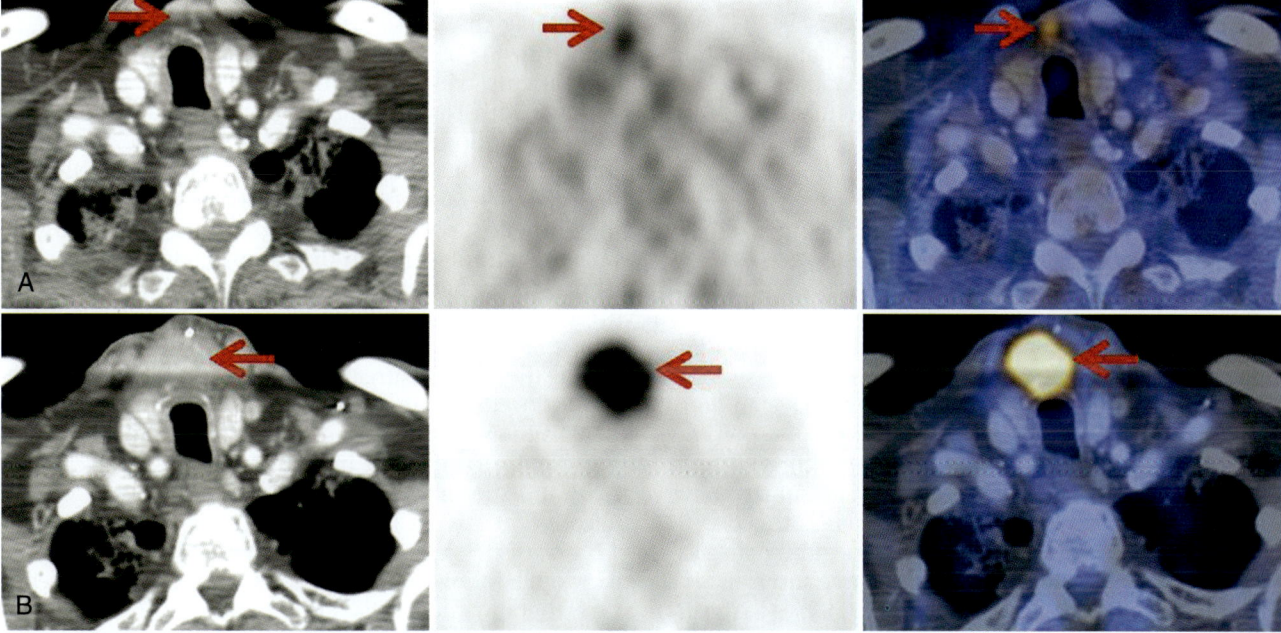

Figure 4-60 A 65-year-old woman with left base of tongue/tonsil squamous cell carcinoma, with local recurrence 9 years after primary definitive chemoradiation, treated with composite resection, total laryngectomy, and left selective node dissection. **A:** Three-month follow-up PET/CT study with contrast-enhanced high-resolution CT demonstrates mildly increased FDG uptake (SUV_{max} 4.7) in the anterior aspect of the trachea, in the midline. Accompanying CT demonstrates no obvious abnormality; however, there is suggestion of an enhancing nodule situated subcutaneously at the corresponding site (*arrows*). These findings may represent postsurgical inflammatory changes; however, the focal nature of FDG uptake corresponding to an enhancing mass seen in the right ill-defined soft tissue nodule raises suspicion for recurrent/residual disease. **B:** Six-month follow-up PET/CT with contrast-enhanced CT shows interval increase in size and metabolic activity (SUV_{max} 18.4) within the aforementioned soft tissue mass in the right subglottic region anteriorly, extending through the lateral margin of the laryngeal cartilage and lies in close proximity to surgical clips within the right neck (*arrows*), consistent with extensive tumor recurrence.

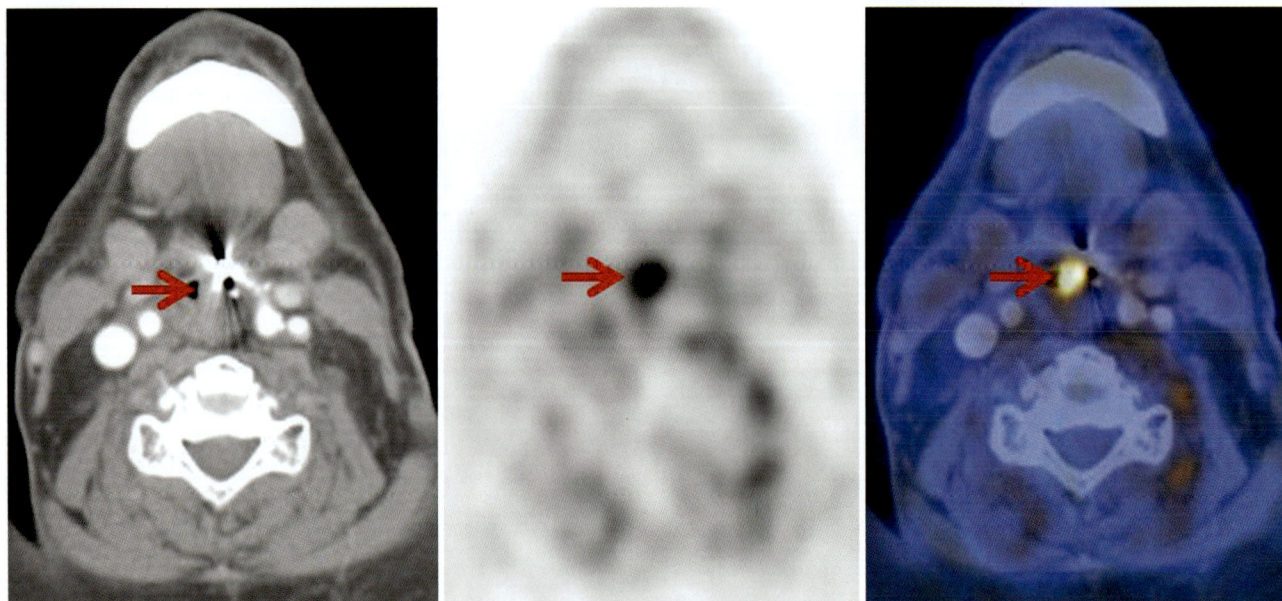

Figure 4-61 A 64-year-old man with a history of recurrent transglottic squamous cell carcinoma (SCC), status post total laryngectomy with creation of neopharynx. Four-month follow-up PET/CT study with contrast-enhanced high-resolution CT demonstrates focally increased FDG uptake (SUV_{max} 7.7) corresponding to an area associated with a surgical clip and thickening of the neopharynx/esophagus superiorly (*arrows*). Although no separate discrete mass is appreciated in this region, the focal and intense nature of FDG uptake is most consistent with tumor recurrence/residual tumor. In addition, evaluation of the CT study is limited by metallic artifacts obscuring the region for the presence of an associated soft tissue. Subsequent endoscopic biopsy revealed recurrent poorly differentiated SCC, and the patient was started on chemotherapy.

inflammatory changes usually induced by repeat manipulations (Figure 4-62). Patients can also present with recurrent disease outside the head and neck because chemoradiation followed by surgery is effective in local control but cannot prevent distant metastasis (Figure 4-63). In a retrospective study, Gourin et al found that the incidence of distant metastases in patients with suspected recurrent disease was approximately 25%, with sensitivity and specificity of FDG PET/CT of 86% and 84%, respectively.

■ DOES FDG PET/CT HAVE A ROLE IN SURVEILLANCE OF HNSCC AFTER THERAPY?

One controversial issue is the application of FDG PET/CT in a surveillance setting. Conceivably, a survival benefit can be achieved for patients who have an early asymptomatic recurrence following primary therapy. Goodwin et al reported that patients with recurrent, early-stage HNSCC who undergo salvage surgery have a 70% 2-year relapse-free survival, whereas those with recurrent, advanced-stage HNSCC undergoing surgical salvage have just a 22% 2-year relapse-free survival.

Hence, early detection of recurrent HNSCC is critically important for achieving a successful surgical salvage. Second primary malignancies can also be detected early by frequent follow-up. Early recurrence in HNSCC may be asymptomatic in nearly 50% of patients, and FDG PET/CT may improve early detection of recurrence (Figures 4-64 through 4-67). A systematic review revealed that the pooled sensitivity, specificity, PPV, and NPV of PET for detecting residual or recurrent HNSCC were 94%, 82%, 75%, and 95%, respectively.

What Is the Optimal Timing for Sequential Evaluation in Detection of Recurrent Disease?

In general, the 5-year risk for both locoregional recurrence (30%–50%) and distant metastases (20%–30%) for patients with head and neck SCC is fairly high. Patients with HNSCC should be followed closely both clinically and radiographically for the first 2 years after treatment because most recurrences present within this period. However, debate still exists over the optimal timing of the first surveillance imaging study. Early PET/CT imaging within 1 month of therapy yields low sensitivity due to the paucity of viable tumor cells as well as the presence of transient fluctuations in FDG uptake early after treatment. Specificity is also negatively impacted during the early posttreatment period secondary to therapy-induced inflammatory changes (Figures 4-49, B, 4-68, and 4-69). PET scans performed 3 months after completion of therapy have high sensitivity exceeding 82% and specificity close to 90%. The majority of PET negative cases recur after median follow-up of more than 12 months (Figures 4-64 through 4-67). It is acceptable to adopt a follow-up policy of ceCT 1 month after definitive therapy, then FDG PET/ceCT every 3 months for the first year, then every 6 months for the second year, and annually thereafter for 5 years or until recurrence (Figures 4-51, 4-54, 4-56, 4-57, 4-60, 4-62, and 4-64). Patients with scans highly suggestive of recurrence should undergo tissue confirmation, whereas patients with questionably abnormal findings should undergo additional PET/CT 3 months later. Posttherapy baseline PET/CT should be performed 2 to 3 months after the conclusion of therapy.

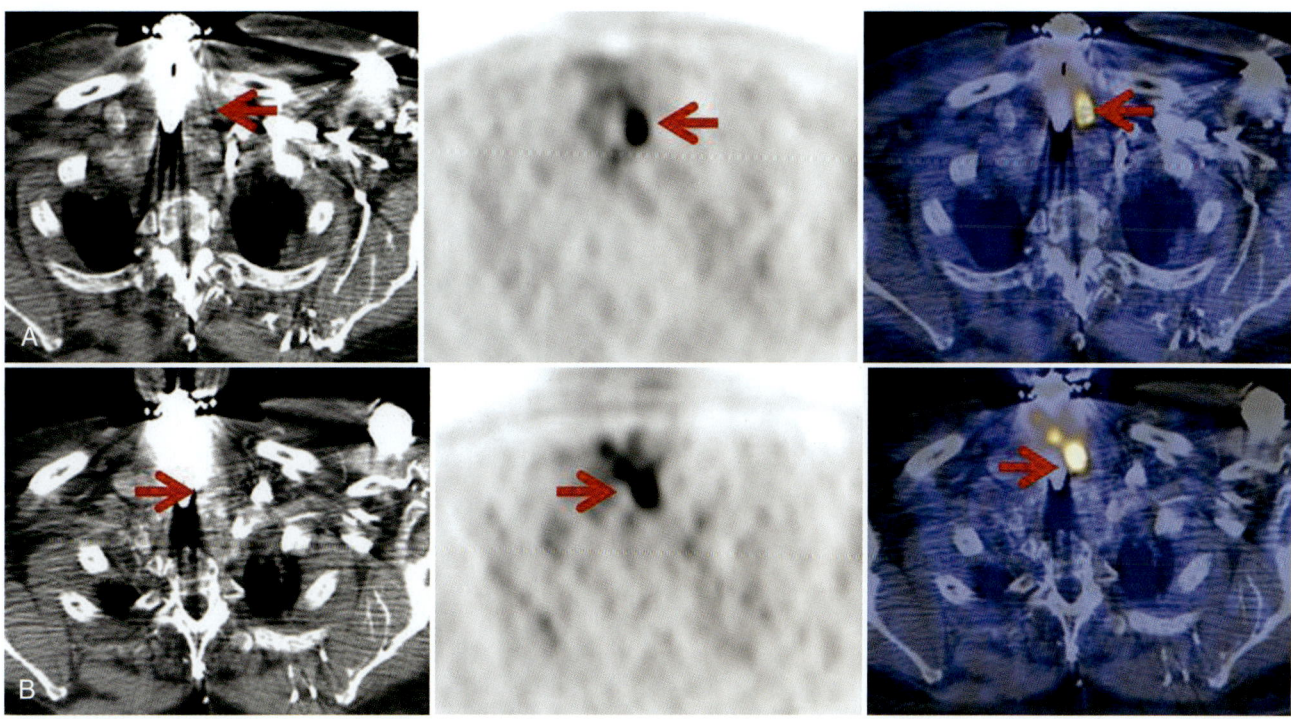

Figure 4-62 A 55-year-old man status post chemoradiation for treatment of advanced laryngeal and hyperpharyngeal squamous cell carcinoma. The patient had undergone attempted decannulation in the past but because of severe chronic granulation tissue and stenosis has been tracheostomy dependent since 6 months ago. **A:** Six-month follow-up PET/CT study performed with contrast-enhanced high-resolution CT demonstrates increased FDG uptake (SUV_{max} 5.2) in the left posterior aspect of the tracheostomy site (*arrows*). Accompanying CT study demonstrates no obvious abnormality. However, significant metallic artifacts hamper the evaluation by CT. These findings may represent postsurgical inflammatory changes. However, the focal nature of the FDG uptake prompted close follow-up. **B:** Nine-month follow-up PET/CT with contrast-enhanced CT shows persistently increased FDG uptake near the tracheostomy site (*arrows*), somewhat more prominent and extensive compared to the prior study (SUV_{max} 6.4). Again, the findings on the accompanying CT are hampered by metallic artifacts. A recurrent tumor could not be ruled out because these findings are nonspecific for both recurrence and inflammatory changes. Subsequent biopsy revealed granulomatous changes with acute and chronic infection. False-positive FDG PET findings are common in the presence of significant inflammation.

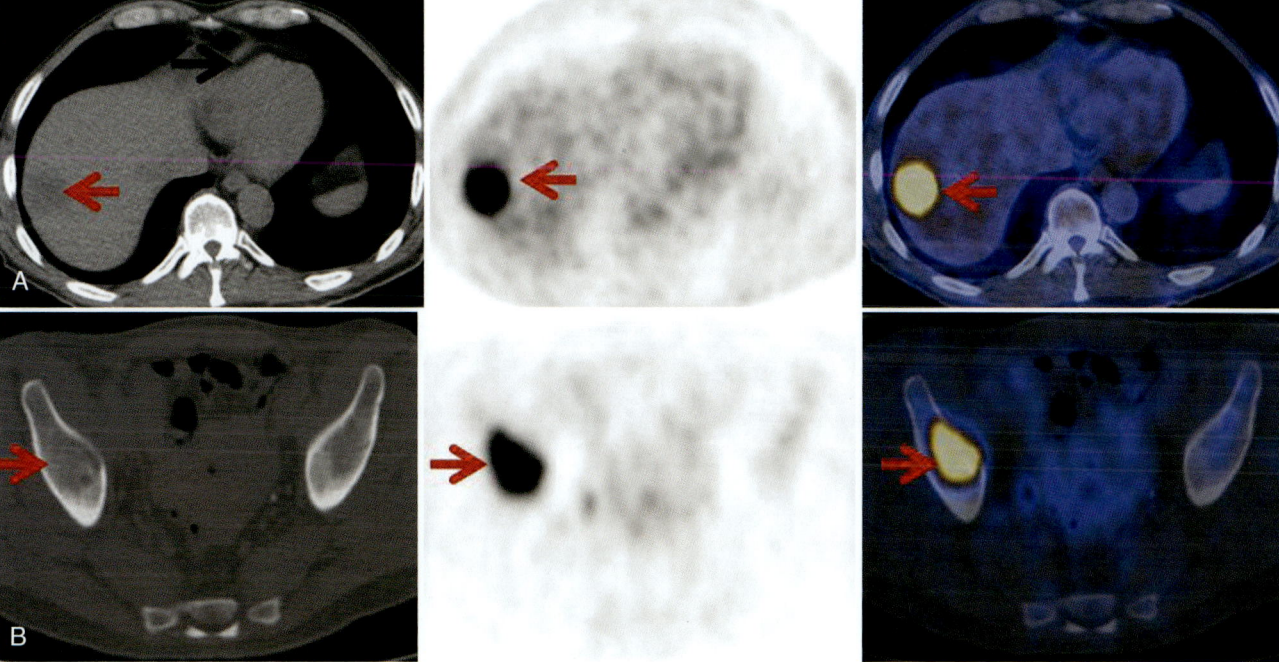

Figure 4-63 A 57-year-old man with tonsillar squamous cell carcinoma, status post pharyngectomy, partial base of tongue resection, and radiation therapy. **A:** Fifteen-month follow-up PET/CT study with low-dose CT demonstrates increased FDG uptake (SUV_{max} 9.5) corresponding to a large hypodense mass in the dome of the liver (*arrows*) new since the prior study (not shown), consistent with hepatic metastasis. **B:** There is a large lytic lesion with significant FDG uptake (SUV_{max} 17) in the right acetabulum (*arrows*), consistent with distant osseous metastatic disease.

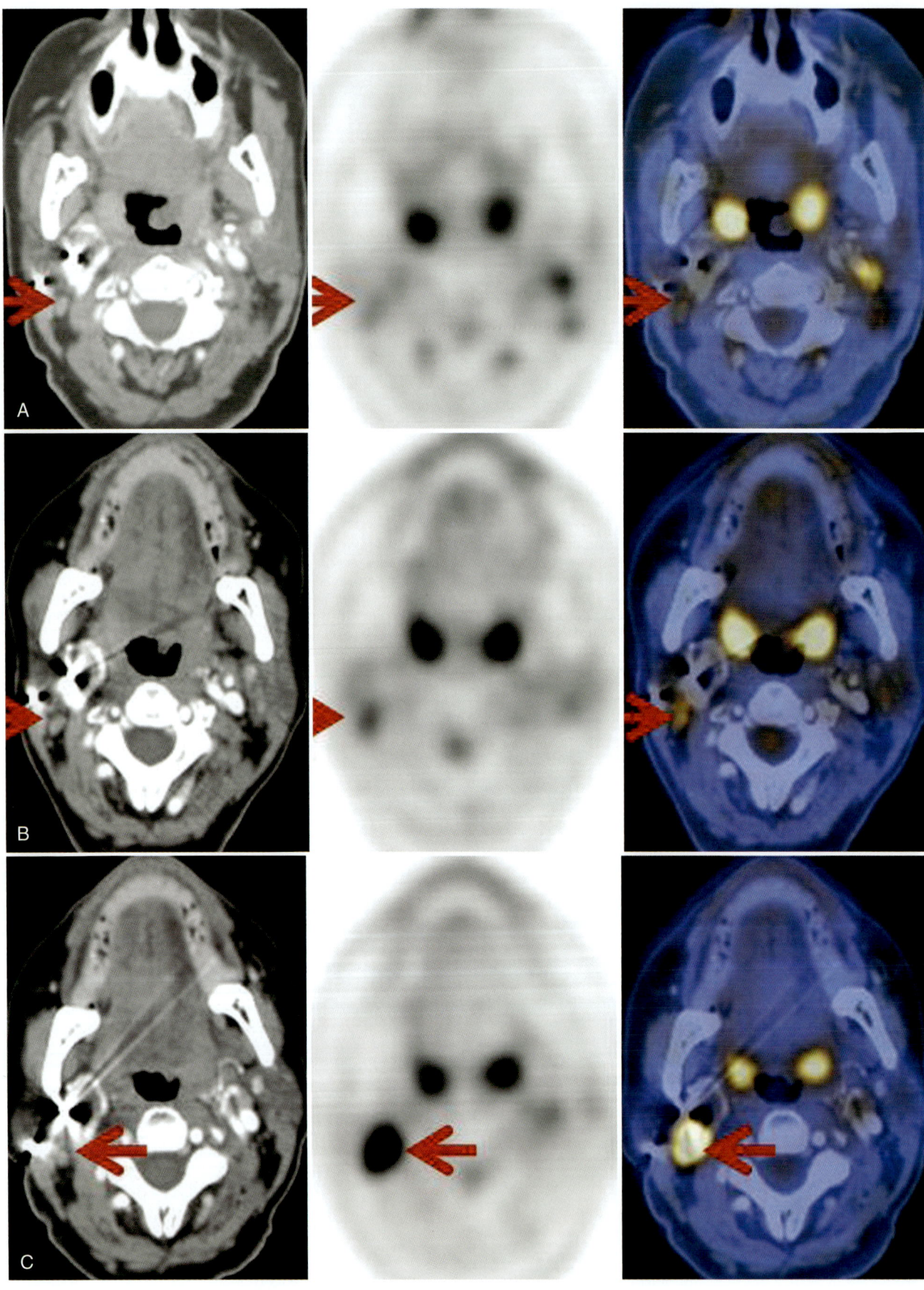

Figure 4-64 A 72-year-old man with a history of right base of tongue squamous cell carcinoma, status post base of tongue resection, right neck dissection, and radiation therapy. **A–C:** Follow-up PET/CT studies performed with contrast-enhanced high-resolution CT at 3, 6, and 9 months, respectively, demonstrate gradually increasing FDG uptake in the right level IIB region with no obvious CT abnormality except for a small lymph node that shows normal morphology (*arrows*). Due to multiple surgical clips, evaluation of CT is suboptimal, and a dominant mass cannot be appreciated even on the last follow-up PET/CT study when the SUV$_{max}$ of the level IIB lesion reaches 11.5 **(C)** from 3.2 **(B)** on the prior study. These findings are consistent with recurrent disease, which was proven by subsequent biopsy. Note the value of FDG PET study in identifying recurrent disease preceding pathologic findings on CT.

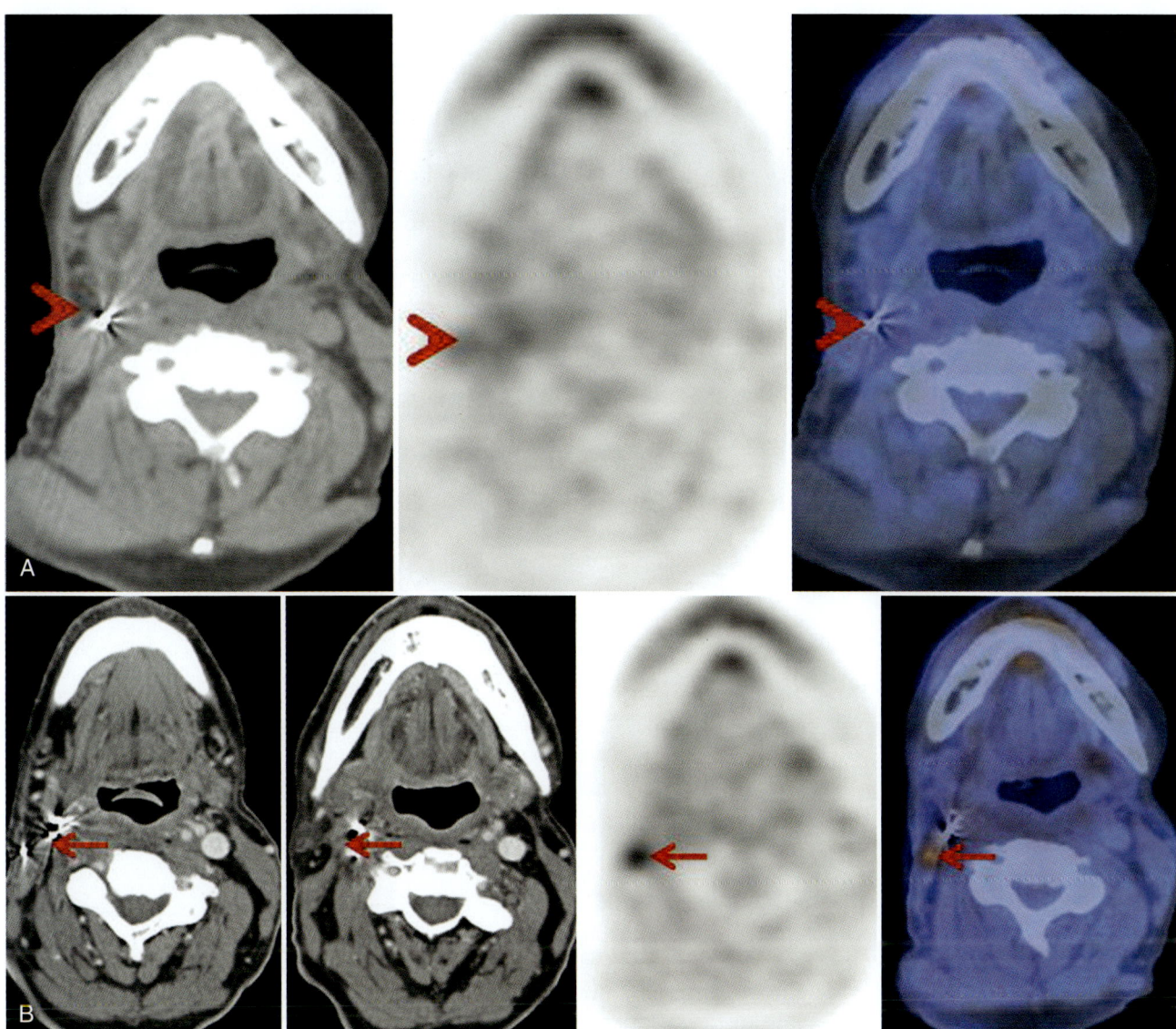

Figure 4-65 A 66 year-old man with a history of right base of tongue squamous cell carcinoma, status post therapy with resection and right neck dissection. **A:** Nine-month PET/CT study with low-dose CT demonstrates no abnormal finding except for diffuse uptake corresponding to surgical clips (*arrowheads*) probably representing physiologic changes and/or muscle tension of tissue inflammation. **B:** Twelve-month follow-up PET/CT study performed with contrast enhanced high-resolution CT reveals focal increased FDG uptake (SUV$_{max}$ 4.3) near the clips but now corresponds to a subtle soft tissue nodule (*arrows*), which is highly suspicious for recurrent disease. Subsequent biopsy confirmed recurrence, and the patient underwent salvage therapy. Early recurrence in squamous cell carcinoma of the head and neck may be asymptomatic in nearly 50% of patients, and FDG PET/CT may improve early detection of recurrence.

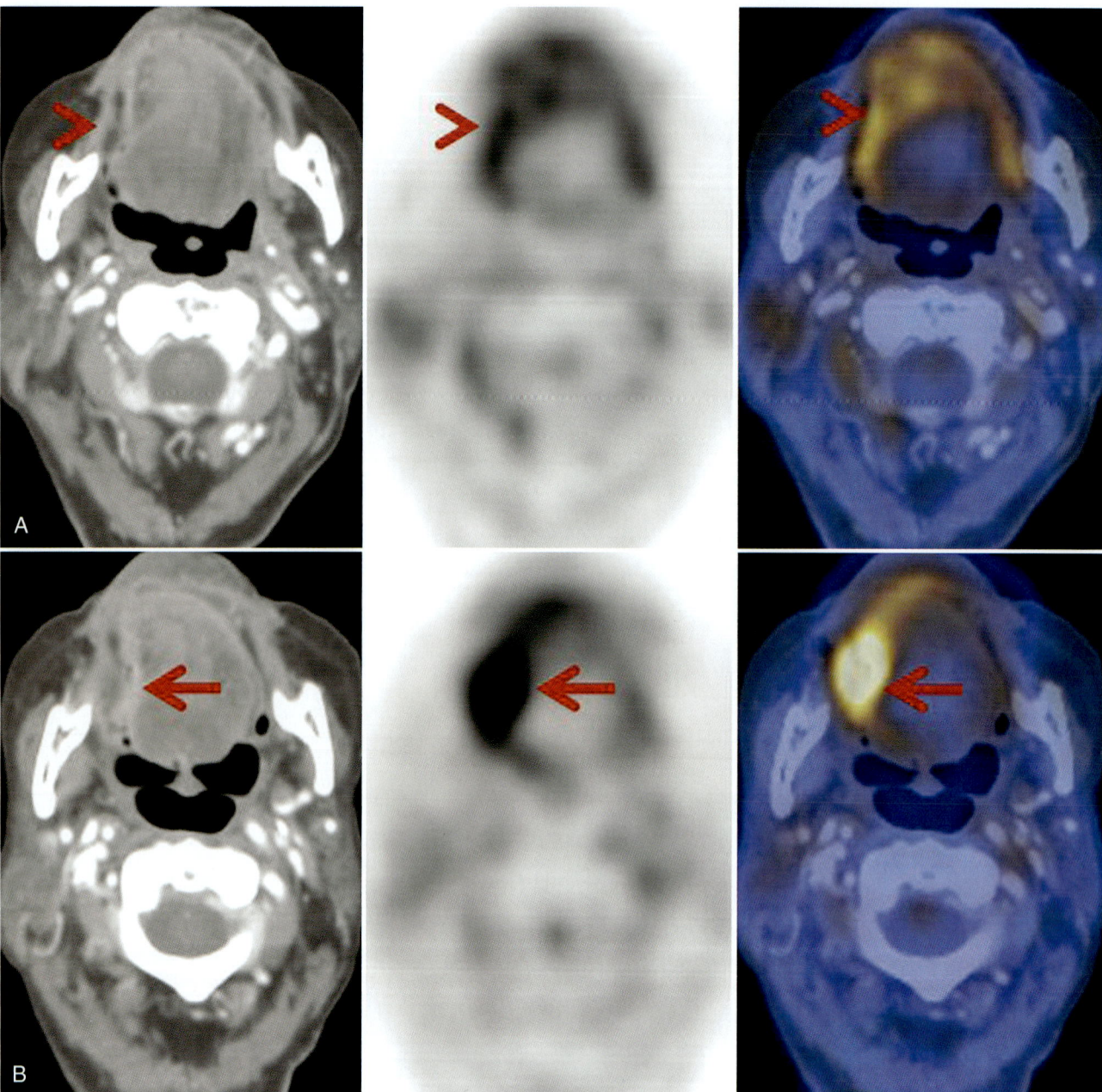

Figure 4-66 A 69-year-old man with a history of recurrent tongue squamous cell carcinoma, status post hemiglossectomy **A:** Six-month follow-up PET/CT study performed with contrast-enhanced high-resolution CT demonstrates diffusely increased symmetric FDG uptake in the oral cavity with no focal uptake, probably representing postsurgical changes. Note tissue heterogeneity on the right side of the oral cavity that represents surgical changes (*arrowheads*). **B:** Twelve-month follow-up PET/CT study performed with contrast-enhanced high-resolution CT demonstrates increased FDG uptake (SUV$_{max}$ 11) in the region of the right tongue along the previously resected tongue (*arrows*), corresponding to a streaky and slightly enhancing soft tissue density, consistent with recurrent tumor. Subsequent biopsy of this region confirmed recurrent tumor.

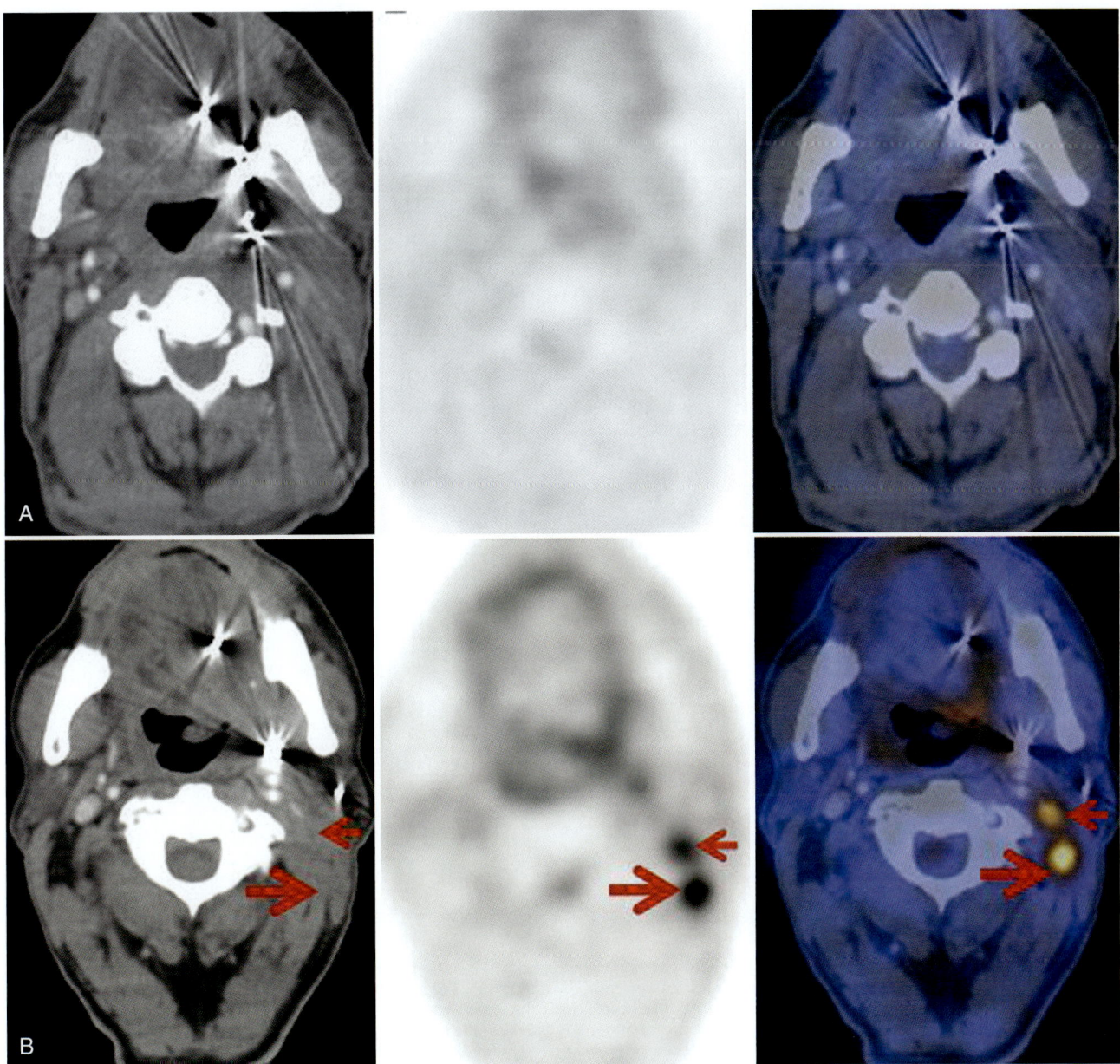

Figure 4-67 A 72-year-old woman with a history of tongue squamous cell carcinoma, status post partial glossectomy, left selective lymph node dissection, and flap reconstruction. **A:** Six-month follow-up PET/CT study with contrast-enhanced CT demonstrates no abnormal increased FDG uptake in the head and neck region. **B:** Nine-month follow-up PET/CT study with contrast-enhanced CT demonstrates interval development of two discrete foci of radiotracer uptake (SUV_{max} 13.4) in the left posterior lateral neck in the level IIB region associated with increased soft tissue density (small and large *arrows*), likely representing metastatic lymph nodes. Artifacts from the clips limit evaluation of the soft tissues of the left neck and tongue. Note the value of FDG PET imaging in the identification of recurrent disease and the development of recurrence within a rather short interval, which would require frequent follow-up PET/CT imaging to detect recurrence at an earlier period than by conventional methods.

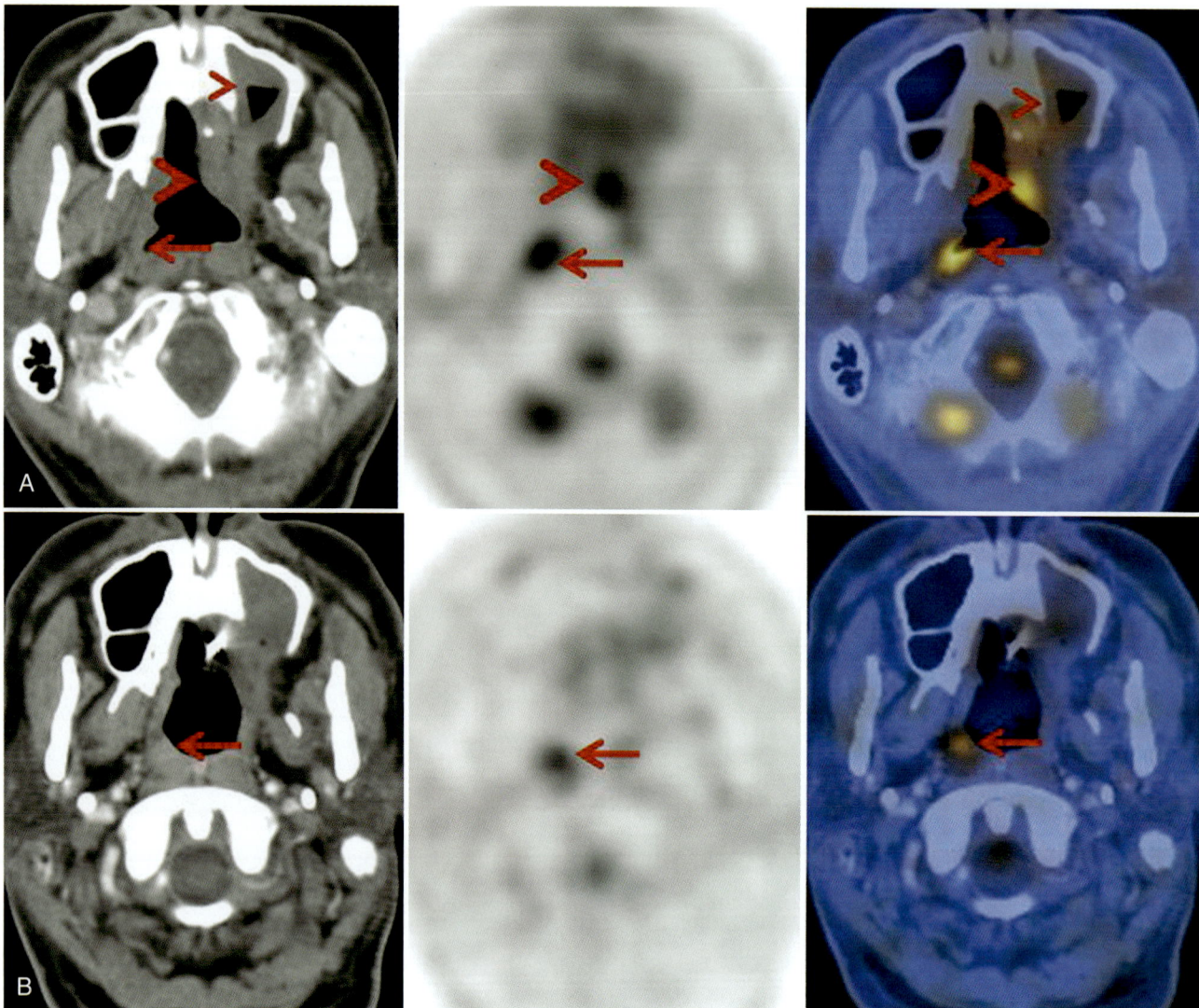

Figure 4-68 A 50-year-old man with a history of left hard palate squamous cell carcinoma, status post resection and reconstruction with free flap. **A:** Six-month follow-up PET/CT study with contrast-enhanced high-resolution CT demonstrates mildly increased FDG uptake (SUV_{max} 3.5) in the posterior margin of the surgical bed corresponding to mild soft tissue thickening at the resection margin and along the posterior left maxillary and palatal walls (*arrowheads*). There is also asymmetric uptake (SUV_{max} 3.0) in the right nasopharyngeal wall with no soft tissue abnormality (*arrows*). These findings probably represent postsurgical changes. However, recurrent disease cannot be excluded. Note the opacification in the left maxillary sinus (small *arrowheads*). Subsequent biopsy revealed inflammatory changes. **B:** Nine-month follow-up PET/CT with contrast-enhanced CT demonstrates resolution of uptake in the palate with persistence of opacification in the left maxillary sinus, consistent with resolution of the inflammatory change. Note the interval decrease in FDG uptake in the right nasopharyngeal wall, which probably represents asymmetric lymphoid tissue secondary to treatment changes on the contralateral site (*arrows*) and resolution of previous lymphoid hyperplasia, which might be due to ongoing inflammation in the palate.

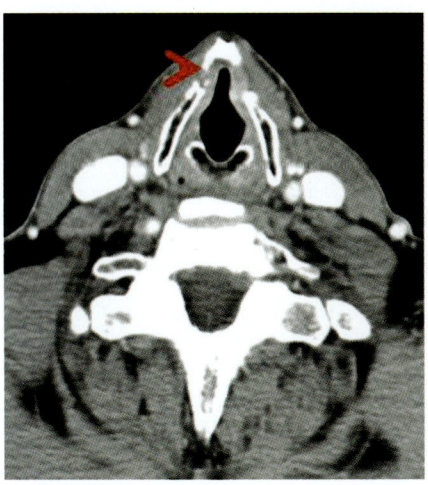 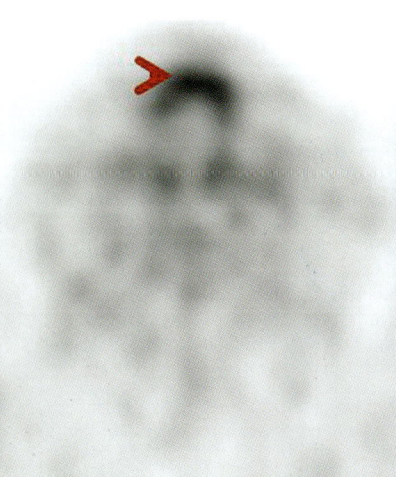 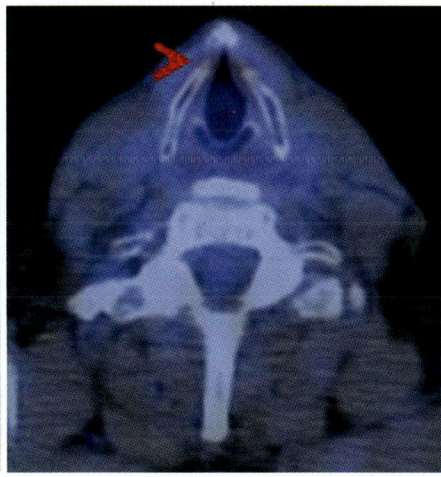

Figure 4-69 A 67-year-old man with a history of left vocal cord squamous cell carcinoma, status post laser excision. Four-month follow-up PET/CT study performed with low-dose CT (low-dose CT slice not shown) and separately acquired contrast-enhanced high-resolution CT demonstrate increased FDG uptake (SUV_{max} 2.2) in the anterior commissure of the larynx, probably representing posttherapy inflammatory changes, particularly, in the absence of a soft tissue density on the accompanying CT study. Subsequent laryngoscopic examination was unremarkable, and the patient has been recurrence free for a follow-up period of 12 months. Note that the uptake localized in the anterior commissure in untreated patients is almost invariably associated with malignant causes, however, in the posttherapy setting, inflammatory changes may also occur in this region (compare with Figure 4-78).

Local recurrence rates for laryngeal SCC can be substantially high, ranging from 15% to 50%. Recurrence of advanced compared to early-stage laryngeal carcinomas is approximately twice as high (10%–25% vs 25%–50%). Once recurrence occurs, treatment options are dictated by the mode of treatment previously given, tumor volume of recurrent disease, and performance status and comorbidities of the patient. The gold standard for diagnosing recurrent laryngeal tumor is direct laryngoscopy. However, laryngoscopy is invasive and is not conducive to evaluation of lymph nodes or distant metastases. A systematic review laryngeal carcinoma by Brouwer et al revealed sensitivity of 89% and specificity of 74% for FDG PET in the detection of recurrent tumor after radiotherapy. In a retrospective study of 78 patients by Martin et al revealed different results for sensitivity and specificity of 82% and 95%, respectively, in detecting residual disease after treatment with chemoradiotherapy for mucosal carcinoma of the head and neck.

■ WHAT ARE THE PITFALLS IN EVALUATION OF HNSCC?

Interpretation of the posttreatment neck can be challenging due to alterations in anatomic spaces and planes, development of postradiation inflammatory changes, and ensuing fibrosis. Surgical resection, flap reconstruction, radiation, and frequent use of adjunctive treatments naturally result in significant morphologic and inflammatory changes in the involved regions, including edema, inflammation, fibrosis, distortion of anatomic planes, complex muscle activity resulting from flaps, and loss of symmetry (Tables 4-2 through 4-4).

As a principle, FDG uptake at inflammatory or anatomically altered sites should not be associated with a discrete or dominant mass on CT slices. These changes should decrease with time, so follow-up scans usually increase test specificity. It is preferable to wait 10 to 12 weeks after completion of treatment before performing imaging to reduce false-positive results, particularly after radiation therapy (RT).

What are the Surgically Induced Changes in the Head and Neck?

Postsurgical changes can result in various degrees of FDG uptake ranging from subtle to avid accumulation depending on the procedure and the time between imaging and surgery (Figures 4-70 through 4-76).

Interference from surgical metallic clips and reconstruction hardware are common during the postoperative follow-up period. Although these artifacts usually do not cause false-positive readings, in some cases FDG uptake can be focal and prominent and can prove challenging to the reader and surgeon alike with respect to subsequent management due to the inability to delineate a clear-cut soft tissue association on the CT portion of the study (Figure 4-70). Mandibular reconstructions using titanium mesh with bone and marrow harvested from the iliac bone are performed in a second stage and may present a high complications rate. Another source of false-positive findings is dental interventions, which are frequent due to various therapeutic insults to the osseous structures in this patient population (Figure 4-71). In particular, dentures may cause chronic trauma to the gum line, and the resulting periodontal disease and apical periodontitis demonstrate increased FDG uptake (Figure 4-72). Specific pitfalls in posttreatment imaging of the larynx on FDG PET include mild homogeneous FDG uptake due to tissue healing at the tracheostomy site (Figure 4-73, A and B) and tracheoesophageal puncture for a placement of a voice valve.

Table 4-2 PET/CT Imaging Characteristics of Benign and Malignant Processes in Tumors of the Head and Neck

Organ	Common Anatomic Location for FDG-PET findings	Benign	Malignant
LNs	Levels I–V (levels I-IV most relevant)	Usually SUV<4.0* Morphology: higher short to long axis ratio (longer than wider), contains hilar fat, smooth borders, no stranding in the adjacent fat, may contain calcification Attenuation or enhancement: usually uniform except in areas of fatty content, or vascular flow voids but can give a heterogeneous feature	Usually SUV>4.0 Morphology: length close to its width (round), does not contain fat, may have necrotic or cystic change, irregular or ill-defined margins, stranding or infiltrative changes in the adjacent fat, no calcification Attenuation or enhancement: heterogeneous but can be uniform as well
Lymphoid tissues	Waldeyer's ring	No recommendation for SUV: hyperplastic lymphoid hyperplasia can present with SUVs as high as >10 Usually symmetrical, no discrete mass is seen Lingual tonsils may extend from base of tongue to the anterior portion of the valleculae	Usually asymmetrical* Enhancing mass can be seen on the contrast-enhanced CT
Neck Muscles	Longus colli, pterygoids, temporalis, masseter, extrinsic tongue sternocleidomastoids, scalenes	No recommendation for SUV: asymmetric use of unusual muscle groups can present with SUVs as high as >10 Can be both symmetrical or asymmetrical, no discrete mass is seen	Usually asymmetrical Enhancing mass can be seen on the contrast-enhanced CT
Larynx	Supraglottic and glottic larynx	No recommendation for SUV: phonation during the injection and wait period can cause significant uptake in vocal cords asymmetric uptake can be seen in unilateral vocal cord paralysis Can be symmetrical or asymmetrical, no discrete mass is associated with asymmetrical uptake if contrast-enhanced CT is performed Post therapy edema can accumulate mild degree FDG uptake Base of tongue lymphoid tissue can extend to the level of vallecula	Usually asymmetrical uptake Anterior commissure uptake at initial staging is generally of malignant cause, however, after therapy low grade uptake can be attributable to treatment-related inflammatory changes (radiation therapy or laser surgery) Enhancing mass can be seen on the contrast-enhanced CT
Salivary glands	Parotid submandibular	Can be symmetrical or asymmetrical, usually no discrete mass is associated with symmetrical uptake on the contrast-enhanced CT Can be focal and intense degree of uptake associated with a well-defined/discrete mass/masses in the case of Warthin's tumor, pleomorphic adenoma or intraparotid reactive lymph nodes	Focal asymmetrical FDG uptake associated with a mass/masses, usually ill-defined and demonstrate infiltration into the surrounding tissues. In the presence of enlarged and hypermetabolic lymph nodes, the likelihood of malignancy increases significantly Invariable moderate to high grade FDG uptake except in tumors of minor salivary gland origin which can show low grade or no FDG uptake
Gumline	Alveolar ridge surrounding the mandible and maxilla	No FDG uptake should be seen in the gumline. The diffuse pattern of uptake is usually due to periodontal disease or denture related inflammation, regardless of the degree of uptake	Usually focal intense and associated with a mass. The mass can be unnoticed if noncontrast CT, thus contrast-enhanced CT should be obtained or available at the time of evaluation
Cartilage	Laryngeal trachea	No FDG uptake should be seen.	Focal or diffuse uptake at initial staging should raise suspicion for tumor involvement
Bones		No FDG uptake should be seen except low grade diffuse uptake in the vertebral column	Cortical invasion or destruction with FDG uptake

*No consensus exists with respect to a SUV cut-off to define maligancy. SUV ≥ 4 has been our experience to favor malignancy through a vast number of cases, although false positive results still occur.

Table 4-3 Benign Conditions with Increased FDG Uptake

- Warthin's tumor
- Pleomorphic adenoma
- Inverted papilloma (Schnederian cyst)
- Active granulomas
- Sinus infection
- Lymphoid hyperplasia (Waldeyer's ring)
- Postsurgical unilateral muscle uptake
- Tongue uptake after glossectomy
- Fasciculation of grafts and other inflammatory graft-related changes
- Postradiation or laser therapy inflammation
- Ostomies (e.g., tracheostomy, gastrostomy)
- Dental interventions
- Osteonecrosis
- Cartilage necrosis
- Tracheostomy
- Vocal cord paralysis

Table 4-4 How to Avoid Misinterpretation at Initial Staging?

Stage	Assessment
T staging	Define metabolism/FDG uptake on PET study Define size and location of the primary lesion on associated CT Examine, margins in relation to adjacent organs on CT Look for – surrounding tissue infiltration – signs for invasion of cartilage, bone, adjacent organs – invasion of specific sites important for surgical eligibility
N staging	Define metabolism/FDG uptake on PET study Define level of LNs Define size, eccentricity, examine morphology of lymph nodes Look for – irregular borders and/or surrounding fat infiltration – calcifications, fat in the hila to rule in benign process – heterogeneity in attenuation to rule in malignant process – central necrosis to rule in malignant process – evidence of coalescence
M staging and second primary	Look for focal FDG uptake in the – Remainder of the head and neck organs – Lungs – Bones – Esophagus – Colon – Liver – Other GIT organs

Reconstructive procedures of the head and neck aim to repair soft tissue and bony defects while restoring optimal function and cosmesis. Postresection defects may require reconstruction with prostheses, musculocutaneous-free flap, or pedicled flaps (Figure 4-74). These surgical changes may result in either focal or diffuse FDG accumulation in the involved muscle structures, so false interpretations are common in the posttherapy period. Particularly in patients undergoing partial or total glossectomy with flap reconstruction, the extensive surgery, altered anatomy, compromised functionality of the remnant tongue, lack of mobility of the flap, and fasciculations of the myocutaneous flaps can lead to asymmetric use of muscles or activation of unusual muscle groups; therefore, the physiologic FDG uptake patterns can be unpredictable (Figures 4-53 and 4-75). In the absence of a CT abnormality, increased FGD uptake should be interpreted with caution despite high levels of uptake (Figures 4-51 and 4-56).

In patients with oral cavity and oropharyngeal tumors and composite mandibular resection, healing osteotomies are characterized by increased FDG uptake, but this should not hinder the interpretation if adequate information is provided to the reader (Figure 4-76). Increased FDG uptake increase by free vascularized bone grafts is not commonly reported. Recurrent tumor in the resection bed or flap usually appears as a focal mass, usually at the interface of the operative site and the flap. Any area of soft tissue density within the flap should be considered suggestive of recurrence but also may be simulated by postoperative scan.

What Are the Radiation Therapy-Induced Changes in the Head and Neck?

Radiation therapy usually causes thickening and edema (Figure 4-77) of the mucosal surfaces, which may result in false-positive findings. Any mass associated with uptake should be interpreted as suggestive of recurrence (Figure 4-78). Radiation-induced necrosis of the osseous or cartilaginous structures can also result in false-positive results. Necrosis of the cartilage and bone appears as mixed sclerosis and lucency, sometimes with fragmentation, and can result in marked FDG uptake on PET (Figure 4-59). In the case of osteoradionecrosis, it is difficult to differentiate between persistent or aggravating bone necrosis and tumor recurrence (Figure 4-60). Interval appearance of enhancing lesions on CT and marked cartilage or bony destruction on follow-up imaging may indicate tumor recurrence. Otherwise, either close follow-up or surgical intervention are adopted policies.

What Benign Changes Can Be Seen in the Vocal Cords?

Posttherapy changes in the vocal cords may cause asymmetric uptake following either injury to the recurrent laryngeal nerve or direct therapy to the vocal cord (Figures 4-79 and 4-80). This phenomenon can be the result of compensation by the contralateral vocal cord during phonation or therapy-induced changes, respectively. Localizing asymmetric vocal cord FDG uptake is much less of a diagnostic problem when PET/CT is used. The presence of associated masses on CT in this location suggests a malignant cause (Figure 4-78). In addition, if a patient has unilateral vocal cord paralysis, we have observed that the functioning contralateral cord can appear to have relatively increased FDG uptake compared to the nonfunctional side (Figure 4-80).

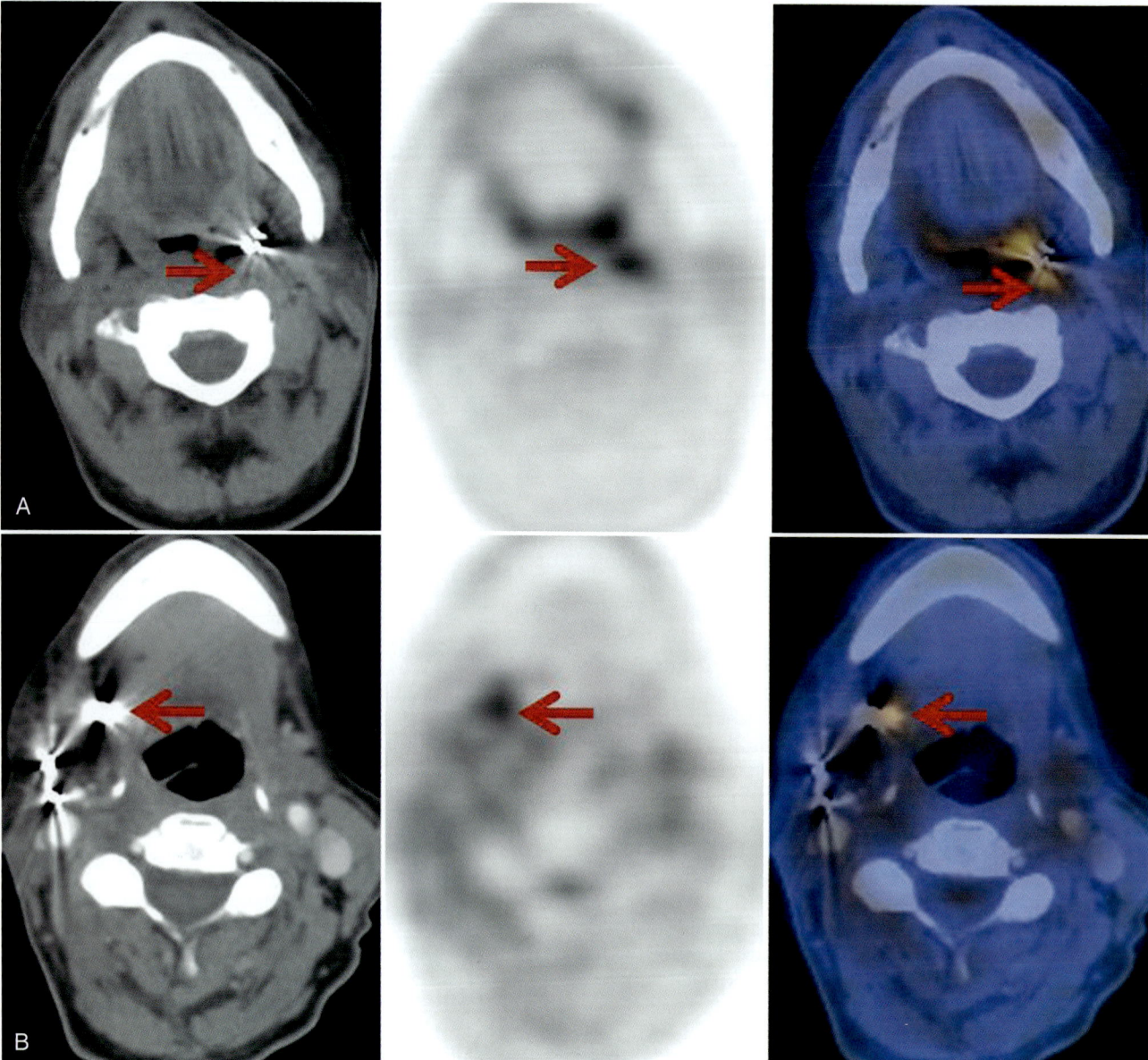

Figure 4-70 Two different patients with 6-month follow-up PET/CT study performed with low-dose CT (**A**) and contrast-enhanced CT (**B**). **A:** Patient with a history of hypoglottic squamous cell carcinoma (SCC), status post left pharyngeal wall resection. **B:** Patient with a history of tonsil SCC, status post resection and right elective neck dissection. There is mildly increased FDG uptake (SUV_{max} 3.0) corresponding to the anatomic planes containing metallic clips (*arrows*). These findings, particularly, in the absence of a soft tissue density, are most consistent with postsurgical changes that may be related to metal artifacts or adjacent muscle uptake. It is difficult to differentiate small volume recurrent disease from inflammatory changes in this setting; thus, frequent follow-up is always recommended to exclude the possibility of recurrence (compare with Figures 4-57 and 4-62).

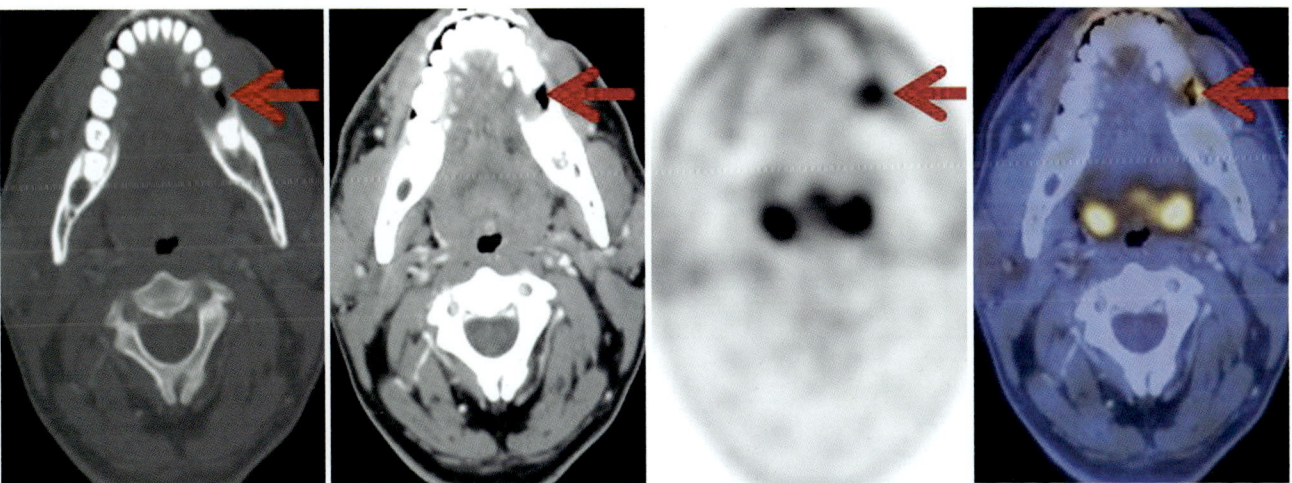

Figure 4-71 A 59-year-old man with a history of left buccal squamous cell carcinoma, status postsurgical resection and radiation therapy. Six-month follow-up PET/CT study performed with contrast-enhanced high-resolution CT, bone **(first from left)** and soft tissue windows **(second from left)**, demonstrates increased uptake (SUV_{max} 5.0) corresponding to the body of the left mandible, which shows a bone defect (*arrows*). The patient has a recent history of tooth extraction in this region. These findings are most consistent with inflammatory changes related to the recent dental manipulation. Note that in the absence of a relevant history, these findings might have been misinterpreted as recurrent disease with bony destruction.

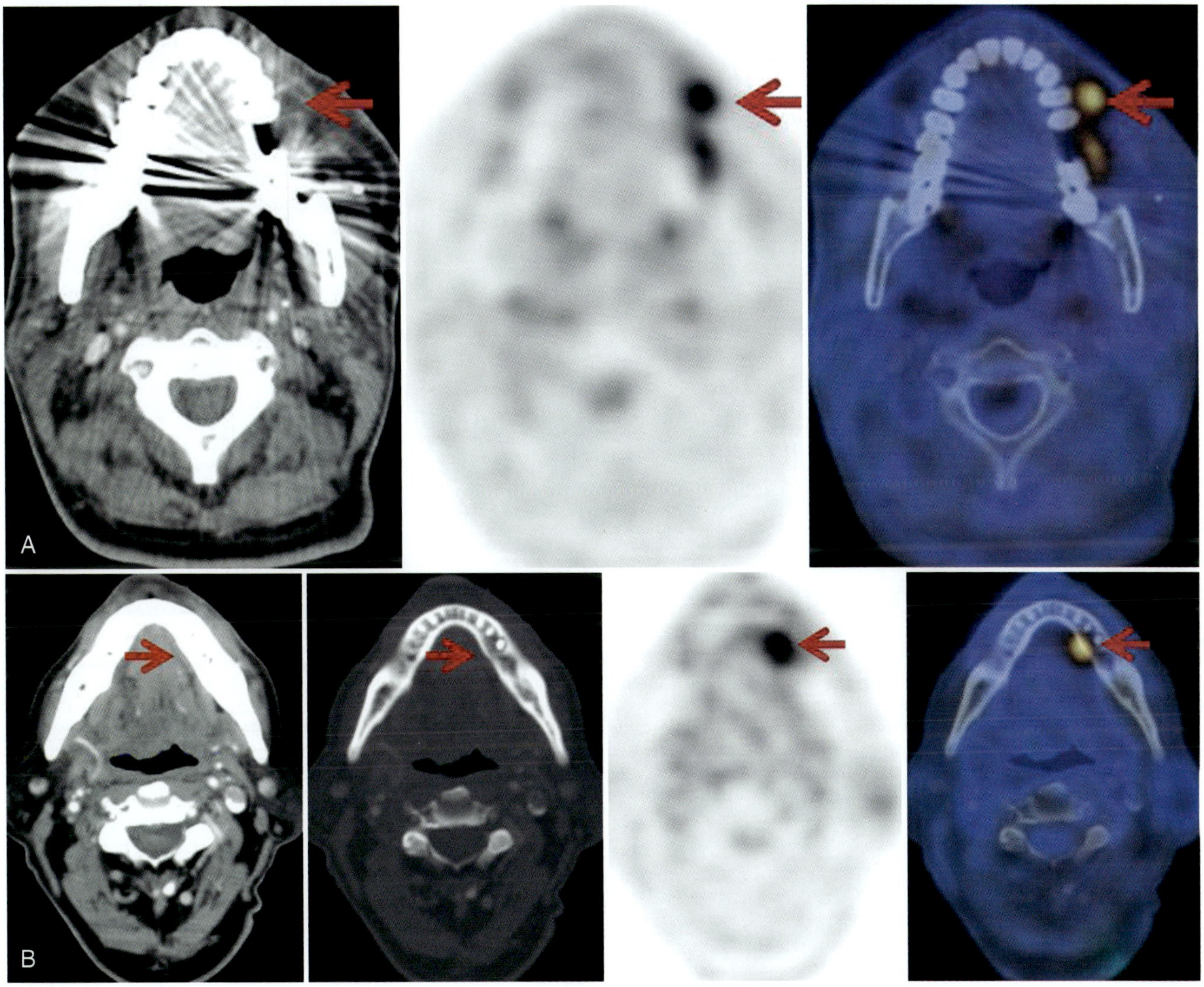

Continued

Figure 4-72 A: A 50-year-old man with a history of left hard palate squamous cell carcinoma (SCC; same patient as shown in Figure 4-68), status post resection and reconstruction with free flap. Six-month follow-up PET/CT study with contrast-enhanced CT shows somewhat focally increased FDG uptake (SUV$_{max}$ 4.5) along the alveolar ridge of the left mandible (*arrows*). The CT portion of the study is limited due to significant metallic artifacts emanating from dental hardware. Although it would be ideal to determine the absence of a soft tissue density in this region to rule out a possible malignant cause, in this patient, these findings probably represent inflammatory gum disease secondary to dentures, which is a common presentation in this patient population. Upon further inquiry, the patient was found to have recent dental manipulation resulting in gum trauma. However, in a patient with a history of buccal SCC, these findings should raise suspicion for recurrent disease. Each patient should be evaluated in the context of the primary diagnosis with a thorough medical history. **B:** A 67-year-old woman with a history of base of tongue SCC, status post partial glossectomy, radiation therapy. Nine-month follow-up PET/CT study with contrast-enhanced CT shows increased FDG uptake (SUV$_{max}$ 6.5) along the medial gum line of the left mandible (*arrows*). No soft tissue mass is appreciated on the corresponding CT slice. These findings probably represent inflammatory gum disease secondary to recent trauma or chronic irritation, which is not infrequent in this population. Upon further inquiry, the patient was found to have started wearing dentures and was complaining about ulceration as a result of irritation.

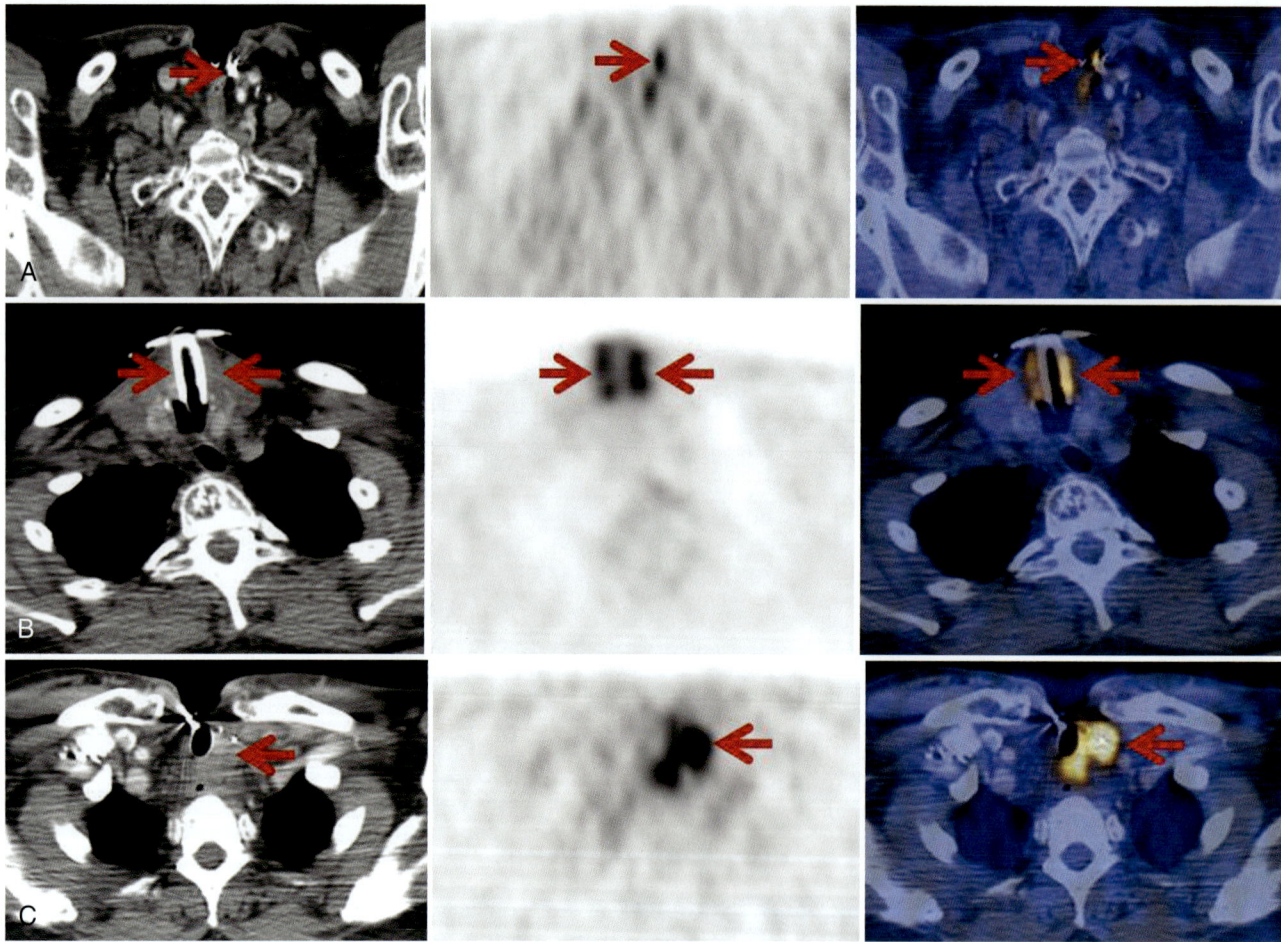

Figure 4-73 A, B: Two different patients with laryngeal squamous cell carcinoma (SCC). **A:** Patient with recent removal of tracheostomy tube (6 weeks prior). **B:** Patient with recent placement of tracheostomy tube (8 weeks prior). Note FDG uptake tracking along the device with no definite evidence of soft tissue density on the companion contrast-enhanced high-resolution CT (*arrows*). This finding is consistent with inflammatory changes. However, close follow-up within 3 to 6 months is recommended to ensure resolution of these findings. **C:** Patient with a history of laryngeal SCC, status post neopharynx reconstruction, tracheostomy removed 6 months ago, presents with progressive difficulty in swallowing and pain. PET/CT study with contrast-enhanced CT shows increased FDG uptake (SUV$_{max}$ 8.5) corresponding to an irregular soft tissue mass posterior to the prior tracheostomy site obliterating the fat planes (*arrows*), most consistent with recurrent disease. Association of a mass on the companion CT study should always increase the suspicion for recurrent disease and should prompt biopsy confirmation. Subsequent biopsy of this mass revealed invasive poorly differentiated SCC.

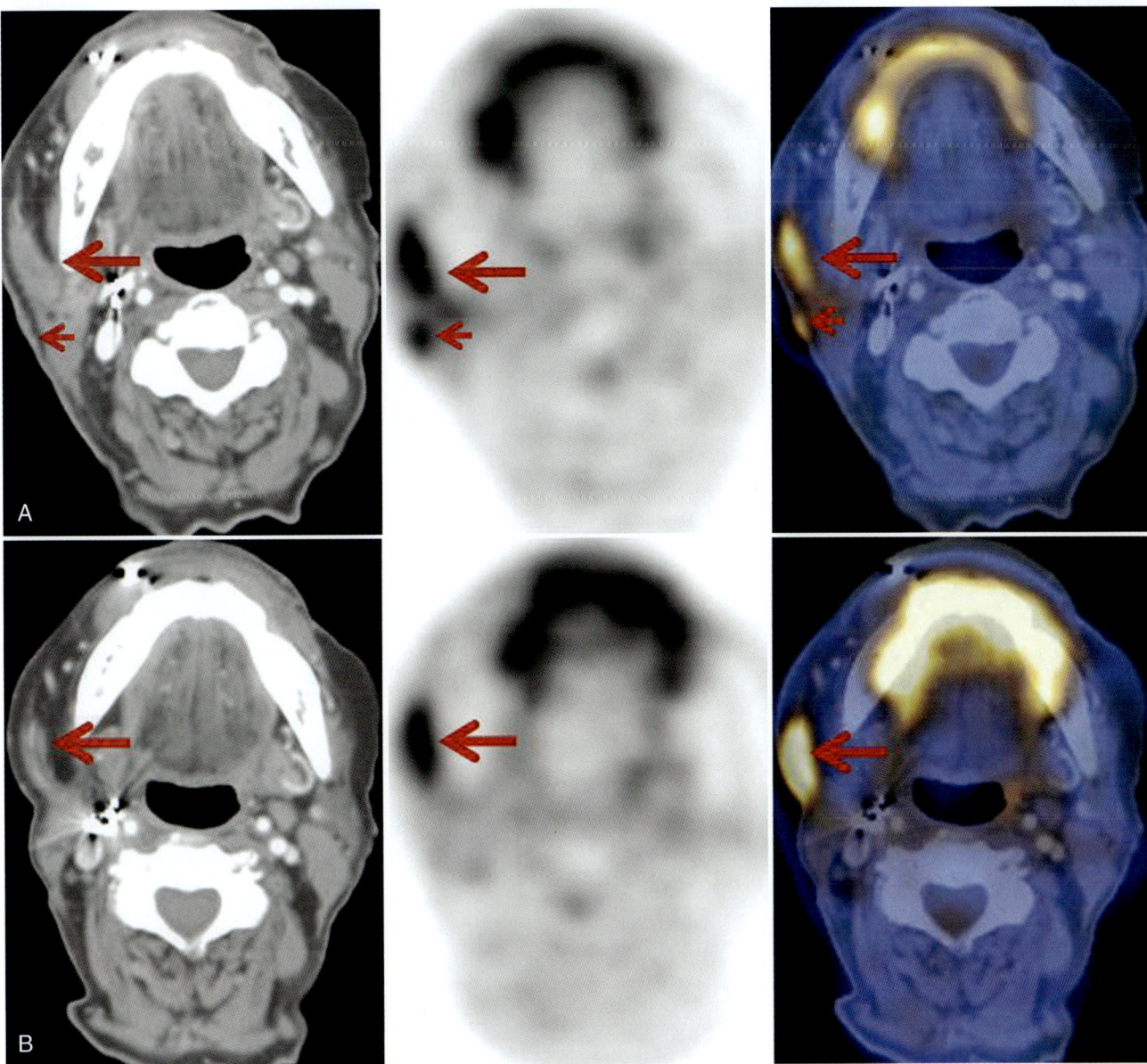

Figure 4-74 A 71-year-old woman with a history of tonsillar squamous cell carcinoma, status neoadjuvant therapy followed by resection, elective right neck dissection, and myocutaneous flap reconstruction. **A:** Six-month follow-up PET/CT study with contrast-enhanced high-resolution CT demonstrates increased FDG uptake (SUV$_{max}$ 5.8) corresponding to the posterior margin of the myocutaneous flap (*arrows*) and overlying skin thickening (*small arrows*) with no associated mass on CT. **B:** Nine-month follow-up PET/CT study with contrast-enhanced CT again shows increased FDG uptake in the same region but a decrease (SUV$_{max}$ 4.1) (*arrows*) and resolution of uptake at the skin surface with no associated mass on CT. These findings are consistent with postsurgical inflammatory changes. The extent and duration of tissue inflammation are dependent on the extent of surgery and the time period between imaging and surgical intervention. These metabolic changes gradually resolve over time but may last as long as 12 months and in some cases even longer. Follow-up imaging is complementary to conventional follow-up to rule out the possibility of residual disease.

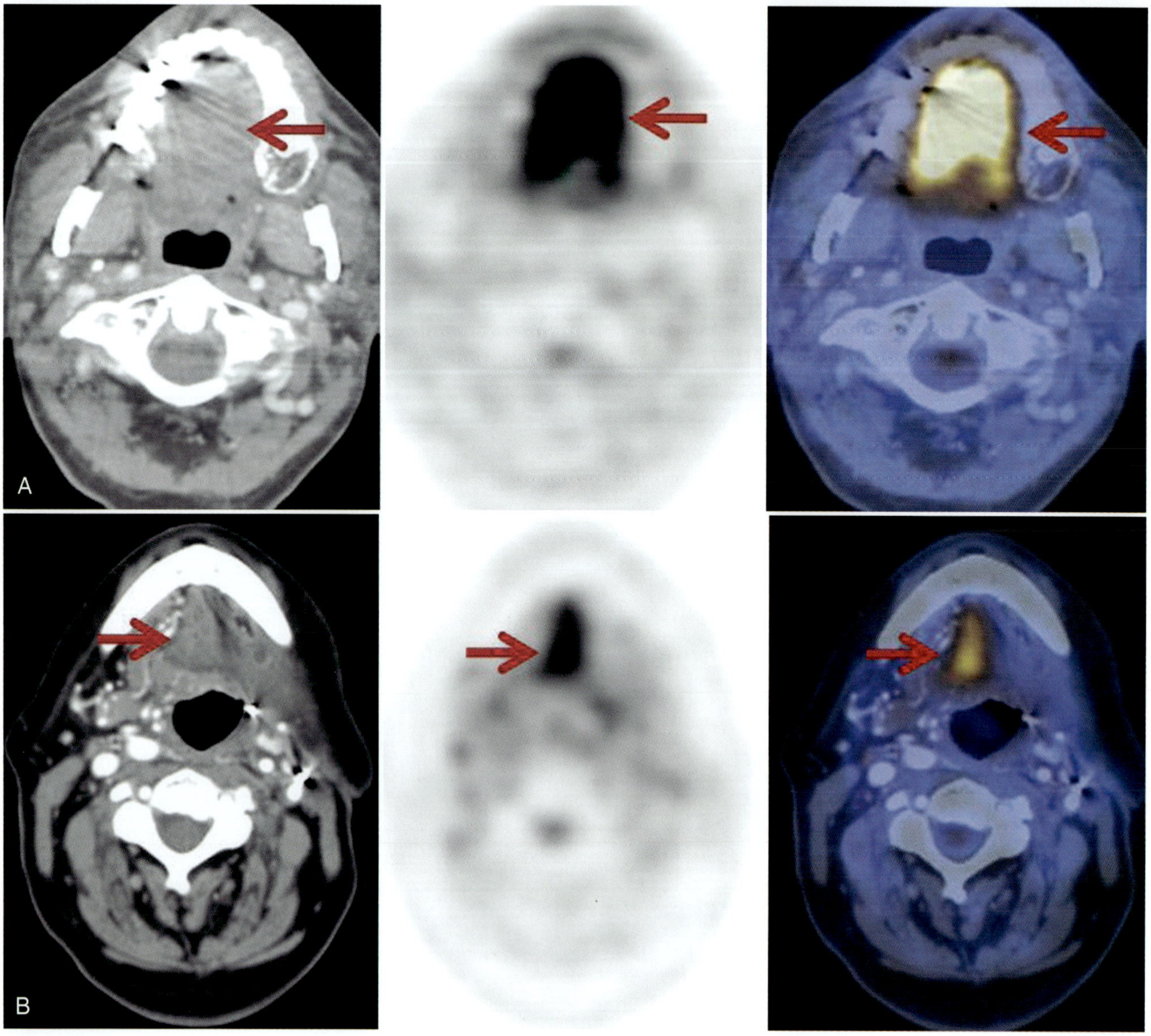

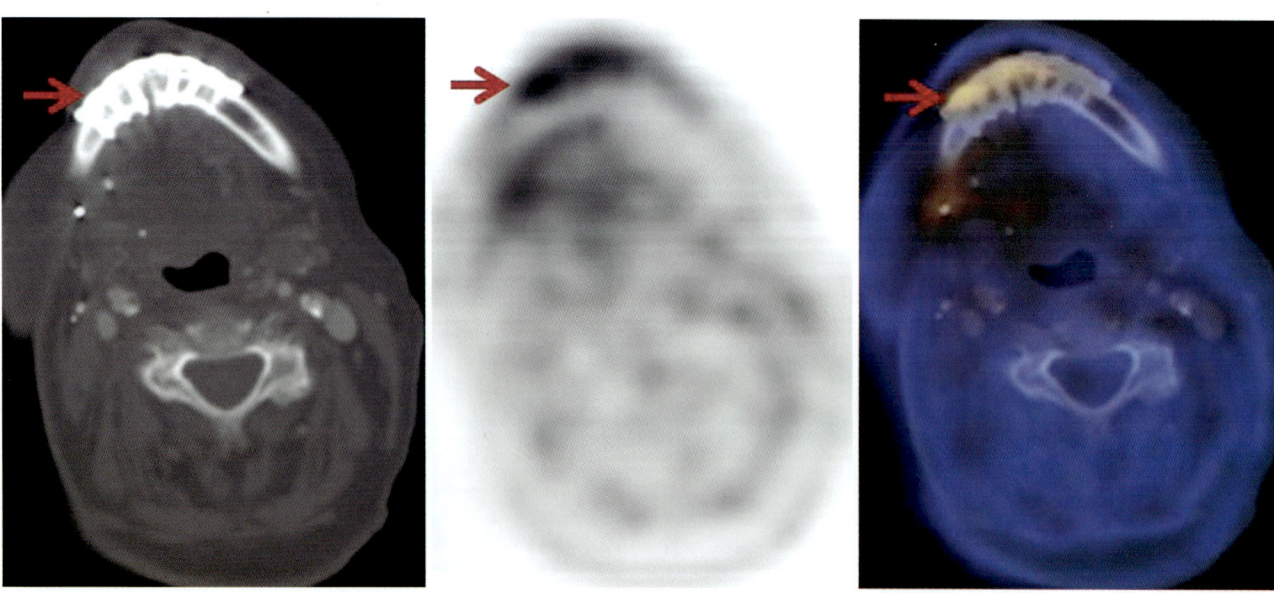

Figure 4-75 Two patients with a history of squamous cell carcinoma of the tongue, status posttreatment with chemoradiation followed by partial glossectomy. Six-month posttherapy PET/CT studies performed with contrast-enhanced high-resolution CT demonstrate significantly increased diffuse uptake (SUV_{max} 8.2) corresponding to the tongue with no appreciable mass on the accompanying contrast-enhanced CT (**A**; *arrows*) and increased uptake (SUV_{max} 4.9) in the genioglossus muscle again with no associated mass (**B**; *arrows*). In the absence of a dominant mass, these findings are consistent with postglossectomy changes related to compensatory use of muscle groups that are not usually involved in speech and swallowing functions, resulting in significantly increased physiologic uptake in the muscles that are utilized.

Figure 4-76 A 67-year-old woman with a history of floor of mouth squamous cell carcinoma, status post treatment with chemoradiation followed by composite resection involving partial mandibulectomy and mandibuloplasty with titanium rod placement. Six-month posttherapy PET/CT study performed with contrast-enhanced high-resolution CT (bone window) demonstrates diffusely increased FDG uptake (SUV_{max} 4.2) corresponding to the site of mandibuloplasty and associated rods with no appreciable destructive change (*arrows*). It is challenging to note erosive or destructive changes in the presence of extensive surgical change associated with surgical hardware on the accompanying contrast-enhanced CT. Titanium rods are not known to cause increased uptake, but bone remodeling may result in this pattern of diffuse uptake.

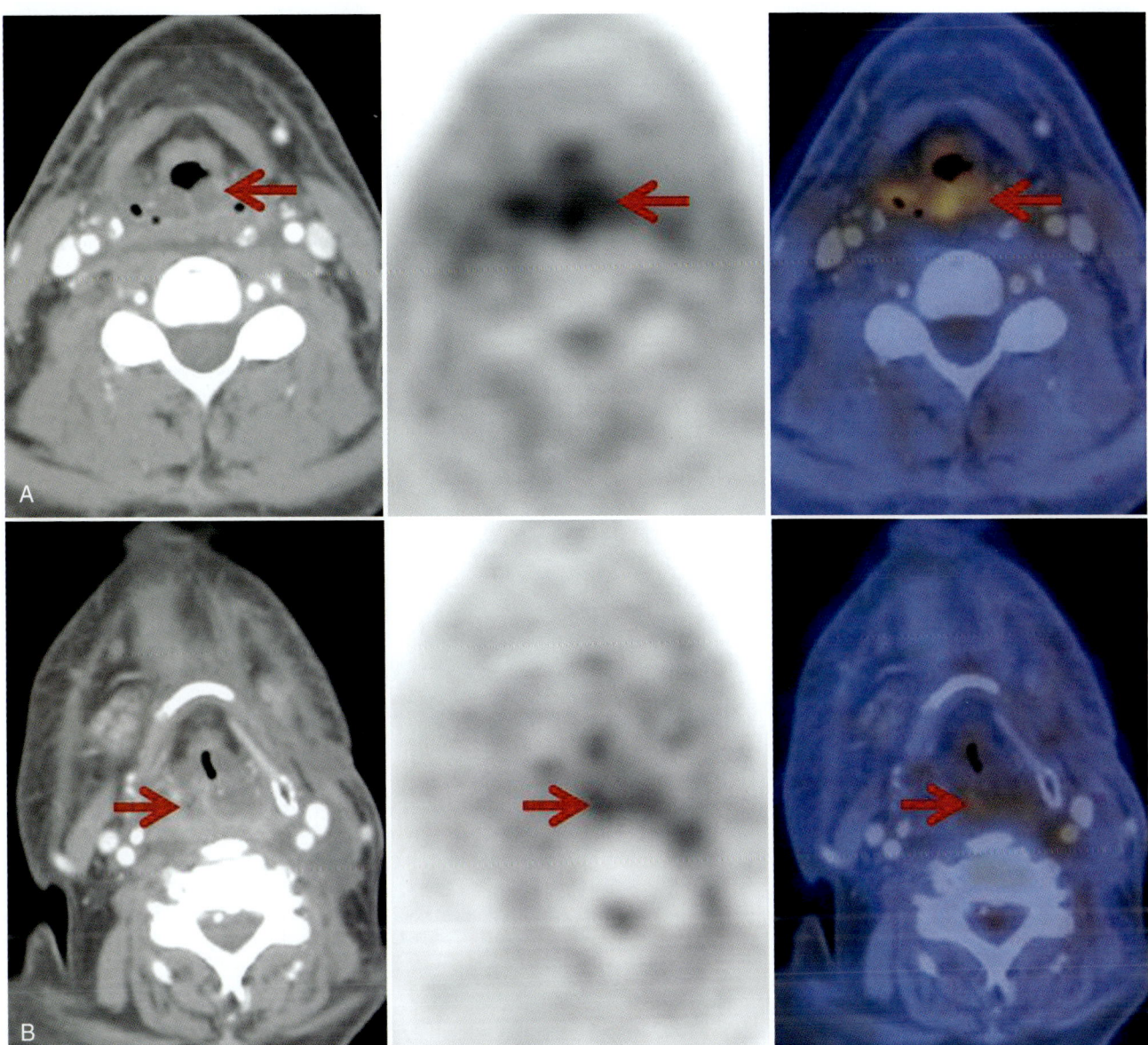

Figure 4-77 Two patients with a history of tongue supraglottic squamous cell carcinoma, status post treatment with chemoradiation. Three-month posttherapy PET/CT studies performed with contrast-enhanced high-resolution CT demonstrate edematous changes (*arrows*) and mucosal thickening of the supraglottic larynx with diffuse low-grade and irregular FDG uptake (SUV_{max} 3.2). These metabolic changes gradually resolve over time, usually preceding the resolution of edema; however, they may last longer than a year in some cases. It is not difficult to recognize the pattern of low-grade uptake; however, in cases with high risk of recurrence, these findings may lead to equivocal readings. In most of these cases biopsy is contraindicated due to the possibility of aggravation of inflammation and necrosis in the radiotherapy field. Follow-up imaging is significantly helpful and complementary to conventional follow-up to rule out the possibility of recurrence.

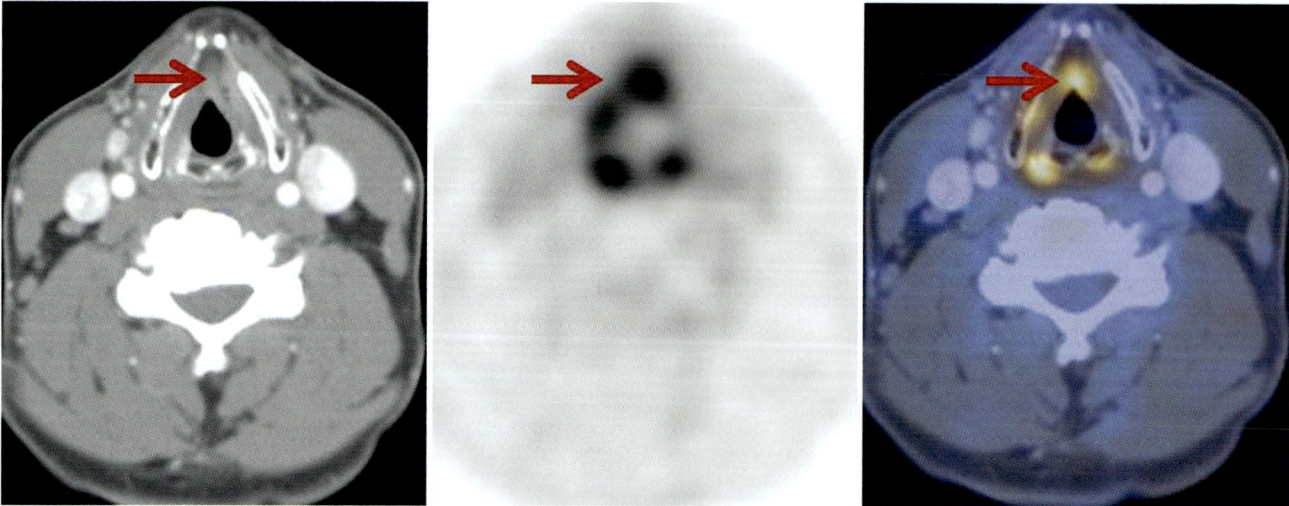

Figure 4-78 A 58-year-old man with a history of left vocal cord squamous cell carcinoma, status post laser excision. Twelve-month follow-up PET/CT study performed with contrast-enhanced high-resolution CT demonstrates increased uptake (SUV_{max} 7.6) corresponding to a soft tissue nodule in the anterior commissure (*arrows*), consistent with recurrent disease, which was subsequently proven by biopsy. Note that association of FDG uptake with a mass significantly increases the likelihood of recurrent disease (compare with Figure 4-69).

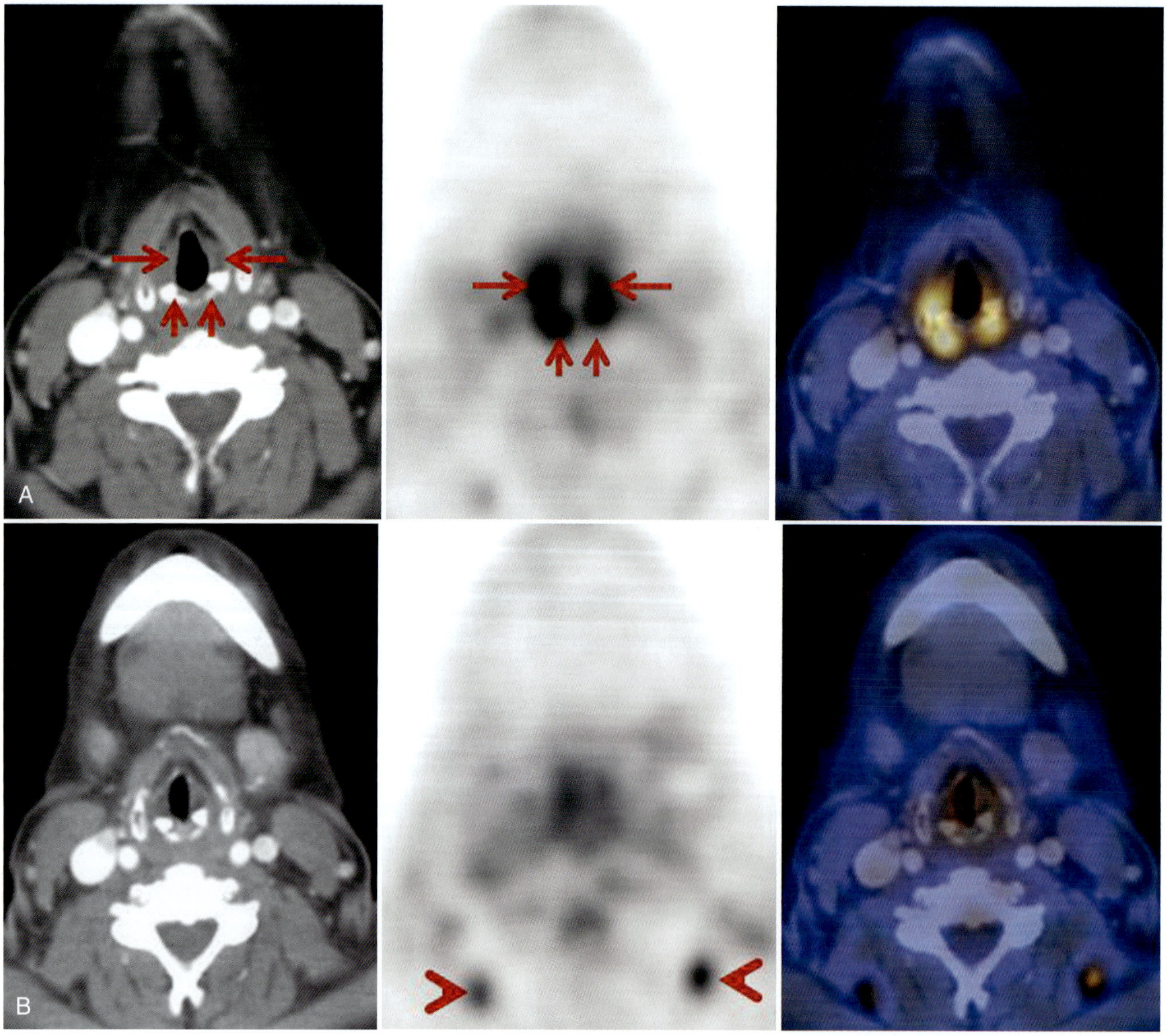

Figure 4-79 A 64 year-old patient with a history of left vocal cord squamous cell carcinoma, status postradiation therapy 9 month prior to PET/CT imaging. **A:** PET/CT study performed with contrast-enhanced high-resolution CT reveals FDG uptake in both vocal cords (*small horizontal arrows*) and cricoarytenoid muscles (*small vertical arrows*), slightly more prominent in the right vocal cord. There is no appreciable nodule or mass on the vocal cords on the associated CT slice. The patient was noted to speak loudly during the FDG injection and uptake period. This uptake pattern probably reflects the activation of intrinsic laryngeal muscles during phonation. Subsequent laryngoscopy was unremarkable. **B:** At 3-month follow-up study, the patient kept silent during the FDG injection and uptake period. The previously noted uptake in the vocal cords had resolved, proving the previous uptake to be of physiologic nature. It is essential that patients with a history of head and neck cancer be kept silent during the uptake period of FDG to prevent uptake in the vocal cords, which may lead to false-positive findings.

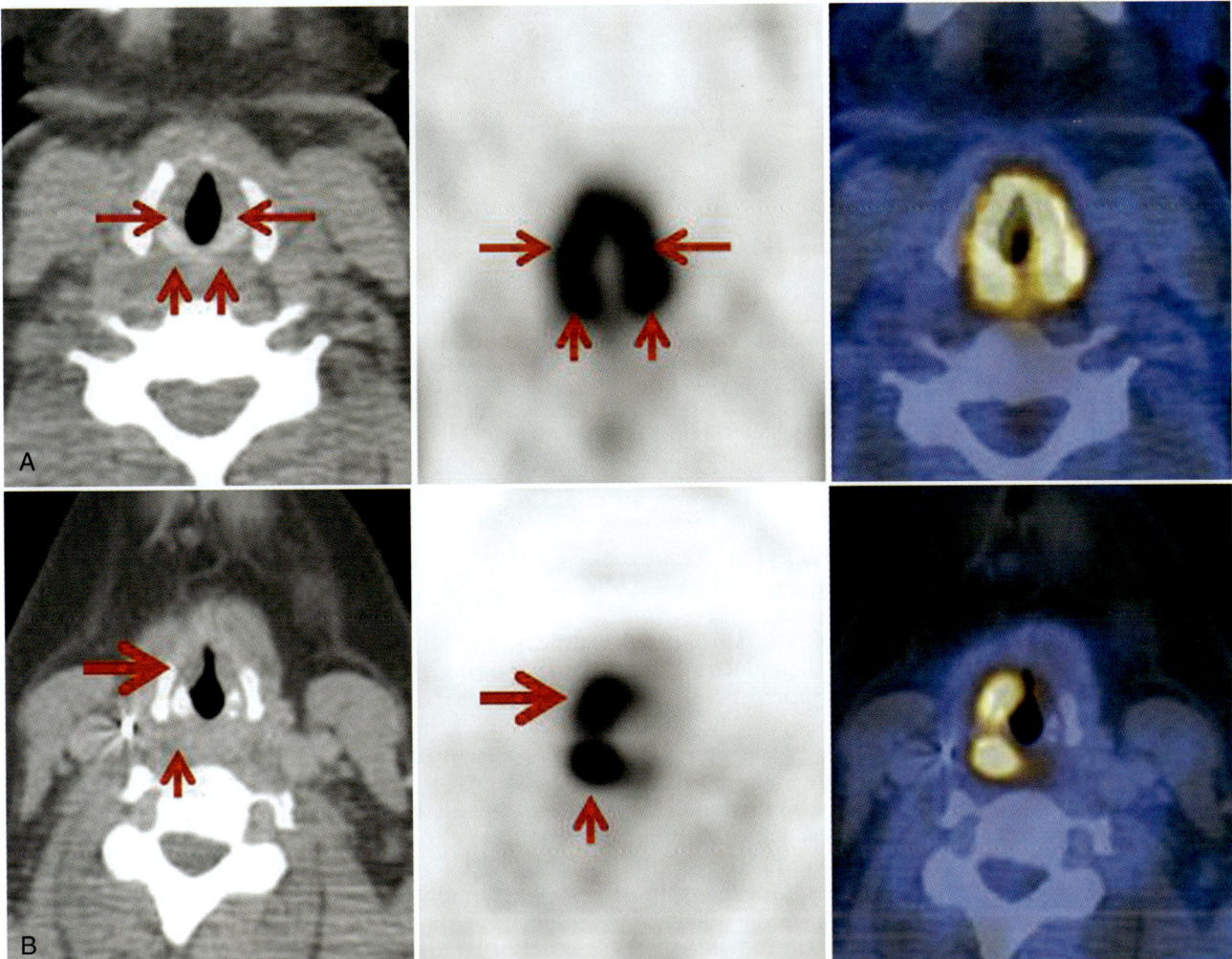

Figure 4-80 Two patients showing various degrees of physiologic vocal cord uptake. **A:** Patient with a history of treated base of tongue squamous cell carcinoma, status post primary therapy, now referred for follow-up study. Axial sections of the FDG PET/CT study with low-dose CT demonstrate symmetric FDG uptake in the thyroarytenoid (*horizontal arrows*) and posterior cricoarytenoid muscles (*vertical arrows*) reflecting activation of intrinsic laryngeal muscles during phonation. **B:** Axial sections of the FDG PET/CT study with low-dose CT demonstrate FDG uptake in the right thyroarytenoid (*horizontal arrow*) and posterior cricoarytenoid muscle (*vertical arrow*) reflecting activation of intrinsic laryngeal muscles during phonation. There is no uptake in the corresponding muscles on the contralateral site, which is consistent with paralysis of the vocal cord at this site. Although this pattern of uptake is characteristic for activated vocal cords, accompanying CT further confirmed the absence of any pathologic mass in this region. It is essential that patients be kept silent during the uptake period of FDG to prevent uptake in the vocal cords, which may lead to false-positive findings.

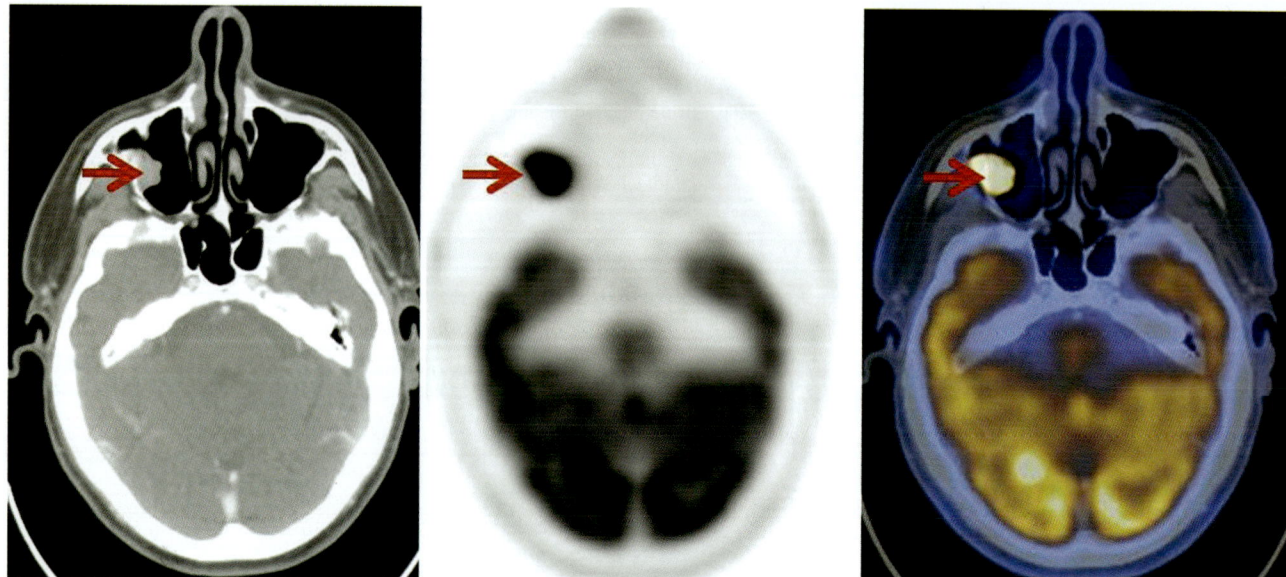

Figure 4-81 A 70-year-old man recently diagnosed with piriform sinus squamous cell carcinoma (SCC), referred for PET/CT study for further evaluation of extent of disease (same patient as shown in Figure 4-26, *B*). PET/CT imaging performed with contrast-enhanced high-resolution CT demonstrates a soft tissue mass projecting off the epithelial surface of the right maxillary sinus (*arrows*), which demonstrated significantly increased FDG uptake (SUV_{max} 28.0). This mass is highly suggestive of a malignant process. However, metastasis is unlikely due to the unusual location. A second primary of the maxillary sinus can be a consideration. Subsequent excisional biopsy of the maxillary sinus mass revealed a sinonasal oncocytic schneiderian papilloma. Based on these findings, the patient's disease was staged as a T3N2bM0 hypopharyngeal carcinoma (primary tumor and metastatic lymph nodes not shown). The patient subsequently underwent chemotherapy and hyperfractionated radiation therapy for hypopharyngeal SCC, followed by selective neck dissection. He responded well to therapy, with no evidence of disease after follow-up of 8 months, which included repeat PET/CT and diagnostic CT studies. The patient is currently without recurrence of maxillary sinus papilloma.

■ HOW DO THE CERVICAL LYMPH NODES CAUSE FALSE-POSITIVE READINGS?

Level I to II lymph nodes can increase their glucose utilization because they are part of an important defense system (Figures 4-13, *B*, 4-35, and 4-36, *B*). Because FDG is not specific to malignancy, it is taken up by inflammatory processes, which may cause false-positive findings in the cervical lymph nodes. In these cases, follicular dendritic cells in germinal centers, which form a system of highly efficient antigen-presenting cells with preferential FDG uptake, were suggested to be the principal cause of false-positive findings in nodal staging. Nonetheless, when CT and MRI data are individually compared to PET results, the specificity is still in favor of FDG PET by 10% at approximately 85%.

■ WHAT BENIGN TUMORS CAN CAUSE AVID FDG UPTAKE?

Some benign tumors, including pleomorphic adenoma, Warthin tumor (Figure 4-81), inverted papilloma (Schneiderian cyst) (Figure 4-82), thyroid adenoma, and Thornwaldt cysts, can accumulate FDG at significant levels. Thus, the expected pattern of distribution should be considered while interpreting imaging, and caution should be exercised when an extraordinary finding is encountered.

The PET/CT reader can avoid errors by recognizing certain common benign physiologic and postoperative presentations. Follow-up studies and a baseline study are important adjuncts for accurate interpretation of PET/CT studies of various challenging settings in patients with head and neck cancer.

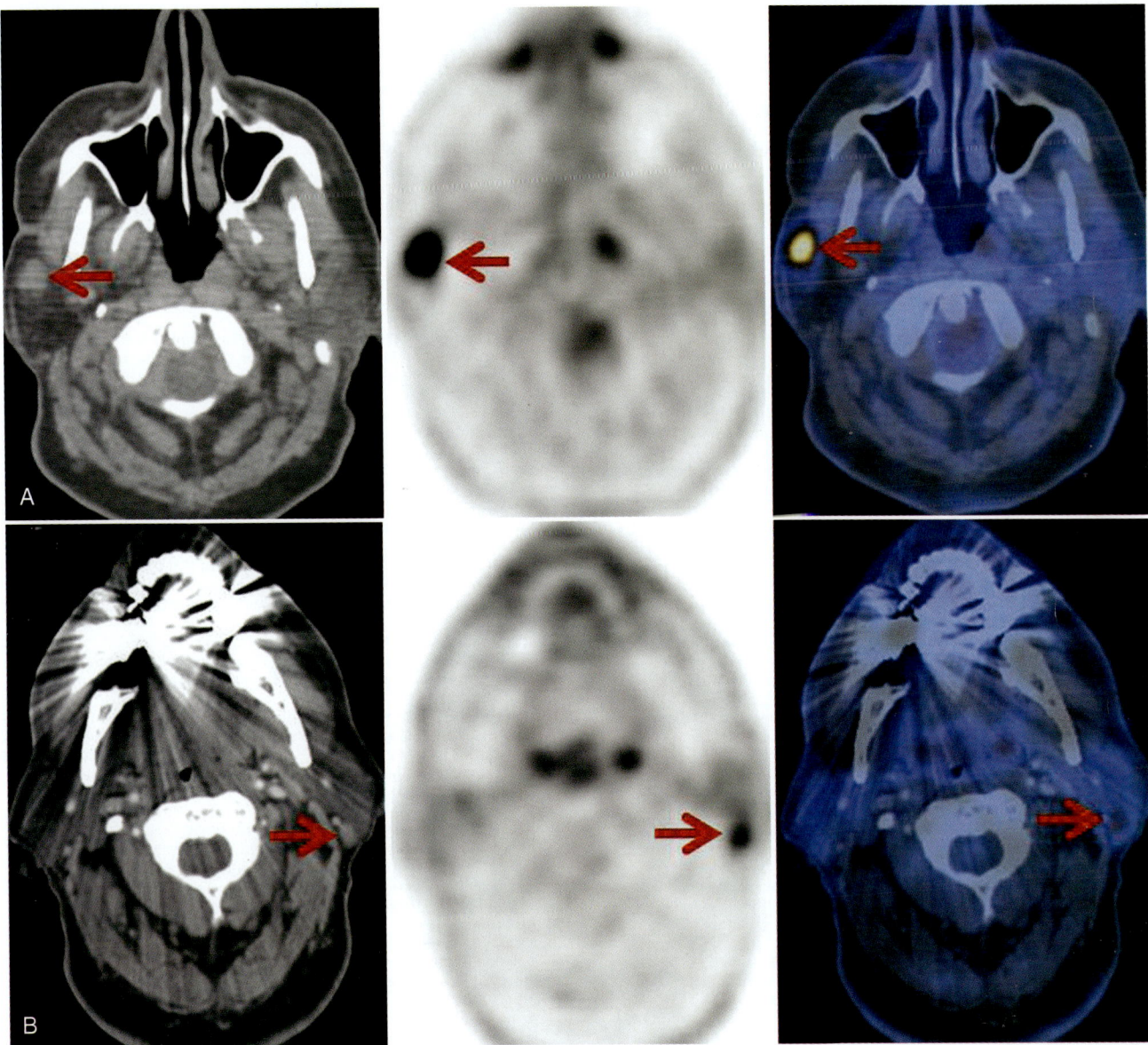

Figure 4-82 Two patients with a history of treated laryngeal (**A**) and tonsillar carcinoma (**B**), respectively, referred for 12-month follow-up FDG PET/CT study. There is no baseline study for comparison. Axial PET/CT images demonstrate a small nodule within the right parotid gland (**A**) and left parotid gland (**B**), both demonstrating smooth borders (*arrows*) and increased FDG uptake (SUV_{max} 6.9 and 3.6, respectively). These findings are consistent with parotid incidentalomas. Subsequent biopsy of the right parotid gland lesion revealed Warthin's tumor, which is a benign neoplasm of the salivary glands. The left parotid gland lesion was not biopsied. However, this finding was persistent on multiple follow-up studies, which may represent either a pleomorphic adenoma or a Warthin's tumor.

Suggested Readings

Abgral R, et al. Does 18F-FDG PET/CT improve the detection of posttreatment recurrence of head and neck squamous cell carcinoma in patients negative for disease on clinical follow-up? *J Nucl Med.* 2009;50(1):24-29.

Agarwal V, Branstetter BFt, Johnson JT. Indications for PET/CT in the head and neck. *Otolaryngol Clin North Am.* 2008;41(1):23-49.

American Cancer Society, Cancer facts and figures. 2007, American Cancer Society (2007). Available at http://www.cancer.org/docroot/STT/stt_0_2007.asp?sitearea=STT&level=1.

Andrade RS, Heron DE, Degirmenci B, et al. Posttreatment assessment of response using FDG-PET/CT for patients treated with definitive radiation therapy for head and neck cancers. *Int J Radiat Oncol Biol Phys.* 2006;65:1315-1322.

Babin E, Desmonts C, Hamon M, et al. PET/CT for assessing mandibular invasion by intraoral squamous cell carcinomas. *Clin Otolaryngol.* 2008;33:47-51.

Becker M, Burkhardt K, Dulguerov P, Allal A. Imaging of the larynx and hypopharynx. *Eur J Radiol.* 2008;66:460-479.

Becker M. Neoplastic invasion of laryngeal cartilage: radiologic diagnosis and therapeutic implications. *Eur J Radiol.* 2000;33:216-229.

Bernier J, Domenge C, Ozsahin M, et al. Postoperative irradiation with or without concomitant chemotherapy for locally advanced head and neck cancer. *N Engl J Med.* 2004;350(19):1945-1952.

Bisase B, Kerawala C, Lee J. The role of computed tomography of the chest in the staging of early squamous cell carcinoma of the tongue. *Br J Oral Maxillofac Surg.* 2008;46:367-369.

Bold B, Piao Y, Murata Y, et al. Usefulness of PET/CT for detecting a second primary cancer after treatment for squamous cell carcinoma of the head and neck. *Clin Nucl Med.* 2008;33:831-833.

Bolzoni Villaret A, Piazza C, Peretti G, Calabrese L, Ansarin M, Chiesa F, Pellini R, Spriano G, Nicolai P. Multicentric prospective study on the prevalence of sublevel IIb metastases in head and neck cancer. *Arch Otolaryngol Head Neck Surg.* 2007;133:897-903.

Braams JW, Pruim J, Freling NJ, et al. Detection of lymph node metastases of squamous-cell cancer of the head and neck with FDG-PET and MRI. *J Nucl Med.* 1995;36:211-216.

Braams JW, Pruim J, Kole AC, et al. Detection of unknown primary head and neck tumors by positron emission tomography. *Int J Oral Maxillofac Surg.* 1997;26(2):112-115.

Breau RL, Suen JY. Management of the N(0) neck. *Otolaryngol Clin North Am.* 1998;31:657-669.

Brockstein B, et al. Patterns of failure, prognostic factors and survival in locoregionally advanced head and neck cancer treated with concomitant chemoradiotherapy: a 9-year, 337-patient, multi-institutional experience. *Ann Oncol.* 2004;15(8):1179-1186.

Brouwer J, de Bree R, Comans EF, Castelijns JA, Hoekstra OS, Leemans CR. Positron emission tomography using [18F]fluorodeoxyglucose (FDG-PET) in the clinically negative neck: is it likely to be superior? *Eur Arch Otorhinolaryngol.* 2004;261:479-483.

Brouwer J, de Bree R, Hoekstra OS, Langenijk JA, Castelijns JA, Leemans CR. Screening for distant metastases in patients with head and neck cancer: what is current clinical practice? *Clin Otolaryngol.* 2005;30:438-443.

Brouwer J, Hooft L, Hoekstra OS, et al. Systematic review: accuracy of imaging tests in the diagnosis of recurrent laryngeal carcinoma after radiotherapy. *Head & Neck.* 2008;30(7):889-897.

Brouwer J, Senft A, de Bree R, et al. Screening for distant metastases in patients with head and neck cancer: is there a role for (18)FDG-PET? *Oral Oncol.* 2006;42:275-280.

Brun E, Kjellén E, Tennvall J, et al. FDG PET studies during treatment: prediction of therapy outcome in head and neck squamous cell carcinoma. *Head Neck.* 2002 Feb;24(2):127-135.

Chao KS, Ozyigit G, Blanco AI, et al. Intensity modulated radiation therapy for oropharyngeal carcinoma: impact of tumor volume. *Int J Radiat Oncol Biol Phys.* 2004;59(1):43-50.

Chung TS, Yousem DM, Seigerman HM, et al. MR of mandibular invasion in patients with oral and oropharyngeal malignant neoplasms. *AJNR Am J Neuroradiol.* 1994;15:1949-1955.

Cohan DM, et al. Oropharyngeal cancer: current understanding and management. *Curr Opin Otolaryngol Head Neck Surg.* 2009;17(2):88-94.

Connell CA, Corry J, Milner AD, et al. Clinical impact of, and prognostic stratification by, F-18, FDG PET/CT in head and neck mucosal squamous cell carcinoma. *Head Neck.* 2007;29:986-995.

Cooper JS, Porter K, Mallin K, Hoffman HT, Weber RS, Ang KK, Gay EG, Langer CJ. National Cancer Database report on cancer of the head and neck: 10-year update. *Head Neck.* 2009;31:748-758.

Cooper JS, et al. Postoperative concurrent radiotherapy and chemotherapy for high-risk squamous-cell carcinoma of the head and neck. *N Engl J Med.* 2004;350(19):1937-1944.

Crecco M, Vidiri A, Palma O, et al. T stages of tumors of the tongue and floor of the mouth: correlation between MR with gadopentetate dimeglumine and pathologic data. *AJNR Am J Neuroradiol.* 1994;15:1695-1702.

Dammann F, Horger M, Mueller-Berg M, et al. Rational diagnosis of squamous cell carcinoma of the head and neck region: Comparative evaluation of CT, MRI, and 18FDG PET. *AJR Am J Roentgenol.* 2005;184:1326-1331.

Davidson J, Gilbert R, Irish J, et al. The role of panendoscopy in the management of mucosal head and neck malignancy: a prospective evaluation. *Head Neck.* 2000;22:449-454:[discussion: 454-5].

de Braud F, Al-Sarraf M. Diagnosis and management of squamous cell carcinoma of unknown primary tumor site of the neck. *Semin Oncol.* 1993;20:273-278.

Di Martino E, Nowak B, Hassan HA, Hausmann R, Adam G, Buell U, Westhofen M. Diagnosis and staging of head and neck cancer: a comparison of modern imaging modalities (positron emission tomography, computed tomography, color-coded duplex sonography) with panendoscopic and histopathologic findings. *Arch Otolaryngol Head Neck Surg.* 2000;126:1457-1461.

Dietl B, Marienhagen J, Kühnel T, et al. The impact of FDG-PET/CT on the management of head and neck tumours: the radiotherapist's perspective. *Oral Oncol.* 2008;44:504-508.

Ellis JR, Gleeson FV. New concepts in lung cancer screening. *Curr Opin Pulm Med.* 2002;8:270-274.

Elsheikh MN, Mahfouz ME, Elsheikh E. Level IIb lymph nodes metastasis in elective supraomohyoid neck dissection for oral cavity squamous cell carcinoma: a molecular-based study. *Laryngoscope.* 2005;115:1636-1640.

Fakhry N, Jacob T, Paris J, et al. Contribution of 18-F FDG PET for detection of head and neck carcinomas with an unknown primary tumor. *Ann Otolaryngol Chir Cervicofac.* 2006;123:17-25.

Fakhry N, Lussato D, Jacob T, et al. Comparison between PET and PET/CT in recurrent head and neck cancer and clinical implications. *Eur Arch Otorhinolaryngol.* 2007;264:531-538.

Feinmesser R, Miyazaki I, Cheung R, et al. Diagnosis of nasopharyngeal carcinoma by DNA amplification of tissue obtained by fine-needle aspiration. *N Engl J Med.* 1992;326:17-12.

Fleming Jr AJ, Smith Jr SP, Paul CM, et al. Impact of [18F]-2-fluorodeoxyglucose-positron emission tomography/computed tomography on previously untreated head and neck cancer patients. *Laryngoscope.* 2007;117:1173-1179.

Freudenberg LS, Fischer M, Antoch G, et al. Dual modality of 18F-fluorodeoxyglucose-positron emission tomography/computed tomography in patients with cervical carcinoma of unknown primary. *Med Princ Pract.* 2005;14:155-160.

Fukui M, Blodgett T, Snyderman C, et al. Combined PET-CT in the Head and Neck. Part 2. Diagnostic Uses and Pitfalls of Oncologic Imaging. *RadioGraphics.* 2005;25:913-930.

Galer CE, Kies MS. Evaluation and management of the unknown primary carcinoma of the head and neck. *J Natl Compr Canc Netw.* 2008;6:1068-1075.

Gil Z, Even-Sapir E, Margalit N, et al. Integrated PET/CT system for staging and surveillance of skull base tumors. *Head Neck.* 2007;29:537-545.

Goerkem M, Braun J, Stoeckli SJ. Evaluation of clinical and histomorphological parameters as potential predictors of occult metastases in sentinel lymph nodes of early squamous cell carcinomas of the oral cavity. *Ann Surg Oncol.* 2010:(in press).

Goerres GW, Schmid DT, Gratz KW, et al. Impact of whole body positron emission tomography on initial staging and therapy in patients with squamous cell carcinoma of the oral cavity. *Oral Oncol.* 2003;39:547-551.

Goerres GW, Schmid DT, Bandhauer F, et al. Positron emission tomography in the early follow-up of advanced head and neck cancer. *Arch Otolaryngol Head Neck Surg.* 2004;130(1):105-109:[discussion: 120-1].

Goldenberg D, Sciubba J, Koch WM. Cystic metastasis from head and neck squamous cell cancer: a distinct disease variant? *Head Neck.* 2006;28(7):633-638.

Goodwin WJ. Salvage surgery for patients with recurrent squamous cell carcinoma of the upper aerodigestive tract: When do the ends justify the means? *Laryngoscope.* 2000;110(suppl 93):1-18.

Gordin A, Daitzchman M, Doweck I, et al. Fluorodeoxyglucose-positron emission tomography/computed tomography imaging in patients with carcinoma of the larynx: diagnostic accuracy and impact on clinical management. *Laryngoscope.* 2006;116:273-278.

Goshen E, Davidson T, Yahalom R, et al. PET/CT in the evaluation of patients with squamous cell cancer of the head and neck. *Int J Oral Maxillofac Surg.* 2006;35:332-336.

Gourin CG, Watts TL, Williams HT, Patel VS, Bilodeau PA, Coleman TA. Identification of distant metastases with positron-emission tomography-computed tomography in patients with previously untreated head and neck cancer. *Laryngoscope.* 2008 Apr;118(4):671-675.

Gourin CG, Watts T, Williams HT, Patel VS, Bilodeau PA, Coleman TA. Identification of distant metastases with PET-CT in patients with suspected recurrent head and neck cancer. *Laryngoscope.* 2009 Apr;119(4):703-706.

Gourin CG, Williams HT, Seabolt WN, Herdman AV, Howington JW, Terris DJ. Utility of positron emission tomography-computed tomography in identification of residual nodal disease after chemoradiation for advanced head and neck cancer. *Laryngoscope.* 2006;116:705-710.

Gutzeit A, Antoch G, Kuhl H, et al. Unknown primary tumors: detection with dual-modality PET/CT initial experience. *Radiology.* 2005;234:227-234.

Ha PK, Hdeib A, Goldenberg D, et al. The role of positron emission tomography and computed tomography fusion in the management of early-stage and advanced-stage primary head and neck squamous cell carcinoma. *Arch Otolaryngol Head Neck Surg.* 2006;132:12-16.

Hafidh MA, Lacy PD, Hughes JP, et al. Evaluation of the impact of addition of PET to CT and MR scanning in the staging of patients with head and neck carcinomas. *Eur Arch Otorhinolaryngol.* 2006;263:853-859.

Halpern J. The value of chest CT scan in the work-up of head and neck cancers. *J Med.* 1997;28:191-198.

Hannah A, Scott AM, Tochon-Danguy H, et al. Evaluation of 18 F-fluorodeoxyglucose positron emission tomography and computed tomography with histopathologic correlation in the initial staging of head and neck cancer. *Ann Surg.* 2002;236:208-217.

Harnsberger HR. The Larynx and Hypopharynx *Handbook of Head and Neck Imaging.* 2nd ed. St. Louis: Mosby; 1994:224-259.

Harnsberger HR. Squamous Cell Carcinoma: Nodal Staging. In: ed. *Handbook of Head and Neck Imaging.* 2nd ed. St. Louis: Mosby; 1994:283-298.

Henschke CI, Shaham D, Yankelevitz DF, et al. CT screening for lung cancer: past and ongoing studies. *Semin Thorac Cardiovasc Surg.* 2005;17(2):99-106.

Hermans R, Van den Bogaert W, Rijnders A, et al. Value of computed tomography as outcome predictor of supraglottic squamous cell carcinoma treated by definitive radiation therapy. *Int J Radiat Oncol Biol Phys.* 1999;44:755-765.

Holmstrup P, Thorn JJ, Rindum J, Pindborg JJ. Malignant development of lichen planus-affected oral mucosa. *J Oral Pathol.* 1988;17:219-225.

Horiuchi C, Taguchi T, Yoshida T, et al. Early assessment of clinical response to concurrent chemoradiotherapy in head and neck carcinoma using fluro-2-deoxy-d-glucose positron emission tomography. *Auris Nasus Larynx.* 2008 Mar;35(1):103-108.

Houghton DJ, Mcgarry G, Stewart I, Wilson JA, Mackenzie K. Chest computerized tomography scanning in patients presenting with head and neck cancer. *Clin Otolaryngol.* 1998;23:348-350.

Hudgins PA. Flap reconstruction in the head and neck: expected appearance, complications, and recurrent disease. *Semin Ultrasound CT MR.* 2002 Dec;23(6):492-500.

Isles MG, McConkey C, Mehanna HM. A systematic review and meta-analysis of the role of positron emission tomography in the follow up of head and neck squamous cell carcinoma following radiotherapy or chemoradiotherapy. *Clin Otolaryngol.* 2008 Jun;33(3):210-222.

Jalisi M, Jalisi S. Advanced laryngeal carcinoma: surgical and non-surgical management options. *Otolaryngol Clin North Am.* 2005;38(1):47-57:viii.

Jereczek-Fossa B, Jassem J, Orecchia R. Cervical lymph node metastases of squamous cell carcinoma from an unknown primary. *Cancer Treat Rev.* 2004;30:153-164.

Jemal A, Siegel R, Ward E, et al. Cancer statistics, 2006. *CA Cancer J Clin.* 2006;56:106-130.

Jeong HS, Baek CH, Son YI, et al. Use of integrated 18F-FDG PET/CT to improve the accuracy of initial cervical nodal evaluation in patients with head and neck squamous cell carcinoma. *Head Neck.* 2007;29:203-210.

Jeong HS, Chung MK, Son YI, et al. Role of 18F-FDG PET/CT in management of high-grade salivary gland malignancies. *J Nucl Med.* 2007;48:1237-1244.

Johansen J, Buus S, Loft A, et al. Prospective study of 18FDG-PET in the detection and management of patients with lymph node metastases to the neck from an unknown primary tumor. Results from the DAHANCA-13, study. *Head Neck.* 2008;30:471-478.

Johansen J, Eigtved A, Buchwald C, Theilgaard SA, Hansen HS. Implication of 18F-fluoro-2-deoxy-D-glucose positron emission tomography on management of carcinoma of unknown primary in the head and neck: a Danish cohort study. *Laryngoscope.* 2002;112:2009-2014.

Johnson JT. Carcinoma of the larynx: selective approach to the management of cervical lymphatics. *Ear Nose Throat J.* 1994;73(5):303-305.

Jones J, Farag I, Hain SF, et al. Positron emission tomography (PET) in the management of oro-pharyngeal cancer. *Eur J Surg Oncol.* 2005;31:170-176.

Kao J, et al. The diagnostic and prognostic utility of positron emission tomography/computed tomography-based follow-up after radiotherapy for head and neck cancer. *Cancer.* 2009;115(19):4586-4594.

Kau RJ, Alexiou C, Laubenbacher C, Werner M, Schwaiger M, Arnold W. Lymph node detection of head and neck squamous cell carcinomas by positron emission tomography with fluorodeoxyglucose F 18 in a routine clinical setting. *Arch Otolaryngol Head Neck Surg.* 1999;125:1322-1328.

Keberle M, Strobel P, Relic A. Simultaneous pleomorphic adenomas of the parotid and of the submandibular gland. *Fortschr Rontgenstr.* 2005;177:436-438.

Kim MR, Roh JL, Kim JS, et al. Utility of 18F-fluorodeoxyglucose positron emission tomography in the preoperative staging of squamous cell carcinoma of the oropharynx. *Eur J Surg Oncol.* 2007;33:633-638.

Kim SY, Roh JL, Kim JS, et al. Utility of FDG PET in patients with squamous cell carcinomas of the oral cavity. *Eur J Surg Oncol.* 2008;34:208-215.

Kim SY, Roh JL, Yeo NK, et al. Combined 18F-fluorodeoxyglucose-positron emission tomography and computed tomography as a primary screening method for detecting second primary cancers and distant metastases in patients with head and neck cancer. *Ann Oncol.* 2007;18:1698-1703.

Kitagawa Y, Nishizawa S, Sano K, et al. Prospective comparison of 18F-FDG PET with conventional imaging modalities (MRI, CT, and 67Ga scintigraphy) in assessment of combined intraarterial chemotherapy and radiotherapy for head and neck carcinoma. *J Nucl Med.* 2003;44:198-206.

Koshy M, Paulino AC, Howell R, et al. F-18 FDGPET-CT fusion in radiotherapy treatment planning for head and neck cancer. *Head Neck.* 2005;27:494-502.

Kothari P, Randhawa PS, Farrell R. Role of tonsillectomy in the search for a squamous cell carcinoma from an unknown primary in the head and neck. *Br J Oral Maxillofac Surg.* 2008;46:283-287.

Krabbe CA, Dijkstra PU, Pruim J, et al. FDG PET in oral and oropharyngeal cancer. Value for confirmation of N0 neck and detection of occult metastases. *Oral Oncol.* 2008;44:31-36.

Kwee TC, Kwee RM. Combined FDG-PET/CT for the detection of unknown primary tumors: systematic review and meta-analysis. *Eur Radiol.* 2009;19:731-744.

Kyzas P, Evangelou E, Denaxa-Kyza D, Ioannidis J. 18 F-fluorodeoxyglucose positron emission tomography to evaluate cervical node metastases in patients with head and neck squamous cell carcinoma: A meta-analysis. *J Natl Cancer Inst.* 2008;100:712-720.

Laubenbacher C, Saumweber D, Wagner-Manslau C, et al. Comparison of fluorine-18-fluorodeoxyglucose PET, MRI, endoscopy for staging head and neck squamous-cell carcinomas. *J Nucl Med.* 1995;36:1747-1757.

Lea J, Bachar G, Sawka AM, Lakra DC, Gilbert RW, Irish JC, Brown DH, Gullane PJ, Goldstein DP. Metastases to level IIb in squamous cell carcinoma of the oral cavity: a systematic review and meta-analysis. *Head Neck.* 2010;32:184-190.

Leemans CR, Tiwari R, Nauta JJP, van der Waal DDS, Snow GB. Recurrence at the primary site in head and neck cancer and the significance of neck lymph node metastases as a prognostic factor. *Cancer.* 1994;73:187-190.

Lim YC, Song MH, Kim SC, Kim KM, Choi EC. Preserving level IIb lymph nodes in elective supraomohyoid neck dissection for oral cavity squamous cell carcinoma. *Arch Otolaryngol Head Neck Surg.* 2004;130:1088-1091.

Lin DT, Cohen SM, Coppit GL, Burkey BB. Squamous cell carcinoma of the oropharynx and hypopharynx. *Otolaryngol Clin North Am.* 2005;38:59-74.

Lin FY, Genden EM, Lawson WL, Som P, Kostakoglu L. High uptake in schneiderian papillomas of the maxillary sinus on positron-emission tomography using fluorodeoxyglucose. *AJNR Am J Neuroradiol.* 2009;30:428-430.

Lin K, Patel SG, Chu PY, et al. Second primary malignancy of the aerodigestive tract in patients treated for cancer of the oral cavity and larynx. *Head Neck.* 2005;27(12):1042-1048.

Ljumanovic R, Langendijk JA, Schenk B, et al. Supraglottic carcinoma treated with curative radiation therapy: identification of prognostic groups with MR imaging. *Radiology.* 2004;232(2):440-448.

Loevner LA, Yousem DM, Montone KT, et al. Can radiologists accurately predict preepiglottic space invasion with MR imaging? *AJR Am J Roentgenol.* 1997;169(6):1681-1687.

Loh KS, Brown DH, Baker JT, et al. A rational approach to pulmonary screening in newly diagnosed head and neck cancer. *Head Neck.* 2005;27(11):990-994.

Lonneux M, Lawson G, Ide C, Bausart R, Remacle M, Pauwels S. Positron emission tomography with fluorodeoxyglucose for suspected head and neck tumor recurrence in the symptomatic patient. *Laryngoscope.* 2000;110:1493-1497.

Magrin J, Kowalski L. Bilateral neck dissection: results in 193 cases. *J Surg Oncol.* 2000;75:232-240.

Marioni G, Marchese-Ragona R, Cartei G, et al. Current opinion in diagnosis and treatment of laryngeal carcinoma. *Cancer Treat Rev.* 2006;32(7):504-515.

Martin RC, Fulham M, Shannon KF, et al. Accuracy of positron emission tomography in the evaluation of patients treated with chemoradiotherapy for mucosal head and neck cancer. *Head Neck.* 2009 Feb;31(2):244-250.

Marur S, Forastiere AA. Head and neck cancer: changing epidemiology, diagnosis, and treatment. *Mayo Clin Proc.* 2008 Apr;83(4):489-501.

McGuirt WF, Williams 3rd DW, Keyes Jr JW, et al. A comparative diagnostic study of head and neck nodal metastases using positron emission tomography. *Laryngoscope.* 1995;105:373-375.

McLeod NM, Jess A, Anand R, Tilley E, Higgins B, Brennan PA. Role of chest CT in staging of oropharyngeal cancer: a systematic review. *Head Neck.* 2009 Apr;31(4):548-555.

Mashberg A, Meyers H. Anatomical site and size of 222 early asymptomatic oral squamous cell carcinomas. *Cancer.* 1976;37:2149-2157.

Medini E, Medini I, Lee CK, Gapany M, Levitt SH. Curative radiotherapy for stage II-III squamous cell carcinoma of the glottic larynx. *Am J Clin Oncol.* 1998;21:302-305.

Mendenhall WM, Mancuso AA, Parsons JT, et al. Diagnostic evaluation of squamous cell carcinoma metastatic to cervical lymph nodes from an unknown head and neck primary site. *Head Neck.* 1998;20:739-744.

Merritt RM, Williams MF, James TH, et al. Detection of cervical metastasis: a meta-analysis comparing computed tomography with physical examination. *Arch Otolaryngol Head Neck Surg.* 1997;123(2):149-152.

Merkx MA, Boustahji AH, Kaanders JH, et al. A half-yearly chest radiograph for early detection of lung cancer following oral cancer. *Int J Oral Maxillofac Surg.* 2002;31(4):378-382.

Miller FR, Hussey D, Beeram M, et al. Positron emission tomography in the management of unknown primary head and neck carcinoma. *Arch Otolaryngol Head Neck Surg.* 2005;131:626-629.

Miller FR, Karnad AB, Eng T, et al. Management of the unknown primary carcinoma: long-term follow-up on a negative PET scan and negative panendoscopy. *Head Neck.* 2008;30:28-34.

Million RR, Cassisi NJ, Mancuso AA. Oral cavity. In: Million RR, Cassisi NJ, eds. *Management of head and neck cancer: a multidisciplinary approach.* Philadelphia: Lippincott; 1994:321-400.

Million RR, Cassisi NJ, Mancuso AA. The oropharynx. In: Million RR, Cassisi NJ, eds. *Management of head and neck cancer: a multidisciplinary approach.* Philadelphia: JB Lippincott; 1994:402-431.

Minn H, Lapela M, Klemi PJ, et al. Prediction of survival with fluorine-18-fluoro-deoxyglucose and PET in head and neck cancer. *J Nucl Med.* 1997;38:1907-1911.

Minn H, Paul R, Ahonen A. Evaluation of treatment response to radiotherapy in head and neck cancer with fluorine-18 fluorodeoxyglucose. *J Nucl Med.* 1988 Sep;29(9):1521-1525.

Moose BD, Greven KM. Definitive radiation management for carcinoma of the glottic larynx. *Otolaryngol Clin North Am.* 1997;30:131-143.

Mukherji SK. Pharynx. In: Som PM, Curtin HD, eds. *Head and neck imaging.* St. Louis: Mosby; 2003:1485-1489.

Mukherji SK, Bradford CR. Controversies: is there a role for positron-emission tomographic CT in the initial staging of head and neck squamous cell carcinoma? *AJNR Am J Neuroradiol.* 2006;27:243-245.

Mukherji SK, Pillsbury HR, Castillo M. Imaging squamous cell carcinomas of the upper aerodigestive tract: what clinicians need to know. *Radiology.* 1997;205(3):629-646.

Murakami R, Furusawa M, Baba Y, et al. Dynamic helical CT of T1 and T2 glottic carcinomas: predictive value for local control with radiation therapy. *AJNR Am J Neuroradiol.* 2000;21(7):1320-1326.

Murakami R, Uozumi H, Hirai T, et al. Impact of FDG-PET/CT imaging on nodal staging for head-and-neck squamous cell carcinoma. *Int J Radiat Oncol Biol Phys.* 2007;68:377-382.

Nabili V, Zaia B, Blackwell KE, et al. Positron emission tomography: poor sensitivity for occult tonsillar cancer. *Am J Otolaryngol.* 2007;28:153-157.

Nahmias C, Carlson ER, Duncan LD, et al. Positron emission tomography/computerized tomography (PET/CT) scanning for preoperative staging of patients with oral/head and neck cancer. *J Oral Maxillofac Surg.* 2007;65:2524-2535.

Nakagawa T, Yamada M, Suzuki Y. 18F-FDG uptake in reactive neck lymph nodes of oral cancer: relationship to lymphoid follicles. *J Nucl Med.* 2008;49:1053-1059.

Nakamoto Y, Tatsumi M, Hammoud D, Cohade C, Osman MM, Wahl RL. Normal FDG distribution patterns in the head and neck: PET/CT evaluation. *Radiology.* 2005;234:879-885.

Ng SH, Chan SC, Liao CT, et al. Distant metastases and synchronous second primary tumors in patients with newly diagnosed oropharyngeal and hypopharyngeal carcinomas: evaluation of (18)F-FDG PET and extended-field multi-detector row CT. *Neuroradiology.* 2008;50:969-979.

Ng SH, Yen TC, Chang JT, Chan SC, Ko SF, Wang HM, Lee LY, Kang CJ, Wong AM, Liao CT. Prospective study of [18F]fluorodeoxyglucose positron emission tomography and computed tomography and magnetic resonance imaging in oral cavity squamous cell carcinoma with palpably negative neck. *J Clin Oncol.* 2006;24:4371-4376.

Ng SH, Yen TC, Liao CT. 18F-FDG PET and CT/MRI in oral cavity squamous cell carcinoma: A prospective study of 124, patients with histologic correlation. *J Nucl Med.* 2005;46:1136-1143.

Oe A, Kawabe J, Torii K, et al. Detection of local residual tumor after laryngeal cancer treatment using FDG-PET. *Ann Nucl Med.* 2007;21(1):9-13.

Ong SC, Schoder H, Leen Y, et al. Clinical utility of 18F-FDG PET/CT in assessing the neck after concurrent chemoradiotherapy for Locoregional advanced head and neck cancer. *J Nucl Med.* 2008 Apr;49(4):532-540.

Padovani D, Aimoni C, Zucchetta P, et al. 18-FDG PET in the diagnosis of laterocervical metastases from occult carcinoma. *Eur Arch Otorhinolaryngol.* 2009;266:267-271.

Parsons JT, Mendenhall WM, Stringer SP, Cassisi NJ. T4 laryngeal carcinoma: radiotherapy alone with surgery reserved for salvage. *Int J Radiat Oncol Biol Phys.* 1998;40:549-552.

Parsons JT, Mendenhall WM, Stringer SP, et al. Squamous cell carcinoma of the oropharynx:surgery, radiation therapy, or both. *Cancer.* 2002;94:2967-2980.

Pavlidis N, Briasoulis E, Hainsworth J, et al. Diagnostic and therapeutic management of cancer of an unknown primary. *Eur J Cancer.* 2003;39:1990-2005.

Pentenero M, Cistaro A, Brusa M, et al. Accuracy of 18F-FDG-PET/CT for staging of oral squamous cell carcinoma. *Head Neck.* 2008;30:1488-1496.

Perlow A, Bui C, Shreve P, Sundgren PC, Teknos TN, Mukherji SK. High incidence of chest malignancy detected by FDG PET in patients suspected of recurrent squamous cell carcinoma of the upper aerodigestive tract. *J Comput Assist Tomogr.* 2004 Sep-Oct;28(5):704-709.

Pfister DG, Laurie SA, Weinstein GS, et al. American Society of Clinical Oncology clinical practice guideline for the use of larynx—preservation strategies in the treatment of laryngeal cancer. *J Clin Oncol.* 2006;24(22):3693-3704.

Pohar S, Brown R, Newman N, Koniarczyk M, Hsu J, Feiglin D. What does PET imaging add to conventional staging of head and neck cancer patients? *Int J Radiat Oncol Biol Phys.* 2007;68:383-387.

Porceddu SV, Jarmolowski E, Hicks RJ, et al. Utility of positron emission tomography for the detection of disease in residual neck nodes after (chemo)-radiotherapy in head and neck cancer. *Head Neck.* 2005;27:175-181.

Quon A, Fischbein NJ, McDougall IR, et al. Clinical role of 18F-FDG PET/CT in the management of squamous cell carcinoma of the head and neck and thyroid carcinoma. *J Nucl Med.* 2007 Jan;48(Suppl 1):58S-67S.

Razfar A, Heron DE, Branstetter 4th BF, et al. Positron emission tomography-computed tomography adds to the management of salivary gland malignancies. *Laryngoscope.* 2010;120:734-738.

Roh JL, Kim JS, Lee JH, et al. Utility of combined (18)F-fluorodeoxyglucose-positron emission tomography and computed tomography in patients with cervical metastases from unknown primary tumors. *Oral Oncol.* 2009;45:218-224.

Roh JL, Pae KH, Choi SH, et al. 2-[18F]-Fluoro-2-deoxy-d-glucose positron emission tomography as guidance for primary treatment in patients with advanced-stage resectable squamous cell carcinoma of the larynx and hypopharynx. *Eur J Surg Oncol.* 2007;33:790-795.

Roh JL, Ryu CH, Kim JS, et al. Clinical significance of intrathoracic lesions detected by 18F-fluorodeoxyglucose positron emission tomography in the management of patients with head and neck cancer. *Oral Oncol.* 2007;43:757-763.

Roh JL, Yeo NK, Kim JS, et al. Utility of 2-[18F] fluoro-2-deoxy-D-glucose positron emission tomography and positron emission tomography/computed tomography imaging in the preoperative staging of head and neck cancer. *Oral Oncol.* 2007;43:887-893.

Ryan WR, Fee Jr WE, Le QT, Pinto HA. Positron-emission tomography for surveillance of head and neck cancer. *Laryngoscope.* 2005 Apr;115(4):645-650.

Schmid DT, Stoeckli SJ, Bandhauer F, et al. Impact of positron emission tomography on the initial staging and therapy in locoregional advanced squamous cell carcinoma of the head and neck. *Laryngoscope.* 2003 May;113(5):888-891.

Schöder H, Carlson DL, Kraus DH, Stambuk HE, Gönen M, Erdi YE, Yeung HW, Huvos AG, Shah JP, Larson SM, Wong RJ. 18F-FDG PET/CT for detecting nodal metastases in patients with oral cancer staged N0 by clinical examination and CT/MRI. *J Nucl Med.* 2006;47:755-762.

Schöder H, Fury M, Lee N, Kraus D. PET Monitoring of Therapy Response in Head and Neck Squamous Cell Carcinoma. *J Nucl Med.* 50 (Suppl 1) 74S-88S.

Schoder H, Yeung HW. Positron emission imaging of head and neck cancer, including thyroid cancer. *Semin Nucl Med.* 2004;34:180-197.

Schoder H, Yeung HW, Gonen M, et al. Head and neck cancer: clinical usefulness and accuracy of PET/CT image fusion. *Radiology.* 2004;231(1):65-72.

Schroeder U, Dietlein M, Wittekindt C, et al. Is there a need for positron emission tomography imaging to stage the N0 neck in T1-T2, squamous cell carcinoma of the oral cavity or oropharynx? *Ann Otol Rhinol Laryngol.* 2008;117:854-863.

Schwartz DL, Ford E, Rajendran J, et al. FDG-PET/CT imaging for preradiotherapy staging of head-and-neck squamous cell carcinoma. *Int J Radiat Oncol Biol Phys.* 2005;61:129-136.

Schwartz DL, Rajendran J, Jueh B, et al. FDG-PET prediction of head and neck squamous cell cancer outcomes. *Arch Otolaryngol Head Neck Surg.* 2004;130:1361-1367.

Schwartz DL, Rajendran J, Jueh B, et al. Staging of head and neck squamous cell cancer with extended-field FDG-PET. *Arch Otolaryngol Head Neck Surg.* 2003;129:1173-1178.

Scott AM, Gunawardana DH, Bartholomeusz D, et al. PET changes management and improves prognostic stratification in patients with head and neck cancer: results of a multicenter prospective study. *J Nucl Med.* 2008;49:1593-1600.

Senft A, de Bree R, Hoekstra OS, et al. Screening for distant metastases in head and neck cancer patients by chest CT or whole body FDG-PET: a prospective multicenter trial. *Radiother Oncol.* 2008 May;87(2):221-229.

Sessions DG, Lenox J, Spector GJ, et al. Analysis of treatment results for base of tongue cancer. *Laryngoscope.* 2003;113:1252-1261.

Shah JP, Medina JE, Shaha AR, et al. Cervical lymph node metastasis. *Curr Probl Surg.* 1993;30(3):273-344.

Shah JP. Patterns of cervical lymph node metastasis from squamous carcinomas of the upper aerodigestive tract. *Am J Surg.* 1990;160(4):405-409.

Shimamoto H, Tatsumi M, Kakimoto N, et al. 18F-FDG accumulation in the oral cavity is associated with periodontal disease and apical periodontitis: an initial demonstration on PET/CT. *Ann Nucl Med.* 2008;22:587-593.

Sigg MB, Steinert H, Grätz K, Hugenin P, Stoeckli S, Eyrich GK. Staging of head and neck tumors: FDG PET compared with physical examination and conventional imaging modalities. *J Oral Maxillofac Surg.* 2003;61(9):1022-1029.

Smoker W. The oral cavity. In: Som P, Curtin H, eds. *Head and Neck Imaging.* St. Louis: Mosby; 2003:1377-1464.

Som PM. Lymph nodes of the neck. *Radiology.* 1987;165(3):593-600.

Spector JG. Distant metastases from laryngeal and hypopharyngeal cancer. *ORL J Otorhinolaryngol Relat Spec.* 2001;63(4):224-228.

Spector JG, Sessions DG, Chao KS, et al. Stage 1 (T1N0M0) squamous cell carcinoma of the laryngeal glottis: therapeutic results and voice preservation. *Head Neck.* 1999;21:707-717.

Spiro RH. Distant metastasis in adenoid cystic carcinoma of salivary origin. *Am J Surg.* 1997;174:495-498.

Spiro RH, Guillamondegui Jr O, Paulino AF, et al. Pattern of invasion and margin assessment inpatients with oral tongue cancer. *Head Neck.* 1999;21(5):408-413.

Spiro RH, Huvos AG, Wong GY, et al. Predictive value of tumor thickness in squamous carcinomaconfined to the tongue and floor of the mouth. *Am J Surg.* 1986;152(4):345-350.

Stalpers LJ, van Vierzen PB, Brouns JJ, et al. The role of yearly chest radiography in the early detection of lung cancer following oral cancer. *Int J Oral Maxillofac Surg.* 1989;18(2):99-103.

Stambuk HE, et al. Oral cavity and oropharynx tumors. *Radiol Clin North Am.* 2007;45(1):1-20.

Stevens MH, Harnsberger HR, Mancuso AA, et al. Computed tomography of cervical lymph nodes: staging and management of head and neck cancer. *Arch Otolaryngol.* 1985;111(11):735-739.

Stoeckli SJ, Steinert H, Pfaltz M, Schmid S. Is there a role for positron emission tomography with 18F-fluorodeoxyglucose in the initial staging of nodal negative oral and oropharyngeal squamous cell carcinoma. *Head Neck.* 2002;24:345-349.

Stokkel MP, Bongers V, Hordijk GJ, van Rijk PP. FDG positron emission tomography in head and neck cancer: pitfall or pathology? *Clin Nucl Med.* 1999 Dec;24(12):950-954.

Strobel K, Haerle SK, Stoeckli SJ, et al. Head and neck squamous cell carcinoma (HNSCC)–detection of synchronous primaries with 18F-FDG-PET/CT. *Eur J Nucl Med Mol Imaging.* 2009;36:919-927.

Suzuki H, Hasegawa Y, Terada A, et al. FDG-PET predicts survival and distant metastasis in oral squamous cell carcinoma. *Oral Oncol.* 2009;45:569-573.

Syms MJ, Birkmire-Peters DP, Holtel MR. Incidence of carcinoma in incidental tonsil asymmetry. *Laryngoscope.* 2000;110:1807-1810.

Teknos TN, Rosenthal EL, Lee D, et al. Positron emission tomography in the evaluation of stage III and IV head and neck cancer. *Head Neck.* 2001;23:1056-1060.

Terhaard CH, Bongers V, van Rijk PP, Hordijk GJ. F-18-fluoro-deoxy-glucose positron-emission tomography scanning in detection of local recurrence after radiotherapy for laryngeal/ pharyngeal cancer. *Head Neck.* 2001;23:933-941.

Terhaard CH, Hordijk GJ, Broek van den P, et al. T3 laryngeal cancer: a retrospective study of the Dutch Head and Neck Oncology Cooperative Group: study design and general results. *Clin Otolaryngol.* 1992;17:393-402.

Thekdi AA, Ferris RL. Diagnostic assessment of laryngeal cancer. *Otolaryngol Clin North Am.* 2002;35(5):953-969.

Thompson LD, Heffner DK. The clinical importance of cystic squamous cell carcinomas in the neck: a study of 136 cases. *Cancer.* 1998;82(5):944-956.

Tucker R, Coel M, Ko J, et al. Impact of fluorine-18, fluorodeoxyglucose positron emission tomography on patient management: first year's experience in a clinical center. *J Clin Oncol.* 2001;19:2504-2508.

van den Brekel MW, Castelijns JA, Stel HV, et al. Modern imaging techniques and ultrasound guided aspiration cytology for the assessment of neck node metastases: a prospective comparative study. *Eur Arch Otorhinolaryngol.* 1993;250(1):11-17.

van den Brekel MW, Runne RW, Smeele LE, et al. Assessment of tumor invasion into the mandible: the value of different imaging techniques. *Eur Radiol.* 1998;8:1552-1557.

Vegers JW, Snow GB, van der Waal I. Squamous cell carcinoma of the buccal mucosa: a review of 85 cases. *Arch Otolaryngol.* 1979;105:192-195.

Veit-Haibach P, Luczak C, Wanke I, et al. TNM staging with FDG-PET/CT in patients with primary head and neck cancer. *Eur J Nucl Med Mol Imaging.* 2007;34:1953-1962.

Wang YF, et al. Positron emission tomography in surveillance of head and neck squamous cell carcinoma after definitive chemoradiotherapy. *Head Neck.* 2009;31(4):442-451.

Wax MK, Myers LL, Gabalski EC, Husain S, Gona JM, Nabi H. Positron emission tomography in the evaluation of synchronous lung lesions in patients with untreated head and neck cancer. *Arch Otolaryngol Head Neck Surg.* 2002 Jun;128(6):703-707.

Wensing BM, Vogel WV, Marres HA, et al. FDG-PET in the clinically negative neck in oral squamous cell carcinoma [erratum in Laryngoscope.2006;116(7, Pt 1):1302]. *Laryngoscope.* 2006;116:809-813.

Wester DJ, Whiteman ML, Singer S, Bowen BC, Goodwin WJ. Imaging of the postoperative neck with emphasis on surgical flaps and their complications. *AJR Am J Roentgenol.* 1995 Apr;164(4):989-993.

Wong RJ, Lin DT, Schoder H, et al. Diagnostic and prognostic value of [(18)F] fluorodeoxyglucose positron emission tomography for recurrent head and neck squamous cell carcinoma. *J ClinOncol.* 2002;20(20):4199-4208.

Yamazaki Y, Saitoh M, Notani K, et al. Assessment of cervical lymph node metastases using FDG-PET in patients with head and neck cancer. *Ann Nucl Med.* 2008;22:177-184.

Yau YY, Samman N, Yeung RW, et al. Positron emission tomography/computed tomography true fusion imaging in clinical head and neck oncology: early experience. *J Oral Maxillofac Surg.* 2005;63:479-486.

Yeager LB, Grillone GA. Organ preservation surgery for intermediate size (T2 and T3) laryngeal cancer. *Otolaryngol Clin North Am.* 2005;38(1):11-20:vii.

Yousem DM, Gad K, Tufano RP. Resectability issues with head and neck cancer. *AJNR Am J Neuroradiol.* 2006;27(10):2024-2036.

Yousem DM, Hatabu H, Hurst RW, et al. Carotid artery invasion by head and neck masses: prediction with MR imaging. *Radiology.* 1995;195:715-720.

Zanation AM, Sutton DK, Couch ME, et al. Use, accuracy and implications for patient management of [18F]-2-fluorodeoxyglucose-positron emission/computerized tomography for head and neck tumors. *Laryngoscope.* 2005;115:1186-1190.

Zbären P, Becker M, Läng H. Pretherapeutic staging of hypopharyngeal carcinoma. Clinical findings, computed tomography, and magnetic resonance imaging compared with histopathologic evaluation. *Arch Otolaryngol Head Neck Surg.* 1997 Sep;123(9):908-913.

Zbaren P, Becker M, Lang H. Pretherapeutic staging of laryngeal carcinoma. Clinical findings, computed tomography, and magnetic resonance imaging compared with histopathologic evaluzation. *Cancer.* 1996;77:1263-1273.

Zimmer LA, Branstetter BF, Nayak JV, Johnson JT. Current use of 18F-fluorodeoxyglucose positron emission tomography and combined positron emission tomography and computed tomography in squamous cell carcinoma of the head and neck. *Laryngoscope.* 2005 Nov;115(11):2029-2034.

SECTION II

PROCEDURES

CHAPTER 5
Diagnostic Angiography
Stephan Meckel and Stephan G. Wetzel

■ INTRODUCTION

In 1927, the intriguing Portuguese neurologist and politician Egas Moniz performed the first diagnostic cerebral angiogram in a 48-year-old male patient with postencephalitic Parkinson disease. He injected a 70% solution of strontium bromide into the surgically exposed carotid artery and produced a series of four angiographic images. The patient died 8 hours later of thromboembolic complications. Since then, the art and science of cerebral angiography have progressively developed as a result of improvements in imaging capabilities and technical equipment and safer contrast media. In the setting of constantly improving, utterly noninvasive computed tomographic angiography (CTA) and magnetic resonance angiography (MRA) capabilities, cerebral catheter angiography remains an important tool for evaluation of the cerebral vasculature today, as in the past. Clearly, if equivalent information can be obtained by noninvasive means, then this method is not indicated. However, even though today it is seldom the first study of choice for imaging of central nervous system (CNS), diagnostic neuroangiography is still considered the reference standard for imaging of a variety of neurovascular diseases that affect the intracranial and extracranial vasculature. Apart from its capability of vessel selective or superselective imaging, the main reason is the unique spatial and time resolution of diagnostic cerebral angiography that still is unbeaten by all current noninvasive means in the armamentarium for neurovascular imaging. Despite technologic advances, a cerebral angiogram still carries a low risk of potentially devastating permanent neurologic damage; hence, this procedure should be undertaken only for strong indications by trained operators. Such training should not only comprise technical competence but also a sound knowledge of relevant neurovascular anatomy and pathology.

■ ANGIOGRAPHIC TECHNIQUE

Aortic Arch

Problem Solving: How and What Are the Reasons for Imaging the Aortic Arch?
The arch aortography is only infrequently required in cerebral angiography if proximal stenosis of the great supraaortic arteries in suspected (e.g., in Takayasu arteritis, dissecting aneurysm, and neurofibromatosis). It usually is performed using a 5F or 6F pigtail catheter that has multiple side holes and an end hole. Therefore, vigorous and frequent flushing is required. The catheter end is placed a few centimeters proximal to the origin of the brachiocephalic trunk with the pigtail loop in the coronal plane. Contrast injections are performed using a power injector (rate 20–30 ml/s, total volume 40–50 ml) and filming is performed in the left anterior oblique projection (30–40 degrees).

Common Carotid Arteries

What Are the Most Optimal Techniques/ Catheters for Accessing the Common Carotid Arteries Routinely and in Difficult Situations?
Selective catheterization of the common carotid arteries in persons younger than 40 years usually can be accomplished using small-diameter standard cerebral catheters (4–5.5F) with simple shapes (e.g., 5F Berenstein/ UCSF-II, Cordis, Bridgewater, NJ, USA) in combination with soft-tipped 0.035-inch guidewires (e.g., Bentson, Cook Medical Inc., Bloomington, IN, USA). In older patients, vessel elongation, tortuosity, and dilatation may require the use of larger-diameter and hence stiffer catheters (e.g., a 7F Berenstein) in combination with stiffer guidewires (e.g., hydrophilic coated 0.035-inch Terumo Glidewire, Terumo Medical Corporation, Somerset, NJ, USA). Alternatively, a reverse-curve catheter may be used. However, selective catheterization beyond the common carotid bifurcation is difficult using this catheter and therefore is not generally recommended.

The basic catheterization technique using a standard cerebral catheter consists of bringing the catheter and inserted guidewire tip to tip within the proximal aortic arch with the tip usually facing downward. Counterclockwise rotation and simultaneous slow backward pulling applied so that the catheter tip is directed cephalad usually will result in engagement of the great vessel ostia. The novice angiographer must be trained on this maneuver, otherwise the applied torque will build up in the shaft of the catheter and then be released suddenly into the tip, causing the catheter to make 360-degree resolutions. For more selective catheterization, the guidewire is then advanced to approximately the level of C7 (above the T1 transverse process), and the catheter is passed over the immobilized guidewire. Advancing the catheter all the way to the guidewire tip should be avoided because this increases the likelihood of vessel dissection or vasospasm. In older patients, it may be necessary to advance a greater length of guidewire to provide sufficient support for catheter advancement, and the tip of the guidewire should be guided fluoroscopically into the external carotid artery (ECA). The guidewire is then withdrawn and the catheter immediately flushed. Before selective catheterization of an internal carotid artery (ICA), the common carotid artery should be routinely injected to view the carotid bifurcation. These views can be documented as either saved roadmap images or an angiographic series.

In cases of a bovine-type arch branching pattern, selective catheterization of the left common carotid artery might require a catheter with a relatively acute angled primary curve or tip such as a 7F Berenstein or a reverse curve catheter.

With increasing age and in the presence of hypertension, unfolding and elongation of the aorta result in the great arteries arising proximal to the arch apex, making selective catheterization with standard 4F or 5F cerebral catheters (e.g., Berenstein) more difficult. This may require the use of reverse-curve catheters such as the Simmons 2/Sidewinder 2 (Angiodynamics, Latham, NY, USA). Various techniques for re-forming their distal shape prior to vessel selection have been described. However, counterclockwise rotation and forward advancement with the catheter tip against the apex of the arch and the guidewire proximal to the major bend of the catheter usually is successful. Once the catheter tip has engaged the vessel ostium, advancement of the tip is accomplished by withdrawing the proximal end. The reverse-curve catheter also may be preferred for evaluation of carotid bifurcation disease because only a short length of leading guidewire is required, thus reducing the likelihood of guidewire impingement against an atherosclerotic plaque.

Standard projections for demonstrating the carotid bifurcation are anteroposterior (AP) and lateral. In cases of suspected ICA stenosis, both oblique views are often necessary to display plaques in their entirety and to detect the maximum area of stenosis. For the bifurcation, a lower injection rate (5–8 ml/s, total volume 5–8 ml) than for intracranial circulation (6–8 ml/s, total volume 7–10 ml) is applied because the distal runoff does not require visualization. A suitable filming rate is four images per second for 4 seconds, followed by 1 image per second for 8 seconds. In the case of presumed ICA occlusion, prolonged filming is necessary, otherwise delayed faint anterograde opacification of the cervical ICA may be missed—a "string sign" of a critical ICA stenosis. Delayed opacification of the carotid siphon does not necessarily imply patency of the cervical ICA, because this is usually due to the ipsilateral ECA collateral vessels anastomosing either directly with the carotid siphon or with the ipsilateral ophthalmic artery (OA).

Internal Carotid Arteries

Problem Solving: What Are the Most Optimal Techniques/Catheters for Accessing the Internal Carotid Arteries Routinely and in Difficult Situations?

Selective catheterization of the ICAs should be performed only by neuroangiographers with sufficient experience and skill. Vessel damage and/or thromboembolism can result in permanent neurologic deficit and even death. Meticulous technique and scrupulous attention to catheter flushing are requisite if serious complications are to be prevented. In young female patients and particularly those with a history of migraine headaches, the likelihood of iatrogenic vasospasm, even with gentle guidewire and catheter manipulations, is increased; therefore, prophylactic application of topical nitropaste may be considered. If significant atherosclerotic bifurcation disease or evidence of arterial dissection is present, then selective ICA catheterization is best avoided. It is generally advised to perform selective ICA catheterization under digital roadmap guidance, particularly if kinking of the proximal or coiling of the distal cervical ICA (tonsillar loop) is present. The tip of the guidewire should be advanced no further than the C2 level because the relatively fixed petrous segment is more prone to dissection. Ideally it should be positioned within a relatively straight vessel segment so that its distal curve conforms to that of a similar curve of the surrounding vessel in order to minimize trauma to vessel intima, as occurs with subintimal injection or dislodgement of atheromatous plaque.

A contrast injection rate of 5 to 7 ml/s for a total of 7 to 9 ml usually is sufficient; however, this rate and volume need to be reduced in the presence of downstream stenosis (e.g., cerebral vasospasm or Moyamoya disease) or alternatively may need to be increased with high-flow states such as arteriovenous malformations or fistulae. Preliminary assessment of intracranial flow with hand injection of contrast is useful if these conditions are suspected or are being investigated. Standard intracranial carotid views include lateral and AP projections (petrous ridges projected midway between orbital roof and floor). A suitable filming rate is three to four images per second for 4 to 5 seconds, followed by one image per second for 7 seconds. The initial filming rate is increased when investigating high-flow vascular malformations.

Vertebral Arteries

Problem Solving: What Are the Most Optimal Techniques/Catheters for Accessing the Vertebral Arteries Routinely and in Difficult Situations?

The vertebral arteries (VAs) usually are the first branches of the subclavian arteries. Prior to vertebral angiography, any previous magnetic resonance imaging (MRI)/MRA/CTA results should be reviewed and the dominant VA indentified. A roadmap image of the subclavian artery should be generally obtained prior to selective catheterization. If there is any suspicion of a VA origin stenosis, then formal angiography is performed. In contradistinction to the common carotid arteries, atherosclerotic narrowing is common at the origins of the VAs. The VA origin usually is best demonstrated using a mild cranial and contralateral oblique projection (Figure 5-1). If a significant stenosis is confirmed, then vertebral angiography is performed using subclavian artery contrast injection (6–8 ml/s, total volume 12–16 ml) with an inflated pressure cuff on the ipsilateral arm. We generally perform selective catheterization of the VAs using digital roadmap guidance. The proximal VA often is tortuous.

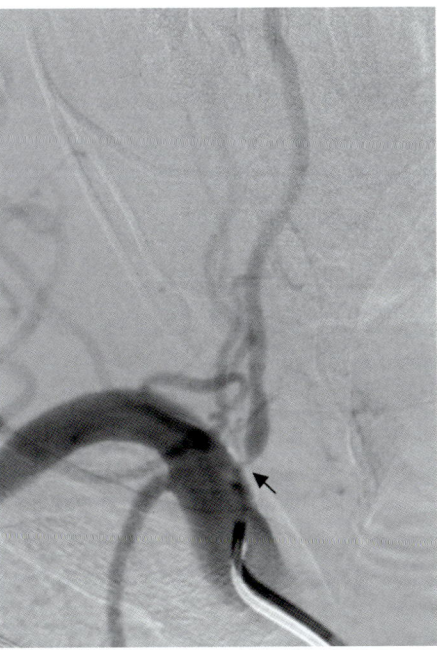

Figure 5-1 Right subclavian artery angiogram, mild Towne and contralateral oblique projection, depicting typical atherosclerotic high-grade stenosis (pinhole) at the origin of the right vertebral artery (*small black arrow*). (Courtesy Dr. Tejinder Pal Singh, Perth.)

In this situation the guidewire and catheter are not passed beyond a sharp bend. Otherwise, the guidewire and catheter usually are not passed beyond the C4 level because the VAs are smaller and more prone to iatrogenic vasospasm than are the carotids. Evaluation of the cervical segment of the VA can be performed in the ipsilateral oblique plane (4–6 ml/s, total volume 4–6 ml). Standard intracranial views include the Towne AP view (petrous ridges projected above the orbital roofs) and the lateral projection. A Waters AP view (petrous ridges projected at the base of the maxillary antra) may be useful for better demonstration of the basilar artery (BA) and its termination (Figure 5-2). The contrast injection rate depends on the vessel caliber (4–6 ml/s, total volume 6–9 ml). The film acquisition rate is three images per second for 4 seconds, followed by one image per second for 7 to 8 seconds. With selective angiography it usually is possible to obtain reflux into the contralateral posterior inferior cerebellar artery (PICA; Figure 5-2, *B*). Prior to any mechanical contrast injection, intracranial runoff should be assessed with preliminary hand injection, because hypoplasia of the distal nondominant VA occurs at a frequency of 5% to 10%.

Basic Safety Advice

What Are the Most Optimal Techniques for Preventing Air Bubbles and Thrombus Formation in Catheters?

Once in the body, a catheter should be flushed using a continuous irrigation system or every 90 to 120 seconds (on average) before and after each wire exchange. It also should be flushed just prior to connecting to a power injector and immediately after disconnecting from a power injector. Generally, a double-flush technique with heparinized saline (1,000 units per liter for pediatric cases, 3,000–6,000 units per liter for adults) is used. A syringe with 5 to 10 ml is attached to a stopcock, which is attached to the hub of the catheter. The syringe is gently aspirated with approximately 2 to 3 ml of blood, checking for clots. After the first syringe is disconnected, a second clean flush syringe with heparinized saline is connected to the end of catheter and aspirated back slightly. The tip of the syringe should be oriented downward so that any air bubbles will rise away from the hub of the catheter. It often is helpful to tap the side of the syringe to force any bubbles toward the plunger. The syringe is then injected with a continuous stream of heparinized saline. The stopcock is turned off midinjection, ensuring that the entire length of the catheter, including the tip, has been filled up with saline. This last point, although seemingly trivial, is very important. If the injection is stopped before the stopcock is turned to the off position, blood could backflow into the tip of the catheter, clot, and produce a thromboembolus.

After the syringe has been removed from the end of a catheter, the hub should be irrigated. This is best performed using a separate syringe filled with heparinized saline with an angiocatheter (20-gauge) attached to the tip. This setup allows injection of a jet of flush directly into the hub for irrigation of any residual blood.

On withdrawal of a guidewire from a catheter, a sucking or hissing sound may be heard. This implies that the end hole of the catheter is obstructed, often because it is resting against the arterial wall. If this occurs, withdraw the catheter 1 cm without concurrent application of suction, which would risk intimal damage. Once stationary, the catheter is gently aspirated until unrestricted back return of blood is confirmed. A gentle hand injection of contrast is performed to ensure free contrast flow from the tip, thus avoiding a forceful wedge injection into a subintimal flap or vessel in spasm. A more vigorous hand injection is then performed to gauge the flow rate and to better view the regional vascular anatomy.

■ COMPLICATIONS AND RISK FACTORS

Every cerebral angiogram carries a potential risk of stroke and even death. The risks may be broadly divided into those associated with the arterial puncture (local), those associated with contrast media or other administered drugs (systemic), and neurologic complications related to endovascular manipulations.

Nonneurologic Complications

What Are Some Common Nonneurologic Complications, and What Are the Best Ways to Prevent Them?

Local complications include groin hematoma, retroperitoneal hemorrhage, pseudoaneurysm formation, arteriovenous fistulae (AVFs), femoral nerve damage (usually self-limiting), arterial dissection, groin infection, sepsis, deep venous thrombosis, and pulmonary embolism. In infants, avascular necrosis of the femoral head as a

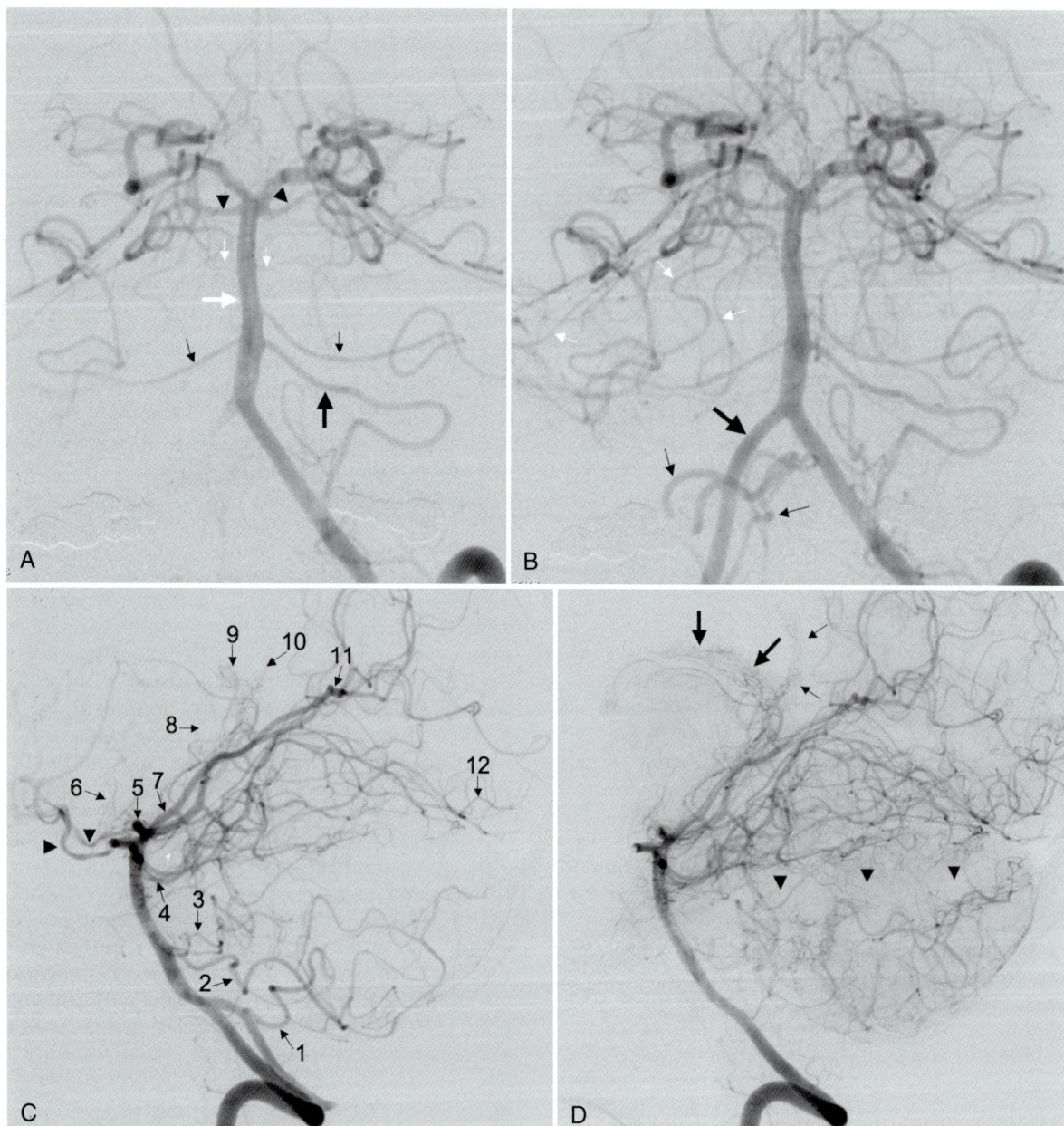

Figure 5-2 Early (**A**) and slightly later (**B**) arterial phases, Waters anteroposterior views, of a left vertebral angiogram showing the basilar artery and its branches. Subsequent reflux into the right V4 segment of the vertebral artery (VA) is shown. **A:** Left posterior inferior cerebellar artery (PICA; *large black arrow*) shows an uncommon high origin from the basilar artery (*large white arrow*). Both anterior inferior cerebellar arteries (AICAs) (*small black arrows*) demonstrate characteristic lateral loops. Multiple fine lateral pontine-perforating arteries arising from the posterolateral basilar artery surface are visualized lateral to the basilar artery (*small white arrows*). Both superior cerebellar arteries (SCAs) are shown to arise just below the basilar artery bifurcation (*black arrowheads*). **B:** Subsequent later arterial phase, Waters anteroposterior view, showing reflux into the right V4 segment (*large black arrow*) with filling of a normally located right PICA (*small black arrows*). The peripheral "stepladder"-configured hemispheric branches of the SCA are shown (*small white arrows*). **C:** Early arterial phase of a left vertebral angiogram, lateral view, showing the cerebellar arteries and the posterior cerebral artery branches. Reflux into the right VA and both posterior communicating arteries (*black arrowheads*) is shown. *1*, Right PICA (originates from VA); *2*, left PICA (originates high from basilar artery); *3*, AICA (typical M-shaped configuration); *4*, SCA; *5*, P1 segment; *6*, perforating branches (anterior and posterior thalamoperforating arteries); *7*, P2 segment; *8*, medial posterior choroidal artery; *9*, lateral posterior choroidal artery; *10*, splenial branches (posterior pericallosal artery); *11*, parietooccipital artery; *12*, calcarine artery. **D:** Subsequent later arterial phase of left vertebral angiogram, lateral view, depicting normal vascular blushes in the choroids plexus (*large black arrows*) and along the dorsal surface of the splenium of the corpus callosum (*small black arrows*). Note faint vascular blushes of the cerebellum with demarcation of the great horizontal fissure of the cerebellum (*black arrowheads*).

consequence of vascular stenoses or occlusions is a rare complication. The risk of significant groin bleeding is dependent on many factors, such as anticoagulation, sheath size, and use of puncture site closure devices. The reported overall rate of serious nonneurologic complications is low (0.6%) in meta-analysis. Permanent disability as a sequela of a nonneurologic complication is extremely rare (0.03%). A groin hematoma requiring medical therapy or surgery occurs very seldom (incidence 0.03%–0.2%). Minor groin hematomas are reported to occur in 0.5% to 8.1%. The rate of groin hematomas was higher in studies of patients receiving heparin as a bolus than in studies that advocated heparinized saline flushing. The most common systemic complications are nausea, vomiting, and/or transient hypotension (1.2%), followed by headaches (0.8%). Severe allergic reactions, such as anaphylaxis (0.03%), are rare. In patients with a suspected history of contrast allergy, a pretreatment regimen with diphenhydramine (e.g., 50 mg given intravenously one hour prior to the procedure) is performed. In high-risk patients (e.g., those with a previous episode of anaphylactoid reaction), additional premedication with corticosteroids (e.g., prednisone 50 mg orally every 6 hours for three doses, ending 1 hour before the procedure) as well as notification of the anesthesiology staff before the case begins is advised.

Acute renal failure is very rarely encountered after a diagnostic angiogram (0.02%). It usually occurs in patients with preexisting renal impairment (particularly in those with a history of diabetes mellitus or multiple myeloma) receiving a relatively large dose (>4 ml/kg) of intravascular contrast media. Adequate hydration of these at-risk patients before, during, and after the procedure is imperative. Life-threatening lactic acidosis is a potential complication in diabetic patients receiving oral metformin. The current recommendation is that this medication not be administered until 48 hours after the procedure assuming normal renal function.

Dion et al. noted that nonneurologic complications are significantly related to age greater than 50 years, hypertension, transient ischemic attack (TIA) as an indication, and the presence of a carotid bruit. Care should be taken that the puncture is below the inguinal ligament, which reduces the likelihood of retroperitoneal hemorrhage. Extra precaution is also required for patients receiving antiplatelet medications and/or anticoagulation or with preexistent coagulopathies, patients receiving long-term steroids or with a history of chronic renal failure, patients who previously have undergone aortofemoral bypass surgery, those with larger sheath sizes, or those in whom repeated arteriotomies have been performed.

Neurologic Complications

What Are Some Common Neurologic Complications, and What Are the Best Ways to Prevent Them?

Neurologic complications are usually, but not always, the result of embolism (clot, plaque, air, or foreign body) or iatrogenic dissection. The most common cause implicated is thromboembolism from catheters or guidewires. Thrombi may most likely develop inside the catheter if the guidewire is withdrawn into the catheter, allowing blood to stagnate within this dead space. Therefore, the importance of avoiding this dead space and keeping the guidewire manipulations to a minimum time is emphasized. Other potential pathophysiologic mechanisms include platelet activation, changes in clotting factors, and neurotoxicity of contrast agents. Vessel rupture may occur if an excessively forceful injection is made into an undersized artery (due to anatomy or spasm). Rare neurologic sequelae include transient cortical blindness, transient global amnesia, involuntary leg movements (monoballismus), and transient sensorineural deafness. The etiologies of these rare phenomena are speculative but in some cases may be related to contrast toxicity. A history of sickle cell anemia may be relevant because contrast media may initiate intravascular sickling, resulting in cerebral ischemia. In addition, patients with Ehlers-Danlos syndrome (particularly type IV) are especially predisposed to significant vessel injury with catheter angiography.

A risk of catheter angiography unique to patients with subarachnoid hemorrhage (SAH) secondary to cerebral aneurysm rupture is that of rebleeding during contrast injection due to increased arterial pressure. The risk of this extremely rare complication is well below the risk of rebleeding following SAH (4% in the first 24 hours, then 1%–2% for the next 4 weeks). Thus, there is no rationale for withholding catheter angiography from patients who suffer from this very serious condition and require accurate and prompt diagnosis and treatment.

Transient and Permanent Neurologic Deficits

In two large-scale prospective studies (19,826 and 2,899 cerebral angiography procedures, respectively), the overall rate of neurologic complications that occurred within 24 hours of the examination varied between 1.3% and 2.63%. The substantial majority of these complications were transient (<24 hours) in 0.7% to 2.09% or were reversible (24 hours to 7 days) in 0.2% to 0.36%. Stroke with permanent disability (>7 days) occurred in only 0.14% to 0.5% of examinations, and death related to a neurologic condition occurred in 0.05%. The indication with the highest rate of neurologic complications was atherosclerotic cerebrovascular disease (4.0%), followed by SAH (3.2%). Patients with a history of frequent TIAs were 67% more likely than those without a history to have a neurologic complication. Other factors for increased risk of neurologic complications include advanced age (>55 years), preexisting cardiovascular disease (coronary artery disease, hypertension, peripheral vascular disease), prolonged fluoroscopic times (>10 minutes), and arteriovenous malformation as the indication. For the pediatric population, cerebral catheter angiography performed by experienced operators has been shown to be a safe procedure.

In a meta-analysis by Cloft et al., the overall neurologic complication rate was lower in patients with SAH, aneurysm, or arteriovenous malformation compared with the rate in patients with ischemic stroke (0.8% vs 3.0%), as was the risk of permanent neurologic complication (0.07% vs 0.7%).

In two large-scale studies that enrolled patients over longer periods of time, the rate of neurologic complications decreased from 2.1% to 0.9% over 5.5 years and from 3.8% to 0.57% over 24 years, respectively. This significant decrease of complication rates in more recent years was attributed to improvement in equipment and angiographer skill and to the introduction of standardized use of heparinized catheter flush systems.

Willinsky et al. noted that the improved complication rate correlated with a lower percentage of patients being examined for carotid stenosis or ischemic stroke and a lower percentage of patients with cardiovascular diseases. Although not yet analyzed by direct comparison, the liberal use of a heparin bolus may be a benefit, as comparison of different studies showed similar overall neurologic complication rates but lower permanent complication rates in studies that used a heparin bolus.

The analysis of risk predictors and complication rates substantiates the argument that patients at higher risk (e.g., those with atherosclerosis, advanced age, vasculitis) should primarily undergo noninvasive imaging. Complications still occur in patients without these risk factors, but at a relatively low rate; therefore, the indications for catheter angiography should be carefully balanced. At our institution, all diagnostic cerebral angiography procedures, except those performed in patients with acute intracranial hemorrhage, usually are performed with a heparin bolus (70 international units per kilogram of body weight) that is given directly after the femoral sheath is inserted. Puncture site closure devices are preferentially used. If these devices cannot be inserted, strict immobilization and local compression are used to prevent the development of hematoma at the puncture site. In rare cases of bleeding at the puncture site, heparin can be reversed with protamine.

Silent Emboli

What Are Silent Ischemic Events, and What are the Best Ways to Minimize Them?

With the advent of diffusion-weighted magnetic resonance imaging has come the realization that clinically apparent stroke may be only the "tip of the iceberg" regarding neurologic complications of cerebral angiography given that clinically silent cerebral microembolism occurs more commonly than overt neurologic complications. The reported incidence of silent microemboli that are visible on diffusion-weighted imaging varies widely (range 9%–26%), depending on the cited source. However, the series that reported higher incidences (18.5%–26%) included both diagnostic and neurointerventional procedures in the analysis, and the latter is associated with a higher risk of thromboembolism. Therefore, a more realistic estimation for the risk of silent emboli from diagnostic catheter angiography alone is likely in the range from 9% to 15%. Similar to the case of overt stroke, preexisting vasculopathy, hypercoagulable state, long fluoroscopic time, high dose of contrast media, difficult vessel catheterization, and use of additional catheters have been identified as risk factors for the development of silent emboli. The exact pathomechanism of silent ischemic events is still subject to debate. Possible causes are air embolism or small blood clots from catheters, arteriosclerotic plaques scraped off from the vessel wall, vessel wall reaction to contrast medium in vasculitis, or even local thrombosis. Bendszus et al. confirmed injected air as a source of silent emboli. Air bubbles can be identified by transcranial Doppler sonography as microembolic signals. Dense showers of such signals are only related to injections of contrast medium and probably are caused by tiny air bubbles dissolved in contrast medium. Cerebral angiographic procedures with systematic use of air filters between the catheter and both the contrast medium syringe and the catheter flushing have shown a significant reduction in silent ischemic events (6% vs 22%). The same study showed that systemic heparin treatment (initial bolus of 50 international units per kilogram of body weight followed by a maintenance dose of 25 international units per kilogram of body weight per hour) resulted in an identical reduction of silent ischemic events.

Level of Experience

What Is the Influence of Operator's Experience on Complication Rates?

The contributing effect of the operator's experience on the procedural neurologic complication rate remains still unclear. Kaufmann et al. found that the involvement of a resident and/or fellow in the procedure was significantly associated with a decreased risk of neurologic outcome. However, other investigators found no difference or demonstrated a nonsignificant increase in neurologic complications if the examination was performed by fellows alone compared to those performed by neuroradiology staff alone. Interestingly, Willinsky et al. found a significantly higher neurologic complication rate when the fellow and staff together performed the cerebral angiogram. The majority of these cases comprised complex procedures with longer fluoroscopic times and consisted of patients who were slightly older and had a higher rate of cardiovascular disease, carotid stenosis, and ischemic stroke. In another study, the incidence of silent ischemic events studied with diffusion-weighted imaging was significantly lower when the angiogram was performed by an experienced senior investigator than when the procedure was performed by a junior neuroradiologist.

■ EVALUATION OF CRANIAL VASCULATURE ON ANGIOGRAPHIC VIEWS

Great Supraaortic Arteries

What Are Common Variants of the Great Supraaortic Arteries?

The typical anatomy of the great vessels that arise from the aortic arch is in branching order of the innominate artery or brachiocephalic trunk, the left common carotid artery, and the left subclavian artery. This anatomy is seen in 65% to 70% of cases. The second most common variant of aortic arch branching occurs when the left common carotid artery has a common origin with the innominate artery (13%) (Figure 5-3). This variant is most often termed a *bovine aortic arch*, which is a misnomer because solely a single great vessel originates from the aortic arch in cattle. A similar but less common variant occurs when the left common carotid artery originates directly from the innominate artery but more distally rather than as a common trunk (9%). These variants of left common carotid artery origin are found more often in blacks compared with whites. Other less common anatomic

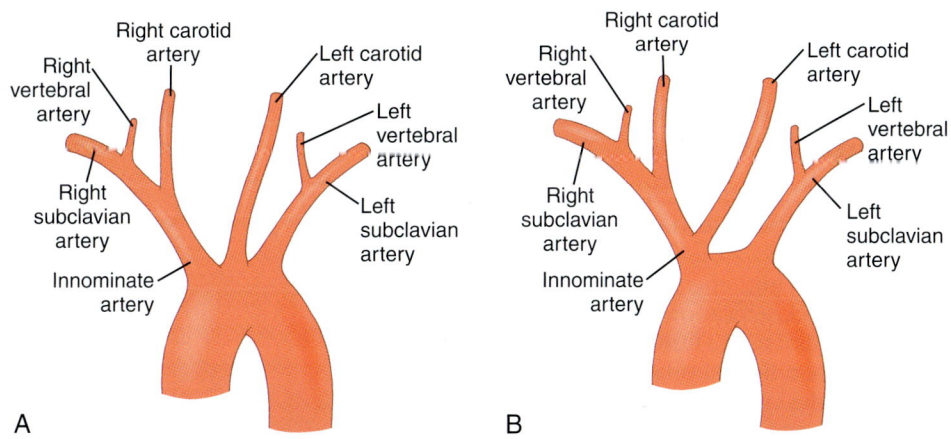

Figure 5-3 The most common aortic arch branching pattern has a separate origin for the innominate, left common carotid, and left subclavian arteries. The second most common pattern of aortic arch branching has a common origin for the innominate and left common carotid arteries. This pattern has been referred to as a "bovine arch". (Redrawn from Layton KF, Kallmes DF, Cloft HJ, Lindell EP, Cox VS. Bovine aortic arch variant in humans: Clarification of a common misnomer. AJNR Am J Neuroradiol 2006;27:1541-1542.)

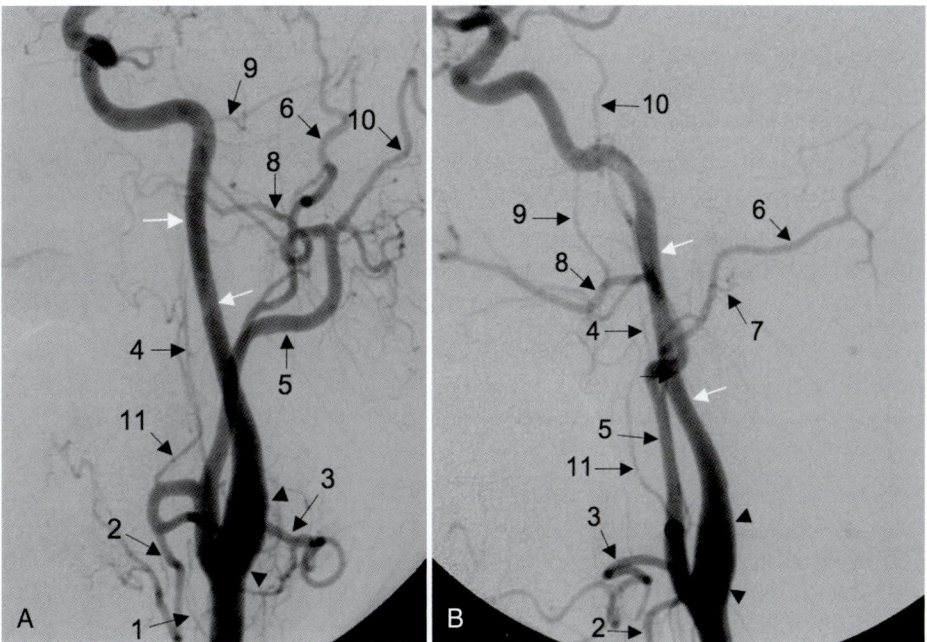

Figure 5-4 Anteroposterior (A) and lateral (B) views of a left common carotid angiogram showing the normal extracranial course of the internal (ICA) and external carotid artery (ECA) and the ECA branches. The carotid bulb is indicated by the *black arrowheads*. The ICA initially lies behind and lateral to the ECA. As the cervical ICA ascends *(white arrows)*, it crosses behind and then courses anteromedially to the main ECA trunk. *1*, Superior thyroid artery; *2*, lingual artery; *3*, facial artery; *4*, ascending pharyngeal artery; *5*, main ECA trunk; *6*, occipital artery; *7*, posterior auricular artery; *8*, maxillary artery; *9*, middle meningeal artery; *10*, superficial temporal artery; *11*, ascending palatine artery (facial artery branch).

variations include a direct origin of the left VA from the aortic arch, usually between the left common carotid and left subclavian arteries (6%) and an aberrant right subclavian artery that arises distal to the left subclavian artery and may course posterior to the esophagus. More than 20 different aortic arch configurations have been described, but those specifically described here are by far the most commonly encountered.

Common Carotid Arteries

What Are the Landmarks for Imaging the Common Carotid Arteries?

The right common carotid artery usually originates at the level of the right sternoclavicular joint. The carotid bifurcation usually is located at the C3–5 level (82%), which fluoroscopically approximates to just below the angle of the mandible. The carotid bifurcation usually is higher in children at C2–4 (80%), and the left side usually is slightly higher than the right. It may occur as high as C1 and as low as T2 as a normal variation. In older patients, a fleck of calcium within a bifurcation plaque can serve as a useful radiographic landmark. The common carotid artery does not have any significant branches and widens near its termination. This bulbous dilatation is carried into the ICA origin and is referred to collectively as the *carotid sinus* (Figure 5-4). The ICA invariably arises posterior to the ECA and, in most cases, laterally. Thus, an ipsilateral anterior oblique or lateral view usually is optimal for displaying the bifurcation;

however, pinhole or web-like high-grade stenoses may be underestimated unless multiple oblique projections are performed.

Internal Carotid Arteries

What Are the Anatomic Segments, Common Variants, and Branches of the Internal Carotid Arteries?

Several systems for classifying the ICA segments have been proposed. The classification proposed by Bouthillier et al. is practical as it uses a numerical scale in the direction of normal blood flow similar to the other major brain supplying arteries, and it takes into account new anatomic information and clinical considerations (Figure 5-5). Seven anatomically distinct segments are described according to their adjacent structures and the compartments they traverse (Figure 5-6):

C1 = Cervical
C2 = Petrous
C3 = Lacerum
C4 = Cavernous
C5 = Clinoid
C6 = Ophthalmic
C7 = Communicating

C1 (Cervical) ICA

The first ICA segment can be divided in two parts: the carotid bulb and the ascending cervical segment (Figure 5-4). The carotid bulb is the most proximal aspect of the cervical ICA, forming a significant dilatation (normal diameter 7.5 mm vs 7.0 mm for the common carotid artery and 4.7 mm for the ICA distal to the bulb). The distribution of blood flow between the ICA and ECA occurs in a ratio of 70:30. In the ascending segment, the ICA courses cephalad within the carotid space, a fascially defined sheath extending from the mediastinum to the skull base. Apart from the ICA, the contents of the carotid space include the internal jugular vein, lymph nodes, sympathetic nerves, and lower cranial nerves IX–XII. This segment usually does not give rise to any branches. The ICA initially lies behind and lateral to the ECA, but, as it ascends, it crosses behind and courses anteromedially to the main ECA trunk (Figure 5-4). Normal variants include a medial origin of the ICA (8%–15%) resulting in a superimposed appearance of the ICA and ECA on the standard lateral projection. If tortuous, this medially projecting ICA can present clinically as a retropharyngeal mass. Tortuosity and even complete looping of the cervical ICA can occur both in young children and older adults (5%–15%) unrelated to hypertension. True agenesis of the ICA is very rare (0.01%), whereas hypoplasia of the ICA has been reported to occur both as an isolated anomaly and in conjunction with other abnormalities (e.g., basal telangiectasia). Both anomalies are associated with a small or absent bony carotid canal. Focal/segmental ICA narrowing is more often acquired (e.g., due to reduced flow, dissecting aneurysm, fibromuscular dysplasia, or segmental stenosis). Duplications and fenestrations of the extracranial ICA and a nonbifurcating carotid artery (common carotid artery extends to the skull base, with

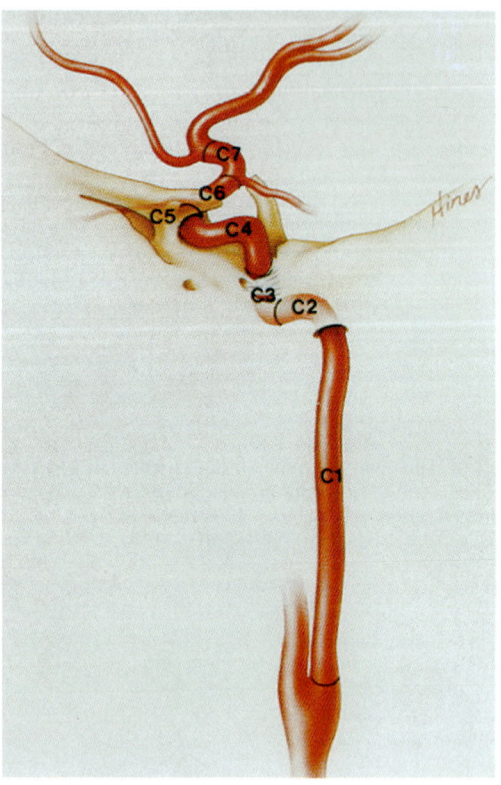

Figure 5-5 According to the classification by Bouthillier et al, the segments of the internal carotid artery are as follows: *C1*, cervical segment (cervical portion); *C2*, petrous segment; *C3*, lacerum segment (C2 and C3 comprise the commonly used petrous portion); *C4*, cavernous segment (cavernous portion); *C5*, clinoid segment (not identified in some earlier classifications); *C6*, ophthalmic, or supraclinoid, segment; *C7*, communicating, or terminal, segment. (From Bouthillier A, van Loveren HR, Keller JT. Segments of the internal carotid artery: a new classification. Neurosurgery 1996;38:425-432; discussion 432-423.)

ECA branches arising separately from this main trunk) are rare anomalies. Anomalous ICA branches include vessels that normally originate from the ECA, such as ascending pharyngeal artery, other ICA segments (vidian artery), or the vertebrobasilar circulation (e.g., cerebellar arteries).

During fetal development, transient segmental anastomoses exist between the primitive carotid and hindbrain circulations. If these connections fail to obliterate, they can persist into adulthood as so-called *carotid–basilar anastomoses*, which are named according to the cranial nerves they parallel, for example, persistent hypoglossal artery (Figure 5-7 and Table 5-1). Most reported examples of persistent carotid–basilar anastomosis are found incidentally at angiography or on cross-sectional imaging modalities. In the cervical ICA, a persistent hypoglossal artery is the most commonly encountered carotid–basilar anastomosis (0.027%–0.26%) that arises usually at the C1–2 level and curves posteromedially toward an enlarged hypoglossal canal (Figure 5-8).

C2 (Petrous) ICA

The C2 segment enters the skull base at the carotid canal and is contained throughout its course by the petrous temporal bone. It is subdivided into the ascending

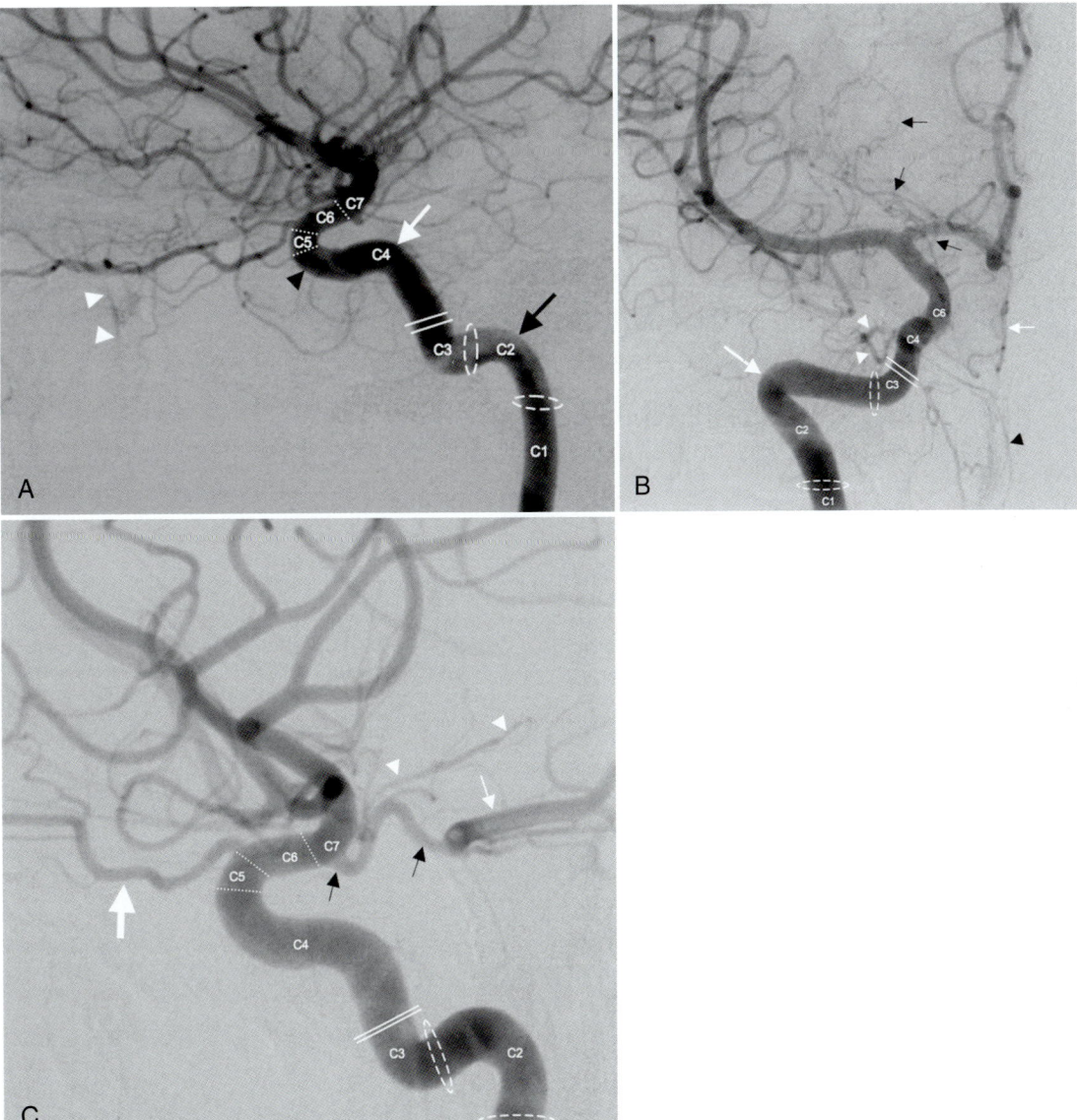

Figure 5-6 Normal selective internal carotid artery (ICA) angiograms in different patients demonstrating the ICA segments. *Circles* indicate positions of exocranial and endocranial openings of the petrous carotid canal. *White lines* denote approximate position of petrolingual ligament. **A:** ICA angiogram, lateral view. *Black arrow* indicates genu of petrous ICA segment; *white arrow* indicates posterior genu of cavernous ICA; *black arrowhead* indicates anterior genu of cavernous ICA; *white arrowheads* point to typical vascular choroid blush of the eye globe. A funnel-shaped infundibular origin of the posterior communicating artery is shown. **B:** ICA angiogram, anteroposterior view. *Large white arrow* indicates genu of petrous ICA segment. The S-shaped carotid siphon is not visualized due to an overlap of the distal cavernous, interdural or clinoid (C5), and proximal supraclinoid (C6) ICA segments. The origin of the ophthalmic artery (*white arrowheads*) is not depicted. The medially orientated ophthalmic artery branches are visualized: the anterior falx artery, which is an extraorbital meningeal branch (*small white arrow*), and the anterior ethmoid arteries (*black arrowhead*). The anterior choroidal artery (*small black arrows*), which originates from the C7 ICA segment, shows its characteristic course overlapped by multiple perforating M1 and A1 branches. **C:** Slightly oblique lateral view (Haughton view) of a selective ICA angiogram opens the carotid siphon and enables excellent visualization of its segments and their branching vessels. The ophthalmic artery is indicated by the *large white arrow*. A medium-sized posterior communicating artery (*small black arrows*) fills the normal-sized P2 segment of the posterior cerebral artery (*small white arrow*). *Small white arrowheads* point to a smaller-caliber anterior choroidal artery.

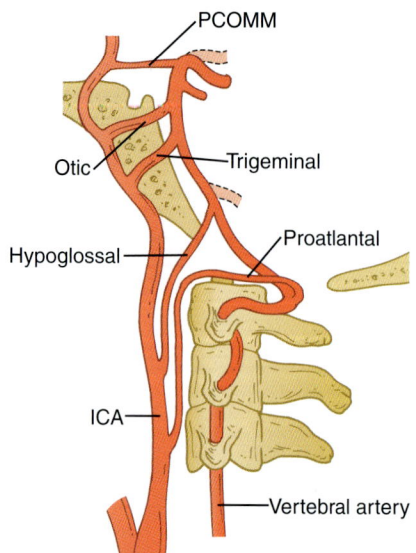

Figure 5-7 Different persistent fetal carotid–vertebrobasilar anastomoses. *ICA*, Internal carotid artery; *PCOMM*, posterior communicating artery. (Redrawn from Luh GY, Dean BL, Tomsick TA, Wallace RC. The persistent fetal carotid-vertebrobasilar anastomoses. AJR Am J Roentgenol 1999;172:1427-1432.)

Table 5-1 Carotid–Basilar Anastomoses

	Embryonic Anatomy	Angiographic Findings and Variants
Posterior communicating artery	From caudal division of primitive ICA to developing vertebro-basilar circulation. Partially regresses	Variants. Fetal origin of posterior cerebral artery. Infundibular origin from ICA
Primitive trigeminal artery	From cavernous ICA to embryonic dorsal longitudinal neural arteries. Normally regresses completely	Most common persistent embryonic carotid–basilar anastomosis
Persistent otic artery	From petrous ICA to embryonic dorsal longitudinal neural arteries. Normally regresses completely	Extremely rare. Almost never identified angiographically
Persistent hypoglossal artery	From cervical ICA to embryonic dorsal longitudinal neural arteries. Normally regresses completely	Second most common persistent embryonic carotid–basilar anastomosis. Origin from C1–2 level of cervical ICA. Passes through enlarged hypoglossal (anterior condyloid) canal
Proatlantal intersegmental artery	From cervical ICA to embryonic dorsal longitudinal neural arteries. Normally regresses completely	Origin from C2–3 level of cervical ICA. Lower origin and more vertical course compared with persistent hypoglossal artery. Horizontal suboccipital course along C1 ring
		Occasionally arises from external carotid artery (less common type)

Adapted from Osborn AG: *Diagnostic Cerebral Angiography.* Lippincott Williams & Wilkins, 1999.
ICA, Internal carotid artery.

(vertical) and horizontal portions. The short 1-cm vertical segment angles sharply at the knee ("genu"), which is angiographically easily identified. The horizontal segment courses anteromedially toward the petrous apex. The intrapetrous ICA has two small and inconstant branches: the vidian and caroticotympanic artery. Both branches may provide collateral blood flow from the ECA if ICA occlusion occurs. The vidian artery passes anteroinferiorly through the vidian (pterygoid) canal and anastomoses with ECA branches. The caroticotympanic artery supplies the middle ear cavity and anastomoses with the inferior tympanic artery, a small branch from the ascending pharyngeal artery. An aberrant petrous ICA is an important anomaly that traverses the middle ear cavity and presents clinically as a retrotympanic mass (Figure 5-9). Noninvasive diagnosis of this important anomaly is established with MRA or CTA. Failure to recognize an aberrant ICA may result in serious complications if it is mistaken for a vascular middle ear neoplasm. Rare anomalies include persistent otic artery and persistent stapedial artery. The latter usually is not visualized at angiography. It arises from the vertical petrous ICA segment, crosses the footplate of the stapes, enlarges the facial nerve canal en route to the middle cranial fossa, and terminates in the middle meningeal artery (Figure 5-10).

C3 (Lacerum) ICA

From the end of the petrous canal, the lacerum segment of the ICA courses above the cartilage-filled foramen lacerum. It then ascends in a posterior extension of the carotid sulcus, part of the basisphenoid. The lacerum segment ends at the petrolingual ligament, a small reflection of periosteum between the lingula of the sphenoid bone anteriorly and the petrous apex posteriorly. This ICA segment has no branches.

C4 (Cavernous) ICA

This segment courses within the cavernous sinus, surrounded by venous channels, and can be divided into three subsegments: a posterior ascending or vertical portion, a longer horizontal segment, and a short anterior vertical portion. The two vertical subsegments form gently rounded curves called the *posterior genu* and the *anterior genu*. The C4 segment exits the cavernous sinus through a dural ring in the superior wall medial to the anterior clinoid process (Figure 5-11). The C4 segment has several small but important branches that are named according to their topographic origins; their divisions are named according to the territories they supply. The posterior trunk (meningohypophyseal artery) arises from the superior aspect of the posterior genu and supplies branches to the pituitary gland (inferior hypophyseal

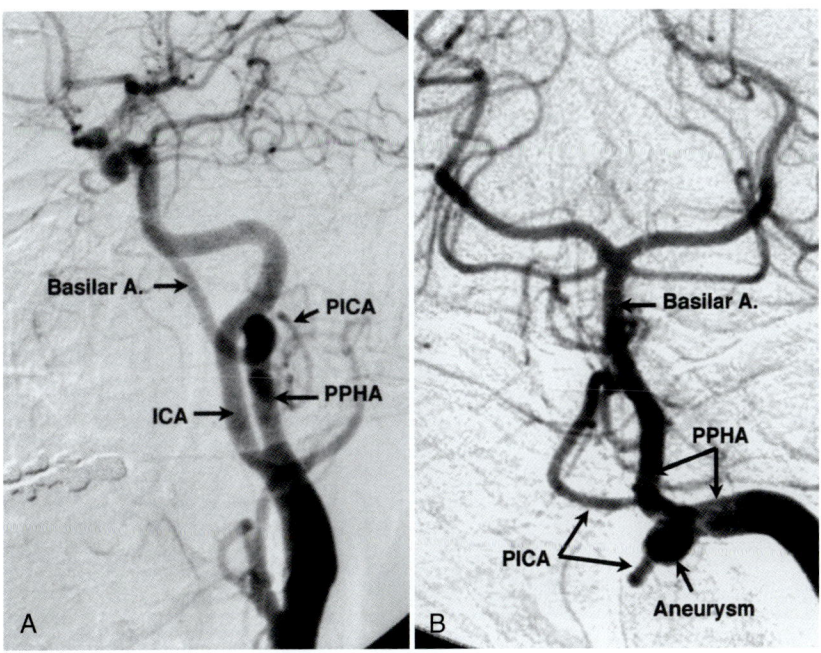

Figure 5-8 A: Preoperative left carotid angiogram, oblique view, showing the persistent primitive hypoglossal artery originating from the internal carotid artery *(ICA)* at the C2 cervical level. **B:** Preoperative selective angiogram of the persistent primitive hypoglossal artery *(PPHA)*, anteroposterior view, demonstrating a saccular aneurysm at the junction of the PPHA and the posterior inferior cerebellar artery *(PICA)*. (From Huynh-Le P, Matsushima T, Muratani H, Hikita T, Hirokawa E. Persistent primitive hypoglossal artery associated with proximal posterior inferior cerebellar artery aneurysm. Surg Neurol 2004;62:546-551; discussion 551.)

artery), tentorium (marginal tentorial artery), and clivus (clival branches) (Figure 5-12). The lateral trunk, also called the *inferolateral trunk*, originates from the lateral aspect of the horizontal portion (found in 66%–84%) and crosses the abducens (VI) nerve within the cavernous sinus (Figure 5-13). It supplies branches to cranial nerves III, IV, and VI as well as to the gasserian ganglion and the cavernous sinus dura. The inferolateral trunk has important anteroinferior anastomoses with the maxillary artery through the artery of the foramen rotundum. A posterior branch supplies the cavernous sinus wall, the gasserian ganglion, and the tentorium (tentorial branch). It anastomoses with branches of the middle meningeal artery (through the foramen spinosum) and the maxillary artery (through the artery of the foramen ovale). Inconstant medial branches (28%) supply the pituitary gland. Normal variants include a tortuous cavernous ICA and a medial course of the C4 segment within the sella turcica instead of laterally along the carotid sulcus. These so-called *kissing ICAs* pose a potential hazard for transsphenoidal surgical approaches to the sella turcica.

A persistent trigeminal artery is the most common and cephalad of the carotid–basilar anastomoses (Figure 5-14). It is found in 0.02% to 0.6% of cerebral angiograms. This vessel anastomosis arises from the posterior genu of C4 and follows either a parasellar (lateral) or an intrasellar (medial) course. The lateral variant follows the trigeminal nerve around the dorsum sellae. The intrasellar variant passes directly posterior through the dorsum sellae. Further variants of the persistent trigeminal artery have been described in relation to their supply of the vertebrobasilar system, which depends on the patency of the posterior communicating arteries. Rarely, aneurysms or direct AVFs to the cavernous sinus *(trigemino-cavernous fistulae)* are found to arise from persistent trigeminal arteries.

C5 (Clinoid) ICA

The C5 segment is the shortest of all ICA segments. It comprises only a small, wedge-shaped area along the superior aspect of the anterior cavernous carotid genu (Figure 5-6). It is an interdural segment that starts at the proximal dural ring and ends at the distal dural ring, where the ICA enters the subarachnoid space. This segment has no branches; only in rare instances does the OA arise from the C5 segment.

C6 (Ophthalmic) ICA

From its junction with the clinoid segment the ICA curves upward and backward to complete the so-called angiographic *carotid siphon*, an S-shaped curve that is formed by the cavernous and supraclinoid ICA segments. This segment is best visualized on lateral angiograms, as on AP views there is often an overlap of the distal intracavernous and proximal intradural ICA segments (Figure 5-6). The absence of a reliable angiographic landmark makes it difficult to distinguish between the end of C5 (interdural) and the beginning of C6 (intradural) segments. Practically speaking, lesions such as aneurysms that are above the OA level usually are at least partially intradural. In this region a loosely adherent, angiographically occult dural evagination called the *carotid cave* is often seen adjacent to the C6 segment. Aneurysms occurring at this location, referred to as *carotid cave aneurysms*, may rupture into the subarachnoid

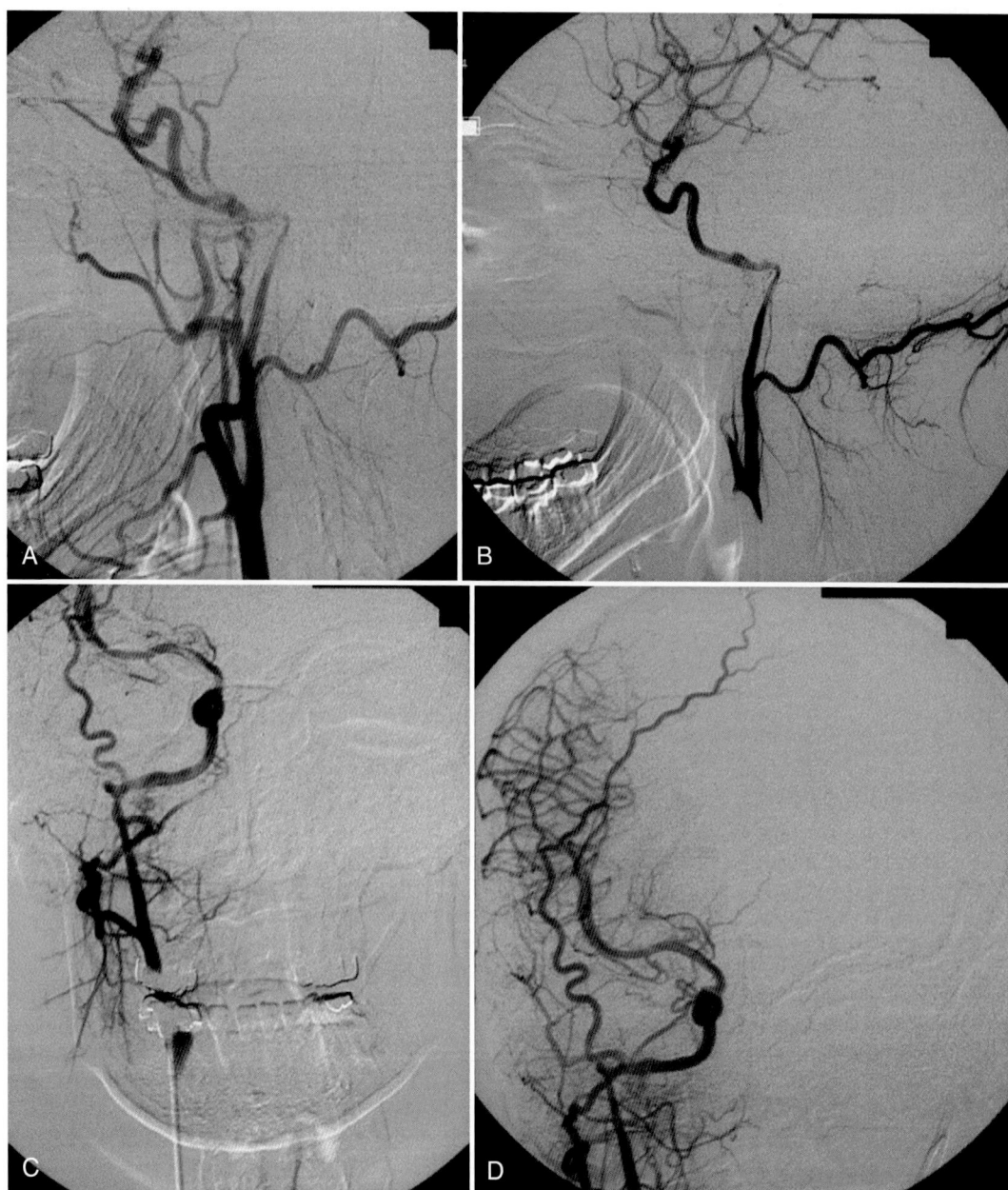

Figure 5-9 Left common carotid artery (CCA) angiograms, anteroposterior (AP) and lateral views (**A, B**), and left internal carotid artery (ICA) angiograms, AP and lateral views (**C, D**), demonstrating typical findings of an aberrant petrous ICA. Instead of a normal ICA, an enlarged inferior tympanic artery anastomosing with a hypertrophied caroticotympanic artery is demonstrated on the CCA injection. In this aberrant arrangement, the ascending pharyngeal artery branch of the external carotid artery gives rise to the inferior tympanic artery, which anastomoses with the caroticotympanic artery to supply the normally located horizontal petrous ICA. The aberrant anastomosis is positioned posteriorly and laterally from the ICA's normal location. An area of narrowing and angulation is demonstrated where the aberrant segment reaches the middle ear. (From Knox WJ, Milburn JM, Dawson R. Bilateral aberrant internal carotid arteries: treatment of a hemorrhagic complication. Am J Otolaryngol 2007;28:212-217.)

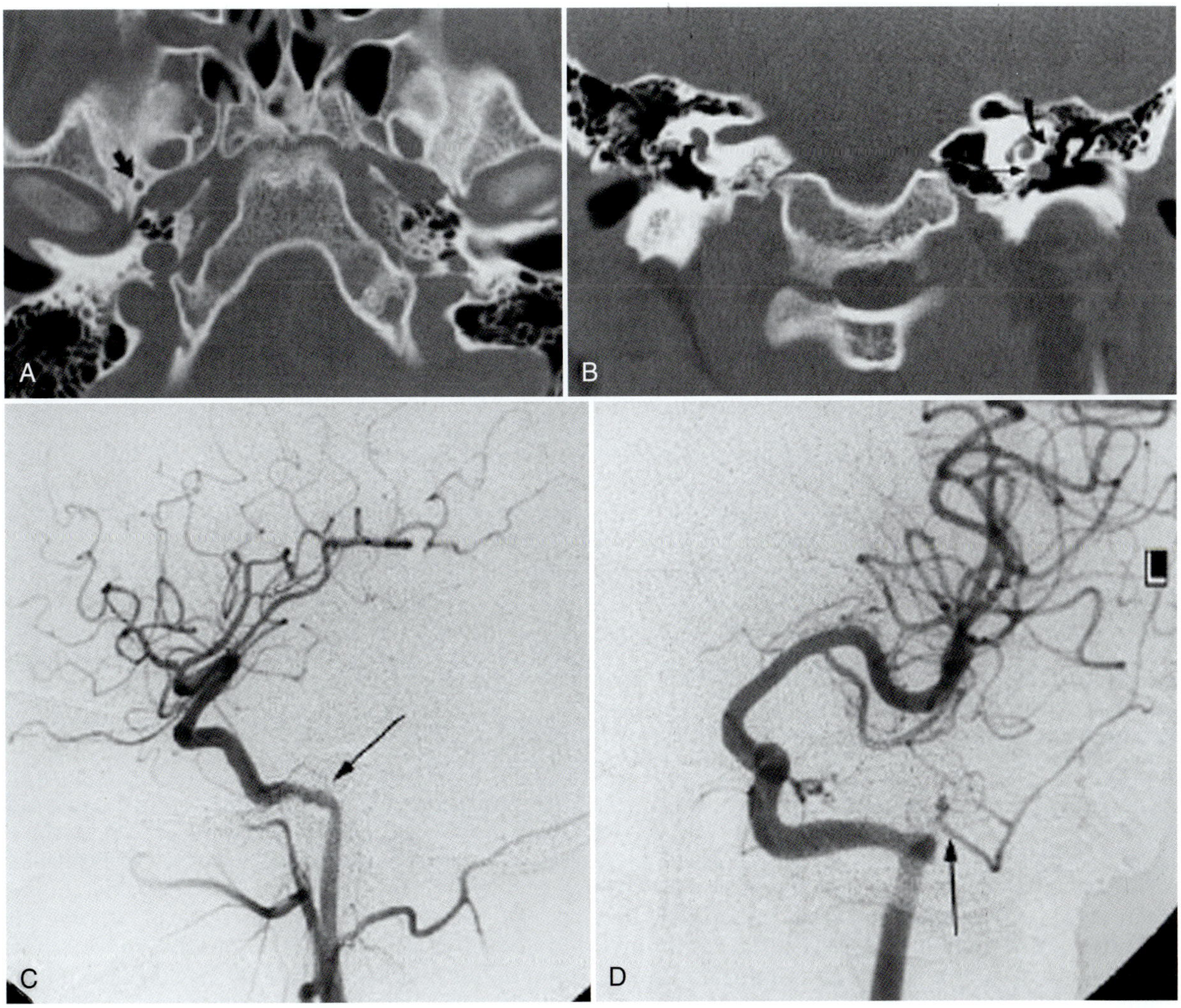

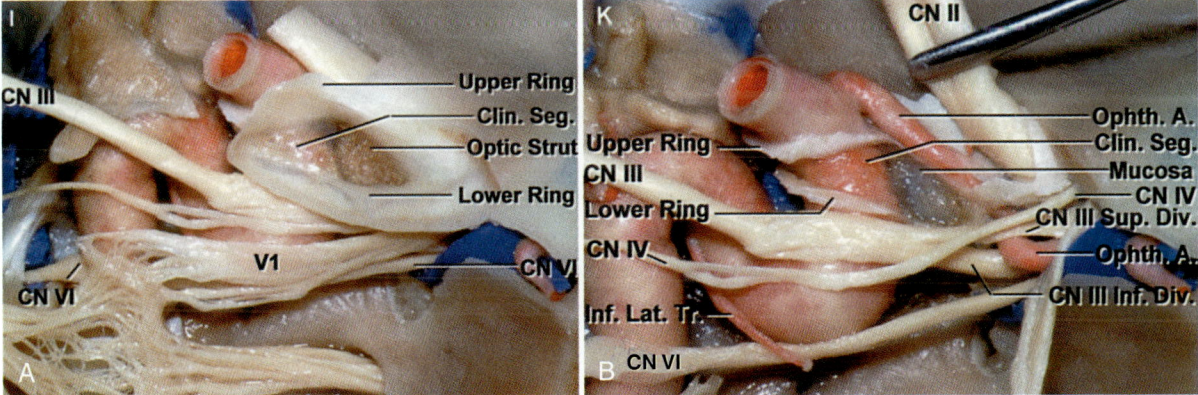

Figure 5-10 A 14-year-old boy with headache, vomiting, dizziness, and ringing in the ear. **A:** Axial computed tomographic (CT) scan showing a normal right foramen spinosum *(arrow)* and absence of the left foramen spinosum. **B:** Coronal CT scan showing the aberrant internal carotid artery (ICA) on the left *(straight arrow)* and the soft-tissue density of a persistent stapedial artery (PSA) *(curved arrow)*. **C, D:** Left carotid arteriograms, lateral and frontal views, showing a PSA arising from the aberrant ICA *(arrow)*. (From Silbergleit R, Quint DJ, Mehta BA, Patel SC, Metes JJ, Noujaim SE. The persistent stapedial artery. AJNR Am J Neuroradiol 2000;21:572-577.)

Figure 5-11 A: Anatomic dissection of the right cavernous sinus. The outer layer of dura has been removed from the lateral wall of Meckel cave and the cavernous sinus. The venous plexus surrounding the nerves has been removed to expose the trigeminal divisions and cranial nerves III and VI coursing in the wall of the cavernous sinus. The anterior clinoid process has been removed. The optic strut separates the optic canal and superior orbital fissure. The dura extending medially off the upper surface of the anterior clinoid forms the upper dural ring around the internal carotid artery, and the dura lining the lower margin of the clinoid extends medially to form the lower dural ring. The clinoid segment of the carotid artery, located between the upper and lower ring, is enclosed in the dura sheath referred to as the carotid collar. **B:** The optic nerve has been elevated to expose the ophthalmic artery coursing within the optic sheath. At the orbital apex, the artery penetrates the optic sheath and enters the orbital apex on the lateral side of the optic nerve. Removal of additional optic strut exposes the mucosa lining the sphenoid sinus on the medial side. The shortest of all the internal carotid artery segments, the clinoid segment, is exposed between the lower (proximal) and upper (distal) dural rings. (From Rhoton AL Jr. The cavernous sinus, the cavernous venous plexus, and the carotid collar. Neurosurgery 2002;51:S375-S410.)

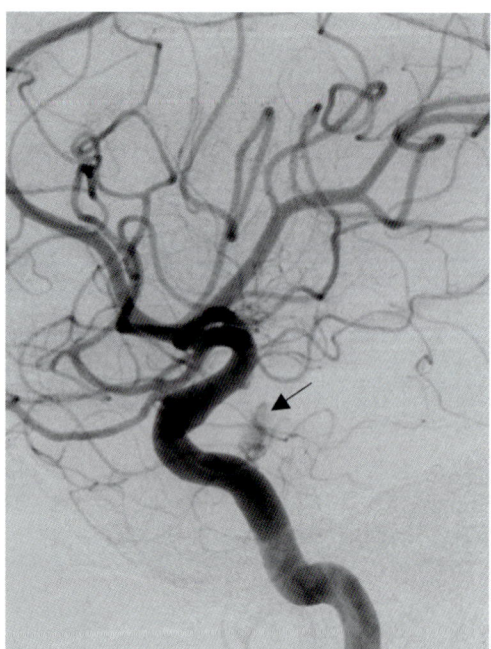

Figure 5-12 Late arterial phase of selective left internal carotid artery angiogram, lateral view, showing a prominent but normal posterior pituitary blush *(black arrow)*. The posterior trunk (so-called *meningohypophyseal trunk* or *artery*) can frequently give rise to such vascular blush, which should not be mistaken for a tumor blush. Alternatively, it can be seen as a small vessel arising from the superior aspect of the posterior genu.

space. Angiographically, this subtype of paraclinoid ICA aneurysm arises at the anterior ICA and points medially and superior. A more accurate way of determining the location of aneurysms in the paraclinoid location (extradural vs interdural vs intradural) can be provided by CTA, which enables the visualization of more reliable bony landmarks (e.g., optic strut, anterior clinoid process). Two important branches arise from the C6 segment: the OA and the superior hypophyseal artery.

The OA is typically the first major intradural ICA branch originating from the anteromedial or superomedial surface of the ICA near the junction of the C5/C6 segments (90% intradural origin) (Figure 5-15). It courses superiorly, then turns and runs directly anteriorly through the optic canal into the orbit. Its ocular branches include the central retinal artery (rarely visualized) and the ciliary arteries. The vascular plexus of the ocular choroid can almost always identified as a distinct crescent-shaped vascular blush on midarterial phase views of ICA angiograms (Figures 5-6, *A*, and 5-15, *B*). A prominent meningeal branch, the anterior falx artery, arises from the anterior ethmoidal branches of the OA, following a relatively straight course then curving superiorly to supply part of the falx (Figure 5-16). Major orbital branches are the lacrimal artery and unnamed muscular branches that supply the extraocular muscles. A number of extraorbital branches arise from the OA: supraorbital, anterior and posterior ethmoidal, dorsal nasal, palpebral, medial frontal, and supratrochlear arteries, which have extensive anastomoses with branches of the ECA. These anastomoses may become an important source of collateral blood flow to the intracranial circulation in the event of proximal ICA occlusion. A rare variant is the ophthalmic origin of the middle meningeal artery (0.5% of cases) that arises from the recurrent meningeal branch of the OA. The OA itself, on the other hand, may anomalously originate from the middle meningeal artery passing into the orbit through the superior orbital fissure or a foramen in the greater sphenoid wing instead of through the optic canal. In 8% of cases, the OA shows a lower, cavernous origin (Figure 5-17).

Although one or more superior hypophyseal arteries arising from the posteromedial aspect of the C6 segment are rarely visualized, even on high-resolution digital subtraction angiography (DSA) studies, they may be a site for aneurysm formation.

C7 (Communicating) ICA

The C7 segment begins just proximal to the origin of the posterior communicating artery (PCoA) and ends as the ICA bifurcates into its terminal branches, the anterior and middle cerebral arteries (MCAs).

The first major branch, the PCoA arises from the posterior aspect of the intradural ICA, courses posteriorly, runs above the oculomotor (cranial nerve III) nerve, and anastomoses with the posterior cerebral artery (PCA), a branch of the BA. It gives rise to several small branches, the anterior thalamoperforating arteries that supply the medial thalamus and walls of the third ventricle. The PCoA varies greatly in size (from absent to very large). If the P1 PCA segment is hypoplastic or absent, the PCoA may supply the entire PCA territory, which is then termed *fetal origin* of the PCA. A funnel-shaped dilatation called the *PCoA infundibulum* is seen at the PCoA origin in 6% to 17% of cases. It is typically round or conical shaped, 2 mm or less in diameter, and has a wide base at its origin from the ICA. The PCoA arises from its apex (Figure 5-6, *A*). It is considered a normal variant but must be distinguished from an ICA–PCoA aneurysm.

The second branch of the C7 segment is the anterior choroidal artery (AChA), which is a small but relatively constant and very important vessel (Figure 5-6, *B* and *C*). It arises from the posteromedial aspect of the C7 segment a short distance above the PCoA origin either as a single trunk or as a plexus of small vessels. The proximal (cisternal) AChA segment courses posteromedially below the optic tract through the crural cistern, curves around the cerebral peduncle, and ends in a definite lateral angulation where the AChA enters the temporal horn through the choroidal fissure (angiographic plexal point). The distal (intraventricular) AChA segment continues posteriorly within the supracornual cleft of the temporal horn following the choroid plexus, typically curving around the pulvinar of the thalamus and then running anteriorly for a variable distance. The choroid plexus of the lateral ventricle may appear as a dense homogeneous stain or blush persisting well into the capillary or early venous phase of carotid angiograms.

The AChA territory is variable but may include many important structures in an arc-shaped zone lying between the corpus striatum anterolaterally and the thalamus posteromedially: the optic tract, posterior limb of the internal capsule, cerebral peduncle, choroid plexus, and medial temporal lobe. The AChA exists

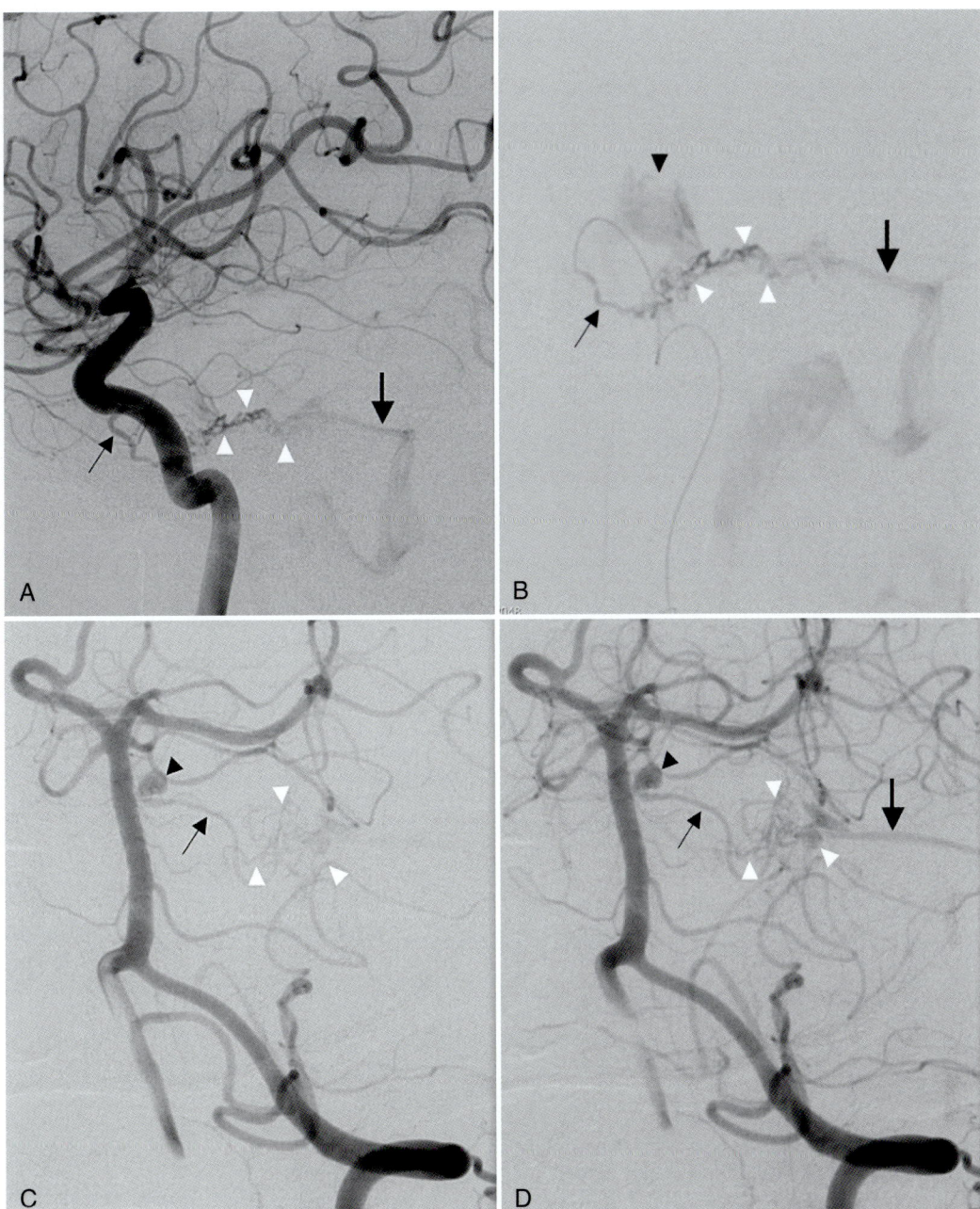

Figure 5-13 Right internal carotid artery angiogram, lateral view. **A:** Enlarged inferolateral trunk (ILT, *small black arrow*) originating from horizontal portion of the cavernous (C4) internal carotid artery (ICA), which has formed a dural arteriovenous fistula (DAVF, *white arrowheads*) with drainage into the superior petrosal sinus *(large black arrow)*. Subsequent anterograde venous drainage is shown into the sigmoid sinus. **B:** Superselective angiogram, lateral view, obtained from microcatheter injection into right ILT *(small black arrow)* better illustrates the fine fistulous network of dural vessels *(white arrowheads)* that shunt into superior petrosal sinus *(large black arrow)* as well as retrogradely into the posterior portion of the cavernous sinus *(black arrowhead)*. Left vertebral angiogram, oblique Waters view, early arterial **(C)** and subsequent later arterial **(D)** phases showing further arterial supply to DAVF from enlarged right lateral pontine artery *(small black arrow)* with numerous fistulous connections *(white arrowheads)* to draining superior petrosal sinus *(large black arrow)*. At the origin of this arterial feeder from the basilar artery a posteriorly directed flow-related aneurysm is disclosed *(black arrowhead)*. (Courtesy Dr. William McAuliffe, Perth.)

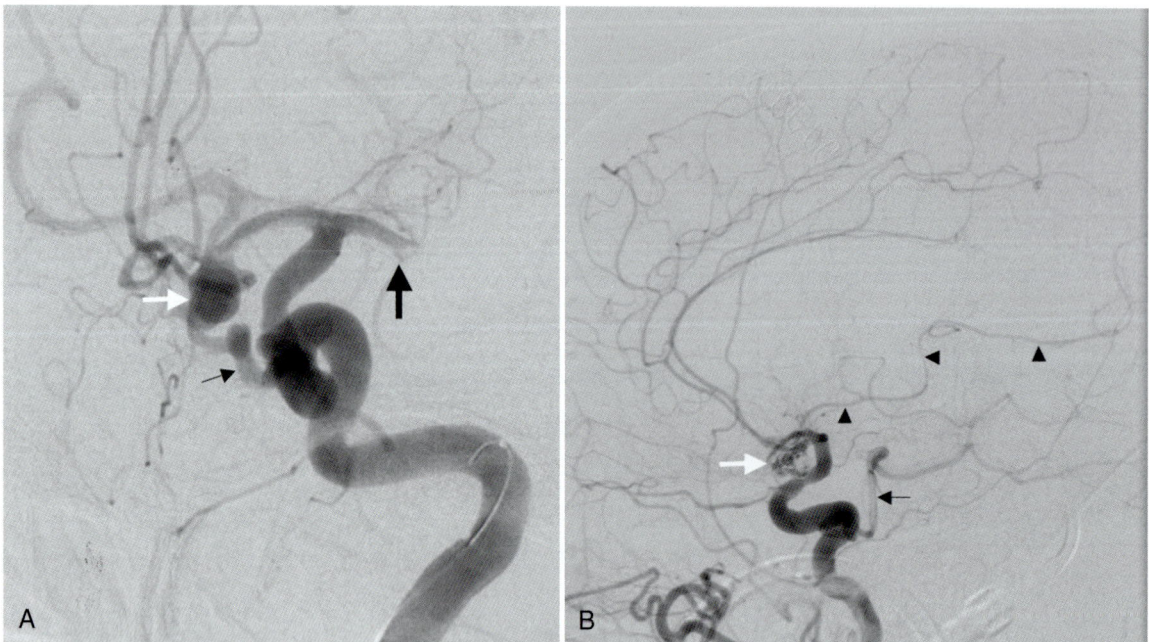

Figure 5-14 **A:** Left internal carotid artery (ICA) angiogram, anteroposterior view, showing an abrupt termination of the contrast column in the mid-M1 portion of the left middle cerebral artery (MCA) consistent with an occlusion. A meniscus of contrast outlines the proximal clot *(large black arrow)*. The lateral lenticulostriate arteries arising from the proximal M1 segment show normal opacification, but there is no filling of branches beyond the thrombus. This acute thromboembolic arterial occlusion complicated endovascular treatment of a ruptured anterior communicating artery aneurysm *(large white arrow)*. A persistent trigeminal artery that arises from the left cavernous ICA portion and contributes to the basilar artery circulation is also identified *(small black arrow)*. **B:** Left common carotid artery angiogram, lateral view, showing large bare area in the MCA distribution only with filling of the posterior M2 division *(black arrowheads)*. This injection was performed after partial coil embolization of the ruptured anterior communicating artery aneurysm *(large white arrow)* had been achieved and subsequent intraarterial thrombolysis of the M1 occlusion had been initiated. In addition, a persistent trigeminal artery with a typical appearance arising from the cavernous ICA is disclosed *(small black arrow)*.

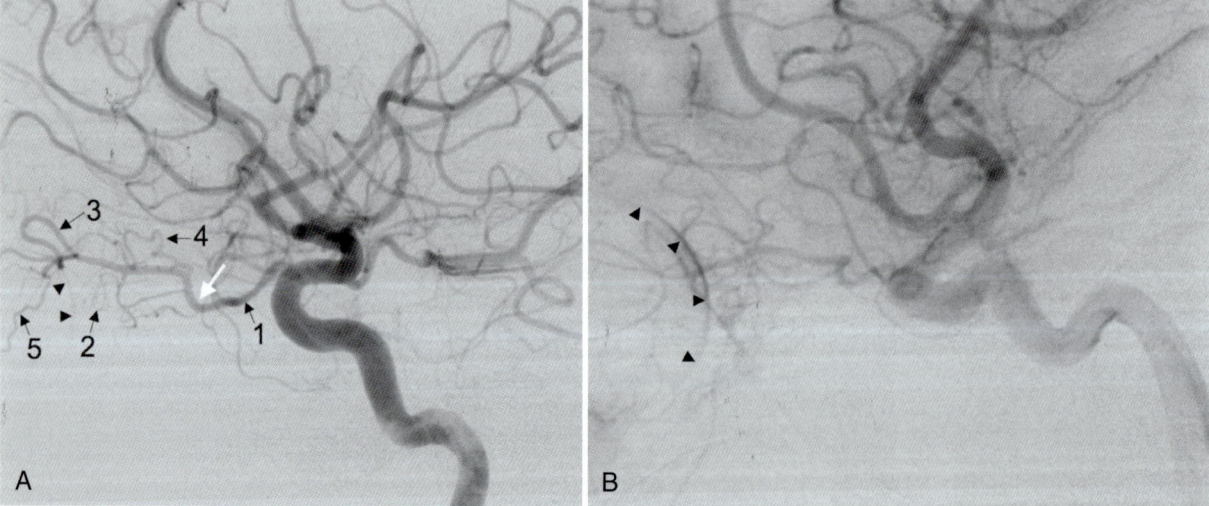

Figure 5-15 **A:** Selective internal carotid artery angiogram, lateral view, of a the ophthalmic artery (OA) and its branches. *White arrow* indicates the abrupt angulation where the OA passes up and over the optic nerve. *1*, OA; *2*, ocular OA branches *(black arrowheads indicate faint vascular choroid blush)*; *3*, orbital OA branches; *4*, lacrimal artery; *5*, anterior ethmoid arteries. **B:** Midarterial phase of an ICA angiogram, lateral oblique view, showing the characteristic crescent-shaped appearance of vascular choroid blush *(black arrowheads)*, which is caused by contrast filling of the ocular vascular choroid plexus. This sign should be actively looked for when performing endovascular embolization procedures in branches of the external carotid artery because the sign may indicate a potential hazard.

in hemodynamic balance with the posterolateral and medial posterior choroidal arteries (PCA branches). Branches of the AChA anastomose freely and frequently with these vessels, resulting in a considerable variation in size and vascular territory of the AChA. Hypoplasia of the AChA is seen in only 3% of cerebral angiograms. In rare cases, the AChA originates from the ICA proximal to the PCoA (instead of distal). This uncommon anomaly needs to be considered preoperatively if a PCoA may be occluded for aneurysm treatment.

Vertebrobasilar System

With minor exceptions, the entire blood supply of the medulla, pons, midbrain, and cerebellum is derived from the vertebrobasilar system. Familiarity with its development, gross anatomy, normal imaging appearance, and vascular territory is a prerequisite for understanding pathologic processes affecting the posterior circulation.

Vertebral Arteries

What Are the Anatomic Segments, Common Variants, and Branches of the Vertebral Arteries?

The VA can be divided into four segments:

1. The V1 (extraosseous) segments extend from the origin of the VAs on the subclavian artery posterosuperiorly to enter the transverse foramen of the sixth cervical vertebrae.
2. The V2 (foraminal) segments ascend vertically passing through the foramina of the C3–6 transverse processes, followed by an inverted L-shaped course through C2. After exiting from the axis, the VAs turn again, running superiorly through the C1 transverse foramen (Figure 5-18).
3. The V3 (extraspinal) segments begin where the VAs exit from C1 to follow a sharp posteromedial bend around the atlantooccipital articulation, producing a prominent grooving along the posterior ring of C1. It then turns sharply forward and upward to pierce the dura at the level of the foramen magnum.

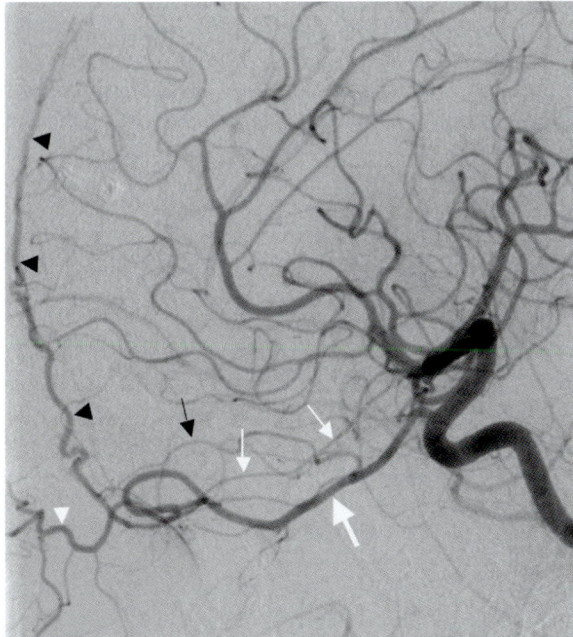

Figure 5-16 Internal carotid artery angiogram, lateral view, of the ophthalmic artery *(large white arrow)* and its orbital and extraorbital branches. *Black arrowheads* delineate a prominent anterior falx artery. This is an extraorbital dural branch that supplies the anterior portions of the falx cerebri. Other extraorbital branches include the anterior ethmoid arteries *(white arrowhead)*. Another important orbital branch is the lacrimal artery *(small black arrow)*, which gives rise to the recurrent meningeal artery *(small white arrows)*. This dural branch courses backward through the superior orbital fissure to anastomose with branches of the middle meningeal artery.

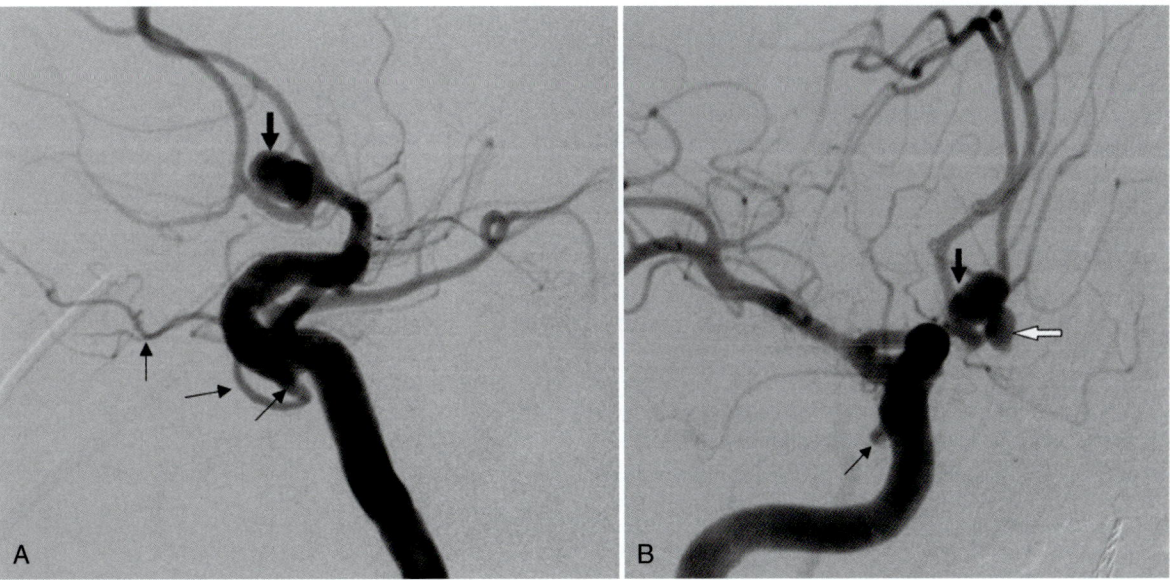

Figure 5-17 Lateral oblique (A) and anteroposterior oblique (B) views of an internal carotid artery (ICA) angiogram demonstrating an anomalous origin of the ophthalmic artery *(small black arrows)* inferiorly from the cavernous ICA segment. In addition, a large, loculated anterior communicating artery aneurysm *(large black arrows)* is noted. The wide-necked aneurysm shows a prominent inferiorly pointing second locule *(white arrow)* that arises from the primary sac. (Courtesy Dr. Tejinder Pal Singh, Perth.)

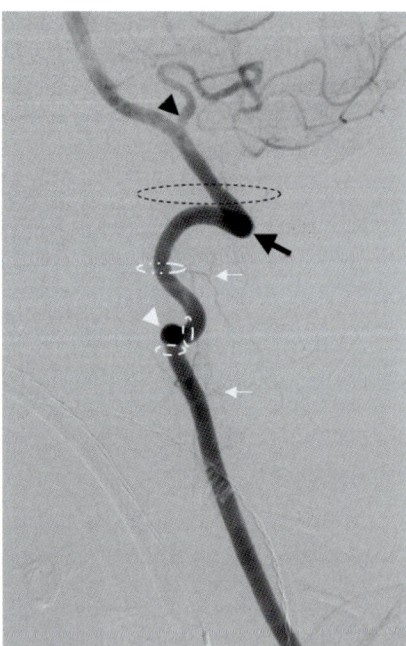

Figure 5-18 Right vertebral angiogram, lateral view, showing the V2 (foraminal), V3 (extraspinal), and V4 (intradural segments). The vertebral artery (VA) shows a nearly vertical course as it passes through the transverse foramina of the C6 to C3 vertebrae. Numerous segmental muscular branches are indicated *(small white arrows)*. The vertebral canal of C2 is indicated by the *lower two white dotted circles*. The VA runs superiorly then turns laterally within C2, forming an inverted L *(white arrowhead)*. After exiting C2, the VA turns cephalad to pass through the transverse foramen of C1 *(upper white dotted circle)*. As it exits the transverse foramen of C1 it curves around the atlantooccipital articulation, turning sharply backward and medially along the upper border of the posterior ring of the atlas. It then bends forward in a tight hairpin turn *(black arrow)* to pierce the dura as it passes through the foramen magnum *(black dotted circle)*. The posterior inferior cerebellar artery is indicated by the *black arrowhead*.

4. The intradural V4 segments first course anteromedially through the foramen magnum and then superomedially behind the clivus to unite at or near the pontomedullary junction.

Each VA has cervical, meningeal, and intracranial branches.

The vascular supply to the neck is organized segmentally according to intervertebral level. Each cervical level is supplied by branches from both the vertebral and the external carotid arteries. The VAs give rise to muscular and spinal cervical branches. Each V2 segment gives off multiple small *unnamed muscular* branches that supply the deep cervical musculature. Segmental *spinal branches* (Figure 5-19) supply the spinal cord and its coverings, anastomosing with spinal arteries from other vessels such as the ascending pharyngeal artery and the thyrocervical trunk.

The meningeal branches supply part of the posterior fossa dura. The *anterior meningeal artery* arises from the distal portion of the V2 segment. This vessel usually is very small and supplies only the dura around the foramen magnum. The *posterior meningeal artery* originates just below the foramen magnum and follows a relatively straight superomedial course to supply the falx cerebelli and the dura along the medial occipital bone (Figure 5-20).

Intracranial VA branches include small meningeal branches, the posterior and anterior spinal arteries, perforating arteries, and the PICA. The *posterior spinal artery* arises from the distal VA or PICA. It descends downward along the dorsal surface of the medulla and spinal cord, forming a vascular network together with numerous spinal radicular branches along the cord all the way down to the cauda equina. The *anterior spinal artery* arises from the distal VA and courses inferomedially to unite with its counterpart from the opposite VA in 50% of cases (Figure 5-19). It gives off a number of small perforating branches to supply the anterior medulla running caudad in the anteromedian sulcus of the spinal cord. The *small perforating arteries* arise directly from the VA to supply the olive and inferior cerebellar peduncle. The *PICA* is the most important, largest, and most variable of all the cerebellar arteries. It arises from the VA at the anterolateral aspect of the brainstem, near the inferior olive. As it courses around the medulla, the main PICA trunk can be divided in four segments and two distinct loops, which are generally best visualized on the lateral projection of a vertebral angiogram (Figure 5-21). It terminates distal the apex of the distal loop by dividing into tonsillohemispheric (lateral) and vermian (medial) branches.

In approximately 75% of patients, the left VA is the same size or larger than the right. However, when the left VA arises directly from the aortic arch (5%–6% of cases), it usually is smaller and may terminate intracranially as the ipsilateral PICA. A shared anterior inferior cerebellar artery (AICA)–PICA trunk is a common normal variant. Occasionally a single trunk supplies both PICAs with a midline crossing anastomotic segment (Figure 5-22). In 0.2% of cases, a small VA terminates in a PICA, and the opposite VA provides most of the posterior fossa blood supply. An extradural origin of PICA is another normal variant (5%–18%) where the PICA origin from the VA lies below the foramen magnum. In one third of cases, the caudal PICA loop extends below the foramen magnum with a normal intradural origin. A duplicated PICA is a rare normal variant (2%). A PICA origin from the posterior meningeal artery or the ICA or a posterior meningeal artery origin from PICA instead of the VA has been described as an uncommon anomaly. Both a bifid and a duplicate VA origin and fenestrated VAs are rare anomalies, found in less than 1% of anatomic dissections (Figure 5-19). The latter is often associated with other anomalies of the brain and spine (e.g., fused vertebrae, aneurysms, and vascular malformations).

Numerous anastomoses exist between muscular extracranial VA branches and ECA branches (e.g., from the occipital and ascending pharyngeal arteries) and may provide an important source of collateral flow in occlusive vascular disease. These anastomoses are regarded as potentially dangerous vessels when endovascular embolization procedures from the ECA system are performed.

Basilar Artery

What Are the Branches of the BA and Its Common Variants?

The BA is a large midline or paramedian vessel that extends from its origin anterior to the pons near the pontomedullary junction to its terminal bifurcation

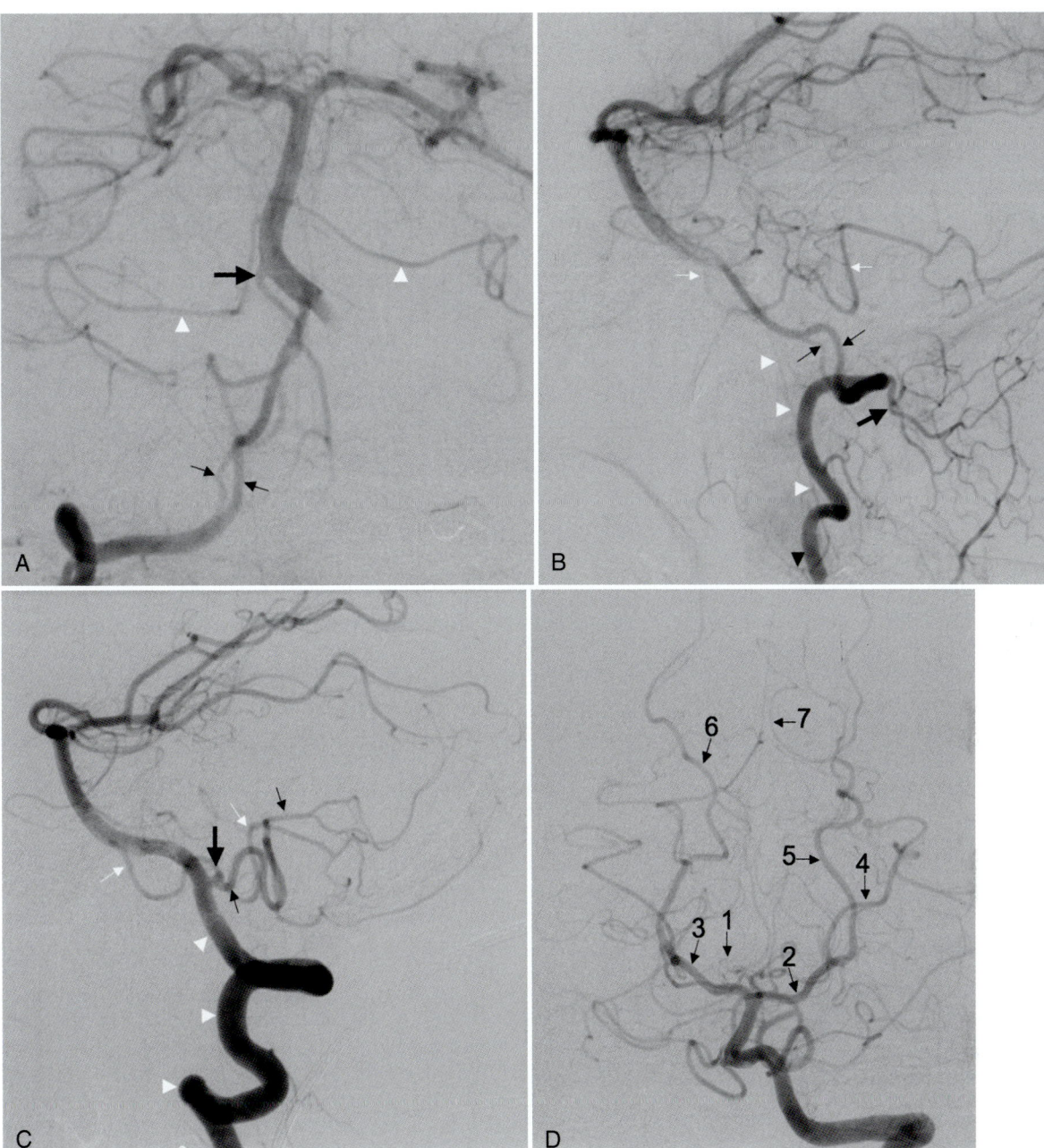

Figure 5-19 A: Right vertebral artery angiogram, Waters anteroposterior view, showing a fenestration of the proximal intradural (V4) segment of the right vertebral artery (VA) *(small black arrows)*. The right V4 segment is mildly hypoplastic, and there is minimal reflux into the distal left VA present at the vertebrobasilar junction. There is an unusual high origin of the right posterior inferior cerebellar artery (PICA) *(large black arrow)* from the proximal basilar artery just below the origin of the anterior inferior cerebellar arteries *(white arrowheads)* as a normal variation. **B:** Same VA angiogram, lateral view, confirms the fenestrated proximal V4 segment of the vertebral artery *(small black arrows)*. The anterior spinal artery *(white arrowheads)* is depicted as a small almost vertically orientated vessel coursing downwards through along the anterior aspect of the cervical cord. Prominent muscular branches originating from the hairpin turn at the C1 level are also shown *(large black arrow)*. A small segmental spinal branch is depicted originating from the V2 segment *(black arrowhead)*. The right PICA originates unusually high from the basilar artery *(small white arrows)* and shows a classical double loop-shaped course. **C:** Left vertebral angiogram, lateral view, of the same patient showing the left dominant VA *(white arrowheads)*. Both PICAs, on the right side *(small white arrows)* originating from the lower basilar artery and on the left side *(small black arrows)* with a normally located origin from the intradural VA, are depicted. A small aneurysm *(large black arrow)* that arises from the left PICA origin is demonstrated. **D:** Left vertebral angiogram, Towne anteroposterior projection, showing the posterior cerebral arteries and their major branches. *1*, Thalamoperforating arteries (small midline blush); *2*, P1 segment; *3*, P2 segment; *4*, posterior temporal artery; *5*, P3 segment; *6*, parietooccipital artery; *7*, calcarine artery.

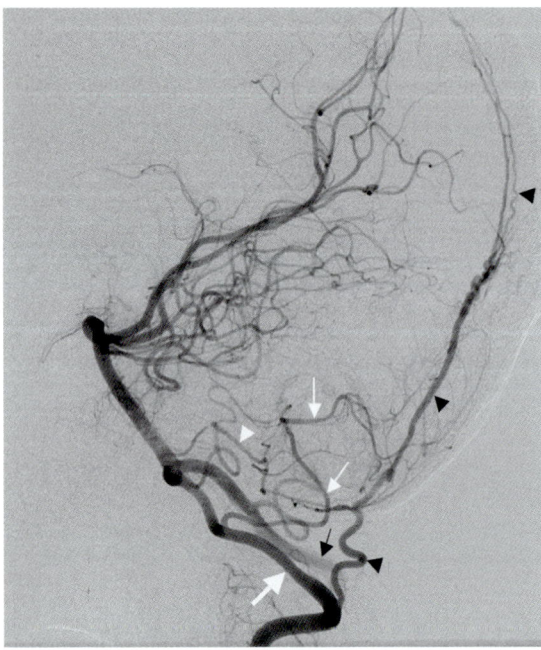

Figure 5-20 Left vertebral artery angiogram, lateral view, showing a prominent posterior meningeal artery *(black arrowheads)* as a normal variant. This dural vessel arises just below the level of the foramen magnum from the posterior bend of the V3 segment and runs in a relatively characteristic course superomedially along the medial aspect of the occipital bone to supply the occipital dura and the falx cerebelli. The left posterior inferior cerebellar artery *(small white arrows)* and low originating anterior inferior cerebellar artery *(white arrowhead)* are depicted as branches of the V4 segment *(large white arrow)* of the left vertebral artery. Reflux into the contralateral right V4 segment is also demonstrated *(small black arrow)*.

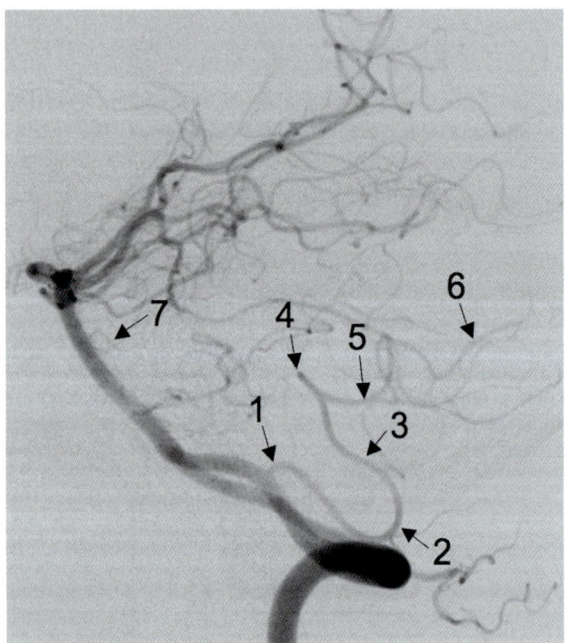

Figure 5-21 Arterial phase of a left vertebral angiogram, lateral view, showing the posterior inferior cerebellar artery (PICA) with its distinct segments and some of its branches. Reflux into the right VA is also demonstrated. *1*, Anterior medullary segment of PICA; *2*, lateral medullary segment of PICA (caudal loop); *3*, posterior medullary segment; *4*, cranial loop of PICA; *5*, supratonsillar segment of PICA; *6*, hemispheric and vermian branches of PICA; *7*, prominent lateral pontine artery.

into the two PCAs. It is located in the interpeduncular cistern adjacent to the dorsum sellae or in the suprasellar cistern below the floor of the third ventricle. The normal BA is 3 to 4 mm in diameter and averages 32 mm in length. Branches of the BA comprise labyrinthine (internal auditory), perforating, and cerebellar arteries and the PCAs. The *labyrinthine arteries* are long slender vessels that arise either directly from the BA (16%) or from the superior (25%) or anterior inferior (45%) cerebellar arteries. They accompany cranial nerves VII and VIII into the internal acoustic meatus. Along its course in the prepontine cistern the BA gives off numerous *pontine perforating arteries,* which can be divided into *median* and *paramedian pontine perforating arteries* and *lateral* or *circumferential pontine arteries* (Figure 5-21).

The BA gives rise to two important cerebellar arteries: the AICA and the *superior cerebellar artery* (SCA).

The AICAs are the smallest of the three cerebellar arteries that arise as single (72%), duplicate (26%), or triplicate (2%) vessels from the proximal BA. They course directly laterally into the cerebellopontine angle cistern lying ventral and medial to cranial nerves VII and VIII. In two thirds of cases, the AICA shows an outward loop that curves into the internal acoustic meatus that has a characteristic single or double (N or M shaped) curve on the lateral angiogram (Figure 5-2, *C*). It terminates by running over the cerebellum to supply its petrosal (anterolateral) surface. The size of the AICA has a reciprocal relationship with that of the PICA, and both arteries may share a common origin, and their hemispheric branches have numerous anastomoses.

The SCAs are the most constant and rostral infratentorial BA branches arising just prior to the BA termination (Figures 5-2 and 5-22). Duplicate (8%) and even triplicate (2%) vessels have been identified as normal variants. In their proximal course, they are separated from the PCAs by cranial nerve III. In their course sweeping around the cerebral peduncles, they lie below cranial nerve IV and above the trigeminal nerve. On AP Towne views they seem to approximate each other behind the brainstem. The superior vermian branches appear very close to the distal PCA on lateral views. The hemispheric SCA branches ramify over the tentorial surface of the cerebellum (Figure 5-2). The vascular territory of the AICA includes the superior surface of the cerebellar hemisphere, superior cerebellar peduncle, upper vermis, dentate nucleus, and part of the brachium pontis.

Numerous anastomoses among the PICA, AICA, and SCA exist over the cerebellar hemispheres and vermis (Figure 5-22).

The perforating arterial supply to the medulla, pons, and tegmentum shows significant variations. The lateral medulla is supplied by the V4 VA segments and the central medulla by perforating BA branches. Except for its upper parts (small SCA branches), the pons is supplied by perforating branches from the BA. The tegmentum typically is supplied by branches of the PCAs and SCAs, but it also receives contribution from perforating arteries directly from the BA.

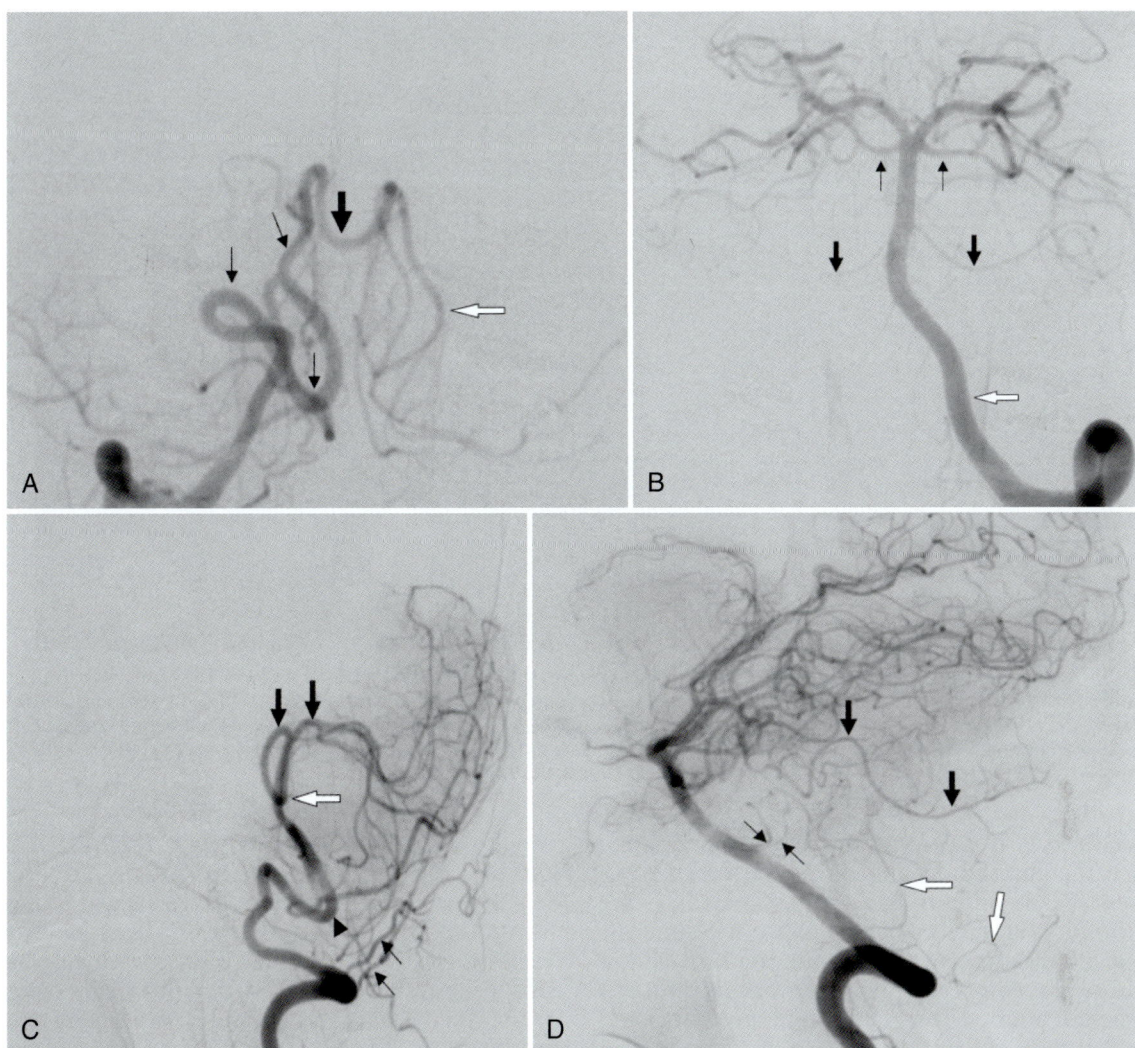

Figure 5-22 A: Angiogram of the right vertebral artery, anteroposterior (AP) view. Bilateral supply of the posterior inferior cerebellar artery (PICA) from the right vertebral artery is demonstrated. The intradural portion of the right vertebral artery terminates in a very prominent right PICA *(small black arrows)*. The cranial loop of the right PICA gives rise to a very prominent midline-crossing bridging segment *(large black arrow)*. This segment then forms the contralateral cranial loop of the left PICA, which divides into its vermian (medial) branches and tonsillohemispheric (lateral) branches *(white arrow)*. **B:** Left vertebral artery angiogram, AP view. No supply of the left PICA from the injected left vertebral artery *(white arrow)* is noted. No reflux into a distal intradural portion of the contralateral vessel is shown, confirming the PICA terminating variant of the right vertebral artery. The basilar artery shows normal supply to the anterior inferior *(large black arrows)* and superior *(small black arrows)* cerebellar arteries. **C:** Right vertebral artery angiogram, lateral view. The V4 (intradural) segment of the right vertebral artery gives rise to a prominent right PICA. The anterior medullary segment, the caudal loop *(arrowhead)*, and posterior medullary segment are nonduplicates. The right supratonsillar PICA segment gives rise to the short interconnecting segment *(white arrow)* with the left PICA, which is depicted en face. The cranial loops are formed as duplicate vessels *(large black arrows)*, giving rise to the terminal PICA branches bilaterally. Note two prominent muscular branches originating from the extradural V3 portion of the right vertebral artery *(small black arrows)*. **D:** Left vertebral artery angiogram, lateral view. No direct PICA supply is demonstrated. The anterior inferior cerebellar arteries are depicted in normal location bilaterally *(small black arrows)*. A very prominent left superior cerebellar artery *(large black arrows)* gives rise to a small collateral hemispheric branch to the territory of the PICA *(white arrows)*. (Courtesy Dr. William McAuliffe, Perth.)

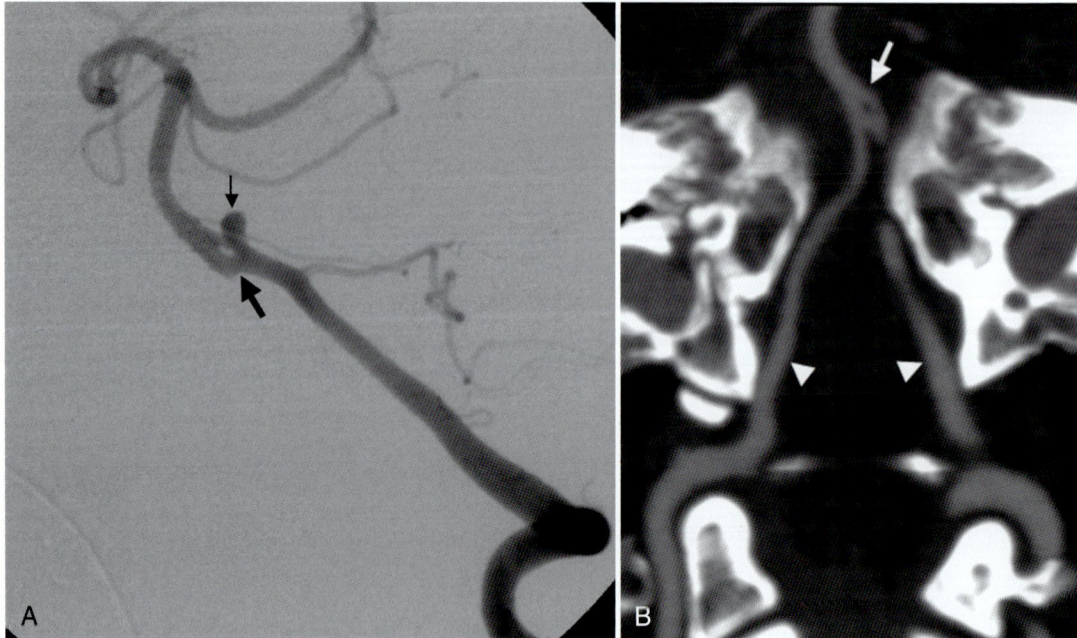

Figure 5-23 **A:** Left vertebral angiogram, oblique view, showing a fenestrated basilar artery *(large black arrow)*. A typical aneurysm is present at the proximal end of the fenestration *(small black arrow)*. **B:** Computed tomographic angiography with targeted, angled anteroposterior, thick maximum intensity projected view allows visualization of the fenestrated basilar artery. Overlying bony structures do not permit complete evaluation of the arterial segments and associated aneurysm on a single reconstructed view. Both proximal intradural portions (V4) of the vertebral arteries *(white arrowheads)* and the fenestrated basilar artery are visualized. (Courtesy Dr. William McAuliffe, Perth.)

If a *fetal-type PCA* is present, this vessel is not opacified when the posterior circulation is studied. In bilateral cases, the BA terminates by bifurcating into the SCAs. Common anomalies of the BA are fenestrations (1.3%) or duplications, which are the result of failure of fusion of the embryonic plexiform primitive longitudinal neural arteries. These are commonly associated with an aneurysm at the proximal end of a fenestration (Figure 5-23). Rarely, the cerebellar arteries arise from the VA, the cavernous ICA, or the PCAs.

Circle of Willis

What Structures Define the Most Important Collateral Pathway at the Base of the Brain, and What Are the Common Variants?

The circle of Willis is an anastomotic ring at the base of the brain providing collateral pathways between the proximal major cerebral arteries. This structure is subject to great individual variation; it is present in its complete or unbroken form in 52% of cases. A complete circle of Willis consists of two ICAs, two anterior cerebral arteries (ACAs; A1 segments), the anterior communicating artery (ACoA), two PCoAs, the BA, and two PCAs (P1 segments) (Figure 5-24). Anatomically the circle of Willis lies above the sella turcica within the interpeduncular and suprasellar cisterns. It surrounds the ventral surface of the diencephalon and lies adjacent to the optic nerves and tracts. It can be easily visualized using noninvasive high-resolution imaging techniques such as CTA or three-dimensional (3D) time-of-flight (TOF) MRA. However, a detailed study of its small but important perforating branches is still largely the domain of conventional cerebral angiography. The entire circle of Willis is rarely seen on a single angiogram (e.g., when three of the four major brain supplying arteries are occluded), but its components usually are visualized sequentially. The anatomic integrity of the circle of Willis can be established using cross-compression angiography. In this technique, a carotid artery is manually compressed while the contralateral carotid or a VA is injected. This information is particularly relevant when deconstructive neurosurgical or endovascular procedures such as carotid sacrifice in the treatment of, for example, giant cavernous aneurysms or life-threatening epistaxis are being contemplated.

The anterior cranial arterial circulation represents the paired terminal ICAs and their terminal branches: the ACAs and the MCAs. The proximal ACA segments, which are also called *precommunicating* or *A1 segments*, are part of the circle of Willis. The ACoA, which lies at the anterior end of the interhemispheric fissure, interconnects both A1 segments. The A1 segment is best visualized on AP or submentovertex views. Because the ACoA typically is orientated in an oblique (rather than strictly anteroposterior) plane, oblique, Waters, or submentovertex views may be required to demonstrate this vessel clearly without the presence of overlapping vessels (Figure 5-25). Temporary cross compression of the contralateral carotid artery is sometimes necessary to demonstrate the ACoA.

The posterior cranial arterial circulation consists of the vertebrobasilar system and the paired PCAs. The two PCoAs provide the major anastomotic link between the anterior (carotid) and posterior (vertebrobasilar) circulations. Each PCoA joins the ipsilateral so-called *precommunicating* or *P1 segment* of the PCA to close the circle of Willis. Transient reflux of contrast into the PCoA during

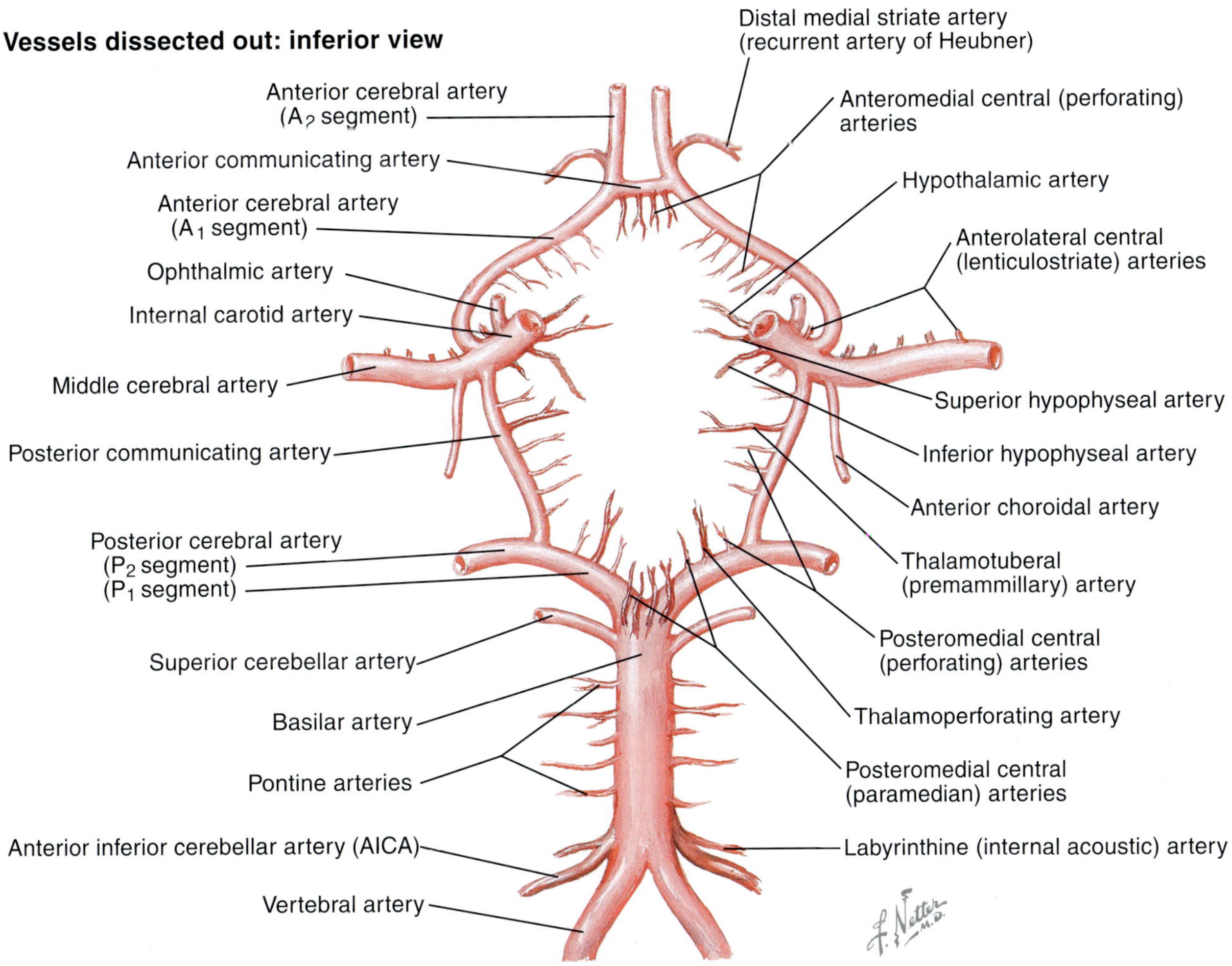

Vessels dissected out: inferior view

Figure 5-24 Anatomic diagram depicts the circle of Willis. Innumerable perforating branches arise from every part of the circle of Willis to supply vital structures at the base of the brain. From Netterimages.com.

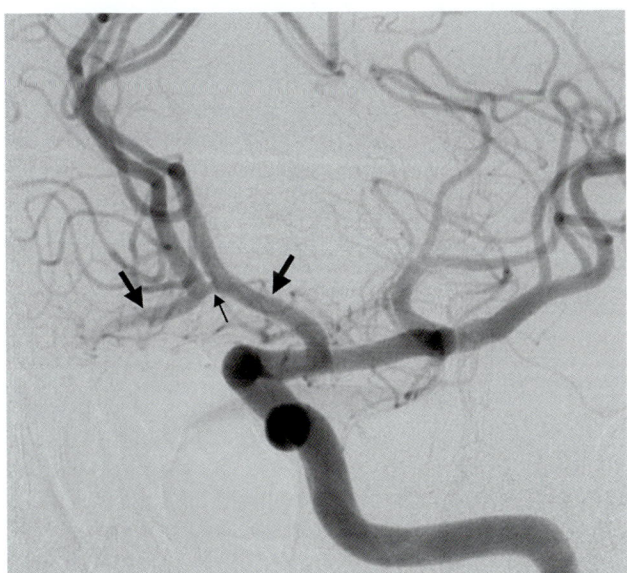

Figure 5-25 Left internal carotid artery angiogram, submentovertex oblique view, depicting the anterior communicating artery *(small black arrow)*. Note cross-flow with filling of the right anterior cerebral artery. The reflux enables depiction of both A1 segments *(large black arrows)*.

injection of either the ICA or a VA often occurs (Figure 5-2, *C*). Ipsilateral carotid cross compression may improve reflux into the PCoA during a VA injection. Lateral or submentovertex views usually best depict the PCoA anatomy, whereas the BA bifurcation and the P1 segments are optimally visualized on steep Towne or shallow submentovertex projections of vertebral angiograms.

Important perforating branches arise from every part of the circle of Willis: the *medial lenticulostriate arteries* and the *recurrent artery of Heubner* supply the caudate nucleus head, anterior limb of the internal capsule, and other parts of the basal ganglia. Several small perforating branches arise from the ACoA, which may have a significant vascular territory including the anterior hypothalamus, optic chiasm, parts of the corpus callosum, columns of the fornix, lamina terminalis, and parolfactory areas. The *anterior thalamoperforating arteries* arise from the PCoA to supply part of the thalamus, the infralenticular limb of the internal capsule, and the optic tracts (Figure 5-24). The distal BA and P1 segments give rise to numerous perforating arteries, the *posterior thalamoperforating arteries*, which course within the interpeduncular fossa to enter the brain behind the mamillary bodies (Figure 5-2, *C*). In 42% of cases, a single

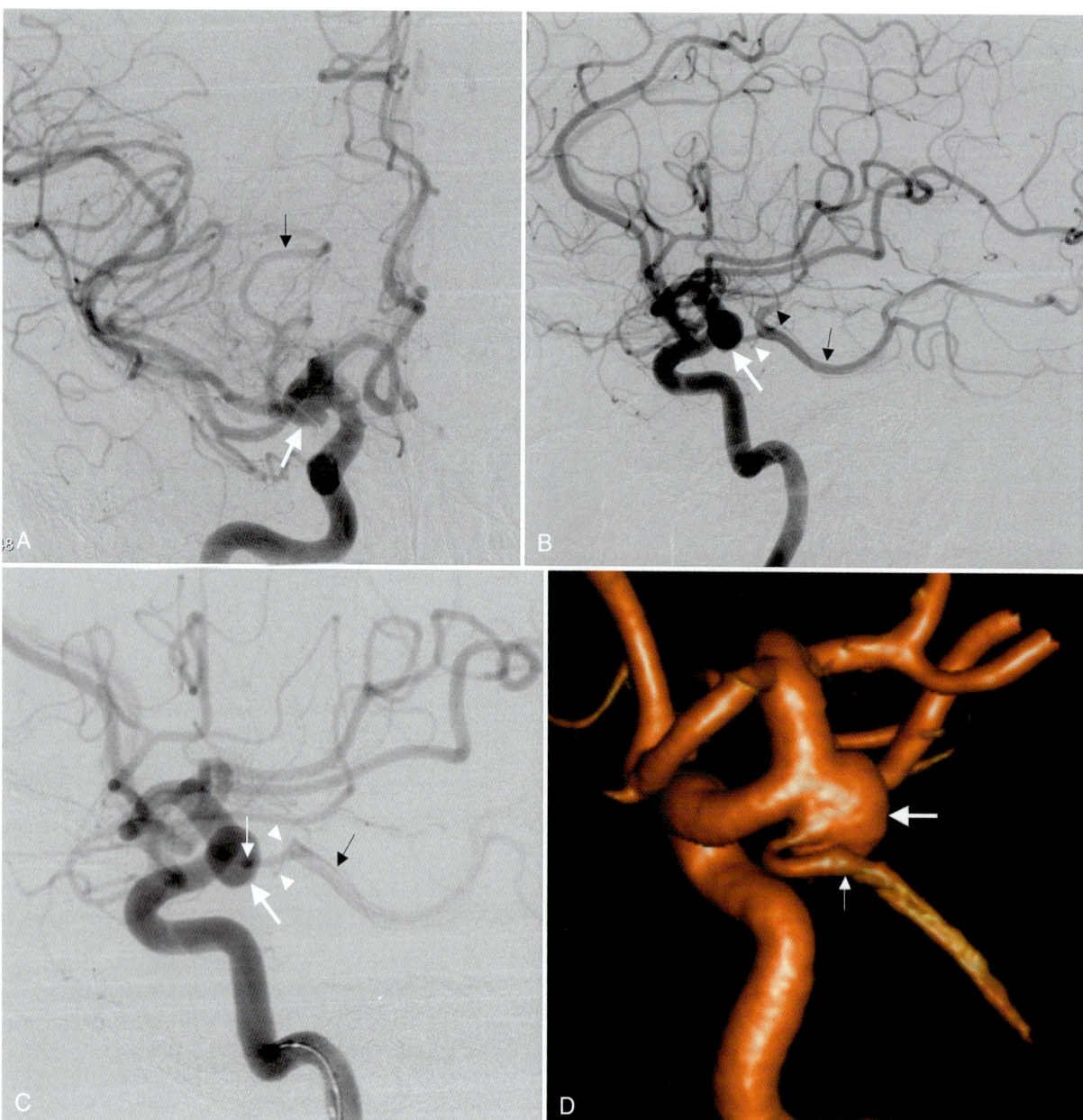

Figure 5-26 Anteroposterior (**A**), lateral (**B**), and lateral oblique (**C**) views of a selective right internal carotid artery angiogram show an inferolaterally pointing aneurysm *(large white arrow)* at the origin of the posterior communicating artery. Filling of the right posterior cerebral artery *(small black arrow)* with temporary short reflux into the right P1 segment *(black arrowhead)* is demonstrated. A prominent anterior thalamoperforating artery *(white arrowheads* in **B** and **C**) arises from the mid-posterior communicating artery. The origin of the posterior communicating artery relative to the vascular anatomy of the aneurysm is not clearly depicted on the standard views (**A, B**). It appears to arise from the aneurysm sac on the oblique working projection view for coiling *(small white arrow)* as demonstrated by double density sign, which projects on the aneurysmal wall (**C**). Note the presence of a microcatheter within the petrous internal carotid artery portion. **D:** The three-dimensional rotational angiographic image of the right internal carotid artery in the same patient better visualizes the origin of the posterior communicating artery *(small white arrow)* with respect to the aneurysm sac *(large white arrow)* as well as the size and configuration of the aneurysm neck. (Courtesy Dr. William McAuliffe, Perth.)

posterior thalamoperforating artery, the so-called *artery of Percheron,* is the largest branch arising from one P1 segment to supply both thalami.

A perfect circle in which all components are present and of adequate and equal size occurs in only 21% of autopsy specimens. The PCoAs usually are smaller than the ICAs and PCAs (Figure 5-26). Some of the more common variations include direct origin of the PCA from the ICAs *(fetal PCA)* in 20% to 30% of cases (Figure 5-27), hypoplastic posterior communicating arteries in 15% to 22% of cases, and hypoplastic A1 segments in 10% of anatomic dissections. A true aplastic A1 segment is found in only 1% to 2% of cases (Figure 5-28). An absent P1 segment is very uncommon. A single ACoA is present in approximately 60% of cases. Multiple vascular channels *(plexiform ACoAs,* 10%–33%) and a *duplicated* (18%) or *fenestrated* (12%–21%) ACoA are considered normal variants of the ACoA. An absent ACoA occurs in only 5% of cases. In the presence of stenoocclusive disease, such normal variations may become very significant prognostic

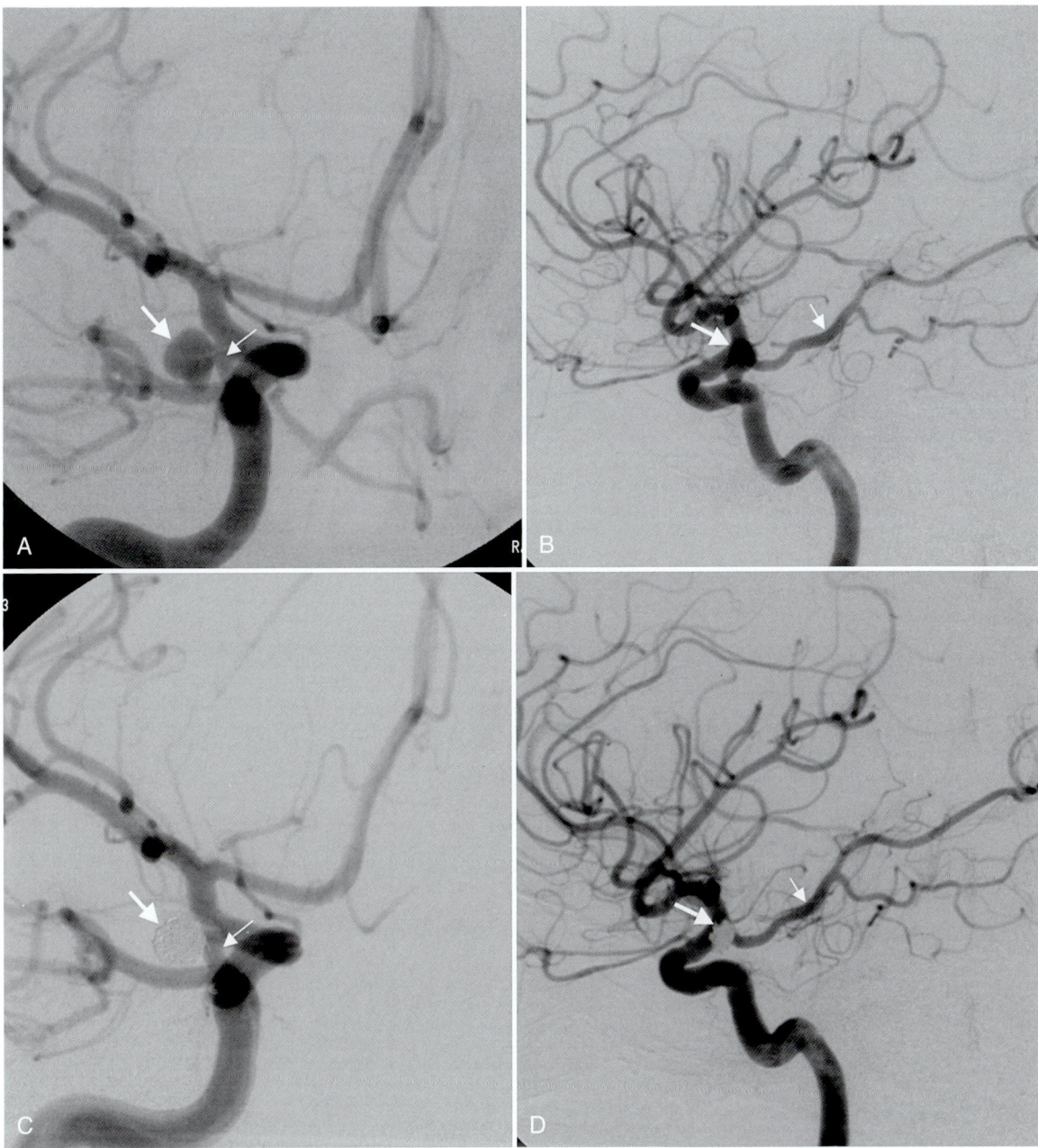

Figure 5-27 Anteroposterior (**A, C**) and lateral (**B, D**) projections of a right internal carotid artery angiogram obtained before and after coil embolization of a lobulated posterior communicating artery aneurysm *(large white arrow)*. The narrow aneurysm neck arises directly from the posterior communicating segment of the posterior cerebral artery *(small white arrow)*, which shows a direct origin from the internal carotid artery, a so-called *fetal variant*. On the control angiogram, which was obtained directly after embolization (**C, D**), complete obliteration of the aneurysm sac by the coil mass *(large white arrow)* and preservation of the parent artery can be noted *(small white arrow)*. (Courtesy Dr. William McAuliffe, Perth.)

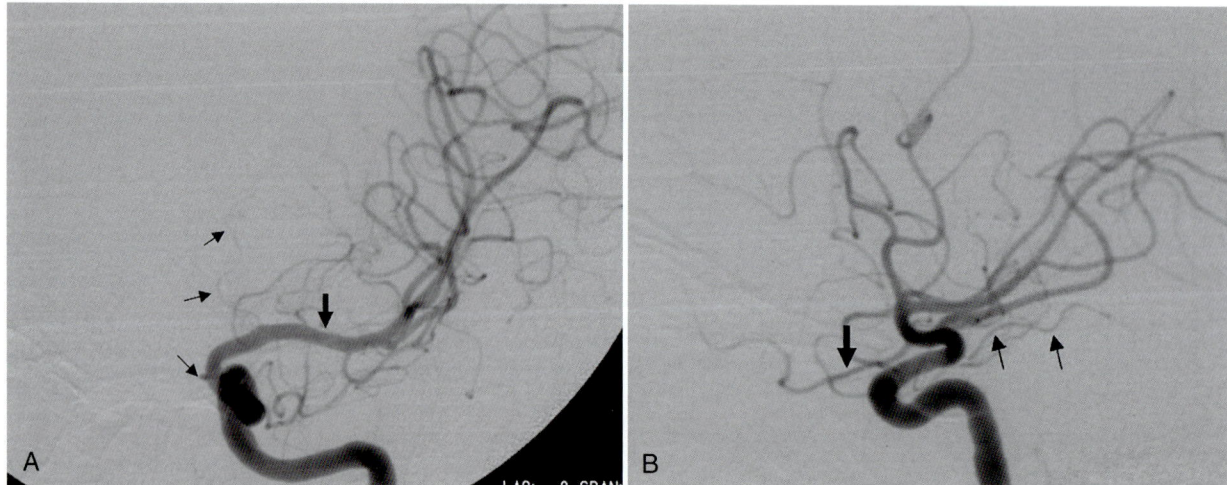

Figure 5-28 A: Anteroposterior view of an internal carotid artery angiogram showing an absent A1 segment of the anterior cerebral artery (ACA). Because the ACA is absent, a prominent anterior choroidal artery is seen *(small black arrows)*. The internal carotid artery essentially terminates in the M1 segment of the middle cerebral artery *(large black arrow)*. **B:** Internal carotid artery angiogram of the same patient, lateral projection, showing absence of the ACA and the posterior communicating artery. The anterior choroidal artery *(small black arrows)* and ophthalmic artery are depicted *(large black arrow)*.

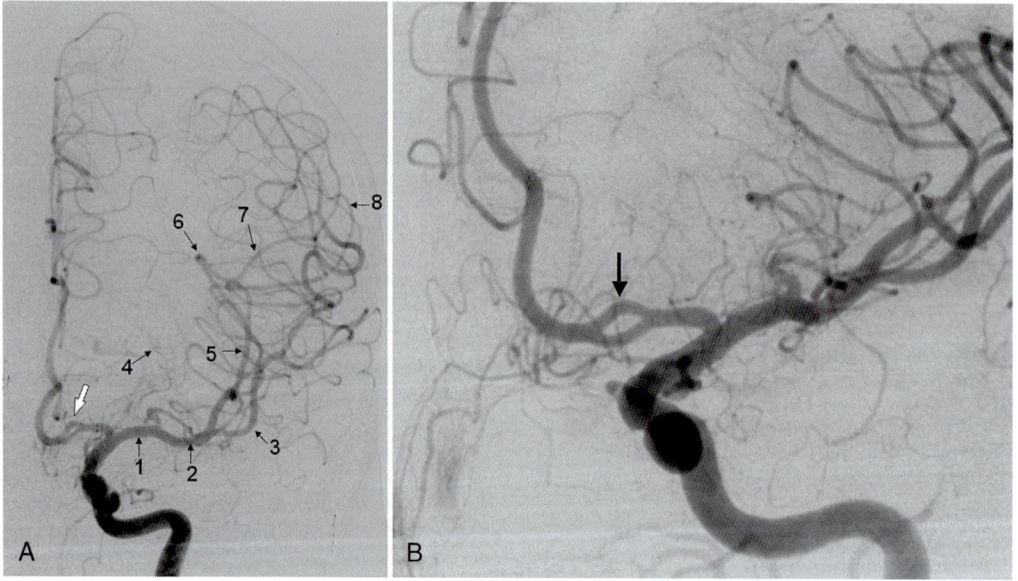

Figure 5-29 A: Left internal carotid artery angiogram, anteroposterior projection, showing a short segmental fenestration of the A1 segment, which is a normal variant *(white arrow)*. The middle cerebral artery (MCA) segments and branches are indicated as follows: *1*, M1 (horizontal) segment; *2*, MCA bifurcation; *3*, MCA genu; *4*, lateral lenticulostriate arteries (penetrating M1 branches); *5*, M2 segment; *6*, apex of sylvian fissure (angiographic sylvian point); *7*, M3 segment; *8*, M4 segment (ramifying cortical hemispheric branches). **B:** Caldwell oblique view best depicts the proximal segments of the anterior cerebral artery. Thereby, the fenestrated A1 segment *(black arrow)* is again visualized. The anterior communicating artery is not seen.

factors, such as a small or absent PCoA that was found to be an independent risk factor for ischemic cerebral infarctions in cases of ICA occlusion. Another example is an *isolated ICA*, which occurs when a fetal PCA and absent A1 segment both are present on the same side. This setup eliminates collateral flow from the contralateral ICA or the vertebrobasilar system in cases of stroke to the vascular ICA territory, which supplies both the ipsilateral MCA and PCA, potentially resulting in a major neurologic deficit.

True anomalies of the circle of Willis are rare. They include an *infraoptic origin of the ACA*, which is located in the ICA near the OA origin, a *fenestration of the ACA* (Figures 5-29 and 5-30), and an *azygos ACA*. The latter is a solitary, unpaired vessel that arises as a single trunk from the confluence of the bilateral A1 segments with an absent ACoA (Figure 5-31). This anomaly is found in various forms of holoprosencephaly. Rare anomalies of the posterior circulation comprise *persistent carotid–basilar anastomoses*, which are described in chapter on the ICA (see Chapter 5, Section "Internal Carotid Arteries"). A detailed discussion of the vessels distal to the circle of Willis is beyond the scope of this article.

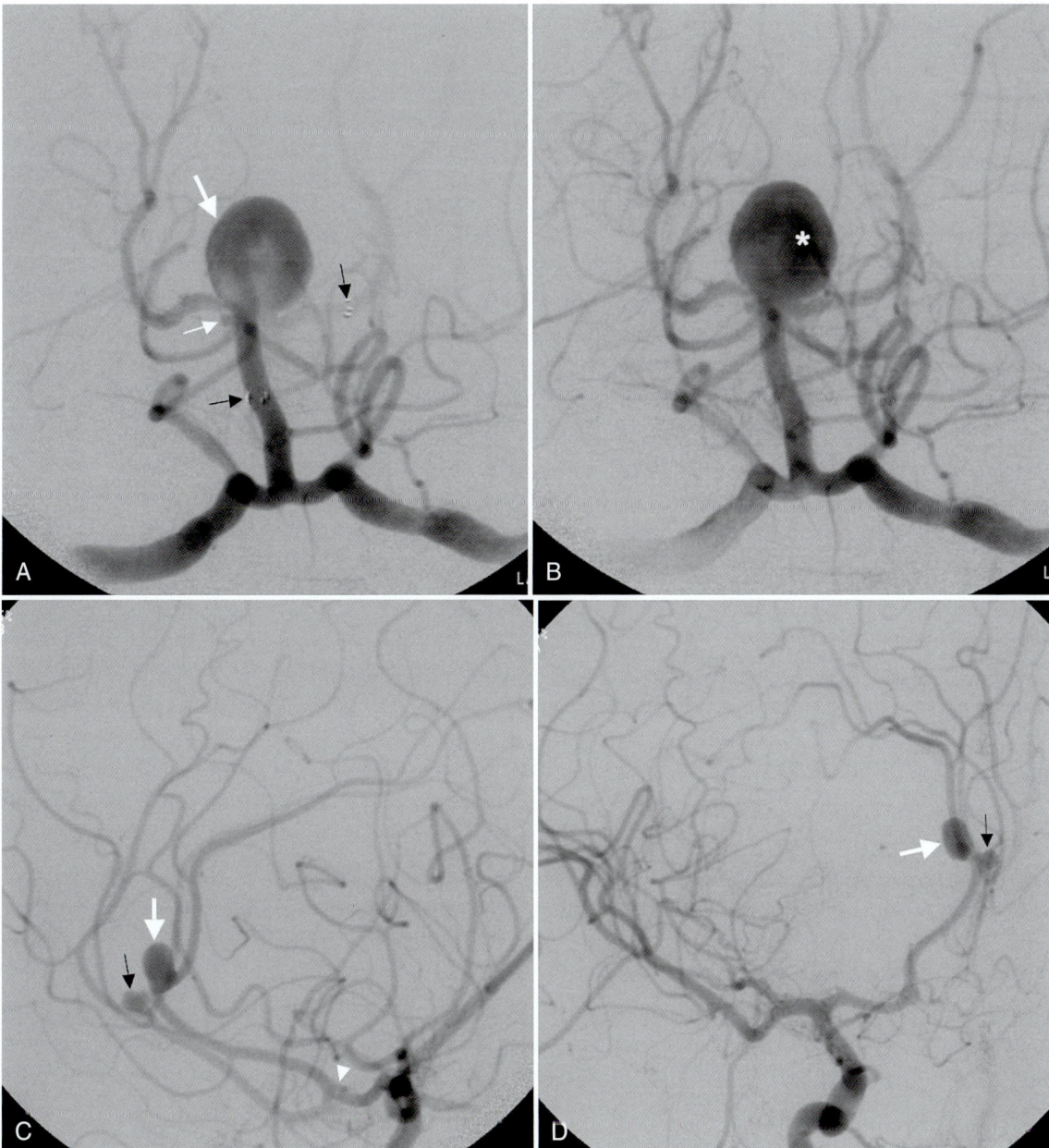

Figure 5-30 Angiograms of different vascular territories from the same patient reveal multiple cerebral aneurysms. Towne anteroposterior projections of selective left vertebral artery angiogram at early (**A**) and subsequent later (**B**) arterial phases demonstrate a large, wide-necked aneurysm at the tip of the basilar artery *(large white arrow)* that incorporates both P1 segments into its neck and intraaneurysmal flow patterns. The inflow contrast jet enters the right paracentral orifice (**A**) and circulates from the right dome in clockwise fashion to the left lateral neck and into the left P1 segment, which shows delayed contrast filling (**A, B**). The central part of this vortex shows slower flow with contrast stasis *(asterisk in **B**)*. Due to symptoms related to mass effect on the mesencephalon, a staged treatment of the basilar tip aneurysm was initiated, with placement of a stent over the wide aneurysm neck. The proximal and distal markers *(small black arrows)* are visualized in the mid-basilar artery and the left posterior cerebral artery, respectively. A second, very small aneurysm *(small white arrow)* arises from the distal basilar artery between the origin of the right superior cerebellar artery and the right P1 segment. Lateral oblique (**C**) and transorbital oblique (**D**) projections of the right common carotid artery angiogram show two other aneurysms at the A2/A3 junction of the right anterior cerebral artery. The larger aneurysm *(large white arrow)* demonstrates a broad neck that incorporates the proximal pericallosal artery over a short distance. The other smaller aneurysm arises from the origin of the callosomarginal artery *(small black arrow)*. A tiny fenestration of the distal A1 segment *(white arrowhead in **C**)* is depicted. (Courtesy Dr. Constantine Phatouros, Perth.)

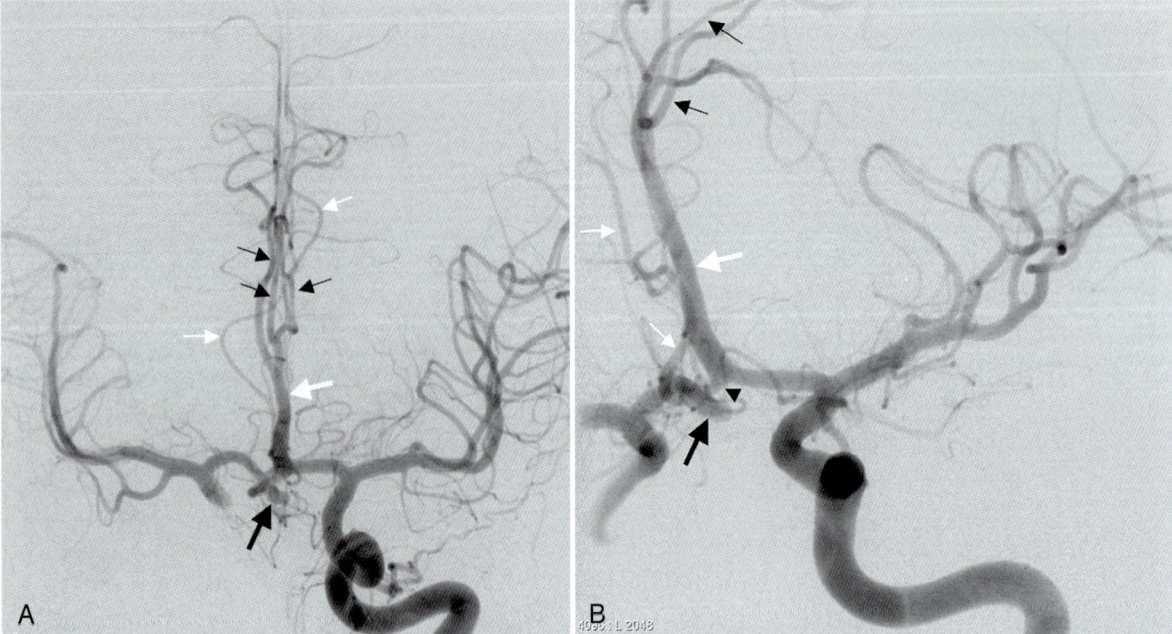

Figure 5-31 Anteroposterior (**A**) and transorbital oblique (**B**) views of left internal carotid artery angiogram show a solitary midline trunk, a so-called *azygos anterior cerebral artery (large white arrow)*, which supplies both the bilateral pericallosal and the right callosomarginal arteries *(small black arrows)*. The right A1 segment gives rise solely to the right orbitofrontal arteries and the left callosomarginal artery *(small white arrows)*, which crosses the midline underneath the anterior falx cerebri. A small inferiorly directed, mildly lobulated aneurysm *(large black arrow)* arises from the right A1/A2 junction at the origin of the anterior communicating artery *(black arrowhead)*. (Courtesy Dr. Tejinder Pal Singh, Perth.)

■ INDICATIONS

Aneurysms

What Are the Characteristics of Intracranial Aneurysms, and What Is the Best Way to Classify Them?

Intracranial aneurysms are classified according to their gross pathologic appearance as saccular or "berry" aneurysms, fusiform aneurysms, and dissecting aneurysms. Saccular aneurysms are round or lobulated focal outpouchings that usually arise from arterial bifurcations. Occasionally they originate directly from the lateral wall of a nonbranching artery. The aneurysmal sac may have a narrow orifice (neck), or it may arise from a more broad-based neck. Most intracranial aneurysms are true aneurysms, that is, they contain at least some layers that are normally found in the arterial wall yet lack other components. Acute thrombi and organized laminated clots are frequently present within the aneurysm lumen.

Intracranial dissecting aneurysms are caused by penetration of circulating blood into the arterial wall with extension between its layers. The opacified false lumen is contained by the vessel adventitia. Once ruptured, intracranial dissecting aneurysms have a high risk of rebleeding (up to 70%) within the first week after initial SAH, with a high mortality rate (46%). Differentiating between dissecting aneurysms from saccular aneurysms is important because the treatment may differ. Angiographically, the signs of intracranial dissection may be subtle, including irregular tapering of the vessel lumen, intraluminal linear filling defects, retention of contrast within the vessel wall, fusiform dilatation interrupted by segments of string-like narrowing ("pearl and string" sign), and/or presence of irregular aneurysm or pseudoaneurysm associated with focal luminal narrowing or irregularity (Figure 5-32) (see section on Intracranial Dissection).

Fusiform intradural aneurysms represent less than 1% of intracranial aneurysms and frequently are associated with vessel tortuosity, atherosclerosis, hypertension, and old age. They typically are located in the supraclinoid ICA and the basilar trunk. They often present with symptoms of mass effect, and rupture is uncommon when the condition is mild. In large aneurysms, stagnation of blood flow may lead to thrombus and subsequent embolic stroke. If ectasia reaches bizarre proportions, the terms *megadolichobasilar anomaly* in the BA or *giant fusiform serpentine aneurysm* are used. The latter subtype typically shows a more malign course due to recurrent SAH, progressive mass effect (e.g., brainstem compression, cranial nerve palsies, or obstructive hydrocephalus), or embolic strokes. MRI has shown some evidence that intracranial dissection may play a role in the growth of these lesions.

The risk of harboring an incidental intracranial aneurysm is 1% to 3% in autopsy series and between 1% and 5% in the general population. The annual risk of rupture is estimated to be 1% to 2%. The reported frequency of multiple aneurysms in large referral centers ranges from 20% to 33% depending on angiographic quality, number of vessels examined, and referral patterns, which all influence the rate of detection of multiple lesions. Up to 30% of patients with SAH have multiple aneurysms. Female gender, cigarette smoking, and vasculopathies such as fibromuscular dysplasia and polycystic kidney disease are recognized risk factors for multiple aneurysm.

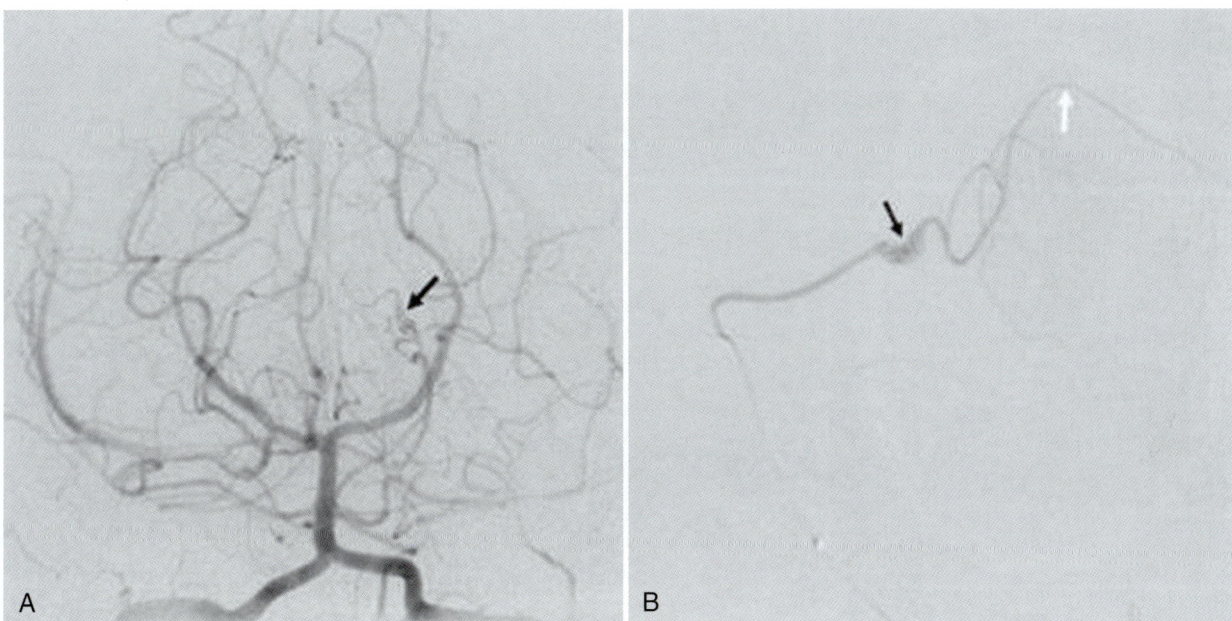

Figure 5-32 **A:** Towne anteroposterior view of left vertebral artery angiogram showing an irregular and fusiform-shaped aneurysm of the peripheral left superior cerebellar artery (SCA; *black arrow*). Flash filling with streaming of the right middle cerebral artery territory via the posterior communicating artery is also demonstrated. **B:** Superselective microcatheter injection of the left SCA, lateral view, better depicts the morphology of this distal dissecting aneurysm with multiple irregular and partially flap-like, filling defects *(black arrow)*. The hemispheric SCA branches that arise distal to the aneurysm are clearly visualized *(white arrow)*. (Courtesy Dr. William McAuliffe, Perth.)

Which Other Types and Causes of Intracranial Aneurysms Exist?

Mycotic aneurysms of infectious origin account for 2% to 4% of all intracerebral aneurysms (5%–15% in children) and have a high risk of rupture. They most often occur in patients with infective endocarditis or a history of drug abuse. The most common causative bacterium is *Streptococcus viridans*, and the most common fungal agent causing aneurysms is *Aspergillus fumigatus*. These lesions typically arise on the smaller arteries distal to the circle of Willis and represent actual pseudoaneurysms caused by distally lodged septic emboli. The latter can either directly destroy the intima or reach the adventitia via vasa vasorum. The inflammation eventually leads to disruption of vessel wall layers and aneurysmal dilatation.

Traumatic aneurysms account for 0.2% to 1% of all intracranial aneurysms (5%–15% in children) and are the most common cause of intracranial pseudoaneurysm (its wall is not composed of normal vessel wall layers but consists of cavitated clot) (Figure 5-33). They usually result from indirect trauma from closed head injury, such as shearing injury or impaction of an artery against a dural fold, such as the distal ACA against the falx cerebri. They may also be caused by direct penetrating trauma or a contiguous skull fracture. The most frequently encountered traumatic aneurysm location is the cavernous ICA segment (48%), which is typically associated with basal skull fractures. These aneurysms might enlarge and produce a cavernous sinus syndrome with nerve compression, or they might secondarily rupture, producing a carotid–cavernous fistula (CCF). Transdural leakage will lead to SAH. The most dangerous form is a medial tear of the ICA with rupture into the sphenoid sinus causing massive and life-threatening epistaxis. Delayed clinical presentation with stroke or hematoma is common (up to 3–4 weeks following the trauma). Angiographic findings in traumatic aneurysms commonly include peripheral or nonbranching locations, delayed filling and emptying of an often irregularly outlined aneurysmal cavity with or without mass effect from hematoma, and absence of a definable neck.

Rarely, neoplastic (oncotic) aneurysms develop as a result of either direct vascular invasion by tumor or implantation of distal tumor emboli (0.1% of all aneurysms). Both primary intracranial (e.g., meningioma, high-grade glioma) and metastatic neoplasms (e.g., atrial myxoma, chorion carcinoma) have been reported to cause neoplastic aneurysms. Occasionally squamous cell carcinomas invade the branches of the ECA and cause an oncotic pseudoaneurysm, which may result in exsanguinating epistaxis.

Which Types of Aneurysms May Be Related to Vascular Malformations?

High-flow states such as arteriovenous malformations (AVMs) and AVFs can increase hemodynamic stress on vessel walls and induce the formation of so-called *flow-related aneurysms* (Figure 5-13, *C* and *D*). The reported association with AVMs are in the range from 5% to 15%. Such aneurysms are thin-walled structures that easily rupture with sudden increase of intravascular pressure. Among patients with ruptured AVMs, 80% harbor flow-related aneurysms. They occur as intralesional (intranidal/perinidal) or feeding artery aneurysms. True intranidal aneurysms may be best detected by superselective angiography.

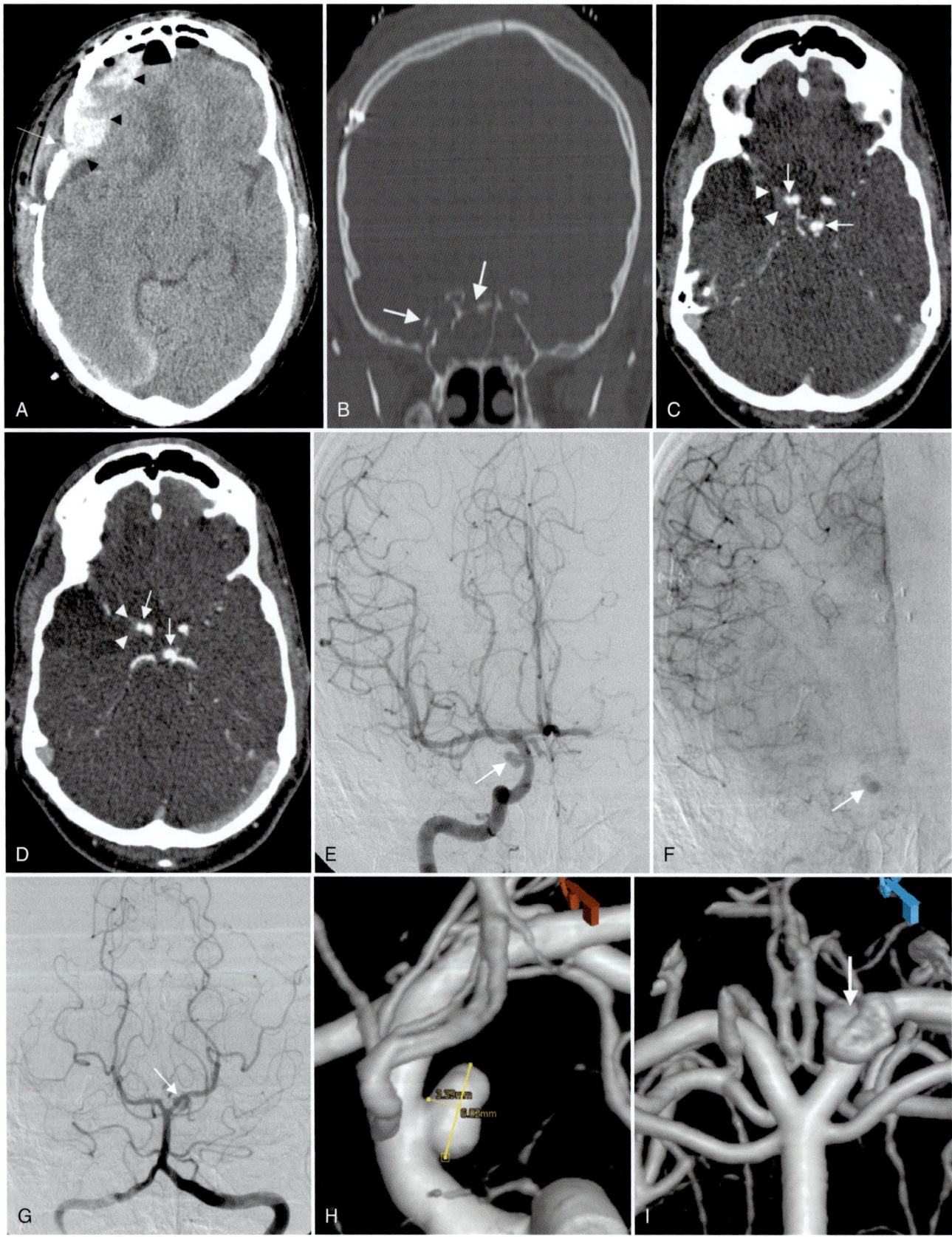

Figure 5-33 Different imaging modalities performed in a 17-year-old patient with severe traumatic head injuries following a motor vehicle accident. **A:** Noncontrast enhanced computed tomographic (CT) image of the head showing a depressed fracture of the right cranial vault in the frontotemporal area *(white arrow)*. An acute extradural hemorrhage is demonstrated *(black arrowheads)*. Mass effect with midline shift as well as bifrontal intracranial air is also shown. **B:** After initial surgical decompression and evacuation of the patient's extradural hematoma, a follow-up CT was performed. The coronally reconstructed image, bone window settings, shows a heavily displaced fracture of the central base of skull with multiple fragments of the walls of the sphenoid sinus *(white arrows)* that partially involve the intracranial segments of the right internal carotid artery (ICA). **C, D:** Axial sources images of CT angiogram revealing two traumatic aneurysms *(white arrows)* located in the supraclinoid (C6) portion of the right ICA and in the left P1 segment of the left posterior cerebral artery, just proximal to the posterior communicating artery junction. The right ICA aneurysm demonstrates marked peripheral thrombus formation *(white arrowheads)*. Selective right ICA angiograms, anteroposterior (AP) view, in early arterial phase **(E)** and later arterial/capillary phase **(F)** show a laterally pointing bilobulated aneurysm located in the superior C6 ICA segment *(white arrow)*. Intraaneurysmal pooling of contrast is noted during the later angiographic phase *(white arrow)*. **G:** Selective left vertebral artery angiogram, Towne AP view, showing large aneurysm in the left P1 segment of the posterior cerebral artery. Volume-rendered reconstructed images derived from three-dimensional rotational angiograms of right ICA **(H)** and left vertebral artery **(I)** show detailed views of both traumatic aneurysms relative to branching vessels and their parent arteries. The left P1 aneurysm reveals a rough and irregular luminal surface *(white arrow)* due to the presence of intrasaccular thrombus.

What Are the Most Important Predisposing Conditions for the Development and Progression of Intracranial Aneurysms?

Under Which Circumstances Is Aneurysm Screening for Individuals Advised?

What Are Important Risk Factors for Rupture of Aneurysms?

The genesis, progression, and rupture of cerebral aneurysms are not well understood. Most intracranial aneurysms are acquired lesions from hemodynamic stresses and degeneration of the vessel wall most pronounced at arterial bifurcations. The understanding of hemodynamic flow patterns as important (co-)factors for the pathogenesis and rupture of cerebral aneurysms has been enhanced by computational flow modeling and MR derived in vivo flow measurements (Figure 5-34). A spectrum of inherited and acquired processes may predispose to aneurysm formation by weakening the vessel wall matrix. Inherited connective tissue disorders are rare (5% of all aneurysms); therefore, the number of patients associated with SAH is small but include those with *Ehlers-Danlos syndrome (EDS) type IV* (large- and medium-sized artery aneurysms, spontaneous CCF, arterial dissection), *Marfan syndrome* (saccular, fusiform, or dissecting aneurysms), and *neurofibromatosis type 1* (NF1) (stenosis, aneurysm, or fistula formation).

The most important unchangeable risk factors are so-called *familial intracranial aneurysms* (10% of cases of SAH) and *autosomal dominant polycystic kidney disease* (ADPKD, <1% of cases of SAH). Approximately 25% of patients with ADPKD have an intracranial aneurysm at autopsy, and the risk of developing de novo aneurysms is increased in ADPKD patients. Familial intracranial aneurysms are a distinct disease entity that affects at least two or more first-degree relatives in the same family with aneurysmal SAH in the absence of other predisposing heritable disorders. The age at onset is late, aneurysms tend to be larger and multiple, multiple modes of inheritance are observed, and genetic testing is not yet available for this disease. If only one first-degree relative is affected, the estimated lifetime risk of SAH remains limited (3.3% vs 0.6% in the general population). However, with two or more affected relatives, a steep rise in risk of SAH is observed, with an absolute lifetime risk of 26%. The prevalence of incidental aneurysms among symptom-free first-degree relatives from families with two or more affected members ranges between 8% and 20.6% depending on the history of cofactors such as smoking and hypertension. Therefore, individuals with two or more first-degree relatives from such families constitute a high-risk group, so noninvasive MRA screening is suggested, particularly in the presence of other modifiable risk factors. Screening for intracranial aneurysms also has suggested in asymptomatic ADPKD patients. When aneurysm screening is undertaken in such individuals, the potential future risk of aneurysm treatment should be taken into consideration. If a first screening is negative, repeated screening should be advised after 5 years (risk of finding an aneurysm is 7%).

Other conditions associated with an increased prevalence of aneurysms are *congenital heart disorders, anomalous vessels, arterial fenestrations* (Figures 5-23 and 5-35), *vasculopathies* (e.g., *fibromuscular dysplasia*), and *sickle cell disease*.

Modifiable risk factors for aneurysm rupture include smoking, arterial hypertension, excessive alcohol consumption, and possibly the use of estrogens.

For unruptured aneurysms, data from the International Study of Unruptured Intracranial Aneurysms (ISUIA) showed that the 5-year cumulative rupture rate was relatively low (0.1%) for small aneurysms (<7 mm) in the anterior circulation in patients without a history of previous SAH. This risk increased to 2.5% to 50% depending on aneurysm size and location (posterior circulation including PCoA artery aneurysms have higher rupture risk than anterior circulation aneurysms). However, these results derived from a large multicenter prospective trial were often criticized for limitations mainly related to sample size asymmetries within groups and a relatively short follow-up period (<5 years in 50%). Other population-based studies confirmed large aneurysm size, posterior circulation location, and history of previous SAH as independent predictors of aneurysm rupture. Slightly higher rupture rates for small aneurysms (<5 mm) were possibly related to racial differences, with Japanese and Finnish descendents having a higher potential for rupture. Other patient characteristics, such as age greater than 60 years, female gender, and aneurysm characteristics (e.g., increasing size and symptoms

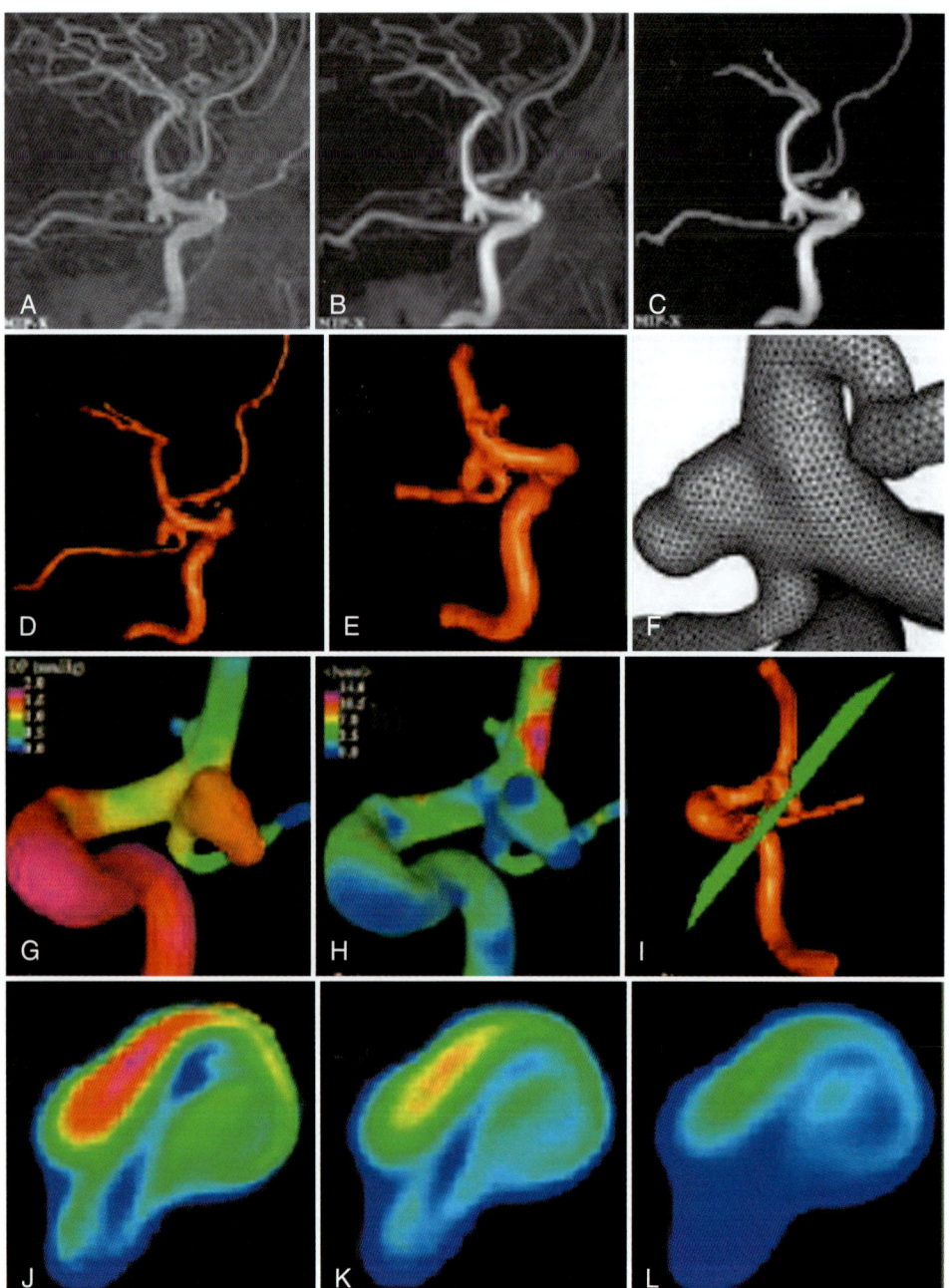

Figure 5-34 Series of images demonstrate the stepwise construction of a patient-specific vascular computational fluid dynamics (CFD) model generated for evaluation of intra-aneurysmal flow dynamics. **A**, Original 3D rotational angiography image. **B**, Smoothed image. **C**, Segmented image. **D**, Initial vascular reconstruction. **E**, Vessel geometry after deformable model and interactive truncation of arterial branches. **F**, Finite element grid. **G**, Peak pressure distribution. **H**, Mean wall shear stress distribution. **I**, Definition of cut plane used to visualize velocity pattern. **J–L**, Intra-aneurysmal flow velocity on cut plane at different instants during the cardiac cycle. (From Cebral JR, Castro MA, Burgess JE, Pergolizzi RS, Sheridan MJ, Putman CM. Characterization of cerebral aneurysms for assessing risk of rupture by using patient-specific computational hemodynamics models. AJNR Am J Neuroradiol 2005;26:2550-2559)

other than SAH caused by the aneurysm) were found to be associated with a higher risk of rupture in a meta-analysis. Morphologic indicators of rupture risk include the presence of lobulations (Figure 5-36) or daughter aneurysms ("blebs") and a high aspect ratio (defined as the ratio of depth to neck size of a cerebral aneurysm) (Figure 5-37).

Studies have addressed the question of aneurysm enlargement of nonruptured aneurysms under serial MRA or CTA imaging surveillance. The yield of short-term follow-up by CTA or MRA (1-year interval) of small (<5 mm) unruptured aneurysms in high-risk patients (history of previous SAH or familial intracranial aneurysms) is very low (growth rate 3.2%). Large aneurysm size (>8 mm) was the only independent predictor for further aneurysm enlargement, with a frequency of aneurysm enlargement of 10% (mean observation period approximately 4 years) in other studies.

Where Are Intracranial Aneurysms Commonly Located, and What Is Their Clinical Presentation?

Intracranial aneurysms usually arise on the circle of Willis or at the MCA bifurcation (Figure 5-38). Approximately 90% are located in the anterior circulation and only 10% in the vertebrobasilar circulation. Specific common sites include the ACoA complex (30%–35%), internal carotid–posterior communicating artery (30%–35%), MCA bifurcation or trifurcation (20%), and tip of the BA (5%). Aneurysms typically are lesions in adults (peak presentation at age 40–60 years). The most common clinical manifestation of symptomatic intracranial aneurysm is SAH. In 85% to 95% of

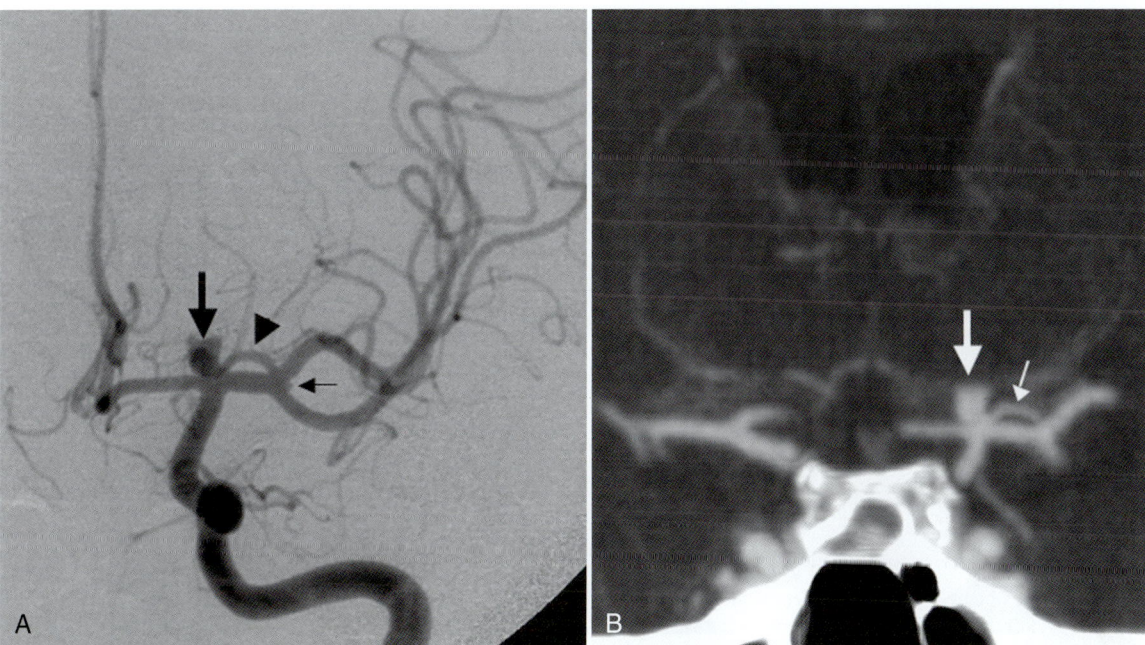

Figure 5-35 **A:** Left internal carotid artery angiogram, anteroposterior view, showing a bilobulated aneurysm at the internal carotid artery (ICA) termination *(large black arrow)*. A short, fenestrated M1 segment is present *(black arrowhead)* as a normal variant. The perforating M1 branches (lateral lenticulostriate arteries) originate from the smaller superior limb of the fenestration. A tiny second aneurysm is evident at the early middle cerebral artery bifurcation *(small black arrow)*. **B:** Computed tomographic angiography, corresponding anteroposterior thick maximal intensity projected image, showing the ICA termination aneurysm *(large white arrow)* and the fenestrated M1 segment *(small white arrow)*. The small second aneurysm is not visualized. (Courtesy Dr. William McAuliffe, Perth.)

patients with SAH, headache is the most common symptom. Much rarer clinical manifestations include cranial neuropathy as the second most common presentation (isolated oculomotor nerve [III] palsy is the most frequent finding), seizure, TIA, and cerebral infarction. Unruptured aneurysms occasionally are misdiagnosed clinically as optic neuritis or migraine headache, sometimes delaying diagnosis of potentially fatal lesions for years.

Intracranial aneurysms are rare in children (<2% of all cases) and have different characteristics in the pediatric group compared to adults: male predominance (3:1); aneurysms are more common in posterior circulation or distal to circle of Willis (nearly 20%) and at terminal ICA bifurcation (25%–50%); giant aneurysms (>2.5 cm) are common in children; mass effect is a common presenting symptom (approximately 20% of cases); and aneurysms are more frequently associated with trauma (up to 20%) and infection.

What Is the Patient's Clinical Status in Acute SAH, and How Does It Determine the "Hunt and Hess" Clinical Classification?

The most widely used method for clinical grading of SAH is the Hunt and Hess Scale (Table 5-2). Imaging of acute SAH usually is performed using nonenhanced CT scans, although MR sequences such as FLAIR imaging also can be used for diagnosis. The severity of SAH on nonenhanced CT is assessed using the Fisher Scale (Table 5-3). However, this score does not necessarily correlate with patient clinical symptoms or aneurysm size. The location of SAH can sometimes suggest the site of a ruptured aneurysm: focal hematomas in the sylvian fissure suggest MCA location; interhemispheric SAH may occur with ACoA aneurysms; and hemorrhage in the fourth ventricle and cerebellopontine angle cisterns is often associated with a ruptured PICA aneurysm. A pattern of perimesocephalic SAH can be associated with vertebrobasilar aneurysms but also with nonaneurysmal hemorrhage.

What Are the Most Important Factors that Determine Clinical Outcome after Aneurysmal Rupture?

The short-term outcome of an aneurysm rupture is generally dismal, with an overall 30-day survival of 40% to 57%. The long-term outcome of aneurysm rupture is variable, with permanent neurologic disability occurring in a significant number of survivors. Besides higher grades on the Hunt and Hess and Fisher CT scales, aneurysm size greater than 10 mm, patient age greater than 50 years, giant aneurysm, and posterior circulation aneurysm are other factors that are associated with a poor outcome. Data from the International Subarachnoid Aneurysm Trial (ISAT) showed that in patients with a ruptured aneurysms, for which endovascular coiling and neurosurgical clipping are therapeutic options, the outcome in terms of survival free of disability at 1 year is significantly better with endovascular coiling.

If a patient survives the initial hemorrhage from an aneurysm rupture, a number of delayed complications can develop that still may be devastating, such as focal hematoma with mass effect, including cerebral herniation syndromes, hydrocephalus, and cerebral ischemia with stroke. The latter may be caused by thromboembolic events from the aneurysm sac or most commonly

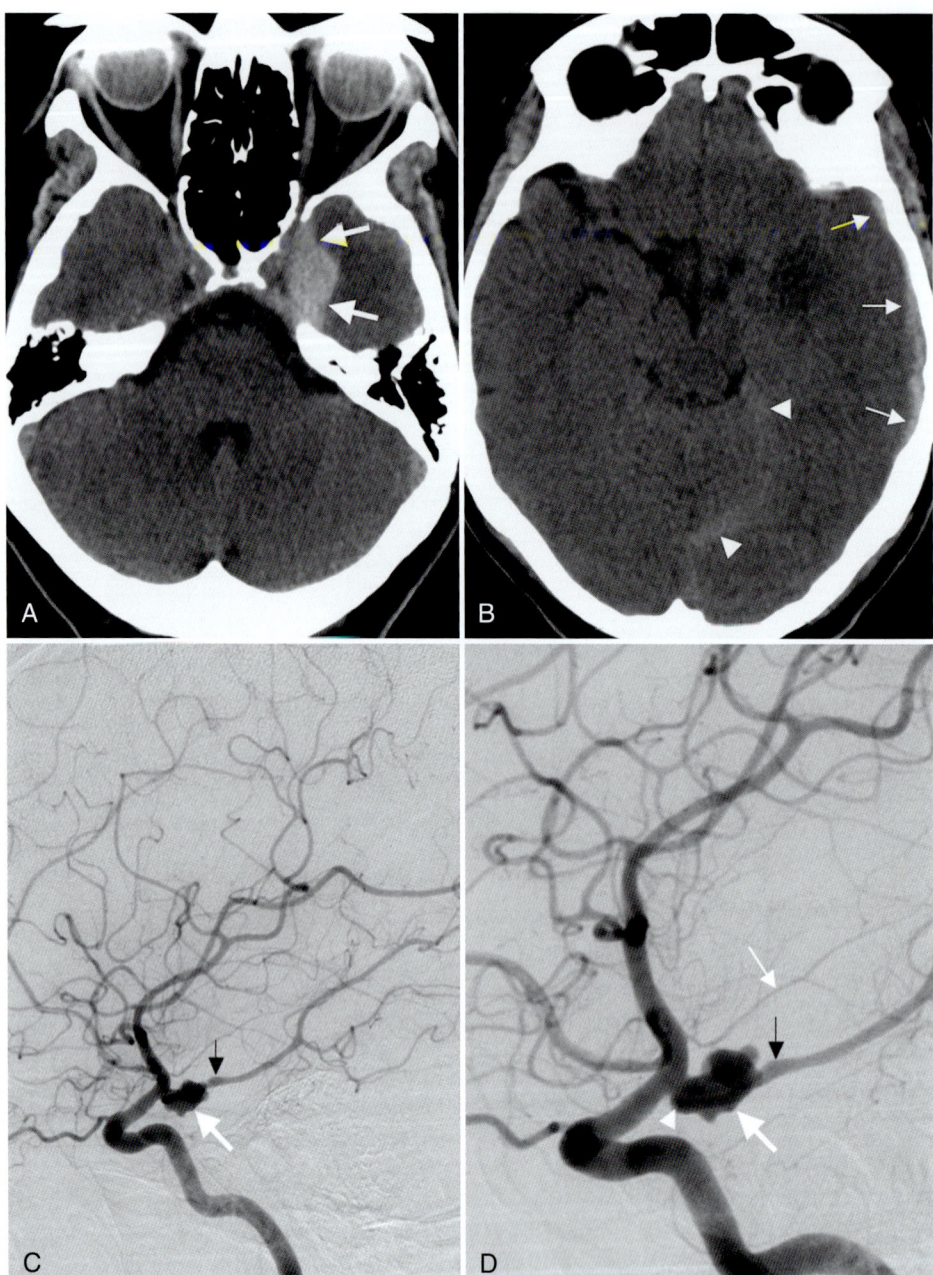

Figure 5-36 Noncontrast computed tomographic (CT) images **(A, B)** in a patient who presented with subacute retroorbital headache and confusion showing an intracranial hematoma located in the middle cranial fossa adjacent to the left cavernous sinus *(large white arrows)*. A history of trauma was denied. In addition, a small left hemispheric subdural hematoma *(small white arrows)* and subdural blood along the left-sided tentorium *(white arrowheads)* is depicted. Subarachnoid blood is not found on CT imaging. Lateral **(C)** and lateral oblique **(D)** projections of selective left internal carotid artery (ICA) angiogram show a multilobulated left posterior communicating artery aneurysm *(large white arrow)*. The origin *(white arrowhead)* of the posterior communicating artery *(small black arrow)* is located in the vicinity of the aneurysm neck. The left anterior choroidal artery *(small white arrow)* arises from the ICA C7 segment clearly separated from the aneurysm neck. Acute subdural hematoma is a rare but well-recognized presentation of ruptured posterior communicating aneurysms, and the presumed mechanism is the formation of arachnoid adhesions from the aneurysmal wall that allow direct bleeding into the subdural space in the absence of subarachnoid hemorrhage. (Courtesy Dr. William McAuliffe, Perth.)

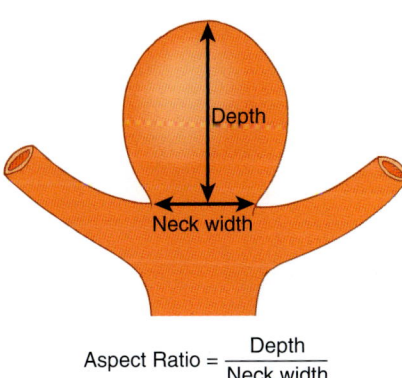

Figure 5-37 Anatomic relationship between neck width and depth (neck to dome distance) of a typical berry-type cerebral aneurysm. The aspect ratio (ratio between depth and neck width) was defined as an anatomic measure and indicator of rupture risk by Ujiie et al. (Redrawn from Ujiie H, Tamano Y, Sasaki K, Hori T. Is the aspect ratio a reliable index for predicting the rupture of a saccular aneurysm? Neurosurgery 2001;48:495-502; discussion 502-493.)

$$\text{Aspect Ratio} = \frac{\text{Depth}}{\text{Neck width}}$$

Table 5-2 Hunt and Hess Clinical Grading Scale for Intracranial Aneurysms

Grade	Clinical Condition
0	Unruptured
I	Asymptomatic or minimal headache, nuchal rigidity
II	Moderate to severe headache, nuchal rigidity, no neurologic deficit other than cranial nerve palsy
III	Drowsiness, confusion, mild focal deficit
IV	Stupor, moderate to severe hemiparesis, possible early decerebrate rigidity and vegetative disturbances
V	Deep coma, decerebrate rigidity, moribund appearance
+1	For vasospasm or systemic disease

As described in Hunt WE, Hess RM: Surgical risks as related to time of intervention in the repair of intracranial aneurysms. J Neurosurg 28:14-20, 1968.

Table 5-3 Density of SAH as Revealed by CT Imaging: Fisher Scale

Score	Description
0	Unruptured
1	No blood detected
2	Diffuse or vertical layers <1 mm thick
3	Localized clot and/or vertical layer ≥1 mm
4	Intracerebral or intraventricular clot with diffuse or no subarachnoid hemorrhage

Adapted from Fisher CM, Kistler JP, Davis JM: Relation of cerbral vasospasm to subarachnoid hemorrhage visualized by computerized tomographic scanning. Neurosurgery 1980;6(1):1-9.

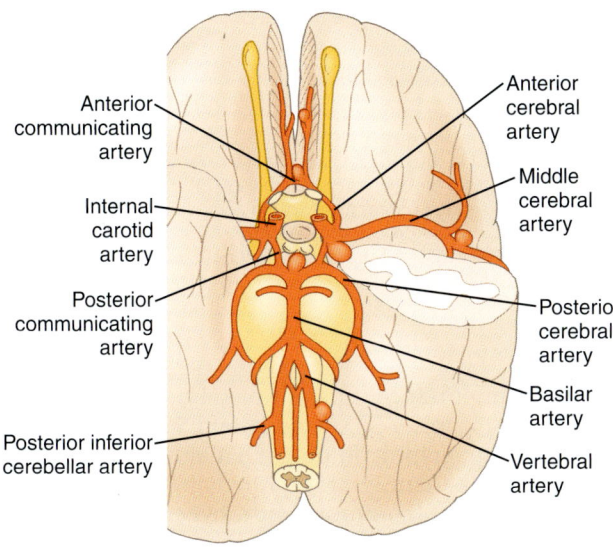

Figure 5-38 Common sites of intracranial aneurysms on the circle of Willis at the base of the brain. (Redrawn from Schievink WI. Intracranial aneurysms. N Engl J Med 1997;336:28-40.)

as a result of cerebral hypoperfusion due to vasospasm. Untreated ruptured aneurysms carry a high risk of rebleeding (at least 50% of untreated aneurysms rehemorrhage within 6 months).

Angiographic Evaluation of Intracranial Aneurysms

What Are the Optimal Angiographic Views and Modalities (2D vs 3D Rotational DSA) for Visualization of Intracranial Aneurysms?

A technically adequate and complete cerebral angiogram in patients with a possible intracranial aneurysm includes evaluation of the complete intracranial circulation with multiple projections of each vessel studied. All components of the circle of Willis, the MCA, and both PICAs must be visualized. At a minimum, standard AP, lateral, and both 30-degree transorbital oblique views should be included, but additional views (e.g., submentovertex projection) are often needed. If the ACoA does not fill spontaneously, injection of one ICA during temporary cross compression of the contralateral carotid may be required to visualize this important potential site of aneurysm. In cases of a hypoplastic PCoA, temporary ipsilateral carotid compression during the vertebrobasilar study may show transient reflux of the PCoA. If reflux from the dominant VA into the contralateral VA is not sufficient to completely visualize both PICAs, a separate injection of the nondominant vessel may be required (Figure 5-2). Assessment of cross-flow patterns between different circulations is most helpful if temporary or permanent occlusion of the parent vessel becomes necessary during therapy.

For decision making (endovascular vs surgical therapy) and planning of therapy (e.g., simple coil embolization of aneurysm vs balloon-assisted coiling procedure), delineation of the aneurysm neck is most important. Second, defining the presence of branches that may arise from the aneurysm or near the neck of the aneurysm is essential (Figure 5-39). Instead of obtaining multiple projections, most centers currently perform a 3D rotational angiogram directly after the angiographic standard projections (Figures 5-26, D). This study can facilitate the determination of the optimal

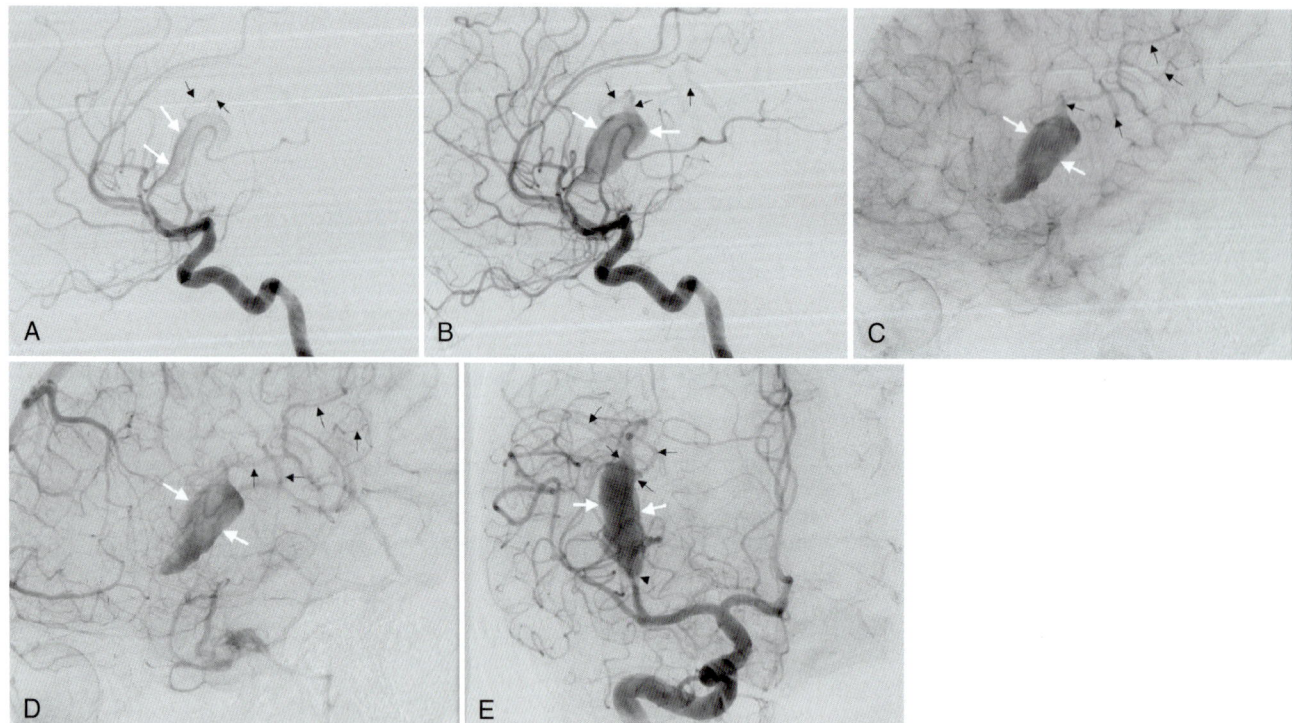

Figure 5-39 Serial lateral views (**A-D**) and anteroposterior (AP) view (**E**) of the right internal carotid artery angiogram in a patient harboring a giant fusiform distal middle cerebral artery (MCA) aneurysm. A slow pattern of inflow into the large aneurysm sac *(large white arrows)* and outflow from the aneurysm sac into two small M3 branches *(small black arrows)* of the MCA are noted at the early (**A**) and late (**B**) arterial phases. The sluggish flow within these two arterial branches *(small black arrows)* persists during the capillary (**C**) and early venous phases (**D**). Such hemodynamic information may be essential for therapy planning in order to determine the safety of anticipated parent artery occlusion, which was successfully performed in this patient (images not shown). **E:** Selective right internal carotid artery angiogram, AP view, demonstrating a tapered narrow aneurysmal neck *(black arrowhead)* arising from a large sylvian (M2) branch of the MCA. The origins of the two M3 arteries *(small black arrows)* are located on the aneurysmal dome *(large white arrows)*. (Courtesy Dr. Tejinder Pal Singh, Perth.)

working projection and thereby decrease the total number of DSA exposures. Moreover, a clear benefit compared to 2D DSA projections is better visualization and understanding of complex anatomic vascular patterns (e.g., relationship of aneurysm to parent/branching vessel in ACoA complex or MCA bifurcation/trifurcation) as well as better visualization of the aneurysm neck. With 2D DSA imaging, small aneurysms may be obscured by overprojection of adjacent vessels. Studies have demonstrated that 3D rotational angiography can depict considerably more small additional aneurysms than 2D DSA. It also can detect small treatable ruptured aneurysms in a high proportion of cases with DSA-negative aneurysmal SAH. For these reasons, 3D rotational DSA has been proposed as the new gold standard for detection of aneurysms. Disadvantages of 3D rotational DSA compared to 2D DSA are the higher contrast load per acquisition run (18-24 ml vs 6-8 ml), its tendency to overestimate aneurysmal neck width, and the longer acquisition time (6-8 seconds), which makes the examination more prone to degraded image quality by motion artifacts in uncooperative patients. Under such circumstances, it preferentially should be performed under general anesthesia directly preceding endovascular therapy of the targeted aneurysm. Another benefit of 2D DSA projections is its capability to evaluate intraaneurysmal and parent vessel flow patterns that are of particular importance if parent vessel occlusion is contemplated (Figures 5-30, *A* and *B*, and 5-39).

Other angiographic findings that should be actively looked for in patients with ruptured aneurysms include vasoconstriction (common with hyperacute SAH or delayed in cerebral vasospasm), ischemia and infarction (unusual in the setting of acute SAH but occur as delayed complications in cerebral vasospasm), and mass effect (from focal hematoma or partially/completely thrombosed aneurysm). Avascular mass effect is demonstrated by stretching and draping of adjacent vessels.

It is important to screen the complete basal cerebral circulation for the presence of multiple aneurysms (Figure 5-30). When more than one aneurysm is present, identifying which aneurysm likely ruptured is essential for treatment planning. The only true but very rare sign of contrast extravasation indicates active bleeding from an aneurysm. Other helpful but not reliable signs include size (the larger aneurysm is more likely to have ruptured), irregularity (presence of "blebs," "daughter aneurysms," and/or a multilobulated dome) (Figures 5-17 and 5-35), and focal mass effect from a hematoma. Most helpful, however, is a correlation of aneurysm sites with the pattern of SAH distribution on head CT.

In giant aneurysms (>25 mm, 5% of all aneurysms), exact delineation of the aneurysm neck relative to its parent vessel may be difficult due to the presence of multiple layers of organized thrombus or obscuring lobulations on standard 2D DSA. A 3D rotational angiogram or a rapid-sequence 2D DSA acquisition may be helpful in such instances.

Small saccular aneurysms that are completely thrombosed may be invisible on DSA. True aneurysm must be distinguished from aneurysm mimics such as vascular loops (differentiated by multiple projections or 3D rotational DSA) and infundibuli (most commonly located at the PCoA origin, less commonly at the AChA origin) as described earlier (see section on Internal Carotid Arteries) (Figure 5-6, A).

Angiogram-Negative SAH

What Is the Best Way to Follow Up on Patients with Acute SAH and Initially Negative Angiogram?

It is important to ensure that any angiographic examination of patients with nontraumatic SAH is complete because an incomplete angiogram is the most common cause of negative findings. In 10% to 20% of patients with verified SAH, the initial technically adequate catheter angiogram is negative. Possible causes include so-called *nonaneurysmal perimesencephalic hemorrhage*, thrombosed aneurysm, vascular lesions of the spine, spinal neoplasms, pregnancy-induced hypertension, sympathomimetic drug abuse, bleeding disorders, and anticoagulants/antiplatelets. Investigators have demonstrated that repeat angiography performed approximately 1 week after the ictus is the most sensitive imaging modality for detecting a lesion causing the hemorrhage, the most common being an aneurysm that has been thrombosed during the initial angiogram. The yield of a second angiogram is best for patients with a classic SAH pattern (8%–46%), followed by a perimesencephalic hemorrhage pattern (0%–7%), and is worst in patients with a negative CT scan and positive lumbar puncture (0%). Contrast-enhanced MRI of the brain and spine may only be occasionally helpful in detecting hemorrhagic tumors such as cervical ependymoma, spinal cavernous angioma, or AVM in patients with an atypical presentation for aneurysmal SAH. The value of performing a third angiogram several weeks after the ictus is debatable due to a low overall yield, but it may have a role in the management of selected patients (e.g., those with a dense classic SAH pattern or suspicious wall irregularity on second angiogram). The role of noninvasive CTA or MRA as a follow-up test has not been established in the setting of an initially negative angiogram. However, its use has been suggested for subpopulations of patients for whom the risk-to-benefit ratio favors a noninvasive test, such as those with perimesencephalic hemorrhage.

Noninvasive Evaluation of Intracranial Aneurysms

Noninvasive methods of assessing the intracranial circulation for the presence of an unruptured intracranial aneurysm or for follow-up of treated intracranial aneurysms include MRA and CTA.

Problem Solving: What Are the Benefits and Shortcomings of CTA for Imaging Cerebral Aneurysms?

Problem Solving: Can CTA Study Replace the Invasive Catheter Angiogram in Case of Acute SAH?

Based on the recent advances in CT technology that have resulted in the outstanding accuracy of the latest 16- and 64-row multidetector CTA technique, many institutions have changed their diagnostic imaging algorithm for patients presenting with SAH and now routinely apply CTA for this indication. Furthermore, management decisions (e.g., endovascular vs surgical treatment of an acutely ruptured aneurysm) may be solely based on CTA findings, with direct progression to craniotomy in some cases. However, the sensitivity of CTA for the diagnosis of a cerebral aneurysm is still imperfect compared to catheter angiography, mainly owing to its inferior maximum spatial resolution (0.35–0.5 mm vs 0.1 mm in conventional DSA and 0.2–0.3 mm in 3D rotational angiography). Along with the implementation of new diagnostic algorithms, a discussion has emerged in the scientific literature as to the optimal diagnostic test for patients presenting with acute SAH. Our current practice is to apply CTA as the first-line investigation that is performed immediately after plain CT study in patients with proved SAH. This is followed by a conventional catheter angiogram, including a 3D rotational angiography study. Characterization of aneurysms and the further management plan are derived from the two imaging modalities in a side-by-side analysis as we consider them complementary examinations for the following reasons.

First, a valuable benefit of an initial noninvasive workup includes obtaining knowledge of the vascular anatomy before invasive catheterization or endovascular therapy, which can help in tailoring a DSA examination or avoid the risks of difficult catheterizations in the individual patient (e.g., in the case of severe atheromatous disease at the neck arteries). For example, if a ruptured aneurysm has been confirmed on DSA in the anterior circulation and the CTA study is of optimal quality allowing for accurate evaluation of the vertebrobasilar arteries, a full "four-vessel" DSA may not be conducted. Therefore, potentially risky catheter maneuvers can be avoided if access to the VAs is complex. Second, apart from luminographic details, CTA can provide more precise information on intraaneurysmal thrombus and calcified components of the aneurysm/vessel walls compared to DSA. Third, CTA can demonstrate reliable bony landmarks that can differentiate between intradural or extradural aneurysms involving the (para-)clinoid ICA segment, such as the optic strut, which may facilitate treatment decisions (Figure 5-40).

However, DSA is still required because its higher spatial resolution enables better characterization of the neck and identification of smaller but often crucial vessels relative to the aneurysm/parent artery complex, such as the AChA or recurrent artery of Heubner. Second, any negative CTA warrants further DSA investigation

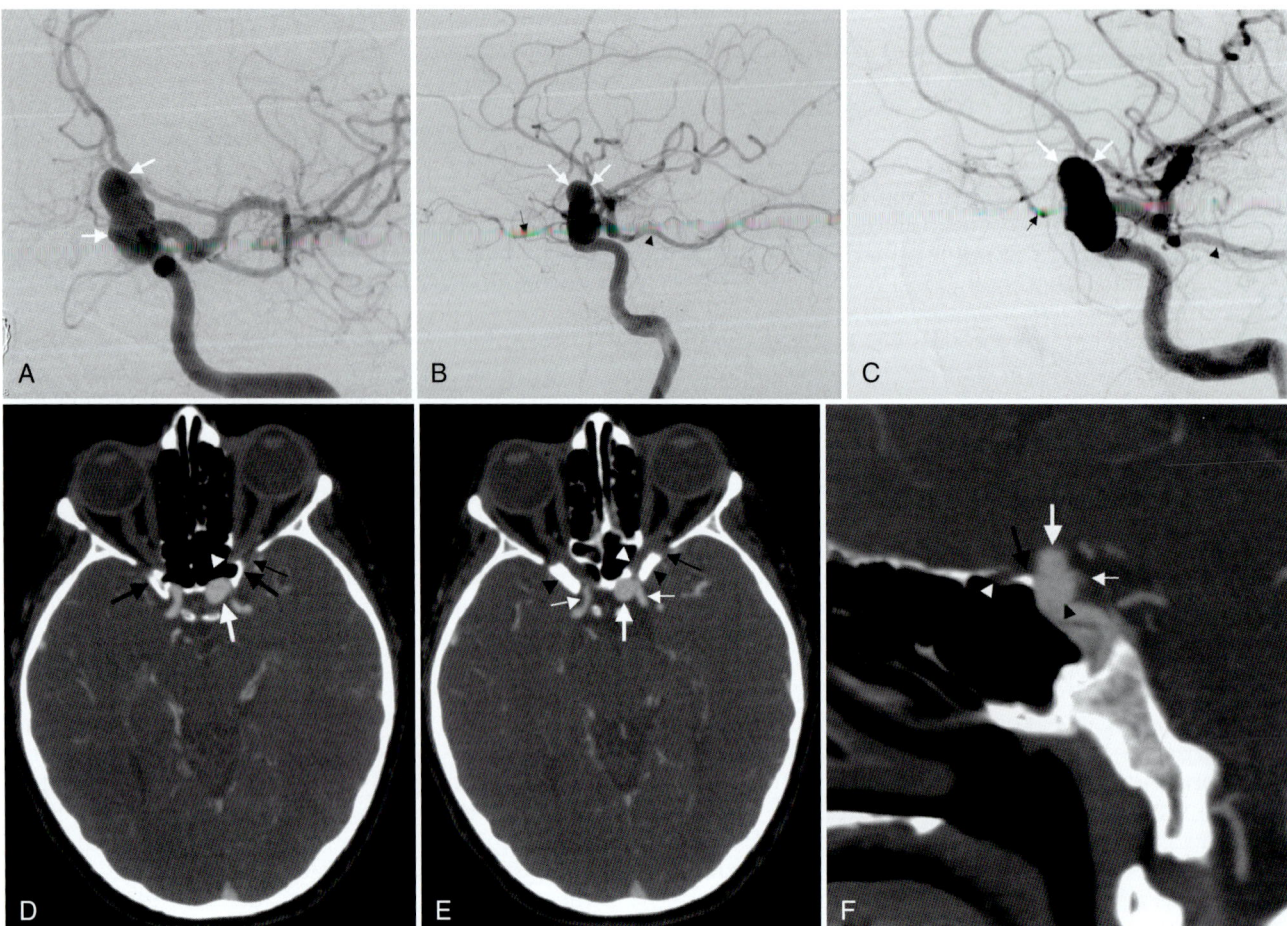

Figure 5-40 Anteroposterior oblique (**A**), lateral (**B**), and Haughton lateral oblique (**C**) views of the left internal carotid artery angiogram show a large multilobulated aneurysm *(large white arrows)* in the paraclinoid region of the internal carotid artery, which points superomedially. It is impossible to determine the relationship to its apparent broad neck to the clinoid segment of the internal carotid artery (extradural vs intradural vs transitional location) on the different angiographic views. Moreover, the origin of the ophthalmic artery *(small black arrow)* cannot be separated from the aneurysm neck. The presence of a fetal variant of posterior cerebral artery *(black arrowhead)* is demonstrated. Computed tomographic angiography (CTA) (**D–F**) can be useful for determining exactly the location of the aneurysm neck with respect to bony landmarks, which can serve as reliable indicators for the dural rings. **D:** Axial source image at level of partially pneumatized optic strut *(large black arrows)* showing the inferior portion of the broad-necked aneurysm pointing medially into the sella *(large white arrow)*. **E:** Subsequent higher axial image at level of anterior clinoid process *(black arrowheads)* showing further neck parts of the aneurysm neck *(large white arrow)* involving the ophthalmic portion of the internal carotid artery *(small white arrows)*, which is clearly in a subarachnoid location. The optic strut *(large black arrows)*, which is the inferior bony root of the anterior clinoid process *(black arrowheads)*, separates the superior orbital fissure *(small black arrow)* from the optic canal *(white arrowhead)*. The anterior boundary of the clinoid segment of the internal carotid artery and its inferior boundary accurately localizes the point at which the internal carotid artery pierces the proximal dural ring (oculomotor membrane) and exits the cavernous sinus. This serves as a very useful landmark for determining the partially subarachnoid location of the neck in this aneurysm. **F:** Sagittally reconstructed CTA image showing the relationship of the whole wide aneurysm neck. It is defined as transitional because it is mostly located in the clinoid (C5) segment at the level of the optic strut *(large black arrow)* but also involves the cavernous segment (C4) with an inferior locule *(black arrowhead)* and the ophthalmic segment (C6, *small white arrow*) with the larger superior locule *(large white arrow)*. The optic canal *(white arrowhead)* is demonstrated superior to the optic strut. (Courtesy Dr. Tejinder Pal Singh, Perth.)

because CTA alone may give a false-negative result (negative predictive value of CTA ranges between 82% and 96%). These mostly relate to aneurysms smaller than 3 to 4 mm or aneurysms in arteries adjacent to bone or venous structures (cavernous, clinoid, and ophthalmic ICA segments). Interestingly, many small aneurysms that are first missed on CTA become evident after review of the DSA examination. This fact points to the importance of the reading radiologist's awareness of potential CTA pitfalls and interpretation errors (e.g., infundibulum vs small aneurysm), the use of a good workstation/software for 3D and multiplanar reconstructions, and the need for sufficient time to review CTA images. In addition, distinct sources of SAH, such as a blood blister-like aneurysm, pial AVMs, or AVFs with pial drainage, and intracranial dissection may not be visible on CTA. There also is a remote possibility that an aneurysm detected on CTA may not be the source of hemorrhage if a patient harbors other smaller aneurysms that can only be resolved on DSA.

Hence, we suggest to solely skip the DSA examination in patients with ruptured aneurysms who present with extensive intraparenchymal hemorrhage and mass effect requiring immediate craniotomy for decompression and hematoma evacuation. In addition, there is significant potential for CTA in cases where aneurysms are of low likelihood, such as subarachnoid blood in patients after significant trauma or in patients without hemorrhage but with severe headaches and a family history of aneurysm.

Angiographic Follow-up of Treated Aneurysms

Problem Solving: What Is the Role of MRA in the Follow-up of Coiled Aneurysms?

With the increasing use of endovascular therapy as primary treatment of ruptured and unruptured intracranial aneurysms, continued angiographic surveillance of aneurysms after coil embolization has become standard practice. This is mainly because recurrence after coil embolization due to compaction of the original coil mass or migration of the coil mass into intraaneurysmal thrombus has been estimated to occur in 10% to 40% of patients. Some investigators have recommended that at least two follow-up examinations should be performed within the first year after treatment. However, minimizing morbidity related to angiographic follow-up is particularly important in the context of the very low risk of rerupture after successful coil embolization, which is estimated between 0.11% and 0.21%. MRA is very attractive for this purpose because platinum alloys used in aneurysm coils create relatively little distortion of local magnetic field. The resultant images are minimally affected by coil-induced artifacts in comparison to CT/CTA images, which usually are severely degraded by streak and beam hardening artifacts that typically obscure not only the aneurysm but also the adjacent parent/branching vessels and the surrounding brain parenchyma. Despite the application of different MRA techniques (e.g., 3D TOF and contrast-enhanced MRA), the reported sensitivity and specificity rates for detection of residual aneurysms range between 90% and 100%. The initial MRA study should be performed in close temporal proximity to the initial endovascular treatment (24-48 hours) in order to provide a direct correlation with the immediate posttreatment DSA (Figure 5-27) and the baseline examination for subsequent comparison with serial MRA studies. In addition, the baseline MRA indicates whether MRA can be used effectively as a follow-up technique in the future, because the initial baseline MRA–DSA correlation in some patients may be unreliable (e.g., artifact related to the presence of aneurysm clips, aneurysms with particularly complex anatomy, or complex stent and coil constructs). In these patients, follow-up is performed primarily by conventional angiography, which remains the gold standard for evaluation of treated aneurysms. Moreover, DSA should be liberally used to resolve any cases of diagnostic uncertainty on the noninvasive imaging test or to verify the diagnosis of small aneurysm recurrences identified by MRA and to ensure an accurate estimation of the size. In patients not requiring retreatment, these small recurrences may be subsequently followed noninvasively.

Problem Solving: What Is the Role of CTA in the Follow-up of Clipped Aneurysms?

Although not useful for the evaluation of coiled aneurysms, CTA is far superior to MRA for the evaluation of aneurysms after surgical clipping because of the substantial artifacts on MR images created by the available surgical clips, which usually completely obscure the immediate perianeurysmal region. Using the latest technology CT scanners (16- to 64-section multidetector row CT scanners) and optimized imaging parameters (optimal scanning pitch to minimize clip-related artifacts is approximately 0.6 mm), CTA often can effectively depict and follow small aneurysm remnants; demonstrate patency, stenosis, or vasospasm in the adjacent parent vessels; and provide surveillance of the entire cerebrovasculature for de novo aneurysms after surgical clipping. In the intraoperative or immediate postoperative period, CTA imaging may be required to evaluate aneurysm residual and parent vessel compromise. Although the risk for recurrence of a clipped aneurysm is low, evidence indicates that aneurysm recurrence as well as de novo aneurysm formation with subsequent SAH can occur even after successful surgical treatment. This evidence supports the use of routine periodic imaging surveillance after successful surgical clipping. However, extensive artifacts due to multiple clips, older-generation cobalt-containing clips, or unfavorable clip position relative to the area of interest, as well as arterial segments encased within osseous structures (e.g., near the skull base) and poor examination quality (e.g., suboptimal timing of contrast bolus) may obscure the aneurysm and adjacent parent vessel and preclude the noninvasive evaluation with CTA. In these cases, conventional catheter angiography, which remains the standard of reference for follow-up of clipped aneurysms, should be used to resolve any cases of diagnostic uncertainty.

Cerebral Vascular Malformations

Problem Solving: How to Classify Cerebral Vascular Malformations?

Is AV Shunting Present? If Not, Could the Cerebral Vascular Malformation Be a Developmental Venous Anomaly, Cavernoma, or Capillary Telangiectasia?

Cerebral vascular malformations have been classified according to a combination of anatomic and histopathologic features, clinical presentation, biologic behavior, and imaging characteristics. The presence or absence of AV shunting within a cerebral vascular malformation is the fundamental distinguishing feature (Table 5-4). Noninvasive vascular imaging studies such as CTA or MRI/MRA usually are the initial investigations and are sufficient to diagnose cerebral vascular malformations without AV shunting, such as cavernoma, capillary telangiectasis, or developmental venous anomaly (DVA). However, diagnostic catheter angiography remains the gold standard for delineating the detailed angioarchitecture of a vascular malformation and planning the appropriate therapy.

Table 5-4 Classification of Cerebral Vascular Malformations

Cerebral vascular malformations with arteriovenous shunting
    Arteriovenous malformation
        Plexiform nidus
            Mixed (plexiform–fistulous) nidus
    Arteriovenous fistula
        Single or multiple fistulae
        Monopedicular or multipedicular

Cerebral arteriovenous malformations without arteriovenous shunting
    Capillary telangiectasis
    Developmental venous anomaly
    Venous varix without associated arteriovenous malformation or arteriovenous fistula
    Cavernous malformation (cavernoma)

Modified from Osborn AG: *Diagnostic Cerebral Angiography.* Lippincott Williams & Wilkins; 1999.

Table 5-5 Spetzler-Martin Arteriovenous Malformation Grading System

Feature	Points Assigned
Size of arteriovenous malformation (cm)	
Small (<3)	1
Medium (3–6)	2
Large (>6)	3
Eloquence of adjacent brain	
Noneloquent	0
Eloquent	1
Venous drainage	
Superficial only	0
Deep	1

Grade is total of assigned points for size and eloquence plus venous drainage (grade 6 is reserved for inoperable lesions).
Modified from (Hamilton MG, Spetzler RF: The prospective application of a grading system for arteriovenous malformations. *Neurosurgery* 34(1):2-6; discussion 6-7, 1994.

Arteriovenous Malformations

Problem Solving: What Are the Characteristics of AVMs, and Which Factors Determine Their Risk of Hemorrhage?

Problem Solving: What Features Determine the Spetzler-Martin Grading: Is the AVM 3 Cm or More? Is the Nidus Located in Eloquent Brain? Is Deep or Superficial Venous Drainage Present?
AVMs are most common type of cerebrovascular malformations that exhibits AV shunting. They are composed of a collection of dysplastic plexiform vessels that are supplied by one or more arterial feeders and drained by one or more venous channels. AVMs may have a pure plexiform nidus or contain a mixed plexiform–fistulous nidus. On gross pathology, they appear as tightly packed masses of abnormal vascular channels and may contain small amounts of gliotic brain, dystrophic calcification, and blood products. Other abnormalities associated with AVMs include flow-related aneurysms and endothelial remodeling with resulting angiopathy in both the feeding arteries and the draining veins. Chronic regional arterial hypoperfusion and venous hypertension may cause cerebrovascular steal with resulting atrophy in otherwise normal brain at a distance from AVMs. The majority of AVMs are located in the cerebral hemispheres, and 15% occur in the posterior fossa. Depending on their location, they can be classified as *superficial* (convexity) or *deep* (ratio 2:1 to 3:1). A combination of high-resolution MRI and selective angiography is required for complete anatomic localization and delineation of AVMs. Only 2% of AVMs are multiple; these occur almost exclusively in the setting of neurocutaneous syndromes such as hereditary hemorrhagic telangiectasis or Wyburn-Mason syndrome. The incidence of sporadic solitary AVMs in the general population is estimated between 0.04% and 0.52% (autopsy series data).

Approximately 50% of patients with AVMs present with symptoms caused by hemorrhage. Other than seizure (25%), nonhemorrhagic focal neurologic syndromes such as ischemia are relatively infrequent. The majority of AVMs become symptomatic by age 50 years (peak age at initial presentation 20–40 years), but 25% of AVMs hemorrhage by age 15 years. Reports indicate that the risk of hemorrhage of an AVM can be widely variable (from 0.9% to 34.4% per year), depending on various clinical and morphologic characteristics. In a single-center cohort study that evaluated the natural history of AVM, the highest hemorrhage rates per year were found for AVMs with initial hemorrhagic presentation (7.5%), associated aneurysms (5.4%), and presence of deep venous drainage (6.9%). These factors were demonstrated to be independent risk factors for future hemorrhage from AVMs. Furthermore, lesions that present with hemorrhage or have associated aneurysms have a risk of rebleeding twice that of AVMs without these characteristics, and the risk is highest in the first years after diagnosis. AVMs with associated aneurysms have a higher risk of hemorrhage even 5 years after diagnosis. A study disclosed a lower morbidity from spontaneous AVM hemorrhage either at initial presentation or during follow-up of untreated patients compared to intracranial hemorrhage from other causes. Data from the most recent studies suggest that the natural history risk for patients with unruptured AVMs is far more benign than for those who present with rupture, and concerns were raised about the actual benefit of invasive treatment strategies, particularly for this cohort of patients. A large international, randomized controlled multicenter trial (A Randomized Trial of Unruptured Brain AVMs [ARUBA]) is currently underway to determine the natural history versus treatment-related risks of best interventional therapy in nonruptured AVMs.

A widely used grading system to guide patient management and determine the treatment-related risk and prognosis of an AVM is the *Spetzler-Martin grading system* (Table 5-5), which was introduced in 1986 to predict surgical morbidity and mortality. The total grade (1–5) reflects the sum of points assigned for AVM size, eloquence of the adjacent brain, and pattern of venous drainage.

The angiographic evaluation of a cerebral AVM includes a selective and often superselective investigation of the AVM itself as well as the remainder of the

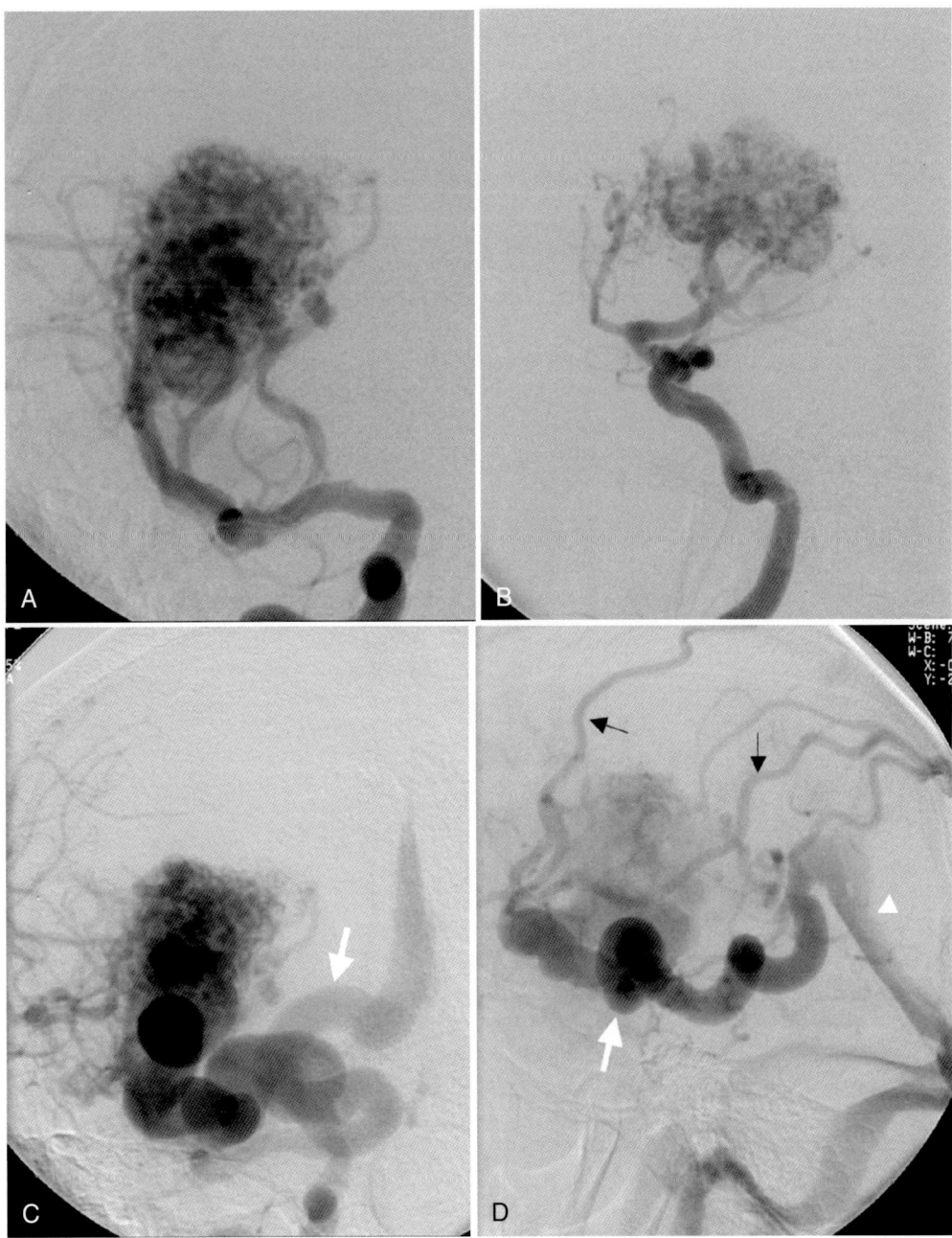

Figure 5-41 Right internal carotid artery angiograms, anteroposterior (**A**) and lateral (**B**) views, with early arterial phase study showing temporal arteriovenous malformation (AVM) supplied by several enlarged middle cerebral artery (M2) branches with a relatively compact nidus structure. **C, D:** Subsequent lateral arterial phase images illustrating venous drainage pattern with enormous varices of deep draining basal vein of Rosenthal *(large white arrow)* leading to early opacification of the straight sinus *(white arrowhead)* and transverse sigmoid sinuses. Superficial drainage occurs via several temporal cortical veins *(small black arrows)*. Findings are consistent with a grade III AVM (Spetzler-Martin scale). (Courtesy Dr. William McAuliffe, Perth.)

cerebral vasculature. A selective, technically complete angiogram of an AVM should provide detailed information on the individual feeding arteries and their vascular territories, the size, shape, and flow conditions of the AVM nidus, as well as delineate the venous drainage pattern (individual veins, deep vs superficial drainage, collaterals, reflux into normal veins/sinus) (Figure 5-41). AV shunting is present when contrast filling of draining veins appears abnormally early in the angiographic sequence. Although this is characteristic of an AVM, it may occur with other pathologies such as ischemia and neoplasm. Identification of both flow-related arterial and venous angiopathy (enlargements, stenoses, occlusions, venous varices) and the presence of an aneurysm (flow-related feeding artery aneurysm or perinidal/intranidal aneurysms) should also be made (Figure 5-42). Venous drainage of the normal brain should be assessed (venous hypertension?). AVMs should be studied using high-resolution DSA with high frame rates. Depending on the planned treatment, consistent magnification factors and calibrated markers may also be suggested.

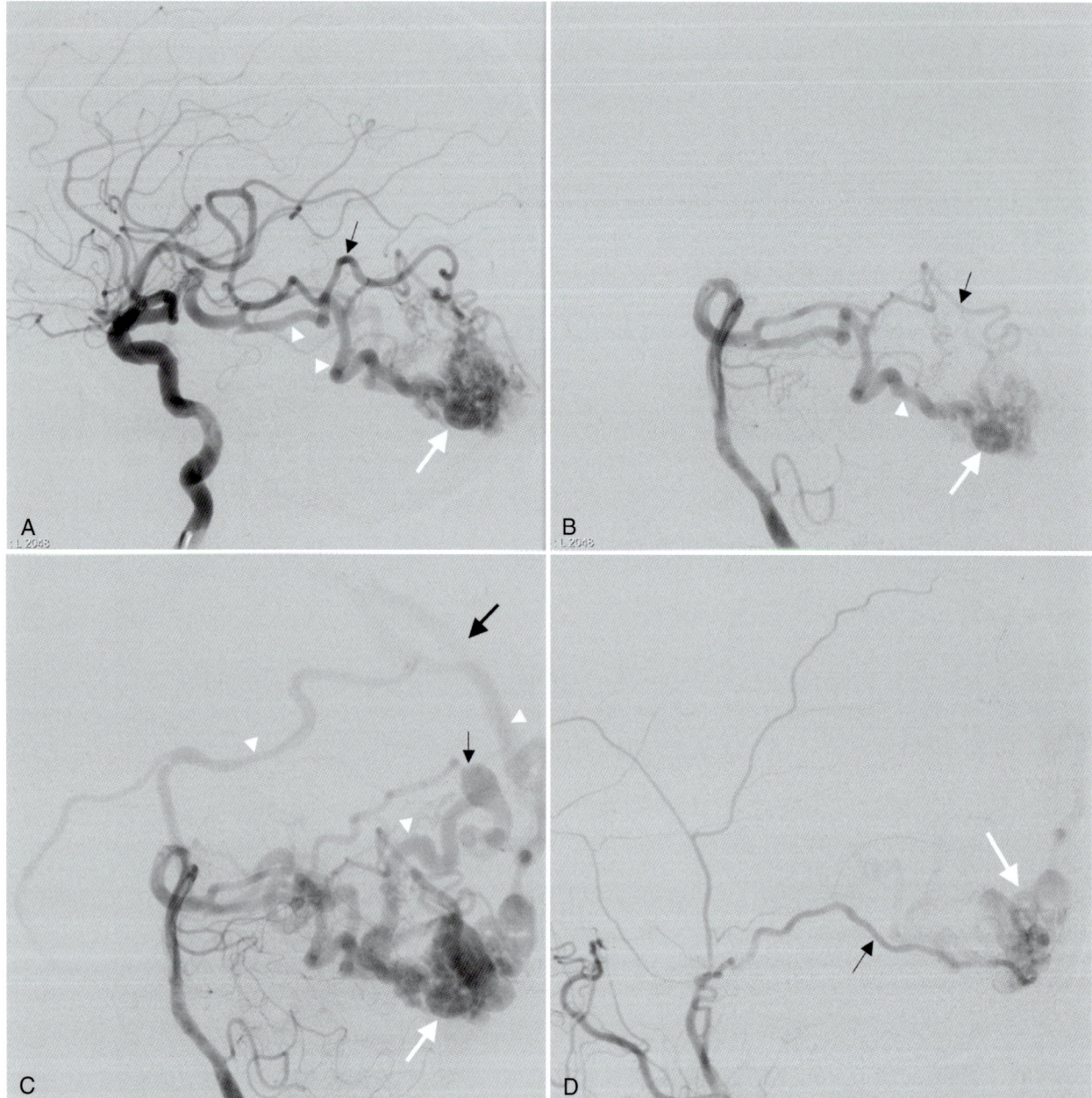

Figure 5-42 **A:** Lateral projection of the left internal carotid artery angiogram showing an arteriovenous malformation (AVM) located on the tentorium in the temporooccipital lobe. It is composed of a relatively compact nidus *(large white arrow)* with major arterial feeders from the left posterior temporal artery *(white arrowheads)* and the posterior temporal branch from the middle cerebral artery *(small black arrow)*. **B:** Lateral view of the selective left vertebral artery angiogram at early arterial phase showing filling of an intranidal aneurysm *(large white arrow)*. In addition to the main posterior temporal artery feeder *(white arrowhead)*, the left calcarine artery *(small black arrow)* shows AVM supply. **C:** Subsequent later arterial phase showing venous drainage from the AVM nidus *(large white arrow)* into enlarged cortical veins *(white arrowheads)* with subsequent early filling of the superior sagittal sinus *(large black arrow)*. Some of these veins demonstrate varicose dilatations *(small black arrow)*. **D:** Selective left external carotid angiogram, lateral view, demonstrating recruitment of transdural arterial supply to the AVM *(large white arrow)* from the posterior division of the left middle meningeal artery *(small black arrow)*. (Courtesy Dr. Tejinder Pal Singh, Perth.)

A superselective angiography of an AVM using microcatheters is often combined with endovascular treatment. This method can provide extensive, detailed information regarding the internal angioarchitecture of an AVM. This includes anatomy, hemodynamics (e.g., flow-related vasculopathy) of the distal segments of feeding arteries, arterionidal junction, compartments of the nidus, plexiform portions, AVFs, intranidal cavities (aneurysm, posthemorrhagic arterial and venous pseudoaneurysms, venous ectasia), veno–nidal junction, and proximal segments of draining veins (stenosis, outlet obstruction, varices).

Occasionally unusual variants of AVMs may be found. A diffuse AVM is an infiltrating lesion that involves an entire lobe or hemisphere of the brain. Angiographically, such lesions appear as a diffuse collection of multiple arterial feeders and draining veins without a compact nidus. They may be very large but cause almost no discernible mass effect. Clinically these lesions often present with intractable seizures rather than symptoms of hemorrhage. Diffuse AVMs may exhibit a "proliferative angiopathy" pattern that continues to recruit additional feeding vessels. Pial AVMs of sufficient size may recruit transdural arterial supply from a dural vessel such as the middle meningeal artery or meningohypophyseal trunk (Figure 5-42). Rarely AVMs are part of a mixed vascular malformation such as AVM–DVA (sometimes called *arterialized venous malformation*) or AVM–capillary telangiectasias.

AVMs may hemorrhage and then thrombose spontaneously, or thrombosis may be induced by stereotactic radiosurgery. Angiograms in patients with completely thrombosed AVMs may appear normal, show an avascular mass effect, or demonstrate only subtle AV shunting (early draining vein without identifiable feeding vessels or nidus). Occasionally, irregular-appearing arteries are present with slow flow that persist into late arterial/capillary phases; these are termed *stagnating arteries*. This subset of AVMs should be referred to as *angiographically occult* AVM (sometimes erroneously termed *cryptic AVM*). Similar findings can be present on postoperative angiograms of surgically excised AVMs.

Arteriovenous Fistulae

Problem Solving: How to Classify Intracranial AVFs?

AVFs are much less common than AVMs and are characterized by direct shunts between pial arteries and venous channels. Two major forms exist: the vein of Galen aneurysmal malformation, which occurs predominantly in neonates and infants, and the pial or subependymal AVF.

Malformations involving the vein of Galen have been classified into four groups: (1) *true vein of Galen aneurysmal malformation* (VGAM); (2) vein of Galen dilatation that occurs secondary to high-flow subpial AVM draining into this vessel; (3) vein of Galen varix that is a varicose dilatation of the vein of Galen in children without an underlying AV shunt and either represents a transient and asymptomatic dilatation of the vein of Galen in neonates presenting with cardiac failure or is associated with complex DVAs draining an entire hemisphere into the deep venous system; and (4) dural vein of Galen dilatation, which is an acquired lesion that develops in the wall of the vein of Galen or at the venous–sinus junction and nearly always is secondary to straight sinus thrombosis in adults or very rarely in children secondary to a complete thrombosis of the vein of Galen or of the falcine sinus.

Problem Solving: What Is the Importance of the Choroidal Arteries and Median Prosencephalic Vein in a True VGAM?

True VGAMs represent an AVF in the wall of a persistent embryonic venous channel called the *median prosencephalic vein*, which lies in the roof of the diencephalon and drains into a primitive accessory sinus, the falcine sinus, which courses posterosuperiorly within the falx to connect to the superior sagittal sinus. Usually the *median prosencephalic vein* regresses by week 10 of fetal development as the definitive internal cerebral veins appear and its caudal remnant remains as the vein of Galen. Angiographically, a typical VGAM consists of one or more enlarged arteries that drain directly into a massively enlarged vein of Galen. On the basis of their angioarchitecture, a *mural form* and a *choroidal form* can be identified in true VGAMs depending on the relationship of the arterial feeders to the prosencephalic vein. *Mural VGAMs* demonstrate a direct fistula in the wall of the prosencephalic vein. The arterial feeder complex usually is less extensive and the rate of flow less severe than in the *choroidal type* (complex feeder network from bilateral sources). Their arterial supply usually involves all the choroidal arteries: the medial and lateral posterior choroidal arteries and the AChAs. In addition, branches from the pericallosal arteries and thalamoperforating branches can contribute to the supply of these lesions. Venous drainage from the aneurysmal dilatation of the vein of Galen (a venous varix) is complicated by thrombosis or absence of the straight sinus with drainage into the falcine sinus in the majority of cases. Distal outlet venous stenosis can occur, and dilated choroidal veins may be present, draining anteroinferiorly into the cavernous sinus. Clinically, neonatal VGAMs usually present with high-output congestive heart failure, tachycardia, respiratory distress, and cyanosis.

Cerebral (pial) AVFs are rare in contrast to dural arteriovenous fistulae (DAVFs). Their angiographic appearance consists of one or more dilated, often bizarre-looking pial arteries that drain directly into a venous channel. Stenosis of the draining vein, which can result in sudden thrombosis and hemorrhage, is commonly seen.

Cerebral Vascular Malformations without AV Shunting

Problem Solving: Is DSA Needed to Diagnose a Cavernoma or a DVA?

Cerebral vascular malformations without evidence of AV shunting arise from postarteriolar vessels and can be categorized into capillary, venous, and cavernous malformations. Because these lesions either represent usually angiographically occult vascular malformations (capillary telangiectasias and cavernous angioma) or can be sufficiently diagnosed and characterized with noninvasive imaging modalities such as CTA or MRI/MRA imaging (DVA, capillary telangiectasias, and cavernous angioma), they are not discussed in detail in this chapter.

Isolated DVAs are generally thought to be congenital and to follow a clinically asymptomatic course. Typically they are diagnosed incidentally during imaging investigations for unrelated symptoms. In contrast to the benign course of isolated DVAs, up to one third of all DVAs are associated with cavernoma, which may present with neurologic symptoms attributable to the cavernoma itself and/or its hemorrhagic complications. Very rare variants are termed *atypical* or *mixed DVAs*. These represent arterialized DVAs or are associated with an AVM nidus that uses the DVA portion of the lesion as a drainage route. Clinically, patients with these lesions often present with intraparenchymal hemorrhage. The appearance of atypical DVA on noninvasive imaging modalities such as CTA and MR/MRA may be very similar to that of nonarterialized DVA. Its angiographic appearance consists of an identifiable arterial component that is either an AVM nidus or multiple tiny dilated arterial feeders, with each vessel acting as a single micro-AVF that drains directly into the medullary veins, which are organized into a classic caput medusae. The etiopathology of DVAs associated with arteriovenous shunting or AVM is still unknown and remains speculative, but it is assumed that these lesions are at greater risk for developing complications than simple DVAs and that their natural history resembles that of classic AVMs.

Dural AVF

Problem Solving: What Is the Definition of a Dural Arteriovenous Shunt and How Best to Classify These Shunts?

AVFs that involve the dura and the epidural space are termed *dural arteriovenous shunts* (DAVSs) or *dural arteriovenous fistulae* (DAVFs). These lesions are much more common than cerebral AVFs. They comprise 10% to 15% of intracranial arteriovenous malformations and can be either congenital or acquired. In general, three types are recognized: dural sinus malformation with arteriovenous shunt, infantile DAVS, and adult DAVF; the latter is the most common type.

Dural sinus malformations are uncommon lesions found in neonates or infants. They usually consist of giant venous pouches or dural lakes involving the superior sagittal sinus with thrombosis, occlusion, or hypogenesis of one jugular bulb. They show slow-flow communications with other venous sinuses or veins. DAVSs are demonstrated within the wall of the venous lake. Infantile DAVSs are rare and often multifocal. They typically are seen as large sinuses with multiple arteriovenous shunts and large arterial feeders. Secondary induced cortico–pial shunts are common. In contrast to adult-type DAVFs, most infantile DAVS have high flow rates and volumes. Spontaneous thrombosis of the venous outflow may lead to increased intracranial pressure hydrocephalus, cerebral venous ischemia, and the so-called *melting brain syndrome*.

Adult-type DAVFs consist of numerous abnormal direct communications, so-called *crack-like vessels*, between dural arteries and veins without an intervening capillary bed. In contrast to AVMs, DAVFs have no true nidus. They are located in the dural wall of a venous sinus, not within the sinus itself. The most common sites are the transverse and sigmoid sinuses; the cavernous sinus is also a frequent location. With the exception of bilateral cavernous sinus lesions, most DAVFs are solitary lesions. Their precise etiology is still debated, but many of these lesions seem to be acquired secondary to venous hemodynamic compromise, such as stenosis, thrombosis, or occlusion of a dural venous sinus. Recanalization of the compromised vessel lumen leads to an enlargement, and microscopic arteriovenous shunts, which normally are present in the sinus wall, may enlarge and form numerous small microfistulae, resulting in a DAVF. Due to the common association with a previous sinus thrombosis, investigators have stressed the role of activation or stimulation of angiogenesis within the dura in the development of DAVF.

DAVFs may occur at any age and are not uncommon in children, but most become symptomatic between 40 and 60 years of age. Their clinical presentation is highly varied and is primarily determined by the location of the fistula and the subsequent venous drainage pattern. For DAVFs involving the transverse or sigmoid sinuses, headache and bruit are the most common presenting symptoms. Proptosis, chemosis, retroorbital pain, and ophthalmoplegia are commonly associated with cavernous sinus lesions. Other manifestations include pulse-synchronous tinnitus, cranial neuropathy, and even potentially reversible vascular dementia due to venous hypertensive encephalopathy. Although most DAVFs have a benign natural history even with reported spontaneous involutions, lesions with aggressive behavior resulting in neurologic deterioration and oftentimes intracranial hemorrhage can occur and be fatal.

Table 5-6 Cognard Classification Scheme of Venous Drainage in Dural Arteriovenous Fistulas

Type	
Type I	Anterograde drainage into a sinus
Type IIa	Reflux into the sinus (retrograde flow)
Type IIb	Reflux into cortical veins
Type IIa + IIb	Reflux into both sinus and cortical veins
Type III	Direct cortical venous drainage without venous ectasia
Type IV	Direct cortical venous drainage with venous ectasias
Type V	Spinal venous drainage

Modified from Cognard C, Gobin YP, Pierot L, Bailly AL, Houdart E, Casasco A, Chiras J, Merland JJ: Cerebral dural arteriovenous fistulas: clinical and angiographic correlation with a revised classification of venous drainage. *Radiology* 194(3):671-680, 1995.

Problem Solving: What Determines the Prognosis in DAVFs and How to Classify Their Venous Drainage Patterns?

The pattern of venous drainage is the single most important determinant of clinical presentation, neurologic status, and long-term prognosis of DAVFs. Therefore, the most useful and modern classification schemes that were proposed by Cognard et al. and Borden et al. focus on the different venous drainage patterns (Table 5-6). Reflux into cortical veins or direct cortical venous drainage with or without venous ectasias worsens the prognosis of DAVF. Stenosis or thrombosis of venous drainage is also associated with an indicator of a bad prognosis. For DAVFs near the cavernous sinus, the Barrow classification system based on the arterial supply is widely used (see section on Traumatic Arterial Injuries: Traumatic AV Fistulae).

Angiographically, most DAVFs have multiple dural arterial feeders (Figure 5-43). The most commonly involved vessels that supply a DAVF are transmastoid branches of the occipital artery and meningeal branches of the ECA (e.g., neuromeningeal branch of ascending pharyngeal artery, branches of middle meningeal artery). Tentorial and dural branches of the ICAs and VAs are other frequently contributing feeders (Figure

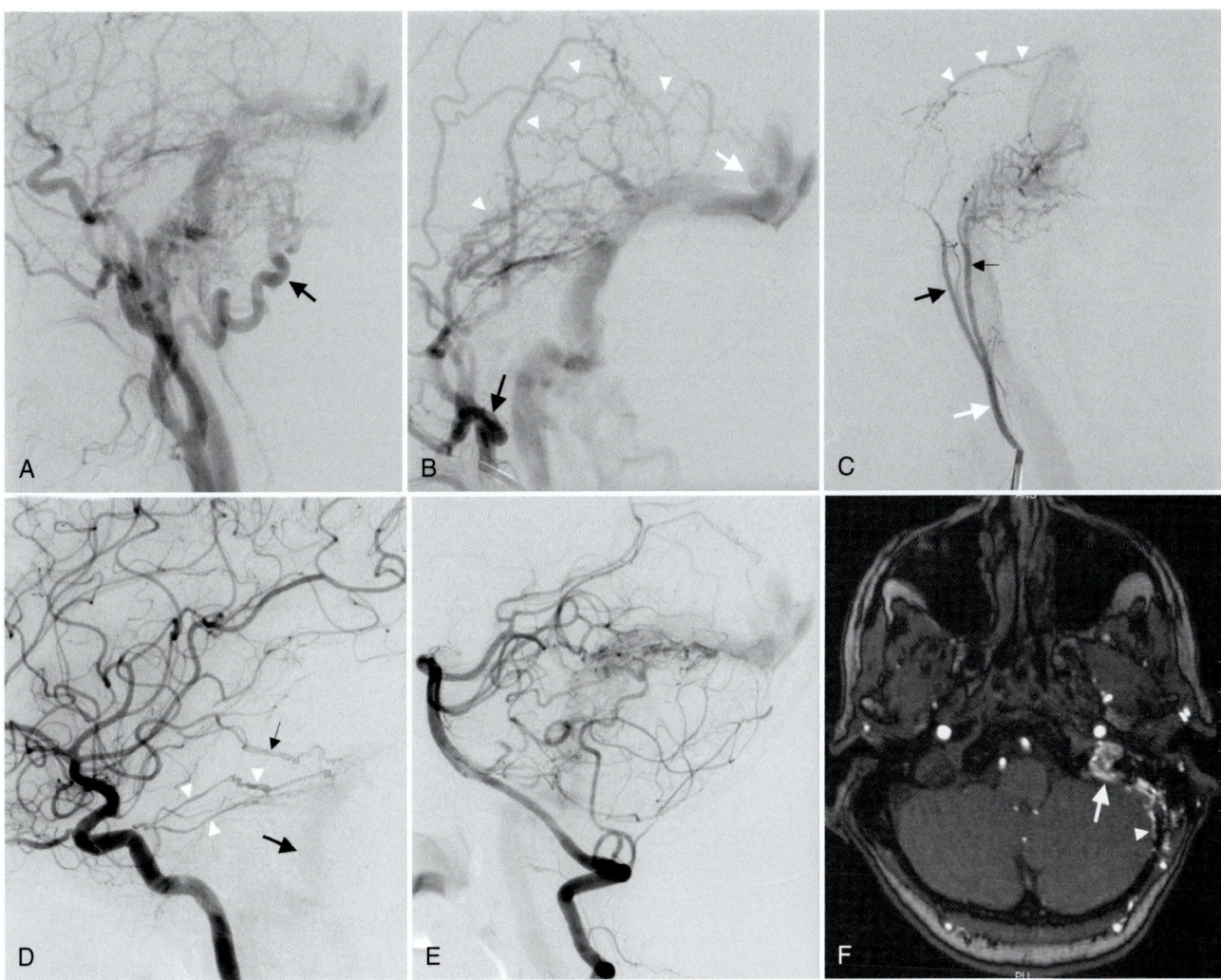

Figure 5-43 A, B: Left common carotid artery angiogram, lateral view, in arterial phase showing abnormal early venous contrast filling of left transverse sigmoid sinus consistent with dural arteriovenous fistula (DAVF) (A). Major arterial supply originates from transmastoid branches of enlarged left occipital artery (large black arrows). B: Superselective left occipital artery angiogram, lateral view, illustrating typical arterial network consisting of numerous small transmastoid and dural crack-like vessels that supply multiple tiny micro-AVFs within wall of dural sinus (white arrowheads). Venous reflux into contralateral transverse sinus is depicted (large white arrow). This is a type IIa DAVF (Cognard scale). C: Superselective left ascending pharyngeal artery angiogram, lateral view, showing additional arterial feeders from both anteriorly located pharyngeal trunk (large black arrow) and posterior neuromeningeal trunk (small black arrow) of ascending pharyngeal artery (large white arrow). Posteriorly the neuromeningeal trunk supplies large network of shunts to jugular bulb through its jugular branch. Anteriorly, fine lateral clival and superior pharyngeal artery (via foramen lacerum) branches anastomose with dural internal carotid artery (ICA) branches (tentorial branches of meningohypophyseal artery and inferolateral trunk) to give additional fistula supply (white arrowheads). These anastomoses are potentially dangerous collateral vessels toward the ICA system when performing transarterial embolization procedures. D: Left ICA angiogram, lateral view, demonstrating enlarged tentorial branches of the meningohypophyseal trunk (white arrowheads) as well as small pial temporal middle cerebral artery branches that supply the DAVF (small black arrow), resulting in faint opacification of left sigmoid sinus (large black arrow). E: Selective left vertebral artery angiogram, lateral view, illustrating numerous other small pial feeding vessels from left superior cerebellar artery and anterior inferior cerebellar artery branches. F: Axial three-dimensional time-of-flight magnetic resonance image showing typical hyperintensities within the left sigmoid sinus/jugular bulb (large white arrow) as well as hyperintensities adjacent to these veins (white arrowhead), which correspond to high-flow signal derived from arterialized sinuses and feeding arteries. (Courtesy Dr. William McAuliffe, Perth.)

5-13). Numerous arteriovenous microfistulae form a fine vascular network in the wall of the affected dural sinus. Determining the type of DAVF (e.g., Cognard I–V) depends on accurate assessment of the venous drainage pattern and hemodynamics. Delineation of the flow (anterograde vs retrograde) within the involved sinuses or cortical veins (e.g., vein of Labbé) is important. Reflux into cortical or spinal perimedullary veins (Figure 5-44) and venous ectasias must be noted. Dural sinus stenosis or occlusion is a common but invariably seen finding.

Noninvasive Imaging Modalities

Problem Solving: What Is the Role of Modern CTA and MRA Imaging Modalities in Vascular Malformations with AV Shunting?

Modern high-resolution multidetector CTA imaging and fast time-resolved 3D MRA techniques have been shown to reliably enable the diagnosis of cerebral AV shunting lesions such as AVM and DAVF.

Static CTA techniques appear advantageous in the emergent setting with patients presenting acutely with

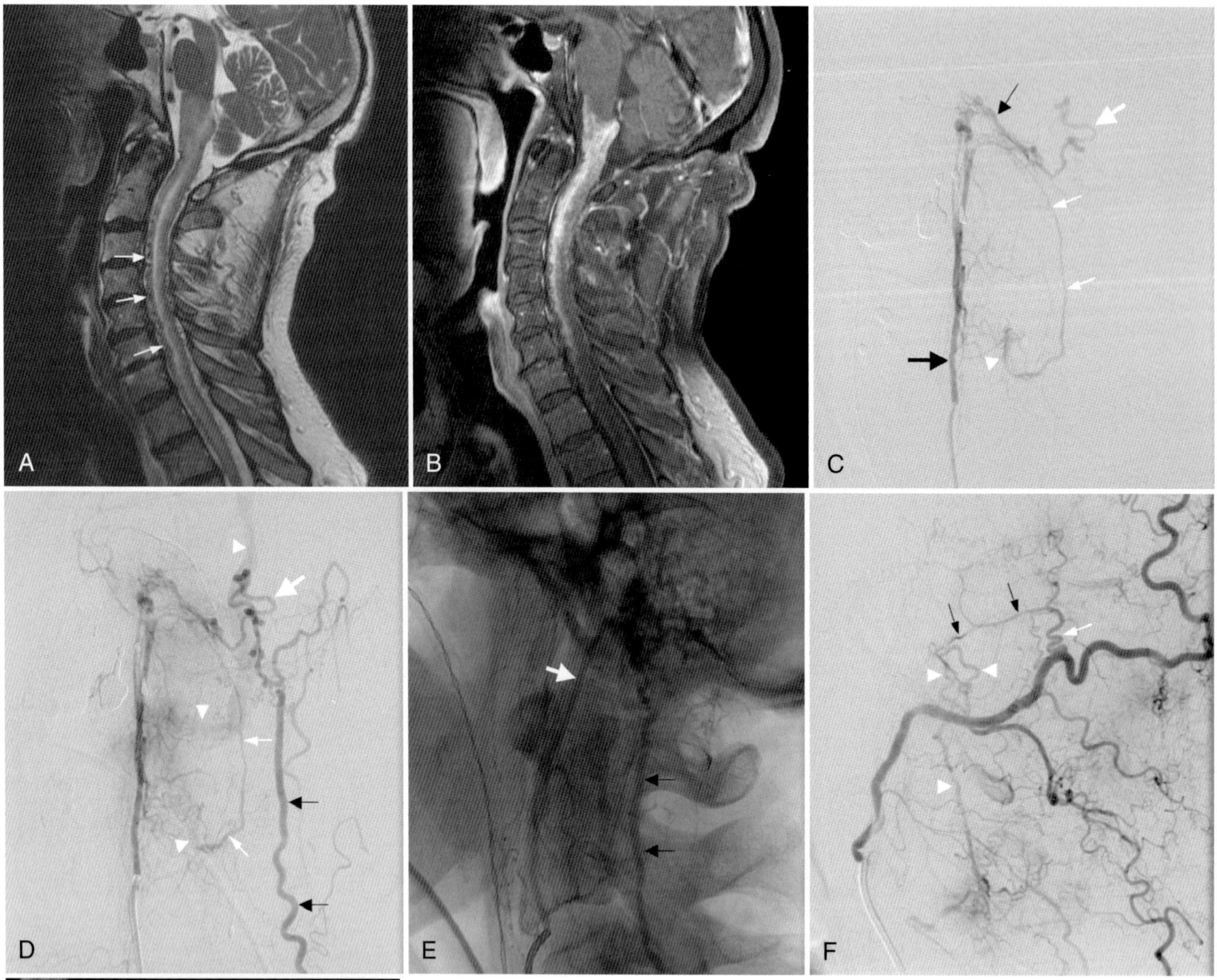

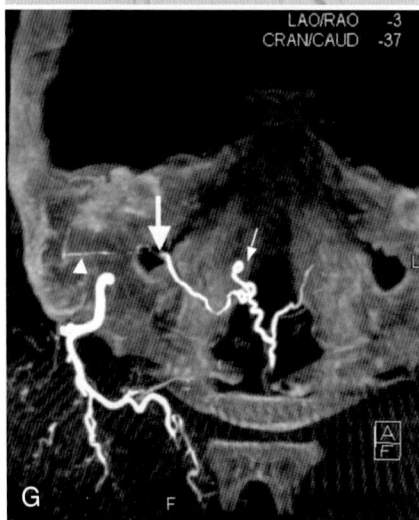

Figure 5-44 **A:** T2-weighted magnetic resonance image of the cervical spine in sagittal orientation showing extensive central intramedullary edema involving the medulla oblongata as well as cervical and upper thoracic cord with prominent epimedullary flow voids *(small white arrows)*. **B:** Corresponding T1-weighted image (with sat saturation) after gadolinium administration showing massive intramedullary contrast enhancement in these areas. **C:** Early arterial phase image, lateral view, of superselective angiogram with catheter tip located in right ascending pharyngeal artery *(large black arrow)*. A dural arteriovenous shunt is located at the right craniocervical junction and is supplied by small jugular *(small black arrow)* and hypoglossal branches of the neuromeningeal trunk of the ascending pharyngeal artery. Venous drainage is directed into dilated veins of the anterior medullary venous (AMV) system *(large white arrows* in **C** and **D**). **D:** Subsequent later arterial phase image showing further inferior drainage into the grossly enlarged anterior spinal vein *(small black arrows)* (corresponding to grade V dural arteriovenous fistula on Cognard scale). The odontoid arch system, an important arterial arcade surrounding the dens, is filled via the hypoglossal branch of the neuromeningeal trunk of the ascending pharyngeal artery *(small white arrows* in **C** and **D**). At the C2–3 intervertebral space it anastomoses with the vertebral artery, which shows faint opacification *(white arrowheads* in **C** and **D**). This anastomosis poses an important potential hazard when performing embolization procedures for this arteriovenous shunt. **E:** Unsubtracted lateral view of superselective right ascending pharyngeal angiogram showing location of fistula at craniocervical junction with feeding neuromeningeal trunk *(white arrow)* and anterior spinal venous drainage *(small black arrows)* posterior to odontoid peg. **F:** Superselective angiogram of right occipital artery, lateral view, demonstrating additional arterial supply of fistula from a small transmastoid branch of occipital artery *(small white arrow)* via tiny meningeal vessel *(small black arrows)* to shunt into AMV/anterior spinal vein *(white arrowheads)*. **G:** Targeted maximal intensity projected reconstructed image of superselective right occipital artery three-dimensional rotational angiogram (DynaCT) is useful for accurate anatomic localization of the fistula point relative to overlaid bony landmarks at the skull base. The fistula point is confined by a transition in vessel caliber from a tiny transmastoid arterial feeder *(white arrowhead)* to the retroclival convoluted bridging vein *(thin white arrow)*. This can be identified at the right jugular foramen *(large white arrow)*. Subsequent caudal venous drainage through the foramen magnum into the midline anterior spinal vein is also delineated. (Courtesy Dr. Tejinder Pal Singh, Perth.)

Table 5-7 Classification of Intracranial Nonatheromatous Vasculopathies

Inflammatory Vasculopathy—Vasculitis

Primary angiitis of the CNS	Systemic vasculitis with CNS involvement	Systemic diseases with secondary CNS angiitis	CNS diseases with secondary vasculitis
	Polyarteritis nodosa	Systemic lupus erythematosus	Meningitis (pyogenic, fungal, parasitic, tuberculous, syphilitic)
	Hypersensitivity granulomatosis (Churg and Strauss)	Antiphospholipid syndrome	
	Wegener granulomatosis	Scleroderma	
	Behçet's disease	Rheumatoid arthritis	Septic emboli
	Giant cell arteritis	Sjögren's syndrome	Sarcoid
	Takayasu arteritis		
	Temporal arteritis		

Noninflammatory Vasculopathy

Inherited disorders	Oncotic vasculopathy	Radiation-induced vasculopathy	Idiopathic progressive arteriopathy of childhood
Neurocutaneous syndromes	Tumor emboli		Moyamoya disease
Neurofibromatosis type 1	Pseudoaneurysm		
Tuberous sclerosis	Intravascular lymphoma		
Menkes kinky hair disease			
Ehlers-Danlos type IV			
Sickle cell disease			

Reversible Vasculopathy Syndromes

Reversible cerebral vasoconstriction syndrome	Posterior cerebral encephalopathy syndrome may coexist with reversible cerebral vasoconstriction syndrome		
Pregnancy and puerperium			
Vasoactive drug and blood product exposure			
Miscellaneous			
Headache disorders (e.g., migraine)			
Idiopathic			

CNS, Central nervous system.

intracranial hemorrhage or clinical suspicion of a vascular malformation. However, precise assessment of arterial feeders, fistula points, and grading of venous drainage still is impossible on static CTA images. The newest generation of multirow CT scanners (64 or 320 rows) offers the possibility of generating dynamic images of the cerebrovascular circulation covering a large area of interest (e.g., entire head), and reported preliminary results for the diagnosis and classification of cranial arteriovenous shunts appear promising.

Dynamic, contrast-enhanced MRA methods that generate images at high spatial and temporal resolutions can be used to diagnose and characterize AVMs with regard to main arterial feeders, nidus size, major draining veins, and the Spetzler-Martin grading. They can be used for image-guided radiosurgery of intracranial AVMs or during follow-up of treated AV shunts to reduce radiation exposure to patients. However, they are not capable of replacing DSA for comprehensive characterization of AVMs and DAVFs. The relatively lower spatiotemporal resolutions and nonselective mode of vascular visualization are limitations for a robust depiction of small or low-flow AV shunting lesions, intranidal/feeding artery aneurysms, and feeding arteries/pedicles. For these reasons, the catheter angiogram is still considered the standard of reference for diagnosis, grading, and therapy planning in AV shunting lesions. Equivocal findings on noninvasive CTA or MRA studies should directly prompt further investigation with DSA.

The application of dynamic intraarterial CTA (DynaCT digital angiography), which uses a biplane C-arm flat-panel detector angiography system, provides additional information in the evaluation DAVFs compared to 2D DSA. This method especially enhances detailed visualization of fistulous points and small vessels in relation to fine osseous structures, which may be very useful for planning endovascular or surgical treatment of DAVFs (Figure 5-44, *G*).

Vasculitis, Reversible Cerebral Vasoconstriction Syndromes, and Noninflammatory Vasculopathies

Problem Solving: What Is the Role of Catheter Angiography in Suspected Cerebral Vasculitis?

How Specific Are Vasculitis-like Changes on DSA, and What Conditions Other than Cerebral Vasculitis May Show Similar Findings?

Atherosclerosis is by far the most common cause of a vasculitis-like angiographic pattern in adults. However, a large variety of congenital and acquired nonatheromatous disorders or conditions can produce cerebral inflammatory vasculopathies, noninflammatory vasculopathies, or reversible vasculopathy syndromes (Table 5-7).

Neurocutaneous Syndromes and Inherited Vasculopathies

A number of inherited disorders can involve the intracranial arteries. NF1 and tuberous sclerosis are the two phakomatoses that most often cause cerebral vascular manifestations. Slowly progressive stenotic or occlusive lesions of the supraclinoid ICAs may cause an angiographic moyamoya pattern to develop in NF1. Less commonly aneurysms (see section on Indications/Aneurysms), ectasias, or fistulae in the large- and medium sized arteries are encountered in NF1. *Ehlers-Danlos syndrome (type IV)* is characterized by spontaneous vessel ruptures, dissections, aneurysm formation of large- and medium sized arteries, or spontaneous direct CCFs. *Sickle-cell disease* causes vascular occlusions or endothelial damage from sickled red cells, and neurologic complications including stroke are commonly encountered (25% of cases). Angiographically, stenosis of the supraclinoid ICAs and the proximal ACA/MCA segments may result in a moyamoya pattern often seen in *sickle cell disease*. Multiple aneurysms in this disorder also have been reported (see section on Indications/Aneurysms).

Moyamoya Disease

Idiopathic progressive arteriopathy of childhood, also called *moyamoya disease*, is an arteriopathy of unknown etiology that has two peak ages of presentation in Japan and Pacific rim countries: childhood (early onset) and adulthood (late onset). Children usually present with ischemic symptoms, whereas adults also commonly present with intracranial hemorrhage. The prognosis in this disorder depends on the rapidity and extent of vessel occlusions as well as the development of effective collaterals. The classic angiographic pattern consists of stenosis or occlusion of the distal ICAs with collateral circulation from multiple enlarged lenticulostriate and thalamoperforating arteries that resemble a "puff of smoke," which is the translation of the Japanese word "moyamoya." Widespread dural, leptomeningeal, and pial collaterals also may develop. This so-called angiographic *moyamoya pattern* is nonspecific and has been reported in a number of disorders other than idiopathic progressive arteriopathy of childhood, such as NF1, radiation therapy, sickle cell disease, and atherosclerosis. Moyamoya disease is also associated with other vascular anomalies (e.g., aneurysms, AVMs, ectasias, fenestrations).

Inflammatory Vasculopathy— Vasculitis

Inflammatory vasculopathies (true vasculitides) can be subdivided into primary (isolated) angiitis of the CNS and systemic vasculitic diseases with secondary CNS involvement (Table 5-7). The angiographic imaging appearance of the intracranial vasculitides is nonspecific and similar, regardless of specific etiology. Multiple segmental smooth or slightly irregularly shaped stenosis alternating with dilated segments is typical (Figure 5-45).

Primary angiitis of the CNS is characterized pathologically by inflammation of the media and adventitia of preferentially small arterioles and venules (<300 μm in diameter, which is below the resolution of conventional DSA); however, vessels of any size can be affected. Invasive brain or leptomeningeal biopsy usually is the only test that allows for definite diagnosis, although the result may be negative in some cases owing to a patchy distribution of histologic involvement. Studies have shown that typical angiographic features of vasculitis do not reliably identify patients with primary angiitis of the CNS proved on biopsy by neuropathologic criteria. The sensitivity of these findings was reported as low as 10% to 20% when small-vessel involvement was present, and the ability to distinguish vasculitis from other disorders ranged between 24% and 60%.

Several types of systemic necrotizing vasculitides may involve the cerebral vasculature with nonspecific angiographic findings. The most common types are *polyarteritis nodosa* and *hypersensitivity (allergic) angiitis and granulomatosis (Churg-Strauss)*. In systemic lupus erythematosus, neurologic involvement with stroke is common, but true cerebral vasculitis is rare; the angiogram is most commonly normal. The causes of stroke in systemic lupus erythematosus include thrombosis secondary to hypercoagulopathy from antiphospholipid syndrome, emboli from Libman-Sacks endocarditis, accelerated atherosclerosis, and cerebral vasculitis (primary lupus vasculitis or secondary to CNS infection). Antiphospholipid syndrome is characterized clinically by strokes at an unusually early age, recurrent arterial and venous thromboses, infertility and spontaneous fetal loss, and thrombocytopenia. The most commonly encountered angiographic abnormalities are solitary stem or distal branch occlusions; however, vasculitic patterns and nonatherosclerotic great vessel origin stenosis also may occur.

Other systemic diseases that may cause CNS vasculitis include *scleroderma, rheumatoid disease,* and *Sjögren syndrome*. Behçet disease, which is classically characterized by recurrent oral and genital ulcers and uveitis, may also cause CNS vasculitis involving small- and medium-sized vessels. Parenchymal lesions in the basal ganglia, brainstem, and cerebellum are typical on MRI, but cerebral venous thrombosis and meningitis also may occur.

Infective pyogenic, granulomatous, fungal, and parasitic *meningitis* as well as sarcoidosis have a predilection for the basal cisterns and commonly narrow the terminal ICA and the proximal MCA and ACA segments. Other infectious causes of intracranial vasculopathy include human immunodeficiency virus, cysticercosis, Lyme disease, and meningovascular syphilis.

Neoplasms with tumor emboli may cause pseudoaneurysms and intracranial vascular stenosis. Lymphoproliferative diseases such as angiocentric large cell lymphoma may present initially with vasculitis.

Noninvasive Imaging Alternatives

Contrast-enhanced, flow-compensated high-resolution T1-weighted MRI has been reported to demonstrate thickening and contrast enhancement of vessel walls in patients with different types of inflammatory CNS vasculitis affecting the large arteries of the brain. Although the value and diagnostic accuracy of this sign is still unclear and warrants additional studies, MRI including MRA may be advantageous. Besides visualization of vessel wall changes, it is capable of showing parenchymal

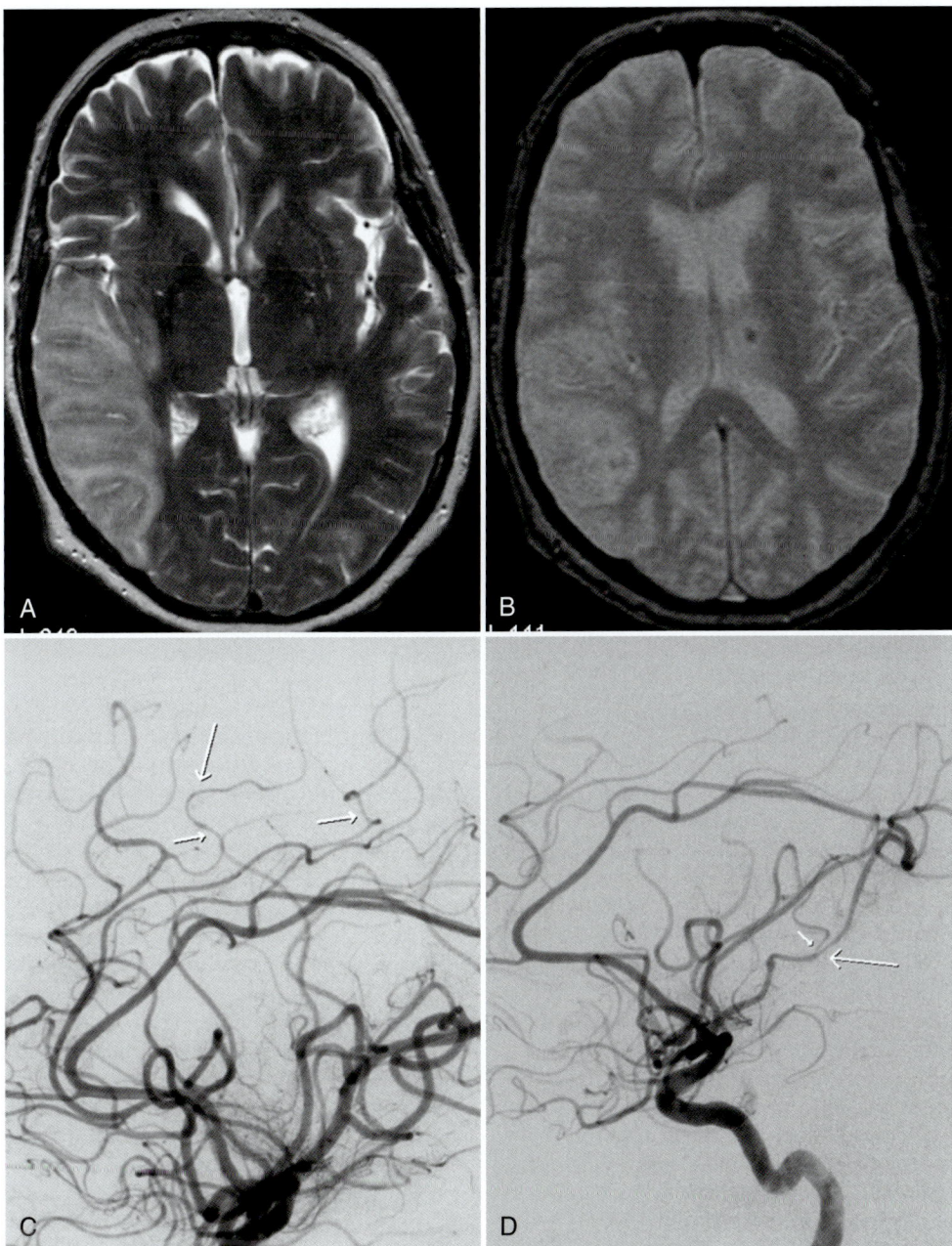

Figure 5-45 Axial T2-weighed (**A**) and gradient-recalled echo (**B**) magnetic resonance (MR) images obtained from a patient with new onset of headaches and left-sided hemiparesis. Imaging findings are consistent with multiple areas of cortical ischemia involving the right temporoparietal lobe, left thalamus, and left occipital lobe. Contrast-enhanced MR images (not shown) revealed partially enhancing and nonenhancing infarcts consistent with different age of these lesions. **B:** Petechial hemorrhages involving infarcted and noninfarcted areas are visualized. A subsequently performed catheter angiogram revealed typical findings of vasculitis. **C:** Left internal carotid artery angiogram, lateral view, during arterial phase showing multiple areas of alternating constrictions and dilatations in the anterior cerebral artery branches *(thin white arrows)*. **D:** Right internal carotid artery angiogram, lateral view, during arterial phase showing similarly affected vessels in the middle cerebral artery territory *(thin white arrows)*. Right frontal brain/leptomeningeal biopsy disclosed mixed inflammatory vessel wall infiltrates with small amounts of fibrinoid necrosis involving small and large vessels and secondary ischemic brain damage. No evidence of systemic vasculitis was present (negative on screenings for hypercoagulable disorders and autoantibodies). These findings were consistent with primary CNS vasculitis.

abnormalities (mainly stroke and/or hemorrhages) that are very common in different types of inflammatory vasculopathies. However, caliber changes of medium- and small-sized arteries can be reliably depicted only by catheter angiography compared to current MRA techniques.

Despite this potential advantage, the invasive catheter angiogram is considered useful only when the pretest probability for vasculitis is high (e.g., in case of multiple infarcts in different vascular territories on MRI, positive clinical findings such as headaches, and positive cerebrospinal fluid analysis) due to the low sensitivity and specificity of this method. The combination of normal MRI and cerebrospinal fluid is regarded a very powerful negative predictor in excluding the possibility of CNS vasculitis in many patients.

Table 5-8 Conditions Associated with Reversible Vasculopathy Syndromes

Reversible Cerebral Vasoconstriction Syndromes

Pregnancy and puerperium, early pregnancy, late pregnancy, eclampsia, preeclampsia, delayed postpartum eclampsia	Vasoactive drugs and blood products Phenylpropanolamine, pseudoephedrine, ergotamine, tartrate, Methergine, bromocriptine, lisuride, selective serotonin reuptake inhibitors, sumatriptan, isometheptine, cocaine, ectasy, amphetamine derivatives, marijuana, lysergic acid diethylamide, tacrolimus (FK-506), cyclophosphamide, erythropoietin, intravenous immune globulin, red blood cell transfusions	Miscellaneous Hypercalcemia, porphyria, pheochromocytoma, bronchial carcinoid tumor, unruptured cerebral aneurysm, head trauma, spinal subdural hematoma, postcarotid endarterectomy, neurosurgical procedures	Headache disorders- Migraine, primary thunderclap headache, benign exertional headache, benign sexual headache, primary cough headache

Posterior Reversible Encephalopathy Syndrome May Coexist with Reversible Cerebral Vasoconstriction Syndrome

Toxemia of pregnancy (preeclampsia/eclampsia) Autoimmune diseases Systemic lupus erythematosus, scleroderma, Wegener, polyarteritis nodosa	Posttransplantation Allogeneic bone marrow transplantation, solid organ transplantation Status post chemotherapy Combination high-dose chemotherapy, cytarabine, cisplatin, gemcitabine, tiazofurin, bevacizumab (Avastin), kinase inhibitor BAY 34-9006	Immune suppression Cyclosporine, tacrolimus (FK-506) Miscellaneous Hypomagnesemia, hypercalcemia, hypocholesterolemia, intravenous immune globulin, Guillain-Barré syndrome	Infection/sepsis/shock Systemic inflammatory response syndrome, multiorgan dysfunction syndrome

Modified from Calabrese LH, Dodick DW, Schwedt TJ, Singhal AB: Narrative review: reversible cerebral vasoconstriction syndromes. *Ann Intern Med* 146(1):34-44, 2007; and Bartynski WS: Posterior reversible encephalopathy syndrome, part 1: fundamental imaging and clinical features. *AJNR Am J Neuroradiol* 29(6):1036-1042, 2008.

Reversible Cerebral Vasculopathy Syndromes

Reversible cerebral vasoconstriction syndromes (RCVSs) has been introduced as a descriptive term that summarizes a group of diverse disorders characterized by prolonged but reversible angiographic vasoconstriction of the cerebral arteries. In the past, RCVSs have been given various eponymic or syndromic labels, including Call syndrome (or Call-Fleming syndrome), benign angiopathy of the CNS, postpartum angiopathy, thunderclap headache with reversible vasospasm, migrainous vasospasm or migraine angiitis, and drug-induced cerebral arteritis or angiopathy. Clinically these disorders typically present with acute-onset severe, "thunderclap headaches" that recur for a few days, with or without additional neurologic signs and symptoms. Although most patients experience complete resolution of headache and neurologic symptoms within days to weeks, others may be left with permanent neurologic deficits secondary to ischemic or hemorrhagic stroke.

The characteristic angiographic findings in RCVS are nonspecific (vasculitis-like), with alternating areas of arterial constriction and normal vascular caliber or dilatation, often called *beading*, in multiple vascular beds involving the large and medium cerebral arteries (anterior and posterior circulation). Although rare exceptions exist, the reversibility of vasoconstriction over days to weeks is the feature that best distinguishes this disorder from true cerebral vasculitis, particularly primary angiitis of the CNS, which is the most important differential diagnosis. The distinction of these conditions is important because the treatment differs for both. Although catheter angiography is considered the gold standard technique, some angiographic features can also be demonstrated on serial CTA or MRA.

Understanding of RCVS has been limited by the lack of a unique underlying pathologic basis and validated diagnostic criteria. Currently a large number of associated conditions have been described, including uncomplicated pregnancy or puerperium, eclampsia/preeclampsia, exposure to certain medications or drugs (e.g., cocaine, ecstasy, methamphetamines, and a spectrum of sympathomimetic drugs), and the setting of catecholamine-secreting tumors. RCVS also can occur without an identifiable course or in association with other headache disorders (Table 5-8). Uncertainty exists in the distinction of RCVS from migraine attacks and posterior reversible leukoencephalopathy syndrome (PRES) due to overlapping clinical and imaging features. The latter syndrome is characterized by reversible gray matter and white matter lesions on MRI that often occur in the setting of hypertensive encephalopathy. However, these lesions have also been described in patients with presentations or associated conditions typical of RCVS (Table 5-8). Angiographically, PRES findings are consistent with what is typically described as vasospasm or arteritis, but again reversibility of vasculopathy can be observed on repeat angiographic studies. Therefore, the suggestion has been made that RCVS and PRES may coexist or that RCVS may even be the cause of PRES due to a common pathophysiologic basis consisting of disturbances in cerebral arterial tone with subsequent cerebral hypoperfusion in the two syndromes.

Cerebral Vasospasm

Cerebral vasospasm following SAH may appear angiographically identical to RCVS but can be differentiated clinically based on the history and the absence of subarachnoid blood. Rarely hyperacute or acute vasoconstriction occurs after SAH, which may cause extensive global ischemia. Pathologically altered cerebral arterial tone is the source of vasoconstriction with alternating areas of stenosis that affect the proximal as well as the distal

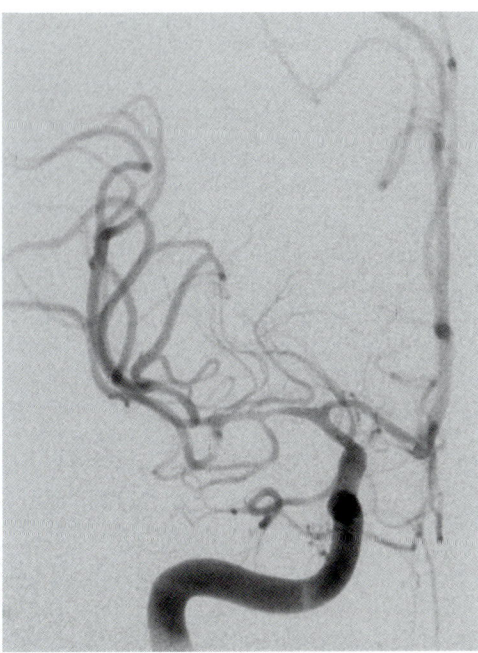

Figure 5-46 Right internal carotid angiogram, anteroposterior view, obtained 9 days after subarachnoid hemorrhage secondary to a ruptured middle cerebral artery aneurysm that had been coil embolized prior to this angiogram. Multiple areas of segmental narrowing in the M1 segment and M1/M2 junctions of the middle cerebral artery, the A1 segment of the anterior cerebral artery, and the suraclinoid internal carotid artery are seen. These findings are typical of severe cerebral vasospasm.

vasculature, which typically is not multifocal but may mimic a vasculitis-like pattern after SAH (Figure 5-46). This is often disclosed on angiography in patients who develop secondary neurologic deterioration or ischemic symptoms with a peak between 4 and 11 days after rupture of an intracranial aneurysm. This condition is a major cause of morbidity and mortality secondary to SAH.

■ CAROTID DISEASE, INTRACRANIAL ARTERIAL STENOSIS, AND TRAUMA

Carotid Stenosis

Problem Solving: What Is the Current Role of DSA in Atherosclerotic Disease of the Carotid Arteries? Is the Gold Standard Imaging Technique Still Required?

Imaging of the carotid artery for screening of critical stenosis (>70%– 99%) is a very common investigation that is performed for primary or secondary prevention of stroke in patients with TIAs or who suffered from previous stroke. For decision making regarding potential carotid endarterectomy or stenting, quantification of carotid stenosis according to North American Symptomatic Carotid Endarterectomy Trial (NASCET) is the most widely accepted method, although various different methods have been used in the past. This trial was based on conventional angiography, so the percentage decrease in residual carotid lumen is estimated by using ratio calculations from the angiographic projection showing the "narrowest" stenosis (Figure 5-47).

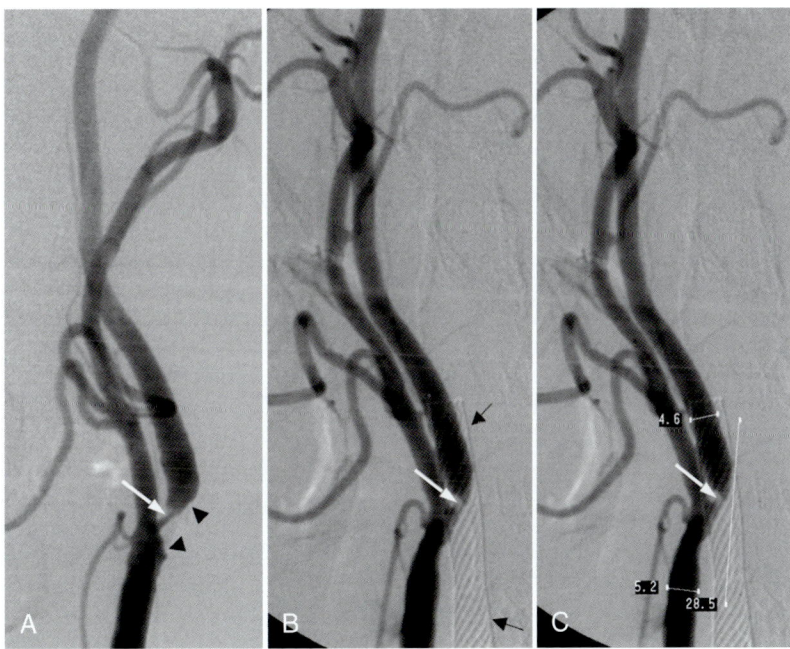

Figure 5-47 Left common carotid artery (CCA) angiogram in oblique (**A**) and lateral (**B, C**) views showing a high-grade eccentric stenosis of the proximal internal carotid artery (ICA). **A:** Eccentric atherosclerotic plaque involving the carotid bifurcation on oblique view of CCA angiogram. Note subtraction artifact from plaque calcification *(black arrowheads)*. A high-grade stenosis of the proximal ICA *(white arrow)* is demonstrated. **B:** On the lateral view, a carotid stent that was inserted previously into the contralateral ICA is visible *(small black arrows)*. Again, the high-grade proximal stenosis of the left ICA *(white arrow)* is shown. **C:** CCA angiogram, lateral view, is used to measure the diameter of the CCA proximal to the stenosis and the ICA distal to the stenosis as well as the vessel length to tailor the appropriate size of the carotid stent before treatment of the ICA stenosis *(white arrow)*. (Courtesy Dr. William McAuliffe, Perth.)

Apart from determining stenosis severity (moderate vs high grade), the angiographic workup needs to provide other important information, including the following. (1) Identify and accurately discriminate a true occlusion from a near occlusion, also called a *pseudoocclusion*. The latter is defined as a very-high-grade stenosis (99%) with distal luminal collapse that may cause very slow anterograde flow with delayed contrast washout. This so-called *string sign* occurs when only a trickle of anterograde flow can be detected on late phases of carotid angiograms or color flow Doppler ultrasound. (2) Identify tandem stenotic lesions (e.g., in the carotid siphon or intracranial circulation) and evaluate existing and potential pathways for collateral circulation. (3) Identify coexisting atherosclerotic disease (aortic arch, great vessels, intracranial vessels). (4) Identify intraluminal thrombus, which usually occurs at the site of greatest luminal compromise and increases the risk of periprocedural thromboembolism during carotid stenting. (5) Identify vessel tortuosity, configuration, and variants of the aortic arch that may interfere with access for endovascular stenting. (6) Identify plaque ulceration and plaque content/morphology, which may be used in the future for risk stratification in asymptomatic patients or in patients with moderate stenosis (concept of "plaque vulnerability"). For characterizing plaque morphology (e.g., intraplaque hemorrhage), noninvasive techniques such as high-resolution MRA or carotid ultrasound have shown promising results in published studies and may be applied clinically in the future. Catheter angiography is still considered the gold standard for imaging of carotid stenosis but has been widely eliminated as a screening method for carotid disease. This is mainly due to its invasiveness and associated risks of stroke, which are particularly high for this subgroup of patients (see section on Complications and Risk Factors). Instead, a wide range of noninvasive imaging modalities with their own distinct advantages and drawbacks is currently in use. The techniques most often used are carotid duplex and color Doppler flow ultrasonography, TOF and contrast-enhanced MRA, and CTA.

The major benefit of CTA is the acquisition of isotropic 3D image data at relatively high spatial resolution that allows for accurate measurement of luminal dimensions of both carotid arteries in a multiplanar fashion. It also may provide additional information on plaque content in the arterial wall with or without mural calcifications, and extravascular tissues. Another advantage is a high sensitivity for the detection of distal or tandem lesions. For first-generation single-slice CTA, the sensitivity and specificity for detection of 70% to 99% stenosis and of occlusion were 85% and 93%, and 97% and 99%, respectively. Using multidetector CTA technology, very high sensitivity and specificity for detection of carotid stenosis (>50%) was demonstrated. However, compared with 2D DSA, a mild underestimation of stenosis measurements seems to be more common than overestimation, but misclassification is reported rare in careful assessment of images. In fact, the overestimation on CTA may be partly related to limited and suboptimal DSA views that can lead to an underestimation of stenosis degree on DSA.

A meta-analysis of MRA demonstrated a high diagnostic accuracy of TOF and contrast-enhanced MRA techniques for the detection of high-grade ICA stenosis and occlusions, with contrast-enhanced MRA having the edge over TOF MRA. However, the sensitivity of both methods for identifying moderate-degree stenosis was markedly reduced (50%–69%). The distinction of near occlusion (pseudoocclusion) from true occlusion of the carotid artery may be critical for determining patients eligible for carotid endarterectomy or stenting. This has often been a diagnostic dilemma for noninvasive imaging modalities, and a combination of two different modalities, such as carotid ultrasonography as a screening test and MRA and/or DSA for confirmation, has been applied to solve this problem. In this particular subgroup, DSA may be required under rare circumstances to diagnose a true "string sign," which represents diffuse luminal narrowing or distal ICA stenosis/occlusion (e.g., in the siphon) with collapsed proximal lumen and cannot be differentiated from near occlusions when ultrasound and MRA fail to demonstrate a focal high-grade lesion. Alternatively, multidetector CTA, which has proven excellent correlation with DSA for the diagnosis of carotid near occlusion, may be applied. The accuracy of MRA for detecting lower-degree stenosis is likely to increase in the future with the use of modern high-field (3 T) MR scanners with dedicated multichannel neurovascular array coils. In a report using contrast-enhanced MRA with highly accelerated parallel imaging techniques at 3 T on an extended field of view (circle of Willis included), the whole supraaortic arterial tree was imaged at very high spatial resolution (voxel size 0.44 mm^3), resulting in diagnostic values comparable to DSA for arterial stenosis detection.

Whether small differences in the performance of modern CTA and MRA techniques for carotid stenosis are important for patient outcome and in which cases DSA or a combination of noninvasive methods would produce the best result are unclear. However, the potential risks of DSA should be considered when determining the diagnostic method of choice. After all, the present situation is notably different from the time of the major studies on carotid endarterectomy, with advances in the best medical treatment as well as carotid stenting being evaluated as an alternative therapy in ongoing randomized multicenter trials (International Carotid Stenting Study [ICSS] and Carotid Revascularization Endarterectomy vs. Stenting Trial [CREST]).

Intracranial Atherosclerosis

Problem Solving: Under Which Conditions Is DSA Necessary in Intracranial Arterial Stenoocclusive Disease?

Atherosclerotic disease in large intracranial arteries is an important and often underrecognized cause of stroke. It is estimated to account for approximately 5% to 10% of ischemic strokes in the United States and 33% to 67% in Asia. Moreover, the overall risk of recurrent ischemic events may be as high as 15% to 38% per year among persons with intracranial atherosclerotic disease.

The diagnostic accuracy of CTA for evaluation of intracranial atherosclerotic arterial stenosis has been reported to be very high (97.1% sensitivity, 99.5% specificity for >50% stenosis) compared to DSA. Furthermore, CTA detected large arterial occlusion with 100% sensitivity and specificity. Another study demonstrated that CTA has a higher sensitivity than MRA for intracranial stenosis and occlusion. TOF MRA, which is routinely performed for visualization of the intracranial arteries, is limited by a lower spatial resolution than DSA and CTA and by flow-related artifacts. Particularly in stenotic lesions, proton spin dephasing, and consequently flow signal intensity loss, commonly occurs secondary to complex, slow, or in-phase flow. Therefore, TOF MRA is considered more inaccurate in grading stenosis and tends to overestimate high-grade stenoses.

The major limitation of CTA is its inferior spatial resolution compared to DSA; however, this is likely to improve in the future with advancing multidetector CT technology. Using current CTA technology for the detection of stenosis in smaller vessels (diameter <2 mm, which is typical for ACA and distal MCA branches), a slight difference in measurement could potentially result in a significant difference in the degree of stenosis. Because CTA is essentially a vessel cast technique, it also provides no significant flow hemodynamic information as does DSA, which may be very important in determining related risks and guiding decisions for treatment of such lesions.

DSA is considered the gold standard in the evaluation of intracranial stenosis and occlusion. It provides images with high spatial resolution. However, mainly owing to its procedural risks, costs, and limited availability, noninvasive CTA and MRA are more desirable for screening for stenosis in the larger intracranial arteries and for following patients with such conditions. Of interest, false-positive findings of arterial occlusion in the vertebrobasilar system can rarely occur with DSA compared to CTA and are related to low- or balanced-flow states in the setting of severe stenosis.

With increasing use of intracranial stents for treating intracranial stenosis, symptomatic or asymptomatic in-stent restenosis is a common delayed complication that is reported in up to 30% of cases. The clinically more concerning complication of delayed stent thrombosis may occur under much rarer instances. To diagnose and differentiate these conditions, a vigorous angiographic follow-up is suggested. Noninvasive angiographic imaging techniques appear not advantageous for this indication due to stent-related artifacts. Current case series suggest that current CTA techniques may be prone to misinterpretation of in-stent stenosis and in-stent thrombus, which may result in inappropriate management. Mainly owing to its comparable less artifact-affected visualization of stent struts and stent lumen, angiographic CT with intravenous contrast application may be a noninvasive alternative technique in the future. This new technique provides cross-sectional CT-like images based on 3D rotational radiography performed with a rotating C-arm–mounted flat-panel detector. However, to date only case reports have shown promising results with this new technique. In the meantime, DSA should be considered a method of choice for follow-up imaging after intracranial stent placement.

Ischemic Stroke

Problem Solving: What Are the Indications for Cerebral Angiography and Typical Angiographic Findings of Ischemic Stroke?

Imaging of acute ischemic stroke including visualization of intracranial arterial vasculature is not the domain of invasive diagnostic catheter angiography. Besides early signs of stroke on CT imaging of the brain, CTA and CT perfusion imaging can reliably demonstrate major extracranial and intracranial arterial occlusions, high-grade stenosis or intravascular thrombus, and potentially salvageable tissue indicated by a penumbra. These examinations are widely available, and they are easy and fast to perform on a helical CT scanner. MRI, particularly diffusion weighted imaging, more accurately detects cerebral ischemia within minutes of its onset. MR can also be used to detect hemorrhage as well as determine the status of the extracranial and intracranial arteries on MRA. A mismatch between findings on diffusion and perfusion MR images may be used to predict the presence of a penumbra. These techniques are mainly applied in the setting of acute ischemic stroke to rule out hemorrhage and to determine the stroke pattern as well as the risks, benefits, and prognosis of potential candidates for thrombolysis. The so-called *therapeutic time windows* that allow safe administration of intravenous or intraarterial thrombolysis therapy are very narrow in these patients. Classically, revascularization treatments for acute ischemic stroke are generally restricted to within 3 hours of symptom start for intravenous tissue plasminogen activator or 6 to 8 hours for intraarterial thrombolysis and mechanical thrombectomy. The report of the European Cooperative Acute Stroke Study III (ECASS III) trial demonstrated safety and benefit of intravenous thrombolysis between 3 and 4.5 hours after onset of symptoms. As a consequence, the therapeutic window for invasive intraarterial therapies may be further narrowed. Alternate triaging methods for endovascular therapies in patients with acute ischemic stroke have been tested only in small patient collectives and currently still lack validation from large prospective studies.

Outside the setting of intraarterial thrombolysis or endovascular mechanical revascularization procedures, invasive cerebral angiography is not indicated for patients with acute stroke. However, it is important for an interventional neuroradiologist to be familiar with the angiographic signs of acute cerebral infarction. These may occur in the event of a thromboembolic complication when endovascular procedures are performed within a brain-supplying artery (e.g., coiling of a cerebral aneurysm). Early detection of such signs is of particular importance in order to prompt salvage maneuvers such as intraarterial thrombolysis, which may potentially reverse major ischemic damage. The most commonly encountered sign is the presence of *intravascular thrombus*, which is seen as a filling defect within the lumen of an opacified vessel, or *vessel occlusion*. Occlusion can present as a tapered vessel narrowing or abrupt

Table 5-9 Craniocervical Collateral Flow

Intracranial Anastomoses	Extracranial/Intracranial Anastomoses	Extracranial Anastomoses

Circle of Willis
Pial (leptomeningeal) collaterals
Transdural collaterals
	ECA to ICA
	Maxillary artery branches
	    MMA or recurrent meningeal artery to ophthalmic artery
	    MMA to ILT
	    Artery of foramen rotundum to ILT
	    Accessory meningeal artery to ILT
	    Anterior and middle deep temporal arteries to ophthalmic artery
	    Vidian artery to petrous ICA (anterior tympanic artery)
	Facial artery (angular branch) to ophthalmic artery
	Superficial temporal artery to anterior falx artery
	Ascending pharyngeal artery branches
	    Superficial pharyngeal artery to cavernous ICA (foramen lacerum)
	    Superficial pharyngeal artery to ILT
	    Clival rami to cavernous ICA
	    Inferior tympanic artery to petrous ICA (caroticotympanic artery)
	    Jugular branch of neuromeningeal trunk to ICA
	Stylomastoid artery (from occipital or posterior auricular artery) to petrous ICA
	ECA to VA
	Occipital artery branches
	    Transosseous branches
	    C1 anastomotic branch (suboccipital "knot")
	    C2 anastomotic branch
	Ascending pharyngeal artery branches
	    Hypoglossal branch (odontoid arch system)
	    Musculospinal branch
	Subclavian artery to VA
	Ascending cervical artery branches
	    C3 anastomotic branch
	    C4 anastomotic branch
		Subclavian steal (VA to contralateral distal subclavian artery)
		Carotid steal (CCA occlusion with patent ECA and ICA, flow reversal in ECA)
		VA to VA via segmental branches
		ECA to ECA via contralateral branches

Modified from Osborn AG: *Diagnostic Cerebral Angiography*. Lippincott Williams & Wilkins; 1999; and Hacein-Bey L, Daniels DL, Ulmer JL, et al: The ascending pharyngeal artery: branches, anastomoses, and clinical significance. *AJNR Am J Neuroradiol* 23(7):1246-1256, 2002.
ECA, External carotid artery; *ICA*, internal carotid artery; *ILT*, inferolateral trunk; *MMA*, middle meningeal artery; *VA*, vertebral artery.

termination of contrast filling; sometimes meniscal filling defects also occur (Figure 5-14, *A*). Other angiographic abnormalities seen in acute cerebral infarction are *slow anterograde flow* with prolonged circulation time and *delayed arterial contrast "washout"* in the affected area (contrast is still opacifying arteries in the early venous phase of angiogram). Paucity of vessels ("bare areas") in nonperfused or slowly perfused brain may be seen in some cases (Figure 5-14). Another common finding is the presence of pial-to-pial collaterals across the watershed zones with slow retrograde filling (into venous phases) of patent but proximally occluded obstructed branches. "Luxury perfusion" is a misnomer describing a prominent vascular blush that can sometimes be seen within a few hours to days after stroke onset. Different mechanisms such as arteriolar–venular shunting and capillary dilatation have been proposed for this incompletely understood phenomenon. In some cases, AV shunting with early draining veins in the ischemic focus may be observed. Signs of mass effect are uncommon in hyperacute stroke but may develop within the first week after stroke onset.

Collateral circulation plays a crucial role in acute and chronic cervical or intracranial arterial occlusion. The understanding of collateral flow patterns (e.g., through the circle of Willis, pial-to-pial, dural-to-pial, or extracranial-to-intracranial anastomoses) is an important prerequisite for safe cerebral angiography as well as endovascular procedures (Table 5-9). Moreover, it is of significance for planning a revascularization procedure (e.g., carotid stenting) in patients presenting with TIA, stroke, or symptoms of chronic cerebral hypoperfusion (Figure 5-48).

Tumors

Problem Solving: What Is the Role of DSA in Presurgical Evaluation of Intracranial and Extracranial Neoplasms?

Noninvasive studies such as MRI have replaced catheter angiography in the evaluation of extracranial and intracranial masses. Assessment of tumor vascularity or involvement of large arteries, such as the ICA or ACA, or dural venous sinuses in surgical planning can be safely performed using noninvasive angiographic modalities such as CTA/CTV or MRA/MRV. However, diagnostic angiography still may be required for presurgical evaluation of endovascular transarterial embolization of tumor-supplying arteries, as is typical for extraaxial masses supplied by meningeal branches of the ECA (i.e., middle meningeal artery branches in meningiomas). In these cases, knowledge and visualization of potentially dangerous collaterals between the ECA system and the internal carotid or vertebrobasilar system is a crucial prerequisite. Another rare indication for performing cerebral angiography in patients with intracranial mass

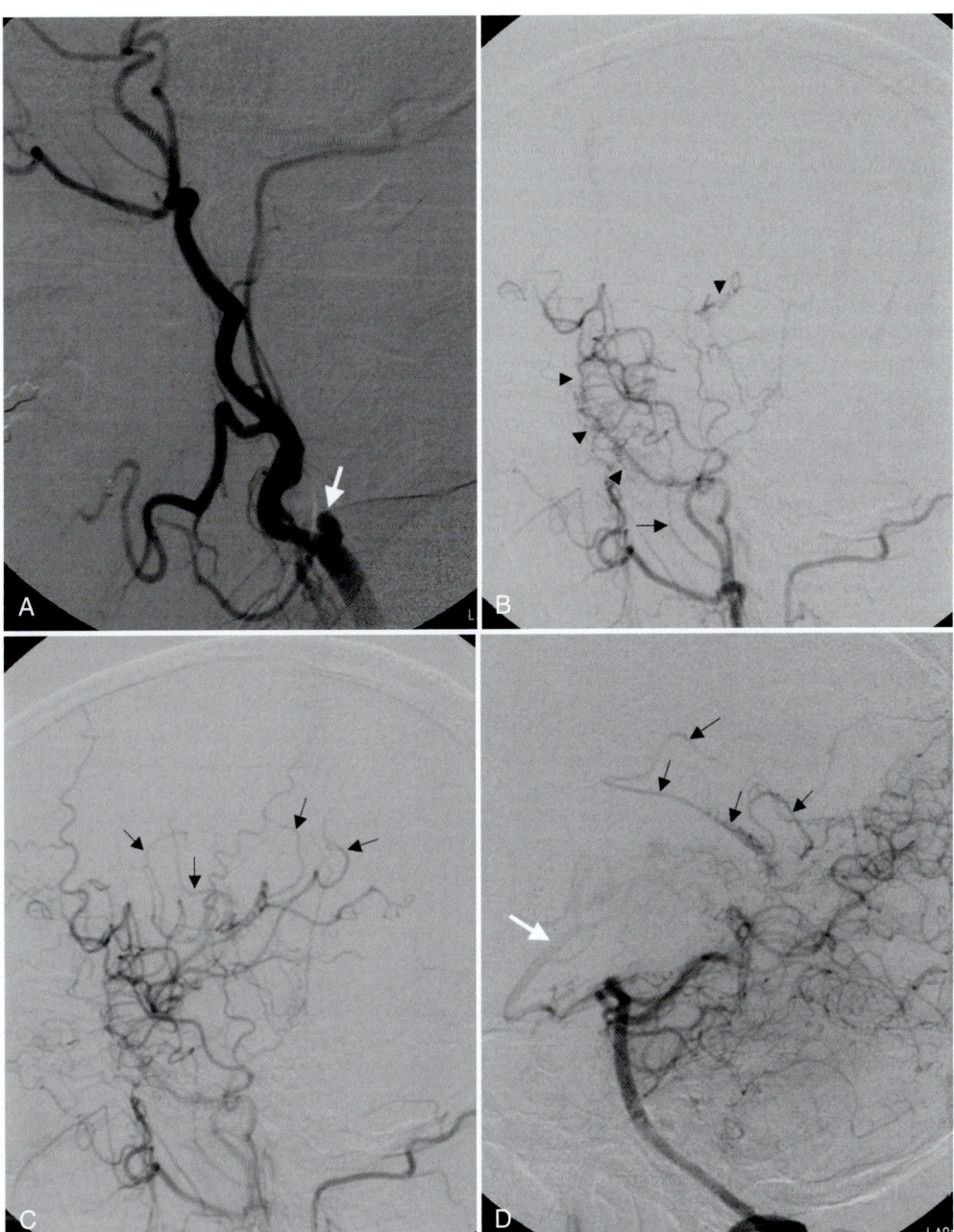

Figure 5-48 Intracranial collateral flow patterns in a patient with right chronic right internal carotid artery (ICA) occlusion. **A:** Right common carotid artery angiogram, lateral view, showing an occlusion of the cervical ICA just distal to the carotid bifurcation. The short vessel stump ends in an rounded outpouching *(large white arrow)*. No anterograde flow was seen on later phase images (not shown). Normal filling of the external carotid artery (ECA) branches is noted. **B:** Right common carotid artery angiogram, lateral view of the cranial circulation, early arterial phase, showing no filling of the intracranial ICA segments. Filling of the ECA branches is noted with multiple small dural-to-pial collaterals *(black arrowheads)* arising from branches of the middle meningeal artery as well as the accessory meningeal artery *(small black arrow)*. **C:** Consecutive midarterial phase showing delayed filling of multiple cortical branches *(small black arrows)* in the right middle cerebral artery (MCA) territory (M3 arteries) via dural-to-pial collaterals. Again, no opacification of the right distal ICA and right proximal MCA is noted. **D:** Left vertebral artery angiogram, lateral view, late arterial phase, showing opacification of the distal right anterior cerebral artery territory (distal pericallosal artery and branches, *small black arrows*) via splenial and choroidal branches from the posterior cerebral artery (pial-to-pial collaterals). Faint collateral filling of the right MCA *(large white arrow)* via the posterior communicating artery is depicted. (Courtesy Dr. Tejinder Pal Singh, Perth.)

lesions is presurgical functional testing for eloquent brain (e.g., a Wada test).

General angiographic features of intracranial masses reflect both their direct and indirect effects on intracranial vessels.

Indirect manifestations of space-occupying lesions include focal or generalized mass effect including herniation syndromes. Small avascular extraaxial or intraaxial neoplasms can be easily overlooked on DSA. When lesions become larger displacement of arterial branches or cortical veins may occur. Cerebral herniations are caused by gross mechanical displacement of brain, cerebrospinal fluid, and blood vessels from one compartment to another. The patterns of herniation are classified according to which anatomic boundaries the herniating structures cross: subfalcine, transtentorial (ascending or descending), transalar, or tonsillar. With larger masses, combinations of these syndromes can occur. Angiographically these syndromes cause classic patterns of vessel displacement (e.g., A2/A3 displacement underneath falx in subfalcine herniation). A detailed description of these characteristic patterns is beyond the scope of this chapter. The identification of these syndromes by catheter angiography has markedly lost its diagnostic relevance over the last decades since CT and MRI have become standard modalities for evaluating intracranial masses. However, the interventional neuroradiologist should be familiar with their appearance because they may indirectly indicate mass effect from expanding hematoma or hydrocephalus during endovascular procedures.

The direct effects of mass lesions include arterial enlargement due to increased tumor supply, angiogenesis with neovascularity, a tumor "blush," blood–brain barrier disruption, intratumoral AV shunts, vascular encasement and occlusion, and rarely oncotic pseudoaneurysms (see section on Indications/Aneurysms). A blush that is an accumulation of contrast during the late arterial and early capillary phases of a cerebral angiogram is not pathognomonic for neoplasm. It occurs normally in some relatively vascular areas such as the basal ganglia and simply reflects increased capillary density. An abnormal blush is a nonspecific finding that may occur with trauma, infection, cerebral ischemia, and prolonged seizures. A spectrum of both benign and malignant intracranial neoplasms demonstrates a prolonged vascular blush that represents increased vessel density secondary to neoplastic vascular proliferation.

The most common tumor for which angiograms are sometimes required to assess the possibility of presurgical endovascular embolization is meningioma, including all three histologic variants (benign, atypical, anaplastic). Angiographically, most meningiomas are highly vascular lesions that are supplied by multiple radiating vessels from hypertrophied meningeal arteries ("sunburst pattern"), such as the middle meningeal artery (Figure 5-49). A homogeneous prolonged tumor blush from late arterial to capillary phases is called the *mother-in-law sign:* it comes early and stays late. ICA or VA angiograms often demonstrate only avascular mass effect due to a lack of pial supply. In larger lesions, the periphery of the tumor may also be supplied by pial branches. Evaluation of the venous phase is crucial because growth into dural venous sinuses with secondary occlusion is a typical phenomenon. Other tumors that may be evaluated for presurgical planning or potential embolization include invasive skull base tumors such as pituitary adenoma (uniform tumor blush), hemangioblastoma (very intense vascular mural nodule), and hemangiopericytoma (Figure 5-50).

Neovascularity (irregular and bizarre-appearing vessels, laking, pooling of contrast) is a common but not entirely specific finding in primary malignant brain tumors such as glioblastoma multiforme. Neoplastic intratumoral AV shunts (early draining veins) are usually seen in high-grade gliomas and metastases. Vascular displacement or encasement is often seen in large skull base tumors such as pituitary adenoma, meningioma, and chordoma. Arterial occlusions and strokes are uncommon manifestations of intracranial neoplasms. Cortical vein occlusions or dural venous sinus invasion classically occurs in extraaxial tumors such as meningioma or dural metastasis.

A diagnostic angiogram may sometimes be obtained in patients with extracranial/cervical neoplasms. Such neoplasms include juvenile nasopharyngeal angiofibroma (intense and prolonged vascular stain from internal maxillary artery branches), meningioma, schwannoma, and paraganglioma. The latter has a strikingly similar angiographic appearance regardless of location (glomus caroticum, glomus jugulare, glomus tympanicum, glomus jugulotympanicum): a well-delineated round or lobulated vascular mass with dense, prolonged contrast staining is typical (cave: rare risk of hypertensive crisis precipitated by angiography in paragangliomas). AV shunts occur, glomus jugulare tumors typically occlude the jugular vein, and carotid body tumors splay apart the ECA and ICA. A detailed description of angiographic patterns of head and neck tumors and their mimics (reactive lymphadenopathy) is beyond the scope of this chapter.

Angiographic evaluation may be required in cases of difficult surgical access, skull base invasion, vascular encasement/invasion that requires larger vessel sacrifice (e.g., for temporary ICA balloon test occlusion), or for presurgical embolization in highly vascular lesions. Delineating vascular supply and collateral vessels that include the identification of potentially dangerous collateral flow patterns (Figure 5-51 and Table 5-9) is essential when performing and interpreting angiograms from these patients.

Cerebrovascular Trauma and Dissection

Problem Solving: What Different Types of Head and Neck Vessel Injuries May Occur in Trauma?
What Circumstances Require a Cerebral Angiogram in Patients with Sustained Head or Neck Trauma?
Traumatic injury to the vessels of the head and neck can result in potentially devastating neurologic sequelae. Because of the associated substantial morbidity and

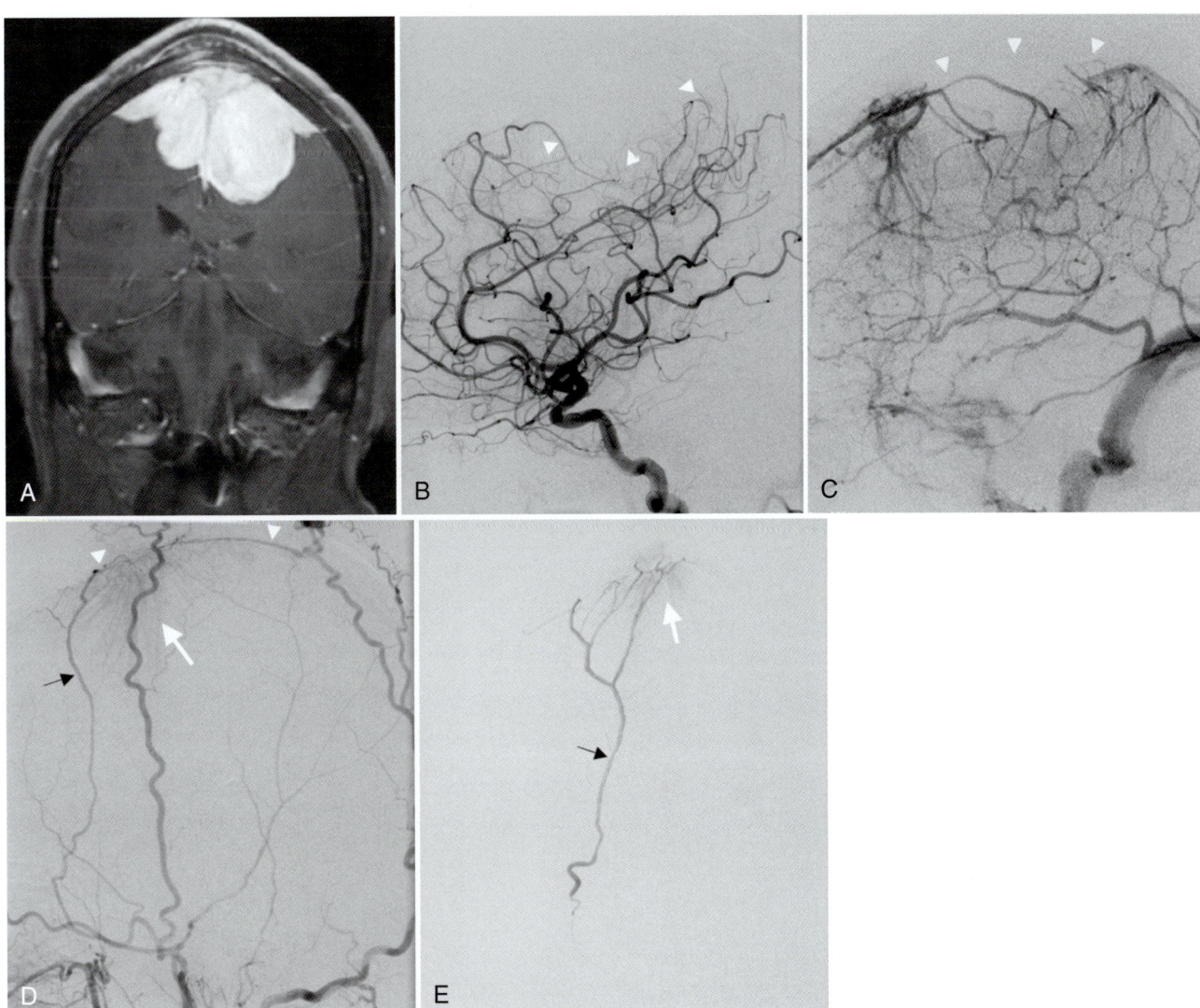

Figure 5-49 T1-weighted magnetic resonance image postgadolinium, coronal view (**A**), showing large multilobulated bilateral parasagittal extraaxial mass that is homogeneously contrast enhancing and involves the superior sagittal sinus, cranial vault, and overlying scalp. Right internal carotid artery angiogram with late arterial (**B**) and venous (**C**) phase images, lateral view, show no relevant tumor supply from pial arteries but avascular mass effect *(white arrowheads* in **B**) with stretching and draping of distal pial arteries. Segmental occlusion of the superior sagittal sinus *(white arrowheads* in **C**) with draping of cortical veins is also demonstrated. **D:** Selective left external carotid artery angiogram, lateral view, late arterial phase, showing an enlarged frontal branch of the middle meningeal artery *(small black arrow)* that supplies the dural-based tumor with a typical "sunburst" tumor blush *(large white arrow)*. Additional supply predominantly to the bony and scalp components is depicted from branches of the superficial temporal artery *(white arrowheads)*. **E:** Superselective angiogram from a microcatheter inserted into the frontal branch of middle meningeal artery *(small black arrow)* again shows radial tumor blush *(large white arrow)* before presurgical embolization. A typical meningioma was subsequently found after surgical resection. (Courtesy Dr. Constantine Phatouros, Perth.)

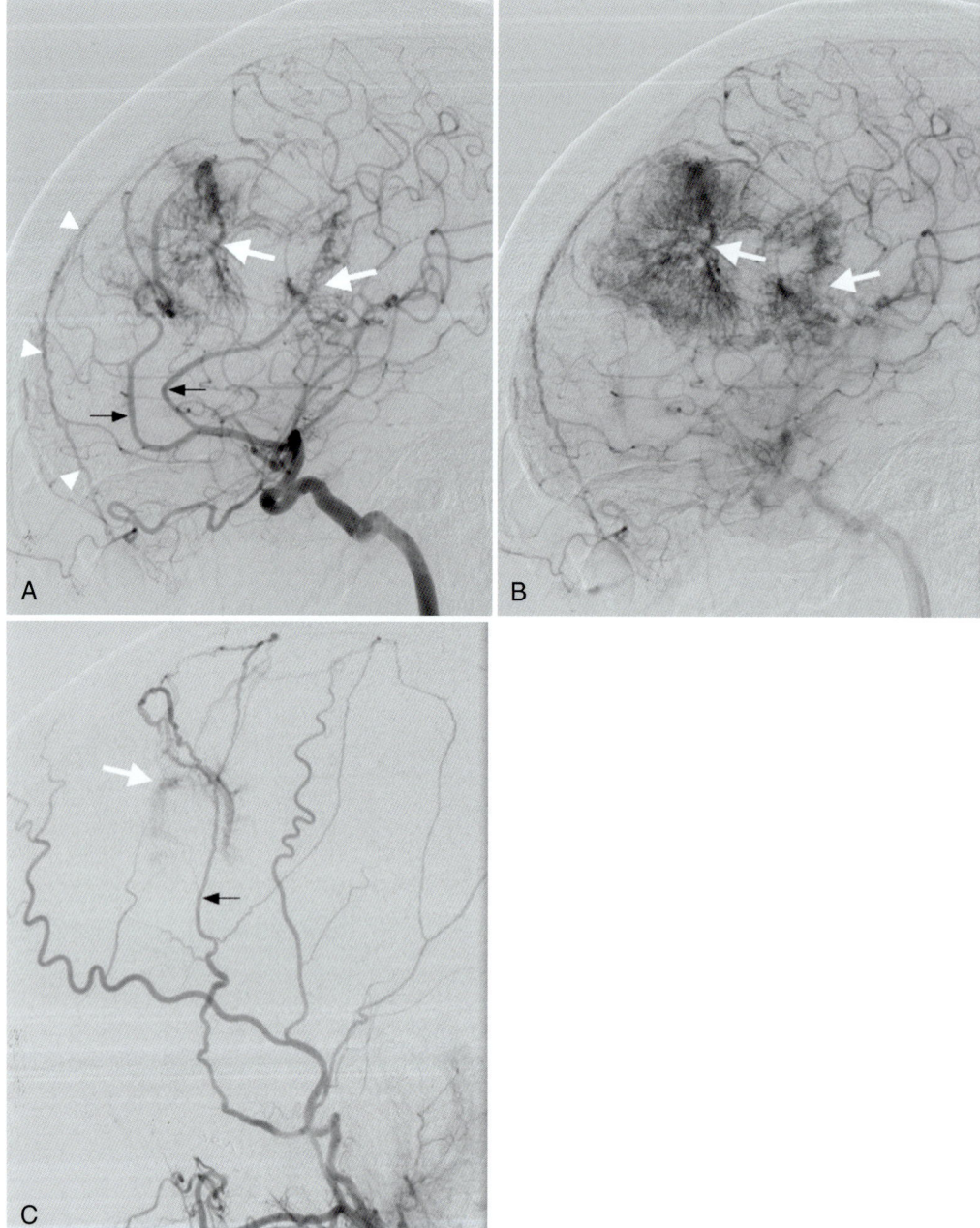

Figure 5-50 Left internal carotid artery angiogram, lateral view, early (**A**) and late (**B**) arterial phase, showing an irregularly configured, highly vascular mass with pial supply from the pericallosal and callosomarginal arteries *(small black arrows* in **A**). The large tumor blush *(large white arrows* in **A** and **B**) consists of multiple small "sunburst" vessels as well as bizarre-appearing vessels with pooling of contrast representing signs of neovascularity. Additional meningeal feeders to the tumor are derived from an enlarged anterior falx artery *(white arrowheads* in **A**). **C:** Selective external carotid angiogram, lateral view, showing further meningeal arterial supply to the tumor *(large white arrow)* from enlarged frontal branch of middle meningeal artery *(small black arrow)*. The patient underwent subsequent endovascular embolization of middle meningeal artery branches and pial anterior cerebral artery branches. Surgical removal of a highly vascularized parasagittal extraaxial mass revealed a hemangiopericytoma. (Courtesy Dr. William McAuliffe, Perth.)

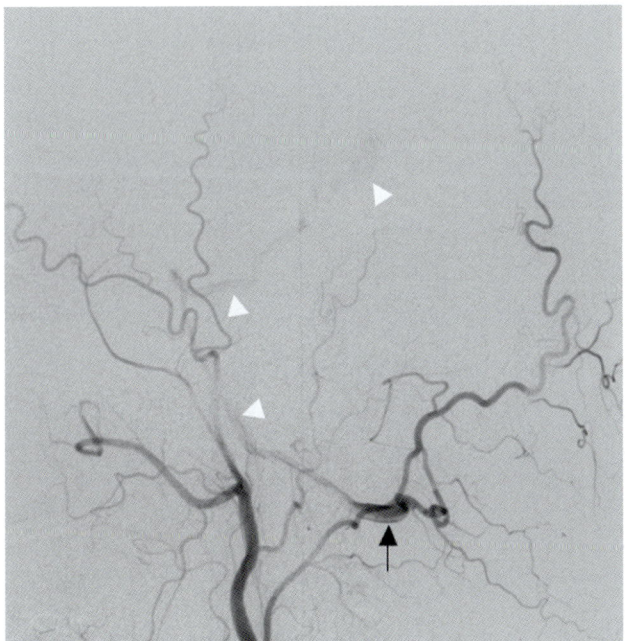

Figure 5-51 Right external carotid artery angiogram, lateral projection, illustrating a typical suboccipital craniocervical anastomosis between muscular branches of the occipital artery and vertebral artery at the level of C1 (so-called suboccipital Carrefour or knot). The V3 segment of the right vertebral artery is transiently opacified with contrast *(small black arrow)*. The patient has an arteriovenous malformation (AVM) supplied by branches of the posterior cerebral artery. There is evidence of faint filling of the vertebrobasilar system and the AVM *(white arrowheads)*. This collateral pathway poses a significant potential risk for stroke in the vertebrobasilar territory when performing neurointerventional embolization procedures.

mortality, it is important to diagnose this rare complication of head and neck trauma. The incidence of cerebral vascular trauma ranges from 0.18% to 1.55% of all trauma patients, with an approximate ratio of 2:1 for ICA involvement compared to VA involvement. Motor vehicle accidents account for the majority of these lesions, and there is a male dominance with a mean age less than 30 years in most series. A high risk of neurovascular injury showed a strong tendency to be associated with fractures of the sella turcica–sphenoid sinus complex. The two major pathomechanisms are penetrating trauma and blunt trauma, with blunt trauma being by far the more common. For traumatic artery injuries, the three major anatomic substrates are dissections, pseudoaneurysms, and AVFs.

Traumatic Arterial Injuries

Traumatic Cervical Artery Dissections

Dissections account for the majority of cerebrovascular trauma sequelae. An *arterial dissection* is defined as an intramural hematoma that might produce a stenosis of the vessel, a luminal irregularity, and occasionally an aneurysmal dilatation. Most dissections are associated with an intimal defect if the dissection does not arise from ruptured vasa vasorum. The intimal tear that is associated with the primary injury may allow propagation of circulating blood into the vessel wall. Further distal, rerupture can occur through the intima into the vessel lumen, creating a flap or double lumen, or through the adventitia outside the vessel wall.

Traumatic dissections typically involve both the cervical and petrous parts of the ICA and spare the bulb. The most common cause of traumatic ICA dissections are motor vehicle accidents with associated hyperextension/flexion injuries of the neck. VA dissections can occur when the head is rotated in extension, leading to stretching of the artery between C1 and C2, or can occur due to direct vessel wall injury from a fracture of the transverse foramen.

Although delayed cerebral ischemia is the most frequently encountered clinical presentation, 20% to 33% of patients are clinically asymptomatic. Other clinical presentations include carotodynia (i.e., neck pain along the course of artery), headaches, Horner syndrome, and cranial neuropathies. Spontaneous dissections commonly show improvement or resolution of stenotic lesions on follow-up angiography (85% of cases). In contrast, traumatic dissections resolve or improve in only 55%, while 25% progress to complete occlusion.

Conventional angiography has historically been considered the gold standard for dissection diagnosis. The angiographic appearance of dissection is variable but often characteristic: smooth tapering of the vessel lumen that may lead to an occlusion of the artery (string sign); luminal stenosis that may or may not be followed by aneurysmal dilatation (pearl and string sign); or vessel wall irregularity. An intimal flap is only rarely encountered on angiographic images (Figure 5-52). However, catheter angiography lacks assessment of the vessel wall for intramural hematoma; therefore, dissections in unusual locations or having atypical morphology may be misclassified or attributed to other processes. A combination of MRI/MRA and multidetector CT/CTA have emerged as viable alternatives for both diagnosis and follow-up of dissection. In general, the two techniques have different strengths and weaknesses. MRI is the ideal method for detecting acute infarction or hemorrhage as possible sequelae of dissection. Axial T1 weighted fat-suppressed images can detect the methemoglobin of intramural hematoma within the false lumen (crescent sign). Multidetector CT/CTA is faster and more widely available, and it provides greater spatial resolution than MRI/MRA. Vertinsky et al. compared both methods and slightly favored CT/CTA, particularly for VA dissections, because of visualization of more features (e.g., intimal flaps, stenoses, pseudoaneurysms) in the affected arterial segment. Although the two, often complementarily used, noninvasive modalities are the preferred methods for diagnosis of dissection, conventional angiography may help in rare instances of confusing or ambiguous cases.

Traumatic Aneurysms

Traumatic intracranial aneurysms are discussed in the section on Indications/Aneurysms Traumatic extracranial carotid (pseudo-)aneurysms may be the result of penetrating trauma or blunt trauma (e.g., rotatory hyperextension, strangulation, fractures of the mandibular angle). Extradural carotid aneurysms due to

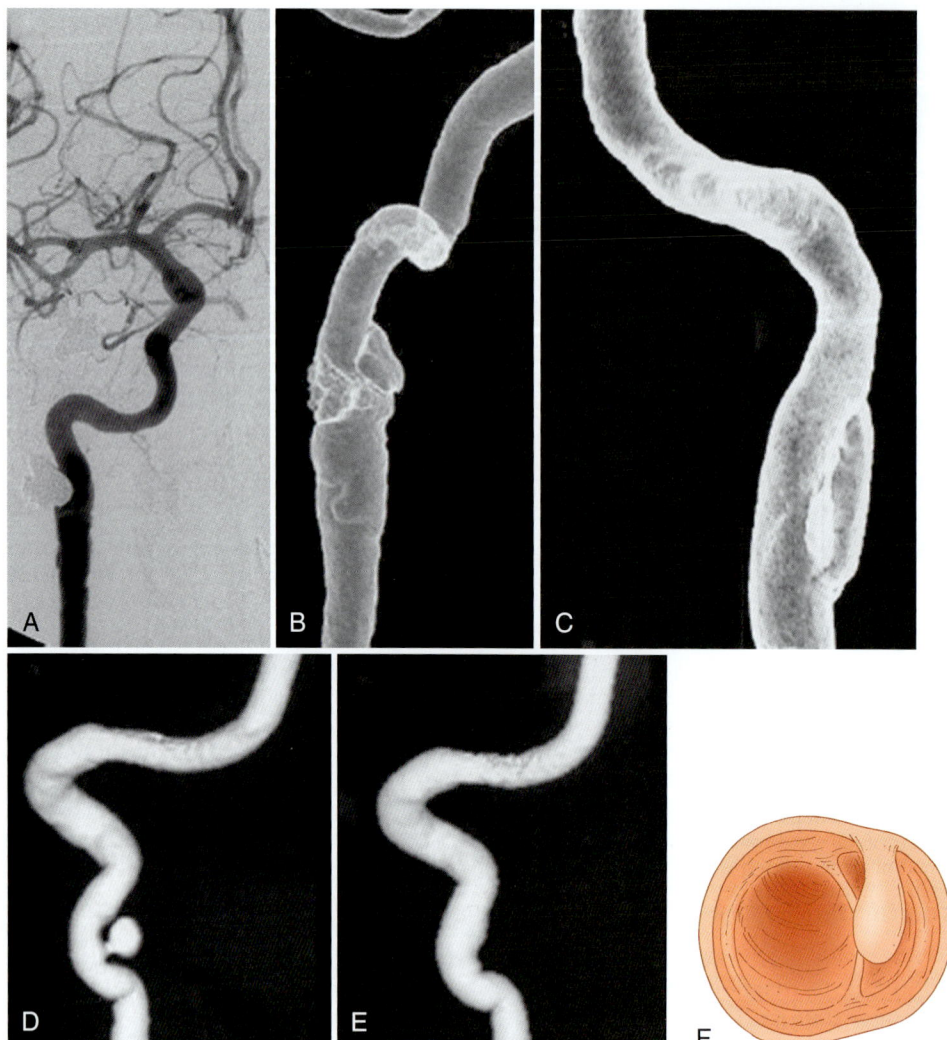

Figure 5-52 Spectrum of traumatic dissections in three patients. Dissecting processes of the internal carotid artery can go along with vessel wall irregularities (**A, B**), with a flap and double-lumen sign (**C, F**) or with an aneurysmal dilatation (**D**) that in this case spontaneously completely regressed on follow-up 3 months later (**E**). (From Krings T, Geibprasert S, Lasjaunias PL. Cerebrovascular trauma. Eur Radiol 2008;18: 1531-1545.)

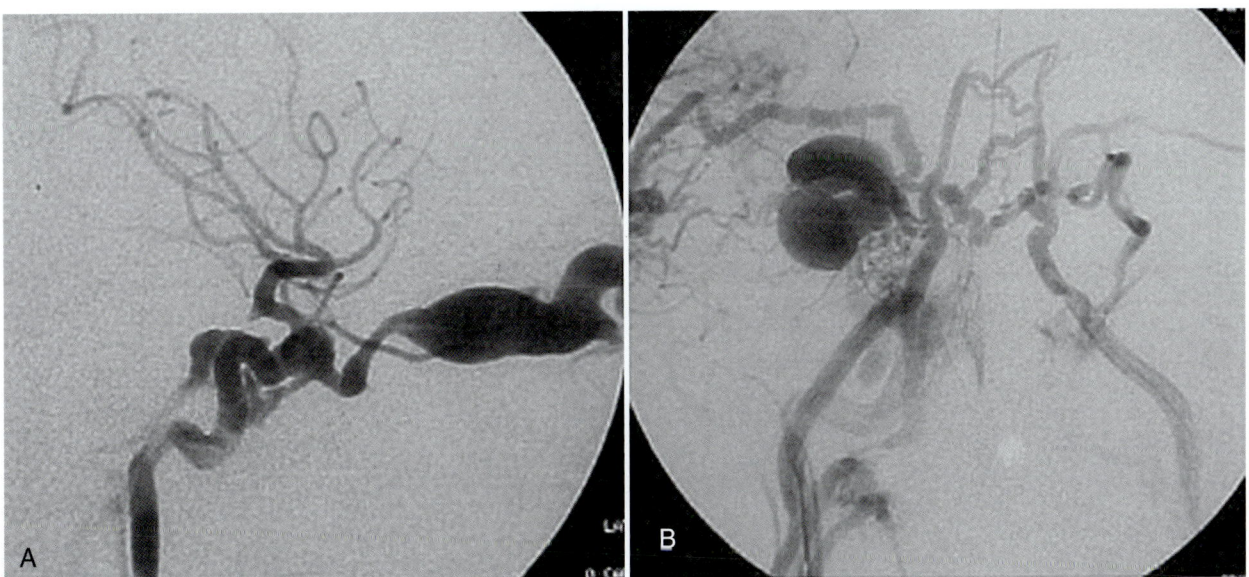

Figure 5-53 Traumatic carotid–cavernous fistula (CCF) following a motor vehicle accident. **A:** Lateral view of internal carotid artery (ICA) angiogram. Direct filling of the ophthalmic vein via the cavernous sinus is the most frequently encountered venous drainage route. **B:** Anteroposterior view of ICA angiogram at later phase filling of ophthalmic veins but also via the intercavernous sinus, contralateral cavernous sinus, sphenoparietal veins bilaterally, and inferior petrosal sinus. (From Krings T, Geibprasert S, Lasjaunias PL. Cerebrovascular trauma. Eur Radiol 2008;18:1531-1545.)

penetrating injuries (more common) typically result from stabbing or gunshot wounds. Iatrogenic trauma (following endarterectomy, tracheostomy, radical neck dissection, intraoral surgery, biopsy of the middle ear mass in the presence of an intratympanic course of the carotid artery) also may cause such lesions.

Traumatic AVFs

The most common traumatic AVFs are CCFs. They occur as a result of a tear in the ICA that is fixed within the cavernous sinus by fibrous trabeculae and small meningeal arteries. CCFs may be classified by cause (traumatic or spontaneous) or by flow velocity (high vs low). However, the most common classification is based on arterial supply. Type A CCFs are direct shunts between the cavernous sinus and the ICA. Indirect CCFs are dural fistulae between the cavernous sinus and dural branches of the ICA (type B), the ECA (type C), or both (type D). Traumatic CCFs are almost always direct high-flow fistulae between the ICA and the cavernous sinus (type A). The typical etiology of such lesions is a skull base fracture; however, iatrogenic fistulae following transsphenoidal surgery also might be encountered.

Traumatic CCFs usually present a few days to a few weeks after injury. Typical clinical findings include immediate objective vascular bruit, pulsating exophthalmos, and chemosis. Ophthalmoplegia is another common finding; it is caused by mass or pulsation effects from the arterialized venous pouches. Blindness related to CCF always occurs with a delay following secondary glaucoma in which is related to venous congestion. Delayed neurologic deficits due to intracranial venous congestion and subsequent hemorrhagic events are exceedingly rare. If the venous pouches extend beyond the cavernous sinus into the suprasellar region, rupture may lead to devastating SAH. In cases of massive trauma, the fistula may be associated with additional epistaxis due to widespread laceration of the ICA.

DSA is regarded the method of choice for evaluation of CCFs prior to treatment. Traumatic high-flow lesions require rapid frame rates as well as high-contrast volumes and injection rates. In some cases with very rapid flow, the cavernous sinus is immediately opacified and the precise fistula point is obscured. Injection of the contralateral ICA or a VA with temporary ipsilateral carotid artery compression may successfully demonstrate the site of fistulation. The route of venous drainage affects prognosis and therefore requires careful evaluation. Possible drainage routes are anteriorly via the superior and inferior ophthalmic veins (the most frequently encountered route) (Figure 5-53), via the superior and inferior petrosal sinuses, which usually connect to the transverse and sigmoid sinuses but may also have connections with the posterior fossa veins, via the pterygoid plexus, via sylvian veins into cortical veins, or via the basal vein of Rosenthal into the vein of Galen. Dangerous signs associated with increased morbidity or mortality include cortical or deep venous drainage, associated pseudoaneurysms cavernous sinus varices, and venous outflow obstruction.

Traumatic AVFs other than CCFs are uncommon. Fistulae from the ECA constitute approximately 7% of head and neck AVFs, most commonly supplied from the middle meningeal and occipital arteries. Close spatial relation between the branches of the ECA and the emissary veins in some areas of the skull may lead to an AVF secondary due to fractures. Such lesions can be classified into intracranially and extracranially draining fistulae. The former, which are usually supplied by a meningeal ECA branch, may demonstrate cortical venous drainage

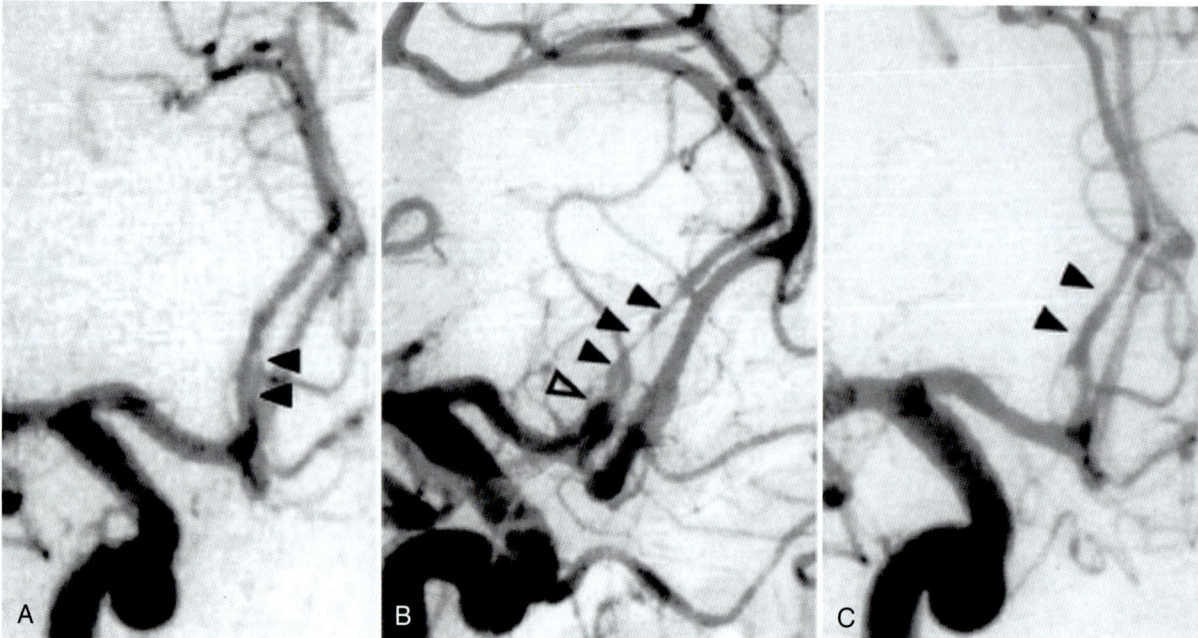

Figure 5-54 Representative findings of serial changes of the lesion in a case of anterior cerebral artery (A2 segment) dissection. **A:** Angiogram of the right carotid artery, oblique view, obtained at admission, showing mild stenosis accompanied by double lumen *(arrowheads)* at A2. **B:** Angiogram of the right carotid artery, oblique view, showing progression to severe stenosis *(closed arrowheads)* with aneurysmal dilation *(open arrowhead)* 2 weeks after onset. **C:** Angiogram of the right carotid artery, oblique view, showing resolution 5 months after onset *(arrowheads)*. (From Ohkuma H, Suzuki S, Kikkawa T, Shimamura N. Neuroradiologic and clinical features of arterial dissection of the anterior cerebral artery. AJNR Am J Neuroradiol 2003;24:691-699.)

(risk of hemorrhage), drain into the cavernous sinus (mistaken for CCF), or manifest with a sole diploic or dural drainage. Extracranially draining AVFs typically present with a pulsatile mass, a bruit, or cranial nerve deficit depending on the location of the fistula (most commonly cranial nerve XII). Traumatic AVFs affecting the VA are 10 times less common than CCFs and are constituted by an abnormal communication between the extracranial VA or its muscular branches and the surrounding venous plexuses. Clinical symptoms are pulsatile tinnitus or a cervical bruit (present each in 30%–40% of patients). Enlarged venous pouches may cause myeloradiculopathy or even quadriparesis. Blurred vision resulting from posterior fossa venous congestion is rare and indicates emergency treatment. In rare instances, reflux into the spinal perimedullary veins leads to progressive congestive myelopathy. Neck or facial pain and a torticollis may be present. Symptoms of posterior circulation TIAs, lower cranial nerves deficit, and decreased distal pulse of the ipsilateral upper extremity may point to a steal phenomenon of a VA fistula.

Intracranial Dissection

Not long ago intracranial dissection was considered as an extremely rare disease, but it has become increasingly recognized. Clinicopathologically it can be classified into two categories: (1) dissections between the intima and media, causing luminal narrowing or stenosis (simply termed *dissections*); and (2) dissections between the media and adventitia, or at the media, causing aneurysmal dilatation (termed *dissecting aneurysms*). The mean age of onset is 51 years (range 8–86 years). Headache is a common prodrome and presenting symptom. Neurologic deficits are caused by ischemia or stroke, are due to stenosis or occlusion, or are the result of SAH. SAH due to rupture of a dissecting aneurysm is believed to occur in 1% to 10% of patients. In some cases, a (minor) trauma preceding dissection is found. Many predisposing factors including hypertension and fibromuscular dysplasia have been proposed, but often no history of trauma and no underlying disease can be identified.

On DSA, the only pathognomonic finding suggesting a dissection—the double-lumen appearance with an intimal flap—is rarely encountered in intracranial dissections. The presence of the "pearl and string sign" (i.e., focal narrowing with a distal site of dilatation) is considered a reliable sign. In contrast, the string sign and tapered narrowing are less reliable signs because these changes might also be seen in arteriosclerotic disease and in the presence of vasospasm. Serial changes of angiographic findings are often seen during follow-up angiograms and reflect the dynamic nature of a dissection (Figure 5-54). The vast majority of spontaneous intracranial dissections are found in the posterior circulation, most commonly involving the V4 segment of the VA. Bilateral involvement as well as extension of an extracranial to an intracranial dissection are not uncommon. Dissection might also occur in the ICA, MCA, or ACA.

Besides visualization of the sequela of intracranial dissection (e.g., stroke, hemorrhage), CT/CTA and MRI/MRA are capable of raising the suspicion or definitively establishing the diagnosis of intracranial dissection in many cases. For recognition of intracranial dissection, these modalities require use of an additional feature: direct assessment of the vessel wall. Chen et al. reported a high diagnostic accuracy (98.5%) of CTA in detecting intracranial VA dissections. The principal findings are increased external arterial diameter (100%) and a crescent-shaped mural thickening (79%). However, differentiating an intramural hematoma in an occluded dissection from a mural thrombus in an occluded vessel may not be possible. On TOF MRA, suppression of flow signal in venous plexus surrounding the arteries can be problematic and limiting. Direct visualization of intramural hematoma on T1-weighted MRI is incomplete at the subacute stage. In contrast, contrast-enhanced MRA has been shown to be effective in depicting a double lumen in dissections of the intracranial vertebrobasilar arteries. Because of these limitations and the incomplete sensitivities of noninvasive imaging methods, DSA is still considered necessary for the definite diagnosis of intracranial artery dissection.

Suggested Readings

Abe T, Hirohata M, Tanaka N, et al. Clinical benefits of rotational 3D angiography in endovascular treatment of ruptured cerebral aneurysm. *AJNR Am J Neuroradiol.* 2002;23:686-688.

Agid R, Willinsky RA, Farb RI, Terbrugge KG. Life at the end of the tunnel: Why emergent CT angiography should be done for patients with acute subarachnoid hemorrhage. *AJNR Am J Neuroradiol.* 2008;29:e45:author reply e46-e47.

Altaf N, Morgan PS, Moody A, MacSweeney ST, Gladman JR, Auer DP. Brain white matter hyperintensities are associated with carotid intraplaque hemorrhage. *Radiology.* 2008;248:202-209.

Alvarez H, Garcia Monaco R, Rodesch G, Sachet M, Krings T, Lasjaunias P. Vein of Galen aneurysmal malformations. *Neuroimaging Clin N Am.* 2007;17:189-206.

Anxionnat R, de Melo Neto JF, Bracard S, et al. Treatment of hemorrhagic intracranial dissections. *Neurosurgery.* 2003;53:289-300:discussion 300-301.

Barrow DL, Spector RH, Braun IF, Landman JA, Tindall SC, Tindall GT. Classification and treatment of spontaneous carotid-cavernous sinus fistulas. *J Neurosurg.* 1985;62:248-256.

Bartynski WS. Posterior reversible encephalopathy syndrome, part 1: Fundamental imaging and clinical features. *AJNR Am J Neuroradiol.* 2008;29:1036-1042.

Bartynski WS. Posterior reversible encephalopathy syndrome, part 2: Controversies surrounding pathophysiology of vasogenic edema. *AJNR Am J Neuroradiol.* 2008;29:1043-1049.

Bartynski WS, Boardman JF. Catheter angiography, MR angiography, and MR perfusion in posterior reversible encephalopathy syndrome. *AJNR Am J Neuroradiol.* 2008;29:447-455.

Bash S, Villablanca JP, Jahan R, et al. Intracranial vascular stenosis and occlusive disease: Evaluation with CT angiography, MR angiography, and digital subtraction angiography. *AJNR Am J Neuroradiol.* 2005;26:1012-1021.

Bendszus M, Koltzenburg M, Bartsch AJ, et al. Heparin and air filters reduce embolic events caused by intra-arterial cerebral angiography: A prospective, randomized trial. *Circulation.* 2004;110:2210-2215.

Bendszus M, Koltzenburg M, Burger R, Warmuth-Metz M, Hofmann E, Solymosi L. Silent embolism in diagnostic cerebral angiography and neurointerventional procedures: A prospective study. *Lancet.* 1999;354:1594-1597.

Beneficial effect of carotid endarterectomy in symptomatic patients with high-grade carotid stenosis. North American Symptomatic Carotid Endarterectomy Trial Collaborators. *N Engl J Med.* 1991;325:445-453.

Berg M, Zhang Z, Ikonen A, et al. Multi-detector row CT angiography in the assessment of carotid artery disease in symptomatic patients: Comparison with rotational angiography and digital subtraction angiography. *AJNR Am J Neuroradiol.* 2005;26:1022-1034.

Bloem BR, Van Buchem GJ. Magnetic resonance imaging and vertebral artery dissection. *J Neurol Neurosurg Psychiatry.* 1999;67:691-692.

Bor AS, Rinkel GJ, Adami J, et al. Risk of subarachnoid haemorrhage according to number of affected relatives: A population based case-control study. *Brain.* 2008;131:2662-2665.

Borden JA, Wu JK, Shucart WA. A proposed classification for spinal and cranial dural arteriovenous fistulous malformations and implications for treatment. *J Neurosurg.* 1995;82:166-179.

Bouthillier A, van Loveren HR, Keller JT. Segments of the internal carotid artery: A new classification. *Neurosurgery.* 1996;38:425-432:discussion 432-423.

Brinjikji W, Cloft H, Lanzino G, Kallmes DF. Comparison of 2D digital subtraction angiography and 3D rotational angiography in the evaluation of dome-to-neck ratio. *AJNR Am J Neuroradiol.* 2009;30:831-834.

Britt PM, Heiserman JE, Snider RM, Shill HA, Bird CR, Wallace RC. Incidence of postangiographic abnormalities revealed by diffusion-weighted MR imaging. *AJNR Am J Neuroradiol.* 2000;21:55-59.

Broderick JP, Brown Jr RD, Sauerbeck L, et al. Greater rupture risk for familial as compared to sporadic unruptured intracranial aneurysms. *Stroke.* 2009;40:1952-1957.

Brouwer PA, Bosman T, van Walderveen MA, Krings T, Leroux AA, Willems PW. Dynamic 320-section CT angiography in cranial arteriovenous shunting lesions. *AJNR Am J Neuroradiol.* 2010;31:767-770.

Brown Jr RD, Huston J, Hornung R, et al. Screening for brain aneurysm in the Familial Intracranial Aneurysm study: Frequency and predictors of lesion detection. *J Neurosurg.* 2008;108:1132-1138.

Buhk JH, Wellmer A, Knauth M. Late in-stent thrombosis following carotid angioplasty and stenting. *Neurology.* 2006;66:1594-1596.

Burger IM, Murphy KJ, Jordan LC, Tamargo RJ, Gailloud P. Safety of cerebral digital subtraction angiography in children: Complication rate analysis in 241 consecutive diagnostic angiograms. *Stroke.* 2006;37:2535-2539.

Burns JD, Huston 3rd J, Layton KF, Piepgras DG, Brown Jr RD. Intracranial aneurysm enlargement on serial magnetic resonance angiography: Frequency and risk factors. *Stroke.* 2009;40:406-411.

Butler WE, Barker 2nd FG, Crowell RM. Patients with polycystic kidney disease would benefit from routine magnetic resonance angiographic screening for intracerebral aneurysms: Decision analysis. *Neurosurgery.* 1996;38:506-515:discussion 515-506.

Calabrese LH, Dodick DW, Schwedt TJ, Singhal AB. Narrative review: Reversible cerebral vasoconstriction syndromes. *Ann Intern Med.* 2007;146:34-44.

Cebral JR, Castro MA, Burgess JE, Pergolizzi RS, Sheridan MJ, Putman CM. Characterization of cerebral aneurysms for assessing risk of rupture by using patient-specific computational hemodynamics models. *AJNR Am J Neuroradiol.* 2005;26:2550-2559.

Chaloupka JC, Huddle DC. Classification of vascular malformations of the central nervous system. *Neuroimaging Clin N Am.* 1998;8:295-321.

Chaves C, Estol C, Esnaola MM, et al. Spontaneous intracranial internal carotid artery dissection: Report of 10 patients. *Arch Neurol.* 2002;59:977-981.

Chen CJ, Tseng YC, Lee TH, Hsu HL, See LC. Multisection CT angiography compared with catheter angiography in diagnosing vertebral artery dissection. *AJNR Am J Neuroradiol.* 2004;25:769-774.

Choi JH, Mast H, Sciacca RR, et al. Clinical outcome after first and recurrent hemorrhage in patients with untreated brain arteriovenous malformation. *Stroke.* 2006;37:1243-1247.

Clarke G, Mendelow AD, Mitchell P. Predicting the risk of rupture of intracranial aneurysms based on anatomical location. *Acta Neurochir (Wien).* 2005;147:259-263:discussion 263.

Cloft HJ, Joseph GJ, Dion JE. Risk of cerebral angiography in patients with subarachnoid hemorrhage, cerebral aneurysm, and arteriovenous malformation: A meta-analysis. *Stroke.* 1999;30:317-320.

Cognard C, Gobin YP, Pierot L, et al. Cerebral dural arteriovenous fistulas: Clinical and angiographic correlation with a revised classification of venous drainage. *Radiology.* 1995;194:671-680.

Cognard C, Weill A, Spelle L, et al. Long-term angiographic follow-up of 169 intracranial berry aneurysms occluded with detachable coils. *Radiology.* 1999;212:348-356.

da Costa L, Wallace MC, Ter Brugge KG, O'Kelly C, Willinsky RA, Tymianski M. The natural history and predictive features of hemorrhage from brain arteriovenous malformations. *Stroke.* 2009;40:100-105.

Debrey SM, Yu H, Lynch JK, et al. Diagnostic accuracy of magnetic resonance angiography for internal carotid artery disease: A systematic review and meta-analysis. *Stroke.* 2008;39:2237-2248.

Dion JE, Gates PC, Fox AJ, Barnett HJ, Blom RJ. Clinical events following neuroangiography: A prospective study. *Stroke.* 1987;18:997-1004.

El-Saden SM, Grant EG, Hathout GM, Zimmerman PT, Cohen SN, Baker JD. Imaging of the internal carotid artery: The dilemma of total versus near total occlusion. *Radiology.* 2001;221:301-308.

Flis CM, Jager HR, Sidhu PS. Carotid and vertebral artery dissections: Clinical aspects, imaging features and endovascular treatment. *Eur Radiol.* 2007;17:820-834.

Furlan A, Higashida R, Wechsler L, et al. Intra-arterial prourokinase for acute ischemic stroke. The PROACT II study: A randomized controlled trial. Prolyse in Acute Cerebral Thromboembolism. *JAMA.* 1999;282:2003-2011.

Gasparotti R, Grassi M, Mardighian D, et al. Perfusion CT in patients with acute ischemic stroke treated with intra-arterial thrombolysis: Predictive value of infarct core size on clinical outcome. *AJNR Am J Neuroradiol.* 2009;30:722-727.

Gonzalez LF, Walker MT, Zabramski JM, Partovi S, Wallace RC, Spetzler RF. Distinction between paraclinoid and cavernous sinus aneurysms with computed tomographic angiography. *Neurosurgery.* 2003;52:1131-1137:discussion 1138-1139.

Hacein-Bey L, Daniels DL, Ulmer JL, et al. The ascending pharyngeal artery: Branches, anastomoses, and clinical significance. *AJNR Am J Neuroradiol.* 2002;23:1246-1256.

Hacke W, Kaste M, Bluhmki E, et al. Thrombolysis with alteplase 3 to 4.5 hours after acute ischemic stroke. *N Engl J Med.* 2008;359:1317-1329.

Hadizadeh DR, von Falkenhausen M, Gieseke J, et al. Cerebral arteriovenous malformation: Spetzler-Martin classification at subsecond-temporal-resolution four-dimensional MR angiography compared with that at DSA. *Radiology.* 2008;246:205-213.

Hamilton MG, Spetzler RF. The prospective application of a grading system for arteriovenous malformations. *Neurosurgery.* 1994;34:2-6:discussion 6–7.

Heiserman JE, Dean BL, Hodak JA, et al. Neurologic complications of cerebral angiography. *AJNR Am J Neuroradiol.* 1994;15:1401-1407:discussion 1408–1411.

Hill MD, Demchuk AM, Frayne R. Noninvasive imaging is improving but digital subtraction angiography remains the gold standard. *Neurology.* 2007;68:2057-2058.

Hiu T, Kitagawa N, Morikawa M, et al. Efficacy of DynaCT digital angiography in the detection of the fistulous point of dural arteriovenous fistulas. *AJNR Am J Neuroradiol.* 2009;30:487-491.

Hochmuth A, Spetzger U, Schumacher M. Comparison of three-dimensional rotational angiography with digital subtraction angiography in the assessment of ruptured cerebral aneurysms. *AJNR Am J Neuroradiol.* 2002;23:1199-1205.

Hosoya T, Adachi M, Yamaguchi K, Haku T, Kayama T, Kato T. Clinical and neuroradiological features of intracranial vertebrobasilar artery dissection. *Stroke.* 1999;30:1083-1090.

Ishibashi T, Murayama Y, Urashima M, et al. Unruptured intracranial aneurysms: Incidence of rupture and risk factors. *Stroke.* 2009;40:313-316.

Janjua N, El-Gengaihy A, Pile-Spellman J, Qureshi AI. Late endovascular revascularization in acute ischemic stroke based on clinical-diffusion mismatch. *AJNR Am J Neuroradiol.* 2009;30:1024-1027.

Kadkhodayan Y, Alreshaid A, Moran CJ, Cross 3rd DT, Powers WJ, Derdeyn CP. Primary angiitis of the central nervous system at conventional angiography. *Radiology.* 2004;233:878-882.

Kallmes DF, Layton K, Marx WF, Tong F. Death by nondiagnosis: Why emergent CT angiography should not be done for patients with subarachnoid hemorrhage. *AJNR Am J Neuroradiol.* 2007;28:1837-1838.

Kaufmann TJ, Huston 3rd J, Mandrekar JN, Schleck CD, Thielen KR, Kallmes DF. Complications of diagnostic cerebral angiography: Evaluation of 19,826 consecutive patients. *Radiology.* 2007;243:812-819.

Kaufmann TJ, Kallmes DF. Diagnostic cerebral angiography: Archaic and complication-prone or here to stay for another 80 years? *AJR Am J Roentgenol.* 2008;190:1435-1437.

Kern R, Ringleb PA, Hacke W, Mas JL, Hennerici MG. Stenting for carotid artery stenosis. *Nat Clin Pract Neurol.* 2007;3:212-220.

Koelemay MJ, Nederkoorn PJ, Reitsma JB, Majoie CB. Systematic review of computed tomographic angiography for assessment of carotid artery disease. *Stroke.* 2004;35:2306-2312.

Krings T, Geibprasert S, Lasjaunias PL. Cerebrovascular trauma. *Eur Radiol.* 2008;18:1531-1545.

Krings T, Willmes K, Becker R, et al. Silent microemboli related to diagnostic cerebral angiography: A matter of operator's experience and patient's disease. *Neuroradiology.* 2006;48:387-393.

Kuker W, Gaertner S, Nagele T, et al. Vessel wall contrast enhancement: A diagnostic sign of cerebral vasculitis. *Cerebrovasc Dis.* 2008;26:23-29.

Kuroda S, Houkin K. Moyamoya disease: Current concepts and future perspectives. *Lancet Neurol.* 2008;7:1056-1066.

Lasjaunias PL, Landrieu P, Rodesch G, et al. Cerebral proliferative angiopathy: Clinical and angiographic description of an entity different from cerebral AVMs. *Stroke.* 2008;39:878-885.

Layton KF, Kallmes DF, Cloft HJ, Lindell EP, Cox VS. Bovine aortic arch variant in humans: Clarification of a common misnomer. *AJNR Am J Neuroradiol.* 2006;27:1541-1542.

Levy EI, Turk AS, Albuquerque FC, et al. Wingspan in-stent restenosis and thrombosis: Incidence, clinical presentation, and management. *Neurosurgery.* 2007;61:644-650:discussion 650–641.

Little AS, Garrett M, Germain R, et al. Evaluation of patients with spontaneous subarachnoid hemorrhage and negative angiography. *Neurosurgery.* 2007;61:1139-1150:discussion 1150–1131.

Livingston RR. Regarding the risk of death from CT angiography in patients with subarachnoid hemorrhage. *AJNR Am J Neuroradiol.* 2008;29:e44:aut hor reply e46–e47.

Lubicz B, Levivier M, Francois O, et al. Sixty-four-row multisection CT angiography for detection and evaluation of ruptured intracranial aneurysms: Interobserver and intertechnique reproducibility. *AJNR Am J Neuroradiol.* 2007;28:1949-1955.

Mast H, Young WL, Koennecke HC, et al. Risk of spontaneous haemorrhage after diagnosis of cerebral arteriovenous malformation. *Lancet.* 1997;350:1065-1068.

Matsubara S, Hadeishi H, Suzuki A, Yasui N, Nishimura H. Incidence and risk factors for the growth of unruptured cerebral aneurysms: Observation using serial computerized tomography angiography. *J Neurosurg.* 2004;101: 908-914.

Matsumoto M, Kodama N, Endo Y, et al. Dynamic 3D-CT angiography. *AJNR Am J Neuroradiol.* 2007;28:299-304.

McKenzie JD, Dean BL, Flom RA. Trigeminal-cavernous fistula: Saltzman anatomy revisited. *AJNR Am J Neuroradiol.* 1996;17:280-282.

Meckel S, Lovblad KO, Abdo G, et al. Arterialization of cerebral veins on dynamic MDCT angiography: A possible sign of a dural arteriovenous fistula. *AJR Am J Roentgenol.* 2005;184:1313-1316.

Meckel S, Maier M, Ruiz DS, et al. MR angiography of dural arteriovenous fistulas: Diagnosis and follow-up after treatment using a time-resolved 3D contrast-enhanced technique. *AJNR Am J Neuroradiol.* 2007;28:877-884.

Meckel S, Mekle R, Taschner C, et al. Time-resolved 3D contrast-enhanced MRA with GRAPPA on a 1.5-T system for imaging of craniocervical vascular disease: Initial experience. *Neuroradiology.* 2006;48:291-299.

Meckel S, Stalder AF, Santini F, et al. In vivo visualization and analysis of 3-D hemodynamics in cerebral aneurysms with flow-sensitized 4-D MR imaging at 3 T. *Neuroradiology.* 2008;50:473-484.

Mizutani T. A fatal, chronically growing basilar artery: A new type of dissecting aneurysm. *J Neurosurg.* 1996;84:962-971.

Mizutani T, Aruga T, Kirino T, Miki Y, Saito I, Tsuchida T. Recurrent subarachnoid hemorrhage from untreated ruptured vertebrobasilar dissecting aneurysms. *Neurosurgery.* 1995;36:905-911:discussion 912–903.

Molyneux A, Kerr R, Stratton I, et al. International Subarachnoid Aneurysm Trial (ISAT) of neurosurgical clipping versus endovascular coiling in 2143 patients with ruptured intracranial aneurysms: A randomised trial. *Lancet.* 2002;360:1267-1274.

Moniz EL. *L'Angiographie Cérébrale.* Paris: Masson & Cie; 1934 142–214.

Morita A, Fujiwara S, Hashi K, Ohtsu H, Kirino T. Risk of rupture associated with intact cerebral aneurysms in the Japanese population: A systematic review of the literature from Japan. *J Neurosurg.* 2005;102:601-606.

Morris P. *Practical Neuroangiography.* Philadelphia: Lippincott Williams & Wilkins; 2007.

Nael K, Villablanca JP, Pope WB, McNamara TO, Laub G, Finn JP. Supraaortic arteries: Contrast-enhanced MR angiography at 3.0 T—Highly accelerated parallel acquisition for improved spatial resolution over an extended field of view. *Radiology.* 2007;242:600-609.

Nguyen-Huynh MN, Wintermark M, English J, et al. How accurate is CT angiography in evaluating intracranial atherosclerotic disease? *Stroke.* 2008;39:1184-1188.

Ogilvy CS, Carter BS. A proposed comprehensive grading system to predict outcome for surgical management of intracranial aneurysms. *Neurosurgery.* 1998;42:959-968:discussion 968–970.

Ohkuma H, Suzuki S, Kikkawa T, Shimamura N. Neuroradiologic and clinical features of arterial dissection of the anterior cerebral artery. *AJNR Am J Neuroradiol.* 2003;24:691-699.

Ohkuma H, Suzuki S, Shimamura N, Nakano T. Dissecting aneurysms of the middle cerebral artery: Neuroradiological and clinical features. *Neuroradiology.* 2003;45:143-148.

Oran I, Kiroglu Y, Yurt A, et al. Developmental venous anomaly (DVA) with arterial component: A rare cause of intracranial haemorrhage. *Neuroradiology.* 2009;51:25-32.

Osborn AG. *Diagnostic Cerebral Angiography.* Philadelphia: Lippincott Williams & Wilkins; 1999.

Papke K, Kuhl CK, Fruth M, et al. Intracranial aneurysms: Role of multidetector CT angiography in diagnosis and endovascular therapy planning. *Radiology.* 2007;244:532-540.

Pelkonen O, Tikkakoski T, Leinonen S, Pyhtinen J, Sotaniemi K. Intracranial arterial dissection. *Neuroradiology.* 1998;40:442-447.

Phatouros CC, Higashida RT. Diagnostic cerebral angiography. *Carotid and Neurovascular Intervention.* 1998:1.

Qureshi AI, Suarez JI, Parekh PD, et al. Risk factors for multiple intracranial aneurysms. *Neurosurgery.* 1998;43:22-26:discussion 26–27.

Rates of delayed rebleeding from intracranial aneurysms are low after surgical and endovascular treatment. *Stroke.* 2006;37:1437-1442.

Rhoton Jr AL. The cavernous sinus, the cavernous venous plexus, and the carotid collar. *Neurosurgery.* 2002;51:S375-S410.

Rinkel GJ. Intracranial aneurysm screening: Indications and advice for practice. *Lancet Neurol.* 2005;4:122-128.

Ronkainen A, Hernesniemi J, Puranen M, et al. Familial intracranial aneurysms. *Lancet.* 1997;349:380-384.

Ronkainen A, Miettinen H, Karkola K, et al. Risk of harboring an unruptured intracranial aneurysm. *Stroke.* 1998;29:359-362.

Roy D, Raymond J, Bouthillier A, Bojanowski MW, Moumdjian R, L'Esperance G. Endovascular treatment of ophthalmic segment aneurysms with Guglielmi detachable coils. *AJNR Am J Neuroradiol.* 1997;18:1207-1215.

Sandvei MS, Romundstad PR, Muller TB, Vatten L, Vik A. Risk factors for aneurysmal subarachnoid hemorrhage in a prospective population study: The HUNT study in Norway. *Stroke.* 2009;40:1958-1962.

Schomer DF, Marks MP, Steinberg GK, et al. The anatomy of the posterior communicating artery as a risk factor for ischemic cerebral infarction. *N Engl J Med.* 1994;330:1565-1570.

Silberstein M, Tress BM, Hennessy O. Selecting the right technique to reform a reverse curve catheter (Simmons style): Critical review. *Cardiovasc Intervent Radiol.* 1992;15:171-176.

Silvennoinen HM, Ikonen S, Soinne L, Railo M, Valanne L. CT angiographic analysis of carotid artery stenosis: Comparison of manual assessment, semiautomatic vessel analysis, and digital subtraction angiography. *AJNR Am J Neuroradiol.* 2007;28:97-103.

Siva A. Vasculitis of the nervous system. *J Neurol.* 2001;248:451-468.

Smith WS, Sung G, Saver J, et al. Mechanical thrombectomy for acute ischemic stroke: Final results of the Multi MERCI trial. *Stroke.* 2008;39:1205-1212.

Srinivasan A, Goyal M, Al Azri F, Lum C. State-of-the-art imaging of acute stroke. *Radiographics.* 2006;26(Suppl 1):S75-S95.

Stapf C, Mohr JP, Choi JH, Hartmann A, Mast H. Invasive treatment of unruptured brain arteriovenous malformations is experimental therapy. *Curr Opin Neurol.* 2006;19:63-68.

Taschner CA, Gieseke J, Le Thuc V, et al. Intracranial arteriovenous malformation: Time-resolved contrast-enhanced MR angiography with combination of parallel imaging, keyhole acquisition, and k-space sampling techniques at 1.5 T. *Radiology.* 2008;246:871-879.

Tissue plasminogen activator for acute ischemic stroke. The National Institute of Neurological Disorders and Stroke rt-PA Stroke Study Group. *N Engl J Med.* 1995;333:1581-1587.

Topcuoglu MA, Ogilvy CS, Carter BS, Buonanno FS, Koroshetz WJ, Singhal AB. Subarachnoid hemorrhage without evident cause on initial angiography studies: Diagnostic yield of subsequent angiography and other neuroimaging tests. *J Neurosurg.* 2003;98:1235-1240.

Turk AS, Rowley HA, Niemann DB, et al. CT angiographic appearance of in-stent restenosis of intracranial arteries treated with the Wingspan stent. *AJNR Am J Neuroradiol.* 2007;28:1752-1754.

Ujiie H, Tamano Y, Sasaki K, Hori T. Is the aspect ratio a reliable index for predicting the rupture of a saccular aneurysm? *Neurosurgery.* 2001;48:495-502:discussion 502-493.

van Rooij WJ, Peluso JP, Sluzewski M, Beute GN. Additional value of 3D rotational angiography in angiographically negative aneurysmal subarachnoid hemorrhage: How negative is negative? *AJNR Am J Neuroradiol.* 2008;29:962-966.

van Rooij WJ, Sprengers ME, de Gast AN, Peluso JP, Sluzewski M. 3D rotational angiography: The new gold standard in the detection of additional intracranial aneurysms. *AJNR Am J Neuroradiol.* 2008;29:976-979.

Vertinsky AT, Schwartz NE, Fischbein NJ, Rosenberg J, Albers GW, Zaharchuk G. Comparison of multidetector CT angiography and MR imaging of cervical artery dissection. *AJNR Am J Neuroradiol.* 2008;29:1753-1760.

Wallace RC, Karis JP, Partovi S, Fiorella D. Noninvasive imaging of treated cerebral aneurysms, part I: MR angiographic follow-up of coiled aneurysms. *AJNR Am J Neuroradiol.* 2007;28:1001-1008.

Wallace RC, Karis JP, Partovi S, Fiorella D. Noninvasive imaging of treated cerebral aneurysms, Part II: CT angiographic follow-up of surgically clipped aneurysms. *AJNR Am J Neuroradiol.* 2007;28:1207-1212.

Wermer MJ, Rinkel GJ, van Gijn J. Repeated screening for intracranial aneurysms in familial subarachnoid hemorrhage. *Stroke.* 2003;34:2788-2791.

Wermer MJ, van der Schaaf IC, Algra A, Rinkel GJ. Risk of rupture of unruptured intracranial aneurysms in relation to patient and aneurysm characteristics: An updated meta-analysis. *Stroke.* 2007;38:1404-1410.

Wermer MJ, van der Schaaf IC, Velthuis BK, Majoie CB, Albrecht KW, Rinkel GJ. Yield of short-term follow-up CT/MR angiography for small aneurysms detected at screening. *Stroke.* 2006;37:414-418.

Wiebers DO, Whisnant JP, Huston 3rd J, et al. Unruptured intracranial aneurysms: Natural history, clinical outcome, and risks of surgical and endovascular treatment. *Lancet.* 2003;362:103-110.

Willinsky RA, Taylor SM, TerBrugge K, Farb RI, Tomlinson G, Montanera W. Neurologic complications of cerebral angiography: Prospective analysis of 2,899 procedures and review of the literature. *Radiology.* 2003;227:522-528.

Wills S, Ronkainen A, van der Voet M, et al. Familial intracranial aneurysms: An analysis of 346 multiplex Finnish families. *Stroke.* 2003;34:1370-1374.

Woo HH, Masaryk TJ, Rasmussen PA. Treatment of dural arteriovenous malformations and fistulae. *Neurosurg Clin N Am.* 2005;16:381-393:x.

Yamaura A, Ono J, Hirai S. Clinical picture of intracranial non-traumatic dissecting aneurysm. *Neuropathology.* 2000;20:85-90.

Yoon DY, Lim KJ, Choi CS, Cho BM, Oh SM, Chang SK. Detection and characterization of intracranial aneurysms with 16-channel multidetector row CT angiography: A prospective comparison of volume-rendered images and digital subtraction angiography. *AJNR Am J Neuroradiol.* 2007;28:60-67.

CHAPTER 6
Neurointerventional Radiology
Ruth Thiex, Ajit Puri, and Darren B. Orbach

■ BRIEF HISTORICAL BACKGROUND

Therapeutic endovascular occlusion predates Egas Moniz's development of cerebral angiography and was first described in 1904 by James Dawbarn, a general surgeon, who injected liquid paraffin into surgically exposed external carotid artery branches in malignant head and neck tumors. In 1930, Brooks et al. introduced a piece of muscle into the internal carotid artery to treat a traumatic cavernous carotid fistula. In 1960, Luessenhop and Spence described embolization of brain arteriovenous malformations (AVMs) by open arteriotomy of the carotid artery followed by introduction of small emboli (pellets), initially handmade methacrylate spheres and later silicone, that preferentially made their way into the AVM via passive flow. Improvements in the efficacy and safety of brain AVM embolization were made by Djindjian et al., Kricheff et al., Wolpert and Stein, and Doppman et al. in the late 1960s and 1970s. A few years later, Zanetti and Sherman introduced cyanoacrylate as an adhesive embolic agent.

In the 1960s and early 1970s, Serbinenko developed a nondetachable, flow-directed balloon that was used for selective catheterization of circle of Willis branches. He described using his balloons for treating cavernous carotid fistulae while preserving the parent internal carotid artery, and he proposed using balloon occlusion for treatment of saccular aneurysms of cerebral arteries. For many years, balloon techniques remained the only option for treatment of endovascular aneurysm occlusion.

In the 1980s, tremendous technical innovation occurred in materials science and design, with the variable stiffness microcatheter that tremendously improved the utility, efficacy, and safety of superselective intracranial angiography. In 1986, Target Therapeutics introduced their tracker microcatheter and associated microguide wire (Boston Scientific/Target, Fremont, CA), allowing controlled navigation that was less dependent on the influence of blood flow and vascular geometry. In the following years, a panoply of microcatheters became available, with refined properties (braided walls, surface coatings) optimized for specific anatomic configurations. Flow-guided microcatheters, such as the Magic (Boston Scientific), are designed with a proximal shaft for support and pushability, a supple midshaft, and an extra supple 1.2F, 1.5F, or 1.8F shapeable distal segment for flow-guided catheterization. Whereas these microcatheters are navigated using a combination of torquability and blood flow, guidewire-directed microcatheters such as the Prowler (Codman & Shurtleff, Inc., Raynham, MA), Excelsior SL-10 (Boston Scientific), and Echelon microcatheters (ev3, Irvine, CA), are manually advanced over a guidewire. Safer access, refined embolic agents, and a better understanding of functional anatomy all developed in tandem, allowing explosive growth of endovascular options.

The introduction of novel liquid embolic agents, such as N-butyl cyanoacrylate (NBCA, Trufill Liquid Embolic, Cordis Corp.) and Onyx (ev3), enhanced the endovascular treatment of AVMs tremendously. Since the introduction of electrolytically detachable platinum coils by Guglielmi, a plethora of coils from numerous manufacturers has evolved. Attempts to address broad-necked aneurysms, atherosclerotic stenosis, and arterial dissections brought self-expanding stents into play. Higher-coverage stents currently are under active development in attempts to achieve arterial flow redirection, resulting in true endovascular reconstruction of a more optimal arterial lumen.

The pioneering spirit of the early innovators, together with the remarkable technologic achievements of the past two decades in both materials and imaging, has allowed the field of neurointerventional radiology to progress in quantum steps over a remarkably short period of time.

■ CEREBRAL ANEURYSMS

Background

Guido Guglielmi and Ivan Sepetka's development of the detachable platinum coil in 1991 profoundly changed aneurysm therapy, and coil technology continues to evolve. Subsequent developments have included the balloon remodeling technique introduced by Moret et al. to provide a scaffold at the aneurysm neck, allowing coiling of wider-necked aneurysms, and the development of three-dimensional coil shapes. "Bioactive" coated coils, designed to promote aneurysm occlusion via scarring and thrombosis, have yet to convincingly demonstrate superiority over bare metal coils. The introduction of stent technology allowed for endovascular treatment of even more wide-necked aneurysms than was previously feasible. Current clinical research is focused on modifications in stent structure, strut diameter, and configuration to sufficiently redirect flow, lessen shear stress, and result in aneurysm healing. The Pipeline embolization device (Chestnut Medical, Menlo Park, CA), a flexible, self-expanding stent with dense strut coverage, is the first device clinically available in the United States explicitly designed to achieve primary parent vessel reconstruction rather than endosaccular occlusion as a means of aneurysm treatment.

How Were Intracranial Aneurysms Originally Approached Endovascularly?

Permanent exclusion of cerebral aneurysms from the circulation is the main goal of therapy. Endovascular obliteration techniques can be divided into parent artery occlusion with or without preceding bypass procedure (deconstruction), and endosaccular occlusion of the aneurysm, with preservation of the parent vessel (reconstruction).

Deconstruction, or parent vessel occlusion, either surgical or endovascular, continues to be used to treat aneurysms such as nonreconstructable cavernous/petrous/extracranial internal carotid artery aneurysms, extracranial vertebral artery aneurysms, dissecting aneurysms of the internal carotid artery/vertebral artery, fusiform aneurysms without a well-defined neck, and giant saccular aneurysms with an ill-defined neck or inaccessible location.

Surgical ligation of the parent vessel for aneurysms in surgically inaccessible locations was more common before endovascular approaches were devised, but they can be associated with high ischemic stroke morbidity and mortality (Figure 6-1). With the development of detachable balloons, the possibility of endovascular parent artery occlusion for aneurysm treatment became a reality. The most significant advantage of endovascular balloon occlusion over proximal surgical ligation was the possibility of delivering the balloon adjacent to the aneurysm itself, trapping the neck both proximally and distally, thereby preventing backflow and refilling. Another significant advantage was that balloon occlusion can be performed on an awake patient, allowing continuous neurologic assessment during balloon test occlusion, prior to permanent vessel sacrifice. In addition, collateral arterial supply can be evaluated angiographically at the time of balloon test occlusion (Figure 6-2).

The predictive value of balloon test occlusion can be enhanced by qualitative cerebral blood flow imaging by technetium-99m (^{99m}Tc) single-photon emission computed tomographic scanning, where the tracer (typically hexamethylpropyleneamine oxime [HMPAO]) is injected following balloon inflation and vascular occlusion. Hemispheric asymmetries and reductions in tracer uptake have been shown to correlate with the development of neurologic deficits. In cases of failed balloon test occlusion, a bypass graft procedure is required before permanent vessel occlusion. Conversely, if balloon test occlusion is uneventful, permanent vessel sacrifice is performed.

What Are Potential Risks of Detachable Balloons?

Although detachable balloons achieve immediate flow arrest and overall reduction in procedure time, they harbor the following risks: incomplete obliteration of the aneurysm due to fixed, predetermined balloon shape, aneurysm rupture due to wall distension by the balloon or due to other maneuvers during balloon placement, premature detachment of the partially inflated

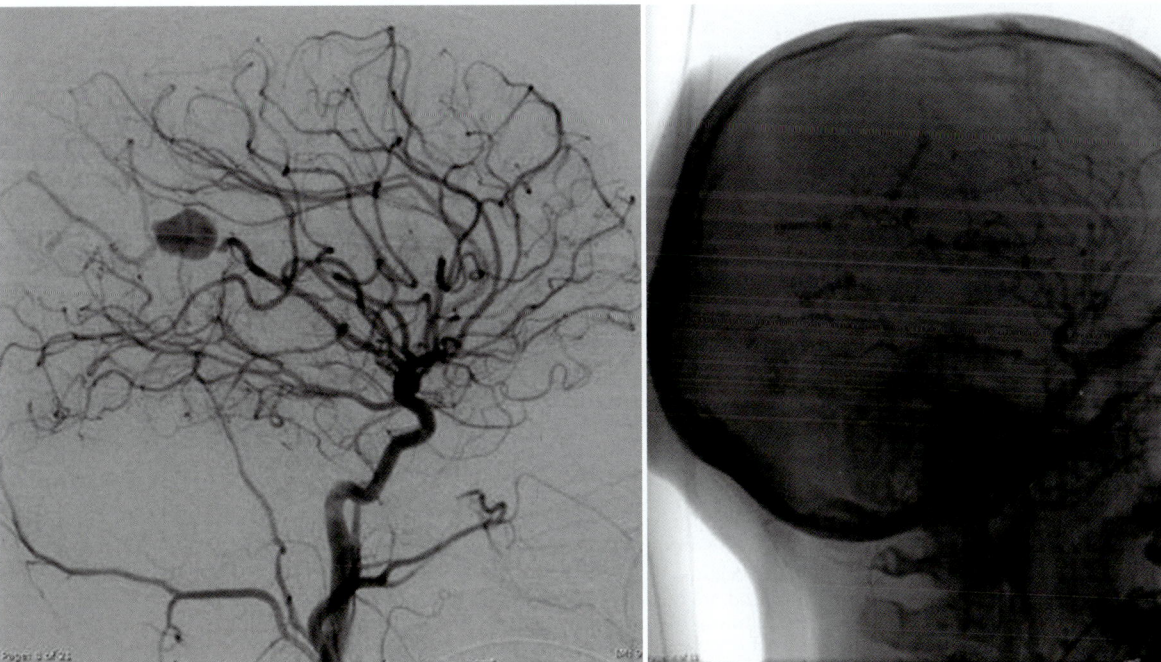

Figure 6-1 Lateral views of a left common carotid artery injection, subtracted *(left)* and unsubtracted *(right)*. The subtracted view shows a middle cerebral artery branch dissecting aneurysm. The unsubtracted view shows parent artery exclusion using surgical clips.

or deflated balloon, and thrombus formation, in cases where the balloon partially projects into the parent vessel (particularly in broad-necked aneurysms).

How Can Endovascular Obliteration of the Aneurysm Alone be Achieved?

The ideal reconstructive goal for intracranial saccular aneurysm treatment is to occlude the aneurysm itself while maintaining parent vessel patency. In 1982, Romodanov and Shchegelov first reported the use of a detachable balloon for occlusion of intracranial aneurysms while maintaining parent vessel patency. However, the definitive breakthrough was Guido Guglielmi's development of the electrolytically detachable coil system for aneurysm treatment, which has revolutionized the endovascular approach to aneurysm management.

Both aneurysm size and neck morphology play critical roles in successful obliteration of the lesion. A number of methods have been reported to measure the size of the aneurysm neck, but the neck typically is categorized as small if it measures ≤4 mm and broad if >4 mm. This distinction is important because it is technically difficult to pack broad-necked aneurysms without the risk of coils prolapsing into the parent vessel, whereas a small neck more readily retains the occlusive coils.

What Is the General Method of Coiling Aneurysms?

General anesthesia is used at most centers to ensure more controlled patient management, better imaging quality, and safer superselective catheterization of the aneurysm. A radial artery line is often placed for continuous monitoring of the arterial blood pressure; this line also facilitates blood draws for measurement of the activated clotting time (ACT). In elective aneurysm coiling, systemic heparinization (ACT target 250–300 seconds) is initiated after groin access. In many centers, for cases of acute subarachnoid hemorrhage, anticoagulation with intravenous (IV) heparin is begun after the first coil is placed, although practice patterns are quite varied in this regard. Preliminary angiographic evaluation is made with standard frontal and lateral views. Three-dimensional angiographic reconstructions facilitate accurate measurement of aneurysm dimensions, identification of perforating vessels originating within the aneurysm region, and selection of the best working projection for embolization (Figure 6-3). In addition to aneurysm size and orientation, the relationship between the aneurysm neck and dome and between the neck and the parent artery, as well as the morphology of the parent artery are evaluated. A roadmap image of the parent vessel and aneurysm is obtained in the best working projection. A microcatheter with two sets of markers (at the tip and 3 cm proximal to the tip) is coaxially advanced into the aneurysm fundus with the aid of a microguide wire. The coaxial catheter system is continuously flushed with heparinized saline to lower the risk of thrombus formation. Once the microcatheter

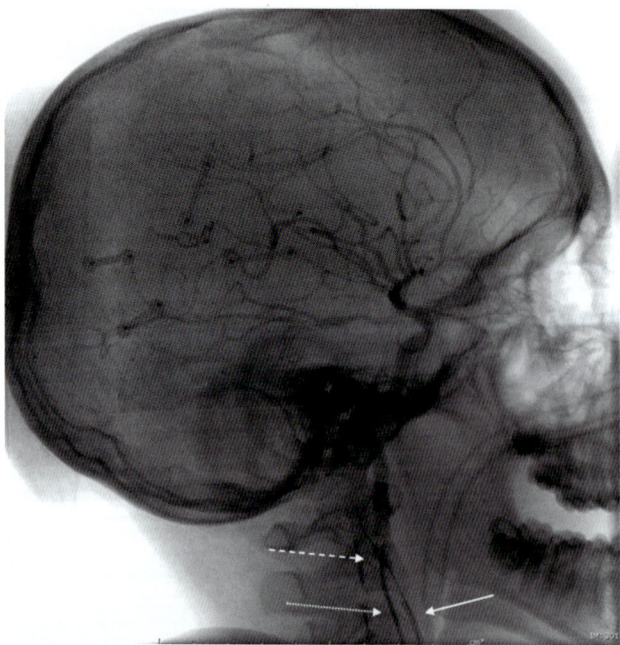

Figure 6-2 Lateral unsubtracted view of a balloon test occlusion. The balloon *(dashed arrow)* is inflated in the external carotid artery, which is supplying a portion of the middle cerebral artery territory via a surgical bypass. The guide catheter in the external carotid is shown with the *solid arrow*. The *dotted arrow* points to a diagnostic catheter in the ipsilateral internal carotid artery, through which contrast was injected to perform the angiogram.

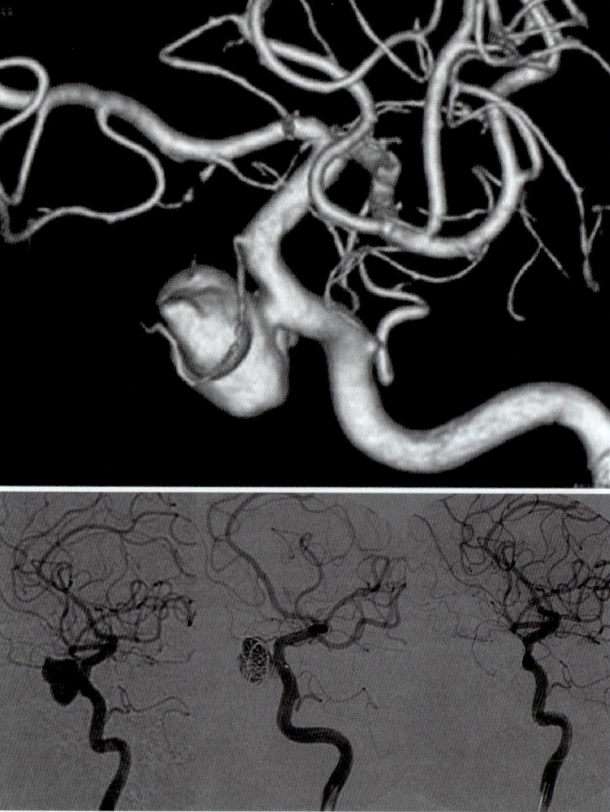

Figure 6-3 Top: Three-dimensional reconstruction from a rotational angiographic run demonstrating an internal carotid artery aneurysm (patient had presented with massive epistaxis due to herniation of aneurysm into sphenoid sinus). The narrow neck of the aneurysm, a favorable configuration for coil retention, is clearly seen. **Bottom:** Progressive packing of the aneurysm volume with detachable coils.

is properly positioned within the aneurysm, a detachable coil is introduced via the microcatheter. When the marker on the delivery mandrel overlaps the proximal platinum marker on the microcatheter, the detachment zone is 2 to 3 mm beyond the tip of the catheter. If coil position is deemed satisfactory, the coil is detached using either an electrolytic or mechanical system. Complete detachment is tested by gently retracting the delivery wire under fluoroscopy while verifying that the coil remains in place.

Most commonly, the first coil deployed is one that takes on a three-dimensional shape as it extrudes from the microcatheter (as opposed to helical coils, which typically are referred to as "2D"). The three-dimensional shape of this initial "framing" coil generates a coil basket within the aneurysm fundus, with one or a few loops of coil preferably bridging the neck. This basket is the structure within which further coils will be packed, as the aneurysm volume is progressively filled (Figure 6-3). The goal of endovascular embolization is complete angiographic obliteration of the fundus, although quantitative analysis reveals that even with no visible angiographic remnant after coiling, at best only 30% to 40% volumetric occlusion is achievable. After embolization, the microcatheter is slowly removed from the aneurysm and a postembolization angiogram performed to assess the final outcome and patency of the parent vessel.

The platinum coil system is a safe and effective treatment option. The suppleness and flexibility of platinum coils allow occlusion of the aneurysm without undue stress on the wall and thus has demonstrated efficacy both for unruptured and ruptured aneurysms. Early treatment of ruptured aneurysms causing subarachnoid hemorrhage both reduces the risk of rebleeding and facilitates the initiation of aggressive management of vasospasm and raised intracranial pressure.

Problem Solving Unfavorable Aneurysm Geometry: What Are Assist Techniques and Some Limitations of Aneurysm Coiling?

One of the most common technical limitations of coil embolization of aneurysms involves the geometry of the aneurysm neck. If the ratio of dome size to neck size is not favorable (usually ratio <2) or the neck itself is very wide (usually >4 mm), the neck will not act as a buttress for the coil mass, and the coils will tend to herniate into the parent artery. Several strategies, all of which are called *assist techniques*, have been developed for facing this challenge. Most (but not all) studies describe an increased complication rate from embolization using assist techniques compared to straightforward coiling. However, a higher complication rate could arise not from the complexity of the techniques themselves but from the fact that the underlying aneurysms requiring such techniques are inherently more dangerous to treat.

Moret and colleagues described the first assist technique, that of *"remodeling,"* in which two microcatheters rather than one are navigated to the aneurysm ostium, one to deploy the coils and the other a balloon microcatheter. The microballoon is inflated at the aneurysm neck during the deployment of each coil, creating a temporary scaffold upon which the loops of the coil can form their three-dimensional shape without parent vessel herniation (Figure 6-4). For balloon-assisted embolization, a potential source of complications is the induction of stasis of blood in the parent artery during balloon inflation, which increases the tendency for thrombi to form and potentially cause ischemia. In order to lower this risk, balloon remodeling is carried out with the patient fully anticoagulated. Some practitioners are reluctant to anticoagulate a patient with an acutely ruptured aneurysm before treatment has started, so in those centers, balloon remodeling is used only in the setting of embolization of unruptured aneurysms.

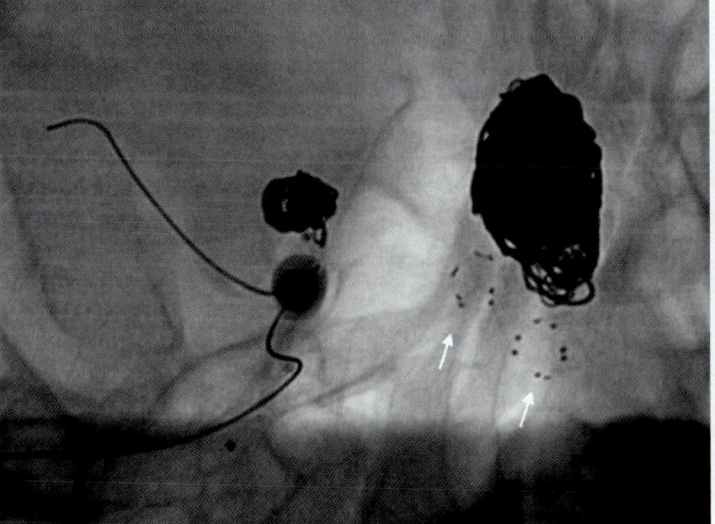
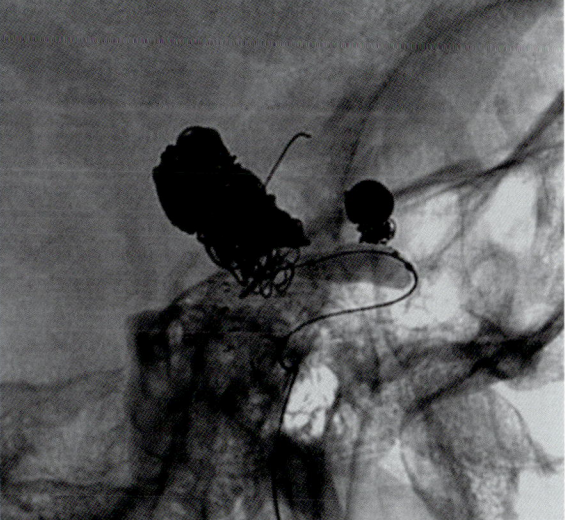

Figure 6-4 Oblique unsubtracted views of balloon-assisted coiling of a cerebral aneurysm. *Left:* Inflated balloon seen en face, with the coil mass seemingly hovering over it. *Right:* Scaffold proved by the balloon allows progressive coiling of the aneurysm neck, eliminating the "hovering coil mass" effect. The patient had a large wide-necked contralateral aneurysm as well coiled using stent assistance. Markers at each end of the stent are delineated by the *white arrows*. (Courtesy Dr. Peter K. Nelson, NYU Medical Center.)

Flexible, self-expanding nitinol stents have become increasingly important in the treatment of wide-necked aneurysms. The stent is deployed in the parent vessel across the ostium of the aneurysm and acts as a baffle to prevent coil herniation. The coil microcatheter is navigated through the struts of the stent into the aneurysm, and the coils are deployed. Alternatively, the coil microcatheter is first introduced into the aneurysm without deployment of coils, the stent is placed, trapping the coil microcatheter against the vessel wall, and then the aneurysm is coiled and the coil microcatheter removed.

In the United States, the two stents most commonly used for this purpose are the Neuroform (Boston Scientific/Target) and the Enterprise (Cordis, Bloomington, IN). Stent-assisted aneurysm embolization can be undertaken either in a single procedure or as a staged procedure, with the stent deployed first and allowed to set into the endothelium for several weeks, after which the patient undergoes a second procedure for aneurysm coiling.

Arterial stents are highly thrombogenic after initial deployment, until they have undergone a period of endothelialization over several weeks to months. Thus, deployment of a stent without pretreatment with a regimen of antiplatelet medications (typically two oral agents, such as clopidogrel and aspirin, given for at least 3 days) would entail a high risk of in situ thrombus formation and potential embolization. Thus, stent-assisted coiling is most straightforward in the setting of elective treatment of unruptured aneurysms. In cases where pretreatment with antiplatelet agents was not possible, a loading dose of antiplatelet agent can be administered intravenously and continued until oral agents have reached therapeutic serum concentration. Although stent-assisted coiling is performed at some centers in cases of ruptured aneurysms, both the thrombotic risks (which are particularly increased in the setting of subarachnoid hemorrhage) and the hemorrhagic risks from antiplatelet medication (particularly in the setting of the potential need for procedures such as ventriculostomy) are high.

In addition to the risk of rupture, giant intracranial aneurysms potentially cause symptoms related to mass effect or arterial pulsation force on adjacent structures, such as cranial nerves. Long-standing cranial neuropathies resulting from compression by a large aneurysm are unlikely to improve, whether treated by surgical clipping or by coiling. However, short-term cranial neuropathies may reverse, although it has proven difficult to predict which aneurysms will respond as well to coil embolization (which does not ameliorate mass effect) as to surgical clipping.

Finally, endovascular embolization may be severely limited in cases where the aneurysm incorporates parent branch vessels into its neck. Although a skilled surgeon may create a clip construct that maintains the patency of such branches while excluding the aneurysm dome, for certain aneurysm geometries no endovascular analogues currently are available.

What Are the Complications of Aneurysm Coiling?

Just as aneurysm rupture may complicate surgical clipping, perforation during embolization may occur and is reported in 2% to 4% of cases, with a higher incidence in recently ruptured and in small aneurysms (Figure 6-5). The cause can be related to fragility of the aneurysm wall, microcatheter instability during coil deployment, or incompatibility between the coil geometry and the aneurysm. Asymptomatic rupture, usually caused by herniation of the microwire, may be suspected only because of contrast extravasation outside the previously defined aneurysm luminal contour. Symptomatic rupture, usually resulting from perforation by coils or by the microcatheter, may cause an immediate spike in intracranial pressure, with accompanying hypertensive bradycardia or even asystole. If rupture is suspected, anticoagulation is immediately reversed using protamine sulfate, and embolization should proceed as rapidly as possible. If available, a balloon may be inflated in the parent vessel to staunch the subarachnoid hemorrhage. If not already in place, immediate external ventricular drainage should be considered.

Thromboembolic complications are reported to occur in approximately 3% of aneurysm embolizations,

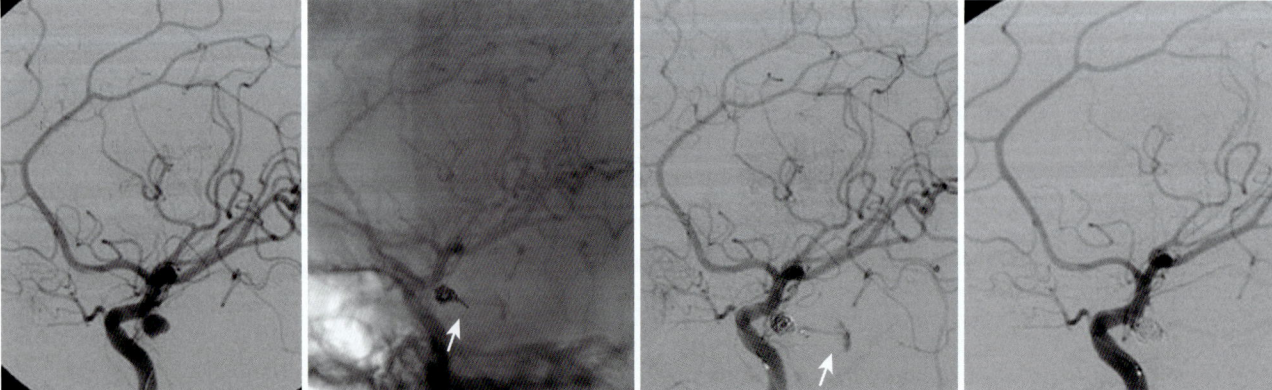

Figure 6-5 First panel: Oblique view of right internal carotid artery communicating segment aneurysm. Second panel: Unsubtracted view during coil embolization demonstrating perforation of the aneurysm by a coil loop, which is seen to protrude beyond the contour of the aneurysm seen in the first panel (white arrow). Third panel: Subtracted view demonstrating contrast extravasation into the subarachnoid space (white arrow), consistent with intraprocedural aneurysm rupture. The patient's heart rate immediately fell and the blood pressure rose. Fourth panel: The aneurysm was rapidly coiled to completion, with no residual filling of the dome. The patient made an uneventful recovery.

with permanent neurologic disability reported in 1.7% to 5% of procedures. Thrombus formation at the aneurysm neck during or immediately after embolization is the likely cause of many such events. Potential etiologies include (1) the hemodynamic effects of the guide catheter in the parent artery slowing flow, possibly due to vasospasm, (2) thrombus formation on the microcatheter or coil mass, (3) stenosis of the parent artery due to protrusion of the coil mass, and (4) displacement of intraaneurysmal thrombus during embolization. Rare causes of thromboembolism are hypercoagulable states, such as antiphospholipid syndrome.

Although aneurysm embolization is almost always performed with anticoagulation, lysis of formed thrombus typically requires additional administration of IV antiplatelet agents such as the IIb/IIIa receptor binders abciximab or eptifibatide. In unruptured cases, fibrinolytic agents such as urokinase or recombinant tissue plasminogen activator (r-tPA) can be used for embolization-related thromboembolism, but their use in the setting of subarachnoid hemorrhage is fraught with risk.

■ ACUTE STROKE

Historical Background

A new era in acute stroke therapy began with publication of the prospective National Institutes of Neurological Disorders and Stroke (NINDS) trial, which was completed in 1995. The study, which led to United States Food and Drug Administration (FDA) approval of tPA for acute ischemic stroke, found that patients treated with IV tPA within 3 hours of symptom onset had a substantially better chance of achieving functional independence, with minimal or no disability at 3 months, than did those given placebo. Additional trials of thrombolysis for acute stroke followed, and a pooled analysis of all 2,775 patients enrolled in the first six IV r-tPA trials demonstrated clear and convincing evidence of a time-dependent benefit of thrombolytic therapy. Treatment within the first 90 minutes of symptom onset increased the odds of a favorable outcome by 2.8-fold, whereas treatment in the 91- to 180-minute window increased the odds by 1.6-fold.

Given the narrow therapeutic window for IV treatment of acute ischemic stroke, timely evaluation and diagnosis of ischemic stroke are paramount. Noncontrast brain-computed tomography (CT) is the minimum CT imaging requirement before proceeding with lytic therapy, with any intracerebral hemorrhage serving as an absolute contraindication to thrombolysis. The history, physical examination, and laboratory exclusion criteria are listed in the guidelines for the early management of adults with ischemic stroke. Early signs of major infarction on initial CT scan (e.g., mass effect, edema, hypodensity involving more than one third of the middle cerebral artery [MCA] territory) are reasons for caution in the use of thrombolytic therapy because of the increased risk of hemorrhage. More sophisticated multimodal approaches to acute stroke imaging include perfusion CT and CT angiography, which provide information about the degree of potentially reversible ischemic injury, intracranial vessel status, and possibly the volume of already infarcted tissue. A multimodal magnetic resonance imaging (MRI) approach includes magnetic resonance angiography (MRA), diffusion-weighted imaging, and perfusion-weighted imaging. Diffusion-weighted imaging allows visualization of ischemic regions within minutes of symptom onset and early identification of lesion size, site, and age. The ischemic penumbra is approximated on MRI as regions of perfusion change without a corresponding diffusion abnormality (diffusion–perfusion mismatch). Multiparametric MRI criteria to differentiate regions with irreversible infarction from regions with potentially reversible ischemia are under investigation.

The major risk of thrombolytic treatment in the NINDS trial was symptomatic intracerebral hemorrhage, which increased 10-fold in treated patients compared with placebo (6.4% vs 0.6%, respectively). Trials of IV r-tPA that included an angiographic component have demonstrated that the rate of recanalization of large-vessel arterial occlusions with IV r-tPA is low, with partial or complete recanalization of only 10% of occluded internal carotid arteries and 25% of occluded proximal MCAs. Therefore, an intraarterial (IA) approach in order to deliver the thrombolytic agent in a high concentration directly into the thrombus has been promoted. More detailed schemes for assessing the initial angiographic data, accounting both for site of occlusion and identification of collateral supply, have been developed in order to stratify patients by the expected rate of recanalization and short-term outcome after IA thrombolysis.

What Are the Benefits of IA Thrombolysis?

IA thrombolysis allows extension of the treatment time window, delivery of a higher concentration of lytic agent to the target thrombus with lower systemic exposure, higher recanalization rates, the potential for salvage therapy for IV r-tPA nonresponders, and combined therapy with other endovascular techniques. The potential benefits of IA lysis were demonstrated early in the Prolyse in Acute Cerebral Thromboembolism II (PROACT II) trial, in which 40% of the 121 subjects treated intraarterially with the lytic prourokinase within 6 hours of symptom onset had a good neurologic outcome (modified Rankin score 0–2) at 3 months, compared to 25% of the 59 subjects who did not receive IA lytic. However, IA thrombolysis requires additional time to initiate therapy, is available only at specialized centers, and involves the risk of potential arterial injury from endovascular manipulation.

Numerous mechanical devices have been used for thrombus extraction and maceration, offering the potential of quick recanalization even in the setting of large clot burden (Figure 6-6). The two FDA-approved devices are the mechanical embolus retrieval in cerebral ischemia (MERCI, Concentric Medical, Inc., Mountain View, CA) system and the Penumbra system (Penumbra, Inc., Alameda, CA), described later, but other techniques, such as balloon angioplasty and stenting, also can be used. However, an IA lytic, deliverable via the most flexible and diminutive microcatheters, still offers the advantage of addressing smaller occlusions in distal arteries not

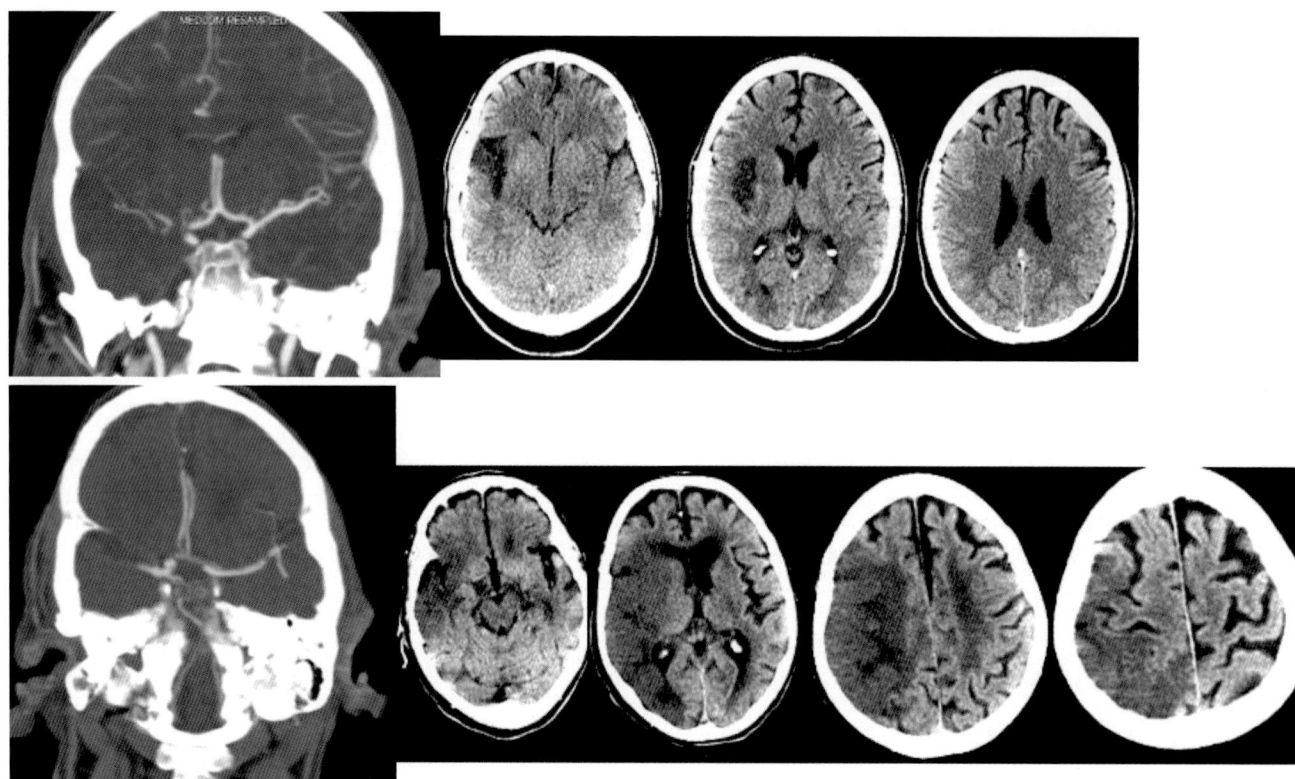

Figure 6-6 Two patients with acute ischemic stroke due to right distal internal carotid and proximal middle cerebral artery occlusion, who presented within several hours of each other. **Top:** This patient was not a candidate for intravenous tissue plasminogen activator (IV tPA) but had a mechanical thrombectomy with the mechanical embolus retrieval in cerebral ischemia (MERCI) device. The patient had an excellent clinical outcome (follow-up computed tomographic scans shown on the *right*). **Bottom:** This patient did receive IV tPA but could not undergo mechanical thrombectomy because of lack of arterial access. The patient had a poor clinical outcome, with a devastating infarct (follow-up computed tomographic scans shown on the *right*).

amenable to mechanical techniques. The Interventional Management of Stroke (IMS) I and II pilot trials demonstrated potential utility in combining IV thrombolysis and its advantages (speed of initiation and widespread availability) with IA techniques for recanalization and their advantages (concentrated local dosing, mechanical techniques for recanalization, and higher rates of recanalization) for the treatment of moderate-to-large strokes (National Institutes of Health Stroke Scale [NIHSS] score ≥10). Moreover, the safety profile for such combined treatment was similar to that of IV tPA alone. Numerous other trials of mechanical and combined mechanical and lytic therapy have been performed, with additional trials underway. It is our practice, and that of many other centers, to administer IA pharmacolysis whenever possible, even in cases where mechanical thrombectomy is attempted. This is done both to increase the efficacy of mechanical thrombus disruption and extraction and to lyse potential small emboli that are dislodged distally in the course of extraction (Figure 6-7). At other centers, however, mechanical thrombectomy is performed without pharmacolysis, with the idea of lessening the risk of hemorrhagic conversion.

What Are Inclusion and Exclusion Criteria for IA Thrombolysis?

At most centers, IA thrombolysis is considered if patients treated with IV r-tPA have experienced no significant neurologic improvement, have radiographic evidence of occlusion of an angiographically approachable vessel (internal carotid artery, MCA M1 or M2 segment, vertebral artery, or basilar artery), and have the potential for delivery of thrombolytic within 6 hours of symptom onset. Primary IA thrombolysis is performed if patients present after 3 hours from symptom onset (i.e., outside the IV window) or had contraindications to IV tPA (e.g., recent history of major surgical procedures). CT exclusion criteria are the same as for IV therapy: hemorrhage of any degree or location, significant mass effect with midline shift, parenchymal hypodensity consistent with ischemic change in a large cortical volume (usually greater than one third of the MCA territory), and the presence of intracranial tumors other than small meningiomas. Potential angiographic exclusion criteria are arterial dissection or stenosis precluding safe microcatheter access to the target vessel or a nonatheromatous arteriopathy, which may increase the risk of inducing hemorrhage with endovascular manipulation.

How Is IA Thrombolysis Carried Out?

It is our practice and that at many centers, to perform IA thrombolysis under general anesthesia in order to lower the risk of vessel injury from movement during endovascular manipulation. At centers where thrombolysis is performed without general anesthesia, the patient's

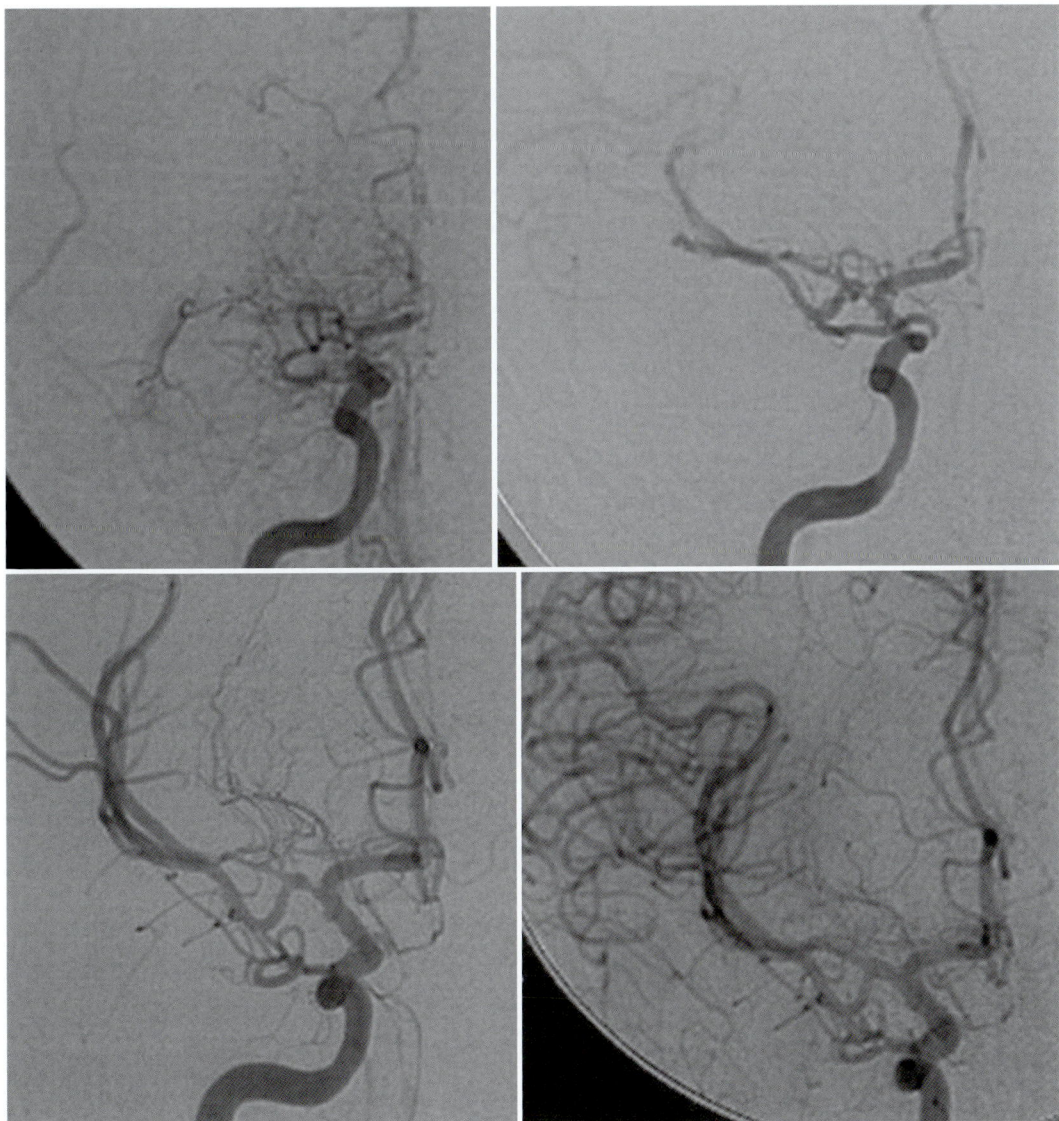

Figure 6-7 Intraarterial thrombolysis in the setting of acute ischemic stroke. **Upper left panel:** Nonopacification of the internal carotid artery (ICA) terminus, M1 segment, and A2 segment, consistent with at least two thrombus fragments. **Upper right panel:** After intraarterial administration of tissue plasminogen activator, recanalization of the ICA terminus, anterior cerebral artery, and inferior division of the middle cerebral artery (MCA), with some filling of the M1 segment, is seen. **Lower left panel:** After one pass of the mechanical embolus retrieval in cerebral ischemia (MERCI) device, filling of both divisions of the MCA and partial filling of the M1 segment are seen. **Lower right panel:** After a second pass of the MERCI device, recanalization of all segments is seen.

neurologic status is ascertained regularly during the case in order to determine potential response to treatment in real time.

IA access is almost always via the femoral artery. If mechanical thrombolysis is contemplated, an 8F or 9F sheath is placed; otherwise, a 5F sheath is adequate. A guide catheter is advanced into the symptomatic artery, and detailed angiographic examination of the vascular anatomy, including the circle of Willis and leptomeningeal collateral circulation, is performed. For carotid cases, the common carotid artery is injected first in order to examine the cervical bifurcation. Continuous heparin flush is administered via the guide catheter.

An angiographic run via the guide catheter delineates the proximal border of the intraluminal occlusion, and delayed images delineate the extent of the collateral circulation. A microcatheter is then advanced over a microguidewire to the level of occlusion. The microwire and microcatheter are gently advanced through the occlusion, along the expected trajectory of the parent vessel, taking care to minimize trauma that might result from this essentially blind navigation. When the microcatheter is believed to be beyond the occlusion, a microcatheter angiographic run is performed, delineating the distal extent of the occlusion. In cases where tPA can be safely administered, small aliquots (e.g., 2 mg) typically are injected slowly into the thrombus, as the microcatheter is gradually withdrawn until it lies just proximal to the occlusion. At some centers, infusion pumps are used for IA tPA administration. Control angiography via the guide catheter is performed, and the process is repeated until the vessel is seen to have recanalized.

Problem Solving: When Are Aggressive Mechanical Clot Disruption Techniques Indicated?

Aggressive mechanical clot disruption provides an advantage over IA pharmacolysis in potentially increasing the recanalization rate and speed and reducing the total thrombolytic dose. Patients with contraindications to tPA are candidates only for mechanical thrombectomy. Mechanical techniques are attempted after IA thrombolysis in patients who had no significant response or persisting occlusion after repeated administration of r-tPA and control angiography. Aggressive mechanical clot disruption is defined as utilization of at least one of the following interventional techniques:

- Aggressive microcatheter/microwire clot maceration
- Percutaneous transluminal angioplasty
- Stent deployment
- Use of a clot extraction device such as the MERCI retrieval system or the Penumbra system

Limited data are available about the use of angioplasty and stenting in the emergency treatment of intracranial lesions in patients with acute ischemic stroke. Percutaneous transluminal angioplasty consists of balloon angioplasty in patients with persisting occlusion in the internal carotid artery and proximal MCA. Balloons are always undersized relative to the estimated lumen diameter of the treated segment. An aggressive combined endovascular approach of intracranial thrombolysis and cervical carotid stent placement during the acute phase has been advocated in patients with acute stroke who had severe ipsilateral cervical internal carotid artery stenosis to timely reestablish intracranial perfusion, effectively prevent early recurrent strokes, and limit the incidence of reperfusion injury. Snare devices are advanced through the microcatheter into the clot matrix with the intention of capturing the clot when pulled. The MERCI device is a flexible, helical-shaped, tapered tip made of nitinol wire. The MERCI comes in three FDA-approved versions: the first generation of five conical helical loops (X5, X6), the L-generation device consisting of cylindrical helical loops with arcading filaments to give greater grip to the clot (L5, L6), and the K-mini helical loops with countertwist to give more tensile strength in smaller target lesions. First-generation MERCI devices achieved recanalization rates of 48%, and, when coupled with IA thrombolytic drugs, recanalization rates of 60% have been reported.

Multi MERCI was an international, multicenter, prospective, single-arm trial of thrombectomy in patients with large-vessel stroke treated within 8 hours of symptom onset. The median NIHSS score was 19. Treatment with the L5 Retriever resulted in successful recanalization in 75 (57.3%) of 131 treatable vessels and in 91 (69.5%) of 131 after adjunctive therapy (IA tPA, mechanical). Overall, favorable clinical outcomes (modified Rankin score [mRS] 0–2) occurred in 36%, and mortality was 34%. Both outcomes were significantly related to vascular recanalization. Symptomatic intracerebral hemorrhage occurred in 16 (9.8%) patients. Josephson et al. identified 68 patients in the MERCI and Multi MERCI trials who would have been eligible for PROACT II. Rates of good outcome (mRS ≤2) and mortality at 90 days were compared, adjusting for differences in baseline NIHSS score and age. Mortality rates did not differ significantly between embolectomy patients and PROACT II control patients (adjusted analysis: MERCI 29.1%, Multi MERCI 18.0%, PROACT II control 27.1%).

Given the differences in study design and baseline characteristics of patients, randomized clinical trials are necessary and currently under investigation (MR RESCUE trial [NIH protocol no. 04-N-0264], IMS III). In the MR RESCUE trial, MRI will be used to compare embolectomy using the Merci Retriever with standard treatment in acute stroke patients and to identify people who might benefit from the device. The primary objective of the NIH-funded, phase III, randomized, multicenter, open-label clinical IMS trial is to determine whether a combined IV/IA approach to recanalization is superior to standard IV r-tPA alone when initiated within 3 hours of acute ischemic stroke onset. Subjects will be randomized in a 2:1 ratio with more subjects enrolled in the combined IV/IA group. If an appropriate thrombus is identified, treatment will continue with either the Concentric MERCI thrombus removal device, infusion of r-tPA, and delivery of low-intensity ultrasound at the site of the occlusion via the EKOS Micro-Infusion Catheter, or infusion of r-tPA via a standard microcatheter. The randomized, multicenter, clinical trial CLOTBUST (Combined Lysis of Thrombus in Brain Ischemia using Transcranial Ultrasound and Systemic tPA) had shown a 49% rate of complete recanalization or dramatic clinical recovery from stroke within 2 hours after tPA bolus when tPA infusion was continuously monitored with transcranial Doppler compared with 30% among patients who received tPA without ultrasound monitoring ($P = .03$).

EXTRACRANIAL CAROTID ATHEROSCLEROTIC DISEASE

Background

Patients with carotid artery stenosis are at increased risk for subsequent stroke, myocardial infarction, and death. The risk of stroke is greatest for persons with neurologic symptoms such as transient ischemic attacks, but it also is increased in patients with asymptomatic lesions. The proportion of all strokes attributable to previously asymptomatic carotid stenosis is small; however, in patients older than 60 years who have cerebral infarction, approximately 15% have ipsilateral carotid stenosis ≥70%. The frequency of hemodynamically significant carotid artery stenosis is higher in symptomatic patients than in asymptomatic patients. In 40% to 50% of patients with a complete stroke, the primary etiology of the stroke is related to extracranial carotid disease.

Carotid endarterectomy (CEA) has been shown to reduce the risk of stroke in patients with moderate-to-severe carotid stenosis (>50% for symptomatic, >60% for asymptomatic) in the North American Symptomatic Carotid Endarterectomy Trial (NASCET) and the Asymptomatic Carotid Atherosclerosis Study (ACAS). The benefits from surgery accrue only if the 30-day rate of perioperative stroke or death rate is 6% or lower for patients with symptomatic and 3% or lower for those with asymptomatic carotid stenosis. Technical or anatomic risks related to the carotid lesion or medical comorbidities render surgery a higher risk for a subgroup of patients.

The perioperative risk of stroke or death has been reported to be elevated in patients with coexistent symptomatic coronary artery disease, congestive heart failure, anatomic variations (high carotid bifurcation) and tandem lesions, ipsilateral intraluminal thrombus, contralateral carotid artery occlusion, postendarterectomy restenosis, and radiation-induced carotid artery stenosis. These patients may be better served by carotid artery stenting, with a potentially lower risk with the endovascular procedure. In 2004, the FDA approved the first carotid artery stenting system (Acculink stent and Accunet embolic protection device, Guidant, Santa Clara, CA) for use in patients with ≥80% asymptomatic carotid stenosis.

Cerebral embolization of friable atheromatous material from the aortic arch and the carotid artery has been found to occur during all stages of the carotid artery stenting procedure and may cause periprocedural neurologic deficits. Several filters for distal embolic protection approved by the FDA include the Accunet, EmboShield (Abbott Vascular, Redwood City, CA), the Spider (ev3), and the EZ filter wire (Boston Scientific, Natick, MA). Devices to arrest or reverse anterograde internal carotid artery flow will soon be widely available.

The Carotid Revascularization Endarterectomy versus Stenting Trial (CREST) is a randomized trial designed to compare the efficacy of CEA with that of carotid artery angioplasty and stent placement with the aid of an embolic protection device in the prevention of stroke, myocardial infarction, and death in symptomatic patients with >50% carotid artery stenosis and asymptomatic patients with >70% stenosis. The Stenting and Angioplasty with Protection in Patients at High Risk for Endarterectomy (SAPPHIRE) trial compared carotid artery stenting with CEA in high-risk patients with ≥50% symptomatic stenosis and ≥80% asymptomatic stenosis. At 1 year, 12.2% of patients undergoing carotid artery stenting had suffered death, stroke, or myocardial infarction within 30 days and death or ipsilateral stroke between 31 days and 1 year compared to 20.1% of the CEA group. Rigorous medical treatment, timely intervention, interventionalists' experience, and analysis of plaque composition may have important influences on the future treatment of patients with carotid artery stenosis.

How Is Carotid Stenting Performed?

Angioplasty and stenting can cause intimal injury that promotes thrombosis, and stents themselves are highly thrombogenic when first deployed. Therefore, patients are pretreated with a dual antiplatelet regimen (aspirin 325 mg daily and clopidogrel 75 mg daily) for at least 3 days before stent placement. Anticoagulation is administered, targeting an ACT of 200-250 seconds throughout the procedure. Head and neck CT angiography or MRA is helpful in the planning phase to estimate the anatomic configuration of the large vessels and to select the devices most appropriate for their specific properties. Selective carotid angiography is then performed to define the severity of stenosis. The common and internal carotid arterial diameters are measured, with special attention paid to the landing zone for the protection device.

After angiography, the lesion is crossed with the protection device. A 3- to 4-mm balloon is advanced to the stenotic segment coaxially over the 0.014 inch wire holding the protection device, and angioplasty is performed. The diameter of the stent is sized to the caliber of the largest segment of the carotid artery in which the stent will be deployed. After stent deployment, poststent dilation typically is performed using a balloon with a diameter matching that of the internal carotid artery distal to the stent. Finally, the embolic protection device is removed, typically using a dedicated retrieval catheter. At most centers, the patient is awake during the entire procedure, enabling continuous neurologic assessment. The patient typically is monitored in an intensive care unit–like setting postprocedure, with tight blood pressure control designed to lower the risk of postreperfusion hemorrhage.

What Are the Most Common Complications of Carotid Stenting, and How Are They Treated?

The various manipulations comprising carotid stenting may result in vessel dissection involving the common, internal, or external carotid arteries. In order to minimize the risk of vessel perforation or dissection, in the process of exchange maneuvers only large branches of the external carotid artery should be used. In cases where symptomatic or flow-limiting dissection occurs, stent deployment at the site usually is warranted. Antiplatelet regimens, initiated in preparation for the carotid stenting procedure, are continued and followed by noninvasive imaging. In asymptomatic and non–flow-limiting dissection, antiplatelet medication and clinical observation usually suffice.

If the patient develops a sudden neurologic change during or after carotid stenting, either hemorrhage or ischemia is likely. Rapid access to the target vessel should be obtained, and, in case of flow obstruction, emergent revascularization should be attempted. In case of neither vessel cutoff nor slow flow on angiography, emergent CT scan should be done to rule out hemorrhage. When hemorrhage is seen, heparin should be reversed with protamine and the blood pressure tightly controlled.

The major long-term complication of carotid stenting is restenosis. The incidence of in-stent recurrent stenosis varies tremendously depending on the duration of follow-up, the type of stent implanted, the implantation technique, and the imaging criteria used to define significant recurrent stenosis. Levy et al. found severe (≥80%) in-stent stenosis based on Doppler criteria in 6 (5%) of 112 high-risk surgical patients. Six patients (three symptomatic) required repeated intervention. The rate of hemodynamically significant restenosis was comparable to published surgical restenosis rates.

At What Intervals and How Should the Patient Be Followed?

Duplex sonography evaluation is most commonly used for follow-up and typically is obtained before discharge, at 6 months, 1 year, and then annually thereafter. In the event of recurrent symptoms or evidence of hemodynamically significant stenosis on Doppler ultrasonography, repeat angiography is performed. Restenosis may require repeated angioplasty, deployment of an additional stent within the first, or a bypass procedure. The dual antiplatelet regimen of clopidogrel and aspirin is maintained for 4 to 6 weeks postprocedure, after which patients typically remain on aspirin therapy alone.

■ CENTRAL NERVOUS SYSTEM ARTERIOVENOUS LESIONS

There are many types of central nervous system (CNS) arteriovenous shunts, that is, lesions with direct transit of arterial blood into the venous system, with distinct pathophysiology and treatment strategies. Cerebral AVMs are the most common, with a prevalence of approximately 0.2% to 0.8%.

Brain AVM

How Are Brain AVMs Commonly Classified?
The widely used Spetzler and Martin classification incorporates the size of the AVM, the pattern of venous drainage, and the "eloquence" of the regions of the brain involved by the AVM. This classification aims at defining the surgical risk of resection rather than the natural history profile of the AVM itself.

What Are Important Features of the Angioarchitecture of AVMs?
Particular architectural features of the vasculature involved by the AVM are noted on angiography, as they may have an impact on the natural history of the lesion. High-flow sequelae, such as kinking, plications, arterial aneurysms, progressive arterial stenosis resulting in a moyamoya pattern, or the development of venous stenosis or venous ectasias, can be associated with an aggressive clinical presentation.

Two types of arterial aneurysms are associated with AVMs: (1) flow-related saccular aneurysms and (2) dysplastic aneurysms, most commonly within the nidus of the AVM. Proximal flow-related aneurysms that appear some distance from the lesion itself, on an arterial pedicle supplying the AVM, have been reported to occasionally regress after occlusion of the AVM. These lesions are more commonly seen in older age groups. In contrast, most practitioners would recommend directly treating dysplastic aneurysms early in the course of AVM treatment in order to lower the risk of bleeding (Figure 6-8). Dysplastic aneurysms have a female preponderance of up to 5:1, can be multiple, and are evenly distributed through the second to sixth decades. Both types of AVM-associated arterial aneurysms are less commonly seen during childhood.

What Symptoms are Caused by Cerebral AVMs?
Intracranial AVMs may cause a number of symptoms, including headaches, seizures, or progressive neurologic deficit, but the most potentially devastating association is intracranial hemorrhage, sometimes causing long-term disability or death. Hemorrhage often occurs due to rupture at a structurally weak point of the lesion, in an arterial, intranidal, or venous location. Small AVMs and deep-seated lesions more frequently present with hemorrhage (86%) compared to large superficial AVMs (46%).

How Are Intracranial AVMs Treated?
Management of intracranial AVMs is a multidisciplinary effort involving neurosurgeons, neurologists, and neurointerventionalists. The ultimate aim of treatment, not always achievable, is complete cure through permanent occlusion of abnormal shunts. AVM can be treated by surgery, embolization, or radiosurgery, as well as through combinations of these modalities. Depending on the local availability of treatment modalities and expertise, different institutions have developed individualized

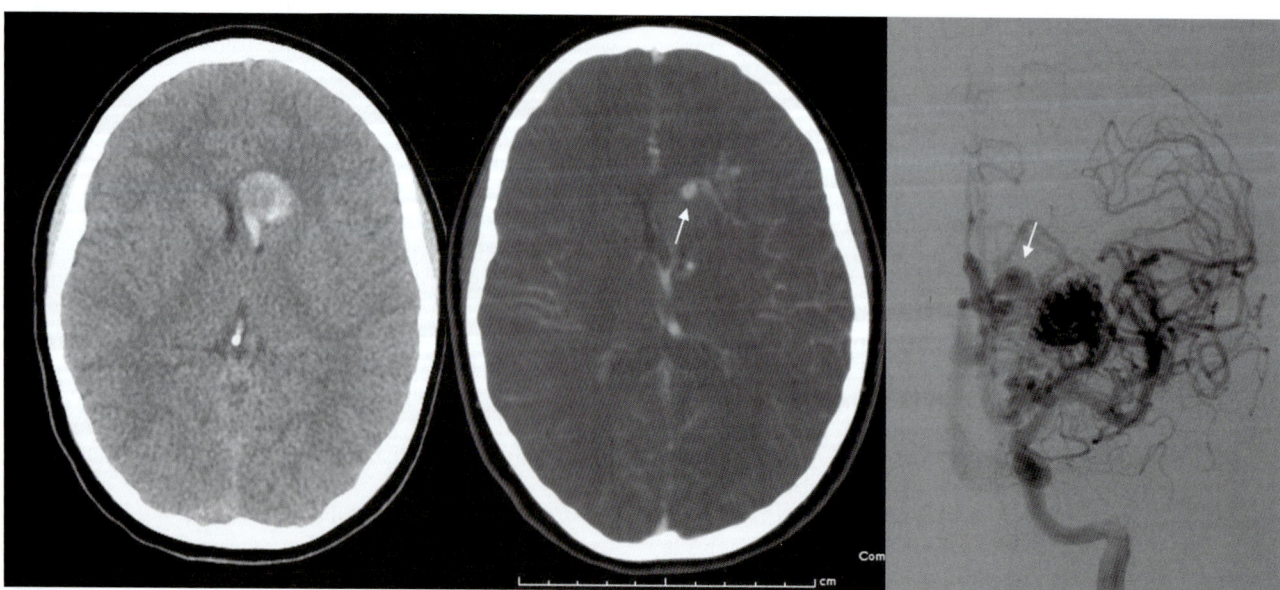

Figure 6-8 Acute hemorrhage associated with basal ganglia arteriovenous malformation (AVM) as seen on noncontrast computed tomography *(left)*, CTA *(middle)*, and catheter angiography *(right)* (left internal carotid artery injection). The hemorrhage occurred precisely at the point in the AVM at which an aneurysm is seen on CTA and DSA *(white arrows)*.

protocols. Generally speaking, surgical resection of the nidus has been the primary mode of therapy in patients with small AVMs located in noneloquent areas, particularly when the patient presents after bleed. Surgery also is useful for larger AVMs after the size of the malformation has been reduced by embolization. Radiosurgery is effective in smaller-sized AVMs, particularly those located in surgically inaccessible areas. However, AVM occlusion after radiosurgery occurs by a biologic cascade that typically requires 2 to 3 years to achieve its endpoint, and the patient may remain exposed to AVM risks during this time period.

Endovascular treatment facilitates neurosurgical intervention, potentially allowing safe resection of otherwise surgically treacherous lesions. Endovascular treatment also can be used in combination with radiosurgery. A minority of AVMs can be treated by endovascular techniques alone, particularly small AVMs and those with simple angioarchitecture (Figure 6-9). AVMs that have recently bled, with angiographically apparent weak points such as intranidal aneurysms or venous obstructions, typically are treated urgently by embolization, surgery, or both in combination.

What Are the Techniques for Endovascular Treatment of AVMs?

Endovascular treatment of cerebral AVMs requires general anesthesia with an arterial line for close monitoring of systemic blood pressure. A guide catheter is introduced into the parent artery supplying the AVM (typically an internal carotid or vertebral artery), through which a microcatheter can be advanced distally to the site of the lesion. The guide catheters allow injection of contrast to create a road map for intracranial navigation and to follow the progress of the procedure. The feeding arteries of the AVM are catheterized using appropriate selections of microcatheters and microwires. The goal of superselective angiography is to achieve a position from which AVM is opacified by contrast and normal brain arterial supply is not seen (Figure 6-9). Embolization can be performed using temporary or permanent embolic material.

Which Embolic Agents are Used for AVM Embolization?

Embolic agents fall into one of four types: liquid, particulate, balloons, and coils. By far, the most commonly used embolic agents are the liquid agents, which have been studied most extensively and provide the maximum protection from AVM bleed/rebleed from vascular malformations. At most centers, particulate agents, balloons, and coils serve only adjunctive roles in the embolization of brain AVMs.

The two most commonly used liquid embolic agents are Onyx and NBCA. Onyx (Micro Therapeutics, Inc., Irvine, CA) is an ethylene vinyl alcohol copolymer dissolved in the organic solvent dimethyl sulfoxide (DMSO). When the material comes into contact with an aqueous solution such as blood, it precipitates over several minutes and forms a spongy cast. In order to prevent early precipitation, the microcatheter dead space is slowly flushed with DMSO prior to injection of Onyx. Because of its slow precipitation, Onyx allows for prolonged injections and aggressive embolization of a large target region from a single arterial pedicle. NBCA, an acrylic glue, is the other most commonly used liquid embolic. It is a low-viscosity liquid that, on contact with hydroxyl ions in blood, rapidly polymerizes to an adherent solid. In order to prevent early polymerization, the catheter is flushed with 5% dextrose prior to injection of NBCA. Unlike the more recently available Onyx, acrylic glues have been used for several decades, with a consequent extensive set of teachings related to the development of technical proficiency with its delivery.

What Are the Various Goals of Embolization of Brain AVMs?

Preoperative Embolization
Preoperative embolization facilitates surgical treatment by reducing the flow in the arteriovenous shunt, decreasing the size of the nidus, and reducing blood loss. High-flow direct arteriovenous shunts, nidal regions supplied by deep arterial feeders not in the pathway of surgical approach, and areas of the AVM with associated aneurysms are the most important targets of embolization.

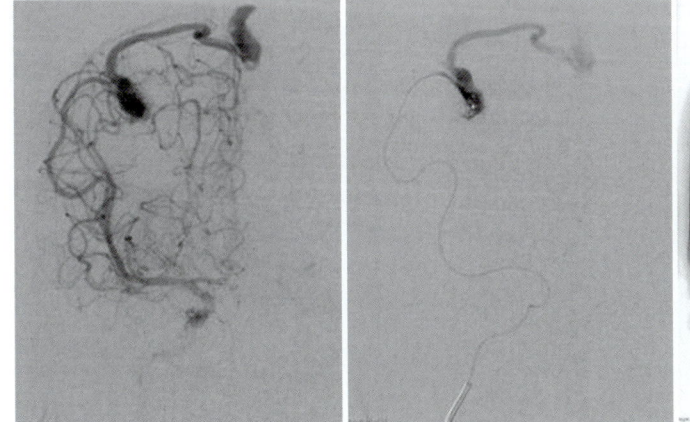
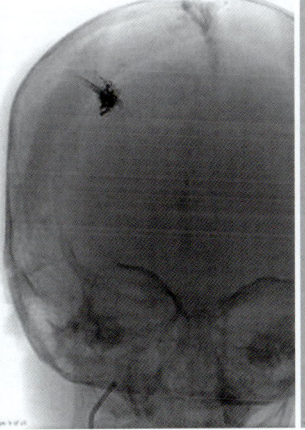
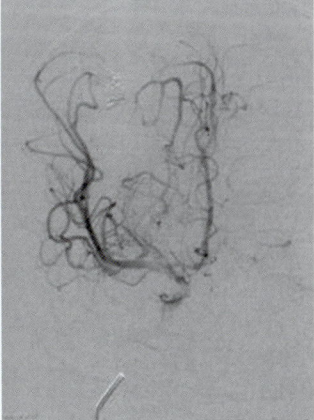

Figure 6-9 **First panel:** Frontal view of right internal carotid artery (ICA) injection in a patient with a focal arteriovenous malformation (AVM) with a compact nidus and a small number of feeding pedicles. **Second panel:** Microcatheter injection from an intranidal position, ideal for embolization. Only the AVM nidus and the draining vein opacify. **Third panel:** Frontal unsubtracted view showing the Onyx cast. **Fourth panel:** Frontal subtracted view, postembolization, showing nonopacification of the AVM.

Pre-Radiosurgery
Embolization can reduce the size of the AVM nidus, making the lesion more amenable to radiosurgery, although there has been recent debate regarding the efficacy of this approach. Nidal areas that contain aneurysms are embolized in targeted fashion to offer added protection from hemorrhage during the several-year latency period after radiosurgery before the AVM is cured.

Curative Embolization
A minority of AVMs have been reported to be cured by embolization alone, with a very wide range of reported percentages. AVMs most amenable to cure by embolization are small lesions with few feeding arteries and a compact nidus.

Targeted Embolization
In patients with AVMs that cannot be definitively treated, targeted embolization of particular regions within the AVM nidus may help in providing symptomatic relief as well added protection from bleeding. However, some evidence suggests that partial embolization of brain AVMs may increase the risk of hemorrhage, so this option is offered only in very particular circumstances.

Staged Embolization
Staged embolization usually is undertaken in large malformations that are not surgically resectable or amenable to radiosurgery in which repetitive hemorrhage has occurred. By staging occlusion of a large AVM, some believe that the hemodynamic consequences of rapid elimination of a large shunt may be prevented.

Dural Arteriovenous Fistulae

Dural arteriovenous fistulae (DAVFs) are arteriovenous shunts that are located within the walls of a dural sinus or involve adjacent cortical veins. Proposed etiologic factors are middle ear and intracranial infections, trauma, surgery, and dural sinus thrombosis. Although the cause-and-effect relationship between dural sinus thrombosis and DAVF appears well established, other mechanisms likely are involved, as most cases of dural thrombosis do not result in development of a dural fistula.

How Are DAVFs Classified?
Djindjian et al. defined four types of DAVF: type 1 draining via the ipsilateral sinus, type 2 draining toward the contralateral sinus, type 3 draining via cortical veins, and type 4 with venous ectasia. This classification system was designed to stratify the severity of the presenting symptoms and the risk of intraparenchymal hemorrhage. A more commonly used classification system has been proposed by Cognard et al.
- I. Venous drainage into dural venous sinus with anterograde flow within the sinus
- IIa. Venous drainage into dural venous sinus with retrograde flow within the sinus
- IIb. Venous drainage into dural venous sinus with anterograde flow within the sinus and cortical venous reflux (Figure 6-10)
- III. Venous drainage directly into cortical veins (cortical venous reflux only) with no shunting into a sinus

How Do DAVFs Clinically Present?
The symptomatology of DAVFs is highly variable, depending on the location of the shunt, the type of venous drainage, and the flow characteristics. Presentation may include exophthalmos, bruit, cranial nerve deficits, focal and global neurologic deficits, increased intracranial pressure, papilledema, and hydrocephalus. The most devastating clinical presentation is intracranial hemorrhage.

Problem Solving: What Are the Therapeutic Options for DAVF?
The therapeutic strategy depends on the clinical presentation and angiographic evaluation. Patients with visual loss, hemorrhage, and infarction and those with cortical

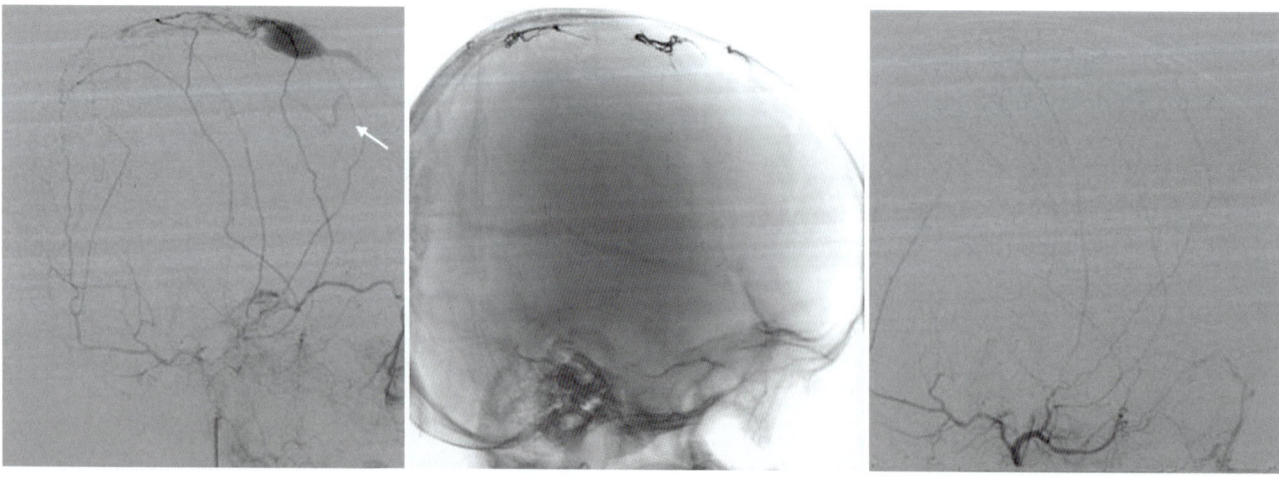

Figure 6-10 *Left:* Lateral view of right external carotid artery (ECA) injection showing opacification of a focally ectatic segment of the superior sagittal sinus during the arterial phase of the injection, diagnostic of a dural arteriovenous fistula. There is reflux into the deep venous system from the sinus *(white arrow)*, imparting a risk of intracranial hemorrhage. *Middle:* Unsubtracted view of the Onyx cast at the fistulous points. *Right:* Postembolization right ECA injection demonstrating nonopacification of the fistula.

venous drainage require prompt therapy. Djindjian type I fistulae on the other end, can be followed conservatively without treatment.

Patients with DAVFs located in the posterior sigmoid or transverse sinus without severe symptoms or high-risk angiographic features are potential candidates for treatment by manual compression of the cervical carotid artery, although the reported efficacy of this technique is quite variable.

Superselective embolization via the external carotid branch feeder to a DAVF can be an effective treatment (Figure 6-10). A variety of agents are available to embolize DAVFs, including polyvinyl alcohol (PVA) particles, liquid adhesive agents such as NBCA, and Onyx. Coils can be used in adjunctive fashion to slow the flow for subsequent injection of permanent liquid embolic agent. Proximal occlusion of a feeding artery should be avoided because future IA access and thus subsequent treatment usually are precluded, while the fistula typically recruits arterial supply from a neighboring collateral vessel.

Transvenous embolization typically involves deployment of coils via a transvenous route under direct fluoroscopic guidance to achieve closure of DAVFs by obstructing outflow. The transvenous route for embolization is tenable only if the sinus is not being used for venous drainage of normal brain. In some cases when the transvenous approach is not technically achievable by endovascular means, direct puncture of the sinus can be performed, followed by occlusion packing with coils.

Because most of the symptoms in DAVF can be related to venous hypertension, recanalization of an occluded or stenosed dural venous sinus using angioplasty or stenting may ameliorate symptoms by reestablishing low-pressure anterograde venous drainage.

The combination of preoperative arterial and subsequent surgical excision of DAVF has been shown to be effective in treating complex lesions. Particulate embolic materials, although nonpermanent, can be used for preoperative embolizations 24 to 48 hours prior to surgical excision. Finally, radiosurgery is increasingly being recognized as an effective modality for treatment of some DAVFs.

SPINAL VASCULAR MALFORMATIONS

Introduction

Vascular malformations of the spine are uncommon lesions that represent potentially treatable causes of myelopathy. Their prevalence, expressed as a percentage of the total number of spinal space-occupying lesions, is reported at 16%. The ratio of spinal to brain AVMs ranges from 1:4 to 1:8. The diagnosis and management of vascular malformations of the spine and spinal cord have undergone significant development since they were first recognized as a clinical entity in 1888. Due to the rarity of these lesions, variable clinical and radiologic presentation, bias of treating centers toward surgery or endovascular therapy, and absence of uniform outcome parameters, a clear set of clinical guidelines has not yet evolved. The gold standard in the diagnosis of spinal vascular malformations remains catheter-based angiography.

What Is the Normal Blood Supply to the Spinal Cord?

The blood supply to the spinal cord is via one anterior spinal artery (ASA) and two or more posterior spinal arteries. The ASA lies in the anterior median sulcus, and the posterior spinal arteries lie on either side of the dorsolateral surface of the spinal cord. The ASA supplies the anterior two thirds of the spinal cord, including the anterior and lateral corticospinal tracts; the posterior spinal arteries primarily supply the posterior third of the cord.

Anterior Spinal Artery

The distal vertebral arteries, typically distal to the origin of the posterior inferior cerebellar arteries, are the typical origin of the ASA. Supply can arise symmetrically from both sides or predominantly from one side. From the cervicomedullary junction to the conus, a single ASA runs within the anterior median sulcus. In the cervical region, the ASA receives further contributions via branches of the vertebral artery as well as the ascending cervical branch of the thyrocervical trunk (Figure 6-11). An important contribution to the ASA axis is a prominent unilateral radicular artery, typically at the C5 or C6 level, known as the *artery of cervical enlargement* (Figure 6-11). In the thoracic and lumbar regions, radiculomedullary branches of the supreme intercostal artery and the thoracic/lumbar segmental arteries join the ASA axis, exhibiting a characteristic hairpin turn as they descend to join the ASA axis in the midline. The most prominent of these radicular vessels is the artery of Adamkiewicz, which commonly arises from the lower intercostal or lumbar arteries, most frequently on the left side, between T9 and L2. The artery of Adamkiewicz should always be identified angiographically before performing thoracic or lumbar embolization or surgical procedures involving the lower thoracic or upper abdominal aorta.

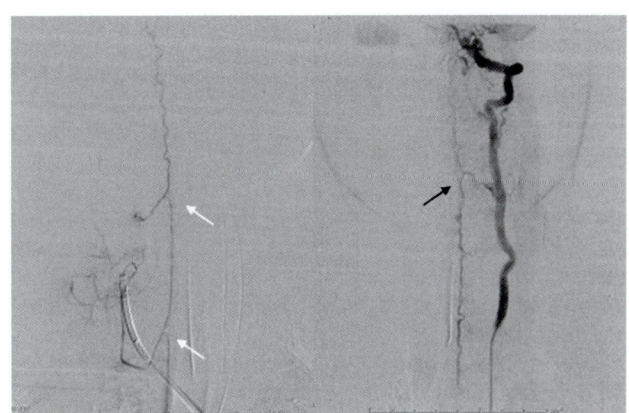

Figure 6-11 Anterior spinal artery (ASA) axis in the cervical region. The ASA runs craniocaudad in the midline. The characteristic hairpin turns of the radiculomedullary feeders are shown by the *white* and *black arrows*. *Left:* Direct injection of a radiculomedullary feeder to the ASA. *Right:* Left vertebral artery injection demonstrating the artery of cervical enlargement *(black arrow)*.

Posterior Spinal Artery

The posterior spinal arteries originate as lateral spinal branches of either the vertebral arteries or the posterior inferior cerebellar arteries. They also receive contributions from the segmental radicular arteries at multiple levels. Although often presented as paired structures, the posterior spinal arteries can be conceptualized as two parallel paramedian craniocaudal networks of vessels on the posterior aspect of the spinal cord. The ASA forms a basket-like anastomosis with the posterior spinal arteries over the surface of the conus medullaris.

How Do We Classify Spinal Arteriovenous Lesions?

Various classification systems have been proposed and have been the subject of fierce debate. Rather than advocate for one system in particular, it is perhaps most useful to consider the precise location of the arteriovenous communication. Thus, spinal arteriovenous lesions may be classified as follows:

- *DAVFs.* These are the most common of the spinal arteriovenous lesions. The nidus typically is located within or on the dura of the proximal nerve root sleeve in the neural foramen, typically at the point where the nerve root sleeve becomes intradural. Flow is from the nidus of the fistula retrograde into the perimedullary veins on the cord surface (coronal venous plexus). These lesions are thought to be acquired, resulting from trauma or venous thrombosis. They are most common in men (with a 5:1 M:F predominance) between the ages of 50 and 70 years and typically present with progressive myelopathy. Regardless of the actual fistula site, symptoms usually are attributable to venous hypertension affecting the most dependent segment of the cord, the conus. MRI typically shows conus signal abnormality as the first parenchymal manifestation.

- *Intradural extramedullary AV fistulae* (Figure 6-12). These are supplied directly by anterior or posterior spinal artery branches and typically have a simple arteriovenous fistula morphology, rather than a nidus, with the fistulous point at a perimedullary location (on the surface of the cord, draining directly into the perimedullary veins). They can present with progressive myelopathy from venous hypertension, myelopathy due to mass effect from massively dilated veins, or spinal hemorrhage.

- *Intramedullary (or "glomus")-type AVMs of the cord.* These lesions are supplied by branches of the anterior and/or posterior spinal arteries. They possess an intramedullary nidus, which drains into the coronal venous plexus on the cord surface and then via medullary veins or extradural veins in an anterograde manner. Patients typically are younger than 50 years. There is no predilection for any part of the cord, and up to half of all patients present with subarachnoid hemorrhage. Treatment, both surgical and endovascular, is particularly challenging.

- *Metameric or "juvenile"-type AVMs with intramedullary, extramedullary, and often extraspinal components.* The nidus in these cases often is quite diffuse. Treatment is very challenging and often is aimed at palliation.

- *Epidural arteriovenous fistulae.* These are extremely rare lesions in which venous drainage occurs is via the epidural venous plexus (Figure 6-13). They have been reported to progress to involve perimedullary venous drainage and thus potentially give rise to myelopathy, with a presentation similar to DAVF.

Problem Solving: Which Spinal Cord Arteriovenous Shunts Should be Treated?

All patients with symptomatic lesions should be considered for treatment because symptoms typically are manifestations of hemorrhage, spinal venous

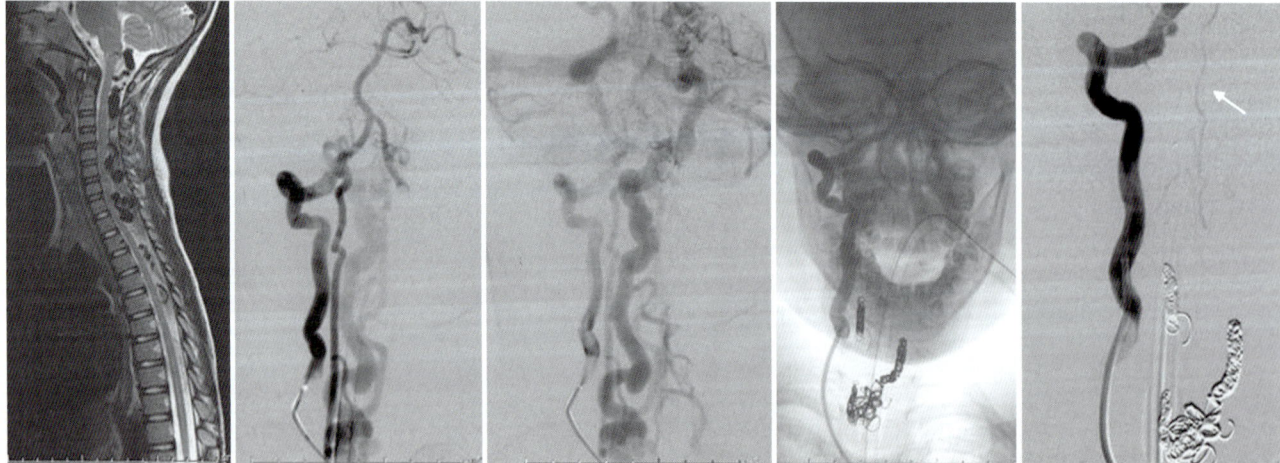

Figure 6-12 Intradural, extramedullary spinal arteriovenous (AV) fistula. The patient presented with severe headaches and motor tics. **First panel:** Sagittal T2-weighted magnetic resonance image demonstrating markedly enlarged intradural flow voids posterior to the spinal cord. Frontal view of a right vertebral artery injection in early arterial **(second panel)** and late arterial **(third panel)** phases demonstrate a posterior spinal AV fistula, with early opacification of massively enlarged perimedullary veins and reflux of arterialized venous blood up the cord to the posterior fossa. **Fourth panel:** Unsubtracted frontal view demonstrating coil masses deposited at the sites of arterial inflow into the venous pouch. **Fifth panel:** Postembolization injection of the right vertebral artery demonstrating nonopacification of the fistula. The anterior spinal artery axis is nicely demonstrated *(white arrow)*.

hypertension, or mass effect, which all are processes that pose a high risk of profound neurologic impairment. Incidentally discovered spinal arteriovenous lesions that show imaging evidence of risk, such as arterialization of perimedullary spinal veins, should be treated prophylactically. If complete obliteration is not feasible, treatment of morphologically high-risk portions of the lesion, such as associated aneurysms, is undertaken.

The potential risk posed by high thoracic or cervical lesions is greater than that posed by more caudal lesions because upper extremity function and respiratory function may be affected. For patients with lower thoracic or lumbar AVMs who have a fixed deficit and in whom no clinical improvement is likely, spinal hemorrhage may not be life threatening, and the indications for aggressive treatment may be less compelling. In some patients with severe pain and spasm, even noncurative embolization may help palliate symptoms.

■ TUMOR EMBOLIZATION

Preoperative embolization of vascular tumors of the head, neck, and CNS has become an important adjunct to the surgical treatment of these tumors. Hypervascular tumors for which embolization may be indicated include hemangioblastomas, intracranial metastases, meningiomas, hemangiopericytomas, neurogenic tumors (e.g., schwannomas), paragangliomas, juvenile nasopharyngeal angiofibromas, hemangiomas, esthesioneuroblastomas, benign bone tumors, malignant bone tumors, and extracranial metastases. The indications for embolization include the following:

- Control surgically inaccessible arterial feeders
- Decrease surgical morbidity by reducing blood loss
- Shorten operative procedure time
- Increase the chances of complete surgical resection
- Decrease the risk of damage to adjacent normal tissue
- Relieve intractable pain

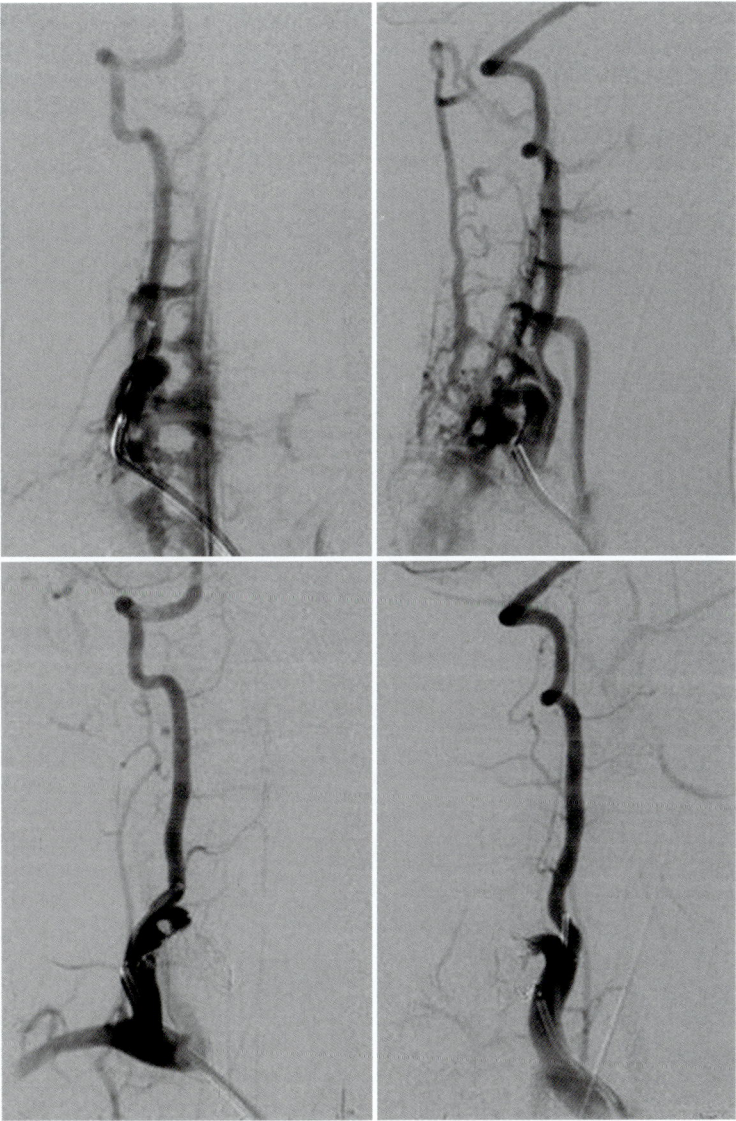

Figure 6-13 Spinal epidural fistula. Frontal *(upper left)* and lateral *(upper right)* views of a right vertebral artery injection demonstrate immediate opacification of the epidural venous plexus. The patient had presented with a new continuous heart murmur. Postembolization views, frontal *(bottom left)* and lateral *(bottom right)*, demonstrate runoff into the vertebral artery, with no opacification of the fistula.

- Decrease expected tumor recurrence
- Allow better visualization of the surgical field with decreased overall surgical complication

Palliative embolization of head, neck, and CNS tumors may be indicated as the sole treatment for patients who present poor surgical risks, patients with intractable hemorrhage, or patients with increasing neurologic deficits from tumor mass effect.

Ideally, an embolic agent is chosen that will devascularize the tumor but spare the adjacent normal tissue. Liquid embolic agents, such as ethanol, acrylic agents, and Onyx, and the smallest-diameter particulate materials can penetrate into the arteriolar tumor supply, but care is needed in their use because their ability to penetrate distally also poses a risk of damage to adjacent normal tissues. Relatively coarser particulate agents, such as large-diameter PVA and Gelfoam, do not penetrate into the tumor as deeply, but they are less likely to damage adjacent normal tissues. Embolic agents, such as liquids and coils, may be permanent or temporary, as is the case for the particulate agents.

How Is Tumor Embolization Carried Out?

MRI is the mainstay of preprocedural noninvasive imaging and typically demonstrates avid enhancement in hypervascular tumors following gadolinium administration. The extent of the tumor is evaluated, including encasement of the internal carotid or vertebral arteries, dural enhancement, and invasion of other vital adjacent structures. In the majority of cases, even if small branches of the internal carotid artery are parasitized to supply the tumor, preoperative embolization is confined to the dominant external carotid artery supply in order to achieve the most favorable risk-to-benefit ratio.

In juvenile angiofibromas, the arterial supply arises from the pterygopalatine portion of the internal maxillary artery. Recruitment of the accessory meningeal, ascending pharyngeal, and ascending palatine arteries is often seen with larger tumors. In paragangliomas, the major supply comes form the ascending pharyngeal artery branches, the stylomastoid branch of the occipital artery, and the temporal branch of the middle meningeal artery. The middle meningeal artery, which supplies the dura of the sphenoid wing, cerebral convexities, and much of the anterior cerebral fossa, is the most dominant feeding vessel of meningiomas, although meningiomas often recruit adjacent meningeal arteries or invade the dura and recruit pial vessels.

It is crucial to search diligently for external carotid–internal carotid anastomoses and anatomic variants, particularly those involving the middle meningeal artery and ophthalmic artery, because these may profoundly impact the ability to safely perform tumor embolization. Superselective injections are necessary to delineate cranial nerve supply or potentially hazardous anastomoses with the internal carotid artery or vertebral artery.

Preoperative embolization is most commonly performed using particles of PVA from 150 to 350 µm in diameter (Contour PVA particles, Boston Scientific, Fremont, CA) suspended in a mixture of contrast and heparinized saline. The microcatheter is advanced into a feeding pedicle and then PVA particles are injected in a pulsatile fashion under fluoroscopic guidance. The particles wedge in the arterioles and accumulate within the tumor bed, inciting necrosis. Some practitioners finish the embolization with coil ligation of the proximal feeder to prevent rapid rerouting and revascularization. Recanalization after PVA particle embolization occurs over weeks and months as the periparticle thrombus resorbs and the particles are phagocytosed.

For permanent embolization, NBCA or Onyx, which forms an occlusive cast in the feeding artery intratumorally, is used.

■ PEDIATRIC VASCULAR LESIONS

Pediatric vascular lesions of the CNS comprise a heterogeneous group of abnormalities such as aneurysms, arteriovenous lesions, and occlusive diseases. Although superficially similar to their corresponding adult lesions, pediatric vascular lesions have crucial differences with regard to clinical manifestations, angioarchitecture, and management strategies. Moreover, limitations related to vascular access, contrast dose, and acceptable radiation dose all play a role in shaping neurointerventional treatment strategy in children. The presentation of CNS vascular lesions in childhood is truly rare, so rigorous natural history data are almost uniformly lacking.

Vein of Galen Malformations

Vein of Galen malformations (VGAMs) are rare intracranial vascular anomalies that constitute only 1% of all intracranial vascular malformations but 30% of vascular malformations presenting in childhood. The lesion is characterized by shunting of arterial flow, typically from anterior and posterior choroidal arteries, into an enlarged persistent embryonic vein dorsal to the tectum, the median prosencephalic vein (the precursor of the true vein of Galen). VGAMs typically are subclassified as either choroidal, with a complex AVM-like nidus, or mural, with direct arteriovenous fistulae in the wall of the median vein. In patients with VGAM, venous drainage of the brain is rerouted via alternative routes, and the median vein does not participate in normal cerebral venous outflow; it is a relatively insulated vascular route. Thus, unlike brain AVMs in which the venous drainage pathway of the brain is exposed to high arterial pressures by virtue of the lesion, the risk of hemorrhage from VGAM is extremely low. With the advent of endovascular neurointerventional techniques, the prospects for successful treatment of these lesions, once dismal, have now much improved.

How Do VGAMs Present, and What Is the Treatment Strategy?

The clinical presentation of VGAMs covers a wide spectrum, ranging from neonatal heart failure to headaches in adulthood. Very-high-flow shunts typically present at birth with right-sided and left-sided heart failure, which if untreated rapidly leads to multiorgan failure and death. Embolization within the first few days of life is performed, targeting the highest-flow components of the lesion. When embolization is effective, almost immediate improvement in the cardiopulmonary status of the patient can be seen, and intraprocedural weaning of pressors becomes feasible. However, intervention at this early age, given the technical challenges associated with vascular access and the friability of the subependymal veins, is fraught with risk.

Lower-flow lesions may present with macrocephaly or mild heart failure at several months of age. Left untreated, these lower-flow lesions may lead to profound impairment of neurologic development or even "melting brain syndrome," with diffuse parenchymal cerebral loss typically accompanied by calcifications. For patients who have a stable cardiac status, a normal neurologic examination, and no macrocephaly, treatment typically is deferred until 5 or 6 months of age, when the risks of intervention are lower but neurodevelopmental setbacks have not yet occurred (Figure 6-14). For all interventions in the first year of life, the goal is not necessarily complete obliteration of the lesion but rather protection from the systemic and neurologic risks posed by untreated lesions.

VGAMs occasionally are detected on prenatal ultrasound scans (from approximately 25 weeks' gestation and later) as a midline vascular mass. When VGAMs are identified, prenatal MRI can be very helpful in demonstrating the location of fistulae, presence of a nidus, the location of arterial feeders, ventricular size, and cerebral parenchymal changes. When diffuse brain parenchymal volume loss is present on imaging or in the setting of multiorgan failure, the prospect of any

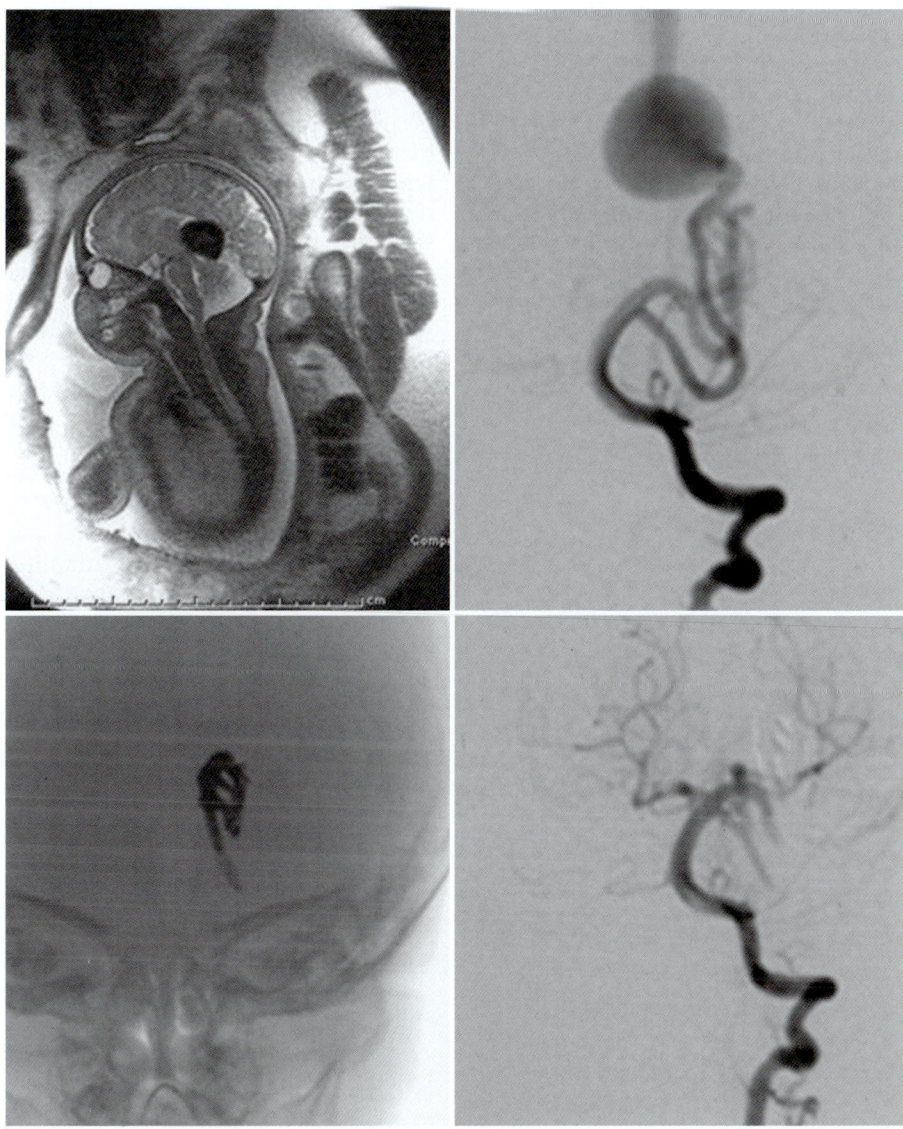

Figure 6-14 Vein of Galen malformation (VAGM), mural type. The lesion was found on routine third-trimester ultrasound. The patient was clinically stable, and embolization was deferred until 5 months of age. *Top left:* Fetal magnetic resonance image demonstrating an enlarged midline vascular structure, corresponding to the median vein of the prosencephalon, and diagnostic of a VGAM. *Top right:* Frontal view of a left vertebral artery injection demonstrating early opacification of the ectatic venous pouch. *Bottom left:* Unsubtracted frontal view demonstrating focal deposit of embolic material (detachable coils followed by Onyx) at the site of arterial inflow into the fistula. *Bottom right:* Postembolization frontal view of a left vertebral artery injection demonstrating normal vertebrobasilar runoff, with nonopacification of the arteriovenous shunt.

intervention leading to good neurologic and systemic outcome is nil.

Most practitioners prefer transarterial embolization as the treatment of choice. Although transvenous and transtorcular embolization have been advocated by some, it may be associated with higher morbidity and usually is reserved for cases where transarterial embolization has failed.

Pediatric Brain AVMs

How Do Cerebral AVMs in Children Differ from Those in Adults?

In most surgical series, children represent 20% of all cerebral AVM cases. Arteriovenous fistulae are more often encountered in neonates; lesions detected in infants are more often nidus-type AVMs. Cerebral AVMs frequently have characteristics in children that differentiate them from their adult counterparts, such as multifocality (Figure 6-15), induced arteriovenous shunts remote from the original lesion, large venous ectasia, venous thrombosis, adjacent brain atrophy, and, particularly in neonates and young infants, systemic phenomena such as cardiac failure. Conversely, other features, such as flow-related arterial aneurysms, are relatively rare in children.

In infants and young children, the clinical expression of cerebral AVM is in many cases related to the remote effects of the AV shunt on hemodynamic and hydrodynamic equilibrium, with signs of congestive heart failure, hydrocephalus, and seizures. After the age of 3 years, more than 50% of AVMs present with intracranial hemorrhage. The next most common presentation is seizure, which occurs in approximately 20% to 25% of cases. Other presentations include headaches in 15% of patients and focal neurologic deficit in fewer than 5% of cases.

Problem Solving: What Are the Treatment Options for Brain AVMs in Children?

Management strategies include single or combined therapy including neurosurgery, transarterial embolization with liquid agents such as NBCA or Onyx, radiosurgery, or a combination of techniques. However, the ability to safely deliver radiation therapy in young children is limited. Wherever possible, surgical resection of brain AVMs in children is a desired endpoint, particularly for lesions that have undergone hemorrhage. Although growing attention is being paid to the possibility of treating brain AVMs in adults with definitive embolization alone, it should be borne in mind that AVMs are evolving lesions, and, particularly in children, residual and dormant segments of the AVM may come to expression at a later date. Periodic clinical and radiologic follow-ups are warranted.

Dural Sinus Malformations

Lasjaunias and colleagues coined the term *dural sinus malformation* to describe congenital dural fistulae that occur early enough to preclude normal development of the venous sinuses, resulting in giant dural lakes, typically involving the torcular, transverse, or superior sagittal sinuses (Figure 6-16). Symptoms often are systemic, with cardiac failure, coagulation disorders, or increased intracranial pressure leading to irritability, macrocrania, neurocognitive delay, and seizures. As opposed to VGAM where the venous sac draining the malformation does not participate in venous drainage of the brain, in dural sinus malformations the cerebral venous system is intrinsically involved. Thus, the prognosis depends on the availability of alternative drainage pathways for cerebral venous blood, most commonly achieved by "capture" of the cavernous sinuses and rerouting of cerebral venous drainage retrograde via the superior ophthalmic veins and emissary veins to the facial and scalp veins. In cases with favorable alternative pathways of venous drainage, early embolization of arteriovenous shunts may allow for normal development.

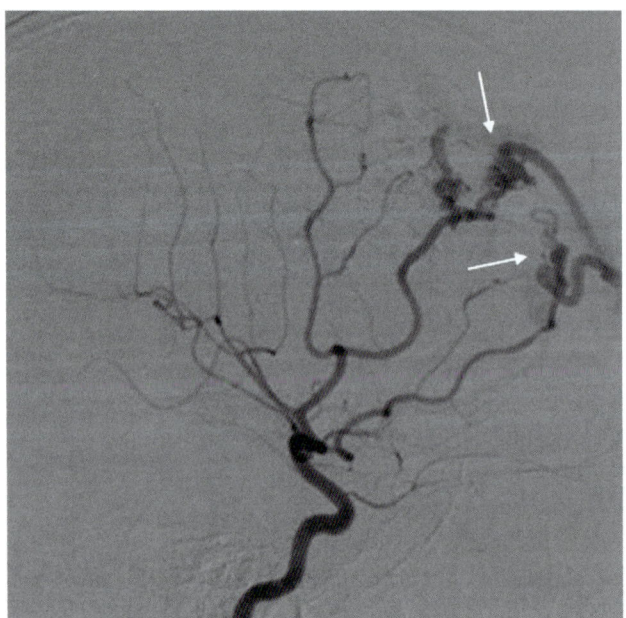

Figure 6-15 Multifocality of brain arteriovenous malformation (AVM) in an infant. Note two discrete foci with AVM nidus *(white arrows)* without a bridge seen angiographically.

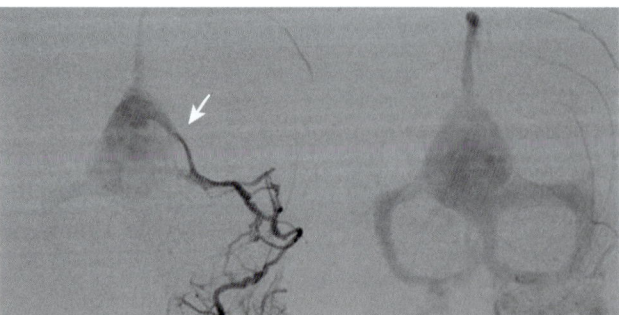

Figure 6-16 Frontal views of a left middle meningeal artery injection in early arterial *(left)* and late arterial *(right)* phases. A direct fistula is seen, with a hole in the massively dilated torcular, through which contrast enters with a "spigot" effect from the middle meningeal artery *(white arrow)*. The dysplastic morphology of the torcular and its incorporation of the medial aspect of the right transverse sinus are apparent on the delayed image.

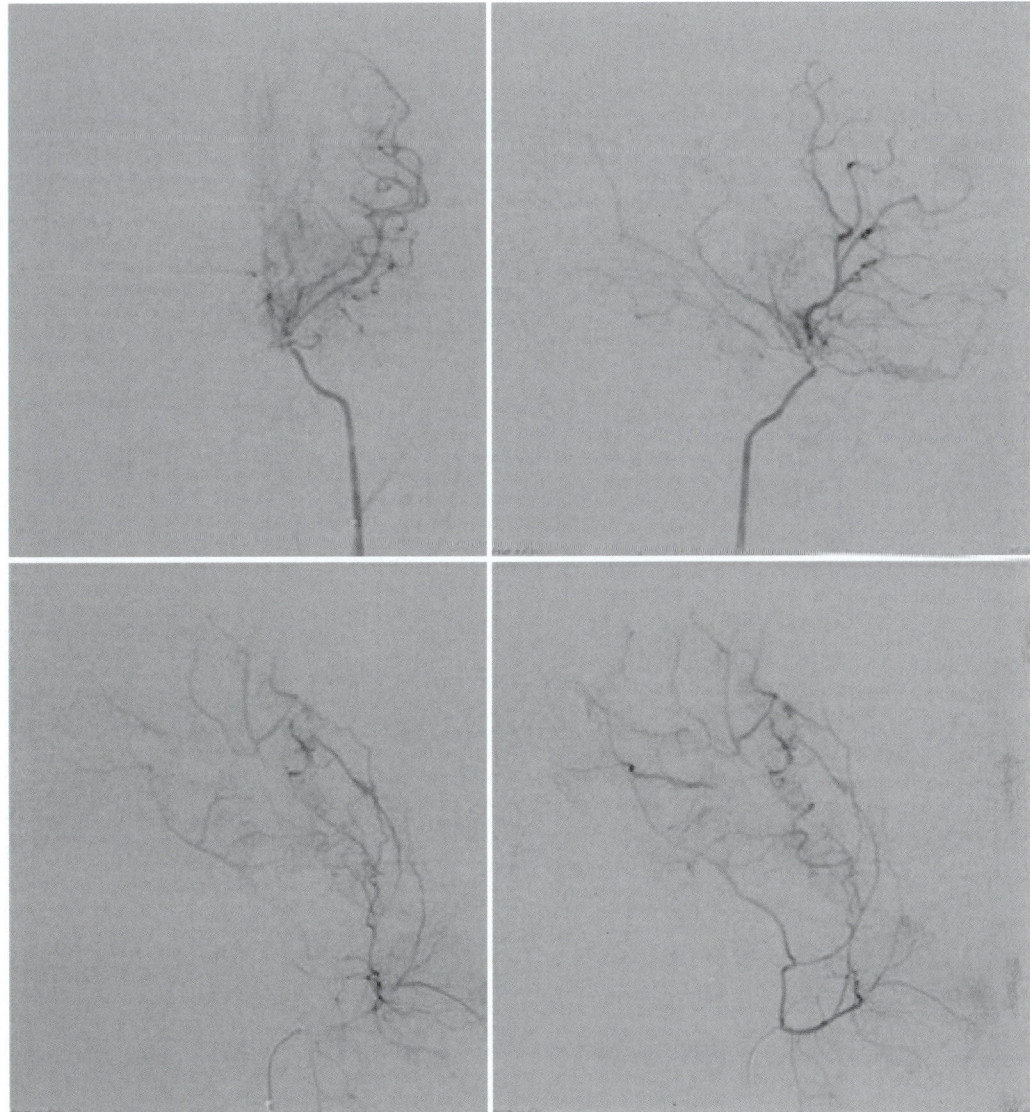

Figure 6-17 Moyamoya disease seen on frontal *(top left)* and sagittal *(top right)* views of left internal carotid artery (ICA) injection. Note stenotic changes involving the terminal ICA and M1 segment as well as severe pruning of the middle cerebral artery (MCA) arterial tree. Postsynangiosis views of left superficial temporal *(bottom left)* and middle meningeal artery *(bottom right)* injection. Note opacification of parts of the MCA candelabra on both of these latter injections.

Pediatric Aneurysms

Intracranial aneurysms in children represent <5% of the total number in the general population. Saccular or "berry" aneurysms constitute 50% to 70% of all cases, are multiple in 2%, and are most commonly located at arterial bifurcations of the circle of Willis, as they are in adults. Infectious or mycotic aneurysms are situated peripherally and comprise 5% to 15% of pediatric aneurysms. Traumatic aneurysms account for approximately 5% to 15% of pediatric aneurysms, of which 40% involve the distal anterior cerebral artery, 35% involve vessels along the skull base, and 25% are cortical in location. A combination of intraluminal, mural, and extravascular factors is responsible for the development of aneurysms, given a clear association with various disease processes that weaken the arterial wall. Conditions such as autosomal dominant inherited polycystic kidney disease, fibromuscular dysplasia, Osler-Weber-Rendu syndrome, coarctation of the aorta, moyamoya syndrome, Marfan syndrome, Ehlers-Danlos syndrome, bacterial endocarditis, fungal infections, neurofibromatosis type 1, and tuberous sclerosis all have been associated with an increased incidence of cerebral aneurysms in children.

How Do Aneurysms Clinically Present in the Pediatric Population?

Cerebral aneurysms present with subarachnoid hemorrhage approximately 70% of the time in children; mass effect (20%), seizure, and stroke are other clinical presentations. In the neonatal period and infancy, males are affected more commonly than are females. Although radiographically, vasospasm after subarachnoid hemorrhage seems to be more prevalent and severe initially, children seem to be less susceptible to delayed ischemic deficits. As in adults, cerebral aneurysms in children can be treated with endovascular coiling or surgical clipping.

■ MOYAMOYA DISEASE

Moyamoya disease is a cerebrovascular occlusive disease of unknown etiology that occurs with highest incidence in Asian populations. The primary pathology consists of progressive occlusion of the main trunks of the cerebral arterial tree, such as the terminal internal carotid arteries and the M1 and A1 arterial segments (Figure 6-17). The name derives from a Japanese term for the cloud-like appearance of pathologically proliferative lenticulostriate perforators. Moyamoya disease has a bimodal age presentation; the first peak occurs in the first decade of life and is associated most commonly with cerebral infarction. Adult patients most often present in the fourth decade with intracranial hemorrhage arising from rupture of the delicate network of collateral vessels. Moyamoya disease may occur as an isolated phenomenon in a previously healthy individual, but it has also been reported in association with sickle cell anemia, Down syndrome, Marfan syndrome, tuberous sclerosis, Turner syndrome, neurofibromatosis type 1, atherosclerotic disease, coarctation of the aorta, fibromuscular dysplasia, and tuberculosis.

Although MRA and magnetic resonance perfusion are invaluable in assessing the arterial tree and perfusion deficits, catheter angiography is frequently used to carefully document progression of disease as well as response to surgical therapy, such as synangiosis and intracranial–extracranial bypass (Figure 6-17).

Suggested Readings

Adams Jr HP, del Zoppo G, Alberts MJ, et al. Guidelines for the early management of adults with ischemic stroke: A guideline from the American Heart Association/American Stroke Association Stroke Council, Clinical Cardiology Council, Cardiovascular Radiology and Intervention Council, and the Atherosclerotic Peripheral Vascular Disease and Quality of Care Outcomes in Research Interdisciplinary Working Groups: The American Academy of Neurology affirms the value of this guideline as an educational tool for neurologists. Stroke. 2007;38:1655-1711.

Alexandrov AV, Molina CA, Grotta JC, et al. Ultrasound-enhanced systemic thrombolysis for acute ischemic stroke. N Engl J Med. 2004;351:2170-2178.

Barnett HJ, Taylor DW, Eliasziw M, et al. Benefit of carotid endarterectomy in patients with symptomatic moderate or severe stenosis. North American Symptomatic Carotid Endarterectomy Trial Collaborators. N Engl J Med. 1998;339:1415-1425.

Barnwell SL, Halbach VV, Dowd CF, Higashida RT, Hieshima GB, Wilson CB. A variant of arteriovenous fistulas within the wall of dural sinuses. Results of combined surgical and endovascular therapy. J Neurosurg. 1991;74:199-204.

Barnwell SL, Halbach VV, Higashida RT, Hieshima G, Wilson CB. Complex dural arteriovenous fistulas. Results of combined endovascular and neurosurgical treatment in 16 patients. J Neurosurg. 1989;71:352-358.

Beneficial effect of carotid endarterectomy in symptomatic patients with high-grade carotid stenosis. North American Symptomatic Carotid Endarterectomy Trial Collaborators. N Engl J Med. 1991;325:445-453.

Berenstein A, Lasjaunias P. Arteriovenous fistulas of the brain. In: Endovascular Treatment of Cerebral Lesions.. Berlin: Springer-Verlag; 1992, 267-317.

Bergstrand A, Hook O, Lidvall H. Vertebral haemangiomas compressing the spinal cord. Acta Neurol Scand. 1963;39:59-66.

Biondi A, Janardhan V, Katz JM, Salvaggio K, Riina HA, Gobin YP. Neuroform stent-assisted coil embolization of wide-neck intracranial aneurysms: Strategies in stent deployment and midterm follow-up. Neurosurgery. 2007;61:460-468:discussion 468–469.

Brisman JL, Niimi Y, Song JK, Berenstein A. Aneurysmal rupture during coiling: Low incidence and good outcomes at a single large volume center. Neurosurgery. 2008;62:1538-1551.

Brooks B. The treatment of traumatic arteriovenous fistula. South Med J. 1930;23:100-106.

Brown Jr RD, Wiebers DO, Torner JC, O'Fallon WM. Frequency of intracranial hemorrhage as a presenting symptom and subtype analysis: A population-based study of intracranial vascular malformations in Olmsted Country, Minnesota. J Neurosurg. 1996;85:29-32.

Carballo RE, Towne JB, Seabrook GR, Freischlag JA, Cambria RA. An outcome analysis of carotid endarterectomy: The incidence and natural history of recurrent stenosis. J Vasc Surg. 1996;23:749-753:discussion 753–744.

Casasco A, Lylyk P, Hodes JE, Kohan G, Aymard A, Merland JJ. Percutaneous transvenous catheterization and embolization of vein of Galen aneurysms. Neurosurgery. 1991;28:260-266.

Chaudhary MY, Sachdev VP, Cho SH, Weitzner Jr I, Puljic S, Huang YP. Dural arteriovenous malformation of the major venous sinuses: An acquired lesion. AJNR Am J Neuroradiol. 1982;3:13-19.

Cogen P, Stein BM. Spinal cord arteriovenous malformations with significant intramedullary components. J Neurosurg. 1983;59:471-478.

Cognard C, Gobin YP, Pierot L, et al. Cerebral dural arteriovenous fistulas: Clinical and angiographic correlation with a revised classification of venous drainage: Radiology. 1995;194:671-680.

Combined intravenous and intra-arterial recanalization for acute ischemic stroke: The Interventional Management of Stroke Study. Stroke. 2004;35:904-911.

Cremonesi A, Manetti R, Setacci F, Setacci C, Castriota F. Protected carotid stenting: Clinical advantages and complications of embolic protection devices in 442 consecutive patients. Stroke. 2003;34:1936-1941.

Dawbarn RH. The starvation operation for malignancy in the external carotid area. JAMA. 1904;17:792-795.

del Zoppo GJ, Higashida RT, Furlan AJ, Pessin MS, Rowley HA, Gent M. PROACT: A phase II randomized trial of recombinant pro-urokinase by direct arterial delivery in acute middle cerebral artery stroke. PROACT Investigators. Prolyse in Acute Cerebral Thromboembolism. Stroke. 1998;29:4-11.

Djindjian R, Cophignon J, Theron J, Merland JJ, Houdart R. Embolization by superselective arteriography from the femoral route in neuroradiology. Review of 60 cases. 1. Technique, indications, complications. Neuroradiology. 1973;6:20-26.

Doppman JL, Di Chiro G, Ommaya A. Obliteration of spinal-cord arteriovenous malformation by percutaneous embolisation. Lancet. 1968;1:477.

Endarterectomy for asymptomatic carotid artery stenosis. Executive Committee for the Asymptomatic Carotid Atherosclerosis Study. JAMA. 1995;273:1421-1428.

Endovascular versus surgical treatment in patients with carotid stenosis in the Carotid and Vertebral Artery Transluminal Angioplasty Study (CAVATAS): A randomised trial. Lancet. 2001;357:1729-1737.

Fiorella D, Woo HH, Albuquerque FC, Nelson PK. Definitive reconstruction of circumferential, fusiform intracranial aneurysms with the pipeline embolization device. Neurosurgery. 2008;62:1115-1120:discussion 1120–1111.

Furlan A, Higashida R, Wechsler L, et al. Intra-arterial prourokinase for acute ischemic stroke. The PROACT II study: A randomized controlled trial. Prolyse in Acute Cerebral Thromboembolism. JAMA. 1999;282:2003-2011.

Gaupp J. Hamorrhoiden der Pia mater spinalis im Geibiet des Lendenmarks. Beitr Pathol. 1888;2:516-518.

Gralla J, Rennie AT, Corkill RA, et al. Abciximab for thrombolysis during intracranial aneurysm coiling. Neuroradiology. 2008;50:1041-1047.

Guglielmi G, Vinuela F, Dion J, Duckwiler G. Electrothrombosis of saccular aneurysms via endovascular approach. Part 2: Preliminary clinical experience. J Neurosurg. 1991;75:8-14.

Guglielmi G, Vinuela F, Sepetka I, Macellari V. Electrothrombosis of saccular aneurysms via endovascular approach. Part 1: Electrochemical basis, technique, and experimental results. J Neurosurg. 1991;75:1-7.

Hacke W, Donnan G, Fieschi C, et al. Association of outcome with early stroke treatment: Pooled analysis of ATLANTIS, ECASS, and NINDS rt-PA stroke trials. Lancet. 2004;363:768-774.

Hacke W, Kaste M, Fieschi C, et al. Intravenous thrombolysis with recombinant tissue plasminogen activator for acute hemispheric stroke. The European Cooperative Acute Stroke Study (ECASS). JAMA. 1995;274:1017-1025.

Hademenos GJ, Massoud TF, Vinuela F. Quantitation of intracranial aneurysm neck size from diagnostic angiograms based on a biomathematical model. Neurol Res. 1995;17:322-328.

Halbach VV, Higashida RT, Hieshima GB, Goto K, Norman D, Newton TH. Dural fistulas involving the transverse and sigmoid sinuses: Results of treatment in 28 patients. Radiology. 1987;163:443-447.

Halbach VV, Higashida RT, Hieshima GB, Hardin CW, Pribram H. Transvenous embolization of dural fistulas involving the cavernous sinus. AJNR Am J Neuroradiol. 1989;10:377-383.

Halbach VV, Higashida RT, Hieshima GB, Mehringer CM, Hardin CW. Transvenous embolization of dural fistulas involving the transverse and sigmoid sinuses. AJNR Am J Neuroradiol. 1989;10:385-392.

Head, neck, and brain tumor embolization. AJNR Am J Neuroradiol. 2001;22:S14-S15.

Horowitz MB, Jungreis CA, Quisling RG, Pollack I. Vein of Galen aneurysms: A review and current perspective. AJNR Am J Neuroradiol. 1994;15:1486-1496.

Jacobs MA, Mitsias P, Soltanian-Zadeh H, et al. Multiparametric MRI tissue characterization in clinical stroke with correlation to clinical outcome: Part 2. Stroke. 2001;32:950-957.

Jahan R, Murayama Y, Gobin YP, Duckwiler GR, Vinters HV, Vinuela F. Embolization of arteriovenous malformations with Onyx: Clinicopathological experience in 23 patients. *Neurosurgery*. 2001;48:984-995:discussion 995–987.

Jones RG, Davagnanam I, Colley S, West RJ, Yates DA. Abciximab for treatment of thromboembolic complications during endovascular coiling of intracranial aneurysms. *AJNR Am J Neuroradiol*. 2008;29:1925-1929.

Josephson SA, Saver JL, Smith WS. Comparison of mechanical embolectomy and intraarterial thrombolysis in acute ischemic stroke within the MCA: MERCI and Multi MERCI compared to PROACT II. *Neurocrit Care*. 2009;10:43-49.

Kak VK, Taylor AR, Gordon DS. Proximal carotid ligation for internal carotid aneurysms. A long-term follow-up study. *J Neurosurg*. 1973;39:503-513.

Kanaan I, Lasjaunias P, Coates R. The spectrum of intracranial aneurysms in pediatrics. *Minim Invasive Neurosurg*. 1995;38:1-9.

Katsaridis V, Papagiannaki C, Skoulios N, Achoulias I, Peios D. Local intra-arterial eptifibatide for intraoperative vessel thrombosis during aneurysm coiling. *AJNR Am J Neuroradiol*. 2008;29:1414-1417.

Katz JM, Gobin YP, Riina HA. Techniques and devices in interventional neuroradiology. In: Hurst RW, Rosenwasser RH, eds. *Interventional Neuroradiology*. New York: Informa Healthcare; 2008:161-182.

Kendall BE, Logue V. Spinal epidural angiomatous malformations draining into intrathecal veins. *Neuroradiology*. 1977;13:181-189.

Khatri P, Hill MD, Palesch YY, et al. Methodology of the Interventional Management of Stroke III Trial. *Int J Stroke*. 2008;3:130-137.

Kidwell CS, Villablanca JP, Saver JL. Advances in neuroimaging of acute stroke. *Curr Atheroscler Rep*. 2000;2:126-135.

Kricheff II, Madayag M, Braunstein P. Transfemoral catheter embolization of cerebral and posterior fossa arteriovenous malformations. *Radiology*. 1972;103:107-111.

Lasjaunias P. Intracranial aneurysms in children. In: *Vascular Diseases of Neonates, Infants and Children*, Berlin: Springer-Verlag; 1997: 373-392.

Lasjaunias P. Pial arteriovenous malformation, In: *Vascular Diseases in Neonates, Infants and Children*, Berlin: Springer; 1997, 203-320.

Lasjaunias PL, Berenstein A, Brugge KG. *Surgical Neuroangiography*. 2nd ed. Berlin: Springer; 2001, 3v.

Lasjaunias P, Rodesch G, Alvarez H. Vascular malformation of the neonatal brain. In: Rutherford MA, ed. *MRI of the Neonatal Brain*. London: WB Saunders; 2002:251-260.

Lasjaunias P, Rodesch G, Terbrugge K, et al. Vein of Galen aneurysmal malformations. Report of 36 cases managed between 1982 and 1988. *Acta Neurochir (Wien)*. 1989;99:26-37.

Lee LJ, Kidwell CS, Alger J, Starkman S, Saver JL. Impact on stroke subtype diagnosis of early diffusion-weighted magnetic resonance imaging and magnetic resonance angiography. *Stroke*. 2000;31:1081-1089.

Levy EI, Hanel RA, Lau T, et al. Frequency and management of recurrent stenosis after carotid artery stent implantation. *J Neurosurg*. 2005;102:29-37.

Lewandowski CA, Frankel M, Tomsick TA, et al. Combined intravenous and intra-arterial r-TPA versus intra-arterial therapy of acute ischemic stroke: Emergency Management of Stroke (EMS) Bridging Trial. *Stroke*. 1999;30:2598-2605.

Lombardi G, Migliavacca F. Angiomas of the spinal cord. *Br J Radiol*. 1959;32:810-814.

Luessenhop AJ, Spence WT. Artificial embolization of cerebral arteries. Report of use in a case of arteriovenous malformation. *JAMA*. 1960;172:1153-1155.

Malisch TW, Guglielmi G, Vinuela F, et al. Unruptured aneurysms presenting with mass effect symptoms: Response to endosaccular treatment with Guglielmi detachable coils. Part I. Symptoms of cranial nerve dysfunction. *J Neurosurg*. 1998;89:956-961.

Mansour N, Choudhari KA. Outcome of oculomotor nerve palsy from posterior communicating artery aneurysms: Comparison of clipping and coiling. *Neurosurgery*. 2007;60:E582:author reply E582.

Massop D, Dave R, Metzger C, et al. Stenting and angioplasty with protection in patients at high-risk for endarterectomy: SAPPHIRE Worldwide Registry first 2,001 patients. *Catheter Cardiovasc Interv*. 2009;73:129-136.

McDougall CG, Deshmukh VR, Fiorella DJ, Albuquerque FC, Spetzler RF. Endovascular techniques for vascular malformations of the spinal axis. *Neurosurg Clin N Am*. 2005;16:395-410:x-xi.

Merland JJ, Riche MC, Chiras J. Intraspinal extramedullary arteriovenous fistulae draining into the medullary veins. *J Neuroradiol*. 1980;7:271-320.

Monsein LH, Jeffery PJ, van Heerden BB, et al. Assessing adequacy of collateral circulation during balloon test occlusion of the internal carotid artery with 99mTc-HMPAO SPECT. *AJNR Am J Neuroradiol*. 1991;12:1045-1051.

Moret J, Cognard C, Weill A, Castaings L, Rey A. [Reconstruction technic in the treatment of wide-neck intracranial aneurysms. Long-term angiographic and clinical results. Apropos of 56 cases]. *J Neuroradiol*. 1997;24:30-44.

Murayama Y, Vinuela F, Tateshima S, Song JK, Gonzalez NR, Wallace MP. Bioabsorbable polymeric material coils for embolization of intracranial aneurysms: A preliminary experimental study. *J Neurosurg*. 2001;94:454-463.

Murphy KJ, Gailloud P, Venbrux A, Deramond H, Hanley D, Rigamonti D. Endovascular treatment of a grade IV transverse sinus dural arteriovenous fistula by sinus recanalization, angioplasty, and stent placement: Technical case report. *Neurosurgery*. 2000;46:497-500:discussion 500–491.

Nelson PK, Sahlein D, Shapiro M, et al. Recent steps toward a reconstructive endovascular solution for the orphaned, complex-neck aneurysm. *Neurosurgery*. 2006;59:S77-S92:discussion S3–S13.

Noser EA, Shaltoni HM, Hall CE, et al. Aggressive mechanical clot disruption: A safe adjunct to thrombolytic therapy in acute stroke? *Stroke*. 2005;36:292-296.

Orbach D, Becske T, Nelson PK. Endovascular management of intracranial aneurysms. In: Hurst RW, Rosenwasser RH, eds. *Interventional Neuroradiology*. New York: Informa Healthcare; 2008:239-261.

Osborn AG. Stroke. In: *Diagnostic Neuroradiology*. St. Louis: Mosby; 1994, 330–400.

Ostergaard JR. Aetiology of intracranial saccular aneurysms in childhood. *Br J Neurosurg*. 1991;5:575-580.

Pia HW, Vogelsang H. [Diagnosis and Therapy of Spinal Angioma.]. *Dtsch Z Nervenheilkd*. 1965;187:74-96.

Pierot L, Condette-Auliac S, Piette AM, Boulin A, Graveleau P, Dupuy M. Thromboembolic events after endovascular treatment of unruptured intracranial aneurysms in two patients with antiphospholipid-antibody syndrome. *Neuroradiology*. 2002;44:355-357.

Piotin M, Spelle L, Mounayer C, Loureiros C, Ghorbani A, Moret J. Intracranial aneurysms coiling with matrix: Immediate results in 152 patients and midterm anatomic follow-up from 115 patients. *Stroke*. 2009;40:321-323.

Qureshi AI. New grading system for angiographic evaluation of arterial occlusions and recanalization response to intra-arterial thrombolysis in acute ischemic stroke. *Neurosurgery*. 2002;50:1405-1414:discussion 1414–1415.

Romodanov AP, Shcheglov VI. Endovascular method of excluding from the circulation saccular cerebral arterial aneurysms, leaving intact vessels patient. *Acta Neurochir Suppl (Wien)*. 1979;28:312-315.

Romodanov AP, Shcheglov VI. Intravascular occlusion of saccular aneurysms of the cerebral arteries by means of detachable balloon catheter. In: Krayenbuhl H, ed. *Advances and Technical Standards on Neurosurgery*. New York: Springer-Verlag; 1982:25-28.

Rosenblum B, Oldfield EH, Doppman JL, Di Chiro G. Spinal arteriovenous malformations: A comparison of dural arteriovenous fistulas and intradural AVMs in 81 patients. *J Neurosurg*. 1987;67:795-802.

Sadasivan C, Cesar L, Seong J, et al. An original flow diversion device for the treatment of intracranial aneurysms: Evaluation in the rabbit elastase-induced model. *Stroke*. 2009;40:952-958.

Serbinenko FA. [Balloon occlusion of saccular aneurysms of the cerebral arteries]. *Vopr Neirokhir*. 1974:8-15.

Smith WS, Sung G, Saver J, et al. Mechanical thrombectomy for acute ischemic stroke: Final results of the Multi MERCI trial. *Stroke*. 2008;39:1205-1212.

Smith WS, Sung G, Starkman S, et al. Safety and efficacy of mechanical embolectomy in acute ischemic stroke: Results of the MERCI trial. *Stroke*. 2005;36:1432-1438.

Spetzler RF, Martin NA. A proposed grading system for arteriovenous malformations. *J Neurosurg*. 1986;65:476-483.

The Interventional Management of Stroke (IMS) II Study. *Stroke*. 2007;38:2127-2135.

Tissue plasminogen activator for acute ischemic stroke. The National Institute of Neurological Disorders and Stroke rt-PA Stroke Study Group. *N Engl J Med*. 1995;333:1581-1587.

Valavanis A. Preoperative embolization of the head and neck: Indications, patient selection, goals, and precautions. *AJNR Am J Neuroradiol*. 1986;7:943-952.

van Rooij WJ, Sluzewski M. Unruptured large and giant carotid artery aneurysms presenting with cranial nerve palsy: Comparison of clinical recovery after selective aneurysm coiling and therapeutic carotid artery occlusion. *AJNR Am J Neuroradiol*. 2008;29:997-1002.

Vinuela F, Fox AJ, Debrun GM, Peerless SJ, Drake CG. Spontaneous carotid-cavernous fistulas: Clinical, radiological, and therapeutic considerations. Experience with 20 cases. *J Neurosurg*. 1984;60:976-984.

Wakhloo AK, Gounis MJ, Sandhu JS, Akkawi N, Schenck AE, Linfante I. Complex-shaped platinum coils for brain aneurysms: Higher packing density, improved biomechanical stability, and midterm angiographic outcome. *AJNR Am J Neuroradiol*. 2007;28:1395-1400.

Wang H, Wang D, Fraser K, Swischuk J, Elwood P. Emergent combined intracranial thrombolysis and carotid stenting in the hyperacute management of stroke patients with severe cervical carotid stenosis. *AJNR Am J Neuroradiol*. 2007;28:1162-1166.

Weber W, Bendszus M, Kis B, Boulanger T, Solymosi L, Kuhne D. A new self-expanding nitinol stent (Enterprise) for the treatment of wide-necked intracranial aneurysms: Initial clinical and angiographic results in 31 aneurysms. *Neuroradiology*. 2007;49:555-561.

Weir B, Amidei C, Kongable G, et al. The aspect ratio (dome/neck) of ruptured and unruptured aneurysms. *J Neurosurg*. 2003;99:447-451.

Wolpert SM, Bruckmann H, Greenlee R, Wechsler L, Pessin MS, del Zoppo GJ. Neuroradiologic evaluation of patients with acute stroke treated with recombinant tissue plasminogen activator. The rt-PA Acute Stroke Study Group. *AJNR Am J Neuroradiol*. 1993;14:3-13.

Wolpert SM, Stein BM. Factors governing the course of emboli in the therapeutic embolization of cerebral arteriovenous malformations. *Radiology*. 1979;131:125-131.

Workman MJ, Cloft HJ, Tong FC, et al. Thrombus formation at the neck of cerebral aneurysms during treatment with Guglielmi detachable coils. *AJNR Am J Neuroradiol*. 2002;23:1568-1576.

Yadav JS, Wholey MH, Kuntz RE, et al. Protected carotid-artery stenting versus endarterectomy in high-risk patients. *N Engl J Med*. 2004;351:1493-1501.

Yamada I, Himeno Y, Suzuki S, Matsushima Y. Posterior circulation in moyamoya disease: Angiographic study. *Radiology*. 1995;197:239-246.

Zanetti PH, Sherman FE. Experimental evaluation of a tissue adhesive as an agent for the treatment of aneurysms and arteriovenous anomalies. *J Neurosurg*. 1972;36:72-79.

CHAPTER 7

Spine Procedures: Biopsies

Wade Wong and Danielle Nanigian

■ CONSIDERING TODAY'S WONDERFUL IMAGING, WHY WOULD ANYONE NEED A BIOPSY?

In spite of today's excellent imaging modalities, imaging diagnoses are still a matter of presenting a reasonable differential diagnosis and then making a best guess based on clinical history, examination, imaging appearance, and other clinical features. No imaging allows visualization of the cellular histology; therefore, tissue sampling is necessary (Figures 7-1 and 7-2).

One of the advantages of image-guided biopsies over open procedures is that image-guided procedures are performed percutaneously with minimal invasiveness, allowing the patient to have rapid recovery with relatively low risk.

Reasons for biopsy include establishment of a pathologic diagnosis when neoplasm is suspected, which is generally necessary prior to treatment. Biopsies can be helpful in differentiating neoplasm from infection because the two processes sometimes appear indistinguishable. When infection is suspected and the patient is undergoing treatment but is not improving, a biopsy can be helpful in establishing the appropriate antibiotic (sensitivity) for treatment.

■ WHAT CONSIDERATIONS SHOULD BE MADE PRIOR TO BIOPSY?

Preoperative biopsy considerations include a review history and physical examination, imaging, laboratory values (particularly coagulation profiles), and patient's medications and allergies. Informed consent should be obtained, and anesthetic requirements (for which the patient may need to be NPO [nothing by mouth] prior to the procedure) should be discussed.

Imaging review is necessary in deciding what needs to be targeted and, if there are multiple targets, the order of priority in which they should be taken. Based on location and risk of biopsy, the method of image guidance is chosen. If the patient is in renal failure, iodine contrast may be contraindicated, and this can be a disadvantage when attempting to stay clear of vascular structures.

Laboratory findings of prime concern include coagulation profiles. Generally an international normalized ratio greater than 1.5 is a reason to delay or defer biopsy. Elevated blood urea nitrogen and creatinine levels may indicate abnormal renal function that may preclude administration of iodine contrast.

Patient medications may alter the timing of biopsy. Typically patients who take warfarin (Coumadin) will

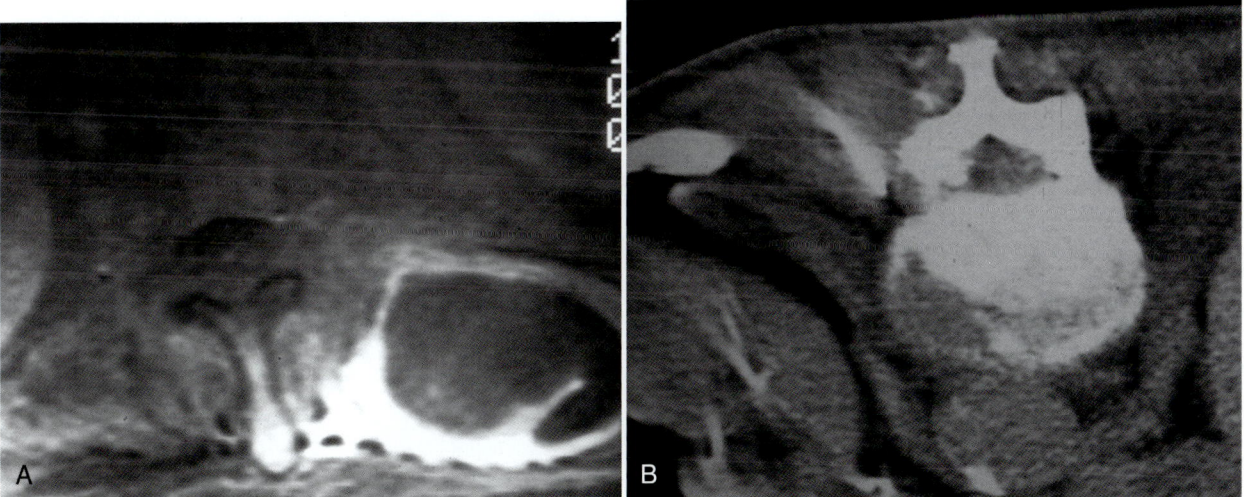

Figure 7-1 **A:** A 56-year-old woman complained of backache and had a low-grade fever of 99.6°F. Her white blood cell count was 9,900. Magnetic resonance imaging reveals paravertebral fluid-filled rim-enhancing mass consistent with abscess. **B:** Computed tomography–guided needle biopsy reveals malignant cells leading to eventual diagnosis of adenocarcinoma metastatic from stomach. This is an excellent example of why tissue sampling is necessary for confirming diagnosis.

stop the drug temporarily 5 days prior to the biopsy. Some patients require a temporary prescription for enoxaparin (Lovenox) in place of Coumadin until 12 hours prior to the biopsy. Other medication considerations include stopping clopidogrel (Plavix) 7 days prior and ticlopidine (Ticlid) 14 days prior to biopsy, particularly if the target is very close to the spinal canal in order to minimize the risk of epidural hematoma. Aspirin and other nonsteroidal antiinflammatory drugs usually are not a problem.

Informed consent should consist of an explanation of the reason for biopsy, other alternatives, a description of the procedure, including a discussion of appropriate anesthesia (usually local and conscience sedation), and an explanation of the risks, which include bleeding, infection, allergy, vascular injury, headache, nerve injury, paralysis, stroke, and even death. In our experience, complication rates are much less than 2%.

Spine Biopsies Lumbar: Problem Solving, How To Do It?

Challenges when performing biopsies of the lumbar spine include avoiding the kidney, bowel, aorta, inferior vena cava, and segmental arteries as well as injury to nerve roots and intraspinal contents.

Image-guided approaches for lumbar biopsies mainly include the posterior oblique approach and the transpedicular approach.

Fluoroscopy or computed tomography (CT) are the common modalities for used for guidance. Operators experienced with fluoroscopy find that fluoroscopic guidance is more efficient and faster than CT, but it requires a familiarity with adjacent unseen soft tissue anatomy relative to osseous landmarks. For those who are not adequately familiar with this anatomy, CT would be safer because adjacent soft tissues can be readily identified and kept out of harm's way. CT is an excellent choice when soft tissue masses distant to osseous landmarks must be biopsied. CT is also advantageous when precise targeting is needed (e.g., adjacent to critical organs, such as the lungs, aorta, or kidney).

For spine biopsies by the posterior oblique approaches, discography needle entry techniques are used. Both disc and bone specimens can be safely retrieved. The procedure usually is performed with the patient in the prone position. The fluoroscope is rotated about 45 degrees to the side through which entry will occur. The superior articular facet of the inferior vertebra is placed in the center of the obliquely visualized disc so that the needle is directed en face directly to the center of the target disc. (The operator can use a set of forceps to thrust the needle swiftly to the target.) The superior margin of the inferior vertebral body is flattened into a straight line appearance. This helps to project the exiting nerve root from the level above superior to the entering needle to avoid injury. Anteroposterior and lateral fluoroscopic views are taken to confirm that the needle is correctly situated in the center of the target. To obtain a sample, move the needle in and out about 1 cm with rotation and aspiration. The same technique can be used to approach osseous lesions of the lumbar spine (Figure 7-3).

For L1-2 and L2-3, the image intensifier may need to be rotated not only obliquely but also caudally. For L5-S1, the image intensifier should be rotated cranially to allow the needle to clear the iliac crest. The operator should visualize a triangle consisting of the bottom

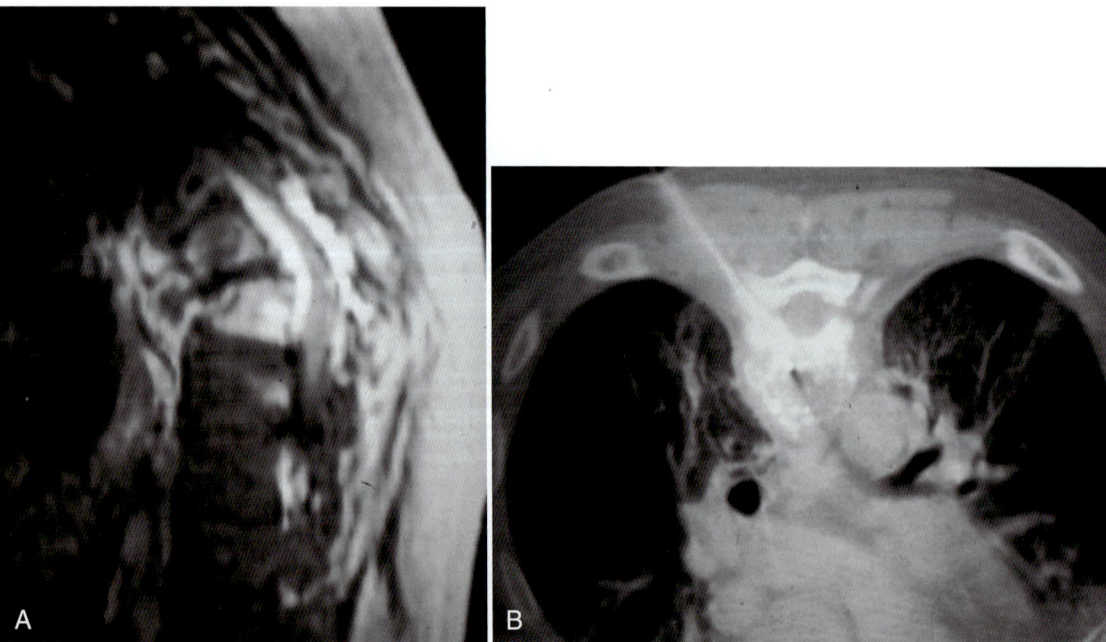

Figure 7-2 A: A 36-year-old man positive for human immunodeficiency virus and PPD (purified protein derivative) complained of back pain and lower-extremity weakness. The presumed diagnosis was tuberculous epidural phlegmon. **B:** Computed tomography–guided needle biopsy reveals *Candida* instead of tuberculosis, which dramatically alters the treatment. This is an example of how imaging without image-guided tissue sampling is relatively nonspecific.

of the L5 vertebral body, the medial border of the iliac crest, and the lateral border of the superior articular facet. The needle must pass through this triangle. A curve on the needle may help the needle to pass up and over the iliac crest. Upon reaching the level of the L5–S1 disc, a twist on the needle will allow it to pass into the disc parallel to the end plates. In cases of very high iliac crests, the triangle may be very difficult to visualize. Side bending the patient away from direction of the needle entry may help to open this space (Figure 7-4). In some situations, entry into the L5–S1 disc may not be feasible. An alternative method would be transpedicular approach through the L5 pedicle. If the disc needs to be sampled in addition to the bone, the trajectory of the needle can be angled superiorly or inferiorly to reach the suspicious disc.

Transpedicular biopsies use the same technique as vertebroplasty and kyphoplasty. The transpedicular entry is an extremely safe means of obtaining tissue samples when done properly. However, you should be careful to avoid a path that enters too medially so as not to breach the spinal canal (lateral recess) or enters too inferiorly so as not to injure the exiting nerve in the neuroforamen (Figures 7-5 through 7-8).

For facet joints biopsies, a posterior oblique approach is taken with the needle directed en face into the slit of the joint. For sacroiliac joint aspirations, a medial to lateral approach usually is taken when performed by fluoroscopy. Remember that the synovial portion of the sacroiliac joint is the more inferior portion, whereas the fibrous portion is the more superior portion.

CT is advantageous over fluoroscopy when the targets are difficult to visualize fluoroscopically or when biopsies must be done with very precise targeting (often to avoid injury to adjacent critical structures such as the kidney, aorta, iliac arteries, or inferior vena cava; Figures 7-9 and 7-10).

Thoracic Spine Biopsies: Problem Solving, How Dangerous? How To Perform?

Challenges to performing thoracic spine biopsies include avoiding the lung, aorta, inferior vena cava, heart, nerve roots, and spinal cord. Other challenges are complications related to extreme kyphotic curvatures, diminished visualization because of large shoulders, and difficult entries because of small pedicles. In addition, the thoracic pedicles are angled more superiorly to inferiorly than are lumbar pedicles, which are oriented more horizontally. This makes it necessary to carefully scrutinize the angle of entry, particularly of upper thoracic pedicles on the lateral fluoroscopic view in order to avoid piercing the exiting nerve root and to set the proper starting point on the skin (usually more superior that expected).

CT is frequently used for thoracic spine biopsies. CT permits clear visualization of adjacent structures that need to be avoided (Figure 7-11).

The typical entries for thoracic biopsies include the costovertebral approach and the transpedicular approach. In the costovertebral approach, the needle passes just lateral to the pedicle and medial to the adjacent rib head (Figure 7-12). This allows the needle pass from posterior to anterior with a lateral to medial angulation for more centralized sampling. When this approach is taken by fluoroscopy, the operator must concentrate on visualizing the pedicle (to stay away from the spinal cord) and the rib head (to keep the needle medial to the rib head so as to avoid injury to the lung) (Figures 7-13 and 7-14).

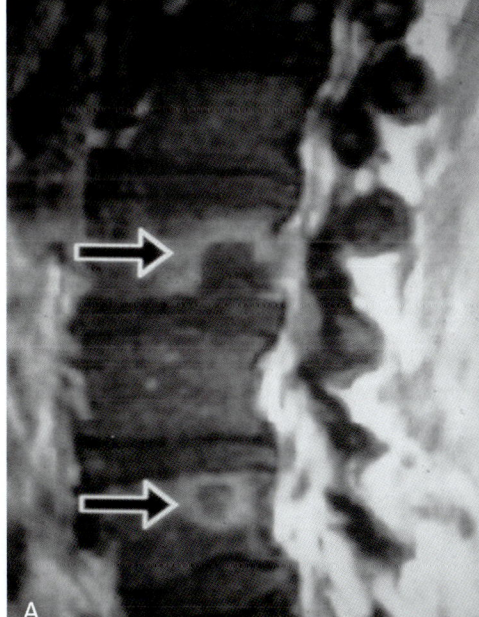
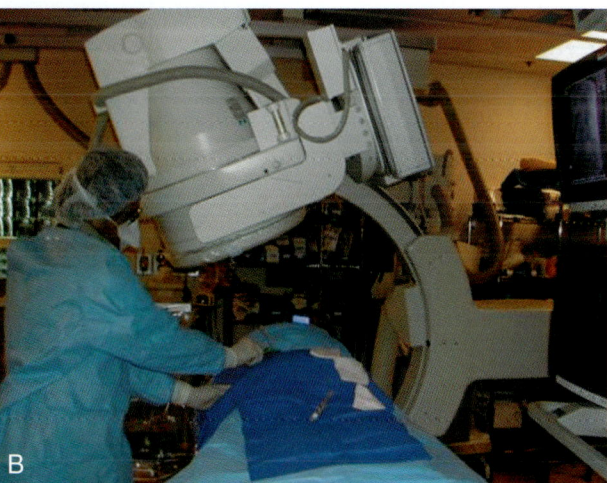

Figure 7-3 **A:** A 43-year-old male with a history of intravenous drug abuse complained of low back pain and had an elevated temperature to 101.3°F. **B:** Prone oblique approach.

continued

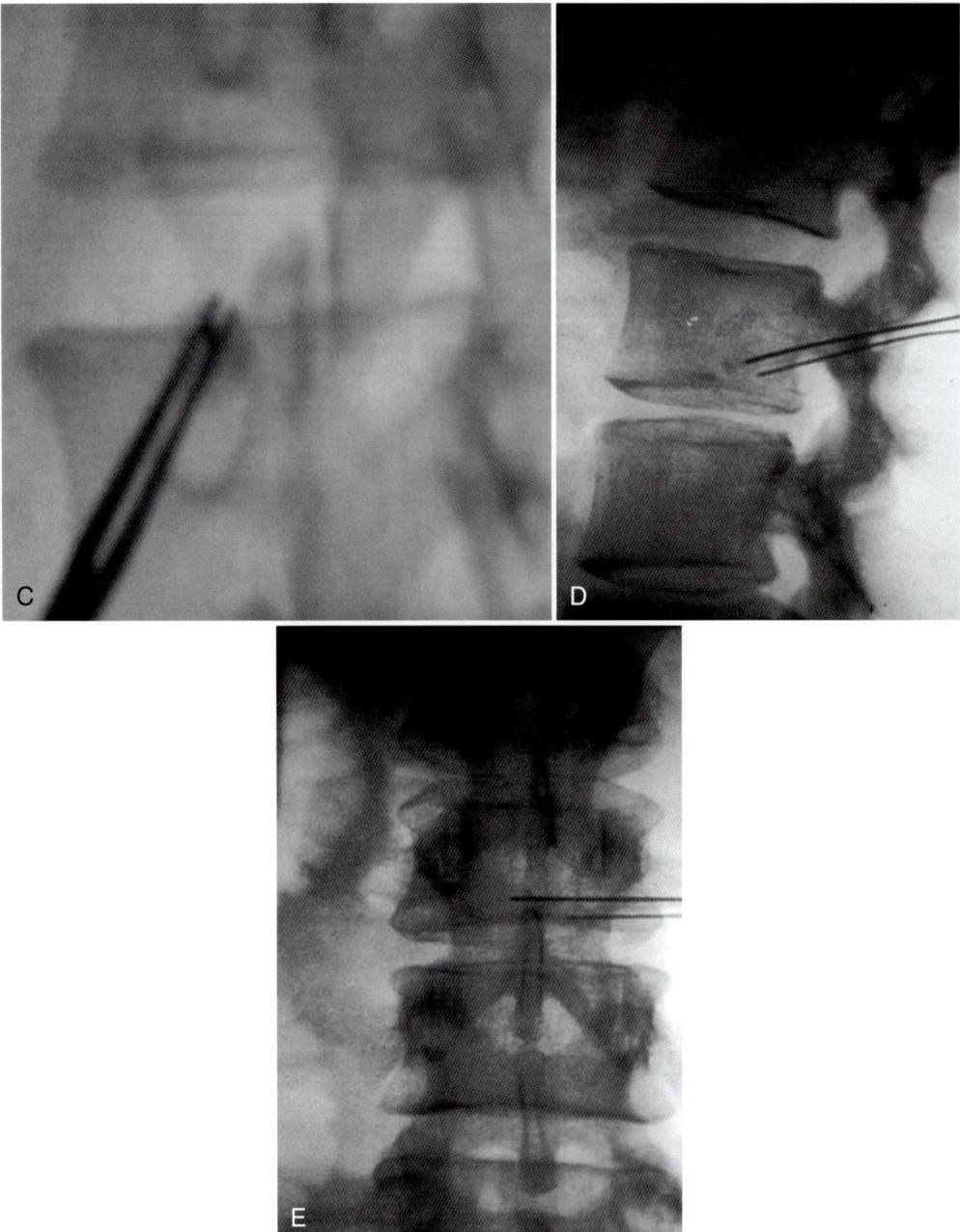

Figure 7-3, cont'd C: En face view of the forceps guiding the needle to the target in typical discographic technique. The superior articular facet bisects the diameter of the disc. The needle is started just anterior to the superior articular facet. This helps to target the needle on the center of the disc. D: Lateral orthogonal confirmatory view. E: Anteroposterior orthogonal view confirms that the needle is centrally located.

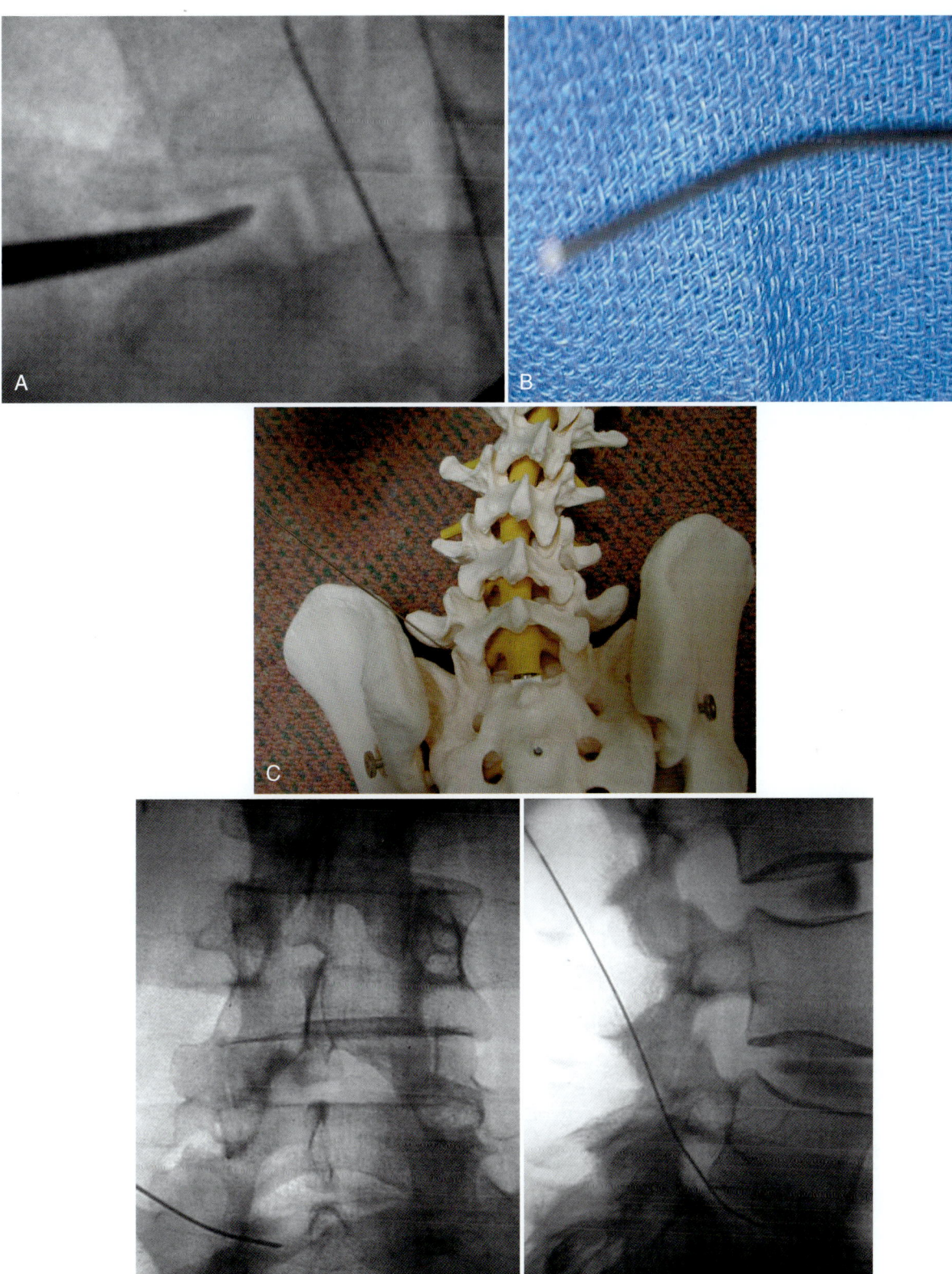

Figure 7-4 A: For L5–S1 disc biopsy, discographic technique is used. In order to visualize the open triangle between the S1 superior articular facet, the iliac crest, and the inferior end plate of L5, the fluoroscope must be turned not only obliquely but also cranially (tip of forceps points to open triangle). **B:** An aid to L5–S1 disc entry is applying a bend on the end of the needle, which allows it to rise over the iliac crest and then level out in the plane of the disc with a final twist of the wrist. **C:** Another aid to clearing the iliac crest is side bending the patient away from the direction of entry. **D:** Anteroposterior view of L5S1 discogram demonstrating L5–S1 disc entry technique with curved needle rotated to parallel the disc margins. **E:** Lateral view of L5–S1 discogram with curve of the needle finally rotated to parallel the axis of the disc after it had been passed over the iliac crest and downward to the L5–S1 disc.

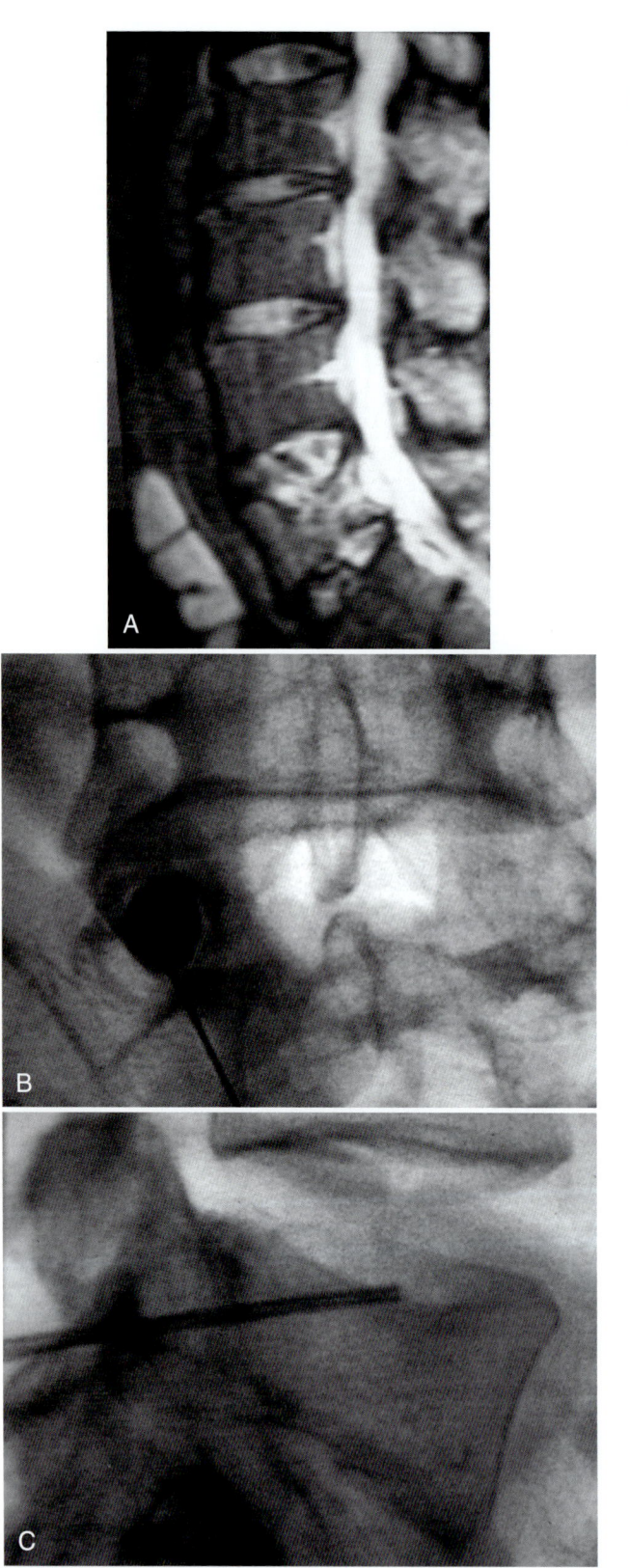
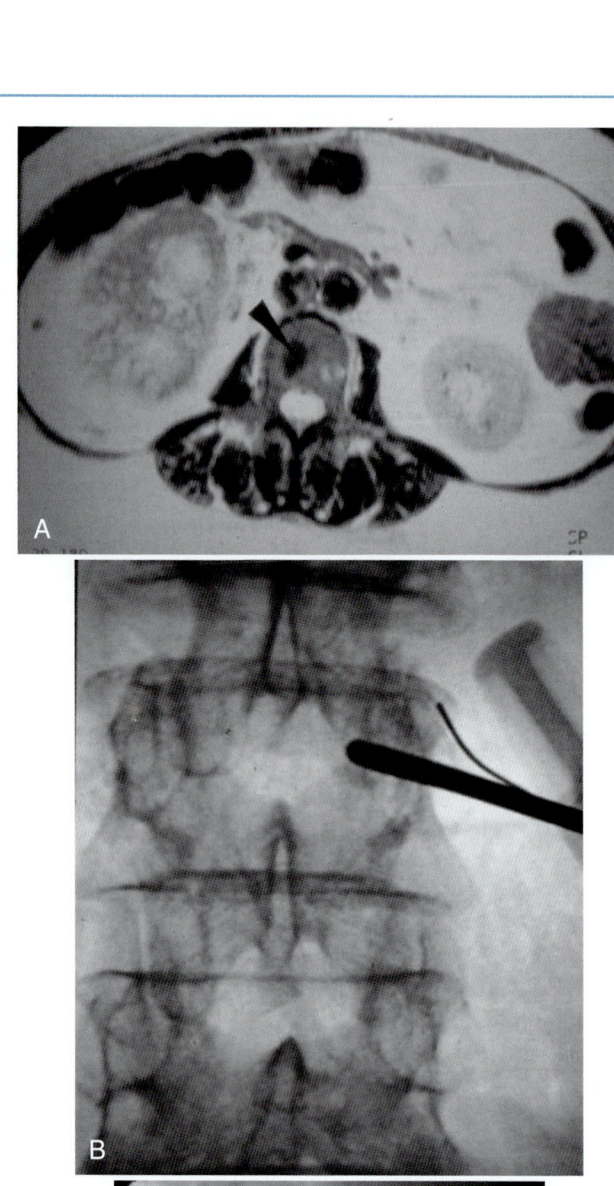
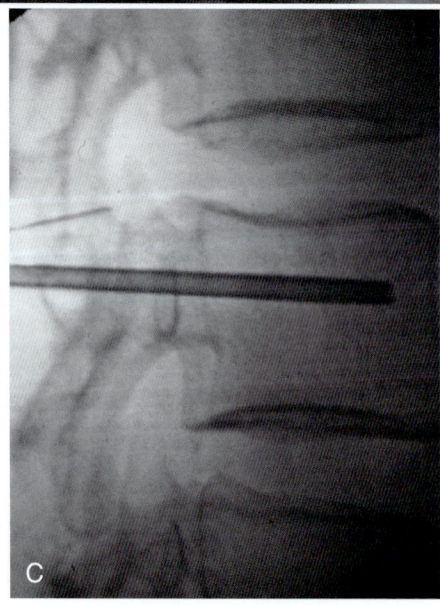

Figure 7-5 A: A 58-year-old man complained of low back pain and had a low-grade fever. He was unable to complete the magnetic resonance imaging examination, so postcontrast scans were not available. He had six lumbar vertebra and very high iliac crests, which made biopsy at L6–S1 difficult. **B:** A transpedicular approach was selected. The needle is directed through the L6 pedicle. **C:** From the transpedicular approach the needle is angled upward to include the L5–6 disc. Pathologic diagnosis is *Escherichia coli* infection.

Figure 7-6 A: A 57-year-old woman complained of back pain and had hematuria. This cases demonstrates a potential problem with the posterolateral approach in that the renal mass might be inadvertently punctured because it cannot be seen fluoroscopically. **B:** An alternative to the posterolateral approach is the transpedicular approach performed fluoroscopically. **C:** Lateral view. Pathologic diagnosis confirmed renal cell carcinoma metastasis. Making this diagnosis led to a less invasive treatment option.

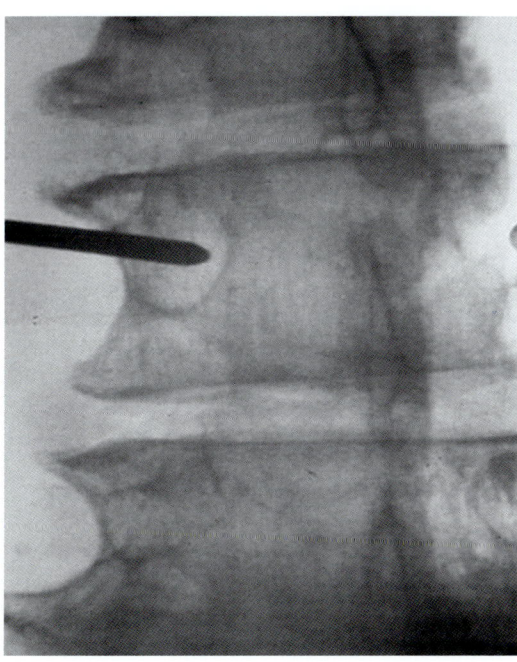

Figure 7-7 Safe technique for transpedicular biopsy involves engaging the pedicle by staying away from the medial border (spinal canal) and inferior border (neuroforamen).

Cervical Spine Biopsies: Problem Solving, Isn't This Risky? How To Perform?

Challenges to performing cervical spine biopsies include avoiding the carotid and vertebral arteries, jugular vein, nerve roots, cranial nerves, spinal cord, esophagus, and trachea.

A variety of approaches for cervical spine biopsies can be used, all of which carry elevated risk compared to thoracic and lumbar approaches. The approaches include posterior oblique (through the pedicle), anterior lateral (similar to cervical discography), or direct anterior to posterior (transoral).

Because of the critical targeting, CT guidance is most frequently relied upon for cervical spine biopsies.

For posterior lateral approaches, a smaller needle may be needed because the pedicles are very small. Be aware of the course of the vertebral artery as it enters the transverse foramen at C6 and exits at C1 to pass into the foramen magnum. The carotid sheath includes the carotid artery, the jugular vein, cervical sympathetics, cranial nerves IX through XII, and internal jugular lymph nodes. The facial nerve and external carotid artery run through the parotid gland and usually are located posterior to the mandible. The cervical nerve roots exit the neuroforamen and take an anterolateral–inferior course. Because of the complex nature of adjacent vascular structures that are frequently difficult to visualize even by CT, iodine contrast may be necessary (Figures 7-15 through 7-18).

Anteroposterior approaches can be performed transorally. Challenges include airway integrity, sterility, and oral access maintenance. For the airway, the patient should be intubated with a sealing cuff to prevent fluids (e.g., secretions, blood, sterilizing fluids) from entering the airway prior to the procedure. Preparation can be done with povidone–iodine (Betadine). We typically use a plastic vaginal speculum to keep the mouth open. CT guidance is required because the targeting must be very precise to avoid penetrating too deeply and injuring the spinal cord (Figure 7-19).

For anterolateral approaches, fluoroscopy can be used similarly to cervical discographic technique. Because the esophagus is situated slightly to the left of the midline, the typical approach starts from the right. The technique consists of pressing firmly along the anteromedial aspect of the sternocleidomastoid muscle in such a way to displace the carotid sheath laterally and the visceral space (trachea and esophagus) medially. This permits a small window of opportunity in which to start the needle toward the center of the spine. In the process of starting the needle, the fluoroscope can be activated momentarily. Once the needle has entered superficially past the carotid sheath and visceral space, a set of forceps can be used to direct the needle either into the targeting disc space or onto the vertebral body. Because the cervical spine components are small, multiple orthogonal planes should be frequently scrutinized in order to avoid injury to vertebral artery, nerve roots, and spinal cord (Figure 7-20).

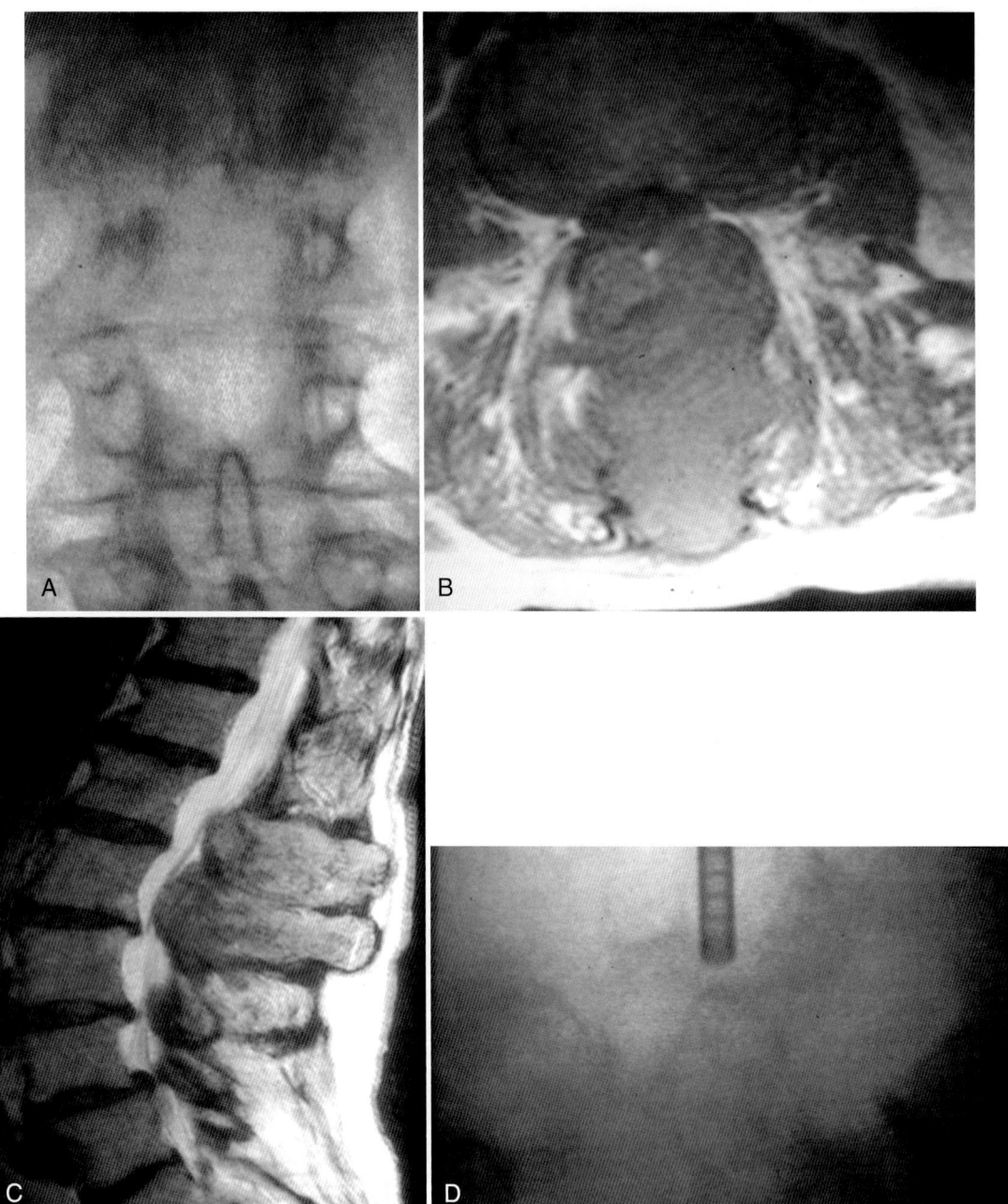

Figure 7-8 A: A 66-year-old male complained of low back pain. Plain films reveal destruction of posterior elements of L1 and L2. **B:** Axial T1 at L2 level showing mass invading posterior elements. **C:** T2-weighted images demonstrating expansile masses of the posterior elements of L1 and L2. **D:** Even though this biopsy would be more clearly guided by computed tomography or magnetic resonance imaging, it still can be safely performed under fluoroscopic guidance by keeping the needle in the midline and staying posterior to the spinal laminar line. Pathologic diagnosis is adenocarcinoma metastatic.

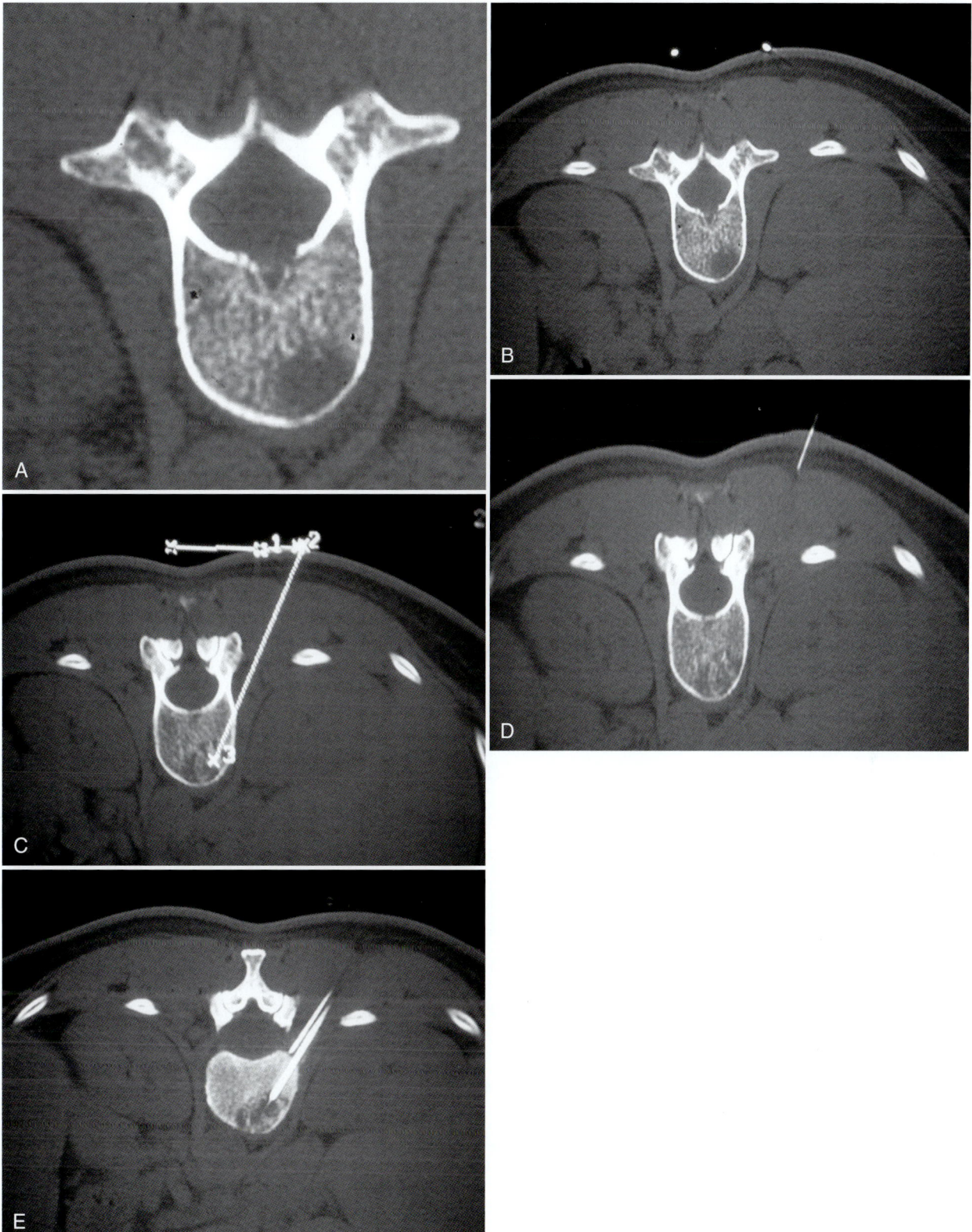

Figure 7-9 **A:** A 48-year-old woman with a history of breast cancer presented with suspicious lesion. **B:** Identifying reference grids on skin surface. **C:** Using the laser light at the cut level referable to the lesion, distances can be measured from the reference marks on the skin to the expected starting point, after which angle of trajectory and depth of needle can be established. **D:** Setting local anesthetic needle along intended course. **E:** Parallel (tandem) technique of guiding the biopsy needle along the course of the already satisfactorily set anesthetic needle to the target point is used in this case. Coaxial passage is another option but requires initial placement of a needle larger than the biopsy needle. Pathologic diagnosis is intraosseous disc (not metastasis).

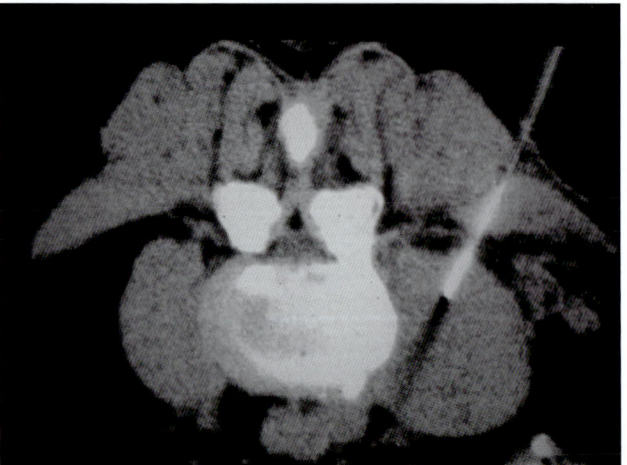

Figure 7-10 A 47-year-old man complained of right lower back pain. The enlarged clinically painful psoas muscle would be difficult to identify on fluoroscopy but can be easily identified and targeted under computed tomographic (CT) guidance. Thus, one of the important considerations favoring CT over fluoroscopy is a soft tissue target without bony landmarks. Biopsy was performed with a 25-gauge thin needle, which retrieved adequate cells to diagnose a transitional cell carcinoma before the primary was found.

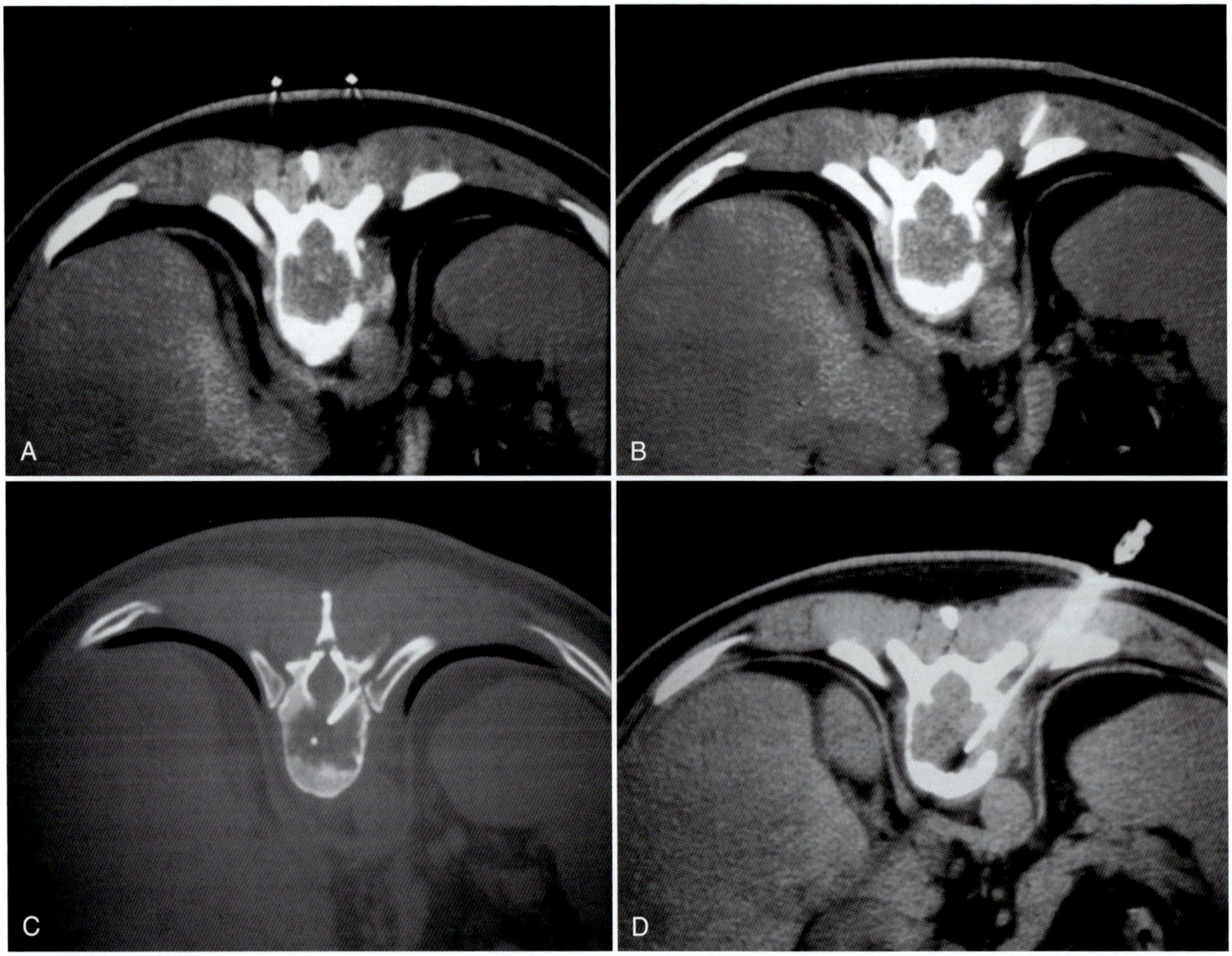

Figure 7-11 A: A 65-year-old man complained of weight loss and upper back pain. Computed tomography (CT) of the thorax reveals lytic lesion of T8. **B:** CT guidance for biopsy is often preferred when precise targeting is needed, such as adjacent to lung or critical blood vessels (e.g., aorta). **C:** For thoracic spine biopsies, a costovertebral approach permits safe needle passage medial to the rib head and along the lateral base of the pedicle. Staying medial to the rib head, whether by CT or fluoroscopy, helps to keep the needle out of the lung. **D:** Pathologic diagnosis is squamous cell carcinoma metastasis.

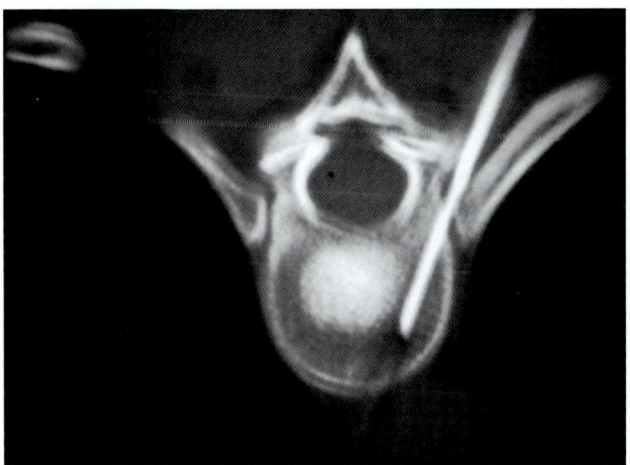

Figure 7-12 Example of computed tomography–guided costovertebral approach. Pathologic diagnosis is prostate cancer.

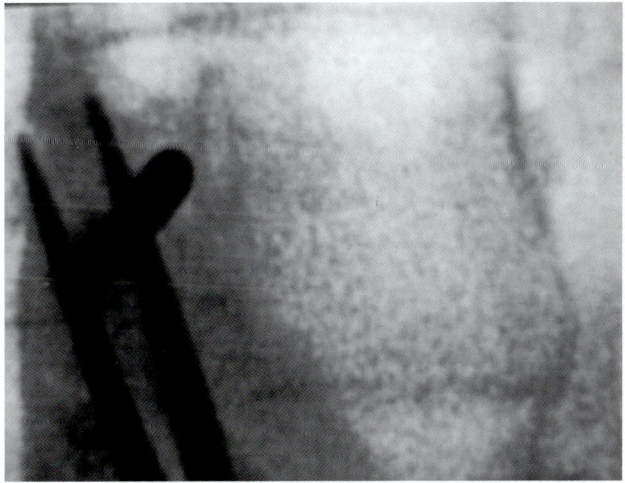

Figure 7-13 Fluoroscopically guided needle biopsy at T5 level using the costovertebral approach. Note how the needle tip is lateral to the pedicle and medial to the rib head. The forceps controls the needle deliberately, preventing the weight of the needle handle from toppling the needle and possibly causing injury to the lung.

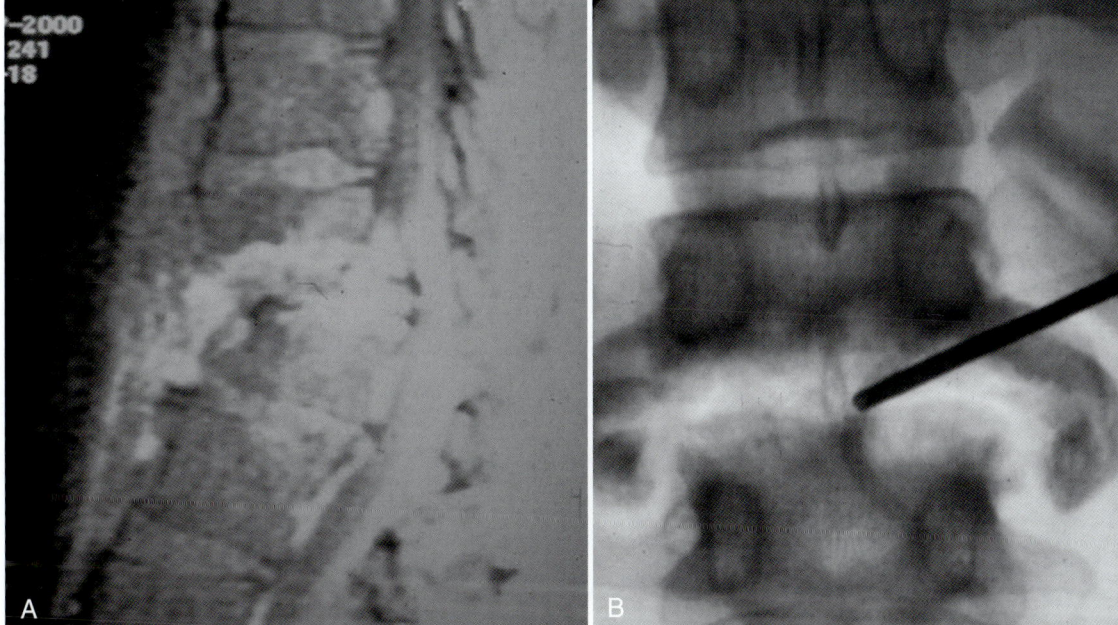

Figure 7-14 A: A 40-year-old paraplegic man in urosepsis. Magnetic resonance imaging reveals worrisome appearance of discitis and osteomyelitis at T12–L1. B: Fluoroscopically guided large-core biopsy was performed at the level of the disc parallel to a costovertebral trajectory. Pathologic diagnosis was fibrosis, aseptic consistent with neuropathic changes.

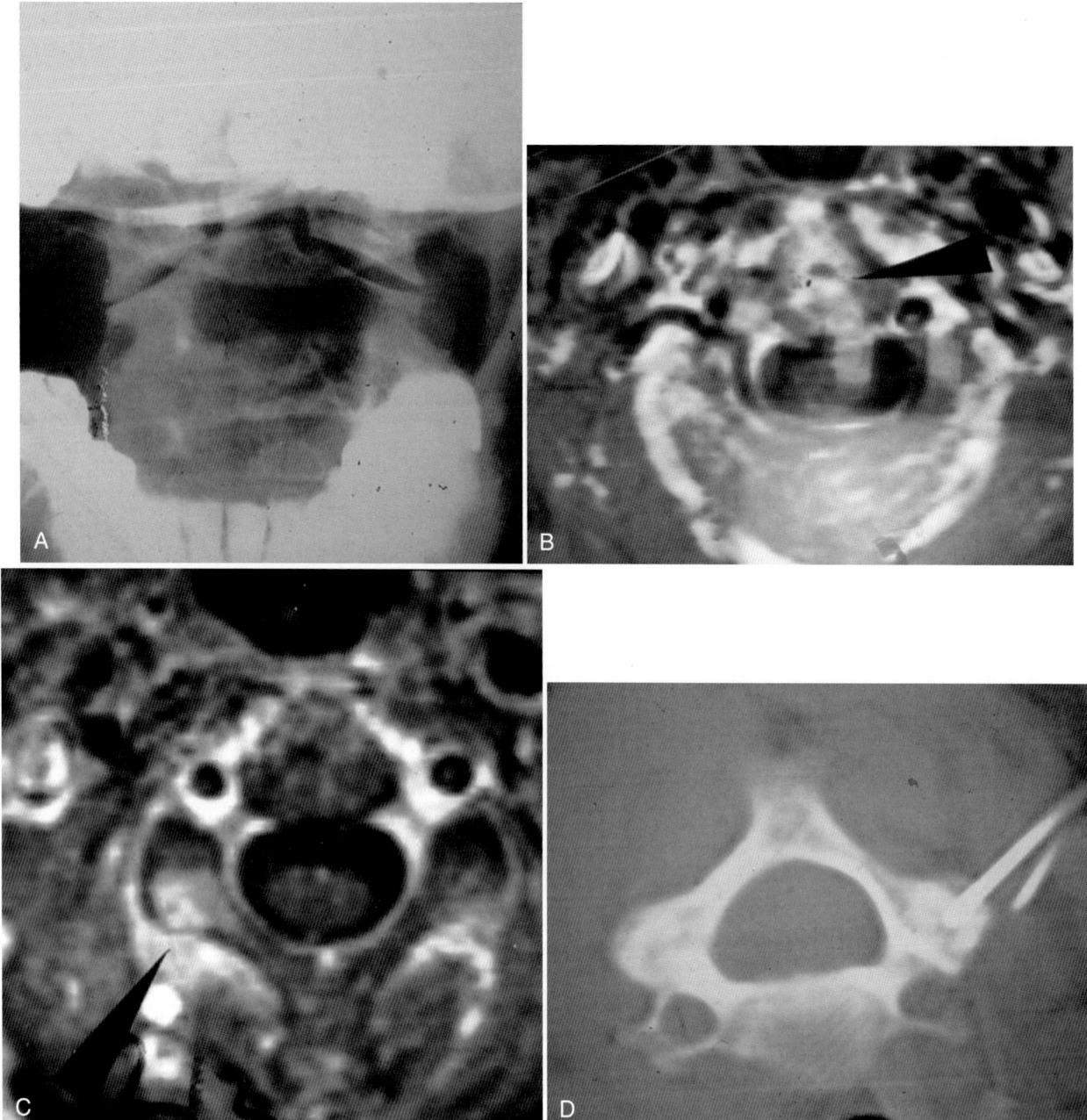

Figure 7-15 A: Odontoid view showing lytic defect at C2 level in a 77-year-old woman who complained of increasing neck pain. She had a history of breast cancer 15 years prior and mycobacterium 5 years prior. She was told that she was cured of both. **B:** Axial T1 postgadolinium demonstrates enhancing mass center of the vertebral body of C2. The trajectory for biopsy of this lesion is precarious with the vertebral artery, carotid sheath, pharynx, spinal cord, and nerve roots surrounding the target. **C:** Axial T1 postgadolinium at the level of the neuroforamen demonstrating a more accessible target on the pedicle–lamina junction. **D:** The most accessible and safest approach is often the best. Pathologic diagnosis is breast cancer metastasis.

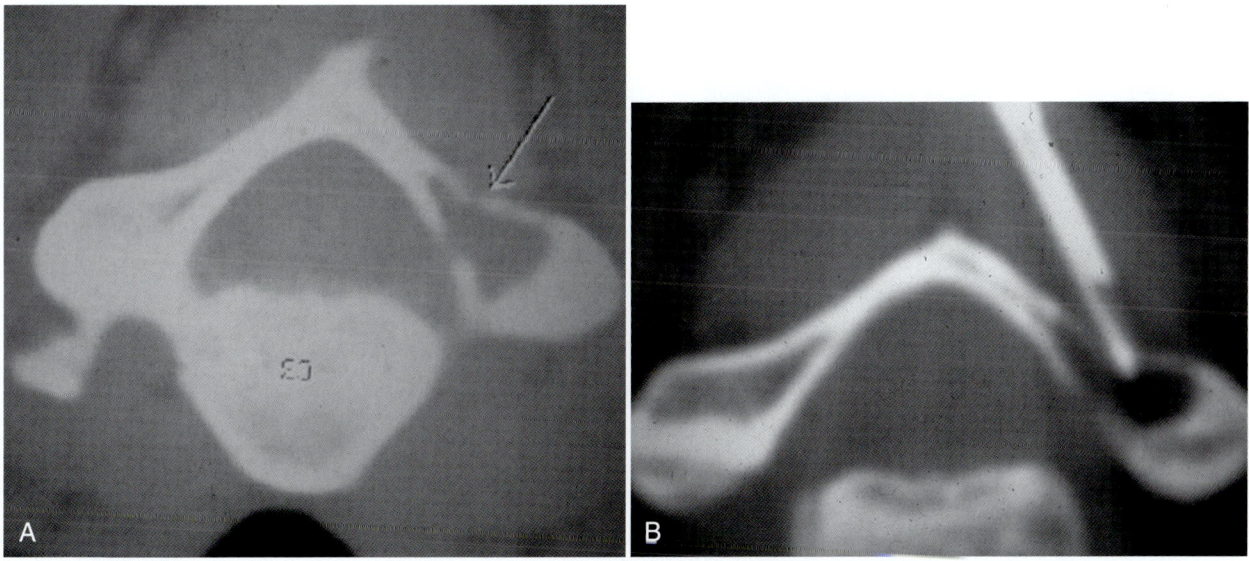

Figure 7-16 **A:** A 42-year-old man complained of upper neck pain. **B:** Biopsy trajectory taken to avoid possible injury to vertebral artery exiting nerve root and spinal cord should needle overshoot the target. Pathologic diagnosis is aneurysmal bone cyst.

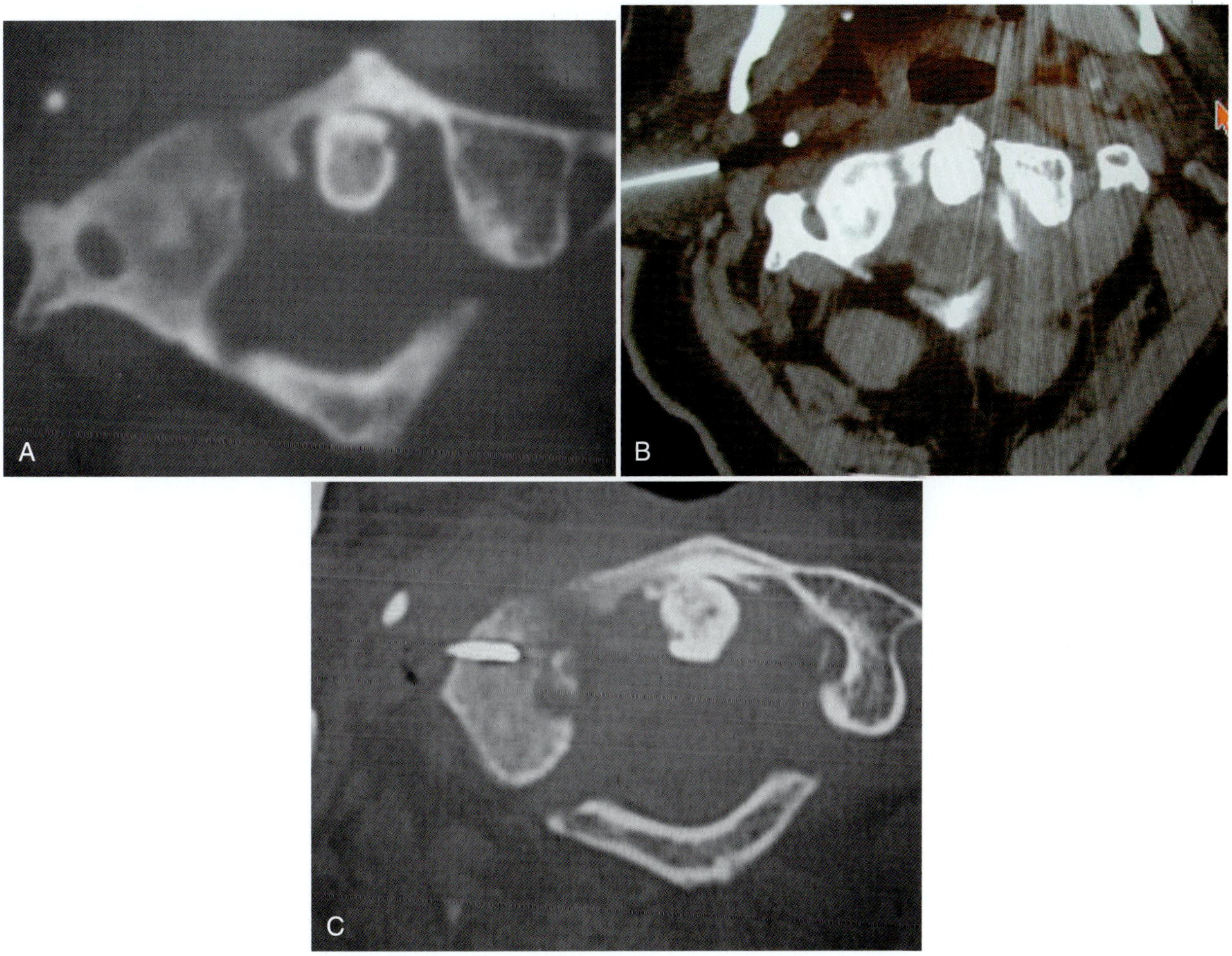

Figure 7-17 **A:** An 84-year-old man complained of upper neck pain. Computed tomographic (CT) scan reveals enlargement and altered mineralization of the right lateral facet of C1. **B:** Obtaining access to this lesion risks causing injury to the vertebral artery, facial nerve, carotid sheath, exiting nerve root, and spinal cord. **C:** The needle is precisely directed through a tight space. Pathologic diagnosis is prostate carcinoma metastasis. This example demonstrates the value of CT for precise targeting.

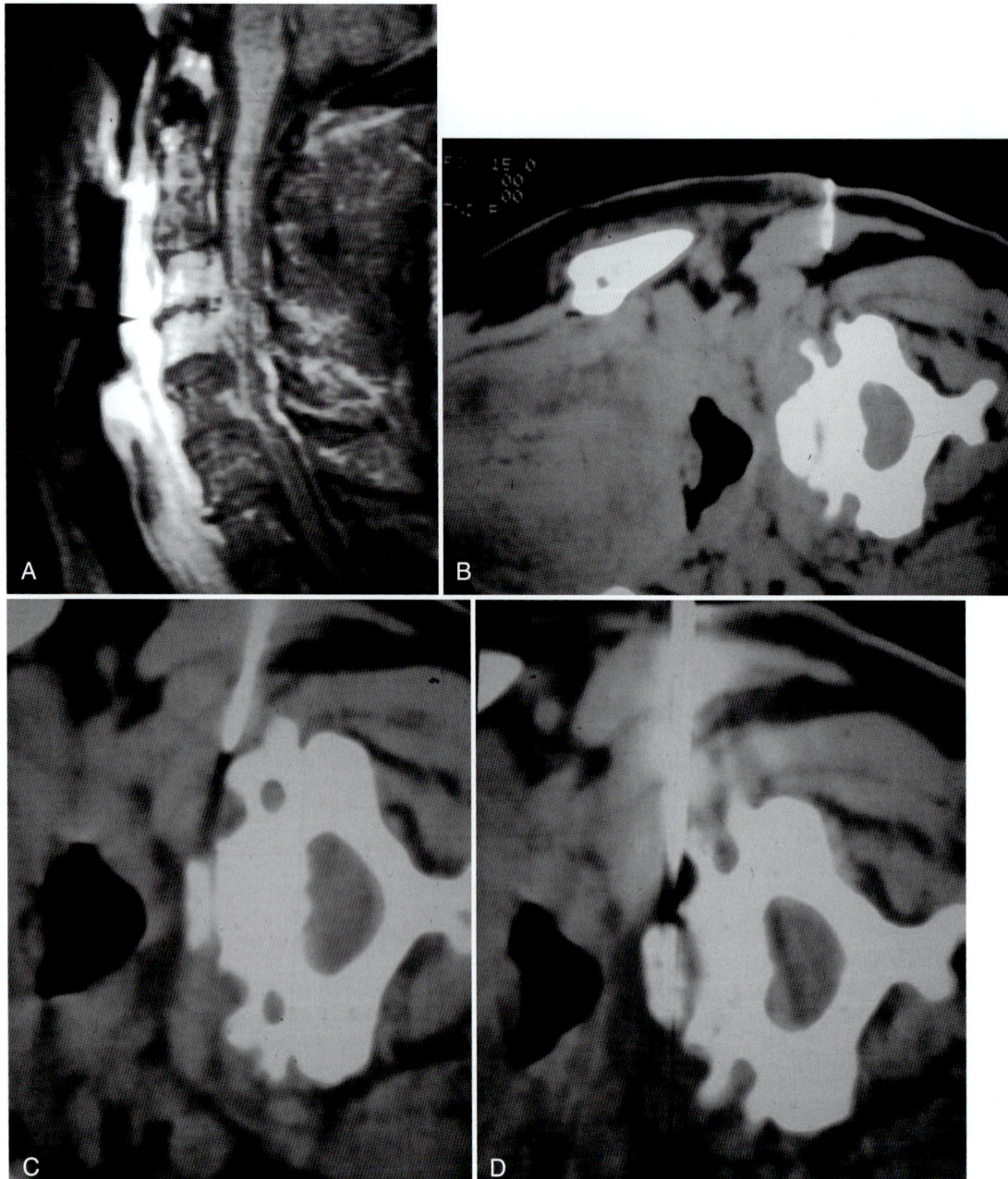

Figure 7-18 A: A 77-year-old woman with a medical history of breast cancer and diabetes. **B:** Targeting challenges include the vertebral artery and carotid sheath. Because the lesion could represent infection, a trajectory through the pharynx is avoided. **C:** A rigid 180-gauge needle is directed posterior to the carotid sheath and then angled anteriorly. **D:** After shoving the carotid sheath anteriorly with the shaft of the needle, the needle is redirected to sample the lesion. Pathologic diagnosis is *Escherichia coli* infection.

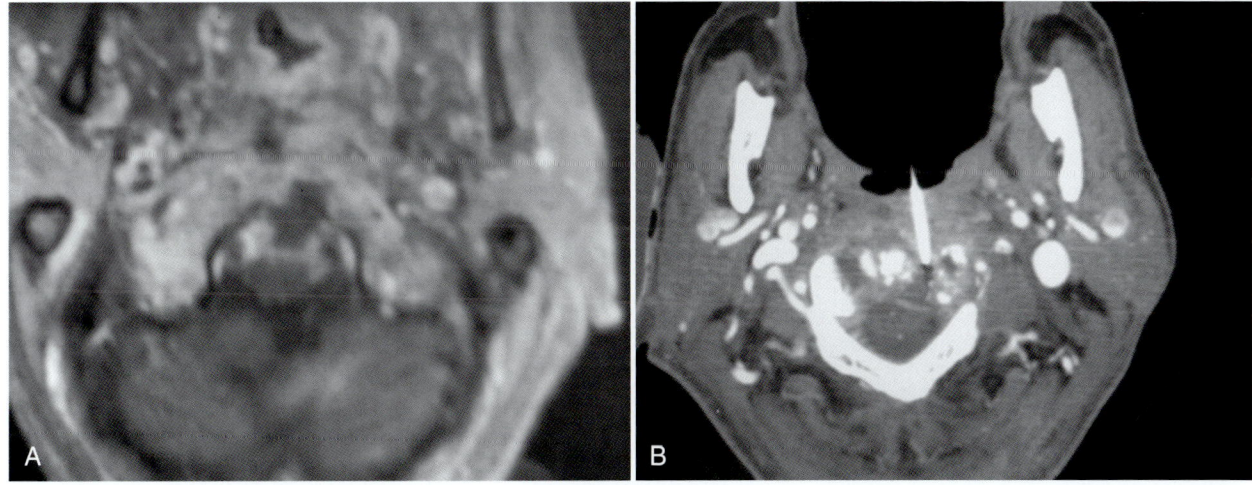

Figure 7-19 A: A 54-year-old man positive for human immunodeficiency virus and with a history of lymphoma complained of neck pain. His temperature was 99.9°F, and his white blood cell count was 9,900. Abnormal enhancement included odontoid, C1, and the clivus. Surgeons were uncomfortable with performing biopsy. **B:** Percutaneous biopsy targeting is difficult from almost any angle. Challenges include the carotid artery, facial nerve, mandible, pharynx, vertebral artery, nerve root, and spinal cord. A transoral approach was taken. Challenges, which include the airway, sterility, and maintaining an open mouth, were resolved by tracheal intubation, use of Betadine preparation, and use of a plastic vaginal speculum. Pathologic diagnosis is *Enterobacter* infection.

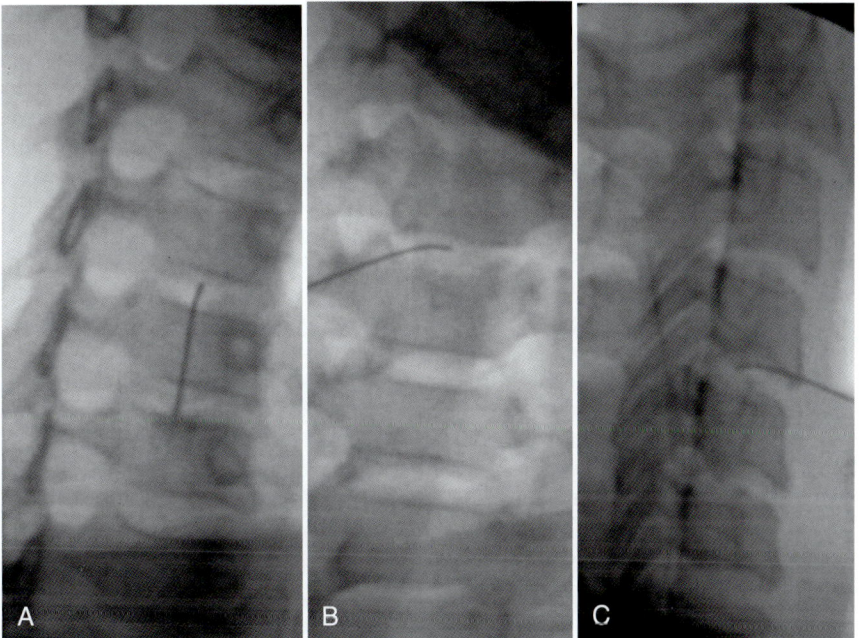

Figure 7-20 A: Anterolateral approaches for cervical spine biopsies can be performed under fluoroscopic guidance using cervical discographic technique. Enter from right side of neck (because esophagus lies left of midline); press down between carotid sheath and visceral space (just anterior to sternocleidomastoid muscle); and direct needle to target, checking on anteroposterior (AP) and lateral views for confirmation. **B:** AP view confirming that needle is correctly positioned in center of target. **C:** Lateral view confirming that needle is correctly positioned in target (and not elsewhere, e.g., in spinal cord).

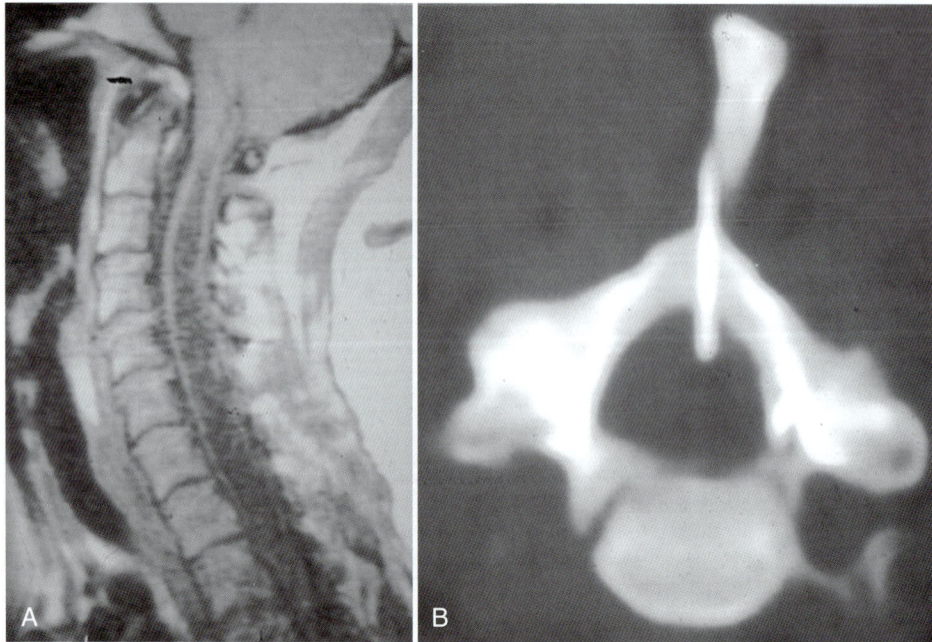

Figure 7-21 **A:** A 27-year-old man complained of increasing weakness and spasticity. Differential diagnosis included syrinx versus neoplasm such as astrocytoma. **B:** Intradural intramedullary needle biopsy was performed with 25-gauge needle and very gentle aspiration. Cerebrospinal fluid (CSF) was acquired and confirmed the diagnosis of syrinx. Subsequently 11 ml of CSF was removed for syringe provocative drainage test. The patient's symptoms improved. This led to intraoperative syrinx drainage for long-lasting decompression.

■ INTRADURAL BIOPSIES: ISN'T THIS FOR NEUROSURGEONS?

Intradural biopsies may be simply a matter of collecting cerebrospinal fluid (CSF) for diagnosis of meningitis. However, if fluid is needed for diagnosis of intradural tumor (e.g., lymphoma or drop metastases), then a large-volume sampling may be required in order to obtain a sufficient cells for diagnosis.

A lumbar puncture is commonly performed under fluoroscopic guidance. A straight down between the spinous processes approach usually works well on young patients. However, in older patients with degenerative bony hypertrophy, a translaminar approach may be more reliable in gaining needle passage. A translaminar approach is taken from a slight lateral to medial angulation with the needle directed to the sublaminar zone of the level above the entry site. Visualization under fluoroscopic guidance is usually accentuated by slight caudal angulation of the image intensifier.

Problem Solving: Canal Stenosis and Lumbar Puncture

Remember that the conus usually is situated about T12–L1, and entry should be below that level. Older patients often have limited flow of CSF below L4–5, not uncommonly because of a higher degree of central canal stenosis at L4–5 and perhaps also at L3–4. Therefore, if CSF fails to flow with a lumbar puncture at L5–S1, a second attempt should be made perhaps at the L2–3 level.

If there is clinical evidence or suspicion of blockage to the flow of CSF, a C1–2 puncture, the needle should be placed in the posterior third of the spinal canals so as to avoid the spinal cord. The patient must remain compliant and still during this procedure. In addition, correct orientation without excessive rotation must be maintained. This may mean aligning the rami of the mandible as a reference so that consistent orientation is maintained. Orthogonal views should be obtained frequently during the procedure.

Intradural biopsies may also involve soft tissue masses intradurally. The introduction of myelographic contrast and/or the use of CT or even magnetic resonance imaging (MRI) may be helpful in visualizing the target. Biopsy of a lesion of the spinal cord is a high-risk procedure that could lead to permanent neurologic injury, particularly if bleeding occurs. If an intradural soft mass must undergo image-guided biopsy, a thin 25-gauge needle with very gentle movements and very conservative aspiration should be considered. In most cases, intradural biopsies should be reserved for those with direct neurosurgical expertise (Figures 7-21 and 7-22).

■ WHAT TO BIOPSY WHEN THERE ARE MULTIPLE TARGETS?

When multiple targets are present, target selection should be considered in order of priority based on relative risk, accessibility, visualization, and operator confidence (competence) (Figures 7-15 and 7-23).

■ WHAT TO DO WHEN THE BIOPSY IS DONE?

Postbiopsy risks include bleeding, vasovagal responses, and anesthetic and sedation recovery. Therefore, patients should be watched either in a holding area or in a

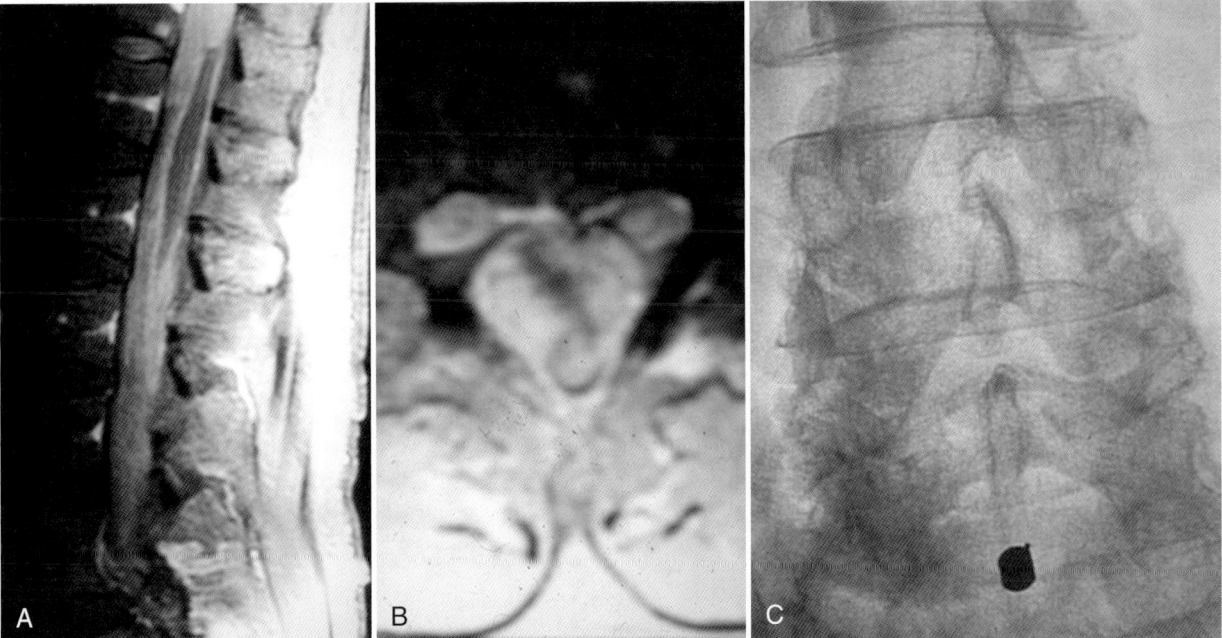

Figure 7-22 T1 postgadolinium images in sagittal (**A**) and axial (**B**) views demonstrating densely enhancing mass surrounding the conus and filling the subconus space in a 27-year-old woman who was progressively developing cauda equina syndrome. **B:** Axial image. **C:** Fine-needle biopsy was gently performed intradurally with a 25-gauge needle. Pathologic diagnosis is chromic lymphocytic leukemia.

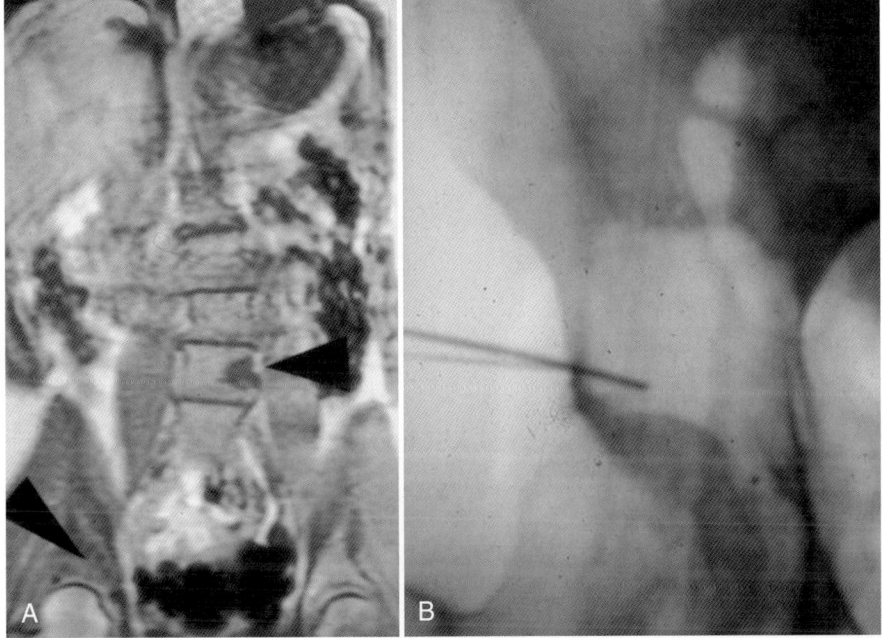

Figure 7-23 A: A 47-year-old woman complained of low back pain. She had a low-grade fever of 100.8°F and a history of intravenous drug abuse. Referring physicians requested a spine biopsy. An additional lesion was observed at the right acetabulum. Because the patient was having difficulty laying still while she demanding more opiates, the more easily accessible and lower-risk target (the acetabular lesion) was chosen. **B:** Biopsy of the acetabulum was performed in less than 5 minutes. Pathologic diagnosis is breast cancer metastasis. Targeting the more easily accessible, lower-risk lesion first often is a better choice.

postanesthesia care unit for a reasonable period of time, possibly 1 to 2 hours, until established discharge criteria are met. If a prebiopsy embolization for a hypervascular mass or an abscess drainage was performed, then a higher level of recovery care, such as inpatient admission or perhaps even ICU admission, should be considered. However, most needle biopsies are performed on an outpatient basis, so postbiopsy patient instructions more commonly include answers to questions such as when it is safe for the patient to eat, drive, bathe, and return to work. Follow-up instructions should be given and appointments made.

■ WHAT ARE THE TOOLS OF THE TRADE?

Depending on the nature of the biopsy, a variety of different types of biopsy needles can be used. In some situations, a thin 25-gauge needle may be all that is necessary, particularly for delicate soft tissue abnormalities. Straight (e.g., Chiba, Francine, Crown) needles in 25, 22, 20, and 18 gauges can be used for sampling cells from soft tissue masses. Crown and Francine needles of similar gauges have teeth at the tip that tend to shred and cut tissue so that a small core of tissue can be obtained (Figure 7-24).

Techniques for MRI-guided biopsies are similar to those for CT, but it is important to ensure that the patient has no contraindication to entering a magnetic field and that the patient does not have any device or product (e.g., ferromagnetic screws) that can cause profound susceptibility artifact and thus obscure imaging of the target. In addition, titanium rather than stainless steel needles (of which the available variety is limited) need to be used.

For osseous lesions, bone biopsy needles from 17 to 11 gauge and even larger may be chosen. For CT

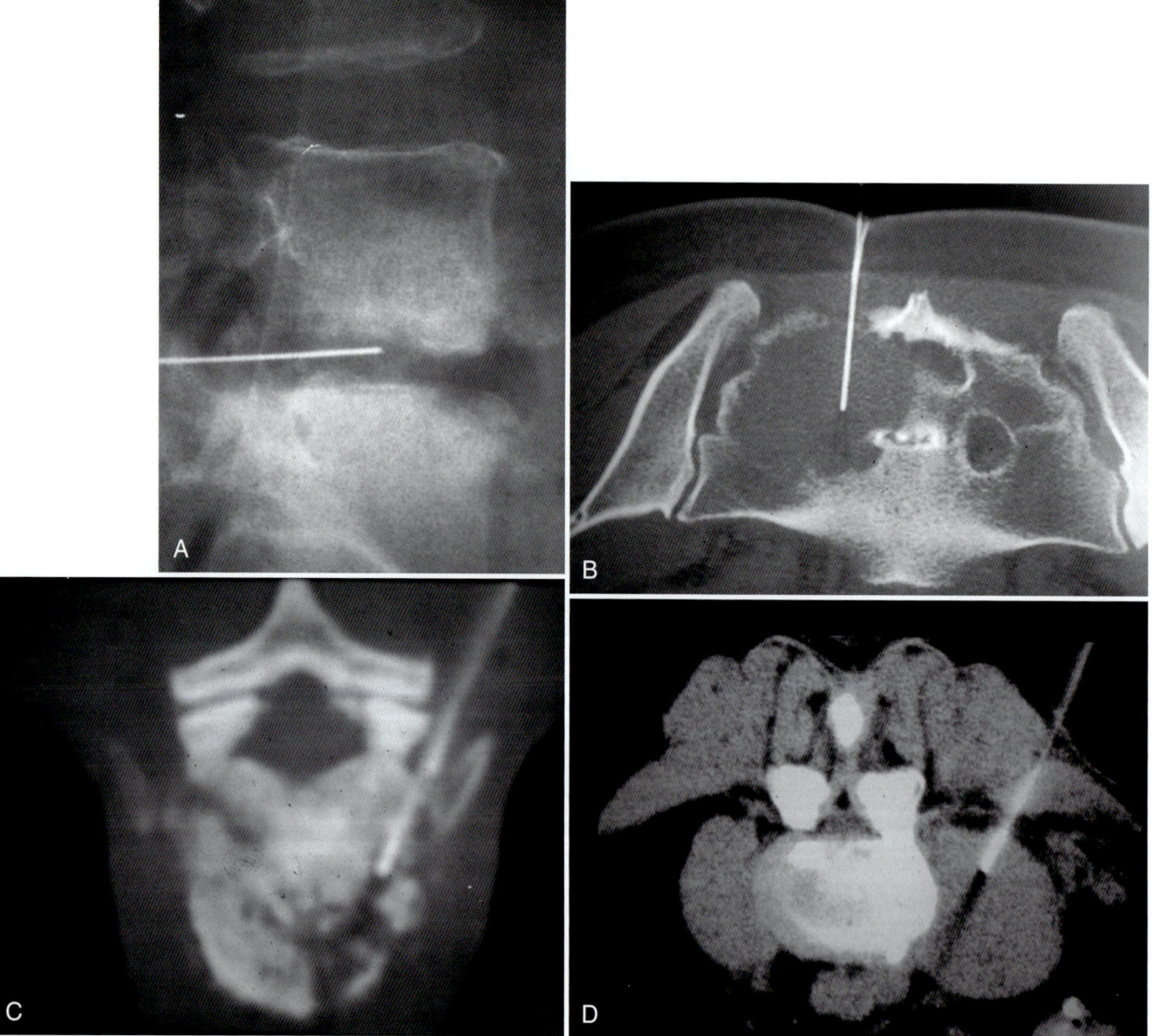

Figure 7-24 A: Straight needles are available in a variety of diameters and lengths. The needle used here was a 20-gauge, 6-inch Chiba needle, which was moved in and out along the disc and angled superiorly and inferiorly to sample the subchondral end plates. Diagnosis is staphylococcal discitis/osteomyelitis. **B:** This lytic lesion was easily sampled using a 20-gauge Crown needle, which has teeth at the tip and tends to yield a core rather than simply cells. Pathologic diagnosis is adenocarcinoma. **C:** An 18-gauge Chiba needle was used to yield the diagnosis of breast cancer metastasis.

guidance, the 17-gauge EZM or 15-gauge Ostycut needles, which do not have heavily weighted handles, may be advantageous because they can be placed in soft tissues under CT guidance without falling out of trajectory when released. For larger sampling of bone, 11-gauge Jamshidi type needles can be used (Figure 7-25).

Bone cores may be difficult to retrieve when the bone is extremely hard, such as osteoblastic bone or very dense bone in young patients. In these situations, placement coaxially of the 17-gauge easy-M needle in the 11-gauge Jamshidi needle may help to loosen the bone core for retrieval. Alternatively, another consideration is use of a drill such as a 3-mm Kyphon drill through a cannula in order to obtain a bone core. When large amounts of material must be retrieved, the 9-gauge Kyphon biopsy device may be selected (Figures 7-26 and 7-27).

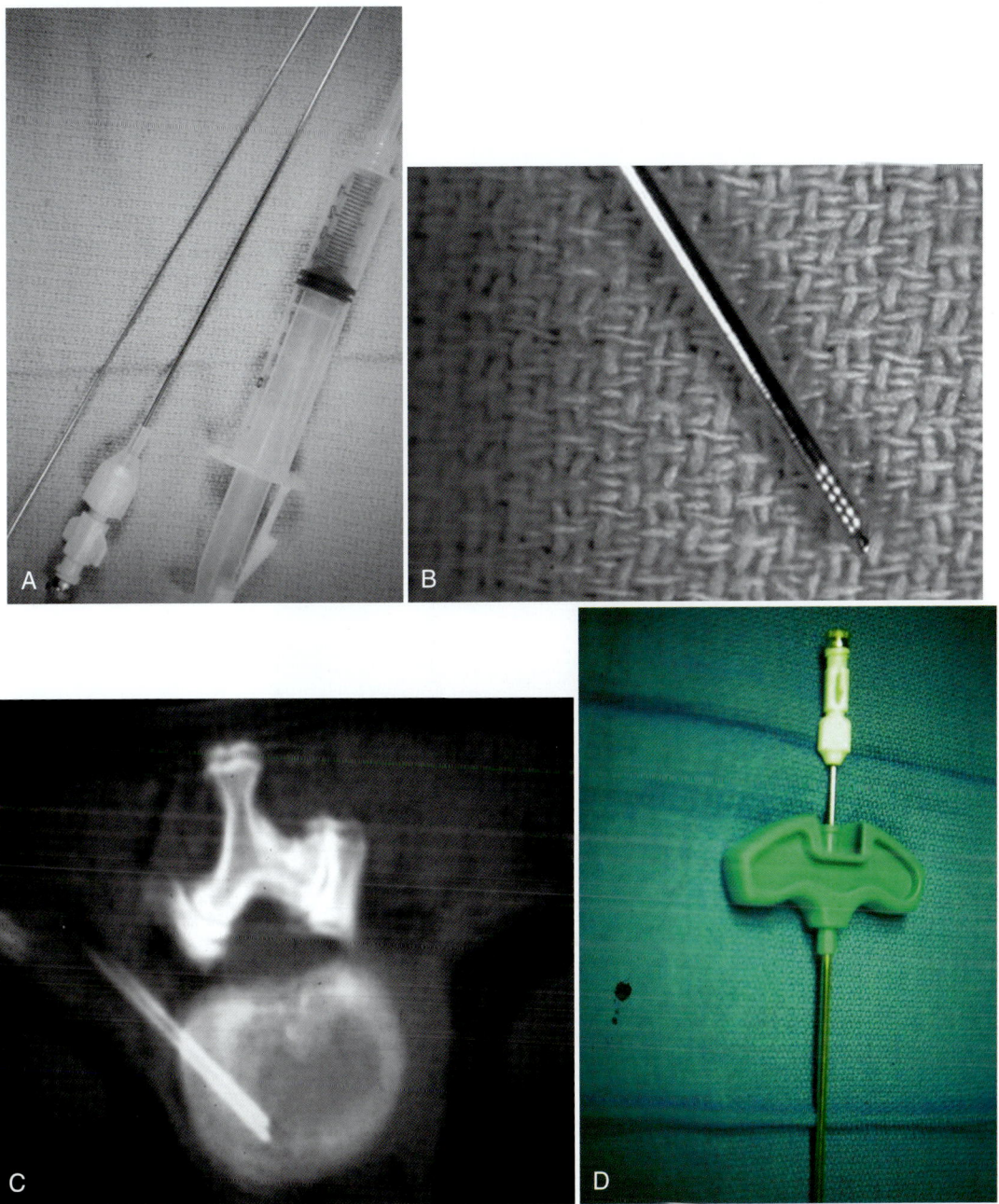

Figure 7-25 **A:** The 17-gauge EZM bone biopsy needle is available in different lengths (5, 7.5, 10, 12.5, 15 cm). It is ideal for computed tomography–guided biopsies because it can be set in soft tissues along its intended trajectory and it does not have a heavy handle that would cause it to fall off course. **B:** The tip of the EZM bone biopsy needle is sharp, constricted, and threaded so that it easily drills into hard bone and reliably retrieves samples. **C:** EZM needles easily drilled into dense bone yield the diagnosis of non-Hodgkin lymphoma. **D:** The EZM bone biopsy needle can be coaxially passed through a larger 11-gauge bone needle during vertebroplasty if a biopsy sample is needed.

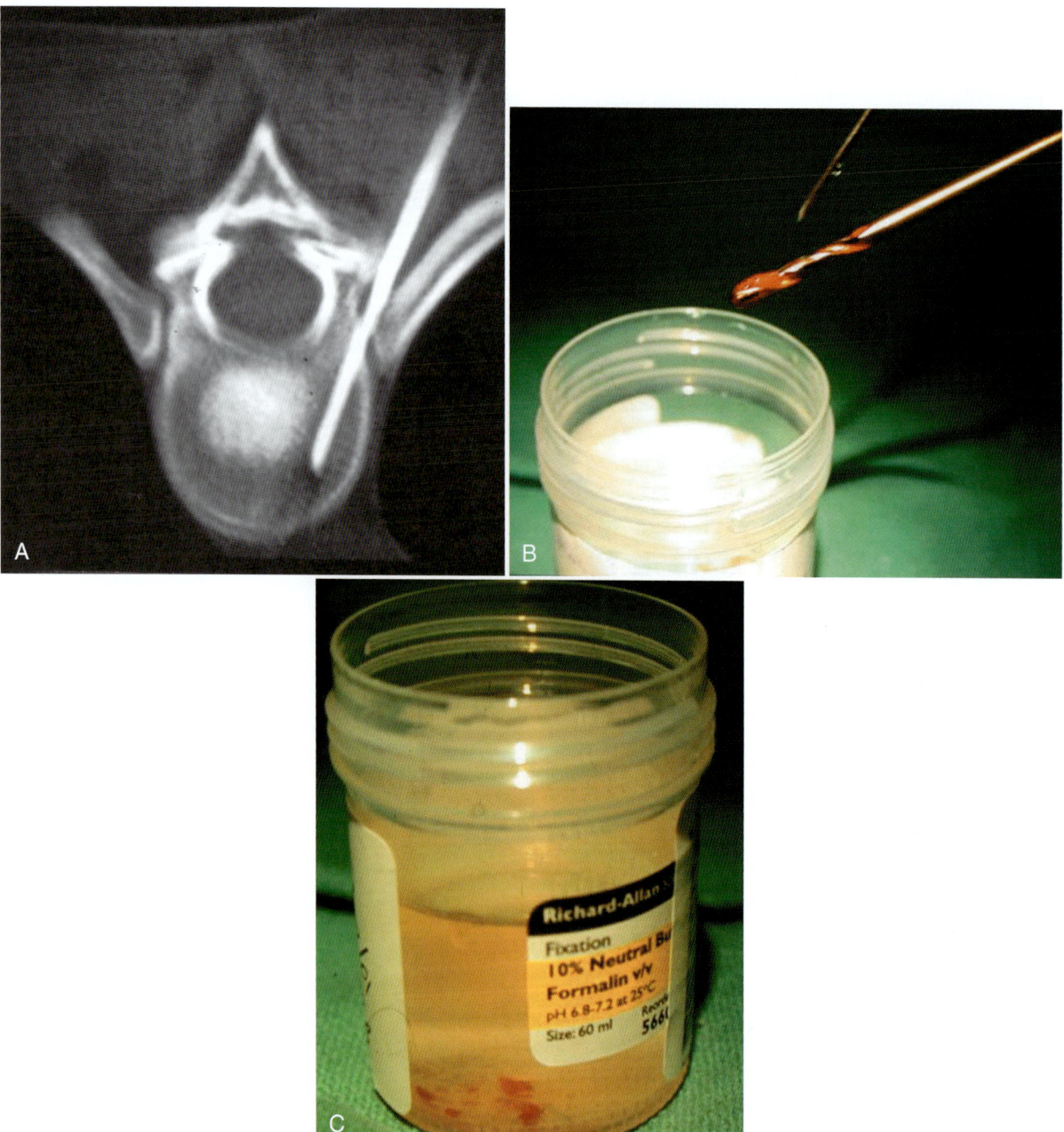

Figure 7-26 A: For blastic bone lesions, the pathologist may require a substantial quantity for diagnosis. An 11-gauge needle may be needed to provide a sufficient sample. However, retrieving a bone core may be difficult in cases with extremely dense bone. **B:** Washing bone out of the grooves of the Kyphon drill. **C:** Numerous bone fragments from the Kyphon drill.

For difficult soft tissue biopsies in paraspinous soft tissue or for soft tissue masses invading bone, spring-loaded cutting-type needles (e.g., Temno) may be selected for more reliable collection of core material. However, these needles have a heavy handle and a cutting extension that protrudes forward such that these needles can be awkward and somewhat risky to use in the spine.

A needle guide for coaxial passage may be necessary (Figure 7-28). For fluid-filled abnormalities, a micropuncture set with placement of a guidewire and subsequent drainage catheter may be considered. For aspirating fluid, usually a large syringe will be chosen over a small syringe because the amount of suction can be quite a bit greater. For drainage of an abscess pocket, a cope-type looping catheter seated within the fluid

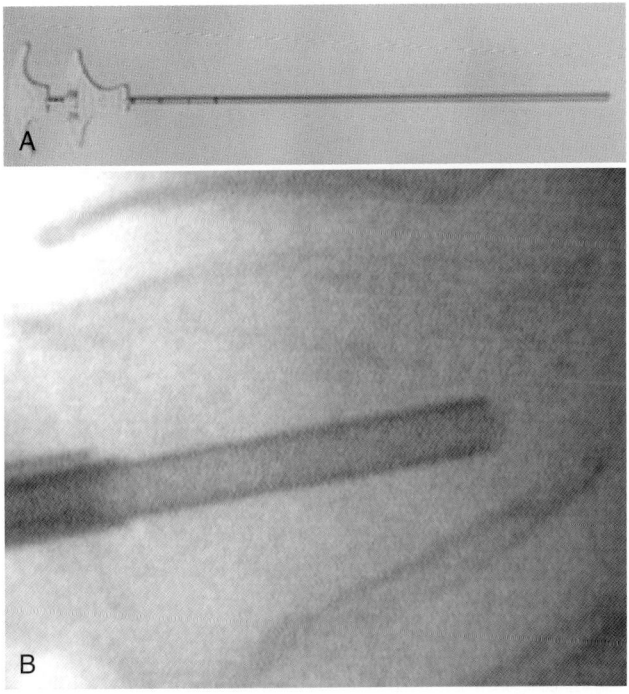

Figure 7-27 A: To obtain very large samples needed by the pathologist for diagnosis, a 9-gauge Kyphon biopsy device can be passed through an 8-gauge canula coaxially. **B:** The 9-gauge Kyphon biopsy device as it is passes through the 8-gauge canula.

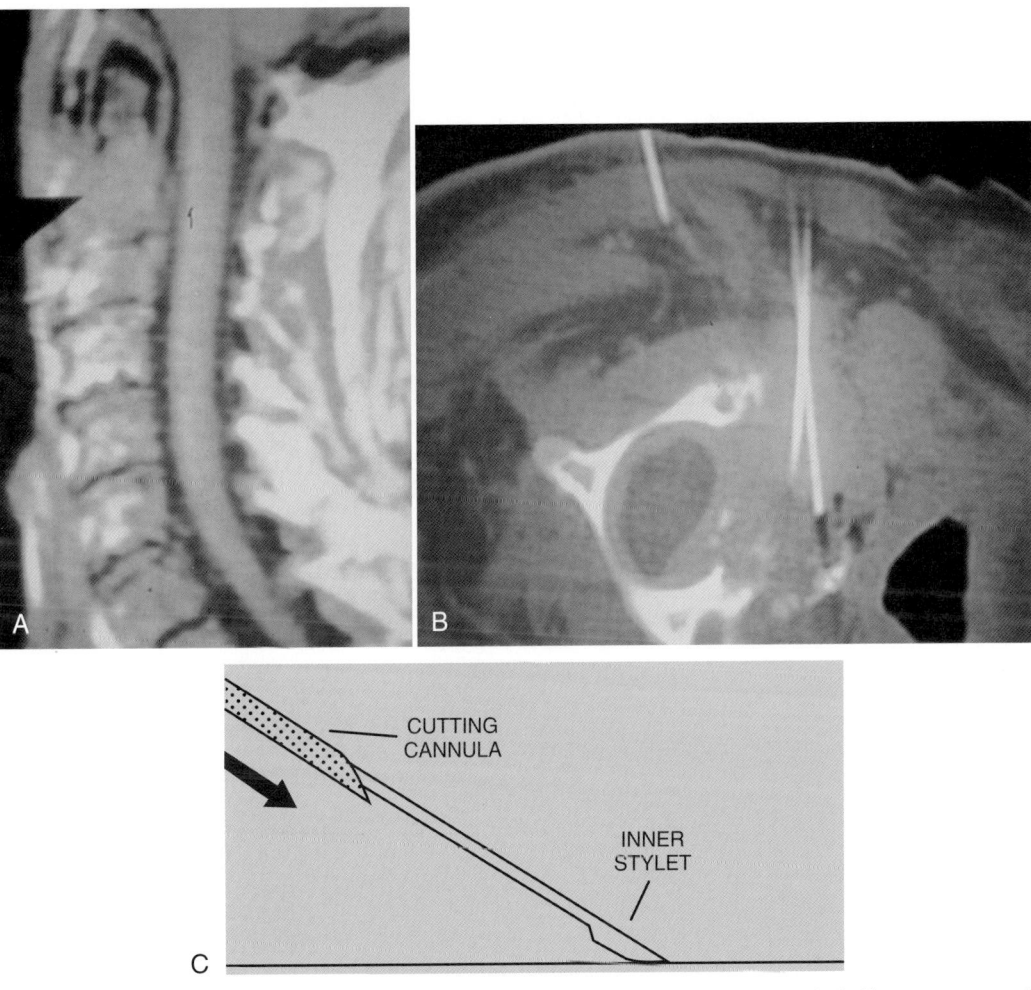

Figure 7-28 A: A 67-year-old woman complained of upper neck pain. She had a medical history that included breast cancer, uterine cancer, and lymphoma. Biopsy is needed because treatment is not the same for all three. **B:** Ten fine-needle passes fail to retrieve an adequate sample. **C:** The spring-loaded cutting needle works well on soft tissue targets. Remember that the inner stylet projects a distance beyond the cutting canula. This must be considered carefully when setting the depth from skin to target so as not to injure critical anatomy, especially in the neck. Also remember that the handle has some weight that can cause the needle to deviate off course if not supported. Usually the safest technique consists of directing the needle coaxially through an already established guiding needle. Pathologic diagnosis is uterine cancer (made on first pass).

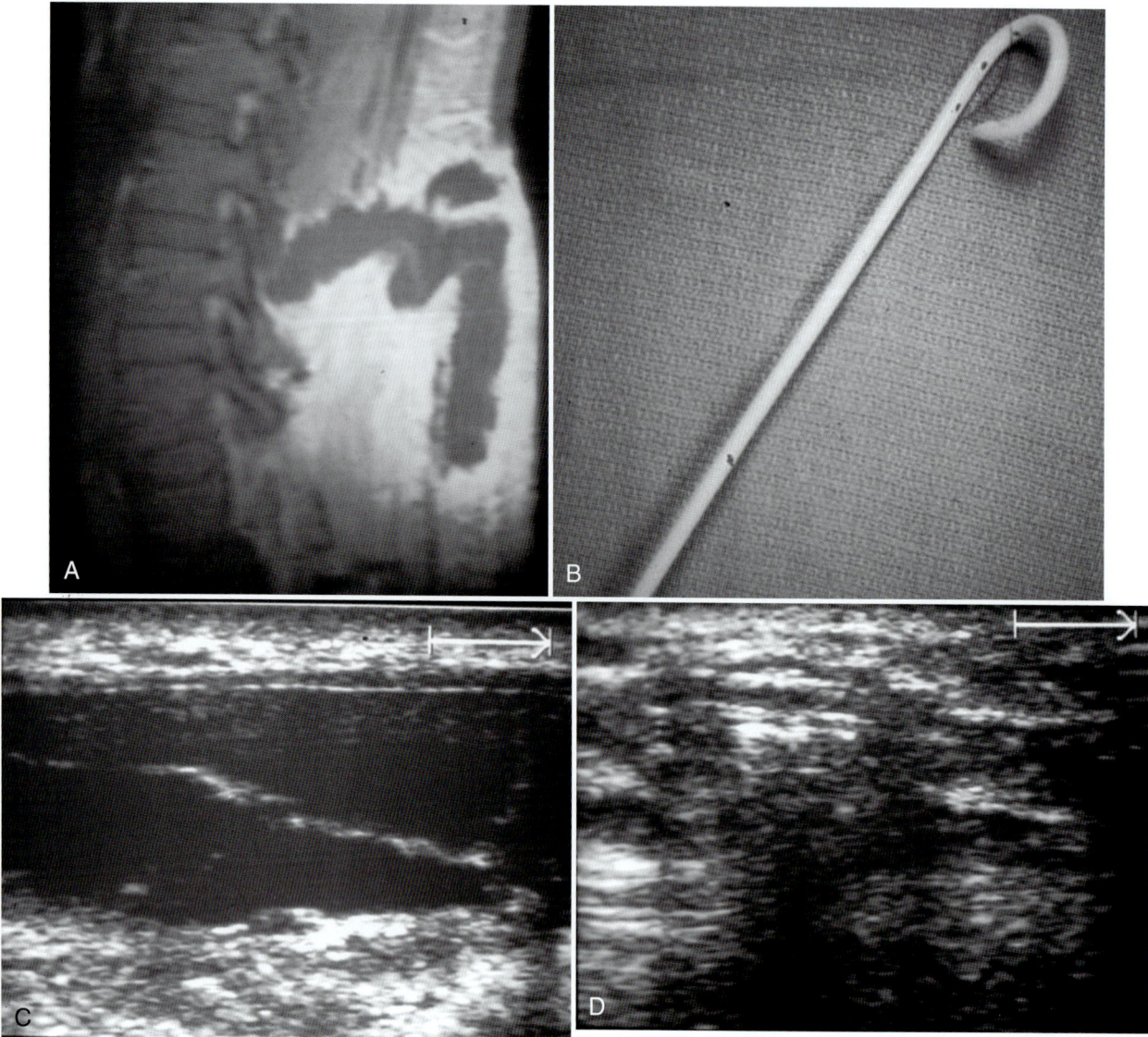

Figure 7-29 **A:** A 36-year-old man 5 days post lumbar laminectomy complained of increased low back pain and fever. Determining the diagnosis was straightforward, but treatment could be effected percutaneously with image guidance. **B:** Cope drainage catheter was placed to drain a large pus pocket. **C:** Cope drainage catheter was placed under ultrasound guidance. **D:** After the fluid was drained, the fever and back pain resolved overnight. Pathologic diagnosis is *Staphylococcus epidermidis* infection.

pocket with drainage to suction (e.g., by Jackson-Pratt bulb) maybe be considered (Figure 7-29).

■ RESULTS: WHAT CAN BE EXPECTED?

Positive results: When infection was suspected
    N = 88 patients
    71 positive (7 delayed up to 7 weeks because of slow growth from underlying granulomatous disease)
   80% positivity
Positive results: When neoplasm was suspected
    N = 92 patients
    85 positive
   92% positivity
Overall 86% positivity
Complication Rate
    2 small hematomas
    1 needlestick to operator
1.6% rate

Problem Solving: What Are the Pitfalls?

Failure to diagnose is one of the more common pitfalls. For neoplasm, this may be due to failure to sample the correct area of abnormality. This is more likely to occur under fluoroscopic guidance than CT guidance, in which case a repeat procedure under CT or even MR guidance may be worthwhile. For situations where infection is suspected, the presence of antibiotics may hinder growth. Therefore, try to obtain a biopsy sample prior to the start of antibiotic therapy or, if antibiotics are present, delay the biopsy, if feasible, until the patient has been off the antibiotics for 1 week (Figure 7-30).

To ensure that an adequate tissue sample is acquired, the presence of a pathologist technician at the procedure to receive samples is recommended. Ideally, the sample is prepared and reviewed with the pathologist at the time of the procedure to determine if the sample is adequate and, in many situations, diagnostic. If this extra step is not taken at the time of the procedure, not infrequently the procedure needs to be repeated at a later time because samples are inadequate and/or nondiagnostic.

Hypervascular neoplasms may pose a danger when performing a biopsy because of potential uncontrollable hemorrhaging. If high vascularity (e.g., renal cell cancer, thyroid metastases) is suspected, then preoperative embolization may be prudent. This usually entails selective transarterial particle embolization, although in some situations coaxial biopsies with final injection of Gelfoam down the outer guiding needle may suffice. If osteoplasty is contemplated, then coaxial biopsy with injection of polymethylmethacrylate will help to cause hemostasis (Figure 7-31 and 7-32).

Needle safety is extremely important for both the operator and the patient. Avoid leaving needles carelessly on the patient or on the work table. Use caution when handling and passing needles so as not to cause needlesticks. Avoid capping needles; a needle holder is worthwhile to prevent inadvertent needlesticks. Dispose of needles properly. When pushing needles into a patient, have adequate control of the needle so as not to inadvertently injure an organ that was not intended for penetration (Figure 7-33).

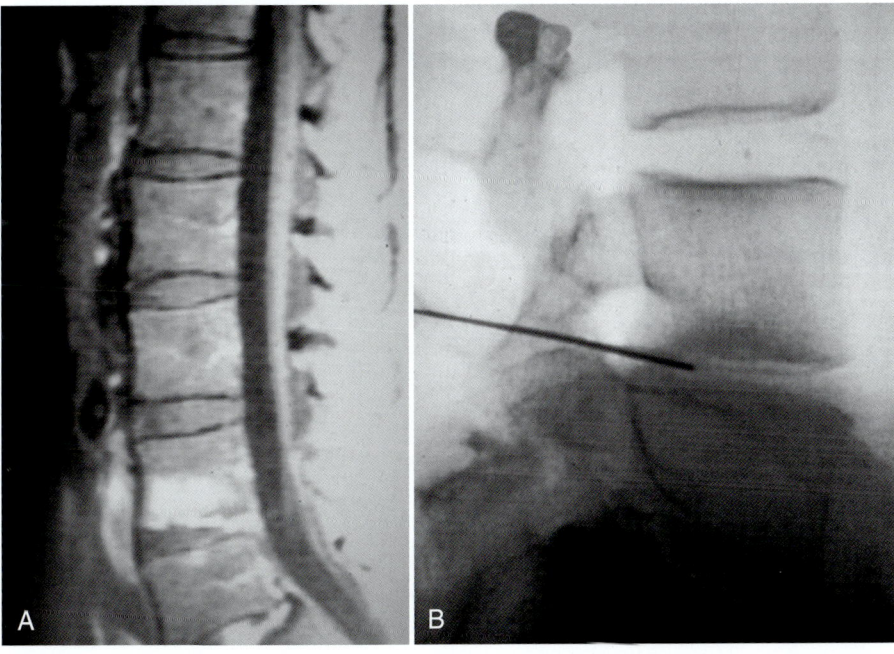

Figure 7-30 A: A 57 year-old man complained of increased low back pain and low-grade fever 10 days post L5–S1 discectomy. He had been started on antibiotics 3 days earlier. B: Biopsies performed at L4–5 and L5–S1 yielded scant *Staphylococcus epidermidis* that could be a contaminant. An infectious disease consultation suggested discontinuing the antibiotics for 1 week. Repeat biopsy 1 week later revealed numerous colonies of *S. epidermidis*. The lesson here is to try to biopsy before antibiotics are given or to discontinue the antibiotics for at least 1 week when biopsies results are negative in the face of suspected spinal infection.

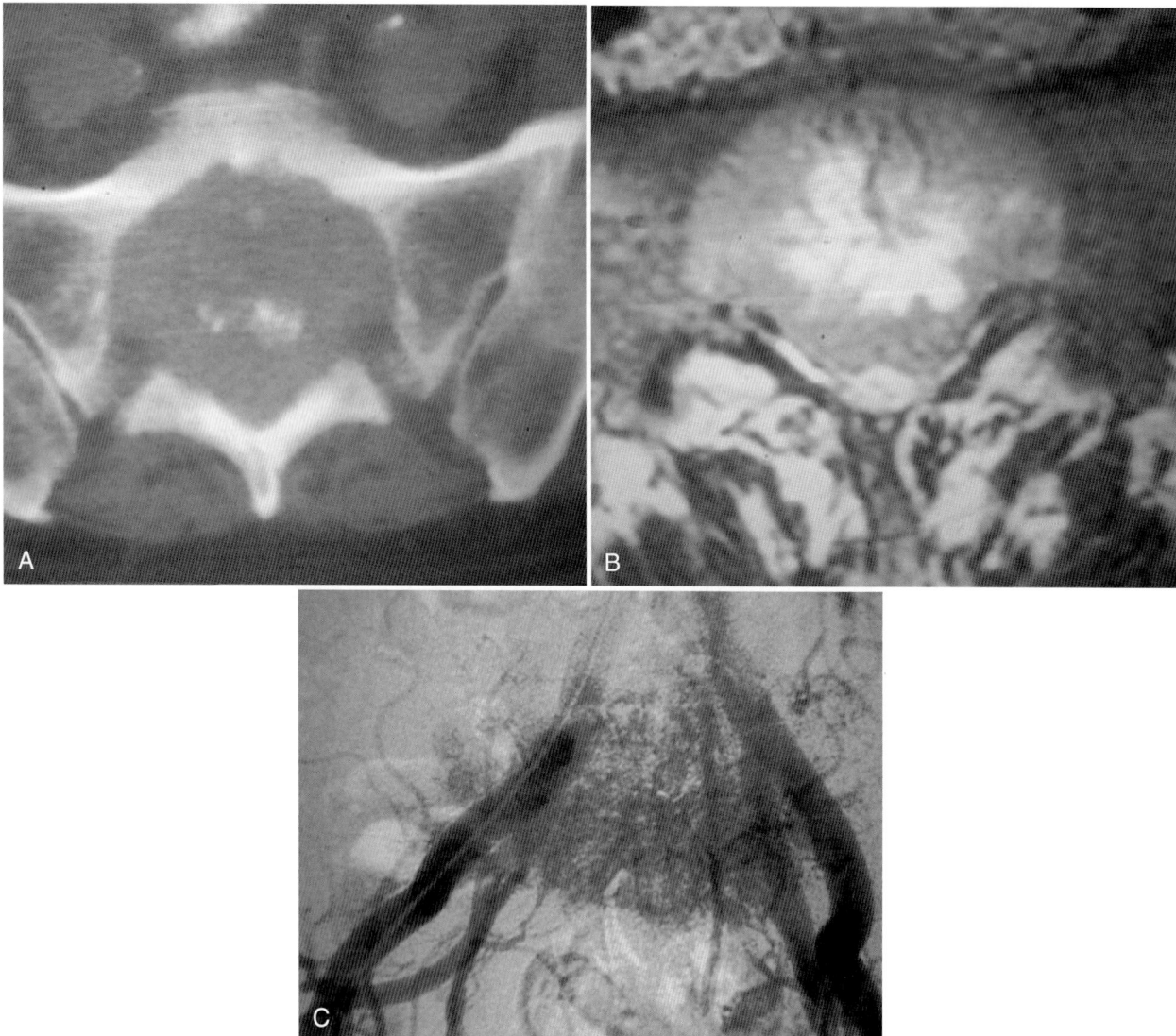

Figure 7-31 A: A 67-year-old man complained of low back pain. Computed tomographic (CT) scan reveals a large area of sacral lysis. **B:** Magnetic resonance imaging reveals numerous serpentine flow voids suggesting considerable hypervascularity of the sacral mass. **C:** Angiogram performed prior to biopsy confirms the hypervascular nature and the need to devascularize prior to biopsy.

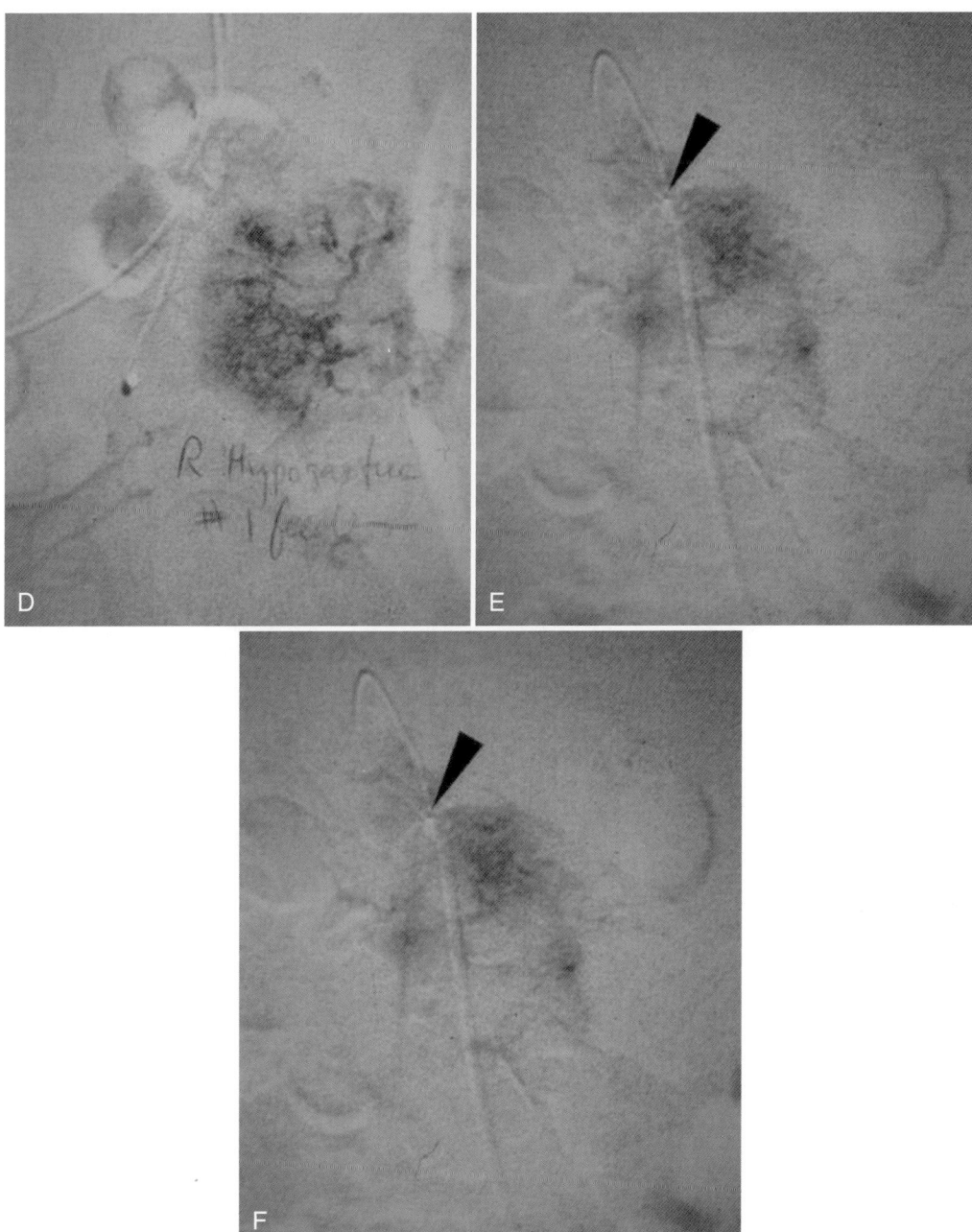

Figure 7-31, cont'd D: Superselective catheterization of feeder from the right internal iliac artery isolates the tumor blush. E: Embolization is performed by flow-directing 200-μm polyvinyl alcohol (PVA) particles until tumor vascularity from this vascular supply ceased. F: Superselective angiogram via microcatheter of feeder subbranch from left internal iliac artery demonstrating contralateral tumor blush prior to embolization with 200-μm PVA particles.

Continued

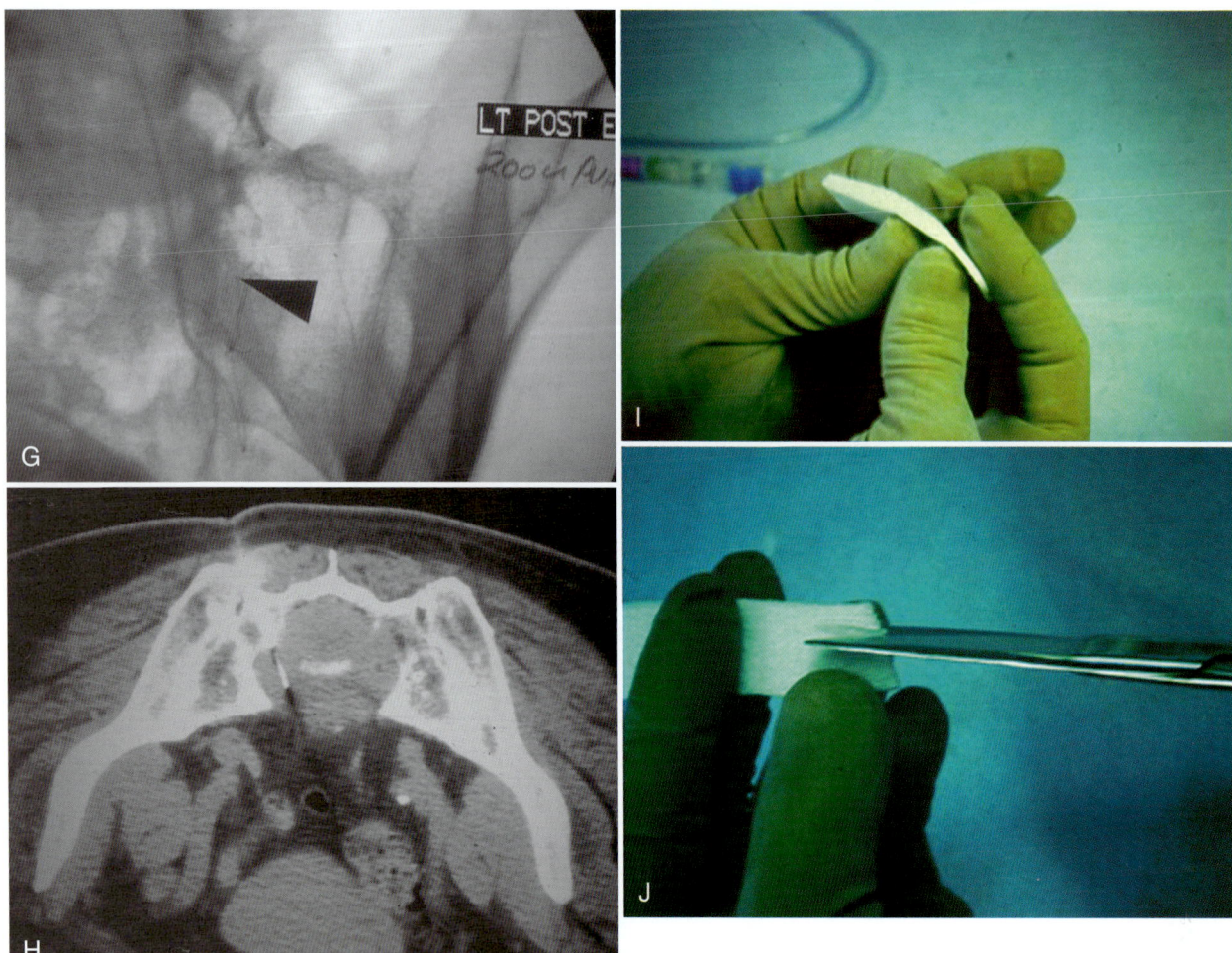

Figure 7-31, cont'd **G**: Postembolization angiogram of left internal iliac artery demonstrating devascularization of tumor mass from this vascular territory. **H**: Biopsy is performed under CT guidance with 17-gauge EZM bone biopsy needle and 22-gauge Crown needle coaxially. Some bleeding continued. **I**: Gelfoam is prepared to stop bleeding along needle tract. Gelfoam is first flattened. **J**: Gelfoam is cut into thin longitudinal strips.

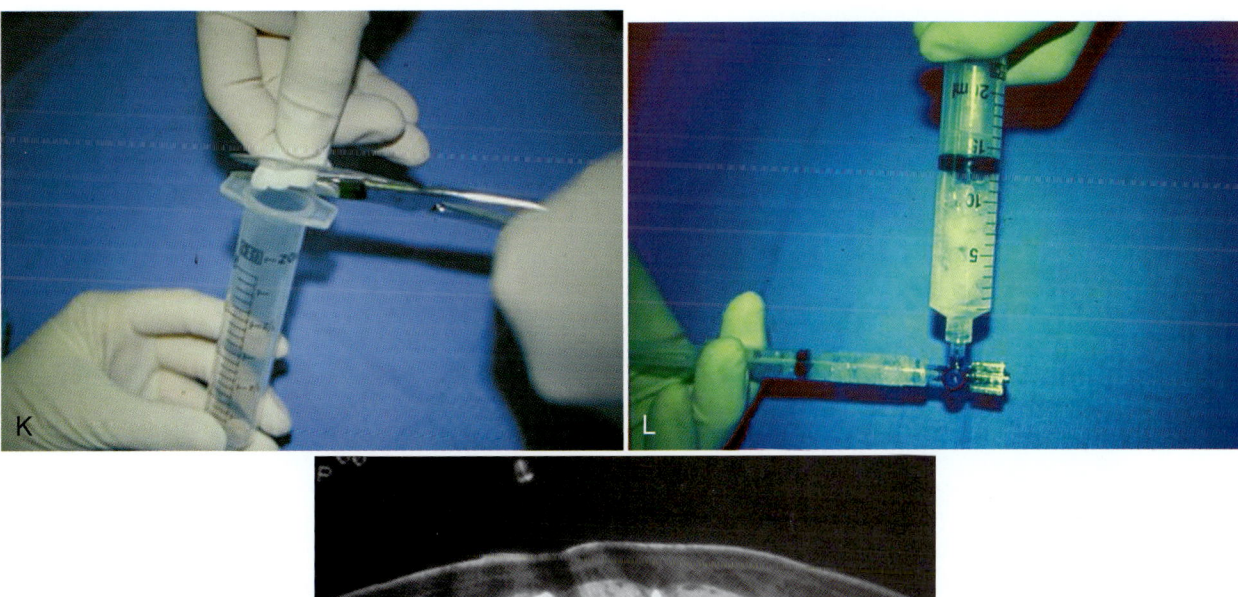

Figure 7-31, cont'd K: Gelfoam is cut horizontally into small squares and dropped into a syringe. L: Gelfoam is mixed with iodine contrast (Omnipaque 240) and injected back and forth through a three-way valve to form a slurry. The needle is replaced back along its original track, and the Gelfoam slurry is injected along the track for hemostasis. M: Gelfoam can be seen post slurry embolization. Bleeding stopped shortly thereafter. Pathologic diagnosis is cordoma of sacrum and renal cell carcinoma of right kidney without metastasis.

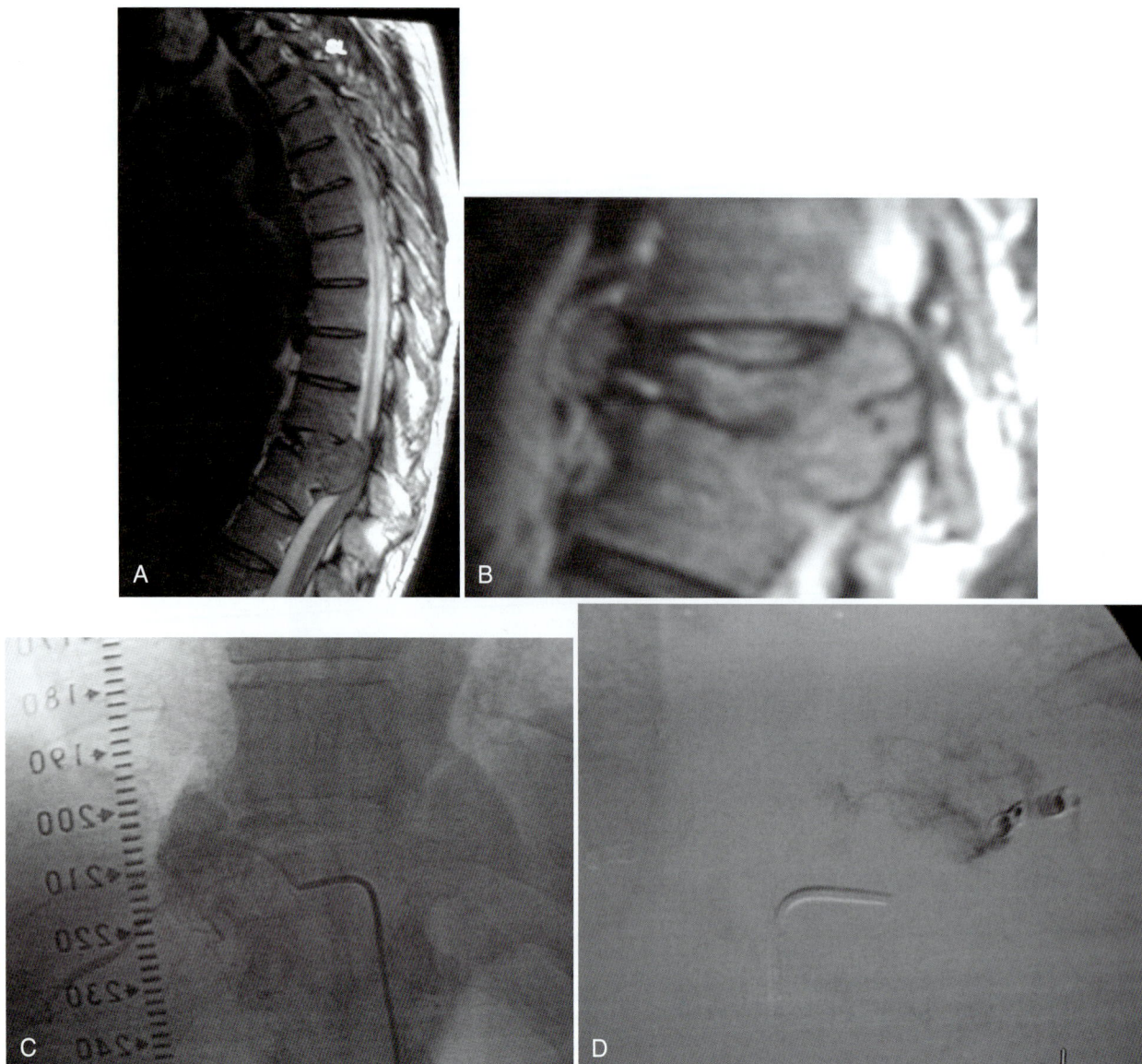

Figure 7-32 A: A 57-year-old man complained of middle back pain and weakness of the lower extremities. T2-weighted sagittal image reveals lower thoracic epidural mass severely compressing the dural sac as well as a suspicious lower cervical mass. B: Magnified image of T10 demonstrating a compression fracture with a retropulsing mass extending posteriorly as well as a flow void suspicious for increased vascularity. C: Spinal angiogram demonstrating hypervascularity of the T10 mass. Embolization prior to biopsy would be prudent. D: Superselective microcatheterization of left T10 intercostal. Coils are placed distally to protect the distal intercostal artery. Polyvinyl alcohol (PVA) particles (200 μm) are flow directed into the tumor feeders until devascularization occurs.

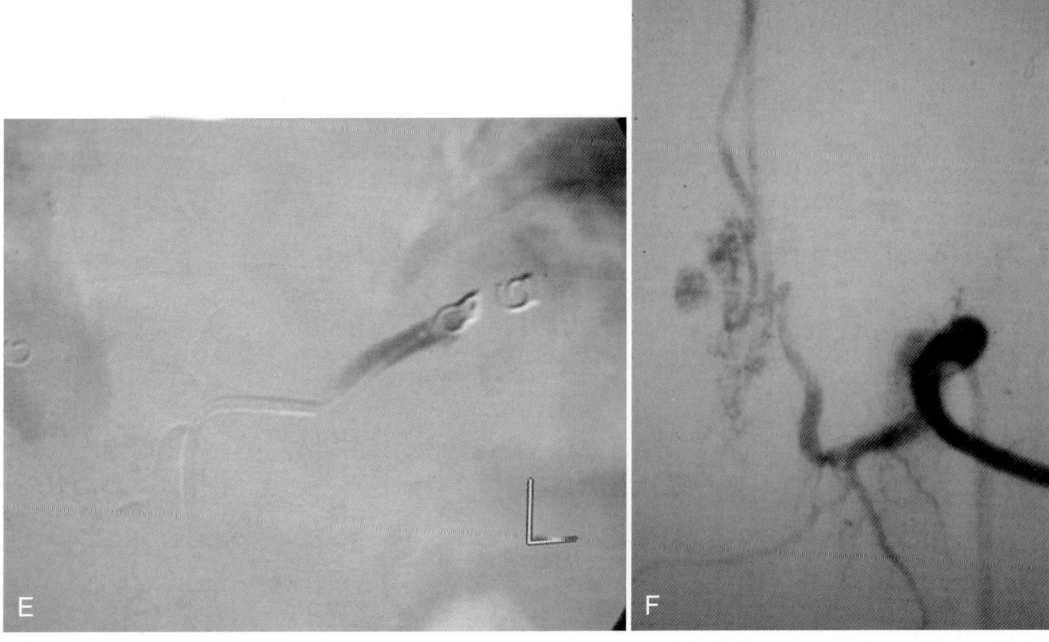

Figure 7-32, cont'd E: Post left T10 intercostal artery embolization image demonstrating absence of tumor vascularity on this side. The contralateral side was subsequently embolized similarly. The biopsy proceeded without incident. Pathologic diagnosis is thyroid carcinoma metastasis to T10. F: Identifying the artery of Adamkiewicz, which has a classic hairpin, is important because inadvertent embolization could cause spinal cord infarction and subsequent paralysis.

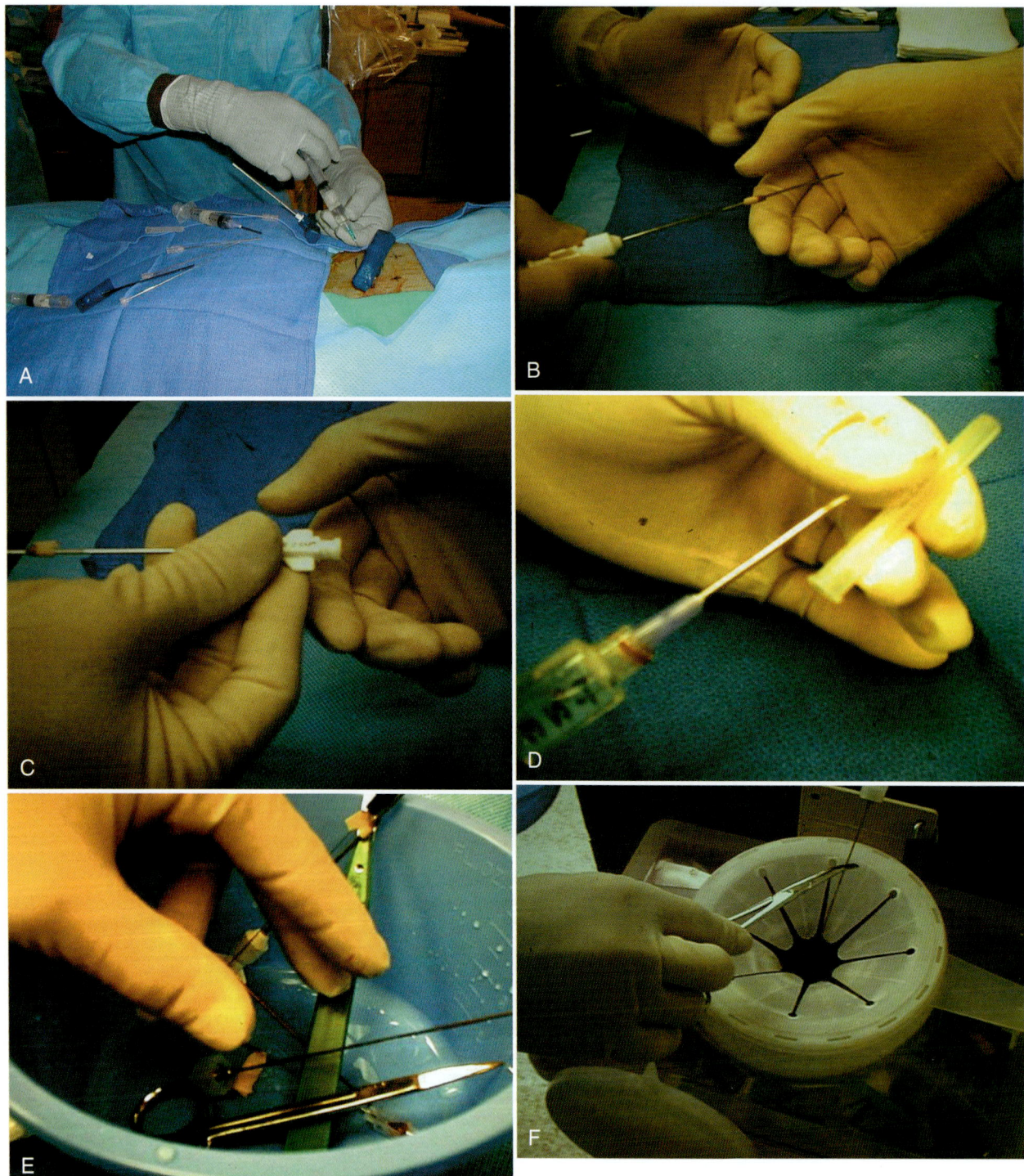

Figure 7-33 A: One the most hazardous aspects of performing spine biopsies is needle injury to the operator. This is hardly the scene conducive to safe practice. Keep sharps neat and orderly to prevent accidents. **B:** Treat needles like firearms. Do not point them where they can cause injury. **C:** When passing needles, hand them off with the nonsharp side first. **D:** Avoid capping needles. **E:** Keep needles in an orderly container. **F:** Dispose of sharps responsibly so that nursing, technical, and janitorial personnel do not suffer injury.

Suggested Readings

Babu NV, Titus VTK, Chittaranjan S, et al. Computed tomographically guided biopsy of the spine. *Spine.* 1994;21:2436-2442.

Cameron DC. Percutaneous coaxial trephine bone biopsy. *Austral Radiol.* 2007;51:370-374.

Chen Y, Chang G, Chen W, Hsu H, Lee T. Local metastases along the tract of the needle: A rare complication of vertebroplasty in treating spinal metastases. *Spine.* 2007;32:E615-E618.

Hadjipavlou AG, Kontakis GM, Gaitanis JN, Katonis PG, Lander P, Crow WN. Effectiveness and pitfalls of percutaneous transpedicle biopsy of the spine. *Clin Orthop Rel Res.* 2003;411:54-60.

Heyer CM, Al-Hadari A, Mueller K, Stachon A, Nicolas V. Effectiveness of CT-guided percutaneous biopsies of the spine: An anaylsis of 202 examinations. *Acad Radiol.* 2008;15:901-911.

Huegli RW, Schaeren S, Jacob AL, Martin JB, Wetzel SG. Percutaneous cervical vertebroplasty in a multi-functional image-guided therapy suite: Hybrid lateral approach to C1 and C4 under CT and fluoroscopic guidance. *Cardiovasc Intervent Radiol.* 2005;28:649-652.

Jelinek JS, Kransdorf MJ, Gray R, et al. Percutaneous transpedicular biopsy of vertebral body lesions. *Spine.* 1996;21:2035-2040.

Layton KF, Thielen KR, Wald JT. A modified vertebroplasty approach for spine biopsies. *AJNR Am J Neuroradiol.* 2006;27:596-597.

Layton KF, Thielen KR, Wald JT. Percutaneous sacroplasty using CT fluoroscopy. *AJNR Am J Neuroradiol.* 2006;27:356-358.

Lis E, Bilsky MH, Pisinski L, Boland P, Healey JH, O'Malley B, Krol G. Percutaneous CT-guided biopsy of osseous lesion of the spine in patients with known or suspected malignancy. *AJNR Am J Neuroradiol.* 2004;25:1583-1588.

Nourbakhsh A, Grady JJ, Garges KJ. Percutaneous spine biopsy: a meta-analysis. *J Boint Joint Surg Am.* 2008;90:1722-1725.

Petsas T, Tsota T, Kalogeropoulou CP, Liatsikos EN. Application of a new guiding system in percutaneous biopsies. *Cardiovasc Intervent Radiol.* 2007;30:276-280.

Pierot L, Boulin A. Percutaneous biopsy of the thoracic and lumbar spine: transpedicular approach under fluoroscopic guidance. *AJNR Am J Neuroradiol.* 1999;20:23-25.

Puri A, Shingade VU, Agarwal MG, Anchan C, Juvekar S, Desai S, Jambhekar NA. CT-guided percutaneous core needle biopsy in deep-seated musculoskeletal lesions: A prospective study of 128 cases. *Skeletal Radiol.* 2006;35:138-143.

Raininko R, Sonninen P. Dorsal CSF space at CI-CII level: technique of cervical myelography. *Neuroradiology.* 1987;29:73-75.

Rankine JJ, Barron DA, Robinson P, Millner PA, Dickson RA. Therapeutic impact of percutaneous spinal biopsy in spinal infection. *Postgrad Med J.* 2004;80:607-609.

Robertson HJ, Smith RD. Cervical myelography: survey of modes of practice and major complications. *Radiology.* 1990;174:79-83.

Rodriguez-Catarino M, Blimark C, Willen J, Mellqvist U, Rodjer S. Percutaneous vertebroplasty at C2: case report of a patient with multiple myeloma and a literature review. *Eur Spine J.* 2007;16:S242-S249.

Sachs DC, Inamasu J, Mendel EE, Guiot BH. Transoral vertebroplasty of renal cell metastasis involving the axis. *Spine.* 2006;31:E925-928.

Schirmer CM, Malek AM, Kwan ES, Hoit DA, Weller SJ. Preoperative embolization of hypervascular spinal metastases using percutaneous direct injection of N-butyl cyanoacrylate: technical case report. *Neurosurgery.* 2006;59:431-432.

Tehranzadeh J, Tao C, Browning CA. Percutaneous needle biopsy of the spine. *Acta Radiol.* 2007;8:860-868.

Uemura A, Matsusako M, Numaguchi Y, Oka M, Kobayashi N, Niinami C, Kawasaki T, Suzuki K. Percutaneous sacroplasty for hemorrhagic metastases from hepatocellular carcinoma. *AJNR Am J Neuroradiol.* 2005;26:493-495.

van de Krats EB, van Walsum T, Verlaan J, Voormolen MH, Mali WPTHM, Niessen WJ. Three-dimensional rotational x-ray navigation for needle guidance in percutaneous vertebroplasty: an accuracy study. *Spine.* 2006;31:1359-1364.

Wong W. *personal experience 1996-97 oral presentation at ASNR "Common Spine Interventions: Percutaneous Biopsies" (Abstract)* Philadelphia, Pennsylvania: American Society of Neuroradiology 36th Annual Meeting; May 17-21, 1998.

Wong W. Lumbar Spine Biopsy. PocketRadiologist: Interventional Top 100 Procedures. Peter Rogers, Anne Roberts, Peter Schloesser, Wade Wong (eds). W.B. Saunders Company, Salt Lake City, Utah, 2003, pps 250-252. Reprinted in: PDA Version: PocketRadiologist: Interventional 100 Procedures. W.B. Saunders Company, Salt Lake City, Utah, 2003, pp 250–252.

Wu L, Li C Chen L, Li C, Qiu X. Magnetic resonance imaging bone biopsies in the iPath-200 system. *Chin Med J.* 2003;116(6):937-940.

Yaffe D, Greenberg G, Leitner J, Gipstein R, Shapiro M, Bachar G. CT-guided percutaneous biopsy of thoracic and lumbar spine: a new coaxial technique. *AJNR Am J Neuroradiol.* 2003;24:2111-2113.

SECTION III

PROBLEM SOLVING: DISEASE CATEGORIES

CHAPTER 8
Neurodegenerative Disorders
Manzoor Ahmed and Michael Phillips

The term *neurodegenerative disease* generally refers to evolving structural neuroanatomic changes with progressive deterioration in the patient's condition. Neurodegenerative disorders (NDDs) would be a relatively simple subject if it comprised only Alzheimer disease (AD) and Parkinson disease (PD). Although NDD clearly is a more complicated topic, AD and PD provide a good basic framework for more complete discussion. They are the predominant dementing and movement disorders, respectively, and serve as an excellent frame of reference for consideration of other processes.

Brain NDDs are primarily a clinical diagnostic domain. Morphologic and functional imaging play a significant role in the diagnosis of NDDs. They (1) complement the clinical diagnosis, (2) act as a problem solver in some difficult cases, (3) exclude treatable mimickers of a specific NDD, and (4) provide one means for further research.

■ DEFINITIONS

As with all fields of endeavor, it helps to know the vocabulary. Following are some useful definitions to keep in mind when thinking about NDDs.

Dementia: Generally means loss of mental functions, such as thinking, memory, and reasoning, which is severe enough to interfere with a person's daily functioning. Dementia is not a disease itself but rather a group of symptoms that might accompany certain diseases or conditions. Diagnostic criteria is "impairment in short and long term memory and at least one other cognitive dysfunction or personality change, significant social and occupational impairment and absence of organic factors causing the mental disorder" (*Diagnostic and Statistical Manual of Mental Disorders*, Fourth Edition). Dementia is clinically divided into cortical and subcortical dementias.

Cortical dementia: Primarily affects cognitive processes such as memory, intellect, and language. AD and Creutzfeldt-Jakob disease (CJD) are two definite forms of cortical dementia. Patients with cortical dementia typically show aphasia, agnosia, and apraxia in addition to severe amnesia. However, the clinical differentiation of cortical from subcortical dementia may be difficult in some cases.

Subcortical dementia: Subcortical dementia contrasts neuropsychologically and anatomically with Alzheimer-type dementia. It occurs in degenerative extrapyramidal disorders as well as in inflammatory, infectious, and vascular conditions. It is a clinical syndrome characterized by slowness and depression. Subcortical dementia is a sequela of processes primarily affecting the thalamus, basal ganglia, and related brainstem nuclei, with relative sparing of the cerebral cortical functions. It typically is seen in PD, Huntington disease, and progressive supranuclear palsy (PSP).

Presenile dementia: Also termed *early-onset dementia*. Onset is before age 65 years. Commonly due to AD and vascular dementia, followed by frontotemporal dementia (FTD) and multiple acquired causes, some of which may be reversible.

Senile dementia: Also termed *late-onset dementia*. Mostly due to AD and other less common NDDs.

Movement disorders: A common but heterogenous group of disorders. In the majority of patients, the clinical diagnosis is not difficult (e.g., idiopathic Parkinson disease [IPD] or essential tremor). PD is the second most common neurodegenerative disease after AD. Our focus is on IPD and its mimickers, clinically termed *atypical Parkinson disorders*. The accuracy of clinical diagnosis of PD and neurodegenerative mimickers is generally very good, but up to 10% to 20% of cases may still be misdiagnosed.

Atypical Parkinson disorders: Several primary NDDs have in common parkinsonian features such as bradykinesia, rigidity, tremor, and gait disturbances. These neurologic conditions are associated with complex clinical presentations that reflect degeneration in various neuronal systems resulting in the term *Parkinson plus*. They include multisystem atrophy (MSA), progressive supra-nuclear palsy (PSP), corticobasal degeneration (CBD), dementia with Lewy bodies (DLB), and PD with amyotrophic lateral sclerosis (ALS). Vascular (usually due to striatal lacunar infarcts), drug-induced, and viral encephalitis-related parkinsonisms are secondary causes of parkinsonism. Importantly, these processes rarely respond to levodopa therapy, which often clinically distinguishes them from IPD.

Synucleinopathies: The term *synucleinopathies* is used to name a group of NDDs characterized by fibrillary aggregates of alpha-synuclein protein in the cytoplasm of selected populations of neurons and glia. These disorders include PD, DLB, pure autonomic failure, and MSA.

Tauopathies: A class of NDDs resulting from the pathologic aggregation of tau protein, a neuronal microtubule stabilizing protein, resulting in a neurofibrillary tangles. In normal brain, tau protein is soluble and nonfilamentous. Tau protein is found in AD and frontotemporal degeneration. Other tauopathies include PSP, CBD, and FTD-parkinsonism linked to chromosome 17. Argyrophilic grain disease, a late-onset dementia, is a tauopathy. It is similar to PSP and CBD on an immunohistochemical analysis but is different clinically, with mild limbic dementia features mimicking AD.

Problem Solving: Is There Normal Aging? (Figure 8-1, A)

Normal brain aging is a relative term with regard to physical and functional abilities, with declining mental functions but no severe compromise of cognitive and motor performance. In general, during normal aging, cognitive functioning declines as cortical gray matter and hippocampus decrease and white matter hyperintensities increase. However, these are general rules that are often difficult to apply directly to individuals. *Successful aging* is a term often applied to subjects who demonstrate relatively preserved functions compared to the age cohort. Although the term has become relatively popular, clear rigorous definitions are not available. Importantly, there is significant overlap in the imaging appearance of normal aging and NDDs, particularly in the early stages of disease progression. We divide the magnetic resonance (MR) appearance of aging brain into three categories:

1. Normal brain except for mild volume loss. No white matter hyperintensities. This may be the imaging marker of "successful aging."

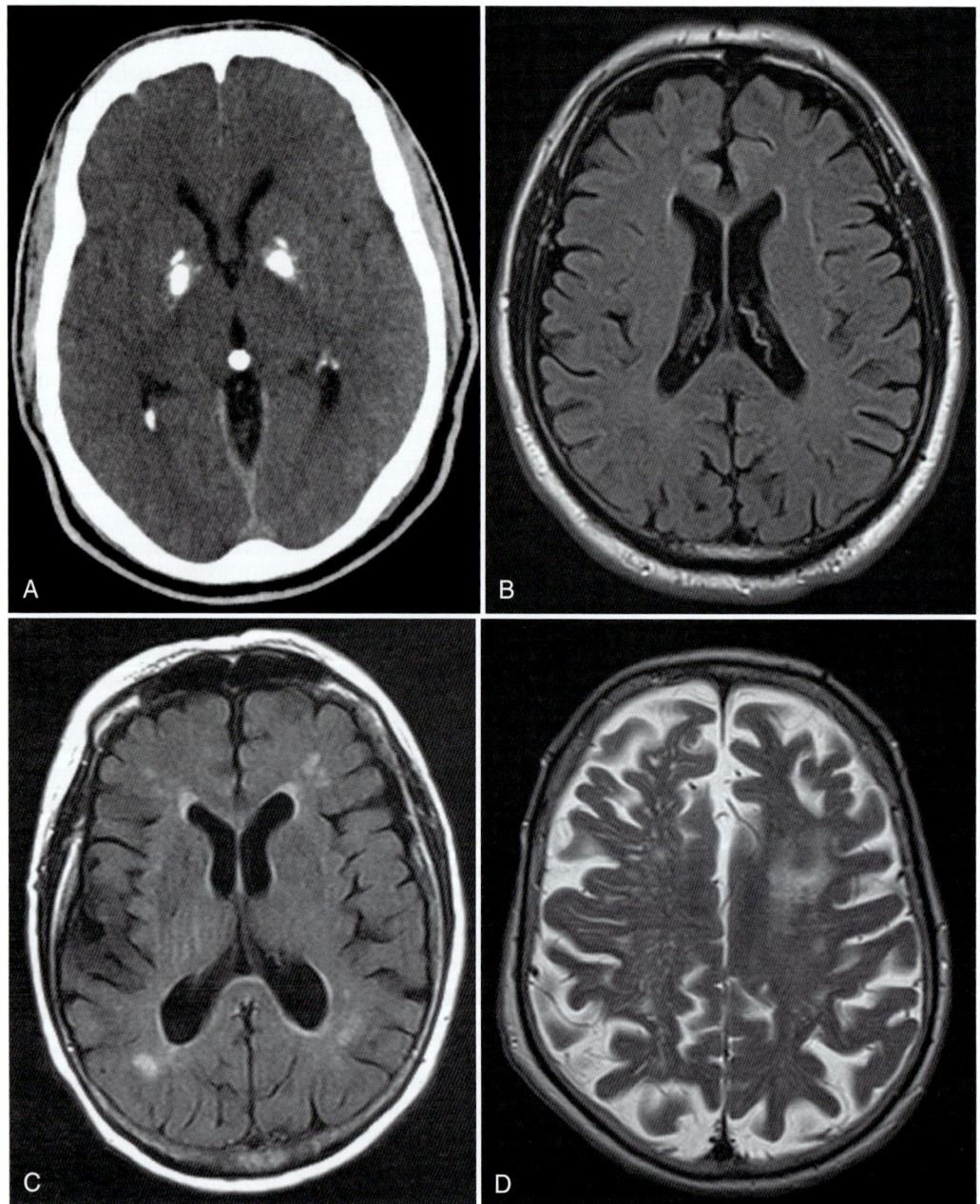

Figure 8-1 Aging. **A:** Axial computed tomography in an asymptomatic case with bilateral dense symmetric globus pallidi calcifications, sparing the putamina. **B:** Axial fluid-attenuated inversion recovery (FLAIR) image showing an unremarkable brain of an 80-year-old man with "successful aging." **C:** Axial FLAIR image of a 78–year-old man with mild diffuse patchy white matter T2 hyperintensities. **D:** Axial T2 image of an octogenarian showing prominent perivascular spaces.

2. Mild to moderate diffuse cerebral volume loss, varying grades of periventricular, and patchy white matter T2 hyperintensities. The majority of elder individuals fall into this category.
3. Profound diffuse cerebral volume loss, and varying grades of periventricular and patchy white matter T2 hyperintensities.

Volume loss "atrophy": We prefer the term *volume loss* to atrophy, although the terms are used interchangeably in this review. Imaging is only capable of determining volume loss at the present level of technology. Atrophy is really a histopathologic term suggesting loss of neurons and axons in glial cells. Although volume loss is often produced by atrophy, other potential causes include hydration status and drug therapy (e.g., steroids). Volume loss clearly correlates with advancing age. Cerebral volume loss is diffuse and generally mild, with more prominent ventricular enlargement. Volumetric magnetic resonance imaging (MRI) analysis is a potential tool for serial longitudinal imaging. Mild diffuse cerebellar hemispheric and posterior vermian volume loss is consistently present in older individuals. The rate of volume loss can vary considerably among individuals.

White matter T2 changes: Aging brain shows grossly two types of white matter changes: (1) white matter hyperintensities in the deep and subcortical white matter, graded as punctuate (grade 1), patchy or beginning confluent (grade 2), and confluent (grade 3); and (2) periventricular hyperintensities surrounding the lateral ventricles. Periventricular hyperintensity is graded as caps surrounding the frontal or posterior horns and pencil-thin lining along the lateral ventricles (grade 1), bands along the lateral ventricles (grade 2), and irregular changes extending into deep white matter (grade 3). These findings are very nonspecific; however, in the absence of other risk factors or known existing conditions, they are suggestive of changes related to underlying vascular processes. T2 hyperintensities can also be seen in the corpus callosum with increasing aging and correlates with periventricular and deep white matter hyperintensities.

Basal ganglia iron deposition and calcifications: The brain progressively accumulates iron in both the gray and white matter. The most prominent increases in iron levels occur in the globus pallidus, dentate, substantia nigra (pars reticulata), and red nuclei. Iron accumulates to a lesser extent in the caudate, putamen, thalamus, cerebral cortex, and white matter after age 30 years. Hypointensity of the putamen usually does not appear until the seventh decade. Iron deposition correlates to T2 hypointensity. T2*-based imaging (e.g., gradient-echo T2 and susceptibility-weighted imaging) is more sensitive to iron deposition. Bilateral basal ganglia calcifications are a common finding related to aging. Physiologic calcification is generally limited to globus pallidi, and the calcification can be asymmetric or present on only one side.

Multifocal microhemosiderin deposits: Manifests as susceptibility foci. They are seen with increasing age but are confounded by hypertension and nonspecific small-vessel disease including amyloid angiopathy. Susceptibility-weighted imaging is more sensitive than conventional axial T2* imaging and should be routinely performed in patients older than 50 years. Multiple cavernous malformations (type IV) as multiple susceptibility foci, typically found in younger patients, can be a diagnostic challenge in rare cases. Similarly, multiple small hemorrhagic metastases presenting as pure hemorrhagic small foci are also very unusual.

Enlarged Virchow-Robin spaces: Virchow-Robin (VR) spaces increase in size and frequency with advancing age. Dilated VR spaces typically occur in three characteristic locations. Type I VR spaces appear along the lenticulostriate arteries entering the basal ganglia through the anterior perforated substance ("subcapsular"). Type II VR spaces are found along the paths of the perforating medullary arteries as they enter the cortical gray matter over the high convexities and extend into the white matter ("subcortical and subinsular"). Type III VR spaces appear in the midbrain ("peduncular"). Enlarged VR spaces is a nonspecific finding; they are seen in all age groups and in multiple neurodegenerative disorders as well as some inflammatory and metabolic storage disorders.

MR spectroscopy: MR spectroscopy demonstrates mild progressive changes in association with normal aging. Allowing for interregion and intersubject variability, there is generally decreased percent N-acetylaspartate (NAA) and its ratios, specifically in the mesial temporal lobes, semiovale, and cortices, representative of diminished neuronal density and dysfunction. In contrast, percent choline and its ratios are increased in these regions, reflecting increased glial activity.

Diffusion tensor imaging: Aging results in a mild but significant increase in the apparent diffusion coefficient (ADC), whereas fractional anisotropy is progressively reduced. These findings appear to accelerate after age 70 years. The declines in fractional anisotropy and the increase in diffusivity reflect a loss of myelin and axonal fibers and an increase in extracellular space.

Problem Solving: Is There a Clinical Diagnosis of NDD?

A common indication for brain imaging is *memory loss*. Memory loss is clinically nonspecific and often reflects the subjective symptoms of the patient rather than the results of formal testing demonstrating memory loss in comparison to age-matched cohort. It is important to interpret the imaging study in light of the provided clinical diagnosis. Morphologic imaging helps in determining the specific diagnosis by complementing the clinical diagnosis but should not be used as a primary initial tool for diagnosis. For example, MRI of the brain of a patient with no history of degenerative disorder interpreted as "unequivocal bilateral temporo-parietal volume loss as suggestive of either mild cognitive impairment or Alzheimer's disease" is appropriate only in the setting of a strong clinical history. If the patient is given a specific diagnosis by a neurologist, the neuroimager's job is fairly easy. It is the group of patients suffering from disorders with overlapping clinical presentations who require supplementary imaging that will assist the clinician with a diagnosis. The categories of

NDDs discussed below, reflects the common indications for acquiring an imaging study, usually as "a problem-solving tool."

Dementia-dominant disorders: Mainly includes AD, vascular dementia, FTD, and dementia with Lewy bodies (DLB). Evaluate the sulcal prominence and associated ventricular dilatation with focus on the selectivity and diffuse feature of the atrophy. If available, voxel-based morphometry or other volumetric measures can be used. Note that the methods require careful correction for calvarial size as well as age. Coronal plane can be used for subjective assessment of hippocampal atrophy. Tools are available for quantitative measures of hippocampal volumes. Specify small- and large-vessel ischemic changes in vascular dementia. Use susceptibility-weighted imaging for detection of hemosiderin parenchymal deposits, a stigmata of small-vessel ischemic disease and/or hypertension and cerebral amyloid angiopathy. Exclude focal frontotemporal focal lesions, which may clinically mimic FTD.

Rapidly progressive dementia: Rapidly progressive dementias develop subacutely over weeks to months, but sometimes over days. The most important role of neuroimaging is to identify signs of prion disease (i.e., CJD). Nonprion disorders constitute about 40% of rapidly progressive dementias, nearly half of which are due to rapidly progressive variants of AD, CBD, LBD, and FTD. CBD and LBD are more commonly confused clinically with CJD. The remainder of the nonprion rapidly progressive dementias either are of unknown origin or are caused by autoimmune or infectious disorders. Autoimmune limbic encephalitis occurs with or without associated malignancy.

Dementia with visual symptoms: The differential diagnosis can be narrowed if a patient with dementia or movement disorders also presents with visual symptoms. The major NDDs in this category include posterior cerebral atrophy (PCA), LBD, PSP, and CBD. Imaging features can be localized in occipital lobes and brainstem. The Heidenhain variant of CJD in a patient who presents with visual symptoms should be remembered because diagnosis can be made by diffusion-weighted imaging (discussed later).

Parkinsonian symptoms: In patients with parkinsonian symptoms, structural imaging is sometimes needed to differentiate PD from Parkinson plus disorders based on certain characteristic imaging features (discussed later). In parkinsonian disorders (e.g., IPD, MSA, PSP, CBD), focus on the deep gray matter, brainstem, and cerebellum, with emphasis on the external capsule, subthalamic nuclei, transverse pontine fibers, and cerebellum. Do not forget associated dementia in these disorders, which is thought to be predominantly subcortical but can have associated cerebral volume loss.

Nonparkinson movement disorders: Examples include Huntington chorea, dystonias, etc.

Progressive atrophy and weakness: Example is ALS. Evaluate the corticospinal tract, including the brainstem and spinal cord, for T2 signal changes.

Spastic paraplegia without amyotrophy: Example is primary lateral sclerosis. Evaluate corticospinal tract for atrophy due to the long-standing course of the disease.

Progressive ataxia: Spinal (e.g., Friedreich ataxia, Machado-Joseph disease). Hereditary cerebellar ataxia (e.g., autosomal dominant or recessive olivopontocerebellar atrophy). Acquired cerebellar ataxia (e.g., paraneoplastic, alcohol-related, idiopathic cerebellar ataxia [usually late onset]).

Problem Solving: Are Cerebral Atrophy, Hypoperfusion, and Hypometabolism Selective or Nonselective?

Generally, we estimate the selectivity of volume loss, for example, bilateral dominant occipital lobe volume loss in PCA or bifrontal volume loss in FTD. We will be correct in most cases if we follow the basic rule (i.e., interpretation in light of clinical diagnosis). If available, volumetric analyses should be used. Note that the routine use of biometric analysis in the clinical setting is somewhat limited due to the relative lack of software approved by the United States Food and Drug Administration. Until recently, software solutions for biometric analysis were largely research tools. The approved packages now available may provide useful information in the evaluation of volume loss. In this section, we focus on diffuse versus localized distribution of atrophy or hypoperfusion and hypometabolism in major NDDs. These changes constitute the core theme of structural and functional imaging in NDDs.

Alzheimer disease (Figures 8-2 through 8-5): AD is the most common cause of dementia. Clinical subtypes (or stages) are (1) mild cognitive impairment (MCI)—mild memory impairment, no cognitive deficits; (2) possible AD—secondary dementia in presence of secondary disease that does impair memory but is not the likely cause; and (3) probable AD—progressive memory loss with two or more cognitive dysfunctions. AD is characterized neuropathologically by the presence of amyloid-beta peptide–containing plaques, neurofibrillary tangles (tau protein aggregates), and amyloid angiopathy. Pathologic stages are (1) transentorhinal—neurofibrillary tangles in parahippocampal gyri (clinically asymptomatic); (2) limbic stage—neurofibrillary tangles increase in parahippocampal gyri and develop in hippocampus (MCI); and (3) neocortical stage—neurofibrillary tangles in temporal and parietal lobes and eventually the rest of the cortex (severe dementia).

MRI shows bilateral parietotemporal volumes loss with disproportionate hippocampal volumes loss, dilated temporal horns, and choroidal fissures. Hippocampal atrophy is a marker of cognitive dysfunction, and the rate of this atrophy is higher in AD than in controls and MCI. Atrophy of the posterior cingulate gyrus is an early finding of AD, and is possibly related to loss of afferent input from associated fibers since it is not a site of primary pathology. MR spectroscopy shows decreased NAA and increased myoinositol and choline in the medial temporal lobes and, to some extent, the parietal lobes. These metabolites are hypothesized to be surrogate markers of neuronal loss and increased glial activity in patients with AD.

Positron emission tomography (PET) is a well-established imaging modality for evaluation of AD.

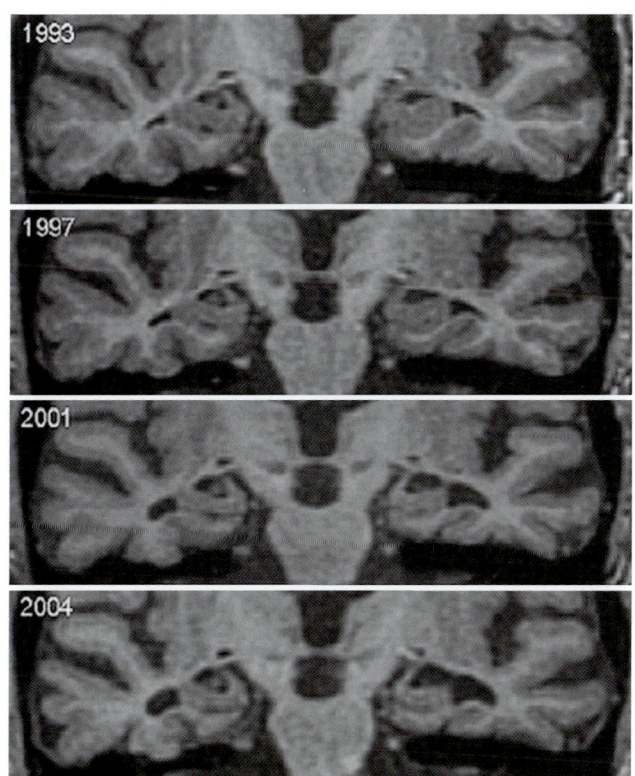

Figure 8-2 Alzheimer disease. Coronal T1 serial imaging showing progressive medial temporal lobe atrophy. (From Whitwell JL, Jack CR Jr. Neuroimaging in dementia. Neurol Clin 2007;25(3):843-857, viii.)

Regional cerebral glucose metabolism using PET ^{18}F-fluorodeoxyglucose (FDG) in AD shows characteristic reductions in neocortical association areas, including the posterior cingulate, precuneus, and temporoparietal and frontal association regions. The primary visual cortex, sensorimotor cortex, basal ganglia, and cerebellum are relatively unaffected. Remember that there is no consistent concordance between PET and histopathologic regional findings suggesting complex pathophysiology, mainly synaptic dysfunction. The sensitivity and specificity for diagnosis of AD is greater than 80% with both single-photon emission computed tomography (SPECT) and PET studies, but the cost effectiveness is debatable. To analyze functional studies on voxel-by-voxel basis, individual brain images need to be transformed into a standard coordinate system with various methods, such as statistical parametric maps, easy Z-score imaging system, and NEUROSTAT. The major advantages of these morphometric methods are better intersubject comparisons and much higher sensitivity and specificity. PET can identify preclinical AD cases with a strong family history, particularly with the apolipoprotein E ε4 allele, which is a risk factor for familial AD.

Amyloid PET imaging is being used for the diagnosis of AD. Multiple radioligands have been introduced, including ^{18}F-FDDNP, ^{11}C-PIB (Pittsburgh B compound), SB13, FPIB, and ^{11}C-BF-227. Pittsburgh B compound and ^{18}FDDNP are more studied and are shown to be more useful in the diagnosis of clinical and preclinical AD. Global increased retention of amyloid ligands occurs predominantly in the frontal and temporoparietal association areas, posterior cingulated gyrus, and caudate nuclei, with no significant increased retention in white matter, cerebellum, brainstem, sensorimotor cortex, and medial temporal lobes compared to the normal controls. Recall that medial temporal lobe atrophy determines cognitive dysfunction rather than amyloid deposition. Also of note, there is not a 1:1 correlation between the presence of brain amyloid and AD. Significant amyloid accumulation can be present in the absence of AD, and not all AD patients have large amyloid deposits. Despite these findings, amyloid binding agents hold great promise as a potential tool for the diagnosis of AD.

Posterior cortical atrophy (Benson's syndrome) (Figure 8-6): A rare early-onset dementing syndrome with predominant and progressive visual symptoms and later development of complex symptoms such as ocular apraxia (Balint syndrome) and agraphia (Gerstmann syndrome). Language, memory, insight, and judgment remain relatively preserved until late in the course of the disease. A number of different neuropathologic disorders are associated with posterior cortical atrophy. PCA is mostly associated with histopathologic changes similar to those found in AD and therefore is considered a subtype of AD. Typically bilateral parietooccipital atrophy is demonstrated on MRI and computed tomography (CT). SPECT and PET show deficits of perfusion and metabolism in both parietal and occipital lobes.

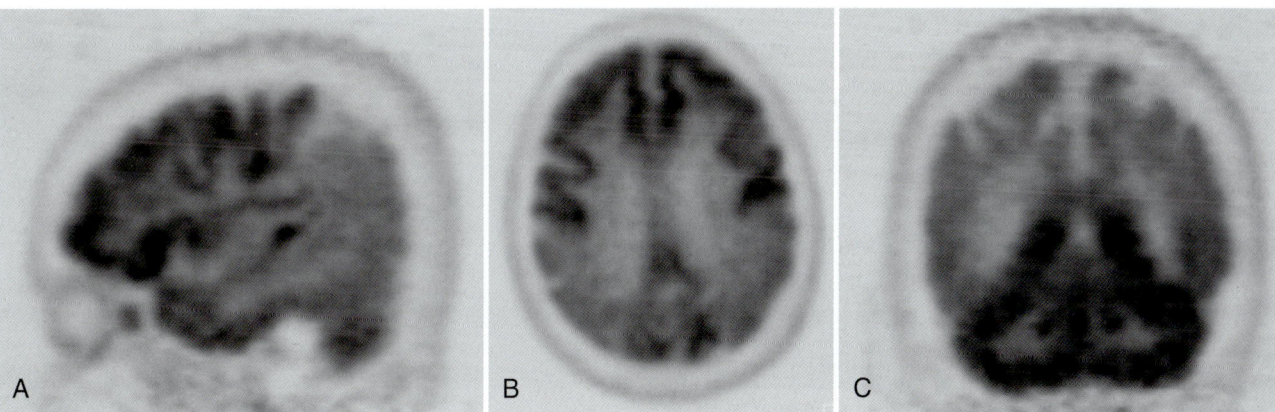

Figure 8-3 Alzheimer disease. Multiplanar ^{18}F-fluorodeoxyglucose positron emission tomographic images showing bilateral symmetric diminished metabolic activity in temporoparietal lobes but normal activity in occipital lobes (partially shown).

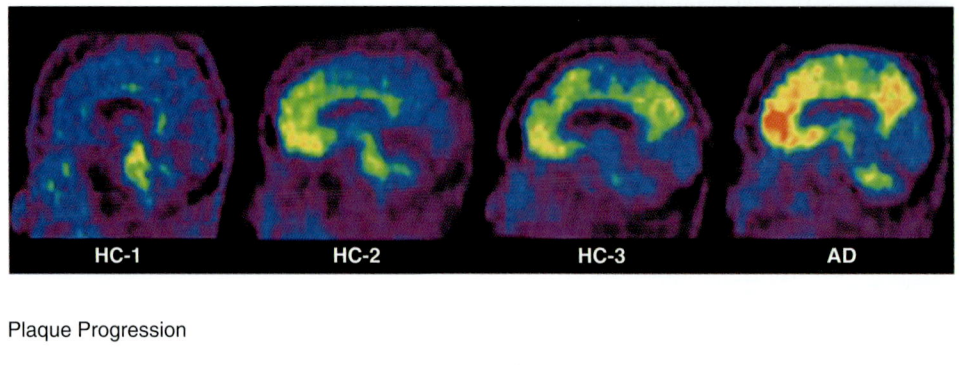

Figure 8-4 Alzheimer disease (AD). Sagittal positron emission tomographic images showing regional uptake of [^{11}C]-Pittsburgh compound B (PIB) reflecting amyloid (A) burden in the brain in three asymptomatic healthy age-matched control subjects (HC1 to 3) and one patient with Alzheimer disease (AD; *top*), and schematics showing the stages of amyloid deposition in the human brain as proposed by Braak and Braak *(bottom)*. All AD subjects matched stage C. About 20% of HC can have A deposition ranging from stage A to C. (From Rowe CC, Ng S, Ackermann U, et al. Imaging beta-amyloid burden in aging and dementia. *Neurology* 2007;68(20):1718-1725.)

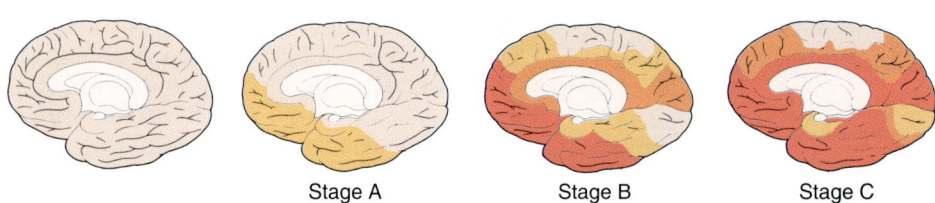

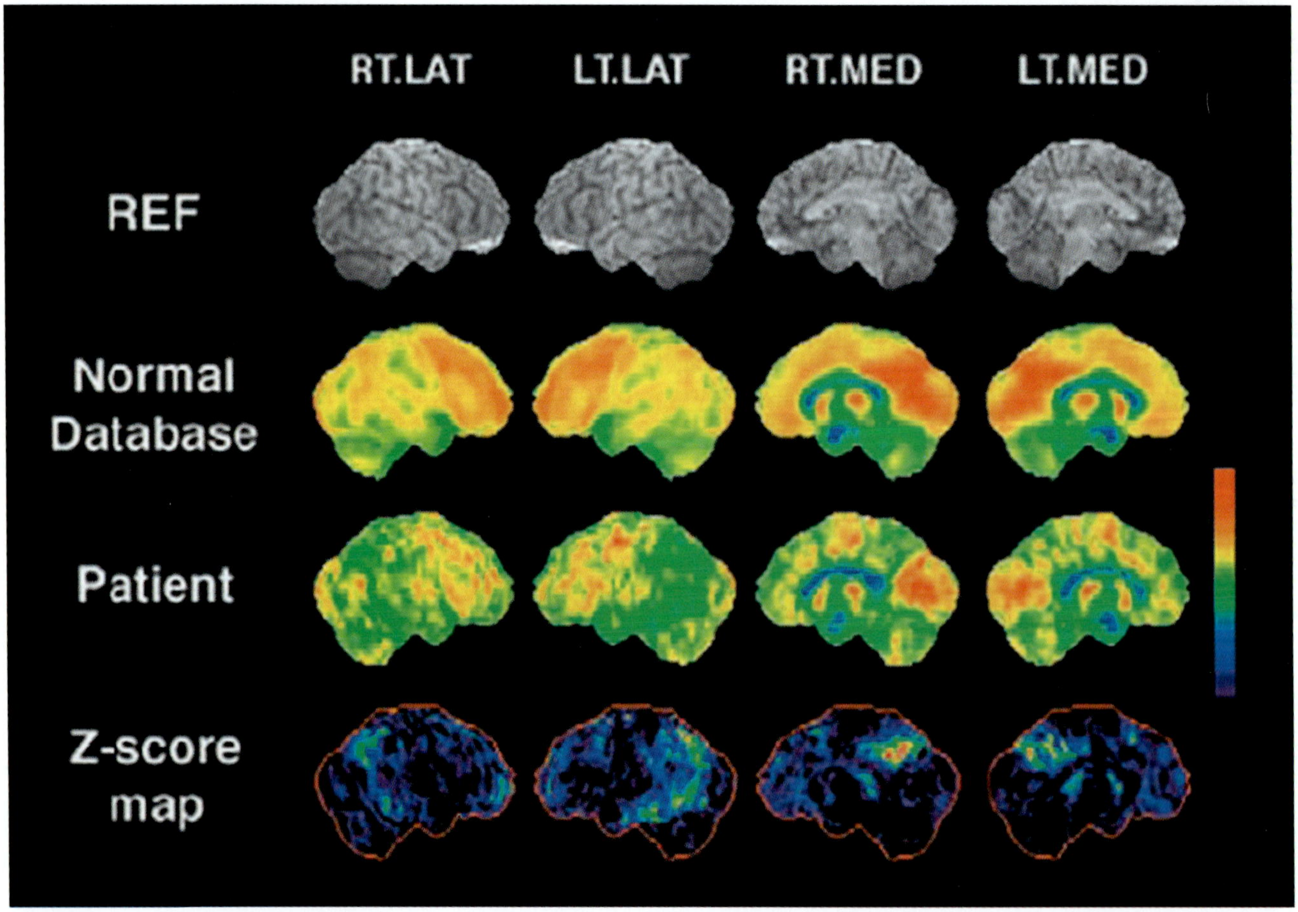

Figure 8-5 Alzheimer disease. Diagnostic Z-score mapping using normal database. Patient's positron emission tomographic image set compared with similarly processed normal patients database. Deviations of regional metabolic activity from normal values is expressed as Z scores *(bottom row)*. (From Minoshima S. Imaging Alzheimer's disease: clinical applications. *Neuroimaging Clin N Am* 2003;13(4):769-780.)

Dementia with Lewy bodies (Figure 8-7): Cortical neurodegenerative disease with established clinical criteria. Generally, more diffuse cerebral volume loss is present compared to AD. The neuropathologic findings in DLB, a condition that may account for up to 15% of dementia, frequently include amyloid beta plaques and neurofibrillary tangles. Therefore, some authors prefer the term *Lewy body variant of AD*. Medial temporal lobe atrophy is less prominent, particularly in the mesial temporal lobes (hippocampus and parahippocampal gyrus). Hypoperfusion and hypometabolism on SPECT and PET imaging are consistently found in the occipital cortex, primarily in association with visual areas, and in the posterior parietal cortex, especially the precuneus. Volume loss in these areas does not account for the hypoperfusion, and demonstration of cholinergic receptor changes in the occipital lobe suggests that cholinergic loss may be important.

Frontotemporal lobar degeneration (FTLD) (Figures 8-8 and 8-9): Commonly referred to as *frontotemporal dementia* (FTD), of which Pick disease is a pathologic variant. Like AD, FTD is a tauopathy. About 20% of cases of presenile dementia are due to FTD. Another type of inclusion is only labeled by anti-ubiquitin antibodies, thus isolating a subgroup of frontotemporal dementia (FTDu, an ubiquitinopathy), which sometimes is familial and sometimes is associated with ALS. FTD is a syndromic diagnosis that includes at least three clinical variants: behavioral variant FTD or the classic FTD; semantic dementia (SD); and progressive nonfluent aphasia.

Behavioral variant FTD causes bifrontal marked atrophy with hypometabolism predominantly in the ventromedial medial frontal region, anterior cingulate gyrus, anterior corpus callosum, and dorsolateral prefrontal cortex. However, the findings may be more widespread or may be within the normal range on the other extreme (the latter subgroup may have a more benign course). Progressive nonfluent aphasia shows dominant perisylvian atrophy. SD typically shows severe bilateral volume loss of the inferolateral temporal pole and parahippocampal regions with sparing of the superior temporal lobe ("temporal dominant FTD"). A new variant called *logopenic progressive aphasia* presents with a slow rate of speech output and word-finding pauses. In addition, the atrophy is more posterior, including angular gyrus and posterior aspects of the middle temporal gyrus and superior temporal sulcus. *Primary progressive aphasia*, a more common term, overlaps with progressive nonfluent aphasia and SD. Some consider primary progressive aphasia to be the primary disorder and the other three its subtypes.

Absence of frontotemporal atrophy does not exclude the diagnosis of FTD. The occipital lobes are almost always spared. Hypometabolism and hypoperfusion seen on functional studies correspond to the atrophy. FDG patterns can vary in the three aphasia subtypes. Typically left temporoparietal hypometabolism is seen in logopenic progressive aphasia, left frontal hypometabolism in progressive nonfluent aphasia, and left anterior temporal hypometabolism in SD.

Neuronal intermediate filament inclusion disease is a neuropathologically distinct, clinically heterogeneous variant of FTD; parkinsonism is one of the presentations. Frontotemporal and caudate atrophy is common.

Vascular dementia (Figure 8-10): Also termed *vascular cognitive disorder*. Generally considered the second most common cause of dementia in the elderly. Diagnosis is dependent on the presence of risk factors for ischemic cerebrovascular disease and temporal relationship of dementia to cerebrovascular events, focal neurologic deficits, and evidence of ischemic changes on imaging. Based on pathophysiology, vascular dementia can be divided into macroangiopathic (large-vessel disease with large cortical infarcts), microangiopathic (small-vessel disease with lacunar infarcts), and microhemorrhagic (multifocal small hemosiderin parenchymal deposits). Sequelae of large-vessel disease result in large discrete defects in the brain parenchyma on structural and functional imaging: multiple infarcts (multiinfarct dementia) or single stroke dementia (strategic stroke vascular dementia).

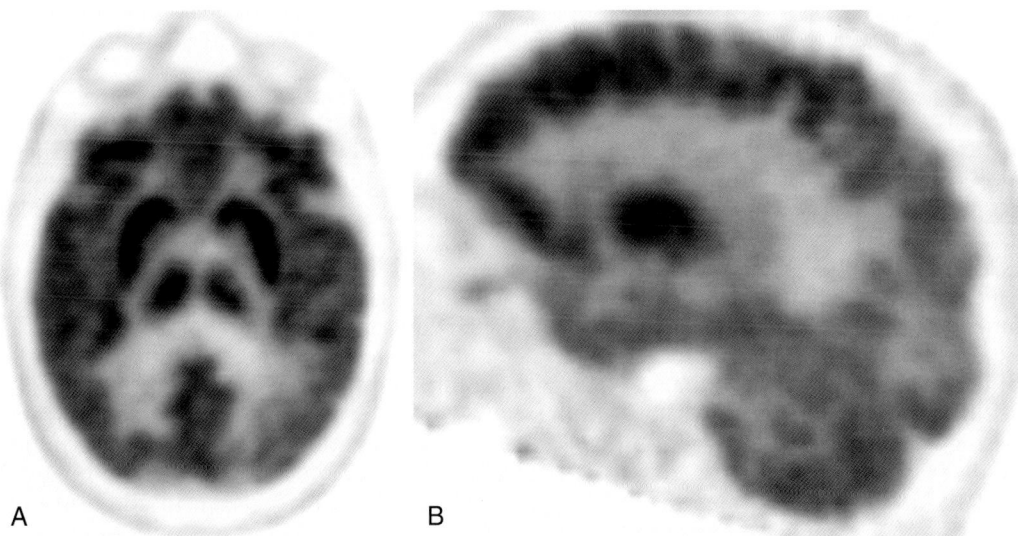

Figure 8-6 Posterior cortical atrophy. Axial and medial sagittal ^{18}F-fluorodeoxyglucose positron emission tomographic images showing bilateral symmetric diffuse hypometabolism in the occipital and adjacent parietal lobes.

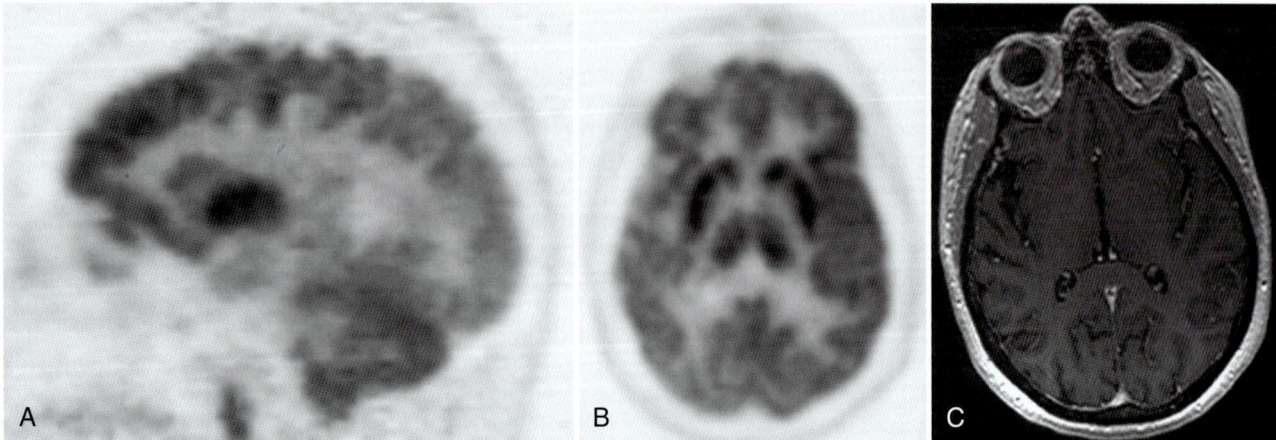

Figure 8-7 Dementia with Lewy body. **A, B:** Global hypometabolism including occipital lobes on ^{18}F-fluorodeoxyglucose positron emission tomographic scan. **C:** Axial T1 magnetic resonance image showing no occipital atrophy.

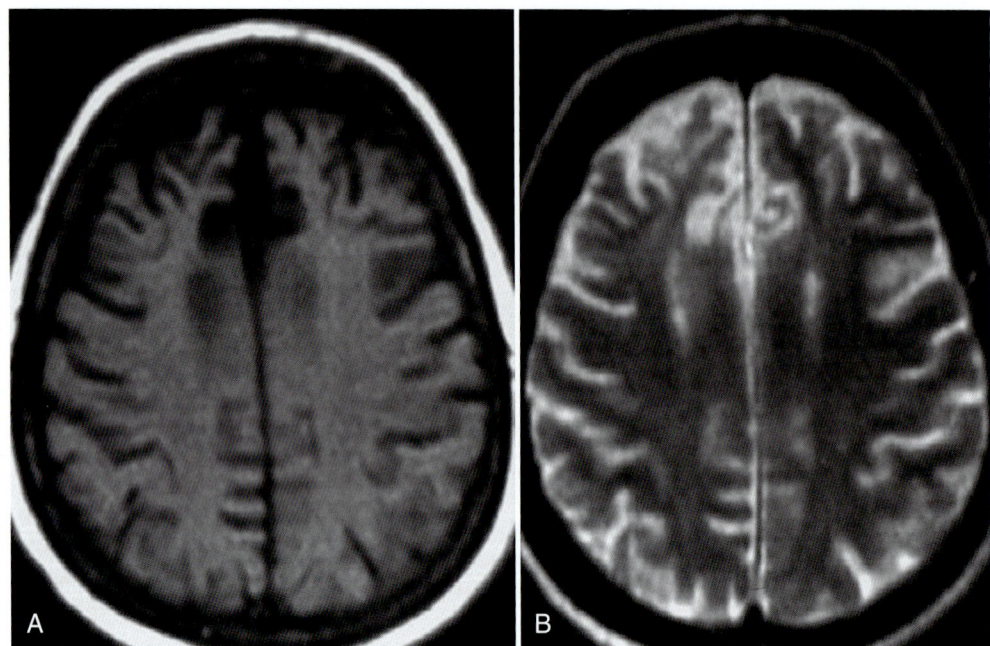

Figure 8-8 Frontotemporal dementia. Axial T1 and T2 images demonstrating bilateral selective anterior frontal cortical atrophy, greater on the right side. (From Gallucci M, Limbucci N, Catalucci A, Caulo M. Neurodegenerative diseases. *Radiol Clin North Am* 2008;46(4):799-817, vii.)

Striatal and particularly thalamic infarcts are easily identified on MRI or CT. They can account for significant cognitive and behavioral dysfunction due to impaired striatocortical and thalamocortical circuitry, particularly in the premotor frontal cortex. Several white matter grading scales for quantitating the degree of vascular disease have been developed. The methods range from very simple assessments to highly detailed regional quantitative measures. Additionally, software methodologies for assessment of the total degree of white matter changes are available. What role these methods will play in the everyday assessment of clinical patients with potential vascular-based dementia is unclear.

Idiopathic Parkinson disease (Figures 8-11 and 8-12): Cognitive impairment and neuropsychiatric symptoms are frequent in PD, with a 70% cumulative incidence of dementia. Parkinson disease with dementia (PDD) is considered a distinct entity from AD. Neuropathologically, it is characterized by the degeneration of populations of nerve cells that develop filamentous inclusions in the form of Lewy bodies and Lewy neurites. These inclusions are made of the tubular filamentous nonsoluble protein alpha-synuclein. PD demonstrates volume loss predominantly in the frontal lobes, whereas PDD affects temoroparietal as well as occipital regions but less prominent medial temporal lobe/hippocampal volume loss than AD and DLB.

The pattern of glucose hypometabolism on FDG PET in PDD resembles AD-dominant hypometabolism in the temporoparietal regions, predominantly in the parietal lobes (angular gyrus), in addition to global hypometabolism.

Presynaptic denervation is the underlying pathogenesis of IPD. ^{18}F-6-Fluorodopa on PET imaging as a

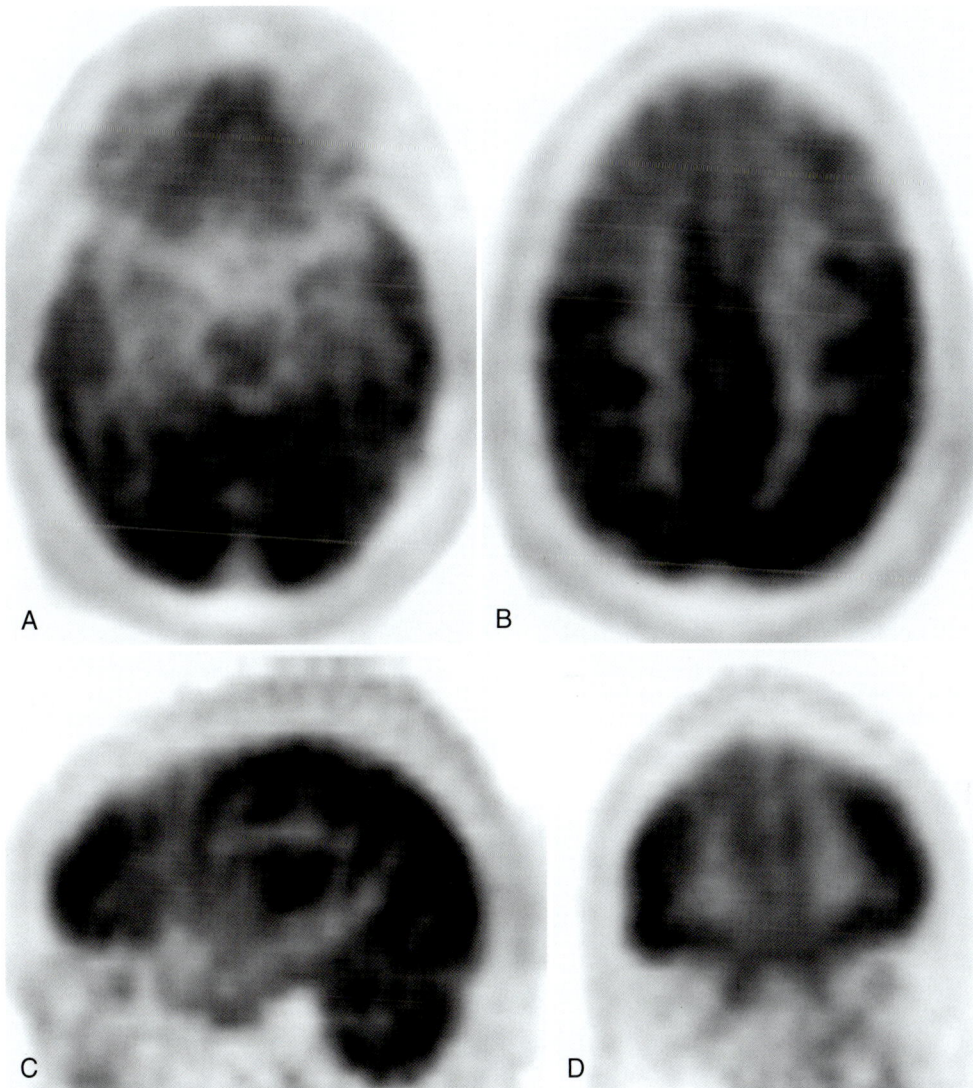

Figure 8-9 Frontotemporal dementia. Multiplanar ^{18}F-fluorodeoxyglucose positron emission tomographic images showing bilateral symmetric frontal and temporal lobes hypometabolism.

marker of dopamine synthesis shows decreased striatal uptake, mainly in the posterior putamina, that is asymmetric early in the course of the disease. Uptake is proportional to the severity of motor deficits. Radiotracer imaging of dopamine transporter (DAT) using SPECT- (FP-CIT, beta-CIT, IPT, TRODAT) or PET-(^{11}C CFT) provides a marker for presynaptic dopamine reuptake. Striatal DAT ligand SPECT uptake is markedly reduced in PD. Brain imaging with DAT ligands helps to determine whether drug-induced parkinsonism is entirely drug induced or is an exacerbation of subclinical PD. About 10% to 15% of the cases diagnosed as early PD may have normal SPECT scans termed as "subjects with scans without evidence of dopaminergic deficit" and generally are determined to be non-PD cases. However, functional imaging has the potential to detect preclinical disease in relatives of PD patients because the clinical manifestations require significantly low levels of dopaminergic dysfunction. Postsynaptic dopaminergic (D2 receptor) imaging with SPECT-IBZM and PET-^{11}C-raclopride also shows decreased striatal uptake but cannot clearly differentiate PD from other parkinsonian disorders.

Multisystem atrophy (Figure 8-13): A sporadic, progressive, neurodegenerative disease of undetermined etiology. Parkinsonian features dominate in more than 80% of patients with MSA, broadly termed as *MSA-P*, whereas cerebellar features dominate in 20% to 50%, termed *MSA-C*. The latter presents with gait ataxia, dysarthria, akinetic limb ataxia, and cerebellar oculomotor disturbance. MSA patients also have autonomic failure in the form of orthostatic hypotension and genitourinary/gastrointestinal disturbances. If autonomic failure predominates, MSA is known as *Shy-Drager syndrome*. If parkinsonism predominates, it is known as *striatonigral degeneration* (SND). If cerebellar ataxia predominates, MSA is known as *sporadic olivopontocerebellar atrophy*. Although cognitive dysfunction may appear minimal, most patients experience frontal system impairment, and many develop dementia late in the course of the disease.

Diffuse progressive cortical atrophy is seen particularly in the SND subtype, with some frontal lobe dominance.

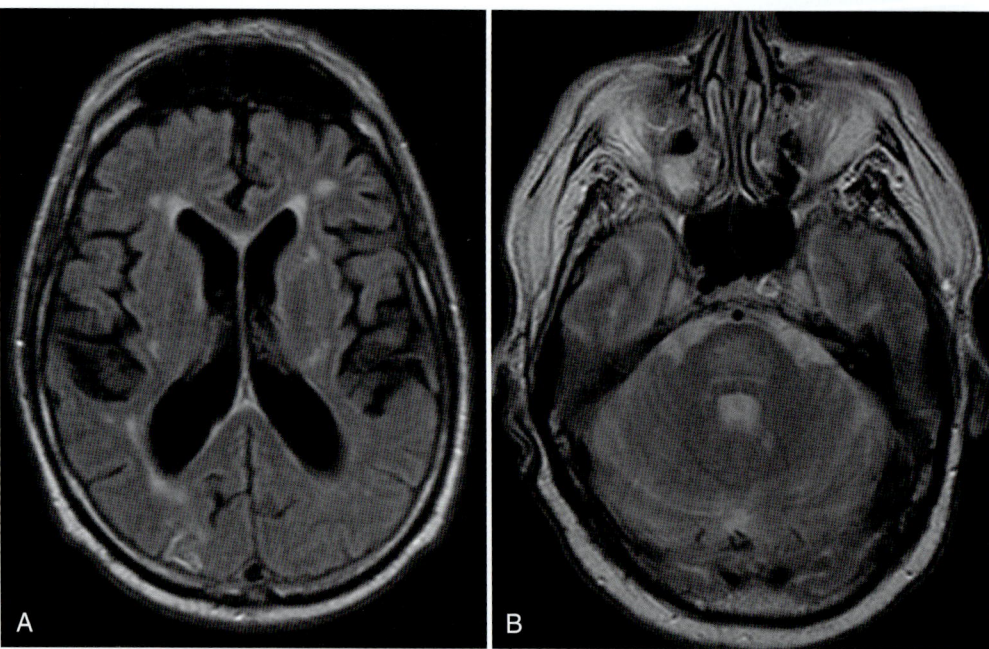

Figure 8-10 Vascular dementia. A: Axial fluid-attenuated inversion recovery image of vasculopathy and clinical diagnosis of multiinfarct dementia showing white matter change and right remote lateral occipital infarct. B: Axial T2 image showing typical pontine small vessel ischemic sequela as well as chronic occlusion of left internal carotid artery lacking normal flow void.

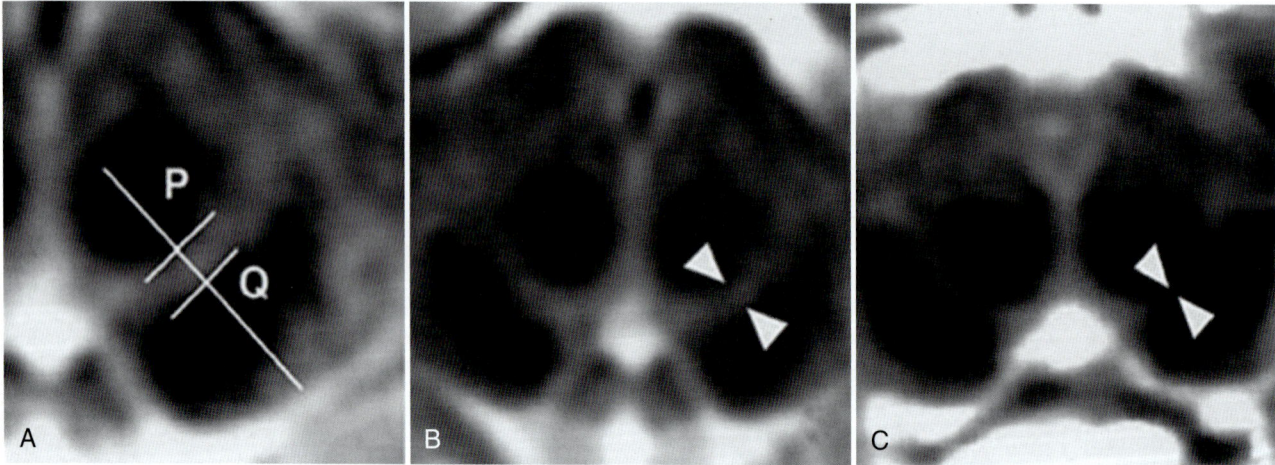

Figure 8-11 Idiopathic Parkinson disease. Magnified axial T2 images showing normal width of substantia nigra (A, B) and marked attenuation (C) in a patient with Parkinson disease.

There is characteristic subcortical and infratentorial atrophy but overlaps in the clinical subtypes and even some overlap with PD. Pontine flattening is seen on sagittal imaging. Decreased anteroposterior diameter of the pons and middle cerebellar peduncles on axial imaging is generally seen. "Hot cross bun sign" is a pontine cruciform hyperintensity on axial T2 imaging that reflects degeneration of transverse pontine fibers. Brachium pontis, cerebellar hemispheric, and vermian atrophy is a dominant feature of sporadic olivopontocerebellar atrophy. Bilateral T2 hyperintensities in the pontine base and brachium pontis is an additional feature relatively specific to MSA compared to PD. Dorsolateral putaminal T2 hypointensity with lateral rim "slit-like" T2 hyperintensity reflects putaminal volume loss and/or gliosis and is more frequent in SND subtype.

Progressive supranuclear palsy (Figure 8-14): PSP is a rare brain disorder that causes serious and permanent problems with control of gait and balance. The prominent clinical manifestation is an inability to aim the eyes properly, resulting in visual symptoms. PSP patients often show alterations of mood and behavior, including depression and apathy, as well as progressive mild dementia. Midbrain atrophy and periaqueductal T2 hyperintensity in the tegmentum and tectum of the brainstem are fairly characteristic features of PSP. Atrophy of the thalamus, striatum, and frontal cortex is also seen. Midbrain structures are more atrophied in PSP than in CBD. Typical (but not pathognomonic) findings in PSP are decreased metabolism and flow in the frontal lobes (hypofrontalism), particularly the medial frontal lobes.

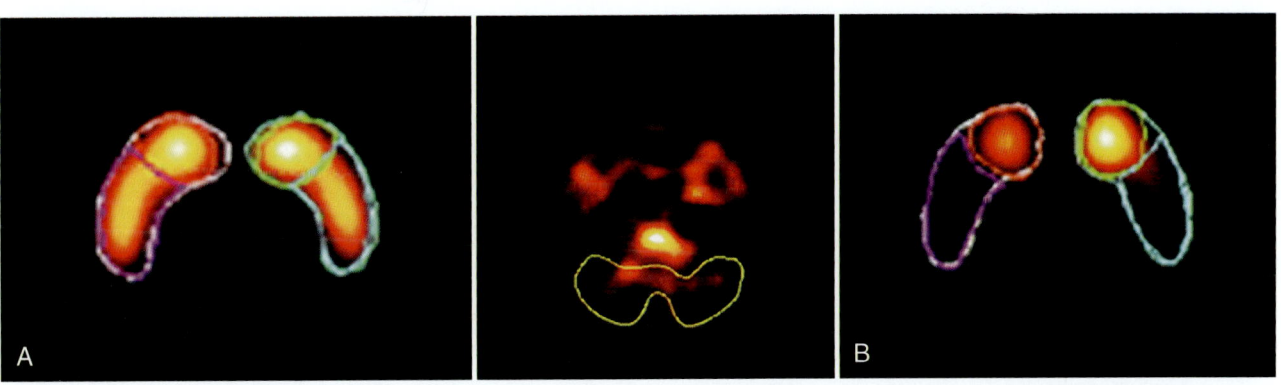

Figure 8-12 Idiopathic Parkinson disease. **A:** Normal striata visualized by ^{123}I-β-CIT SPECT. Regions of interest include the whole striatum as well as the putamen and caudate nucleus separately. Cerebellum used as a reference region. **B:** Striata of a patient with Parkinson disease. Note interstriatal asymmetry and predominance of putaminal degeneration. (From Eerola J, Tienari PJ, Kaakkola S, Nikkinen P, Launes J. How useful is [123I]beta-CIT SPECT in clinical practice? *J Neurol Neurosurg Psychiatry* 2005;76(9):1211-1216.)

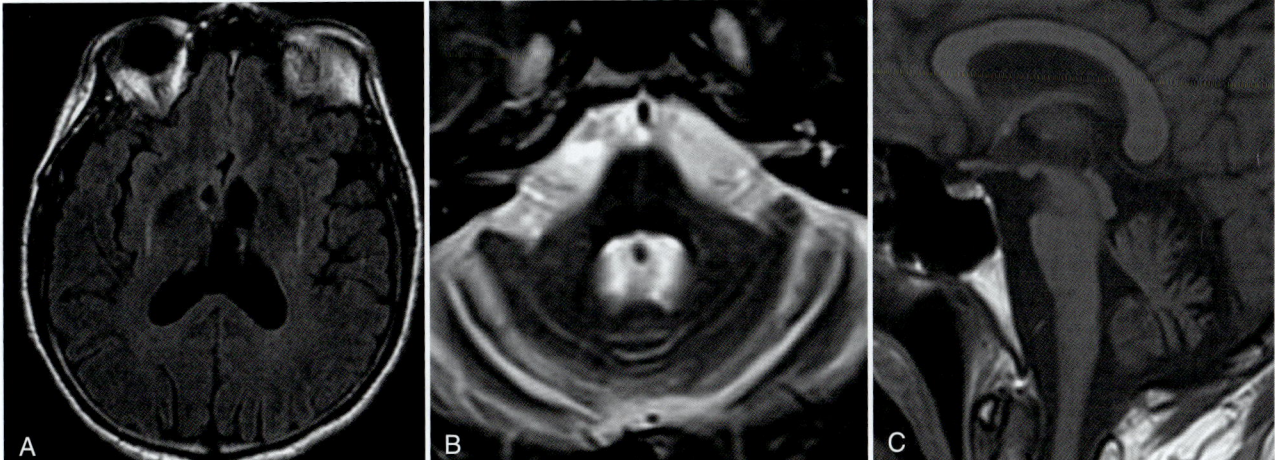

Figure 8-13 Multisystem atrophy. **A:** Lateral putaminal rim T2 hyperintensity on axial fluid-attenuated inversion recovery image. **B:** Axial T2 image showing faintly visualized transverse pontine fibers hyperintensity due to degeneration ("hot cross bun sign"). **C:** Midline sagittal T1 image showing ventral pontine flattening due to atrophy.

Corticobasal degeneration (Figure 8-15): Corticobasal ganglionic degeneration is a rare progressive neurologic disorder characterized by a combination of parkinsonism and cortical dysfunction with strikingly asymmetric features. CBD appears to be closely related to PSP in clinical, pathologic, and genetic terms. In CBD, cognitive symptoms dominate, whereas in PSP, eye movement symptoms dominate. Eye movement abnormalities are common, as in PSP, and a supranuclear gaze palsy can be seen, as in PSP. Parasagittal and paracentral atrophy (perirolandic gyri) is a distinctive feature of CBD and distinguishes it from AD. Asymmetric parietal and dorsal frontal atrophy (contralateral to the side more severely affected), third ventricle dilatation, and lenticular T2 hypointensity are useful aids to careful clinical evaluation. Hyperintensity in the subcortical white matter in the rolandic region on fluid-attenuated inversion recovery (FLAIR) images, asymmetric midbrain, and cerebral peduncle atrophy may be present. Asymmetric glucose hypometabolism and ^{18}F-dopa uptake are seen on PET imaging in the parietal lobe, striatum and thalamus.

Huntington disease (Figure 8-16): Autosomal dominant NDD with loss of γ-aminobutyric acid (GABA)ergic neurons of basal ganglia. Presents with the triad of dementia, choreoathetosis, and psychosis. MRI shows diffuse cerebral atrophy with frontal lobe dominance. The characteristic imaging feature is bilateral caudate nuclear atrophy, which is objectively measured by calculating the ratio of intercaudate distance to the distance between the lateral margins of the frontal horns or inner tables; the latter is more specific and sensitive. Putaminal atrophy is another major imaging feature. Decreased FDG uptake in the basal ganglia can be seen before the development of atrophy and can be used in gene-positive patients at risk for Huntington disease.

Amyotrophic lateral sclerosis (Figure 8-17): Also called *Lou Gehrig disease*. A rapidly progressive, invariably fatal neurologic disease affecting upper and lower motor neurons. The muscles gradually weaken, waste away, and twitch. Degeneration of the corticospinal tract is manifested by posterior limb internal capsule and white matter T2 and FLAIR hyperintensities; internal capsule hyperintensity is a specific sign on PD images. Hypointense line along the posterior rim of the precentral gyri gray matter is seen in patients with ALS. Subcortical white matter T2 hyperintensity

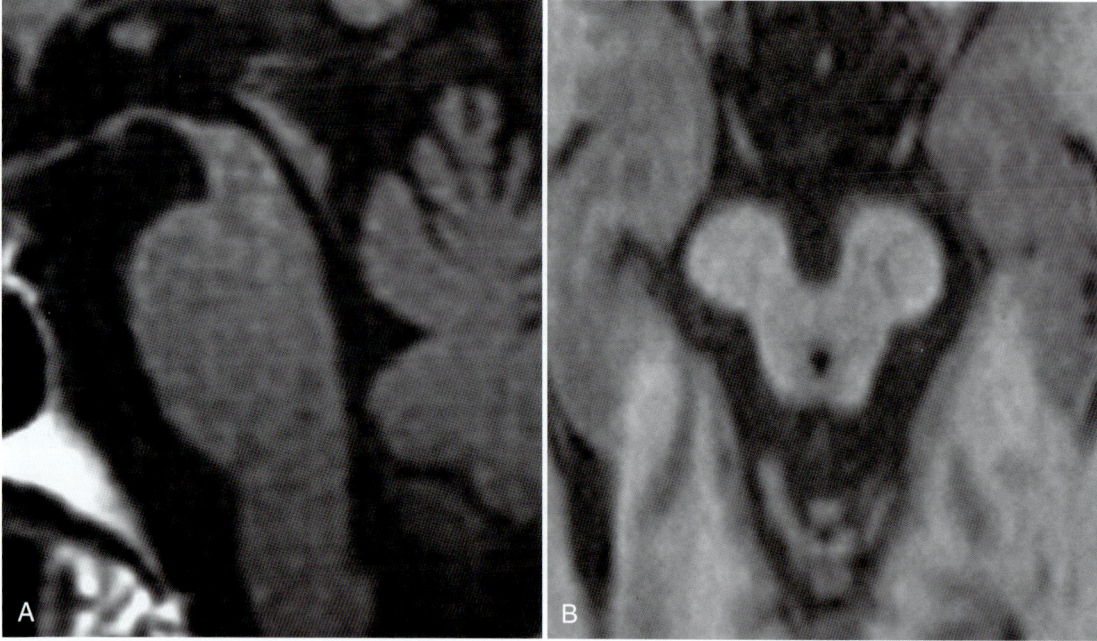

Figure 8-14 Progressive supranuclear palsy. **A:** Midline sagittal T1 image showing pontomesencephalic disproportion with marked midbrain atrophy resulting in a penguin or hummingbird profile. **B:** Mickey Mouse sign on axial T1 midbrain image.

is a useful sign in clinically verified ALS and is better seen on FLAIR images, but both of these signs can also be seen in normal older patients. Hyperintense T2 changes in the body of the corpus callosum represent degeneration of the commissural fibers interconnecting the motor cortices bilaterally. Progressive symmetric frontotemporal atrophy, particularly of the sensorimotor strip, is seen in ALS with or without dementia (termed *ALSD*). Typically, bifrontal but more extensive hemispheric hypometabolism and hypoperfusion can be demonstrated on SPECT and PET studies.

Problem Solving: Reversible versus Irreversible Dementia (Figures 8-18 through 8-21)

One of the most important roles of structural imaging is ruling out dementia mimickers. Reversible dementia is a relative term, because some disorders included in this category may not be completely reversible. The percentages of reversibility in dementia vary, up to 23% for partial reversal and up to 10% for full reversal. Depression, drug intoxication, and metabolic and neurosurgical disorders are the major causes of reversible dementia.

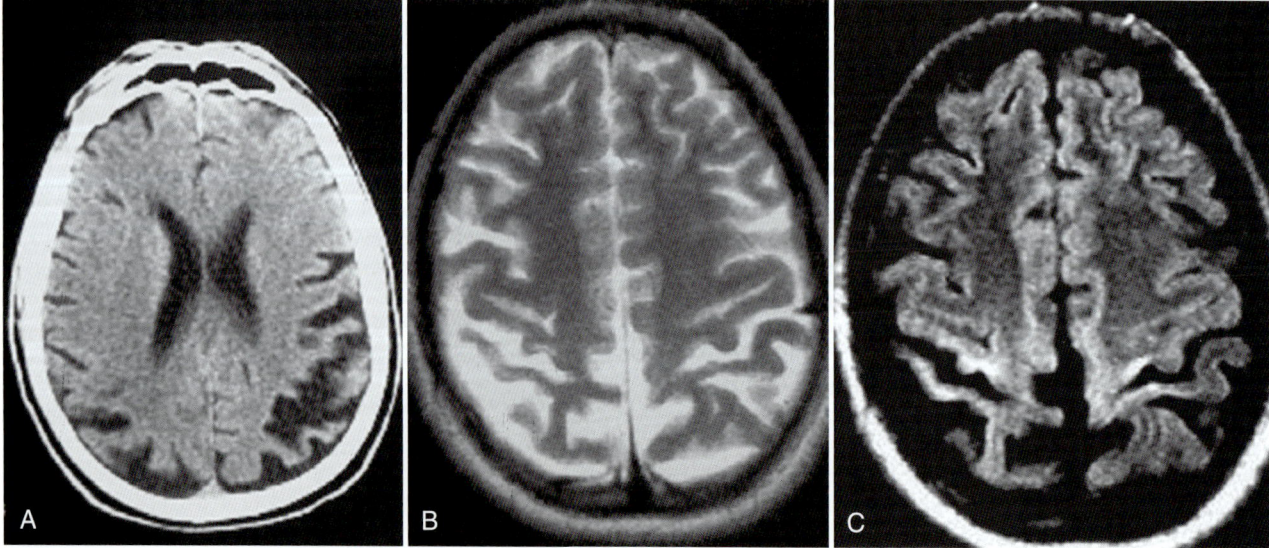

Figure 8-15 Corticobasal degeneration. **A:** Axial computed tomographic image showing asymmetric left parietal cortical atrophy. Axial fluid-attenuated inversion recovery **(B)** and T2 **(C)** images in another patient showing symmetric parietal atrophy. (From Gallucci M, Limbucci N, Catalucci A, Caulo M. Neurodegenerative diseases. *Radiol Clin North Am* 2008;46(4):799-817, vii.)

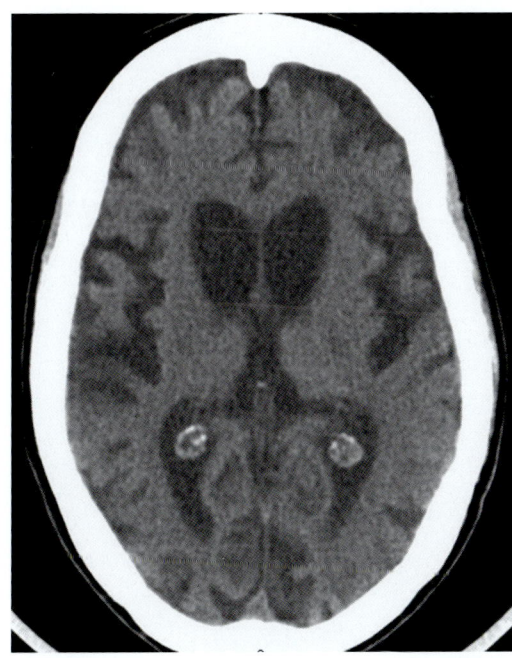

Figure 8-16 Huntington disease. Axial computed tomographic image demonstrating typical bilateral frontal horn lateral flattening due to caudate atrophy.

are seen in dementia due to vitamin B_{12} deficiency and hypothyroidism.

Infectious dementia is seen less frequently now, although a resurgence has taken place in the past three decades with the emergence of acquired immunodeficiency syndrome (AIDS) and variant CJD. Endemic or high-risk groups of dementia at younger ages warrants workup for an infectious etiology. Human immunodeficiency virus (HIV) dementia, also known as *AIDS dementia complex*, an AIDS defining illness, is caused by direct infection of the macrophages and microglia of the central nervous system by the HIV retrovirus, with likely indirect neurotoxic effects on the neurons. The most common imaging feature is a generalized cortical atrophy, which is unusual for younger patients. Diffuse patchy white matter T2 hyperintensity is another prominent feature, mainly in the peritrigonal and subinsular regions. The incidence of HIV dementia is reduced from about 20% to 5% after introduction of highly active antiretroviral therapy (HAART). A severe form of nonspecific leukoencephalopathy can be seen in patients who do not respond to HAART. Neurosyphilis, a somewhat forgotten disease in the western world, is caused by *Treponema pallidum*, which invades the central nervous system early in the course of disease but causes persistent infection in only a subset of infected persons. Individuals with persistent infection or asymptomatic meningitis are at risk for developing symptomatic neurosyphilis. The forms of presentation of neurosyphilis can be grouped in two categories: early (asymptomatic, meningeal, and meningovascular neurosyphilis) and late (progressive general paralysis or dementia paralytica and tabes dorsalis). Meningovascular type manifests as subacute encephalitis syndrome with vasculitis pattern causing infarcts that result in dementia. Dementia paralytica shows diffuse cerebral atrophy predominantly in the mesial temporal lobes. Mesial temporal T2 hyperintensity may be present in addition to nonspecific white matter T2 changes. T2 signal changes improve after penicillin therapy. Lyme disease can result in frontal dementia with subcortical degeneration.

CJD, a rapidly progressive and fatal disease, is caused by a protease-resistant prion protein. A characteristic

Imaging is negative in most of these conditions except for neurosurgical conditions, which comprise subdural hematoma (typically, chronic subdural hematomas with rebleeds and fluctuating mental status), normal pressure hydrocephalus, and intracranial tumors (e.g., anterior fossa large olfactory groove meningioma). This group of disorders also validates the cost effective use of noncontrast CT head for workup of dementias.

Alcohol is a common identifiable cause of cognitive dysfunction. Amnestic syndrome, alcohol dementia, and Wernicke-Korsakoff syndrome (WKS) constitute distinct entities. Diffuse cerebellar atrophy is a consistent marker of alcohol abuse. Specifically, look for mamillary bodies atrophy in chronic cases of Wernicke-Korsakoff syndrome. No specific brain imaging findings

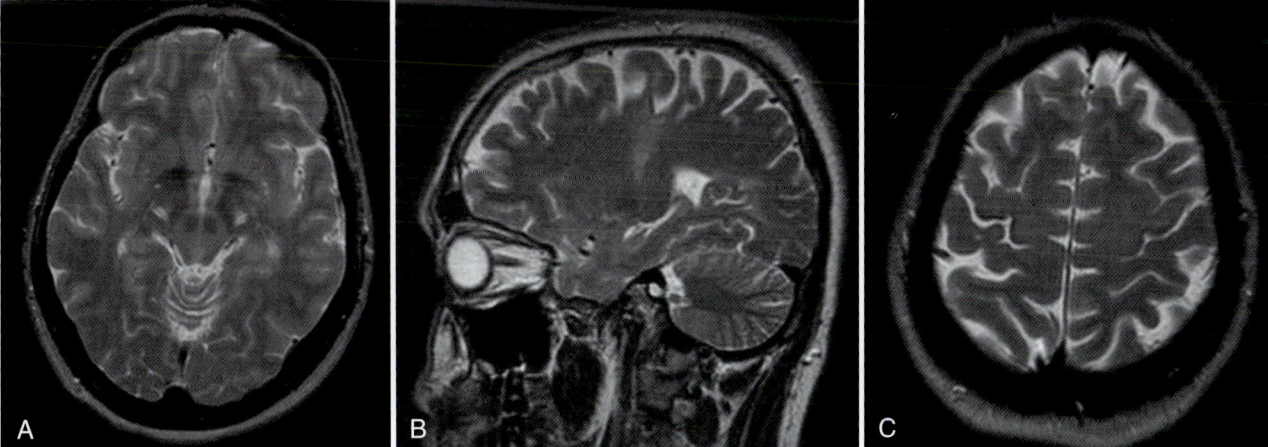

Figure 8-17 Amyotrophic lateral sclerosis. **A:** Axial T2 image showing bilateral corticospinal tract (CST) hyperintensities. **B:** Sagittal T2 image showing subcortical CST hyperintensity. **C:** Axial T2 image demonstrating bilateral motor cortex diffuse hypointensity.

346 SECTION III PROBLEM SOLVING: DISEASE CATEGORIES

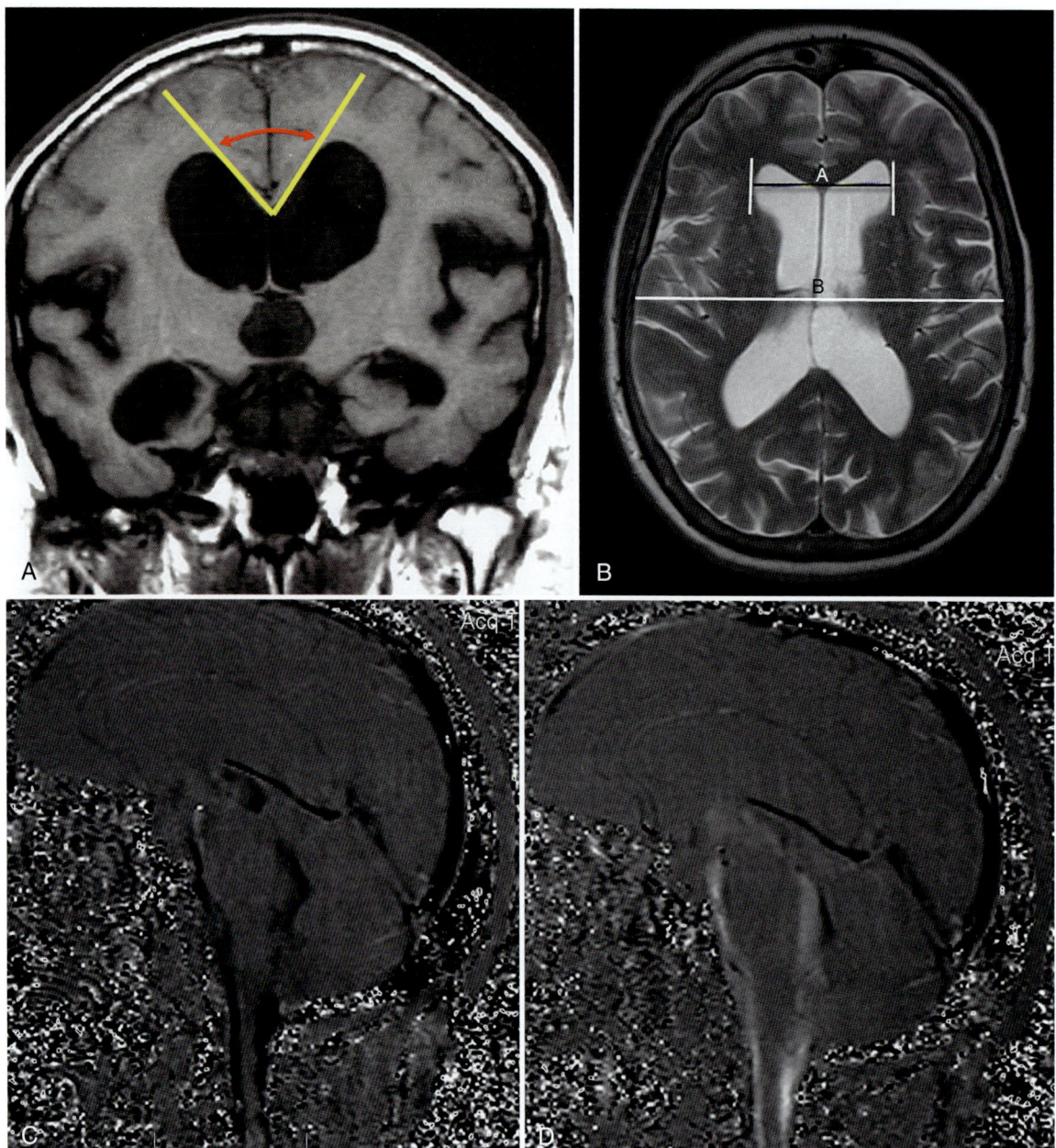

Figure 8-18 Normal pressure hydrocephalus. **A:** Coronal T1 image showing callosal angle (CA <90 degrees). Mean CA is 65 degrees with semantic dementia of 15 degrees compared to 105 degrees in Alzheimer disease. **B:** Axial T2 image demonstrating measurement of the Evan ratio (>0.3). **C, D:** Sagittal midline representative images from cine cerebrospinal fluid (CSF) flow study showing subjective evidence of robust aqueductal CSF flow (alternating phases manifested by black and white colors).

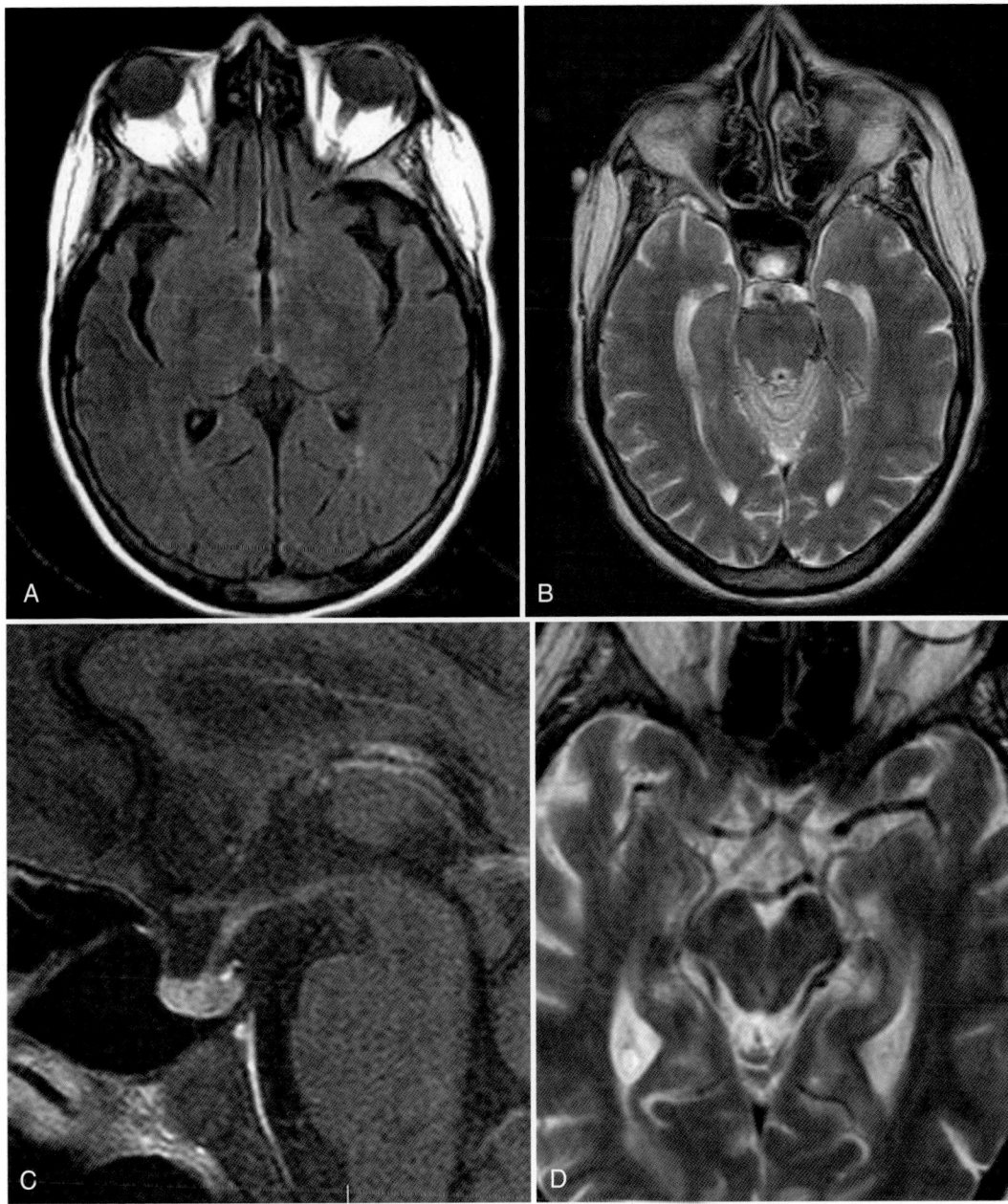

Figure 8-19 Wernicke's encephalopathy. Axial fluid-attenuated inversion recovery image **(A)** showing hypothalamic and axial T2 image **(B)** showing periaqueductal T2 hyperintensity in an acute case of Wernicke encephalopathy. **C, D:** A chronic case showing severe mamillary body atrophy on sagittal and axial imaging. Note that mamillary bodies are consistently seen in normal patients.

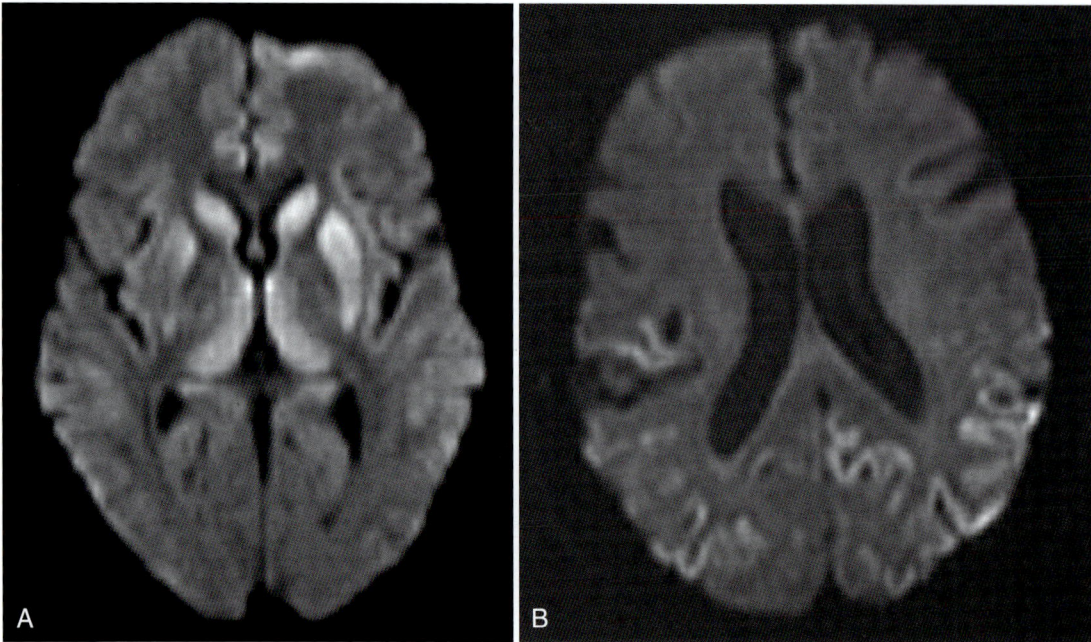

Figure 8-20 Creutzfeldt-Jakob disease. **A:** Axial diffusion tensor image showing bilateral typical striatal and thalamic hyperintensity in a case of variant Creutzfeldt-Jakob disease. **B:** Selective bilateral parietooccipital lobe (posterior) cortical hyperintensity in another patient (Heidenhain variant of Creutzfeldt-Jakob disease).

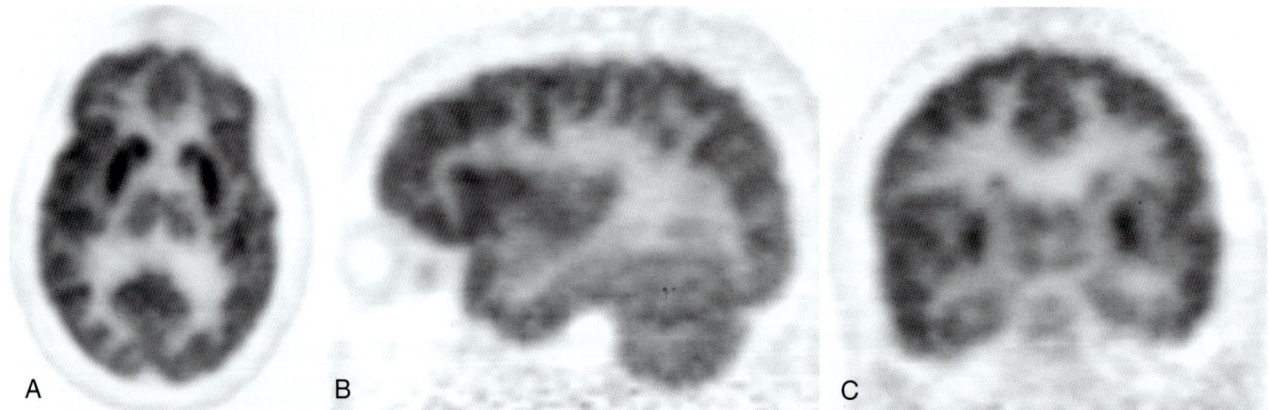

Figure 8-21 Neurosyphilis. Multiplanar ^{18}F-fluorodeoxyglucose positron emission tomographic images showing nonspecific finding of global cortical hypometabolism in a patient with dementia and neurosyphilis.

triad of myoclonus, progressive dementia, and periodic sharp-wave patterns are signs of cortical dysfunction. The course of the disease is the key to suspecting CJD. CJD is classified into sporadic, variant, familial, and iatrogenic types. Diffusion-weighted imaging is the MRI sequence of choice. Interpretation pearls are to: use narrower display windowing for DWI, focus on mesial cortices, think of other disorders if cortical or pial enhancement is present, and recommend follow-up study if the clinical suspicion is high and the current study is negative. Sporadic CJD, the most common type, occurs worldwide and causes hyperintensity of the putamen and caudate nuclei. The variant form typically causes bilateral dorsal thalamic T2 hyperintensity ("pulvinar and hockey-stick signs"). As in PCA, the Heidenhain variant of CJD presents with visual symptoms and dementia with dominant occipital cortical diffusion hyperintensity.

Problem Solving: Mild Cognitive Impairment to Alzheimer Disease
(Figure 8-22)

MCI is an intermediate state between normal cognitive aging and dementia and is a major risk factor for dementia. Diagnosis is based on clinical criteria of a nondemented patient with subjective and objective memory impairment but largely intact cognition and preserved daily activities. MCI is divided into single or multiple domain amnestic MCI (aMCI) and nonamnestic MCI (naMCI). The risk is higher in aMCI progressing to AD, with rates of 10% to 15% per year and 50% at 5 years. Other risk factors are degree of cognitive dysfunction, presence of a specific apolipoprotein E gene allele, and severity of hippocampal atrophy. About 10% to 25% of MCI cases progress to dementia in 10 years;

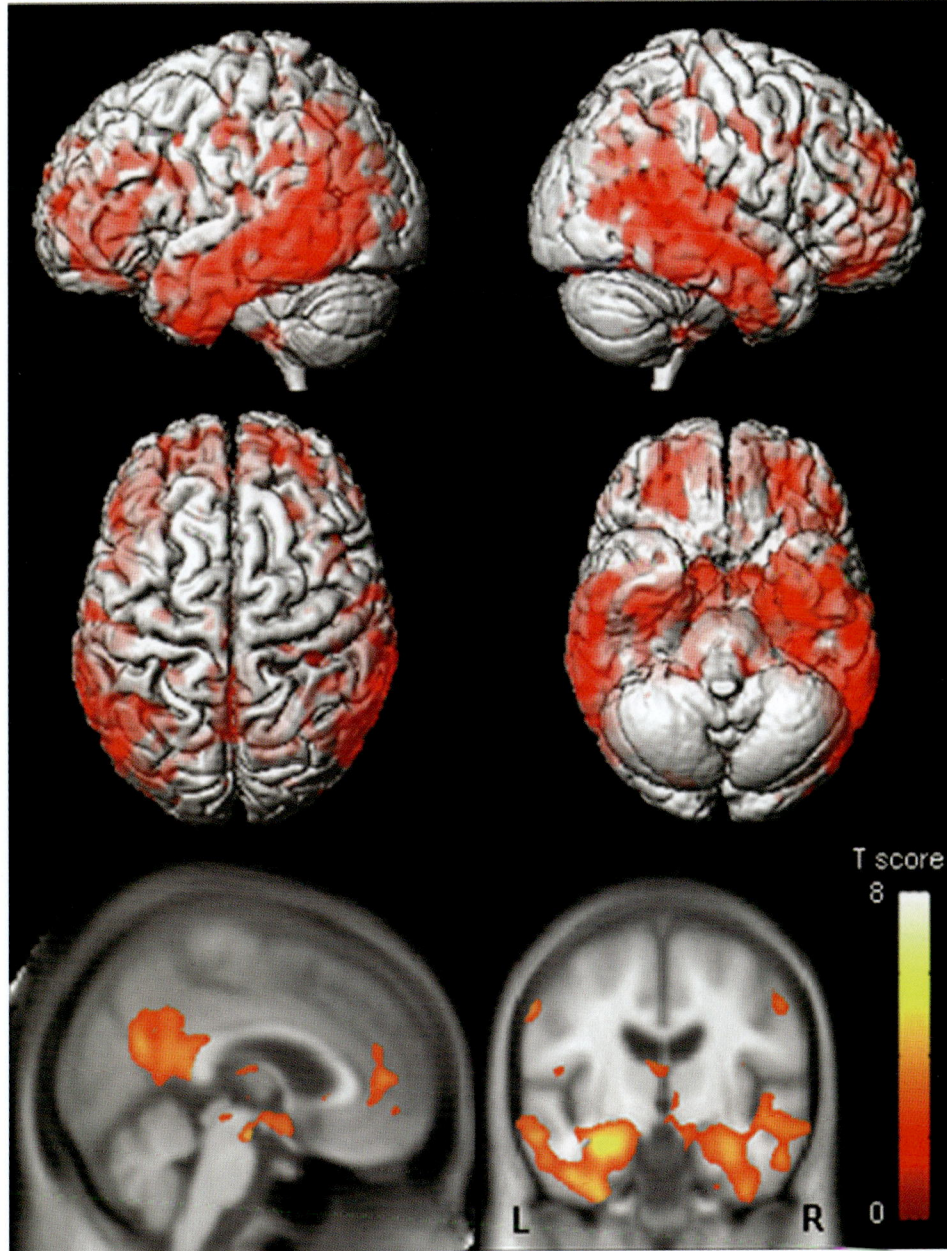

Figure 8-22 Amnestic mild cognitive impairment (aMCI). *Top:* Patterns of cortical atrophy shown on a three-dimensional surface rendering, based on voxel-based morphometry. *Bottom:* Results shown on a sagittal and coronal slice through the customized template, selected to highlight changes in the cingulate cortex and the medial temporal lobes. (From Whitwell JL, Shiung MM, Przybelski SA, et al. MRI patterns of atrophy associated with progression to AD in amnestic mild cognitive impairment. Neurology 2008;70(7):512-520.)

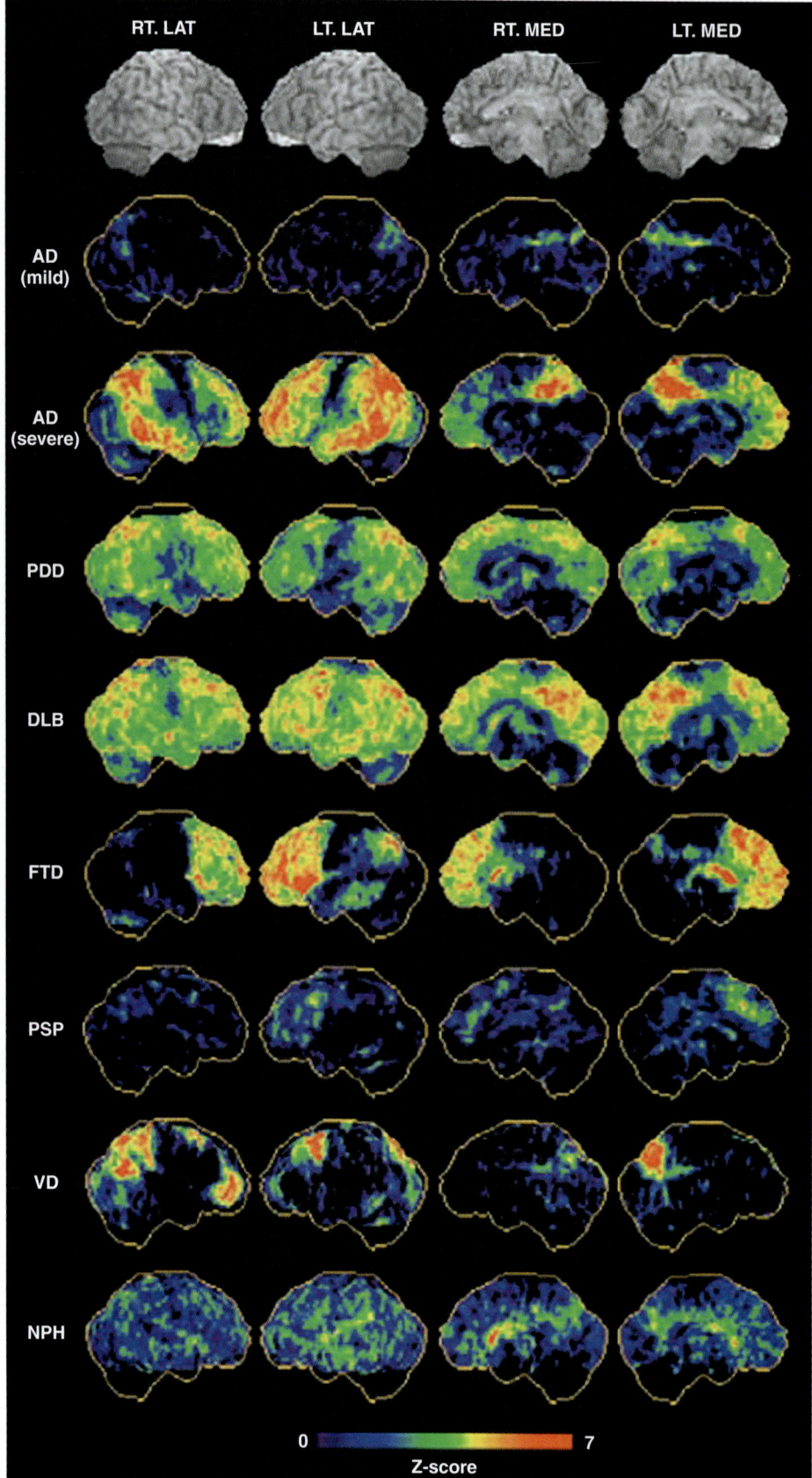

Figure 8-23 Dementias (three-dimensional stereotactic surface projection [3D-SSP] ^{18}F-fluorodeoxyglucose positron emission tomography). Metabolic abnormalities in various dementing disorders as demonstrated by 3D-SSP Z-score maps. Parkinson disease with dementia and dementia with Lewy bodies show metabolic reductions similar to Alzheimer disease in the lateral cortices but additional significant metabolic reduction in the occipital cortex. Frontal dominant reduction in frontotemporal dementia. Mild frontal reduction in progressive supranuclear palsy. Vascular dementia shows patchy reduction related to ischemic foci. Normal pressure hydrocephalus (NPH) shows mild diffuse reduction. (From Minoshima S. Imaging Alzheimer's disease: clinical applications. *Neuroimaging Clin N Am* 2003;13(4):769-780.)

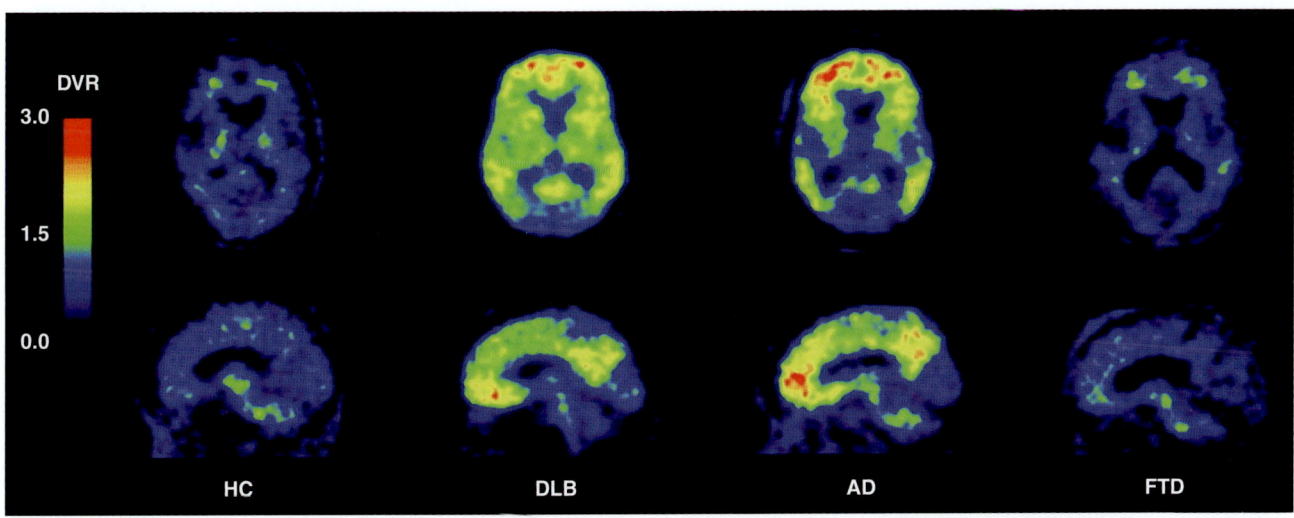

Figure 8-24 Amyloid imaging. Positron emission tomographic images (using distribution volume ratio) showing nonspecific Pittsburgh compound B (PIB) binding in white matter in human control and frontotemporal dementia subjects compared with PIB binding in the frontal, temporal, and posterior cingulate/precuneus cortex of patients with Alzheimer disease and those with dementia with Lewy bodies. (From Rowe CC, Ng S, Ackermann U, Gong SJ, et al. Imaging beta-amyloid burden in aging and dementia. *Neurology* 2007;68(20):1718-1725.)

80% of them are diagnosed with AD. About one fourth of the remaining MCI cases are due to reversible conditions, and the remaining half improve or remain stable. Remember that MCI is an identifiable prodrome for all dementia subtypes rather than just AD (e.g., vascular dementia and Parkinson–LBD).

Voxel-based morphometry is preferably used to detect and objectively measure mesial temporal atrophy. More prominent medial and inferior temporal atrophy is present in aMCI compared to naMCI. More extensive parietotemporal and cingulate atrophy in addition to hippocampal atrophy in aMCI predicts progression to AD. Cortical thinning as a surrogate marker of cognitive impairment is being used in quantitative studies.

High hippocampal diffusivity is associated with a greater risk of progression to AD in aMCI. Mesial temporal metabolite pattern in aMCI is similar to AD (i.e., decreased NAA and elevated ratios of myoinositol to creatine levels).

Both PET and SPECT studies show reduced blood flow and/or glucose metabolism in the temporoparietal lobes, hippocampus, and posterior cingulate gyrus in MCI and represents a higher risk of progressive cognitive decline and thus, development of AD. Pittsburgh compound B (N-methyl-[^{11}C]2-(4'-methylaminophenyl)-6-hydroxybenzothiazole ([^{11}C]PIB) PET uptake is similar to AD, with global increased binding predominantly in frontal association areas. These two groups of functional/molecular studies potentially can be used to identify high-risk patients in the preclinical stage.

Problem Solving: FTD versus AD "Frontotemporal versus Temporoparietal Dementia"
(Figure 8-23 and 8-24)

The average age of onset is younger in FTD than in AD. FTD, unlike AD, lacks cholinergic deficiency, highlighting the clinical significance in differentiating the two disorders. FTD is intermediate between focal disorders of the brain and more generalized neurodegenerative diseases. Some patients experience only aphasia, whereas others progress to dementia within a few years. As alluded to earlier, motor neuron disease develops in a subset of FTD. This subgroup (FTDu) has a higher mortality rate from FTD than other affected patients. Patients with primary progressive aphasia typically have preserved memory and visuospatial functions, whereas those with AD have nearly universal involvement of these functions. In general, the differences between FTD or its variant and AD reflect the pathologic involvement of the frontal and temporal lobes, particularly in the left hemisphere, compared to the early involvement of the hippocampi and parietal lobes in AD. Besides the more common diffuse dementing disorders such as AD, FTD must be differentiated from focal processes such as brain tumors, abscesses, and strokes on conventional structural imaging.

AD can present in the early stage with disproportionate frontal lobe symptoms ("frontal variant of AD") mimicking FTD. FDG PET as metabolic study and SPECT as perfusion study have been useful tools in clinically difficult cases of AD versus FTD, with greater than 80% accuracy. Posterior cingulate atrophy and hypometabolism are specific markers of AD. Remember that AD with associated depression or advanced cases show bilateral frontal lobe deficits on functional studies. Similarly, advanced FTD shows temporoparietal hypometabolism. Amyloid radioligands (e.g., ^{11}C-PIB Pittsburgh B compound and ^{18}F-BAY94-9172) are useful for differentiating FTD and AD. Generally, FTD shows no significant to mild retention of radiotracer.

Structural imaging has a supplementary role with the increasing use of volumetric and quantitative techniques. Atrophic features favoring FTD include asymmetric frontotemporal atrophy, usually on the left side, "knife-edge atrophy" in the anterior temporal lobes (in SD subtype), left perisylvian atrophy (in progressive non-fluent aphasia [PNF]), anterior or diffuse corpus callosum atrophy, and anterior cingulate atrophy. AD is characterized by atrophy of callosal posterior body. Generally, FTD has severe frontotemporal atrophy (left side dominant) and mild hippocampal atrophy compared to moderate hippocampal, temporal, and mild frontal lobe atrophy in AD. Remember that hippocampal atrophy can be present in both FTD and AD.

Problem Solving: Vascular Dementia versus AD "Mixed Dementia" (Figures 8-5, 8-10, and 8-23)

The diagnosis of vascular dementia requires the presence of faster changes and the absence of causes of dementia. Hence, the absence rather than the presence of ischemic changes on imaging is more helpful in distinguishing vascular dementia from AD. Diagnosis of vascular dementia requires the following criteria: cognitive loss, often predominantly subcortical; vascular brain lesions demonstrated by imaging; a temporal link between stroke and dementia; and exclusion of other causes of dementia. Unlike AD, executive functions are dominantly involved, with mild memory impairment. Binswanger disease or subcortical chronic encephalopathy is considered a variant of multiinfarct dementia with periventricular white matter T2 hyperintensities typically due to incomplete infarcts and presenting with dementia, gait, and bladder symptoms. Cerebral amyloid angiopathy is an overlapped condition between vascular diseases and AD.

Large territory infarcts in the middle cerebral artery (MCA) and anterior cerebral artery (ACA) distribution result in dementia in about 30% of stroke survivors. Superficial watershed infarcts such as superior frontal gyrus (MCA–ACA watershed) and inferior temporal gyrus (MCA–posterior cerebral artery watershed) can result in cognitive dysfunction. Single stroke dementia is caused by a single strategically located infarct and usually affects the left hemisphere with thalamic involvement. Small-vessel ischemic disease manifests as patchy deep white matter and deep gray matter T2 hyperintensities (complete and incomplete microvascular infarcts).

The differentiation may be very difficult in some cases due to mixed AD and vascular dementia pathologies, termed *mixed dementia*. Subcortical T2 changes are seen in both vascular dementia and AD; however, in mixed dementia, large/hemispheric infarcts in addition to multiple microinfarcts are more frequent.

Problem Solving: DLB versus AD and PDD (Figures 8-3, 8-5, 8-7, 8-23, and 8-24)

As many as 20% of elderly individuals may suffer from DLB. The consensus criteria for DLB state that the central feature of the condition is a progressive cognitive decline accompanied by two of three additional core features, which include fluctuating cognition, recurrent visual hallucinations, and spontaneous motor features of parkinsonism. LBD has often been misdiagnosed as AD or vascular dementia or confused with idiopathic PDD. Diagnosis of DLB is important for clinicians given the high incidence of adverse response to neuroleptics. DLB in earlier stages is dominated by cognitive symptoms with absent or minimal parkinsonism and therefore is easily confused with AD. Compared to PD, there is progressive cognitive decline with particular deficits of visuospatial ability as well as frontal executive function with less prominent parkinsonism and without the classic parkinsonian rest tremor.

More diffuse cerebral volume loss is seen compared to AD. Relative preservation of medial temporal lobe with less pronounced atrophy is seen compared to AD and vascular dementia. Relatively more atrophy in the midbrain, substantia innominata, hypothalamus, and putamina is seen in DLB compared to AD. However, medial temporal lobe atrophy is present and more pronounced compared to normal controls, PD, and even PDD.

Occipital lobe hypoperfusion and hypometabolism are major differentiating features from AD on SPECT and PET studies. FP-CIT as a marker of presynaptic dopaminergic dysfunction may be used to differentiate DLB from AD with very high accuracy. However, FP-CIT should not be injudiciously used in dementia patients to avoid a high incidence of false positives. Bilateral striatal diminished uptake on FP-CIT is a similar finding to PD and therefore not helpful in differentiating these two disorders. ^{123}I-Meta-iodobenzylguanidine (MIBG) cardiac uptake is significantly reduced in DLB and PD compared to AD. As alluded to before, DLB can have amyloid deposition. Distribution of the amyloid ligands is generally similar to AD but the degree of binding is comparatively mild and varied.

Problem Solving: MSA-P versus PD (Figures 8-12 and 8-25)

PD has a relatively long course compared to the rapid progressive course of MSA, a major component of Parkinson plus syndromes. Generally, a small portion of patients with MSA and vascular parkinsonism show an initial response to levodopa. Clinical differentiation from PD can be difficult if the parkinsonism symptoms are dominant (MSA-P), typically due to SND. Wenning et al. showed the following clinical features suggestive of MSA: poor response to levodopa, autonomic features, speech or bulbar dysfunction, absence of dementia, absence of levodopa-induced confusion, and falls. Misdiagnosis of MSA is usually due to its confusion with PD or PSP.

IPD shows diffuse cerebral volume predominantly in the temporoparietal lobes overlapping with normal aging. In contrast, atrophy and signal changes of the subcortical structures are dominant features of MSA on structural imaging, seen as lateral putaminal slit-like T2 hyperintensity, dorsolateral putaminal T2 hyperintensity, dominant pontine atrophy, transverse pontine fibers degeneration ("hot cross bun sign"), cerebellar atrophy, and middle cerebellar peduncle T2 hyperintensities as described above. Frontoparietal atrophy is seen in MSA. The pathophysiology of PD centers on striatonigral circuitry, but conventional MRI usually is unremarkable. Normal laminated zones of substantia nigra on T2 imaging show hypointense posterior pars reticulata (SNPr) and hyperintense anterior pars compacta (SNPc). Axial T2 imaging can show decreased SNPc width. Characteristic MSA features, such as reduced middle cerebellar

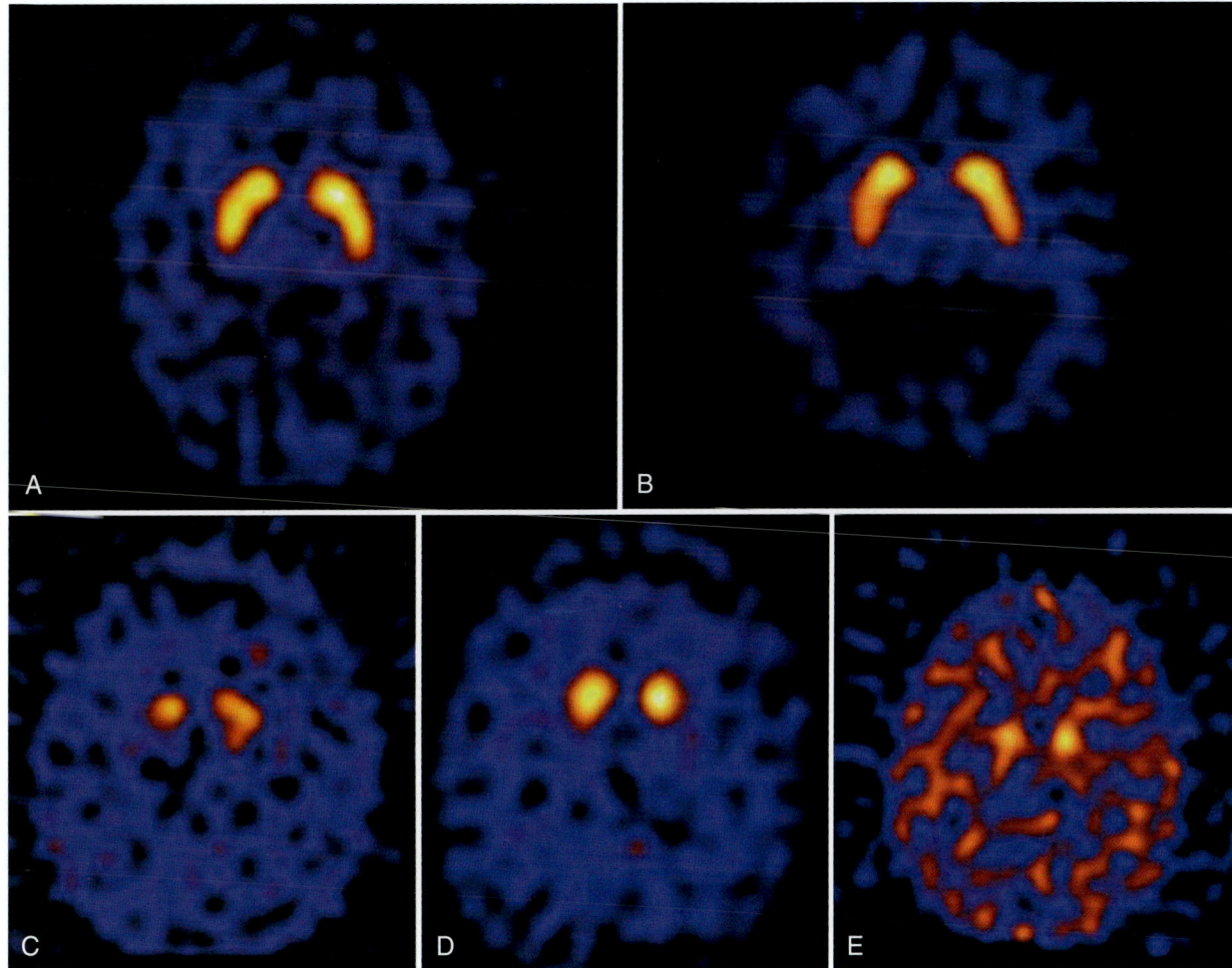

Figure 8-25 Parkinson disease, dementia with Lewy bodies, and Alzheimer disease (FP-CIT)-^{123}I-radiolabeled 2-carbomethoxy-3-(4-iodophenyl)-N-(3-fluoropropyl) nortropane with single-photon emission computed tomographic images. **A:** Healthy older control subject. **B:** Subject with Alzheimer disease. **C:** Subject with dementia with Lewy bodies. **D:** Subject with Parkinson disease. **E:** Subject with Parkinson disease with dementia. (From O'Brien JT, Colloby S, Fenwick J, et al. Dopamine transporter loss visualized with FP-CIT SPECT in the differential diagnosis of dementia with Lewy bodies. *Arch Neurol* 2004;61(6):919-925.)

peduncle width, are useful for distinguishing patients with MSA from those with PD. MR parkinsonian index based on pons and middle cerebellar peduncle area ratios to midbrain and superior cerebellar peduncle has very high accuracy in differentiating MSA from PD. Increased ADC values in middle cerebellar peduncle can add to the differentiation of MSA-P from PD.

Iodine-123 fluoropropyl (FP)-CIT is highly accurate in diagnosing neurodegenerative parkinsonism but usually is not helpful in differentiating MSA from PD. Symmetric or asymmetric decreased striatal uptake is seen in MSA and PD, with more prominent reduction of midbrain uptake in MSA and PSP on advanced volumetric techniques. The tracer can be very helpful in patients with atypical characteristics of parkinsonism (termed *clinically uncertain parkinsonian syndromes* [CUPS]), excluding postsynaptic-like psychogenic, drug-induced, or vascular parkinsonism. ^{18}F-6-Fluorodopa PET shows a greater decrease in caudate relative to putamen in MSA-P compared to PD. ^{123}I-MIBG myocardial scintigraphy is another useful tool because patients with PD and LBD have significantly lower cardiac ^{123}I-MIBG uptake than do patients with MSA and other neurodegenerative PD mimickers. The findings are related to postganglionic cardiac sympathetic nerve denervation in PD and DLB compared to MSA, PSP, CBD, and AD.

Problem Solving: PSP versus PD
(Figures 8-25 and 8-26)

PSP is often misdiagnosed because some of its symptoms are very much like those of PD, AD, and more rare NDDs, such as CJD. The key to diagnosing PSP is identifying early gait instability and difficulty in moving the eyes, the hallmark of the disease. Problems with speech and swallowing are much more common and severe in PSP than in PD. Tremor, almost universal in patients with PD, is rare in those with PSP. Patients with PSP respond poorly and only transiently to levodopa. There is currently no effective treatment of PSP.

Prominent midbrain tegmentum atrophy on midsagittal section ("penguin silhouette sign") compared to pontine atrophy is highly accurate in differentiating PSP from PD and MSA-P; the latter shows more prominent pontine atrophy. Remember the periaqueductal T2 hyperintensity

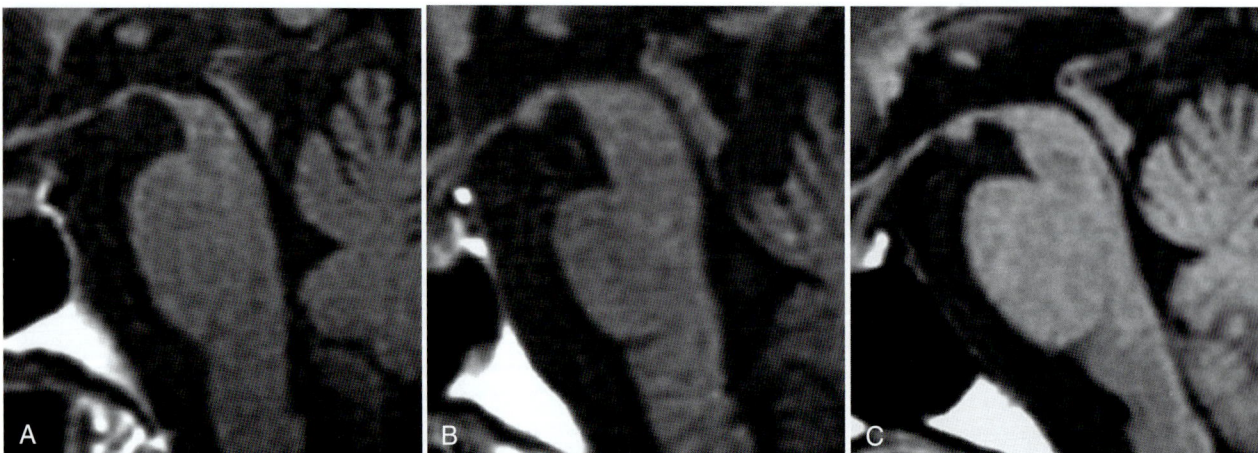

Figure 8-26 Midbrain profiles. Midline sagittal T1 images showing mesencephalic atrophy in progressive supranuclear palsy (A), pontine atrophy and flattening in multisystem atrophy (B), and normal pontomesencephalic profile in Parkinson disease (C).

seen in PSP. Increased ADC values in the putaminal and superior cerebellar peduncles can add to the differentiation of PSP from PD. Increased MR parkinsonian index based on pons and middle cerebellar peduncle area ratios to midbrain and superior cerebellar peduncle has very high accuracy in differentiating PSP from PD and MSA-P.

Typically, decreased FDG metabolism and flow in the frontal lobes (hypofrontalism) plus hypometabolism in the midbrain and thalami are seen compared to dominant parietal hypometabolism in PD. Reduction of medial frontal metabolism may be a valuable diagnostic imaging parameter in distinguishing PSP from PD. Anterior cingulate hypoperfusion seems to be an early, distinct brain abnormality in PSP compared with PD. Using ^{123}I-FP-CIT, PSP patients show more severe and symmetric dopamine transporter loss in the entire striatum compared to patients with PD.

Problem Solving: CBD versus PSP and PD (Figures 8-14 and 8-15)

CBD is difficult to diagnose in the early stages (<50% sensitivity) and more commonly is confused with PSP. CBD shares the same tau haplotype as PSP patients, suggesting that both CBD and PSP share the same genetic background and possibly the same pathologic mechanism. CBD patients do not respond to levodopa treatment. Management is mainly supportive. In CBD, cortical involvement results in dominant cognitive and other cortical dysfunctions compared to impaired eye movement in PSP. Assessment of orofacial apraxias can aid in the clinical differentiation of CBD from PD, PSP, LBD, and MSA, reflecting involvement of supplementary motor areas and the superior parietal lobule. Clinical findings in CBD are more commonly asymmetric.

Asymmetry is also a key imaging feature. Usually asymmetric frontoparietal atrophy is seen and in combination with lack of midbrain atrophy helps in differentiating PSP and PD. Asymmetric atrophy of the cerebral peduncles and midbrain is also seen. Functional studies show asymmetric hemispheric cortical glucose metabolism and decreased ^{18}F-dopa uptake in the parietal lobe, striatum, and thalamus.

Problem Solving: ALS versus Atypical Motor Neuron Diseases (Figure 8-17)

ALS may be mimicked by disorders that affect different levels of the motor system from cortex to muscle. They do not fall into the clinical profile of typical ALS and are collectively termed *atypical motor neuron diseases*. The atypical motor neuron diseases are divided into three groups: (1) upper motor neuron—primary lateral sclerosis, hereditary spastic paresis, and lathyrism; (2) lower motor neuron—progressive muscular atrophy, adult-onset spinal muscular atrophy (spinal muscular atrophy type IV), Kennedy disease, Hirayama disease, multifocal motor neuropathy, and postpolio muscular atrophy; and (3) overlap syndromes—dementia and ALS, dementia parkinsonism and ALS, RPD, CJD, and ALS, and FTD with ALS (FTDu). The distinction is primarily clinical, including electrophysiologic studies, with a limited role of imaging. Primary lateral sclerosis shows more severe bilateral frontoparietal, particularly precentral, atrophy due to a prolonged course of primary lateral sclerosis compared to ALS. FTDu is closely related to ALS, with dominant frontotemporal dysfunction. Dementia is more common in western pacific-type ALS; however, it can also be seen in classic sporadic and familial types (ALS-D). ALS is now grouped together with ALS-D, FTLD-U, and ALS/parkinsonism–dementia complex of Guam and Kii as *TDP-43 proteinopathy*. Pure imaging mimickers of ALS include bilateral wallerian degeneration with atrophy and T2 hyperintensity of the corticospinal tract, typically due to proximal ischemic or demyelinating lesions. A pitfall to remember is normal corticospinal tract hyperintensity on 3-T and higher field systems.

■ SUMMARY OF CHARACTERISTIC IMAGING FEATURES IN NDDS

Atrophy

Diffuse parenchymal volume loss may be seen in any NDD. Imaging characteristics based on symmetry and preferential involvement are enumerated as follows.

Dominant cortical atrophy: AD, LBD, FTLD
Dominant subcortical atrophy: Putamina in MSA, caudate nuclei in Huntington disease
Nonselective diffuse atrophy: Aging, PD, any other NDD in advanced stages
Selective atrophy: Bilateral parietotemporal in AD, bilateral frontotemporal in FTLD and ALS. Localized pontocerebellar atrophy in MSA (sporadic olivopontocerebellar atrophy) or midbrain tegmental atrophy in PSP
Asymmetric atrophy: Asymmetric frontoparietal hemispheric atrophy in CBD; FTLD subtypes can show asymmetric atrophy
Side dominant atrophy: Left side dominant anterior temporal and perisylvian atrophy in SD and progressive non-fluent aphasia (PNFA), subtypes of FTLD, respectively

T2 White Matter Hyperintensities

Common finding in advanced age compromising its specificity for NDDs. Multiple sclerosis is included because of its common incidence and as an important imaging differential diagnosis.
Multiple sclerosis: Pericallosal, perithalamic, callosal, anterior temporal periventricular, brachium pontis, and brainstem surface typical locations. Perpendicular direction relative to corpus callosum. Laminated T2 architecture, also referred to as *surrounding dirty white matter*. Edge enhancement.
Binswanger disease: Overlapped features. Dominant deep white matter patchy T2 hyperintensities compared to well-defined T1 hypointense complete microvascular infarcts (lacunes) mostly in the deep gray matter.
CADASIL (cerebral autosomal dominant arteriopathy with subcortical infarcts and leukoencephalopathy): Confluent white matter T2 hyperintensity in the periventricular white matter, extension into bilateral external capsules, internal capsules, and anterior temporal pole with sparing of frontoorbital white matter. Striatocapsular lacunae. Microhemorrhages.
ALS: Bilateral corticospinal tract hyperintensity including precentral gyrus subcortical white matter and sometimes in ventral spinal cord.

Putaminal T2 Hypointensity

Bilateral putaminal T2/T2* hypointensity in combination with hyperintense putaminal rim (HPR) is a specific marker of MSA in presenile patients. Bilateral putaminal and globus pallidus T2 hypointensity is commonly seen in normal old-age subjects and in other NDDs due to increasing use of susceptibility-weighted imaging.

Hypoperfusion and Hypometabolism

Diffuse hypometabolism and hypoperfusion may be seen in any of the NDDs particularly in the advanced stages.
Temporoparietal: MCI, AD, PD/PDD
Frontotemporal: FTD, ALS, and advanced AD with diffuse hypometabolism and hypoperfusion
Frontal lobes (hypofrontalism): PSP, frontal variants of FTLD and AD
Occipital lobes: DLB and PCA

Specific Radiotracer Uptake

^{18}F-6 Fluorodopa: Marker of presynaptic dopamine synthesis. Bilateral decreased posterior putaminal uptake in IPD, asymmetric in early course, asymmetry can be related to increased uptake due to up-regulation of receptors. Usually similar findings in atypical Parkinson disorders (e.g., MSA, PSP, CBD).
DAT ligands: Marker of presynaptic dopaminergic dysfunction as seen in neurodegenerative Parkinson disorders. Generally does not differentiate IPD from atypical Parkinson disorders. Bilateral striatal decreased uptake in PD (putaminal uptake more reduced than caudate). Uptake may be asymmetric in early course of disease. Striatal reduced uptake (caudate greater than putamina) in MSA and PSP plus more prominent midbrain reduction compared to PD. More extensive diminished uptake in LBD with left hemispheric asymmetry common. Reduced striatal uptake helpful in differentiating from AD. Uptake is generally normal in essential tremor.
Pittsburgh B compound: AD shows global increased retention of amyloid ligands predominantly in frontal and temporoparietal association areas, posterior cingulate gyrus, and caudate nuclei with no significant increased retention in white matter, cerebellum, brainstem, sensorimotor cortex, and medial temporal lobes.
FTD: No significant radiotracer retention.
DLB: Similar to AD but with milder degree of radiotracer retention.

Specific Imaging Signs in NDDs

Hot cross bun sign (Figure 8-13, *A*): Cruciform hyperintensity sign is due to selective loss of myelinated transverse pontocerebellar pontine tegmentum and corticospinal tracts. The sign is highly specific to MSA-C in differential diagnosis from PD and MSA-P.
Hyperintense putaminal rim sign (Figure 8-13, *C*): HPR is a specific sign for MSA in a proper clinical setting and has a high negative predictive value. HPR is commonly seen in normal old-age patients on 3-T systems, attributed to differential putaminal iron deposition rather than true pathologic rim hyperintensity. Rarely seen in other NDDs (e.g., CBD, PSP, old-age PD). HPR is caused by a combination of gliosis and extracellular interstitial fluid due to atrophy. Presence of HPR on FLAIR imaging likely indicates gliosis, differentiating MSA from false positives.
Penguin silhouette and Mickey Mouse signs (Figure 8-14): Signs relatively specific to PSP. Penguin or hummingbird side profile appearance on midsagittal image highlights the hallmark morphologic change in PSP (i.e., midbrain atrophy). Axial image of the midbrain looks like Mickey Mouse and is due to dominant midbrain tegmentum atrophy and sparing of cerebral peduncles and tectum.
Pulvinar and hockey-stick signs (Figure 8-20): Bilateral dorsal thalamic focal hyperintensities on T2, FLAIR, and diffusion-weighted imaging sequences result in

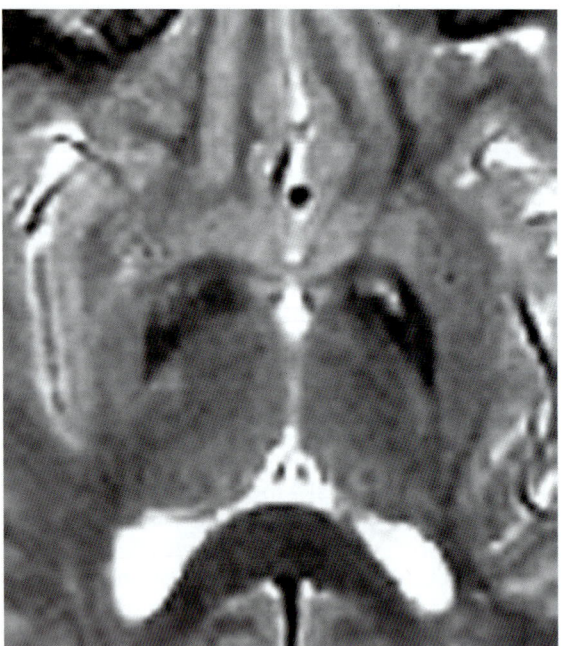

Figure 8-27 Tiger-eye sign. Axial FSE T2 image showing bilateral globus pallidal hypointensity with central hyperintensities, a specific sign for pantothenate kinase deficiency.

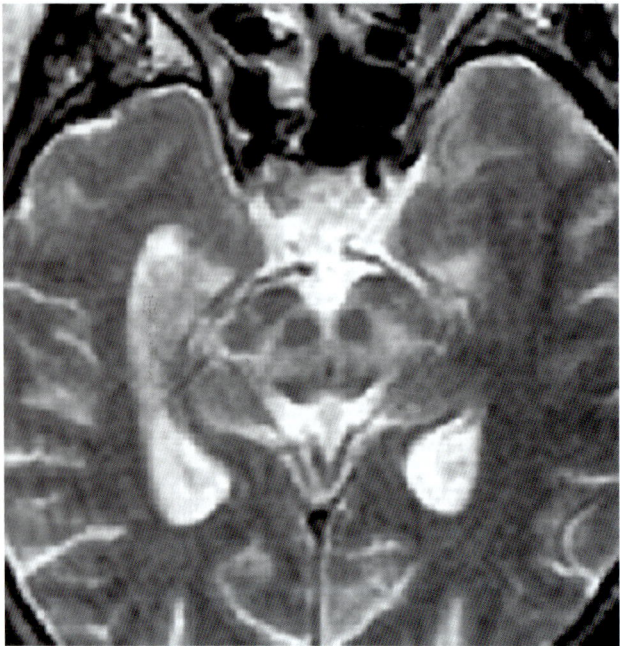

Figure 8-28 Giant panda sign. Magnified axial T2 image of the midbrain showing hyperintense T2 edema around the red nuclei posing as the panda's eyes in Wilson disease.

"pulvinar sign." Presence of the diagnostic test of variant CJD. Dominant bilateral dorsomedial thalamic T2 hyperintensity looks like two hockey sticks against each other and has essentially the same significance as the pulvinar sign.

Tiger-eye sign (Figure 8-27): T2 imaging sign composed of hyperintensities within a hypointense medial globus pallidus. It is absolutely correlated to pantothenate kinase-associated degeneration (PANK2). Parkinsonism is seen predominantly in adult-onset patients whereas dystonia seems to occur more frequently in earlier-onset cases. The pallidal central hyperintensity of the eye sign may develop before rim hypointensity in patients with mutations. The term *neurodegeneration with brain iron accumulation* (NBIA) has replaced the eponym Hallervorden-Spatz disease. NBIA is a heterogeneous group of progressive extrapyramidal disorders characterized by neurodegeneration and excessive focal iron accumulation in the basal ganglia due to spheroid neuronal degeneration. The known causes of NBIA include pantothenate kinase-associated neurodegeneration, neuroferritinopathy, infantile neuroaxonal dystrophy, and aceruloplasminemia.

Face of the giant panda sign (Figure 8-28): Consists of high signal intensity in the tegmentum except for red nucleus, preservation of signal intensity at the lateral portion of the pars reticulata of the substantia nigra, and hypointensity of the superior colliculus. It is one of the specific imaging findings in Wilson disease.

Suggested Readings

Aarsland D, Perry R, Larsen JP, McKeith IG, O'Brien JT, Perry EK, Burn D, Ballard CG. Neuroleptic sensitivity in Parkinson's disease and parkinsonian dementias. *J Clin Psychiatry.* 2005;66(5):633-637.

Amici S, Gorno-Tempini ML, Ogar JM, Dronkers NF, Miller BL. An overview on primary progressive aphasia and its variants. *Behav Neurol.* 2006;17(2): 77-87.

Angelie E, Bonmartin A, Boudraa A, Gonnaud PM, Mallet JJ, Sappey-Marinier D. Regional differences and metabolic changes in normal aging of the human brain: proton MR spectroscopic imaging study. *AJNR Am J Neuroradiol.* 2001;22(1):119-127.

Arahata Y, Kato T, Tadokoro M, Sobue G. [^{18}F-fluorodeoxyglucose positron emission tomography in Parkinson's disease]. *Nippon Rinsho.* 1997;55(1):222-226.

Auchus AP, Chen CP, Sodagar SN, Thong M, Sng EC. Single stroke dementia: insights from 12 cases in Singapore. *J Neurol Sci.* 2002:203-204:85–89.

Avison MJ, Nath A, Berger JR. Understanding pathogenesis and treatment of HIV dementia: a role for magnetic resonance? *Trends Neurosci.* 2002;25(9):468-473.

Barber R, Gholkar A, Scheltens P, Ballard C, McKeith IG, O'Brien JT. Medial temporal lobe atrophy on MRI in dementia with Lewy bodies. *Neurology.* 1999;52(6):1153-1158.

Benamer TS, Patterson J, Grosset DG, Booij J, de Bruin K, van Royen E, Speelman JD, Horstink MH, Sips HJ, Dierckx RA, Versijpt J, Decoo D, Van Der Linden C, Hadley DM, Doder M, Lees AJ, Costa DC, Gacinovic S, Oertel WH, Pogarell O, Hoeffken H, Joseph K, Tatsch K, Schwarz J, Ries V. Accurate differentiation of parkinsonism and essential tremor using visual assessment of [^{123}I]-FP-CIT SPECT imaging: the [^{123}I]-FP-CIT study group. *Mov Disord.* 2000;15(3):503-510.

Berendse HW, Booij J, Stoffers D, Ponsen MM, Hijman R, Wolters E. Presymptomatic detection of Parkinson's disease. *Tijdschr Gerontol Geriatr.* 2002;33(2):70-77.

Beyer MK, Larsen JP, Aarsland D. Gray matter atrophy in Parkinson disease with dementia and dementia with Lewy bodies. *Neurology.* 2007;69(8): 747-754.

Bhattacharya K, Saadia D, Eisenkraft B, Yahr M, Olanow W, Drayer B, Kaufmann H. Brain magnetic resonance imaging in multiple-system atrophy and Parkinson disease: a diagnostic algorithm. *Arch Neurol.* 2002;59(5):835-842.

Bhidayasiri R. How useful is (^{123}I) beta-CIT SPECT in the diagnosis of Parkinson's disease? *Rev Neurol Dis.* 2006;3(1):19-22.

Bobinski M, de Leon MJ, Wegiel J, Desanti S, Convit A, Saint Louis LA, Rusinek H, Wisniewski HM. The histological validation of post mortem magnetic resonance imaging-determined hippocampal volume in Alzheimer's disease. *Neuroscience.* 2000;95(3):721-725.

Boccardi M, Laakso MP, Bresciani L, Galluzzi S, Geroldi C, Beltramello A, Soininen H, Frisoni GB. The MRI pattern of frontal and temporal brain atrophy in fronto-temporal dementia. *Neurobiol Aging.* 2003;24(1):95-103.

Bocti C, Rockel C, Roy P, Gao F, Black SE. Topographical patterns of lobar atrophy in frontotemporal dementia and Alzheimer's disease. *Dement Geriatr Cogn Disord.* 2006;21(5-6):364-372.

Booij J, Habraken JB, Bergmans P, Tissingh G, Winogrodzka A, Wolters EC, Janssen AG, Stoof JC, van Royen EA. Imaging of dopamine transporters with iodine-123-FP-CIT SPECT in healthy controls and patients with Parkinson's disease. *J Nucl Med.* 1998;39(11):1879-1884.

Boxer AL, Geschwind MD, Belfor N, Gorno-Tempini ML, Schauer GF, Miller BL, Weiner MW, Rosen HJ. Patterns of brain atrophy that differentiate corticobasal degeneration syndrome from progressive supranuclear palsy. *Arch Neurol.* 2006;63(1):81-86.

Braffman BH, Zimmerman RA, Trojanowski JQ, Gonatas NK, Hickey WF, Schlaepfer WW. Brain M.R: pathologic correlation with gross and histopathology. 1. Lacunar infarction and Virchow-Robin spaces. *AJR Am J Roentgenol.* 1988;151(3):551-558.

Brass SD, Chen NK, Mulkern RV, Bakshi R. Magnetic resonance imaging of iron deposition in neurological disorders. *Top Magn Reson Imaging.* 2006;17(1):31-40.

Brooks DJ, Ibanez V, Sawle GV, Quinn N, Lees AJ, Mathias CJ, Bannister R, Marsden CD, Frackowiak RS. Differing patterns of striatal ^{18}F-dopa uptake in Parkinson's disease, multiple system atrophy, and progressive supranuclear palsy. *Ann Neurol.* 1990;28(4):547-555.

Burton EJ, McKeith IG, Burn DJ, Williams ED, O'Brien JT. Cerebral atrophy in Parkinson's disease with and without dementia: a comparison with Alzheimer's disease, dementia with Lewy bodies and controls. *Brain.* 2004;127(Pt 4):791-800.

Cairns NJ, Grossman M, Arnold SE, Burn DJ, Jaros E, Perry RH, Duyckaerts C, Stankoff B, Pillon B, Skullerud K, Cruz-Sanchez FF, Bigio EH, Mackenzie IR, Gearing M, Juncos JL, Glass JD, Yokoo H, Nakazato Y, Mosaheb S, Thorpe JR, Uryu K, Lee VM, Trojanowski JQ. Clinical and neuropathologic variation in neuronal intermediate filament inclusion disease. *Neurology.* 2004;63(8):1376-1384.

Chabriat H, Levy C, Taillia H, Iba-Zizen MT, Vahedi K, Joutel A, Tournier-Lasserve E, Bousser MG. Patterns of MRI lesions in CADASIL. *Neurology.* 1998;51(2):452-457.

Chan D, Fox NC, Scahill RI, Crum WR, Whitwell JL, Leschziner G, Rossor AM, Stevens JM, Cipolotti L, Rossor MN. Patterns of temporal lobe atrophy in semantic dementia and Alzheimer's disease. *Ann Neurol.* 2001;49(4):433-442.

Chen ZL. [Deficiency of both Qi (vital energy) and blood]. *Zhong Xi Yi Jie He Za Zhi.* 1982;2(3):185-187.

Cheung G, Gawel MJ, Cooper PW, Farb RI, Ang LC, Gawal MJ. Amyotrophic lateral sclerosis: correlation of clinical and MR imaging findings. *Radiology.* 1995;194(1):263-270.

Cohen CR, Duchesneau PM, Weinstein MA. Calcification of the basal ganglia as visualized by computed tomography. *Radiology.* 1980;134(1):97-99.

Collie DA. The role of MRI in the diagnosis of sporadic and variant Creutzfeldt-Jakob disease. *JBR-BTR.* 2001;84(4):143-146.

Collie DA, Summers DM, Sellar RJ, Ironside JW, Cooper S, Zeidler M, Knight R, Will RG. Diagnosing variant Creutzfeldt-Jakob disease with the pulvinar sign: MR imaging findings in 86 neuropathologically confirmed cases. *AJNR Am J Neuroradiol.* 2003;24(8):1560-1569.

Colloby SJ, Williams ED, Burn DJ, Lloyd JJ, McKeith IG, O'Brien JT. Progression of dopaminergic degeneration in dementia with Lewy bodies and Parkinson's disease with and without dementia assessed using ^{123}I-FP-CIT SPECT. *Eur J Nucl Med Mol Imaging.* 2005;32(10):1176-1185.

Conde-Sendin MA, Hernandez-Fleta JL, Cardenes-Santana MA, Amela-Peris R. [Neurosyphilis: forms of presentation and clinical management]. *Rev Neurol.* 2002;35(4):380-386.

Constantinescu R, Richard I, Kurlan R. Levodopa responsiveness in disorders with parkinsonism: a review of the literature. *Mov Disord.* 2007;22(15):2141-2148;quiz 2295.

Cousins DA, Burton EJ, Burn D, Gholkar A, McKeith IG, O'Brien JT. Atrophy of the putamen in dementia with Lewy bodies but not Alzheimer's disease: an MRI study. *Neurology.* 2003;61(9):1191-1195.

Darby D, Smith C, Woodward M, Merory J, Tochon-Danguy H, O'Keefe G, Klunk WE, Mathis CA, Price JC, Masters CL, Villemagne VL. Imaging beta-amyloid burden in aging and dementia. *Neurology.* 2007;68(20):1718-1725.

Davatzikos C, Resnick SM, Wu X, Parmpi P, Clark CM. Individual patient diagnosis of AD and FTD via high-dimensional pattern classification of MRI. *Neuroimage.* 2008;41(4):1220-1227.

Davies RR, Kipps CM, Mitchell J, Kril JJ, Halliday GM, Hodges JR. Progression in frontotemporal dementia: identifying a benign behavioral variant by magnetic resonance imaging. *Arch Neurol.* 2006;63(11):1627-1631.

Dev KK, Hofele K, Barbieri S, Buchman VL, van der Putten H. Part II alpha-synuclein and its molecular pathophysiological role in neurodegenerative disease. *Neuropharmacology.* 2003;45(1):14-44.

Diehl-Schmid J, Grimmer T, Drzezga A, Bornschein S, Riemenschneider M, Forstl H, Schwaiger M, Kurz A. Decline of cerebral glucose metabolism in frontotemporal dementia: a longitudinal ^{18}F-FDG-PET-study. *Neurobiol Aging.* 2007;28(1):42-50.

Du AT, Schuff N, Kramer JH, Rosen HJ, Gorno-Tempini ML, Rankin K, Miller BL, Weiner MW. Different regional patterns of cortical thinning in Alzheimer's disease and frontotemporal dementia. *Brain.* 2007;130(Pt 4):1159-1166.

Duyckaerts C. [Nosology of dementias: the neuropathologist's point of view]. *Rev Neurol (Paris).* 2006;162(10):921-928.

Erten-Lyons D, Woltjer RL, Dodge H, Nixon R, Vorobik R, Calvert JF, Leahy M, Montine T, Kaye J. Factors associated with resistance to dementia despite high Alzheimer disease pathology. *Neurology.* 2009;72(4):354-360.

Farlow MR, Cummings J. A modern hypothesis: The distinct pathologies of dementia associated with Parkinson's disease versus Alzheimer's disease. *Dement Geriatr Cogn Disord.* 2008;25(4):301-308.

Fazekas F, Chawluk JB, Alavi A, Hurtig HI, Zimmerman RA. MR signal abnormalities at 1.5 T in Alzheimer's dementia and normal aging. *AJR Am J Roentgenol.* 1987;149(2):351-356.

Fazekas F, Kleinert R, Offenbacher H, Payer F, Schmidt R, Kleinert G, Radner H, Lechner H. The morphologic correlate of incidental punctate white matter hyperintensities on MR images. *AJNR Am J Neuroradiol.* 1991;12(5):915-921.

Filippi L, Manni C, Pierantozzi M, Brusa L, Danieli R, Stanzione P, Schillaci O. ^{123}I-FP-CIT in progressive supranuclear palsy and in Parkinson's disease: a SPECT semiquantitative study. *Nucl Med Commun.* 2006;27(4):381-386.

Foster GR, Scott DA, Payne S. The use of CT scanning in dementia. A systematic review. *Int J Technol Assess Health Care.* 1999;15(2):406-423.

Foster NL, Heidebrink JL, Clark CM, Jagust WJ, Arnold SE, Barbas NR, DeCarli CS, Turner RS, Koeppe RA, Higdon R, Minoshima S. FDG-PET improves accuracy in distinguishing frontotemporal dementia and Alzheimer's disease. *Brain.* 2007;130(Pt 10):2616-2635.

Freeman SH, Kandel R, Cruz L, Rozkalne A, Newell K, Frosch MP, Hedley-Whyte ET, Locascio JJ, Lipsitz LA, Hyman BT. Preservation of neuronal number despite age-related cortical brain atrophy in elderly subjects without Alzheimer disease. *J Neuropathol Exp Neurol.* 2008;67(12):1205-1212.

Fujii S, Matsusue E, Kinoshita T, Sugihara S, Ohama E, Ogawa T. Hyperintense putaminal rim at 3T reflects fewer ferritin deposits in the lateral marginal area of the putamen. *AJNR Am J Neuroradiol.* 2007;28(4):777-781.

Galton CJ, Gomez-Anson B, Antoun N, Scheltens P, Patterson K, Graves M, Sahakian BJ, Hodges JR. Temporal lobe rating scale: application to Alzheimer's disease and frontotemporal dementia. *J Neurol Neurosurg Psychiatry.* 2001;70(2):165-173.

Galton CJ, Patterson K, Graham K, Lambon-Ralph MA, Williams G, Antoun N, Sahakian BJ, Hodges JR. Differing patterns of temporal atrophy in Alzheimer's disease and semantic dementia. *Neurology.* 2001;57(2):216-225.

Ganguli M, Dodge HH, Shen C, DeKosky ST. Mild cognitive impairment, amnestic type: an epidemiologic study. *Neurology.* 2004;63(1):115-121.

Gauthier S, Reisberg B, Zaudig M, Petersen RC, Ritchie K, Broich K, Belleville S, Brodaty H, Bennett D, Chertkow H, Cummings JL, de Leon M, Feldman H, Ganguli M, Hampel H, Scheltens P, Tierney MC, Whitehouse P, Winblad B. Mild cognitive impairment. *Lancet.* 2006;367(9518):1262-1270.

Gendelman HE, Lipton SA, Tardieu M, Bukrinsky MI, Nottet HS. The neuropathogenesis of HIV-1 infection. *J Leukoc Biol.* 1994;56(3):389-398.

Geschwind MD, Haman A, Miller BL. Rapidly progressive dementia. *Neurol Clin.* 2007;25(3):783-807;vii.

Geschwind MD, Shu H, Haman A, Sejvar JJ, Miller BL. Rapidly progressive dementia. *Ann Neurol.* 2008;64(1):97-108.

Geser F, Wenning GK, Poewe W, McKeith I. How to diagnose dementia with Lewy bodies: state of the art. *Mov Disord.* 2005;20(suppl 12):S11-S20.

Gilman S, Low PA, Quinn N, Albanese A, Ben-Shlomo Y, Fowler CJ, Kaufmann H, Klockgether T, Lang AE, Lantos PL, Litvan I, Mathias CJ, Oliver E, Robertson D, Schatz I, Wenning GK. Consensus statement on the diagnosis of multiple system atrophy. *J Neurol Sci.* 1999;163(1):94-98.

Gonzalez RG. Imaging NeuroAIDS. *AJNR Am J Neuroradiol.* 2004;25(2):167-168.

Gorno-Tempini ML, Dronkers NF, Rankin KP, Ogar JM, Phengrasamy L, Rosen HJ, Johnson JK, Weiner MW, Miller BL. Cognition and anatomy in three variants of primary progressive aphasia. *Ann Neurol.* 2004;55(3):335-346.

Grafton ST, Mazziotta JC, Pahl JJ, St George-Hyslop P, Haines JL, Gusella J, Hoffman JM, Baxter LR, Phelps M. A comparison of neurological, metabolic, structural, and genetic evaluations in persons at risk for Huntington's disease. *Ann Neurol.* 1990;28(5):614-621.

Groschel K, Hauser TK, Luft A, Patronas N, Dichgans J, Litvan I, Schulz JB. Magnetic resonance imaging-based volumetry differentiates progressive supranuclear palsy from corticobasal degeneration. *Neuroimage.* 2004;21(2):714-724.

Grosskreutz J, Kaufmann J, Fradrich J, Dengler R, Heinze HJ, Peschel T. Widespread sensorimotor and frontal cortical atrophy in Amyotrophic Lateral Sclerosis. *BMC Neurol.* 2006;6:17.

Grossman M, Ash S. Primary progressive aphasia: a review. *Neurocase.* 2004;10(1):3-18.

Guermazi A, Miaux Y, Rovira-Canellas A, Suhy J, Pauls J, Lopez R, Posner H. Neuroradiological findings in vascular dementia. *Neuroradiology.* 2007;49(1):1-22.

Gurses C, Bilgic B, Topcular B, Tuncer OG, Akman-Demir G, Hanagasi H, Baslo B, Gurvit H, Coban O, Emre M, Idrisoglu HA. Clinical and magnetic resonance imaging findings of HIV-negative patients with neurosyphilis. *J Neurol.* 2007;254(3):368-374.

Harris GJ, Pearlson GD, Peyser CE, Aylward EH, Roberts J, Barta PE, Chase GA, Folstein SE. Putamen volume reduction on magnetic resonance imaging exceeds caudate changes in mild Huntington's disease. *Ann Neurol.* 1992;31(1):69-75.

Harvey GT, Hughes J, McKeith IG, Briel R, Ballard C, Gholkar A, Scheltens P, Perry RH, Ince P, O'Brien JT. Magnetic resonance imaging differences between dementia with Lewy bodies and Alzheimer's disease: a pilot study. *Psychol Med.* 1999;29(1):181-187.

Hashimoto M, Kitagaki H, Imamura T, Hirono N, Shimomura T, Kazui H, Tanimukai S, Hanihara T, Mori E. Medial temporal and whole-brain atrophy in dementia with Lewy bodies: a volumetric MRI study. *Neurology.* 1998;51(2):357-362.

Hauser RA, Murtaugh FR, Akhter K, Gold M, Olanow CW. Magnetic resonance imaging of corticobasal degeneration. *J Neuroimaging.* 1996;6(4):222-226.

Hayflick SJ, Hartman M, Coryell J, Gitschier J, Rowley H. Brain MRI in neurodegeneration with brain iron accumulation with and without PANK2 mutations. *AJNR Am J Neuroradiol.* 2006;27(6):1230-1233.

Hecht MJ, Fellner F, Fellner C, Hilz MJ, Heuss D, Neundorfer B. MRI-FLAIR images of the head show corticospinal tract alterations in ALS patients more frequently than T2-, T1- and proton-density-weighted images. *J Neurol Sci.* 2001;186(1-2):37-44.

Hecht MJ, Fellner F, Fellner C, Hilz MJ, Neundorfer B, Heuss D. Hyperintense and hypointense MRI signals of the precentral gyrus and corticospinal tract in ALS: a follow-up examination including FLAIR images. *J Neurol Sci.* 2002;199(1-2):59-65.

Henon H, Pasquier F, Leys D. Poststroke dementia. *Cerebrovasc Dis.* 2006;22(1):61-70.

Henriksen G, Yousefi BH, Drzezga A, Wester HJ. Development and evaluation of compounds for imaging of beta-amyloid plaque by means of positron emission tomography. *Eur J Nucl Med Mol Imaging.* 2008;35(suppl 1):S75-S81.

Herholz K. PET studies in dementia. *Ann Nucl Med.* 2003;17(2):79-89.

Herholz K, Carter SF, Jones M. Positron emission tomography imaging in dementia. *Br J Radiol.* 2007;2:S160-167:80 Spec No.

Hodges JR, Patterson K, Oxbury S, Funnell E. Semantic dementia. Progressive fluent aphasia with temporal lobe atrophy. *Brain.* 1992;115(Pt 6):1783-1806.

Hof PR, Archin N, Osmand AP, Dougherty JH, Wells C, Bouras C, Morrison JH. Posterior cortical atrophy in Alzheimer's disease: analysis of a new case and re-evaluation of a historical report. *Acta Neuropathol.* 1993;86(3):215-223.

Hof PR, Vogt BA, Bouras C, Morrison JH. Atypical form of Alzheimer's disease with prominent posterior cortical atrophy: a review of lesion distribution and circuit disconnection in cortical visual pathways. *Vision Res.* 1997;37(24):3609-3625.

Holland BA, Perrett LV, Mills CM. Meningovascular syphilis: CT and MR findings. *Radiology.* 1986;158(2):439-442.

Hosaka K, Ishii K, Sakamoto S, Sadato N, Fukuda H, Kato T, Sugimura K, Senda M. Validation of anatomical standardization of FDG PET images of normal brain: comparison of SPM and NEUROSTAT. *Eur J Nucl Med Mol Imaging.* 2005;32(1):92-97.

Huang YP, Tuason MY, Wu T, Plaitakis A. MRI and CT features of cerebellar degeneration. *J Formos Med Assoc.* 1993;92(6):494-508.

Huber SJ, Paulson GW. The concept of subcortical dementia. *Am J Psychiatry.* 1985;142(11):1312-1317.

Hughes AJ, Daniel SE, Ben-Shlomo Y, Lees AJ. The accuracy of diagnosis of parkinsonian syndromes in a specialist movement disorder service. *Brain.* 2002;125(Pt 4):861-870.

Ishii K, Sakamoto S, Sasaki M, Kitagaki H, Yamaji S, Hashimoto M, Imamura T, Shimomura T, Hirono N, Mori E. Cerebral glucose metabolism in patients with frontotemporal dementia. *J Nucl Med.* 1998;39(11):1875-1878.

Ishikawa T, Morita M, Nakano I. Brain perfusion imaging in amyotrophic lateral sclerosis with dementia. *Brain Nerve.* 2007;59(10):1093-1098.

Jack Jr CR, Petersen RC, Xu Y, O'Brien PC, Smith GE, Ivnik RJ, Boeve BF, Tangalos EG, Kokmen E. Rates of hippocampal atrophy correlate with change in clinical status in aging and AD. *Neurology.* 2000;55(4):484-489.

Jellinger KA. Neuropathological spectrum of synucleinopathies. *Mov Disord.* 2003;18(Suppl 6):S2-S12.

Jellinger KA. Clinicopathological analysis of dementia disorders in the elderly—an update. *J Alzheimers Dis.* 2006;9(3 suppl):61-70.

Jellinger KA. The enigma of vascular cognitive disorder and vascular dementia. *Acta Neuropathol.* 2007;113(4):349-388.

Jellinger KA. The pathology of "vascular dementia": a critical update. *J Alzheimers Dis.* 2008;14(1):107-123.

Jellinger KA, Attems J. Neuropathological evaluation of mixed dementia. *J Neurol Sci.* 2007;257(1-2):80-87.

Juh R, Kim J, Moon D, Choe B, Suh T. Different metabolic patterns analysis of Parkinsonism on the ^{18}F-FDG PET. *Eur J Radiol.* 2004;51(3):223-233.

Juh R, Pae CU, Kim TS, Lee CU, Choe B, Suh T. Cerebral glucose metabolism in corticobasal degeneration comparison with progressive supranuclear palsy using statistical mapping analysis. *Neurosci Lett.* 2005;383(1-2):22-27.

Kanda T, Ishii K, Uemura T, Miyamoto N, Yoshikawa T, Kono AK, Mori E. Comparison of grey matter and metabolic reductions in frontotemporal dementia using FDG-PET and voxel-based morphometric MR studies. *Eur J Nucl Med Mol Imaging.* 2008;35(12):2227-2234.

Kantarci K. ^{1}H magnetic resonance spectroscopy in dementia. *Br J Radiol.* 2007;2:S146-152:80 Spec No.

Kantarci K, Petersen RC, Boeve BF, Knopman DS, Tang-Wai DF, O'Brien PC, Weigand SD, Edland SD, Smith GE, Ivnik RJ, Ferman TJ, Tangalos EG, Jack Jr CR. ^{1}H MR spectroscopy in common dementias. *Neurology.* 2004;63(8):1393-1398.

Kantarci K, Petersen RC, Boeve BF, Knopman DS, Weigand SD, O'Brien PC, Shiung MM, Smith GE, Ivnik RJ, Tangalos EG, Jack Jr CR. DWI predicts future progression to Alzheimer disease in amnestic mild cognitive impairment. *Neurology.* 2005;64(5):902-904.

Kantarci K, Petersen RC, Przybelski SA, Weigand SD, Shiung MM, Whitwell JL, Negash S, Ivnik RJ, Boeve BF, Knopman DS, Smith GE, Jack Jr CR. Hippocampal volumes, proton magnetic resonance spectroscopy metabolites, and cerebrovascular disease in mild cognitive impairment subtypes. *Arch Neurol.* 2008;65(12):1621-1628.

Kapeller P, Schmidt R, Fazekas F. Qualitative MRI. evidence of usual aging in the brain. *Top Magn Reson Imaging.* 2004;15(6):343-347.

Karner E, Jenner C, Donnemiller E, Delazer M, Benke T. The clinical syndrome of posterior cortical atrophy. *Nervenarzt.* 2006;77(2):208-214.

Kemppainen NM, Aalto S, Wilson IA, Nagren K, Helin S, Bruck A, Oikonen V, Kailajarvi M, Scheinin M, Viitanen M, Parkkola R, Rinne JO. PET amyloid ligand [^{11}C]PIB uptake is increased in mild cognitive impairment. *Neurology.* 2007;68(19):1603-1606.

Kemppainen NM, Aalto S, Wilson IA, Nagren K, Helin S, Bruck A, Oikonen V, Kailajarvi M, Scheinin M, Viitanen M, Parkkola R, Rinne JO. Voxel-based analysis of PET amyloid ligand [^{11}C]PIB uptake in Alzheimer disease. *Neurology.* 2006;67(9):1575-1580.

Keyserling H, Mukundan Jr JS. The role of conventional MR and CT in the work-up of dementia patients. *Magn Reson Imaging Clin N Am.* 2006;14(2):169-182.

Kipps CM, Davies RR, Mitchell J, Kril JJ, Halliday GM, Hodges JR. Clinical significance of lobar atrophy in frontotemporal dementia: application of an MRI visual rating scale. *Dement Geriatr Cogn Disord.* 2007;23(5):334-342.

Kirshner HS, Lavin PJ. Posterior cortical atrophy: a brief review. *Curr Neurol Neurosci Rep.* 2006;6(6):477-480.

Kish SJ, Shannak K, Hornykiewicz O. Uneven pattern of dopamine loss in the striatum of patients with idiopathic Parkinson's disease. Pathophysiologic and clinical implications. *The N Engl J Med.* 1988;318(14):876-880.

Klein RC, de Jong BM, de Vries JJ, Leenders KL. Direct comparison between regional cerebral metabolism in progressive supranuclear palsy and Parkinson's disease. *Mov Disord.* 2005;20(8):1021-1030.

Kojima S. [Clinical types of spinocerebellar degeneration and evaluation with MR imaging]. *Rinsho Shinkeigaku.* 1993;33(12):1294-1296.

Konagaya M, Konagaya Y, Sakai M, Matsuoka Y, Hashizume Y. Progressive cerebral atrophy in multiple system atrophy. *J Neurol Sci.* 2002;195(2):123-127.

Konagaya M, Matsuoka Y, Konagaya Y. Quantitative MRI study of progressive cerebral atrophy in multiple system atrophy. *Rinsho Shinkeigaku.* 2002;42(2):118-125.

Konagaya M, Sakai M, Matsuoka Y, Goto Y, Yoshida M, Hashizume Y. Pathological correlate of the slitlike changes on MRI at the putaminal margin in multiple system atrophy. *J Neurol.* 1999;246(2):142-143.

Konagaya M, Sakai M, Yoshida M, Hashizume Y. An autopsy case of long-course multiple system atrophy (MSA) with remarkable atrophy and numerous NCI in the temporal lobe. *No To Shinkei.* 2006;58(5):430-437.

Koyama M, Yagishita A, Nakata Y, Hayashi M, Bandoh M, Mizutani T. Imaging of corticobasal degeneration syndrome. *Neuroradiology.* 2007;49(11):905-912.

Kramer JH, Duffy JM. Aphasia, apraxia, and agnosia in the diagnosis of dementia. *Dementia.* 1996;7(1):23-26.

Kropp S, Schulz-Schaeffer WJ, Finkenstaedt M, Riedemann C, Windl O, Steinhoff BJ, Zerr I, Kretzschmar HA, Poser S. The Heidenhain variant of Creutzfeldt-Jakob disease. *Arch Neurol.* 1999;56(1):55-61.

Kuipers-Upmeijer J, de Jager AE, Hew JM, Snoek JW, van Weerden TW. Primary lateral sclerosis: clinical, neurophysiological, and magnetic resonance findings. *J Neurol Neurosurg Psychiatry.* 2001;71(5):615-620.

Kuzuhara S. Recent progress in ALS research: ALS and TDP-43. *Rinsho Shinkeigaku.* 2008;48(9):625-633.

Kwee RM, Kwee TC. Virchow-Robin spaces at MR imaging. *Radiographics.* 2007;27(4):1071-1086.

Langford TD, Letendre SL, Marcotte TD, Ellis RJ, McCutchan JA, Grant I, Mallory ME, Hansen LA, Archibald S, Jernigan T, Masliah E. Severe, demyelinating leukoencephalopathy in AIDS patients on antiretroviral therapy. *AIDS.* 2002;16(7):1019-1029.

Lass P, Slawek J, Derejko M, Dubaniewicz M. Regional cerebral blood flow single photon emission tomography (SPECT) and magnetic resonance imaging (MRI) may be useful in the diagnosis of patients with cortico-basal degeneration, progressive supranuclear palsy and multiple system atrophy. *Neurol Neurochir Pol.* 2003;37(suppl 5):263-274.

Lee DY, Choo IH, Jhoo JH, Kim KW, Youn JC, Lee DS, Kang EJ, Lee JS, Kang WJ, Woo JI. Frontal dysfunction underlies depressive syndrome in Alzheimer disease: a FDG-PET study. *Am J Geriatr Psychiatry.* 2006;14(7):625-628.

Lee EA, Cho HI, Kim SS, Lee WY. Comparison of magnetic resonance imaging in subtypes of multiple system atrophy. *Parkinsonism Relat Disord.* 2004;10(6):363-368.

Lee WH, Lee CC, Shyu WC, Chong PN, Lin SZ. Hyperintense putaminal rim sign is not a hallmark of multiple system atrophy at 3T. *AJNR Am J Neuroradiol.* 2005;26(9):2238-2242.

Litvan I, Agid Y, Goetz C, Jankovic J, Wenning GK, Brandel JP, Lai EC, Verny M, Ray-Chaudhuri K, McKee A, Jellinger K, Pearce RK, Bartko JJ. Accuracy of the clinical diagnosis of corticobasal degeneration: a clinicopathologic study. *Neurology.* 1997;48(1):119-125.

Litvan I, Goetz CG, Jankovic J, Wenning GK, Booth V, Bartko JJ, McKee A, Jellinger K, Lai EC, Brandel JP, Verny M, Chaudhuri KR, Pearce RK, Agid Y. What is the accuracy of the clinical diagnosis of multiple system atrophy? A clinicopathologic study. *Arch Neurol.* 1997;54(8):937-944.

Lobotesis K, Fenwick JD, Phipps A, Ryman A, Swann A, Ballard C, McKeith IG, O'Brien JT. Occipital hypoperfusion on SPECT in dementia with Lewy bodies but not AD. *Neurology.* 2001;56(5):643-649.

Lorberboym M, Treves TA, Melamed E, Lampl Y, Hellmann M, Djaldetti R. [^{123}I]-FP/CIT SPECT imaging for distinguishing drug-induced parkinsonism from Parkinson's disease. *Mov Disord.* 2006;21(4):510-514.

Marra CM. Neurosyphilis. *Curr Neurol Neurosci Rep.* 2004;4(6):435-440.

Marshall V, Grosset D. Role of dopamine transporter imaging in routine clinical practice. *Mov Disord.* 2003;18(12):1415-1423.

Marti MJ, Tolosa E, Campdelacreu J. Clinical overview of the synucleinopathies. *Mov Disord.* 2003;18(suppl 6):S21-S27.

Matsuda H. Neurological diseases and SPECT—analysis using easy Z-score imaging system (eZIS). *Brain Nerve.* 2007;59(5):487-493.

Matsusue E, Fujii S, Kanasaki Y, Sugihara S, Miyata H, Ohama E, Ogawa T. Putaminal lesion in multiple system atrophy: postmortem MR-pathological correlations. *Neuroradiology.* 2008;50(7):559-567.

McKeith I, O'Brien J, Walker Z, Tatsch K, Booij J, Darcourt J, Padovani A, Giubbini R, Bonuccelli U, Volterrani D, Holmes C, Kemp P, Tabet N, Meyer I, Reininger C. Sensitivity and specificity of dopamine transporter imaging with $_{123}$I-FP-CIT SPECT in dementia with Lewy bodies: a phase III, multicentre study. *Lancet Neurol.* 2007;6(4):305-313.

McKeith IG, Galasko D, Kosaka K, Perry EK, Dickson DW, Hansexn LA, Salmon DP, Lowe J, Mirra SS, Byrne EJ, Lennox G, Quinn NP, Edwardson JA, Ince PG, Bergeron C, Burns A, Miller BL, Lovestone S, Collerton D, Jansen EN, Ballard C, de Vos RA, Wilcock GK, Jellinger KA, Perry RH. Consensus guidelines for the clinical and pathologic diagnosis of dementia with Lewy bodies (DLB): report of the consortium on DLB international workshop. *Neurology.* 1996;47(5):1113-1124.

McMurtray A, Clark DG, Christine D, Mendez MF. Early-onset dementia: frequency and causes compared to late-onset dementia. *Dement Geriatr Cogn Disord.* 2006;21(2):59-64.

McNeill A, Birchall D, Hayflick SJ, Gregory A, Schenk JF, Zimmerman EA, Shang H, Miyajima H, Chinnery PF. T2* and FSE MRI distinguishes four subtypes of neurodegeneration with brain iron accumulation. *Neurology.* 2008;70(18):1614-1619.

Meyer JS, Huang J, Chowdhury MH. MRI confirms mild cognitive impairments prodromal for Alzheimer's, vascular and Parkinson-Lewy body dementias. *J Neurol Sci.* 2007;257(1-2):97-104.

Minoshima S, Giordani B, Berent S, Frey KA, Foster NL, Kuhl DE. Metabolic reduction in the posterior cingulate cortex in very early Alzheimer's disease. *Ann Neurol.* 1997;42(1):85-94.

Mirzaei S, Knoll P, Koehn H, Bruecke T. Assessment of diffuse Lewy body disease by 2-[^{18}F]fluoro-2-deoxy-D-glucose positron emission tomography (FDG PET). *BMC Nucl Med.* 2003;3(1):1.

Mori H, Yagishita A, Takeda T, Mizutani T. Symmetric temporal abnormalities on MR imaging in amyotrophic lateral sclerosis with dementia. *AJNR Am J Neuroradiol.* 2007;28(8):1511-1516.

Mosconi L, Tsui WH, Herholz K, Pupi A, Drzezga A, Lucignani G, Reiman EM, Holthoff V, Kalbe E, Sorbi S, Diehl-Schmid J, Perneczky R, Clerici F, Caselli R, Beuthien-Baumann B, Kurz A, Minoshima S, de Leon MJ. Multicenter standardized ^{18}F-FDG PET diagnosis of mild cognitive impairment, Alzheimer's disease, and other dementias. *J Nucl Med.* 2008;49(3):390-398.

Nagasawa H, Tanji H, Nomura H, Saito H, Itoyama Y, Kimura I, Tuji S, Fujiwara T, Iwata R, Itoh M, Ido T. PET study of cerebral glucose metabolism and fluorodopa uptake in patients with corticobasal degeneration. *J Neurol Sci.* 1996;139(2):210-217.

Naka H, Ohshita T, Murata Y, Imon Y, Mimori Y, Nakamura S. Characteristic MRI findings in multiple system atrophy: comparison of the three subtypes. *Neuroradiology.* 2002;44(3):204-209.

Naslund J, Haroutunian V, Mohs R, Davis KL, Davies P, Greengard P, Buxbaum JD. Correlation between elevated levels of amyloid beta-peptide in the brain and cognitive decline. *JAMA.* 2000;283(12):1571-1577.

Nicoletti G, Lodi R, Condino F, Tonon C, Fera F, Malucelli E, Manners D, Zappia M, Morgante L, Barone P, Barbiroli B, Quattrone A. Apparent diffusion coefficient measurements of the middle cerebellar peduncle differentiate the Parkinson variant of MSA from Parkinson's disease and progressive supranuclear palsy. *Brain.* 2006;129(Pt 10):2679-2687.

Nicoletti G, Tonon C, Lodi R, Condino F, Manners D, Malucelli E, Morelli M, Novellino F, Paglionico S, Lanza P, Messina D, Barone P, Morgante L, Zappia M, Barbiroli B, Quattrone A. Apparent diffusion coefficient of the superior cerebellar peduncle differentiates progressive supranuclear palsy from Parkinson's disease. *Mov Disord.* 2008;23(16):2370-2376.

Nordberg A. Amyloid imaging in Alzheimer's disease. *Curr Opin Neurol.* 2007;20(4):398-402.

Oba H, Yagishita A, Terada H, Barkovich AJ, Kutomi K, Yamauchi T, Furui S, Shimizu T, Uchigata M, Matsumura K, Sonoo M, Sakai M, Takada K, Harasawa A, Takeshita K, Kohtake H, Tanaka H, Suzuki S. New and reliable MRI diagnosis for progressive supranuclear palsy. *Neurology.* 2005;64(12):2050-2055.

O'Brien JT. Role of imaging techniques in the diagnosis of dementia. *Br J Radiol.* 2007;80(Spec No 2):S71-S77.

Olsen CG, Clasen ME. Senile dementia of the Binswanger's type. *Am Fam Physician.* 1998;58(9):2068-2074.

Orimo S, Amino T, Ozawa E, Kojo T, Uchihara T, Takahashi A, Tsuchiya K, Wakabayashi K, Takahashi H. A useful marker for differential diagnosis of Parkinson's disease—MIBG myocardial scintigraphy. *Rinsho Shinkeigaku.* 2004;44(11):827-829.

Ormerod IE, Harding AE, Miller DH, Johnson G, MacManus D, du Boulay EP, Kendall BE, Moseley IF, McDonald WI. Magnetic resonance imaging in degenerative ataxic disorders. *J Neurol Neurosurg Psychiatry.* 1994;57(1):51-57.

Ortega Lozano SJ, Martinez Del Valle Torres MD, Jimenez-Hoyuela Garcia JM, Gutierrez Cardo AL, Campos Arillo V. Diagnostic accuracy of FP-CIT SPECT in patients with parkinsonism. *Rev Esp Med Nucl.* 2007;26(5):277-285.

Ozsancak C, Auzou P, Dujardin K, Quinn N, Destee A. Orofacial apraxia in corticobasal degeneration, progressive supranuclear palsy, multiple system atrophy and Parkinson's disease. *J Neurol.* 2004;251(11):1317-1323.

Pantoni L, Garcia JH. The significance of cerebral white matter abnormalities 100 years after Binswanger's report. A review. *Stroke.* 1995;26(7):1293-1301.

Peng F, Hu X, Zhong X, Wei Q, Jiang Y, Bao J, Wu A, Pei Z. CT and MR findings in HIV-negative neurosyphilis. *Eur J Radiol.* 2008;66(1):1-6.

Petersen RC, Smith GE, Waring SC, Ivnik RJ, Tangalos EG, Kokmen E. Mild cognitive impairment: clinical characterization and outcome. *Arch Neurol.* 1999;56(3):303-308.

Petersen RC, Stevens JC, Ganguli M, Tangalos EG, Cummings JL, DeKosky ST. Practice parameter: early detection of dementia: mild cognitive impairment (an evidence-based review). Report of the Quality Standards Subcommittee of the American Academy of Neurology. *Neurology.* 2001;56(9):1133-1142.

Pirker W, Asenbaum S, Bencsits G, Prayer D, Gerschlager W, Deecke L, Brucke T. [^{123}I]beta-CIT SPECT in multiple system atrophy, progressive supranuclear palsy, and corticobasal degeneration. *Mov Disord.* 2000;15(6):1158-1167.

Poewe W, Wenning G. The differential diagnosis of Parkinson's disease. *Eur J Neurol.* 2002;9(suppl 3):23-30.

Quattrone A, Nicoletti G, Messina D, Fera F, Condino F, Pugliese P, Lanza P, Barone P, Morgante L, Zappia M, Aguglia U, Gallo O. MR imaging index for differentiation of progressive supranuclear palsy from Parkinson disease and the Parkinson variant of multiple system atrophy. *Radiology.* 2008;246(1):214-221.

Rabinovici GD, Furst AJ, O'Neil JP, Racine CA, Mormino EC, Baker SL, Chetty S, Patel P, Pagliaro TA, Klunk WE, Mathis CA, Rosen HJ, Miller BL, Jagust WJ. ^{11}C-PIB PET imaging in Alzheimer disease and frontotemporal lobar degeneration. *Neurology.* 2007;68(15):1205-1212.

Rabinovici GD, Jagust WJ, Furst AJ, Ogar JM, Racine CA, Mormino EC, O'Neil JP, Lal RA, Dronkers NF, Miller BL, Gorno-Tempini ML. Abeta amyloid and glucose metabolism in three variants of primary progressive aphasia. *Ann Neurol.* 2008;64(4):388-401.

Ravina B, Eidelberg D, Ahlskog JE, Albin RL, Brooks DJ, Carbon M, Dhawan V, Feigin A, Fahn S, Guttman M, Gwinn-Hardy K, McFarland H, Innis R, Katz RG, Kieburtz K, Kish SJ, Lange N, Langston JW, Marek K, Morin L, Moy C, Murphy D, Oertel WH, Oliver G, Palesch Y, Powers W, Seibyl J, Sethi KD, Shults CW, Sheehy P, Stoessl AJ, Holloway R. The role of radiotracer imaging in Parkinson disease. *Neurology.* 2005;64(2):208-215.

Reiman EM, Caselli RJ, Yun LS, Chen K, Bandy D, Minoshima S, Thibodeau SN, Osborne D. Preclinical evidence of Alzheimer's disease in persons homozygous for the epsilon 4 allele for apolipoprotein E. *N Engl J Med.* 1996;334(12):752-758

Rizzo G, Martinelli P, Manners D, Scaglione C, Tonon C, Cortelli P, Malucelli E, Capellari S, Testa C, Parchi P, Montagna P, Barbiroli B, Lodi R. Diffusion-weighted brain imaging study of patients with clinical diagnosis of corticobasal degeneration, progressive supranuclear palsy and Parkinson's disease. *Brain.* 2008;131(Pt 10):2690-2700.

Roman G. Diagnosis of vascular dementia and Alzheimer's disease. *Int J Clin Pract Suppl.* 2001;120:9-13.

Roman GC. Vascular dementia: distinguishing characteristics, treatment, and prevention. *J Am Geriatr Soc.* 2003;51(suppl 5 Dementia):S296-304.

Roob G, Schmidt R, Kapeller P, Lechner A, Hartung HP, Fazekas F. MRI evidence of past cerebral microbleeds in a healthy elderly population. *Neurology.* 1999;52(5):991-994.

Rosas HD, Goodman J, Chen YI, Jenkins BG, Kennedy DN, Makris N, Patti M, Seidman LJ, Beal MF, Koroshetz WJ. Striatal volume loss in HD as measured by MRI and the influence of CAG repeat. *Neurology.* 2001;57(6):1025-1028.

Rowe CC, Ackerman U, Browne W, Mulligan R, Pike KL, O'Keefe G, Tochon-Danguy H, Chan G, Berlangieri SU, Jones G, Dickinson-Rowe KL, Kung HP, Zhang W, Kung MP, Rowe CC, Ng S, Ackermann U, Gong SJ, Pike K, Savage G, Cowie TF, Dickinson KL, Maruff P, Salvarani C, Brown Jr RD, Calamia KT, Christianson TJ, Huston 3rd J, Meschia JF, Giannini C, Miller DV, Hunder GG. Primary central nervous system vasculitis: comparison of patients with and without cerebral amyloid angiopathy. *Rheumatology (Oxford).* 2008;47(11):1671-1677.

Skovronsky D, Dyrks T, Holl G, Krause S, Friebe M, Lehman L, Lindemann S, Dinkelborg LM, Masters CL, Villemagne VL. Imaging of amyloid beta in Alzheimer's disease with ^{18}F-BAY94-9172, a novel PET tracer: proof of mechanism. *Lancet neurology.* 2008;7(2):129-135.

Sasaki M, Ichiya Y, Hosokawa S, Otsuka M, Kuwabara Y, Fukumura T, Kato M, Goto I, Masuda K. Regional cerebral glucose metabolism in patients with Parkinson's disease with or without dementia. *Ann Nucl Med.* 1992;6(4):241-246.

Savage CR. Neuropsychology of subcortical dementias. *Psychiatr Clin North Am.* 1997;20(4):911-931.

Savoiardo M, Strada L, Girotti F, Zimmerman RA, Grisoli M, Testa D, Petrillo R. Olivopontocerebellar atrophy: MR diagnosis and relationship to multisystem atrophy. *Radiology.* 1990;174(3 Pt 1):693-696.

Savoiardo M. Differential diagnosis of Parkinson's disease and atypical parkinsonian disorders by magnetic resonance imaging. *Neurol Sci.* 2003;24(suppl 1):S35-S37.

Scherfler C, Schwarz J, Antonini A, Grosset D, Valldeoriola F, Marek K, Oertel W, Tolosa E, Lees AJ, Poewe W. Role of DAT-SPECT in the diagnostic work up of parkinsonism. *Mov Disord.* 2007;22(9):1229-1238.

Schmidt R, Schmidt H, Kapeller P, Enzinger C, Ropele S, Saurugg R, Fazekas F. The natural course of MRI white matter hyperintensities. *J Neurol Sci.* 2002:203-204:253–257.

Schrag A, Kingsley D, Phatouros C, Mathias CJ, Lees AJ, Daniel SE, Quinn NP. Clinical usefulness of magnetic resonance imaging in multiple system atrophy. *J Neurol Neurosurg Psychiatry.* 1998;65(1):65-71.

Schwarz J, Weis S, Kraft E, Tatsch K, Bandmann O, Mehraein P, Vogl T, Oertel WH. Signal changes on MRI and increases in reactive microgliosis, astrogliosis, and iron in the putamen of two patients with multiple system atrophy. *J Neurol Neurosurg Psychiatry.* 1996;60(1):98-101.

Seppi K, Schocke MF, Wenning GK, Poewe W. How to diagnose MSA early: the role of magnetic resonance imaging. *J Neural Transm.* 2005;112(12):1625-1634.

Seppi K. MRI for the differential diagnosis of neurodegenerative parkinsonism in clinical practice. *Parkinsonism Relat Disord.* 2007;13(suppl 3):S400-S405.

Shim YS, Kim JS, Shon YM, Chung YA, Ahn KJ, Yang DW. A serial study of regional cerebral blood flow deficits in patients with left anterior thalamic infarction: anatomical and neuropsychological correlates. *J Neurol Sci.* 2008;266(1-2):84-91.

Shrivastava A. The hot cross bun sign. *Radiology.* 2007;245(2):606-607.

Small GW, Kepe V, Ercoli LM, Siddarth P, Bookheimer SY, Miller KJ, Lavretsky H, Burggren AC, Cole GM, Vinters HV, Thompson PM, Huang SC, Satyamurthy N, Phelps ME, Barrio JR. PET of brain amyloid and tau in mild cognitive impairment. *N Engl J Med.* 2006;355(25):2652-2663.

Smith AD, Jobst KA. Use of structural imaging to study the progression of Alzheimer's disease. *Br Med Bull.* 1996;52(3):575-586.

Snowden JS, Neary D, Mann DM. Frontotemporal dementia. *Br J Psychiatry.* 2002;180:140-143.

Soliveri P, Monza D, Paridi D, Radice D, Grisoli M, Testa D, Savoiardo M, Girotti F. Cognitive and magnetic resonance imaging aspects of corticobasal degeneration and progressive supranuclear palsy. *Neurology.* 1999;53(3):502-507.

Spillantini MG, Goedert M. Tau protein pathology in neurodegenerative diseases. *Trends Neurosci.* 1998;21(10):428-433.

Spillantini MG, Goedert M. The alpha-synucleinopathies: Parkinson's disease, dementia with Lewy bodies, and multiple system atrophy. *Ann N Y Acad Sci.* 2000;920:16-27.

Strong M, Rosenfeld J. Amyotrophic lateral sclerosis: a review of current concepts. *Amyotroph Lateral Scler Other Motor Neuron Disord.* 2003;4(3):136-143.

Sullivan EV, Pfefferbaum A. Neuroradiological characterization of normal adult ageing. *Br J Radiol.* 2007;2:S99-108:80 Spec No.

Taki J, Yoshita M, Yamada M, Tonami N. Significance of ^{123}I-MIBG scintigraphy as a pathophysiological indicator in the assessment of Parkinson's disease and related disorders: it can be a specific marker for Lewy body disease. *Ann Nucl Med.* 2004;18(6):453-461.

Tam CW, Burton EJ, McKeith IG, Burn DJ, O'Brien JT. Temporal lobe atrophy on MRI in Parkinson disease with dementia: a comparison with Alzheimer disease and dementia with Lewy bodies. *Neurology.* 2005;64(5):861-865.

Tatemichi TK, Desmond DW, Prohovnik I. Strategic infarcts in vascular dementia. A clinical and brain imaging experience. *Arzneimittelforschung.* 1995;45(3A):371-385.

Tatsch K. Imaging of the dopaminergic system in differential diagnosis of dementia. *Eur J Nucl Med Mol Imaging.* 2008;35(suppl 1):S51-S57.

Thal DR, Griffin WS, de Vos RA, Ghebremedhin E. Cerebral amyloid angiopathy and its relationship to Alzheimer's disease. *Acta Neuropathol.* 2008;115(6):599-609.

Thomas LO, Boyko OB, Anthony DC, Burger PC. MR detection of brain iron. *AJNR Am J Neuroradiol.* 1993;14(5):1043-1048.

Thomas M, Hayflick SJ, Jankovic J. Clinical heterogeneity of neurodegeneration with brain iron accumulation (Hallervorden-Spatz syndrome) and pantothenate kinase-associated neurodegeneration. *Mov Disord.* 2004;19(1):36-42.

Tian J, Shi J, Mann DM. Cerebral amyloid angiopathy and dementia. *Panminerva Med.* 2004;46(4):253-264.

Tolnay M, Clavaguera F. Argyrophilic grain disease: a late-onset dementia with distinctive features among tauopathies. *Neuropathology.* 2004;24(4):269-283.

Tolosa E, Wenning G, Poewe W. The diagnosis of Parkinson's disease. *Lancet Neurol.* 2006;5(1):75-86.

Tucker KA, Robertson KR, Lin W, Smith JK, An H, Chen Y, Aylward SR, Hall CD. Neuroimaging in human immunodeficiency virus infection. *J Neuroimmunol.* 2004;157(1-2):153-162.

Tysnes OB, Vilming ST. Atypical parkinsonism. *Tidsskr Nor Laegeforen.* 2008;128(18):2077-2080.

van de Pol LA, Hensel A, van der Flier WM, Visser PJ, Pijnenburg YA, Barkhof F, Gertz HJ, Scheltens P. Hippocampal atrophy on MRI in frontotemporal lobar degeneration and Alzheimer's disease. *J Neurol Neurosurg Psychiatry.* 2006;77(4):439-442.

Varrone A, Marek KL, Jennings D, Innis RB, Seibyl JP. [(123)I]beta-CIT SPECT imaging demonstrates reduced density of striatal dopamine transporters in Parkinson's disease and multiple system atrophy. *Mov Disord.* 2001;16(6):1023-1032.

Varrone A, Pagani M, Salvatore E, Salmaso D, Sansone V, Amboni M, Nobili F, De Michele G, Filla A, Barone P, Pappata S, Salvatore M. Identification by [99mTc]ECD SPECT of anterior cingulate hypoperfusion in progressive supranuclear palsy, in comparison with Parkinson's disease. *Eur J Nucl Med Mol Imaging.* 2007;34(7):1071-1081.

Vataja R, Pohjasvaara T, Mantyla R, Ylikoski R, Leppavuori A, Leskela M, Kalska H, Hietanen M, Aronen HJ, Salonen O, Kaste M, Erkinjuntti T. MRI correlates of executive dysfunction in patients with ischaemic stroke. *Eur J Neurol.* 2003;10(6):625-631.

Vercelletto M, Ronin M, Huvet M, Magne C, Feve JR. Frontal type dementia preceding amyotrophic lateral sclerosis: a neuropsychological and SPECT study of five clinical cases. *Eur J Neurol.* 1999;6(3):295-299.

Verma A, Bradley WG. Atypical motor neuron disease and related motor syndromes. *Semin Neurol.* 2001;21(2):177-187.

Viswanathan A, Chabriat H. Cerebral microhemorrhage. *Stroke.* 2006;37(2):550-555.

Walker Z, Costa DC, Walker RW, Shaw K, Gacinovic S, Stevens T, Livingston G, Ince P, McKeith IG, Katona CL. Differentiation of dementia with Lewy bodies from Alzheimer's disease using a dopaminergic presynaptic ligand. *J Neurol Neurosurg Psychiatry.* 2002;73(2):134-140.

Waniek C, Prohovnik I, Kaufman MA, Dwork AJ. Rapidly progressive frontal-type dementia associated with Lyme disease. *J Neuropsychiatry Clin Neurosci.* 1995;7(3):345-347.

Wenning GK, Ben-Shlomo Y, Hughes A, Daniel SE, Lees A, Quinn NP. What clinical features are most useful to distinguish definite multiple system atrophy from Parkinson's disease? *J Neurol Neurosurg Psychiatry.* 2000;68(4):434-440.

Weytingh MD, Bossuyt PM, van Crevel H. Reversible dementia: more than 10% or less than 1%? A quantitative review. *J Neurol.* 1995;242(7):466-471.

Whitwell JL, Petersen RC, Negash S, Weigand SD, Kantarci K, Ivnik RJ, Knopman DS, Boeve BF, Smith GE, Jack Jr CR. Patterns of atrophy differ among specific subtypes of mild cognitive impairment. *Arch Neurol.* 2007;64(8):1130-1138.

Whitwell JL, Shiung MM, Przybelski SA, Weigand SD, Knopman DS, Boeve BF, Petersen RC, Jack Jr CR. MRI patterns of atrophy associated with progression to AD in amnestic mild cognitive impairment. *Neurology.* 2008;70(7):512-520.

Whitwell JL, Weigand SD, Shiung MM, Boeve BF, Ferman TJ, Smith GE, Knopman DS, Petersen RC, Benarroch EE, Josephs KA, Jack Jr CR. Focal atrophy in dementia with Lewy bodies on MRI: a distinct pattern from Alzheimer's disease. *Brain.* 2007;130(Pt 3):708-719.

Wolf H, Jelic V, Gertz HJ, Nordberg A, Julin P, Wahlund LO. A critical discussion of the role of neuroimaging in mild cognitive impairment. *Acta Neurol Scand Suppl.* 2003;179:52-76.

Yagishita A, Oda M. Progressive supranuclear palsy: MRI and pathological findings. *Neuroradiology.* 1996;38(suppl 1):S60-S66.

Yagishita A. MR imaging of the brain of amyotrophic lateral sclerosis. *Rinsho Shinkeigaku.* 1995;35(12):1554-1556.

Yamamoto A, Miki Y, Tomimoto H, Kanagaki M, Takahashi T, Fushimi Y, Konishi J, Laz Haque T, Togashi K. Age-related signal intensity changes in the corpus callosum: assessment with three orthogonal FLAIR images. *Eur Radiol.* 2005;15(11):2304-2311.

Yuan Y, Gu ZX, Wei WS. Fluorodeoxyglucose-positron-emission tomography, single-photon emission tomography, and structural MR imaging for prediction of rapid conversion to Alzheimer disease in patients with mild cognitive impairment: a meta-analysis. *AJNR Am J Neuroradiol.* 2009;30(2):404-410.

Zabramski JM, Wascher TM, Spetzler RF, Johnson B, Golfinos J, Drayer BP, Brown B, Rigamonti D, Brown G. The natural history of familial cavernous malformations: results of an ongoing study. *J Neurosurg.* 1994;80(3):422-432.

Zeidler M, Sellar RJ, Collie DA, Knight R, Stewart G, Macleod MA, Ironside JW, Cousens S, Colchester AC, Hadley DM, Will RG. The pulvinar sign on magnetic resonance imaging in variant Creutzfeldt-Jakob disease. *Lancet.* 2000;355(9213):1412-1418.

CHAPTER 9
Infection/Inflammation
Majda M. Thurnher, Julia Frühwald-Pallamar, and Stefan B. Puchner

Infection involving the brain is considered an emergency that requires rapid and accurate diagnosis, followed by an appropriate surgical and medical intervention. Because of the potentially devastating neurologic deficits, it is imperative to image patients with clinical suspicion of infectious disease of the central nervous system (CNS). The development of an intracranial infection is dependent on the virulence of the organism and the host's immune system. Some of the CNS infections, such as invasive aspergillosis, are among the most frequent, frightening, and life-threatening opportunistic infections in immunocompromised patients. Although the management of patients with suspected CNS infections has been revolutionized in recent years with new and better antiviral and immunomodulatory therapies, the frequency of CNS infections is not declining. The increasing number of immunocompromised patients who may have CNS infections as a result of acquired immunodeficiency syndrome (AIDS) as well as organ transplantation and bone marrow transplantation (BMT) presents new challenges to clinicians and radiologists.

This chapter outlines the major clinical and key radiologic findings in infections of the CNS.

■ MENINGITIS

Streptococcus pneumoniae is found in 50% of cases of adult meningitis. Other common organisms that cause bacterial meningitis are *Neisseria meningitides* and *Haemophilus influenzae*. *S. pneumoniae* and *N. meningitidis* remain the most common causes of bacterial meningitis in children. In neonates, group B streptococcus is the most common pathogen associated with meningitis, and *Listeria monocytogenes* also causes disease. Physical examination alone is not sufficient to accurately diagnose or rule out meningitis, and lumbar puncture results must be interpreted with care when attempting to differentiate viral from bacterial disease. The classic triad of fever, neck stiffness, and a change in mental status is present in less than 50% of cases; however, 95% of patients will present with at least two of the four symptoms of headache, fever, neck stiffness, and altered mental status. Despite the fears of herniation several or many hours after lumbar puncture, cerebrospinal fluid (CSF) analysis is necessary for the specific diagnosis in a majority of the cases. Computed tomographic (CT) scanning of the head is recommended before lumbar puncture for patients with high-risk factors, such as new-onset seizures, immunocompromised status, papilledema, focal neurologic signs, or impaired consciousness. A CSF absolute neutrophil count greater than 1,000/mm^3 is predictive of bacterial meningitis.

Pyogenic Meningitis

CT and magnetic resonance imaging (MRI) can be normal in early cases of meningitis. Meningeal enhancement usually is seen on postcontrast MR sequences, which are more sensitive than CT. Fluid-attenuated inversion recovery (FLAIR) MRI has proved to be of great value in the detection of meningeal diseases, with high signal in the subarachnoid spaces that reflects a high protein content in the CSF, which causes a decrease in T1 relaxation time and results in hyperintensity (Figure 9-1). The differential diagnosis includes leptomeningeal carcinomatosis and subarachnoid hemorrhage. Communicating hydrocephalus is the most common complication of meningitis, with the inflammatory debris obstructing the flow and reabsorption of CSF. A serious complication of pyogenic meningitis is pyogenic ventriculitis, which can be recognized on imaging as periventricular high signal intensity on FLAIR MRI, ependymal enhancement on postcontrast images, and fluid–fluid levels in the ventricles. The presence of ventricular debris will be seen in the dependent parts of the ventricles as a nonlinear fluid–fluid interface on T1-weighted imaging (T1-WI). In acute blood, a straight level will be seen. In pyocephalus, an irregular level within the ventricle is highly suggestive of pus. Venous thromboses can lead to infarction with an accompanying hemorrhagic component. Due to the infection of small arteries and veins on the surface of the brain, extraaxial fluid collections can occur.

When to Suspect Pyogenic Meningitis
Imaging findings of
    High signal intensity of the subarachnoid spaces on FLAIR MRI
    Meningeal enhancement on postcontrast CT or T1-weighted MRI
    Obstructive hydrocephalus
    Subdural or epidural fluid collections
    Complications (infarcts, venous thrombosis, pyocephalus)

Subdural Empyema

Extraaxial collections can be sterile fluids (effusions) or infected purulent fluids (empyema). Subdural empyemas are infected CSF collections between the dura and

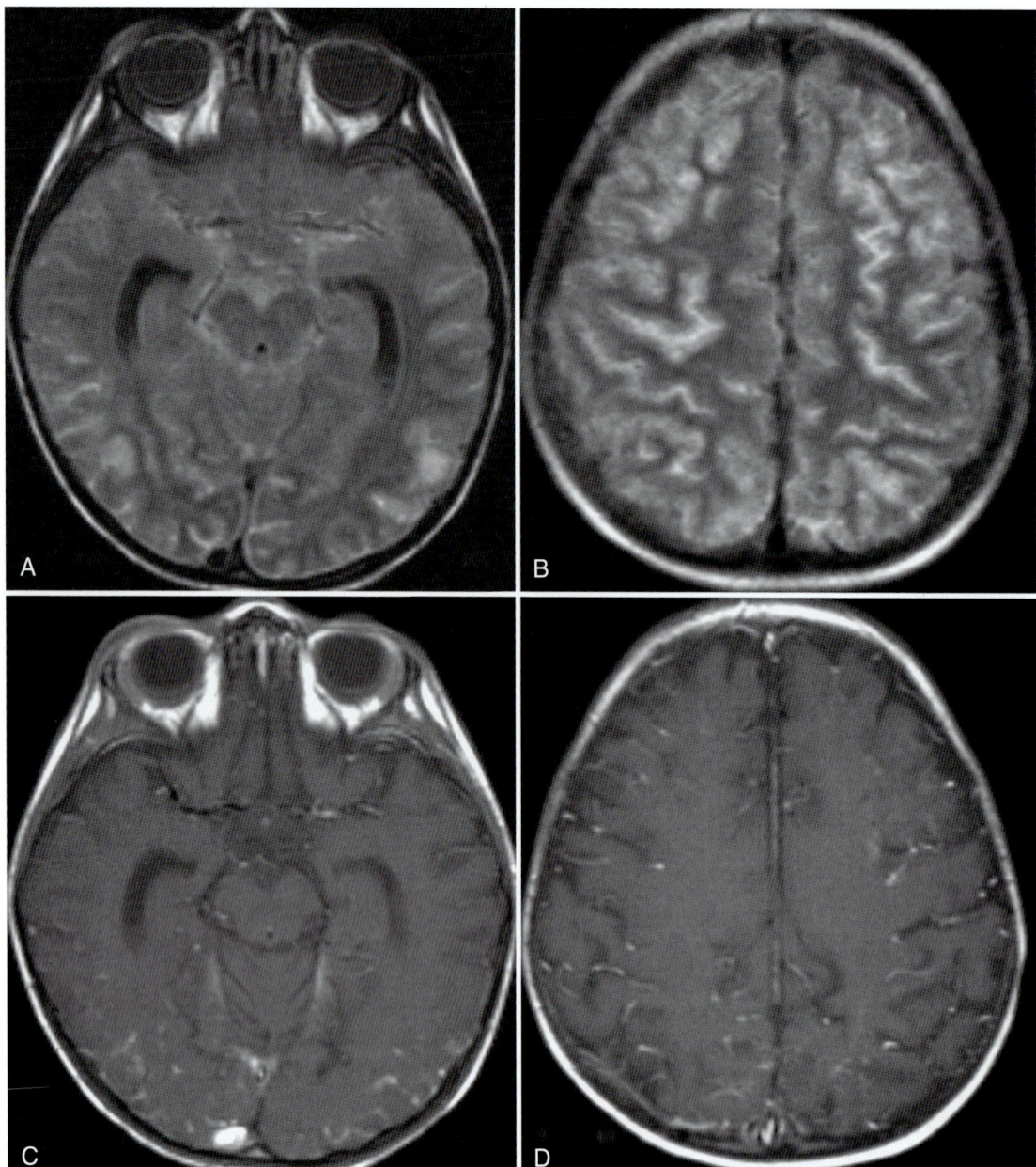

Figure 9-1 Meningitis in a 5-year old child who has suffered from anemia (since her second year of life) and multiple infections. **A, B:** On axial fluid-attenuated inversion recovery images, all subarachnoid spaces have high signal intensity (including the basal cistern). Note dilatation of the temporal horns with a normal-sized fourth ventricle, indicating obstructive hydrocephalus due to the infectious exudates in the basal cistern. **C, D:** Meningeal enhancement is observed on postcontrast T1-weighted images are consistent with meningitis.

arachnoid membranes (subdural space). Clinical signs include fever, vomiting, meningeal signs, and focal neurologic signs (e.g., hemiparesis). Bridging veins can become infected from infected meninges, hematogenous spread may occur, and direct extension of infection from adjacent structures will lead to infection of the superficial veins. On CT, subdural empyemas are isodense to hypodense extraaxial collections with rim enhancement. MRI has a higher sensitivity for detection of small subdural fluid collections and should be performed when subdural collection is suspected. On MRI, subdural empyemas are isointense to the brain parenchyma on T1-WI (increased protein content) and hyperintense on T2-weighted imaging (T2-WI). Diffusion-weighted imaging (DWI) has proved useful in the differentiation between infected collections (empyemas) that are bright, with low apparent diffusion coefficient (ADC) values, and subdural CSF effusions, which have low signal and ADC values similar to CSF (Figure 9-2).

When to Suspect Subdural Empyema
Patients with meningitis, sinus infection, or ear infection
Imaging findings:
    High signal intensity of subdural space on FLAIR MRI
    Rim enhancement on postcontrast images
    High signal of subdural collection on DWI (restricted diffusion)

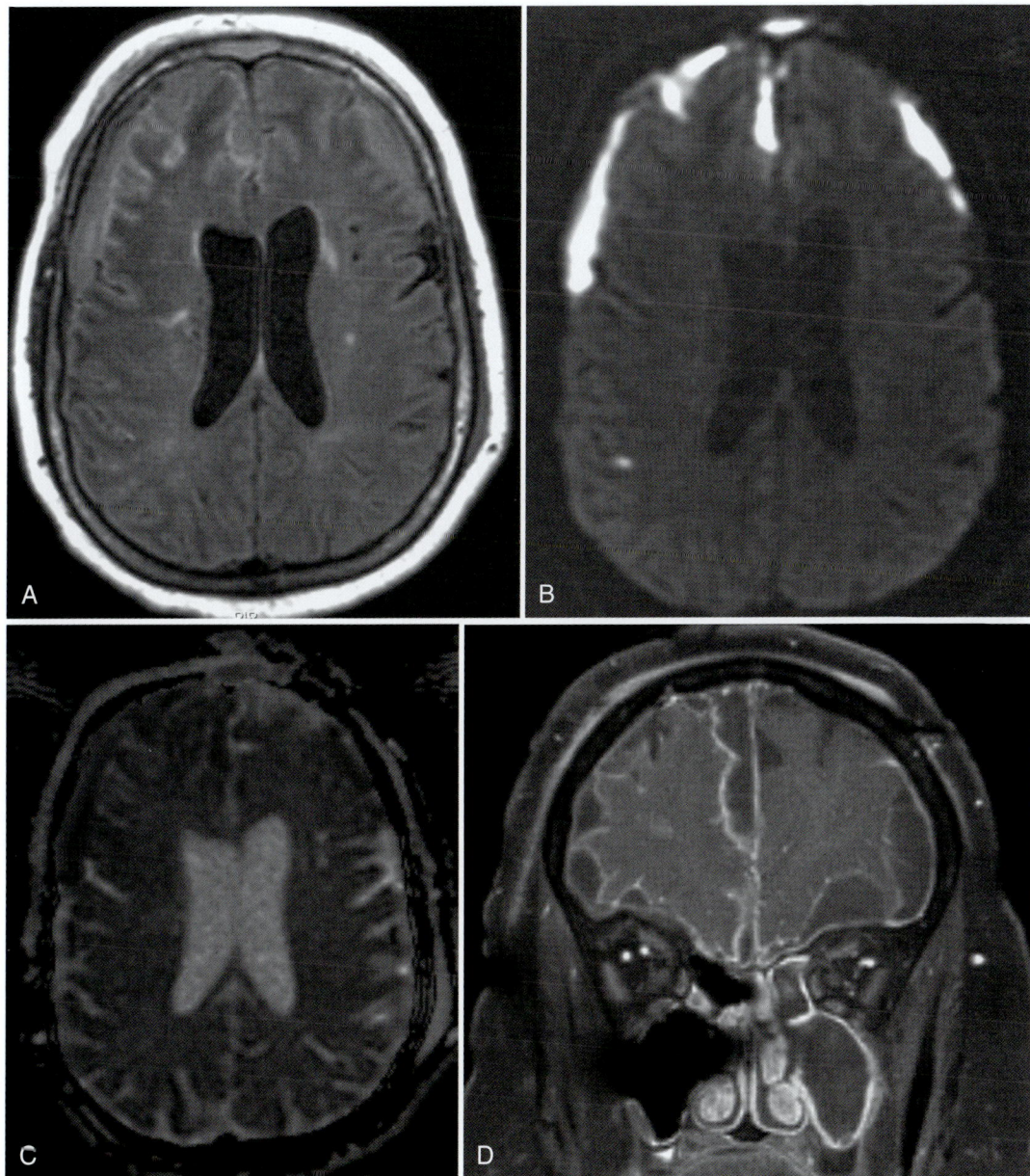

Figure 9-2 Bilateral subdural empyemas in a patient after a tooth implantation procedure. **A:** Bilateral, high signal intensity, extraaxial collections are observed on axial fluid-attenuated inversion recovery in the frontal region. Subarachnoid spaces have high signal intensity indicative of meningeal disease. **B, C:** On trace diffusion-weighted imaging, subdural fluid collections have high signal with low apparent diffusion coefficient values (**C**) representing restricted diffusion due to high viscosity pus in the subdural space. **D:** On coronal postcontrast T1-weighted magnetic resonance image, rim enhancement of the subdural empyemas is demonstrated. Note enhancement and signal intensity changes in the left maxillary sinus and left ethmoid cells (source of infection with contiguous spread to meninges and subdural space).

Epidural Empyema

Epidural abscesses are the result of contiguous spread of infection from mastoids or paranasal sinuses. The infection is located in the epidural space (between the dura and the overlying bone). Patients present with fever, mental status changes, and neck pain. On CT, epidural abscess appears as a hypodense epidural mass of lentiform configuration with midline shift and compression of the brain parenchyma. On MRI, epidural abscesses have iso-signal on T1-WI and high signal on T2-WI, with enhancement of the thickened dural surface. Epidural abscesses will have restricted diffusion with high signal on trace DWI and low ADC values.

Tuberculous Meningitis

The increased incidence of tuberculosis is clearly related to the incidence of AIDS, which is considered the main risk factor for the development of tuberculosis. Tuberculous infection of the CNS starts as tuberculous meningitis (TBM), with a thick gelatinous exudate with a predilection for the meninges covering the base of the brain. Occlusions of the vessels that course through the subarachnoid space result in infarction, most commonly in the region of the basal ganglia. Communicating-type hydrocephalus is the most common complication in meningeal tuberculosis. Hydrocephalus will be seen in 51% of patients with

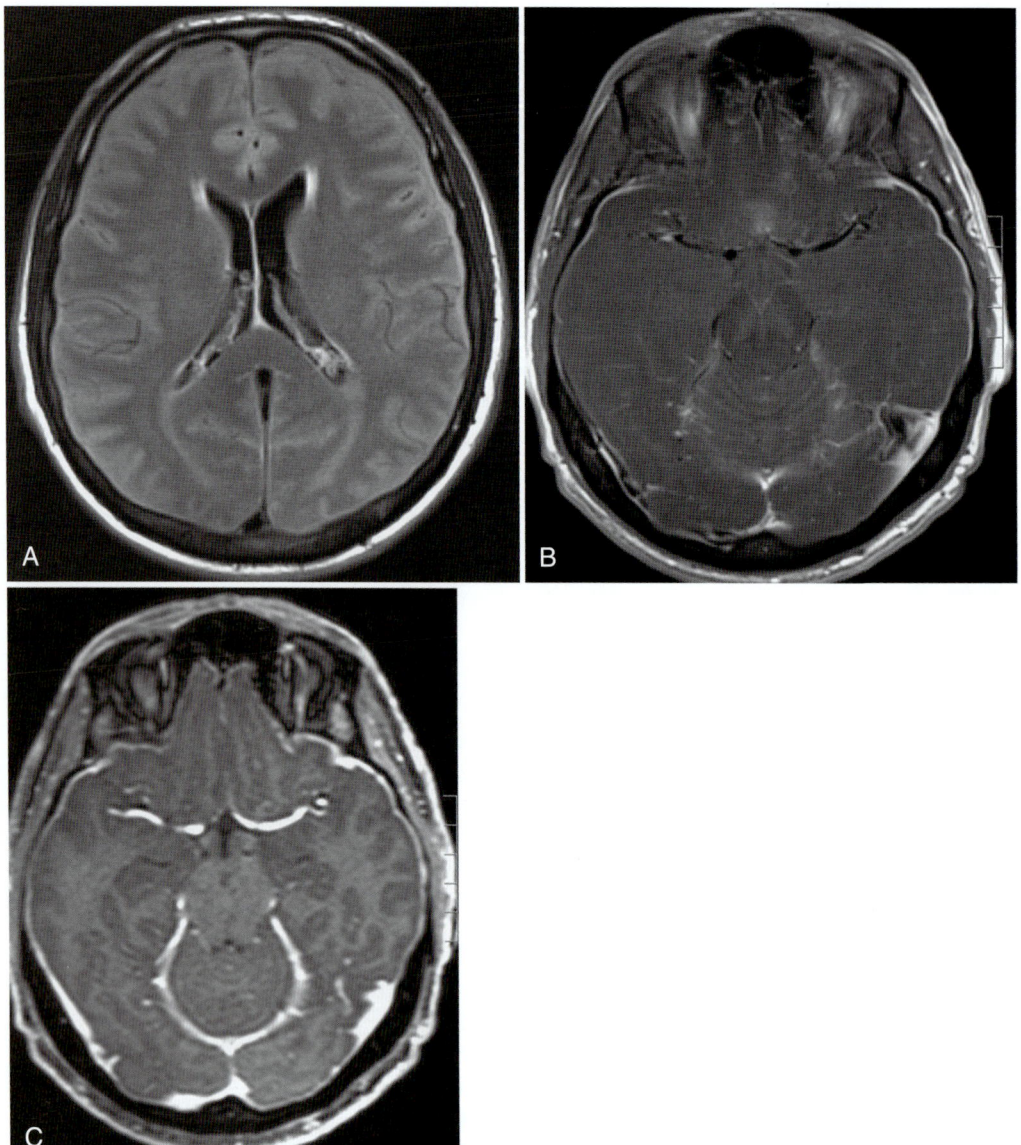

Figure 9-3 Proven tuberculous meningitis in an HIV-positive patient. **A:** Hyperintensity of the subarachnoid spaces is demonstrated on axial fluid-attenuated inversion recovery magnetic resonance image. Bilateral, frontal subdural fluid collections also are seen. **B:** After gadolinium injection, meningeal enhancement in the region of the vermis cerebelli is clearly depicted on postcontrast T1-weighted imaging (T1-WI) with magnetization transfer contrast (MTC). **C:** On postcontrast T1-WI without MTC, no meningeal enhancement can be detected.

AIDS-related CNS tuberculosis. Meningeal enhancement on enhanced CT in the basal cisterns and over the convexity of the brain can be seen in approximately 36% to 61% of TBM cases. Associated tuberculosis ependymitis can be recognized on postcontrast CT scans as abnormal enhancement of the ventricular ependyma. A high prevalence of miliary nodules with a predominantly leptomeningeal distribution will be seen in the CNS of children with TBM. The most common locations of leptomeningeal nodules are between the cerebellar folia (86%) and in the region of the vermis and quadrigeminal cistern (86%) (Figure 9-3). Children with miliary tuberculosis and TBM usually are younger than those with TBM only. Arteries that course through the exudate in the basal cisterns become involved, with spasm and infarction as a consequence (Figure 9-4). Studies using DWI and conventional MRI sequences show that 56.7% of patients with TBM have infarcts. Hydrocephalus occurs in about one third of patients with CNS tuberculosis. The majority of patients have large fourth ventricles with adhesive obstructions in the basal cisterns (Figure 9-4).

When to Suspect TBM

Patients in endemic areas, immunosuppressed patients, human immunodeficiency virus (HIV)-positive patients
Imaging findings:
    Meningeal enhancement (basal regions of the brain)
    Infarcts (most commonly in the basal ganglia region), best depicted with DWI
    Obstructive hydrocephalus
    Enhancement of the cranial nerves
    Miliary pattern of meningeal enhancement in small children

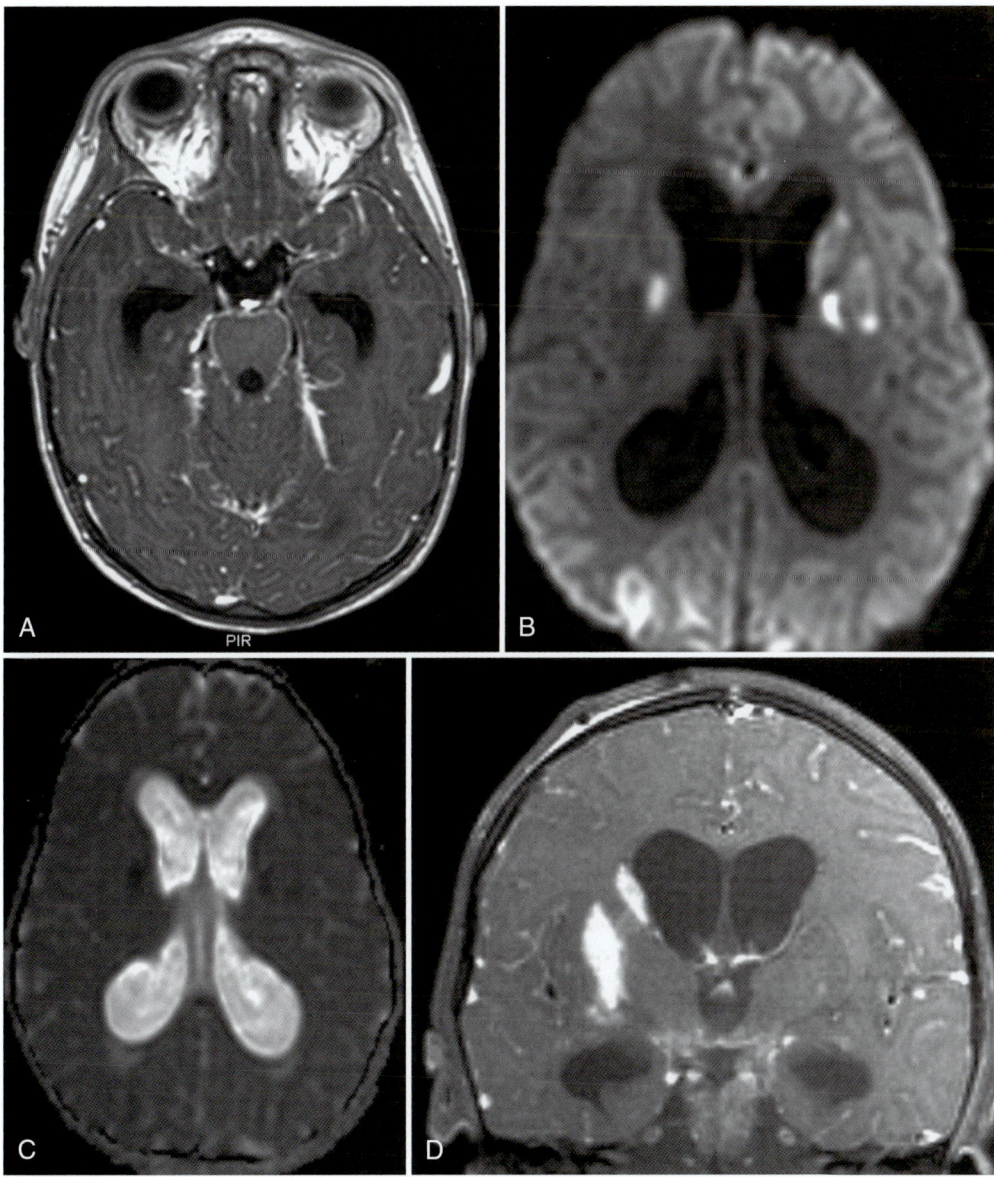

Figure 9-4 Tuberculous meningitis in a 3-year-old child who presented with impairment of consciousness. Computed tomographic scan of the brain showed hydrocephalus. On subsequent magnetic resonance imaging of the brain, meningeal enhancement, hydrocephalus, and bilateral infarcts were detected. **A:** Marked meningeal enhancement is clearly seen on postcontrast T1-weighted imaging (T1 WI) in the axial plane. Note dilatation of the temporal horns as a sign of hydrocephalus. **B:** On axial trace diffusion-weighted imaging, high signal intensity lesions are demonstrated in the basal ganglia region on both sides as well as in the right occipital cortex. **C:** The lesions have low apparent diffusion coefficients indicating restricted diffusion in ischemic lesions. **D:** On T1-WI with fat suppression, enhancement of the subacute ischemic lesion is seen.

Cryptococcal Meningitis

Cryptococcus neoformans is an opportunistic fungus that typically affects HIV-positive and other patients with compromised immune systems. Infection of the CNS is a result of an acquired infection, with hematogenous dissemination of the infection from the lung to the CNS. Immunocompromised patients may present with headache, nausea, vomiting, altered mental status, personality changes, confusion, lethargy, obtundation, or even coma. However, patients may also present with minimal or nonspecific symptoms. Symptoms suspicious for infection, such as fever and nuchal rigidity, are characteristically absent.

The most common form of cryptococcal CNS infection is cryptococcal meningitis. Pathologically, subarachnoid spaces are thickened and filled with multiple organisms and capsular material. Dilatation of the Virchow-Robin spaces is a result of the extension of fungus along the Virchow-Robin perivascular spaces into the basal ganglia, thalami, midbrain, and cerebellum. The Virchow-Robin spaces become dilated. With disease progression, dilated perivascular spaces become confluent and cystic lesions develop called *gelatinous pseudocysts* or *soap bubbles*. These types of lesions do not have a capsule, and they contain mucinous material and fungal organisms. Cryptococcoma is the only parenchymal form of cryptococcal CNS infection. The lesions result from the direct invasion of the brain by the fungus, with the development of a granulomatous reaction. In cases of cryptococcal meningitis, enhanced T1-weighted MRI may demonstrate meningeal enhancement, which usually is nodular. Dilated Virchow-Robin spaces will be recognized on MRI as multiple, bilateral, small round- or oval-shaped lesions, usually located in the basal ganglia, which show high signal on T2-WI and have a signal slightly higher than the CSF on T1-weighted MRI. Gelatinous pseudocysts are slightly bigger in size and do not differ in morphology from the dilated Virchow-Robin spaces on MRI. The most common locations of gelatinous pseudocysts are the basal ganglia and the dentate nucleus. Enhancement and mass effect will not be present.

When to Suspect Cryptococcal Meningitis

HIV-positive patients (especially those with a high viral load level)
Imaging findings:
    Meningeal enhancement (nodular appearance)
    Dilated Virchow-Robin spaces (basal ganglia)
    Cystic lesions without enhancement and mass effect (signal slightly higher than CSF) representing gelatinous pseudocysts

■ ENCEPHALITIS

Viral agents that can cause encephalitis are listed in Table 9-1. The most common viruses that can cause encephalitis are the herpes family viruses (HIV, cytomegalovirus [CMV], herpes-zoster virus). The classic presentation of viral encephalitis is generally characterized by an acute flu-like prodrome that develops into an illness with high fever, severe headache, nausea, vomiting, and altered consciousness, often associated with seizures and focal neurologic signs. In encephalitis, the CSF opening pressure often is slightly raised, and there is usually a mild to moderate CSF pleocytosis of 5 to 1,000 cells/mm^3. An electroencephalogram usually shows nonspecific, diffuse, high-amplitude slow waves of encephalopathy, but it is useful to look for subtle epileptic seizures.

Herpes Simplex Virus Encephalitis

Herpes simplex virus type 1 (HSV-1) is the most common cause of viral encephalitis in adults. Untreated herpes simplex virus encephalitis (HSVE-1) has a high mortality rate, and the prognosis is dependent on early recognition. Pathologically, hemorrhagic encephalitis begins in the inferior and medial temporal lobes and spreads to the frontal lobes in the insular region.

Petechial hemorrhages are present in almost every case at histopathology. The diagnosis can be confirmed by CSF polymerase chain reaction, with sensitivity greater than 95% and specificity approaching 100%.

Approximately 3 to 5 days after onset of symptoms, an area of low attenuation in the temporal lobe may be detected. MRI contributes to early diagnosis, with the earliest imaging findings apparent on FLAIR images 48 hours after onset of symptoms (Figure 9-5). High signal intensity lesions will be observed on T2-WI, with low signal on T1-WI. In the acute phase, the enhancement usually is not present, and gyriform enhancement on enhanced T1-WI will be observed with disease progression (Figures 9-5 and 9-6). On DWI, two distinct

Table 9-1

A. Causative Agents of Acute Viral Encephalitis

1. Herpes viruses
   Herpes simplex virus types 1 and 2, varicella-zoster virus, Epstein-Barr virus, cytomegalovirus, human herpes virus types 6 and 7
2. Enteroviruses
   Coxsackie viruses, echoviruses, enteroviruses 70 and 71, parechovirus, poliovirus
3. Paramyxoviruses
   Measles virus, mumps virus
4. Other
   Influenza viruses, adenovirus, parvovirus, lymphocytic choriomeningitis virus, rubella virus

B. Causative Agents of Acute Viral Encephalitis (Geographically Related)

1. The Americas
   West Nile, La Cross, St. Louis, Rocio, Powassan encephalitis, Venezuelan, eastern and western equine encephalitis, Colorado tick fever virus, dengue, rabies
2. Europe/Middle East
   Tick-borne encephalitis, West Nile, Tosana, rabies
3. Africa
   West Nile (Rift Valley fever virus, Crimean-Congo hemorrhagic fever, dengue, chikungunya), rabies
4. Asia
   Japanese encephalitis, West Nile, dengue, Murray Valley encephalitis, rabies
5. Australasia
   Murray Valley encephalitis, Japanese encephalitis

Modified from Solomon T, Whitley RJ. Arthropod-borne viral encephalitides. In: Scheld M, Whitley RJ, Marra C, eds. *Infections of the central nervous system*. 2nd ed. Philadelphia, PA: Lippincott Williams and Wilkins; 2004.

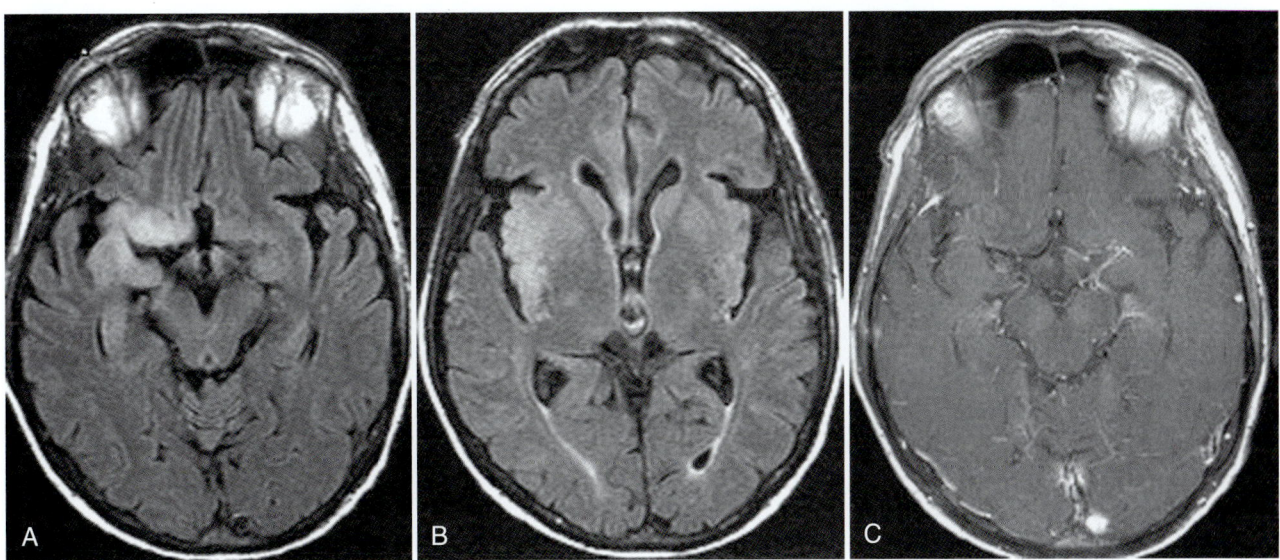

Figure 9-5 Herpes simplex virus encephalitis (HSVE-1) in a patient who presented with seizures and consciousness impairment. **A, B:** Axial fluid-attenuated inversion recovery image showing high signal intensity in the right insular cortex, cingulated gyrus, and right hippocampal region. **C:** No enhancement is observed on postcontrast T1-weighted magnetic resonance image.

types of findings are described in HSVE: lesions similar to cytotoxic edema, and lesions similar to vasogenic edema. In the early stage, the majority of HSV-1 encephalitis cases will have restricted diffusion with high signal (Figure 9-6). DTI analysis has shown slightly reduced mean diffusivity and increased fractional anisotropy values in the earliest phase of HSVE.

When to Suspect HSVE
Seizures, impaired consciousness
Imaging findings:
  Acute stage: Hyperintensity in the temporal lobe on FLAIR images (unilateral or bilateral), nonenhancing, restricted diffusion (high signal on DWI), swollen hypointense cortex on T1-WI
  Subacute stage: Hyperintensity on T2-WI and FLAIR with peripheral gyriform enhancement
Signs of hemorrhage

Human Immunodeficiency Virus

HIV enters the CNS soon after exposure and resides primarily in microglia and macrophages. Pathologic correlates of HIV-related injury include multinucleated giant cell encephalitis and progressive diffuse leukoencephalopathy. Clinically, patients present with dementia, designated as HIV-associated dementia (HAD). The most common reported imaging finding in HIV encephalitis is cerebral atrophy, which is seen in 85% of symptomatic patients. Cortical atrophy is relatively specific to patients with neuropsychological impairment. Enlargement of the ventricular system may be seen in some patients, with or without cortical atrophy. White matter lesions are the second most common MRI finding in patients with HAD, with an average frequency of 78%. These lesions have been described in the supratentorial but also the infratentorial locations, with high signal intensity abnormalities in the pons and cerebellar white matter. Two distinct MRI patterns on T2-WI are observed: (1) diffuse, bilateral, and symmetric high signal intensity involvement of the white matter (butterfly-like); and (2) bilateral, scattering high signal intensity lesions in the white and gray matter (patchy) (Figure 9-7). On T1-weighted MR sequences, the lesions are isointense or slightly hypointense to the white matter. Enhancement and mass effect are not present. Data from recent studies suggest that proton ^{1}H-magnetic resonance spectroscopy (MRS) could potentially be more sensitive than MRI in detecting early CNS involvement in HIV. Decreased N-acetylaspartate (NAA) level and elevated choline (Cho) and myoinositol (MI) levels measured in the basal ganglia region have been observed in patients with HAD (lower NAA/Cr ratio, increased Cho/Cr ratio, increased MI/Cr ratio). Potent antiretroviral combination therapy (highly active antiretroviral therapy [HAART]) in patients with HAD may result in stabilization/regression of white matter abnormalities. First follow-up MR examination will reveal a progression of white matter changes as a result of postinflammatory reactions due to immune reconstitutive effects after the initiation of HAART.

When to Suspect HIV Infection of the CNS
HIV-positive patients (especially those with a high viral load level)
Imaging findings:
  Nonenhancing, bilateral hyperintensities of the white matter (pons, cerebellum, and basal ganglia might be involved)
  Diffuse atrophy
  Patchy, high signal intensity white matter lesions without enhancement and mass effect
  Increased MI/Cr ratio on MRS measured in the basal ganglia
  Initial progression of SI abnormalities after initiation of HAART; regression with time

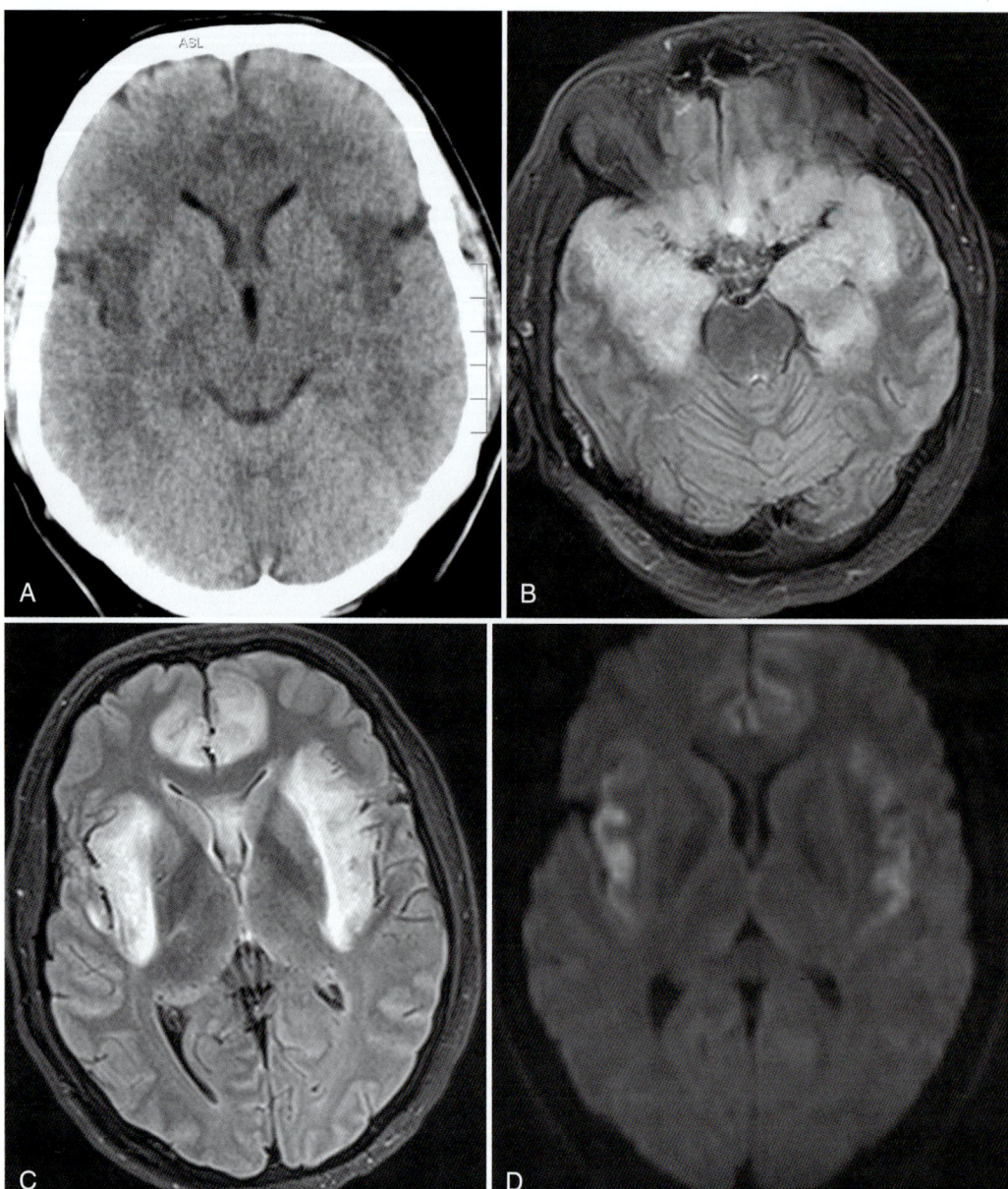

Figure 9-6 A 43-year-old male patient with severe herpes simplex virus encephalitis (HSVE-1). **A:** Axial nonenhanced computed tomographic scan showing bilateral hypodensity of the insular and frontal cortex. **B, C:** Axial fluid-attenuated inversion recovery magnetic resonance images demonstrating extensive high signal intensity changes in the insular region, frontobasal region, and both temporal lobes. **D, E:** On trace diffusion-weighted imaging **(D)**, high signal with low apparent diffusion coefficient values **(E)** is observed in the involved cortex, indicating cytotoxic edema.

Continued

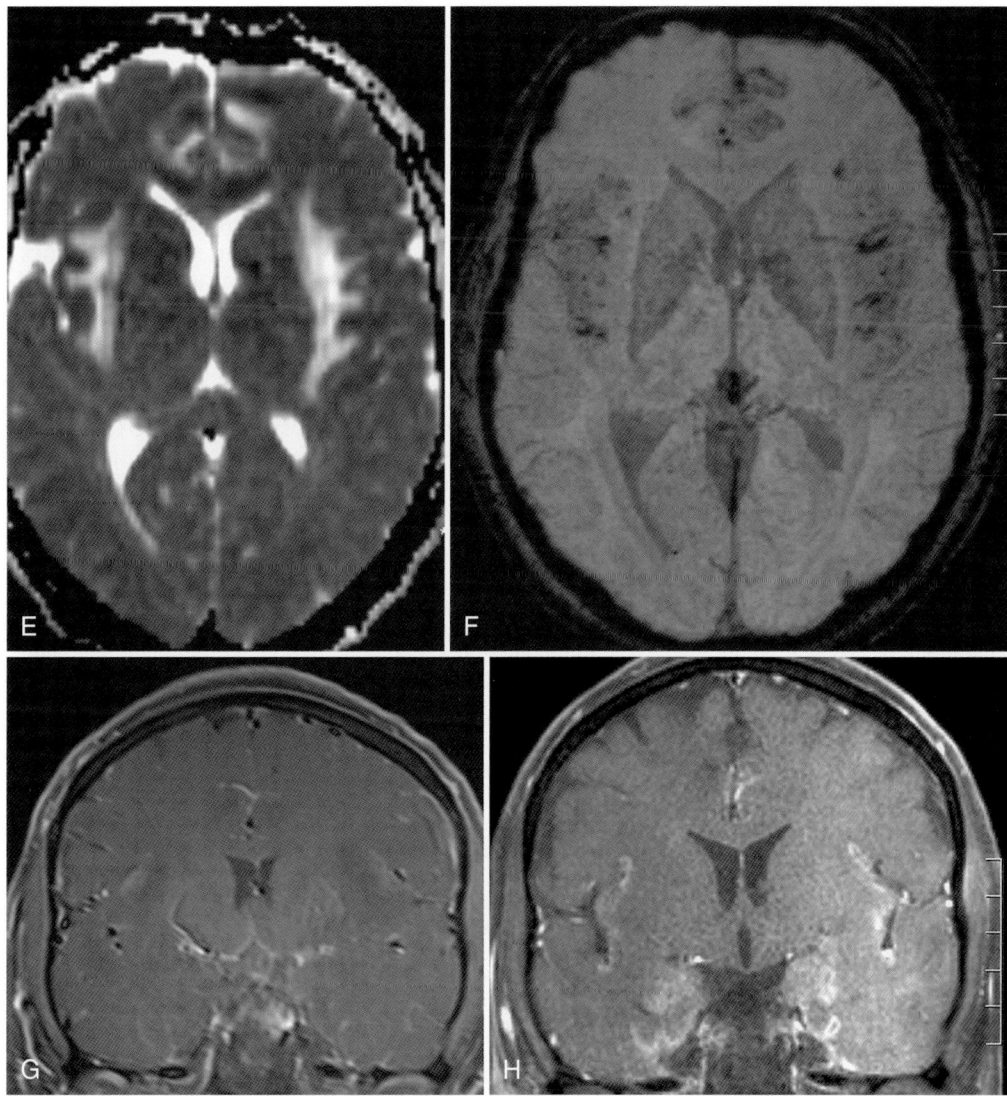

Figure 9-6, cont'd F: On susceptibility-weighted imaging, punctuate low signal intensity changes are shown in the affected regions, representing a hemorrhagic component. G: On postcontrast T1-weighted imaging (T1-WI), no enhancement is observed (acute stage). H: On follow-up magnetic resonance examination 10 days later (subacute stage), gyriform enhancement can be demonstrated on coronal enhanced T1-WI.

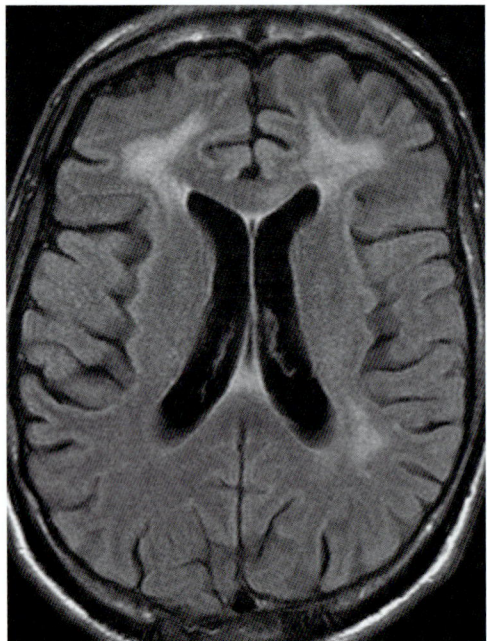

Figure 9-7 Human immunodeficiency virus (HIV) encephalopathy in a 39-year-old male HIV-positive patient who presented with signs of subcortical dementia. Cerebrospinal fluid analysis revealed high viral load level. Axial fluid-attenuated inversion recovery magnetic resonance image showing bilateral, nonenhancing (not shown), high signal intensity abnormalities in the frontal white matter. Subcortical fibers are not involved. Note enlargement of the ventricles and subarachnoid spaces in HIV-associated diffuse atrophy.

Cytomegalovirus

CMV belongs to the family of herpes viruses. In adults, the infection is the result of reactivation of a latent infection. Five distinct neurologic syndromes related to CMV infection are retinitis, myelitis/polyradiculopathy, diffuse micronodular encephalitis, ventriculoencephalitis, and mononeuritis multiplex. In CMV diffuse micronodular encephalitis, small microglial nodules and inclusion-bearing cytomegalic cells are widely distributed in the cortex, basal ganglia, brainstem, and cerebellum. The most common imaging findings in patients with CMV encephalitis are cortical atrophy, periventricular enhancement, and diffuse white matter abnormalities. Generalized atrophy is the most commonly reported CT abnormality. In ventriculoencephalitis, periventricular enhancement has been described. The presence of thin linear enhancement suggests a viral etiology (CMV or varicella-zoster virus), whereas the presence of nodular enhancement suggests a diagnosis of primary CNS lymphoma. In an AIDS patient, a case of cerebral mass lesion due to CMV has been reported. In immunocompromised patients, CMV-induced cerebellitis can occur with swollen cerebellar cortex and linear enhancement (Figure 9-8).

When to Suspect CMV Infection of the CNS

HIV-positive patients, patients after BMT or organ transplantation
Imaging findings:
  Generalized atrophy
  White matter lesions
  Periventricular enhancement

Progressive Multifocal Leukoencephalopathy

Progressive multifocal leukoencephalopathy (PML) is an opportunistic infection caused by the JC *Polyomavirus*. The incidence of PML ranges between 0.7% and 11% in the HIV population. Histopathologic features of PML

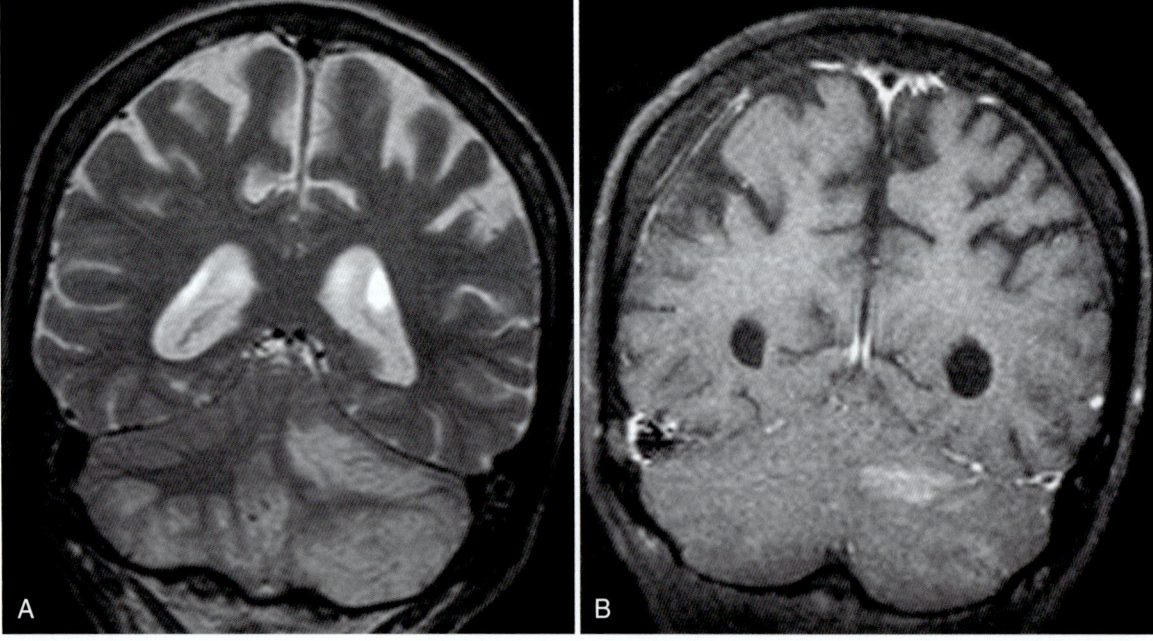

Figure 9-8 Acute viral cerebellitis in an immunocompromised patient 2 months after liver transplantation who presented with nystagmus, dysarthria, and vertigo. Cytomegalovirus was suspected to be the causing agent. **A:** Coronal T2-weighted magnetic resonance image showing diffuse increased signal intensity involving both cerebellar hemispheres. **B:** On coronal enhanced T1-weighted magnetic resonance image, faint enhancement is observed only in the left cerebellar hemisphere.

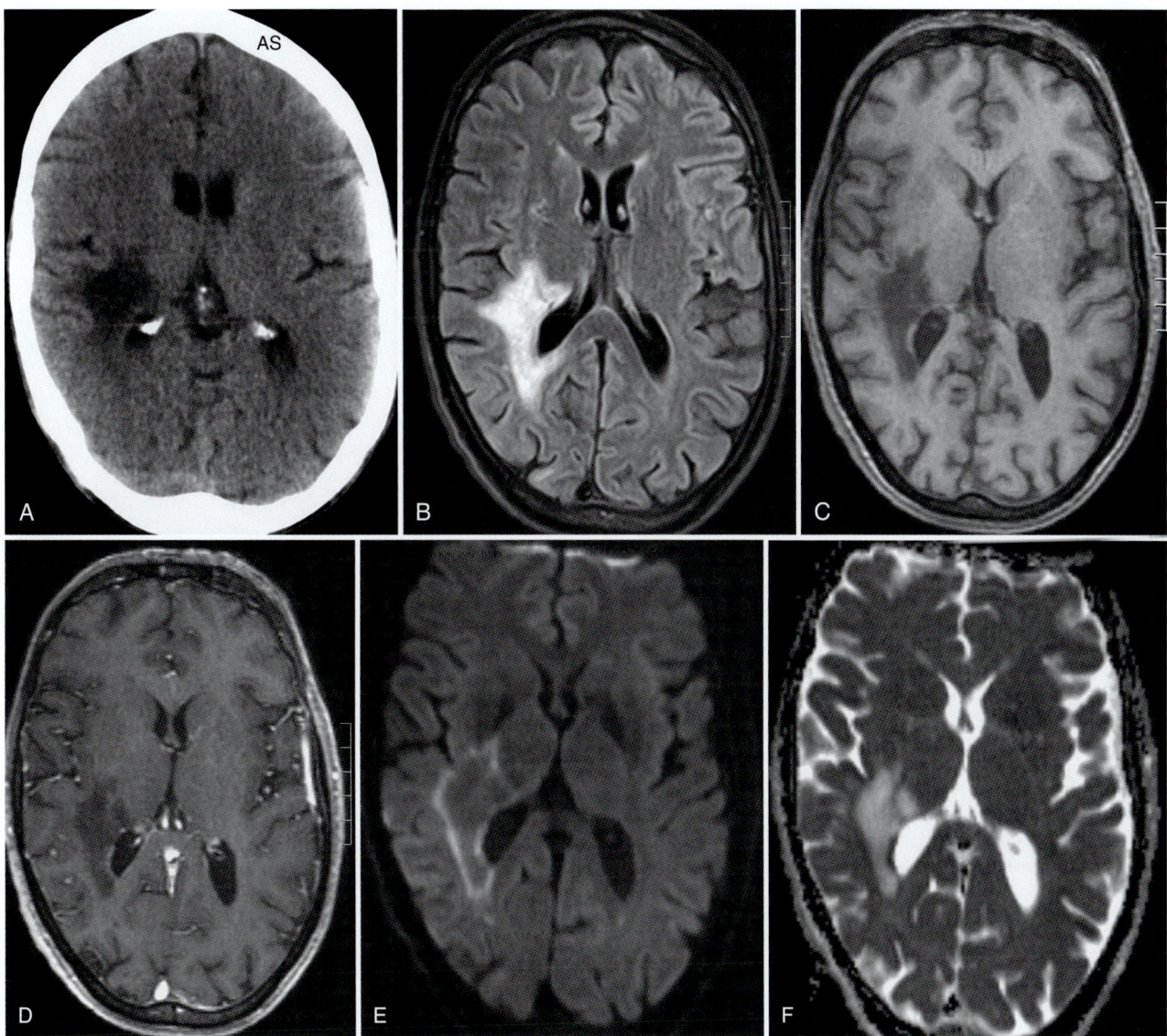

Figure 9-9 Cerebrospinal fluid–proven progressive multifocal leukoencephalopathy (PML) in a 42-year-old male HIV-positive patient. **A:** On nonenhanced computed tomographic scan of the brain, a hypodense area is observed in the right temporal region. Mass effect is not present. **B:** On fluid-attenuated inversion recovery magnetic resonance (MR) image in the axial plane, the scalloped lesion is hyperintense with no mass effect on the right occipital horn. **C, D:** Marked hypointensity is demonstrated on T1-weighted MR image **(C)** with no enhancement on postcontrast T1-weighted image **(D)**. **E, F:** On trace diffusion-weighted imaging, PML lesion has low signal with peripheral high signal outlining the lesion **(E)**. Corresponding apparent diffusion coefficient (ADC) values can be measured on the ADC map **(F)**, indicating higher diffusivity in the demyelinating part of the lesion and restricted diffusion on the border of the lesion where the advancing edge of the lesion occurs.

include demyelination with enlarged oligodendroglial nuclei and bizarre astrocytes. Patients present with any combination of weakness, speech disturbances, limb uncoordination, cognitive deficits, or visual impairment. The disease presents usually with multifocal white matter lesions that occur in any location in the white matter. On CT scans, PML lesions are recognized as patchy, scalloped, low-density lesions located in the white matter. PML lesions are patchy, scalloped, hyperintense lesions on T2-weighted MRI, located in the white matter, with finger-like extension along the white fibers (Figure 9-9). The lesions have marked low signal on T1-weighted MRI and show only rarely peripheral, faint enhancement (Figure 9-9). Subcortical fibers usually are involved, and mass effect is mild or absent. Lesions have been reported in the supratentorial and infratentorial locations. On MRS, PML lesions have significantly reduced NAA, lactate presence, and increased choline and lipids. Without treatment, the prognosis for PML usually is poor. A more benign clinical course has been reported in only a small number of patients. Recent studies have shown clinical and radiologic improvement in patients with PML who underwent potent antiretroviral therapy regimens. On DWI, PML lesions are characterized by a central core of low signal intensity (increased diffusivity) surrounded by a rim of signal hyperintensity (restricted diffusivity) (Figure 9-9). Restricted diffusion has been identified as a characteristic finding in phases of rapid progression in PML.

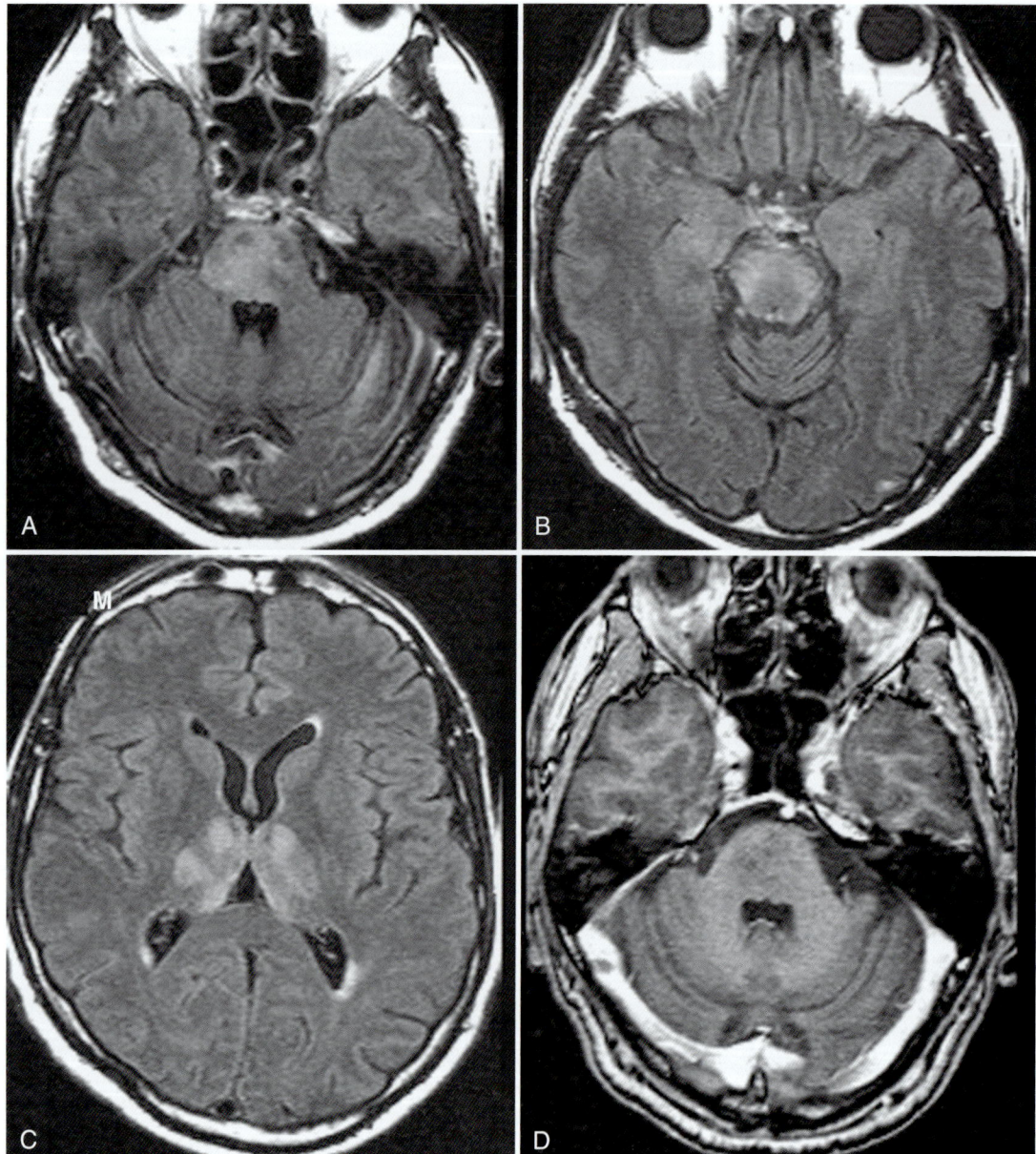

Figure 9-10 *Listeria* brainstem encephalitis in a 60-year-old patient. **A–C:** On axial fluid-attenuated inversion recovery images, high signal intensity abnormalities are seen in the pons, midbrain, and thalamus on both sides. Slightly increased intensity is noted in both hippocampal regions. Pons is not enlarged. **D:** No enhancement is observed on enhanced T1-weighted magnetic resonance image in the axial plane.

When to Suspect PML Infection of the CNS

HIV-positive patients; rarely, patients after BMT or organ transplantation

Imaging findings:
- Multifocal high signal intensity white matter lesions on T2-WI
- Involvement of subcortical arcuate fibers
- No enhancement (rarely faint peripheral enhancement)
- No mass effect
- Fast progression on follow-up images
- Enhancement after initiation of HAART (responders)
- Elevated diffusivity (low signal on DWI and high ADC), with restricted diffusivity of the lesion borders (high signal on DWI with low ADC values)

Brainstem Encephalitis (Mesenrhombencephalitis)

Mesenrhombencephalitis is a form of brainstem inflammation predominantly involving the deep and vital portions of the brain (mesencephalon and rhombencephalon). Suggestive clinical features of brainstem encephalitis are lower cranial nerve involvement, myoclonus, autonomic dysfunction, or even locked-in syndrome. The cause is rarely detected, but potentially causative agents are enteroviruses (especially EV71), flaviviruses, *Listeria*, *M. tuberculosis*, *Brucella*, and *Borrelia*. *L. monocytogenes* and HSV are two known causes of mesenrhombencephalitis that must be treated early to prevent devastating consequences. On MRI, patchy areas of T2

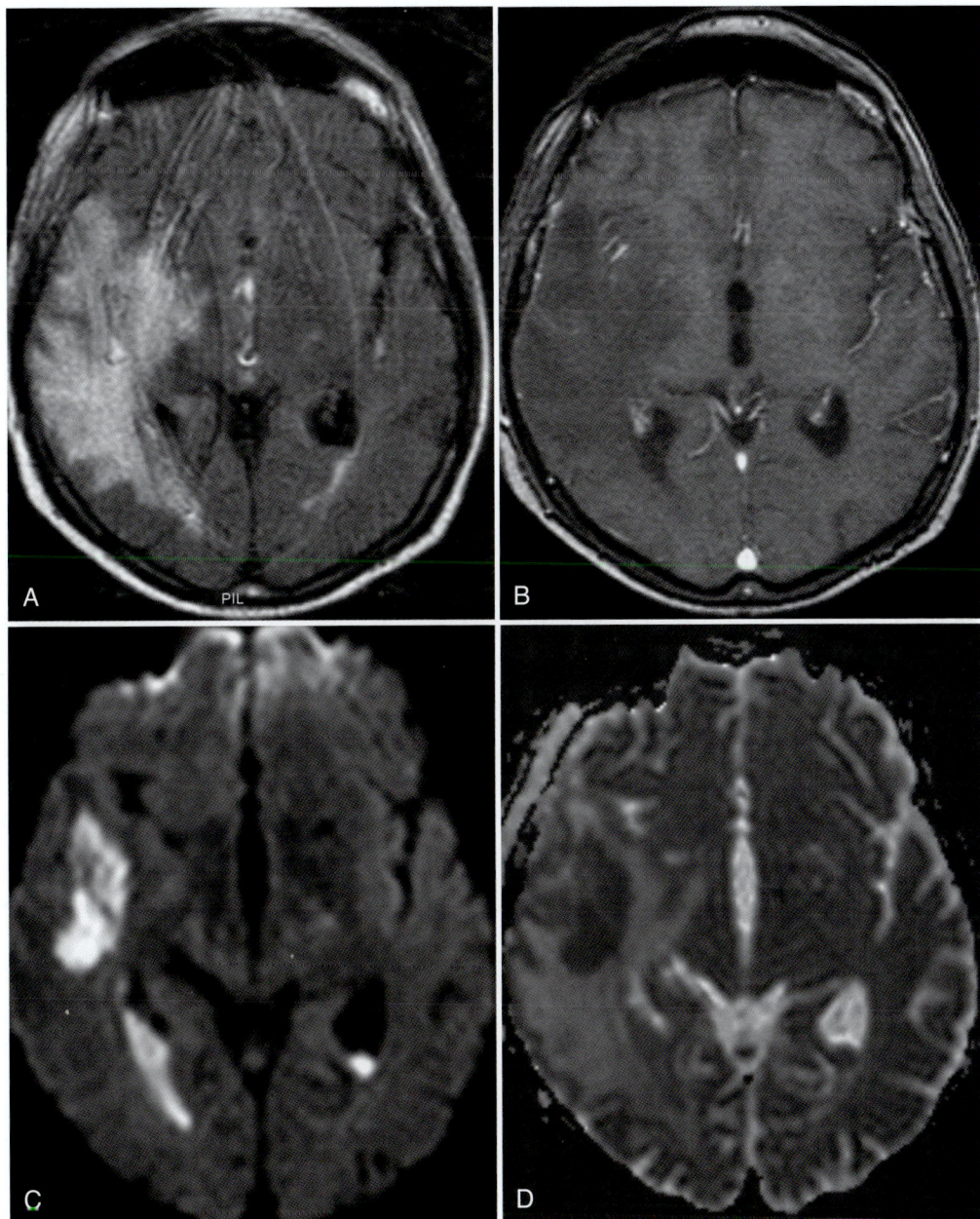

Figure 9-11 Cerebritis and pyocephalus in a 30-year-old patient. **A:** Axial fluid-attenuated inversion recovery image showing large area of high signal intensity in the right temporal lobe. **B:** No enhancement is seen on axial postcontrast T1-weighted magnetic resonance image. **C:** On diffusion-weighted imaging, marked hyperintensity was seen with additional high signal in both occipital horns. **D:** Low apparent diffusion coefficient (ADC) value on an ADC map in the temporal region suggests restricted diffusion in an area of cerebritis. Signal changes in the occipital horns suggest pyocephalus with intraventricular purulent fluid.

signal hyperintensity usually are scattered throughout the affected brainstem regions. Brainstem swelling will be present in only 30% of the cases. Contrast enhancement usually will not be present (Figure 9-10). A pattern of patchy enhancement has been described in cases of *L. monocytogenes* infections.

■ BRAIN ABSCESS

Brain abscess is a life-threatening condition. Approximately 2,500 cases are reported annually in the United States. Contiguous spread of infection from the paranasal sinuses, middle ear, or the mastoid air cells is the most common source of brain abscess. Approximately 10% of all abscesses will be seen after trauma, and in 25% of patients brain abscess is the result of hematogenous dissemination. Otogenic and dental source abscesses usually are caused by anaerobic organisms (*Streptococcus* and *Bacteroides* spp). *Staphylococcus aureus* is the most commonly identified organism after trauma. Fungal brain abscesses are most commonly caused by Aspergillus spp, which usually is detected in severely immunocompromised patients. *Toxoplasma gondii* abscesses are common in patients with AIDS.

Most brain abscesses are the result of a single organism, although 30% to 60% of infections are polymicrobial.

Pyogenic Brain Abscess

Evolution of an abscess in the brain occurs in four stages: (1) early cerebritis stage, characterized by a poorly demarcated area of brain softening with vascular congestion, petechial hemorrhage, and edema; (2) late cerebritis stage; (3) early capsule formation stage; and (4) late capsule formation stage, with a collagenous capsule. In the late cerebritis stage, low attenuation will be recognized on CT scans, with gyral enhancement. On precontrast CT images, formed abscesses may show a smooth, complete capsular ring, which enhances with contrast in a ring-like fashion. Perifocal hypodense edema is always present. On MRI, a hyperintense, ill-defined area will be seen on T2-weighted MRI, without enhancement (Figure 9-11). In the later stage, peripheral enhancement might be seen.

MRI findings of brain abscess will depend on the abscess stage. In the early cerebritis stage, a poorly demarcated area of high signal intensity will be seen on T2-weighted MRI. During the late cerebritis and abscess stages, a thin-walled hypointense ring representing a capsule will be recognized on T2-WI. A mature abscess has a well-defined ring with marked perifocal edema and mass effect delineated on postcontrast images (Figure 9-12).

Untreated pyogenic brain abscesses have a characteristic appearance on DWI, demonstrating a central hyperintensity on trace images and low ADC (Figure 9-13). Restricted diffusion in abscesses has been attributed to the high viscosity of pus due to the presence of inflammatory cells, bacteria, and macromolecules.

When to Suspect Pyogenic Brain Abscess
Young male adult
Imaging findings:
- Intracerebral (intraaxial) mass lesion with smooth ring-like enhancement
- High signal intensity center on T2-WI
- Marked perifocal edema and mass effect
- Homogenously high signal on DWI with low ADC values (restricted diffusion)
- Amino acids (succinate, pyruvate, alanine) and lipid peaks on MRS

Tuberculosis

Tuberculomas, tuberculous abscesses, and focal tuberculous cerebritis are parenchymal forms of CNS tuberculosis. In focal tuberculous cerebritis, intense gyral enhancement will be seen on postcontrast CT scans. Tuberculomas may be solitary or multiple. They can be located anywhere in the brain but predominantly in the supratentorial compartment. On CT, mature granulomas are ring-enhancing lesions. The "target sign" has also been described in CNS tuberculoma, representing central calcification or punctate enhancement surrounded by a zone of hypodensity and a rim of enhancement. However, the target sign on CT can also be seen in other infectious processes. The MRI characteristics of intracranial tuberculoma are extremely diverse. An isointense or hypointense core with a hyperintense rim on T2-weighted and FLAIR images is the most common presentation (Figure 9-14).

Three histologic types of tuberculous granulomas with corresponding radiologic findings on MRI have been described: (1) noncaseating granuloma (T1 hypointense, T2 hyperintense, nodular enhancement); (2) caseating granuloma with a solid center (T1 isointense/hypointense, T2 isointense/hypointense, rim enhancement); and (3) caseating granuloma with a liquid center (T1 hypointense, T2 hyperintense, rim enhancement).

Tuberculomas will have a nonspecific appearance on DWI, with ADC values ranging from 0.406 to 2.64×10^{-3} mm^2/s (Figure 9-14). Lesions with hyperintense centers on T2-WI are likely to have increased signal on DWI, whereas those with hypointense centers on T2-WI will have decreased signal intensity on DWI. DWI and MRS may help to determine the nature of cerebral tubercular lesions; however, they do not help in specific characterization. On MRS, lipids will be present in approximately 86% of cerebral tuberculomas. Calcification might be seen in old tuberculous abscesses.

When to Suspect Tuberculoma
Patients in endemic areas, HIV-positive patients, immunosuppressed patients
Imaging findings:
- Ring-enhancing masses with mass effect and perifocal edema
- Various signal on T2-WI (depending on stage)
- Various signal on DWI
- Lipid peak on MRS
- Additional findings that suggest tuberculous infection of the CNS (meningitis with hydrocephalus, infarcts in basal ganglia region, involvement of cranial nerves)
- Healed tuberculoma may calcify

Aspergillus Brain Abscess

Aspergillus abscesses account for 18% to 28% of all fungal brain abscesses and are the most common CNS complication occurring after BMT. Meningitis, abscess or granuloma, vascular invasion with thrombosis and infarction, and hemorrhage and aneurysm formation are manifestations of cerebral aspergillosis. Pathologically, hyphal elements invade cerebral vessels, resulting in thrombosis and infarctions. Sterile infarctions become septic when the fungus erodes the wall of the vessel, with extension into the brain parenchyma with inflammatory reactions and necrosis. The incidence of aspergillosis in patients after BMT who present with stroke is reported to be 25%.

The most common findings in cerebral aspergillosis are multiple T2-WI homogeneous hyperintense lesions smaller than 1 cm and central hypointensity with surrounding hyperintensity in lesions larger than 1 cm. On MRI, intracerebral lesions in aspergillosis usually

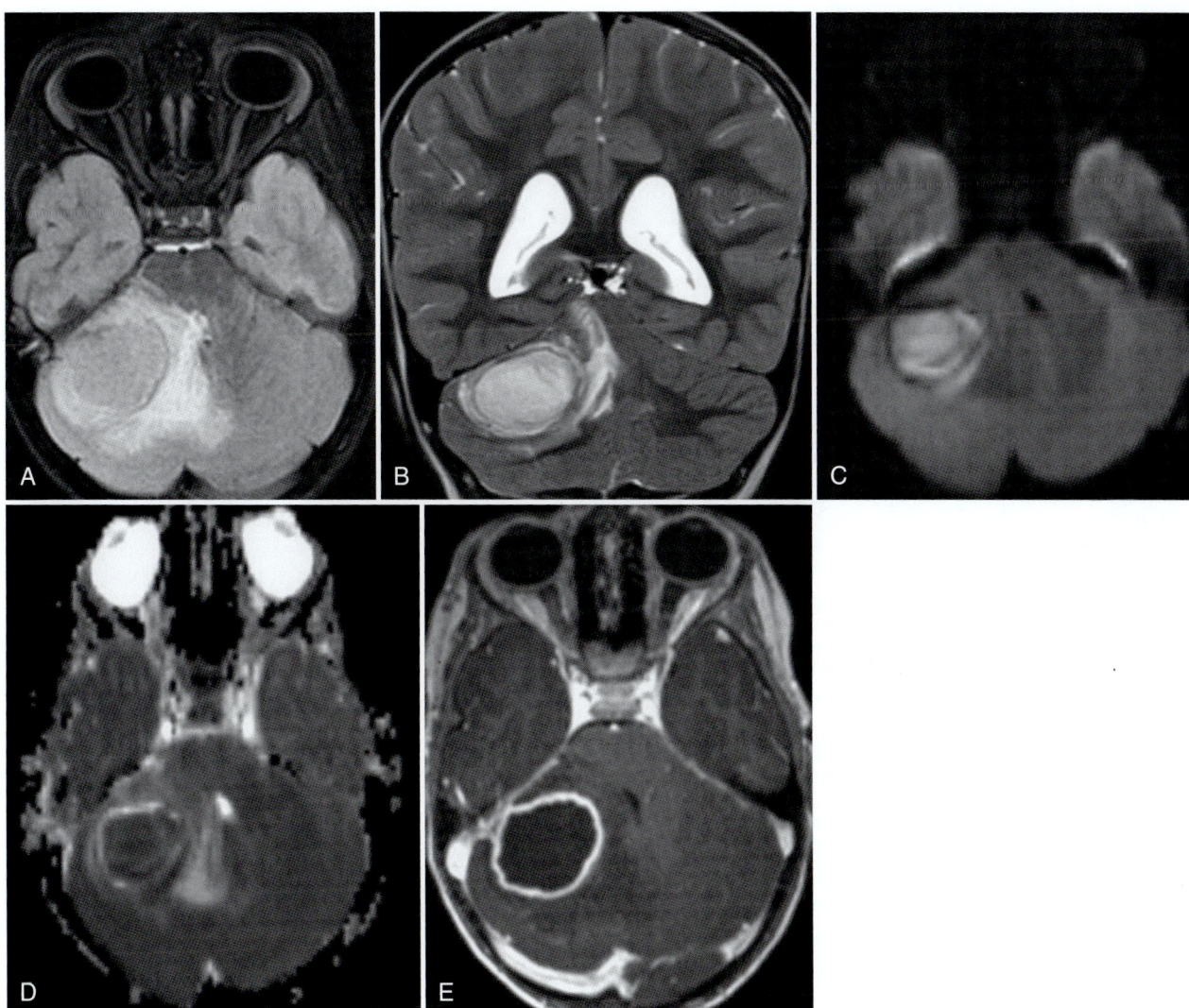

Figure 9-12 Cerebellar brain abscess in a 3-year-old child. The abscess was surgically drained, but no definite organism could be isolated. **A:** Axial fluid-attenuated inversion recovery magnetic resonance image showing intermediate signal intensity mass in the right cerebellar hemisphere, with perifocal edema and mass effect. **B:** The lesion has low signal intensity rim on coronal T2-weighted image, representing an abscess capsule. **C, D:** On trace diffusion-weighted imaging **(C)**, the abscess has high signal, with low apparent diffusion coefficient (ADC) on the ADC map **(D)**. **E:** Smooth enhancement of the abscess capsule is seen on postcontrast T1-weighted imaging.

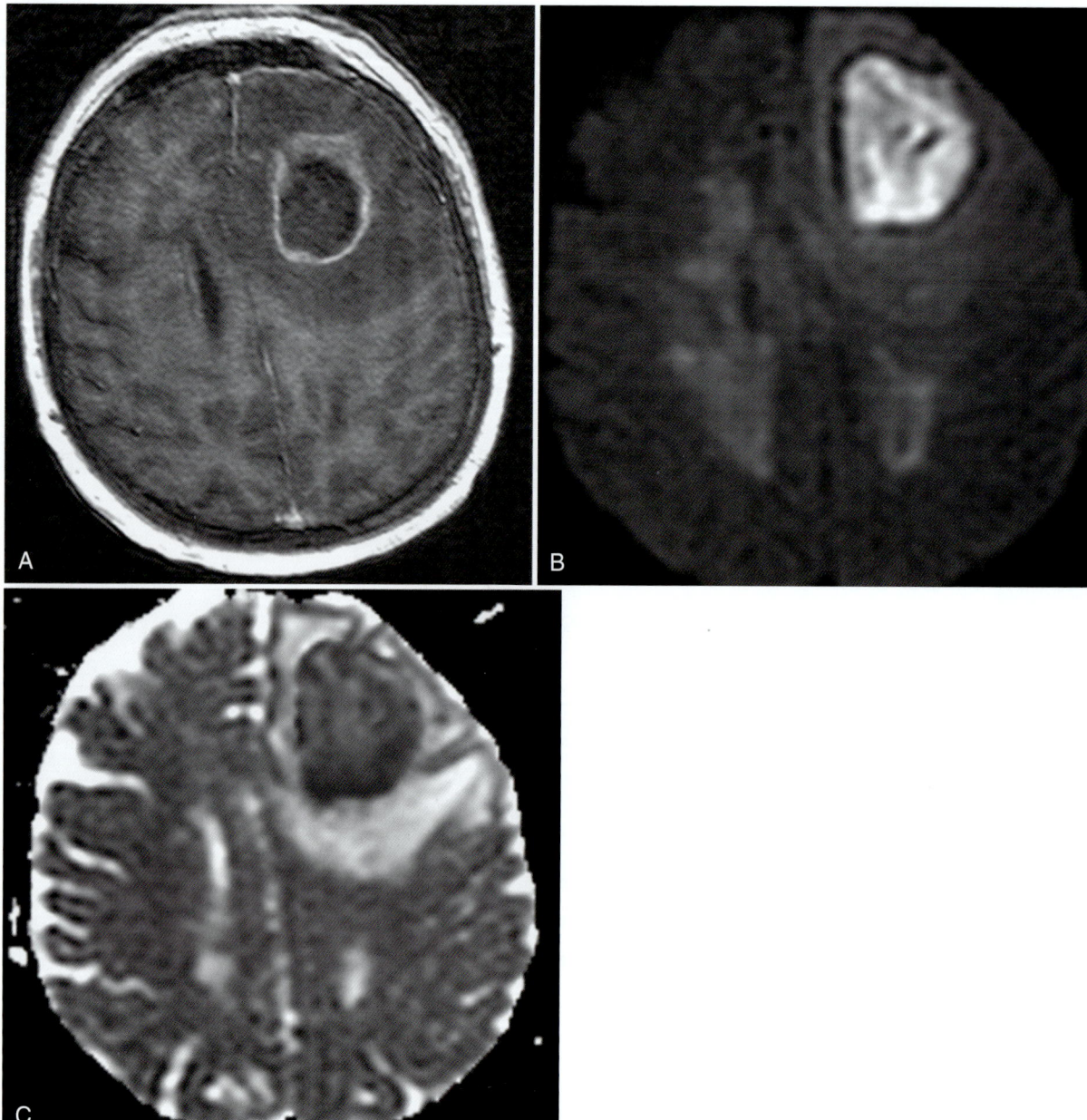

Figure 9-13 Bacterial brain abscess in the left frontal lobe of a 40-year-old female patient who had a stereotactic biopsy of a lesion 2 months before the onset of headache, hallucinations, nausea, and gait disturbances. **A:** On gadolinium-enhanced, T1-weighted axial magnetic resonance image, ring-like enhancing lesion is seen in the left frontal lobe with mass effect and surrounding edema. **B:** Abscess formation has marked high signal on trace diffusion-weighted imaging. **C:** On apparent diffusion coefficient (ADC) map, low ADC values can be measured in the abscess cavity due to restricted diffusion.

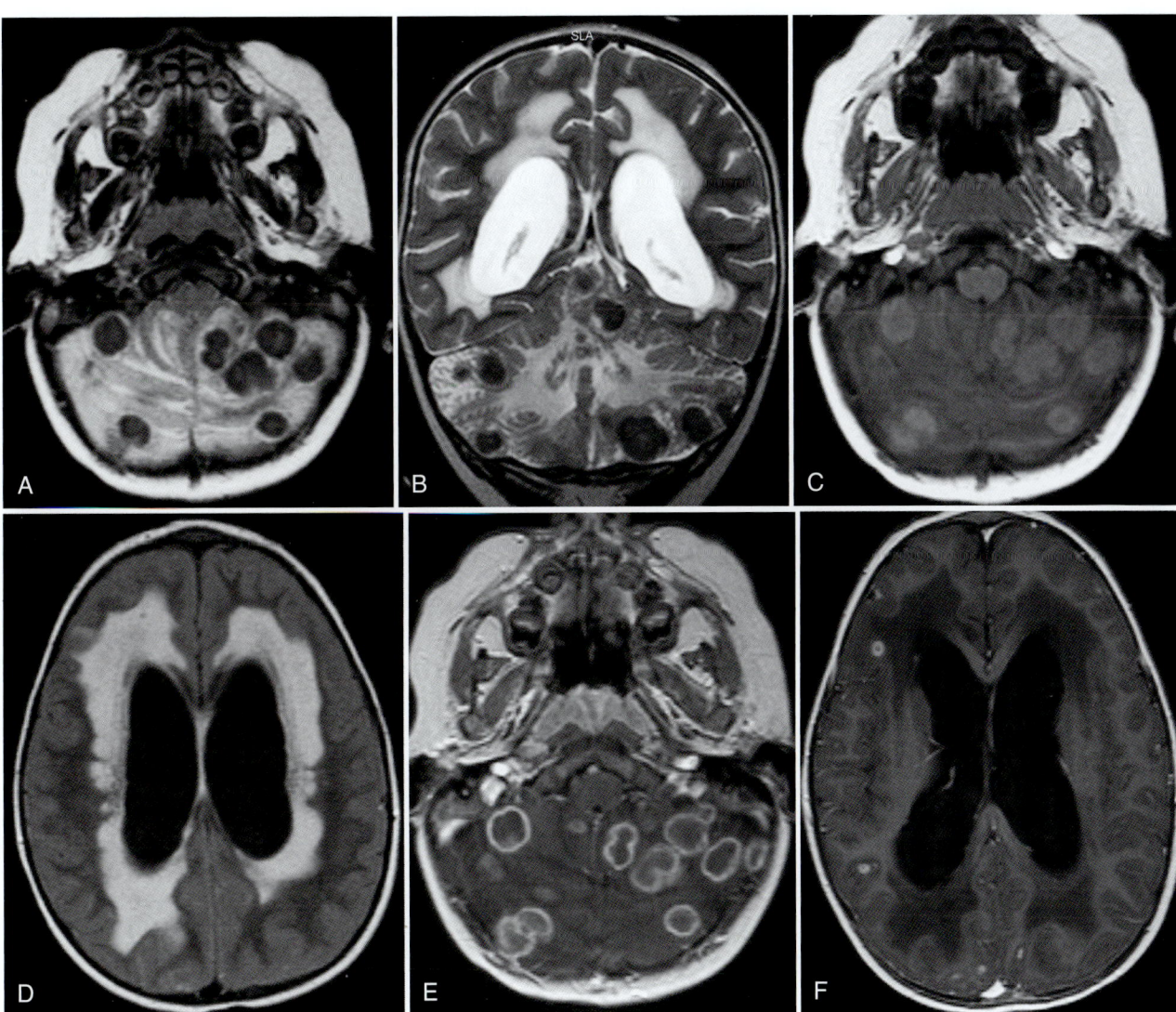

Figure 9-14 Central nervous system tuberculosis in a 5-year-old child with multiple tuberculomas and hydrocephalus. **A:** Multiple low signal intensity lesions with sharp margins are seen in the posterior fossa on axial fluid-attenuated inversion recovery image. **B:** On coronal T2-weighted image, the lesions show marked hypointensity and subsequent hydrocephalus. **C:** On axial T1-weighted image, the lesions are slightly hyperintense. **D:** Marked widening of the ventricles is present due to obstruction of the fourth ventricle. **E:** Ring-enhancing lesions demonstrated on gadolinium-enhanced T1-weighted image represent multiple tuberculomas. **F:** Smaller ring-enhancing tuberculomas are present in the frontal and occipital lobes.

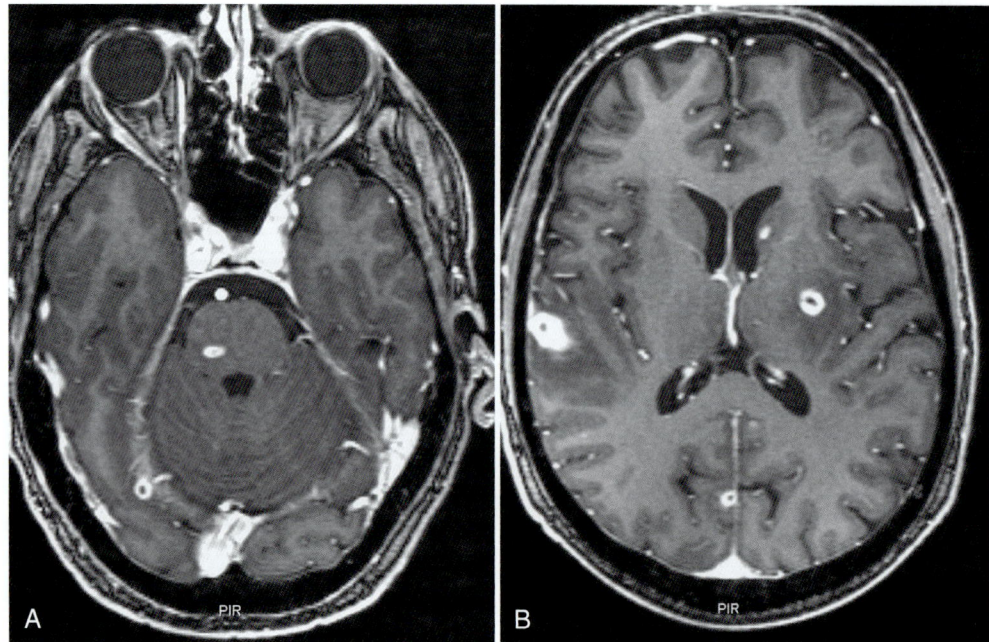

Figure 9-15 Proven cerebral aspergillosis in a patient with acute myelocytic leukemia (**A, B**). Multiple ring-like or nodular enhancing lesions are seen on postcontrast T1-weighted magnetic resonance images.

have low signal centrally or peripherally on T2-WI, probably due to accumulation of fungi containing iron, magnesium, and manganese, as well as blood breakdown products (Figure 9-15). However, low signal on T2-WI is not specific for aspergillosis; it may be seen in various infections (tuberculoma) as well as in neoplastic brain lesions. Contrast enhancement usually is missing and is seen only in patients with relatively preserved immune status. On DWI, aspergillus abscesses might be bright with low ADC values, indicating restricted diffusivity, and are indistinguishable from bacterial abscesses (Figure 9-16). ADC values measured in bacterial abscesses usually are lower than those measured in fungal lesions. This may be due to the lower cell density in fungal abscesses and, to a lesser extent, to the presence of hemorrhage. Some have low signal with high ADC values and can mimic necrotic neoplasms.

Fungal abscesses may also present as microabscesses, which are seen more frequently in candida infection (Figure 9-17).

When to Suspect Aspergillus Brain Abscess
Patients after BMT or organ transplantation, HIV-positive patients
Imaging findings:
    Ring-enhancing masses with mass effect and perifocal edema in an immunocompetent patient
    Nonenhancing lesions in an immunocompromised patient
    High signal on T1-WI or low signal on susceptibility-weighted imaging, indicating hemorrhage
    Cortical location
    Low signal on T2-weighted MRI
    High or intermediate signal on DWI

Cryptococcoma
Cryptococcomas usually are seen in immunocompromised individuals (Figure 9-18). However, isolated cryptococcomas of the CNS have also been described in immunocompetent adults, as occurs in the presence of underlying sarcoidosis. Imaging characteristics of cryptococcomas can overlap with those of tumors and abscesses of other origin. Cryptococcomas are hypodense on CT with high signal on T2-WI and low signal on T1-weighted MRI. On enhanced images, the lesions usually demonstrate a ring-like or nodular enhancement and cannot be distinguished from granulomas of other origin. They occur most commonly in the cerebellum, brainstem, basal ganglia, and temporoparietal regions. Hypointensity on diffusion-weighted MRI scans, with elevated ADC, has been reported in one case.

When to Suspect Cryptococcoma
HIV-positive patients, patients with sarcoidosis
Imaging findings:
    Ring-enhancing masses with mass effect and perifocal edema
    Low signal on DWI (high ADC values)
    In combination with gelatinous pseudocysts or dilated Virchow-Robin spaces

Toxoplasmosis
Cerebral toxoplasmosis results from infection by the intracellular protozoan *T. gondii*. After acute infection, the latent form, called *encysted bradyzoites*, remains in the tissues until a decline in immunity. Rupture of the cysts releases the free tachyzoite, which causes acute illness. In AIDS patients, *Toxoplasma* causes

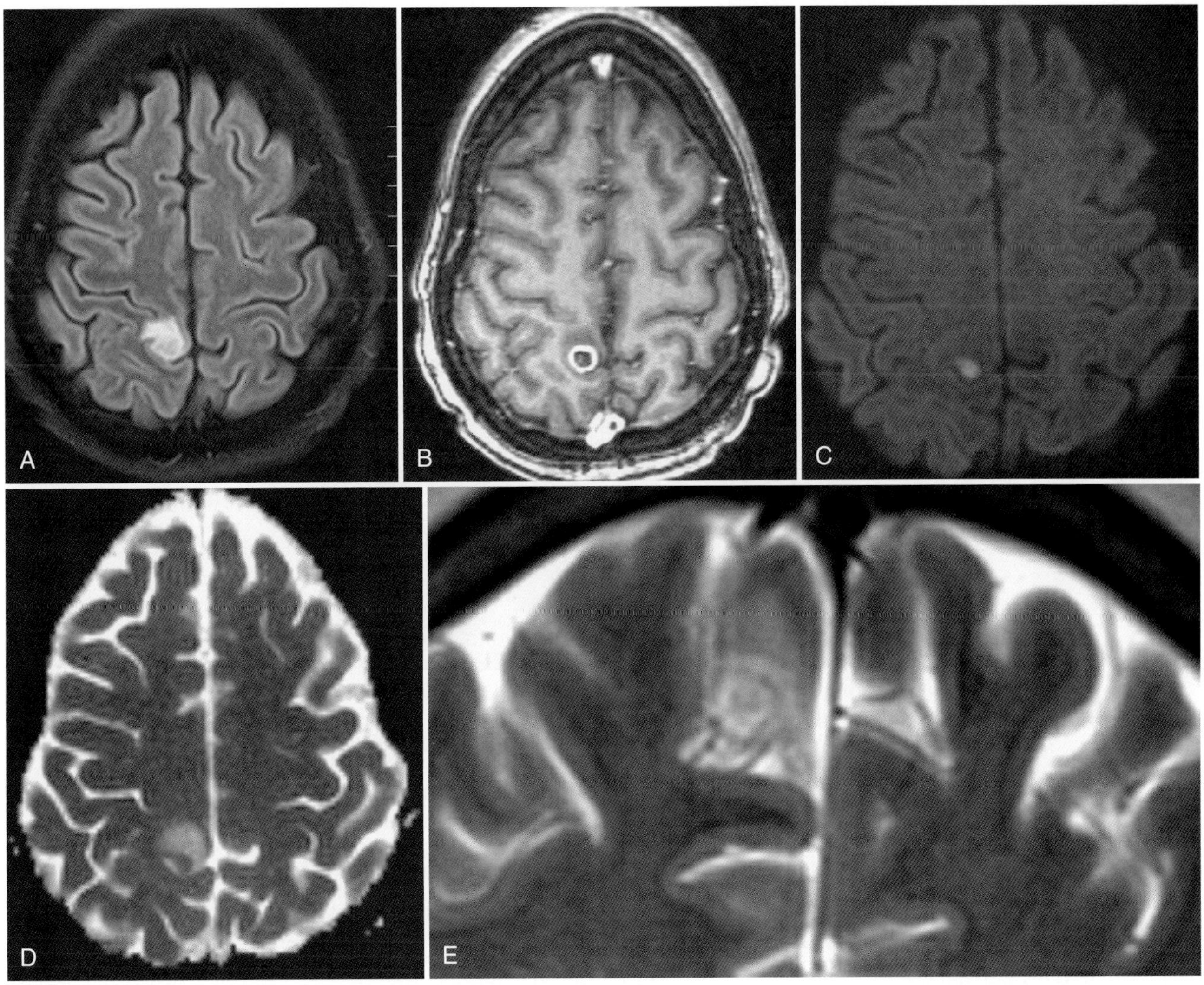

Figure 9-16 Cerebral aspergillosis in 16-year-old girl with acute lymphoblastic leukemia (ALL) who suffered from invasive aspergillosis, with aspergillus granuloma in the lung and liver. **A:** On axial fluid-attenuated inversion recovery magnetic resonance (MR) image, hyperintense cortical lesion is detected in the right parietal region. **B:** The lesion has a ring-like appearance on postcontrast MR images. **C, D:** On trace diffusion-weighted imaging **(C)**, a high signal is seen, with a low apparent diffusion coefficient value **(D)**, indicating restricted diffusivity. **E:** On coronal T2-weighted MR image, a low signal intensity centrally is observed and may be due to iron, magnesium, manganese, or blood products found in the aspergillus fungus.

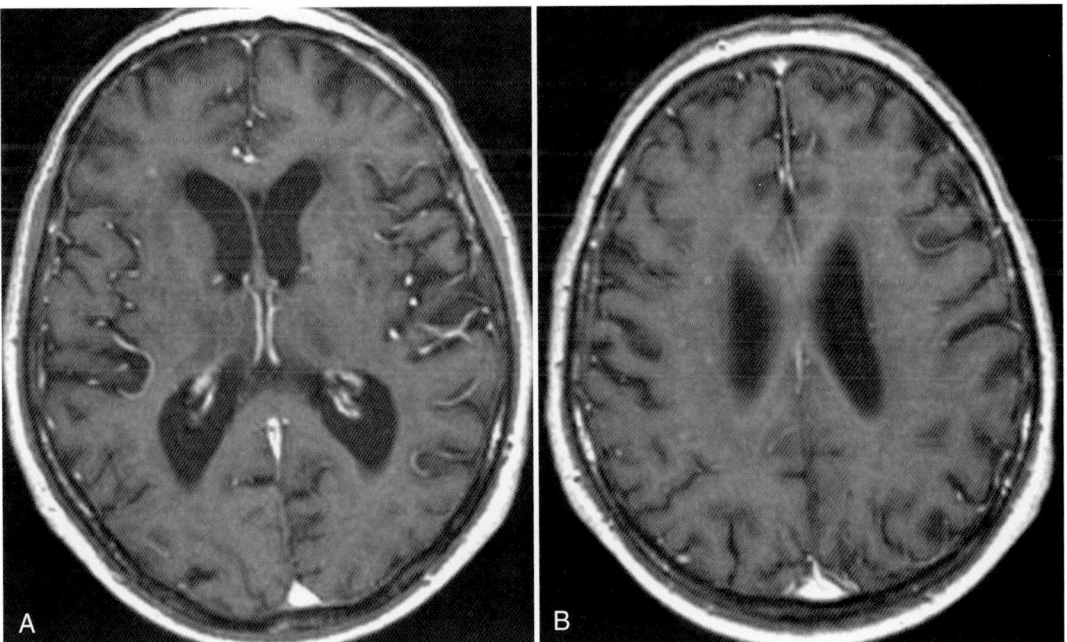

Figure 9-17 Candida brain abscesses in an immunocompromised patient **(A, B)**. Postcontrast T1-weighted magnetic resonance images in the axial plane showing multiple small abscesses (microabscesses) in the white matter of the frontal lobe.

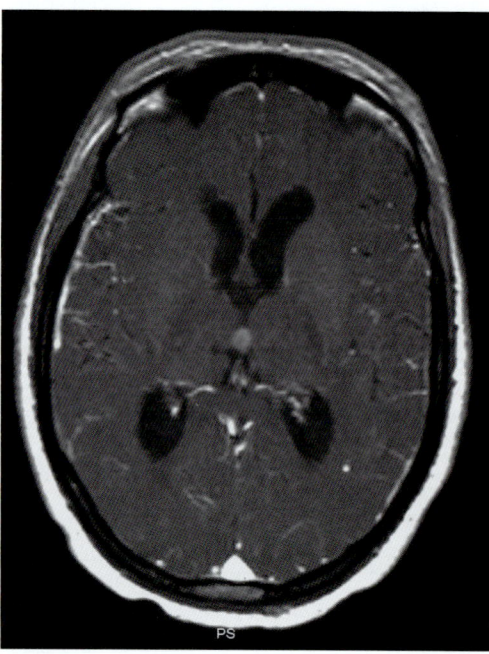

Figure 9-18 Cerebral cryptococcosis in a patient with acquired immunodeficiency syndrome. Axial enhanced T1-weighted magnetization transfer contrast magnetic resonance image showing nodular enhancing lesion (cryptococcoma) in the region of the third ventricle, with slightly enlarged ventricular system.

necrotizing encephalitis. Lesions characteristic of toxoplasma-induced necrotizing encephalitis have three well-defined zones: avascular; necrotic center, with an intermediate zone with intense inflammatory reaction; and peripheral zone with the encyst form of *Toxoplasma*. On nonenhanced CT scans, *Toxoplasma* lesions are hypodense, with edema and mass effect. Solid, nodular, or ring-enhancing lesions typically are observed on postcontrast studies. The most common locations are the basal ganglia and the corticomedullary junction. On T1-weighted MRI, *Toxoplasma* lesions have isointense to low signal centrally. Signal intensity on T2-WI depends on the stage of the lesion, which could be isointense, hypointense, or hyperintense (Figure 9-19). Enhanced T1-WI reveals ring or nodular enhancement. Approximately 10 days after initiation of therapy, a decrease in the number and size of the lesions, with a reduction in edema and mass effect, should be observed on follow-up MR examinations. Calcifications are often seen in healed foci. Toxoplasmosis shows a wide spectrum of diffusion characteristics, with ADC ratios ranging from 0.8 to 2.8, which have significant overlap with those of lymphoma (Figure 9-19). The MRS pattern of *Toxoplasma* lesions is nonspecific, consistent with anaerobic inflammation within the abscess (Figure 9-19). Based on conventional MRI, cerebral toxoplasmosis cannot be distinguished from primary cerebral lymphoma. Use of thallium-201 (^{201}Tl) brain single-photo emission computed tomography (SPECT) in AIDS patients has proved to be helpful in distinguishing toxoplasmosis from lymphoma. A positive ^{201}Tl brain SPECT is suggestive of CNS lymphoma, and negative uptake suggests infection (toxoplasmosis) in AIDS patients. The potential use of ^{18}F-fluorodeoxyglucose (FDG) positron emission tomography (PET) in differentiating lymphoma from toxoplasmosis in AIDS patients also has been examined. The results of the studies have shown that FDG-PET can accurately differentiate lymphoma from infections. The standardized uptake values over cerebral lesions were much higher in lymphomas than in *Toxoplasma* lesions.

When to Suspect CNS Toxoplasmosis

HIV-positive patients; patients after BMT or organ transplantation
Imaging findings:
  Single/multiple ring-enhancing lesions
  Mass effect and marked perifocal edema
  Low signal or isotensity on T1-weighted MRI
  No specific pattern on T2-weighted MRI (low/isointense/high)
  Hemorrhagic after antitoxoplasma therapy
  Nonenhancing or primarily hemorrhagic lesions in patient after BMT
  Varied appearance on DWI and ADC map

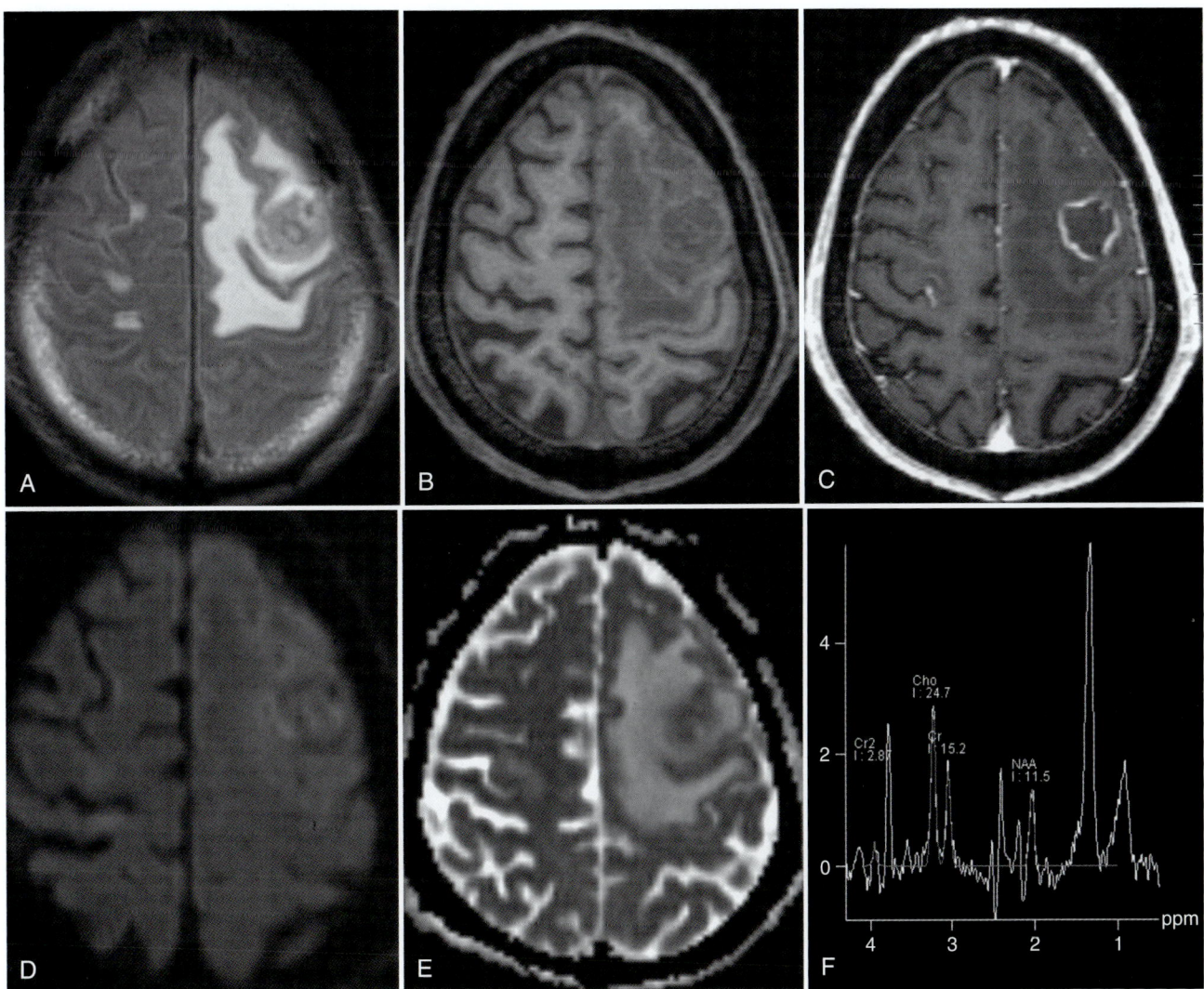

Figure 9-19 Central nervous system toxoplasmosis in a patient with acquired immunodeficiency syndrome. **A:** On axial fluid-attenuated inversion recovery image, cortically located lesion in the left frontal lobe is seen. The lesion has a multilayer (target-like) appearance and marked perifocal edema. Note small subcortical signal abnormalities in the right frontal lobe. **B:** On T1-weighted magnetic resonance (MR) image, the lesions and surrounding edema have low signal. **C:** On postcontrast T1-weighted MR image, peripheral ring-like enhancement is seen. **D, E:** Inhomogeneous signal is observed on trace diffusion-weighted imaging and apparent diffusion coefficient map. **F:** ^{1}H-Magnetic resonance spectroscopy shows low N-acetylaspartate peak, increased choline peak, and large lipid peak.

Suggested Readings

Arnder L, Castillo M, Heinz ER, et al. Unusual pattern of enhancement in cryptococcal meningitis: in vivo findings with postmortem correlation. *J Comput Assist Tomogr.* 1996;20(6):1023-1026.

Batra A, Tripathi RP. Diffusion-weighted magnetic resonance imaging and magnetic resonance spectroscopy in the evaluation of focal cerebral tubercular lesions. *Acta Radiol.* 2004;45:679-688.

Bencherif B, Rottenberg DA. Neuroimaging of the AIDS dementia complex. *AIDS.* 1998;12:233-244.

Bergui M, Bradac GB, Oguz KK, et al. Progressive multifocal leukoencephalopathy: diffusion-weighted imaging and pathological correlations. *Neuroradiology.* 2004;46:22-25.

Bemaerts A, Vanhoenacker FM, Parizel PM, et al. Tuberculosis of the central nervous system: overview of neuroradiological findings. *Eur Radiol.* 2003;13:1876-1890.

Budka H, Constanzi G, Cristina S, et al. Brain pathology induced by infection with the human immunodeficiency virus (HIV). *Acta Neuropathol.* 1987;75:185-198.

Camacho DL, Smith JK, Castillo M. Differentiation of toxoplasmosis and lymphoma in AIDS patients by using apparent diffusion coefficients. *AJNR Am J Neuroradiol.* 2003;24(4):633-637.

Castillo M. Magnetic resonance imaging of meningitis and its complications. *Top Magn Reson Imaging.* 1994;6:53-58.

Chang KH, Han MH, Roh JK, Kim IO, Han MC, Kim C. Gd-DTPA-Enhanced MR imaging of the brain in patients with meningitis: comparison with CT. *AJNR Am J Neuroradiol.* 1990;11:69-76.

Charlot M, Pialat JB, Obadia N, et al. Diffusion-weighted imaging in brain aspergillosis. *Eur J Neurol.* 2007;14:912-916.

Coplin WM, Cochran MS, Levine SR, Crawford SW. Stroke after bone marrow transplantation. *Brain.* 2001;124:1043-1051.

Cosottini M, Tavarelli C, Del Bono L, et al. Diffusion-weighted imaging in patients with progressive multifocal leukoencephalopathy. *Eur Radiol.* 2008;18(5):1024-1030.

Cox J, Murtagh FR, Wilfong A, et al. Cerebral aspergillosis: MR imaging and histopathologic correlation. *AJNR Am J Neuroradiol.* 1992;13:1489-1492.

Demaerel P, Wilms G, Robberecht W, Johannik K, Van Hecke P, Carton H, Baert AL. MRI of herpes simplex encephalitis. *Neuroradiology.* 1992;34(6):490-493.

Dietrich U, Hettmann M, Maschke M, et al. Cerebral aspergillosis: comparison of radiological and neuropathologic findings in patients with bone marrow transplantation. *Eur Radiol.* 2001;11:1242-1249.

Fetter BF, Kintworth GK, Hendy WS. *Mycoses of the central nervous system.* Baltimore: Williams & Wilkins; 1967, pp 87-123.

Fitch MT, Abrahamian FM, Moran GJ, Talan DA. Emergency department management of meningitis and encephalitis. *Infect Dis Clin N Am.* 2008;22:33-52.

Fukui M, Williams RL, Mudigonda S. CT and MR imaging features of pyogenic ventriculitis. *AJNR Am J Neuroradiol.* 2001;22:1510-1516.

Gologorsky Y, DeLaMora P, Souweidane MM, Greenfield JP. Cerebellar cryptococcoma in an immunocompetent child. Case report. *J Neurosurg.* 2007;107:314-317.

Guerini H, Helie O, Leveque C, Adem C, Hauret L, Cordoliani YS. Diagnosis of periventricular ependymal enhancement in MRI in adults. *J Neuroradiol.* 2003;30:46-56.

Hall WA, Truwit CL. The surgical management of infections involving the cerebrum. *Neurosurgery.* 2008;62:519-531.

Hassine D, Gray F, Chekroun R, et al. Encéphalitides a CMV et VZV au cours du SIDA. *J Neuroradiol.* 1995;22:184-192.

Herweh C, Jayachandra MR, Hartmann M, et al. Quantitative diffusion tensor imaging in herpes simplex virus encephalitis. *J Neurovirol.* 2007;13:426-432.

Ho TL, Lee HJ, Lee KW, Chen WL. Diffusion-weighted and conventional magnetic resonance imaging in cerebral cryptococcoma. *Acta Radiol.* 2005;46(4):411-414.

Iranzo A, Moreno A, Pujol J, et al. Proton magnetic resonance spectroscopy pattern of progressive multifocal leukoencephalopathy in AIDS. *J Neurol Neurosurg Psychiatry.* 1999;66:520-523.

Jayasundar R, Singh VP, Raghunathan P, Jain K, Banerji AK. Inflammatory granulomas: evaluation with proton MRS. *NMR Biomed.* 1999;12(3):139-144.

Kanaly CW, Selznick LA, Cummings TJ, Adamson DC. Cerebellar cryptococcoma in a patient with undiagnosed sarcoid: case report. *Neurosurgery.* 2007;60:E571.

Miaux Y, Ribaud P, Williams M, et al. MR of cerebral aspergillosis in patients who have had bone marrow transplantation. *AJNR Am J Neuroradiol.* 1995;16:555-562.

Mishra AM, Gupta RK, Saksena S, et al. Biological correlates of diffusivity in brain abscess. *Magn Reson Med.* 2005;54:878-885.

Morgello S, Cho E, Nielsen S, et al. Cytomegalovirus encephalitis in patients with acquired immunodeficiency syndrome: an autopsy study of 30 cases and a review of the literature. *Hum Pathol.* 1987;18:289-297.

Mueller-Mang C, Castillo M, Mang TG, Cartes-Zumelzu F, Weber M, Thurnher MM. Fungal versus bacterial brain abscesses: is diffusion-weighted MR imaging a useful tool in the differential diagnosis? *Neuroradiology.* 2007;49(8):651-657.

Nelson Jr RP. Bacterial meningitis and inflammation. *Curr Opin Neurol.* 2006;19:369-373.

O´Doherty MJ, Barrington SF, Campbell M, et al. PET scanning and the human immunodeficiency virus-positive patients. *J Nucl Med.* 1997;38:1575-1583.

Olsen WL, Longo FM, Mills CM, et al. White matter disease in AIDS: findings at MR imaging. *Radiology.* 1988;169:445-448.

Ruiz A, Post MJD, Bundschu CC. Dentate nuclei involvement in AIDS patients with CNS cryptococcosis: imaging findings with pathologic correlation. *J Comput Assist Tomogr.* 1997;21:175-182.

Schroeder PC, Post MJ, Oschatz E, Stadler A, Bruce-Gregorios J, Thurnher MM. Analysis of the utility of diffusion-weighted MRI and apparent diffusion coefficient values in distinguishing central nervous system toxoplasmosis from lymphoma. *Neuroradiology.* 2006;48(10):715-720.

Shukla R, Abbas A, Kumar P, Gupta RK, Jha S, Prasad KN. Evaluation of cerebral infarction in tuberculous meningitis by diffusion weighted imaging. *J Infect.* 2008;57(4):298-306.

Singer MB, Atlas SW, Drayer BP. Subarachnoid Space Disease: Diagnosis with fluid-attenuated inversion recovery MR Imaging and comparison with gadolinium-enhanced spin-echo MR imaging-blinded reader study. *Neuroradiology.* 1998;208:417-422.

Solomon T, Whitley RJ. Arthropod-borne viral encephalitides. In: Scheld M, Whitley RJ, Marra C, eds. *Infections of the central nervous system.* 2nd ed. Philadelphia, PA: Lippincott Williams and Wilkins; 2004.

Solomon T, Hart IJ, Beeching NJ. Viral encephalitis: a clinician´s guide. *Pract Neurol.* 2007;7:288-305.

Soo MS, Tien RD, Gray L, Andrews PI, Friedman H. Mesenrhombencephalitis: MR findings in nine patients. *AJR Am J Radiol.* 1993;160:1089-1093.

Teofilo E, Gouveia J, Brotas V, et al. Progressive multifocal leukoencephalopathy regression with highly active antiretroviral therapy. *AIDS.* 1998;12:449.

Thurnher MM, Thurnher SA, Mühlbauer B, et al. Progressive multifocal leukoencephalopathy in AIDS: initial and follow-up CT and MRI. *Neuroradiology.* 1997;39:611-618.

Thurnher M, Schindler EG, Thurnher SA, Pernerstorfer-Schön H, Kleibl-Popov C, Rieger A. Effect of highly active antiretroviral therapy (HAART) on MR imaging findings and clinical course in AIDS dementia complex. *AJNR Am J Neuroradiol.* 2000;21:670-678.

Tien RD, Chu PK, Hesselink JR, Duberg A, Wiley C. Intracranial cryptococcosis in immunocompromised patients: CT and MR findings in 29 cases. *AJNR Am J Neuroradiol.* 1991;12:283-289.

Tsai Y, Chang W, Shen C, et al. Intracranial suppuration: A clinical comparison of subdural empyemas and epidural abscesses. *Surg Neurol.* 2003;59:191-196.

Tsuchiya K, Inaoka S, Mizutani Y, Hachiya J. Fast fluid-attenuated inversion-recovery MR of intracranial infections. *AJNR Am J Neuroradiol.* 1997;18:909-913.

Tsuchiya K, Osawa A, Katase S, Fujikawa A, Hachiya J, Aoki S. Diffusion-weighted MRI of subdural and epidural empyemas. *Neuroradiology.* 2003;45:220-223.

van de Beek D, de Gans J, Spanjaard L, et al. Clinical features and prognostic factors in adults with bacterial meningitis. *N Engl J Med.* 2004;351:1849-1859.

Van Rensburg PJ, Andronikou S, van Toorn R, Pienaar M. Magnetic resonance imaging of miliary tuberculosis of the central nervous system in children with tuberculous meningitis. *Pediatr Radiol.* 2008;38:1306-1313.

Villringer K, Jager H, Dichgans M, et al. Differential diagnosis of CNS lesions in AIDS patients by FDG-PET. *J Comput Assist Tomogr.* 1995;19:532-536.

Von Einsiedel RW, Fife TD, Aksamit AJ, et al. Progressive multifocal leukoencephalopathy in AIDS: a clinicopathologic study and review of the literature. *J Neurol.* 1993;240:391-406.

Von Giesen HJ, Wittsack HJ, Wenserski F, et al. Basal ganglia metabolite abnormalities in minor motor disorders associated with human immunodeficiency virus type 1. *Arch Neurol.* 2001;58:1281-1286.

Wasay M, Kheleani BA, Moolani MK, et al. Brain CT and MRI findings in 100 consecutive patients with intracranial tuberculoma. *J Neuroimaging.* 2003;13(3):240-247.

Weingarten K, Zimmerman RD, Becker RD, Heier LA, Haimes AB, Deck MD. Subdural and epidural empyemas: MR imaging. *AJR Am J Radiol.* 1989;152:615-621.

Whiteman ML, Post MJ, Berger JR, Tate LG, Bell MD, Limonte LP. Progressive multifocal leukoencephalopathy in 47 HIV-seropositive patients: neuroimaging with clinical and pathologic correlation. *Radiology.* 1993;187:233-240.

Yamada K, Zoarski GH, Rothman MI, et al. An intracranial aspergilloma with low signal on T2-weighted images corresponding to iron accumulation. *Neuroradiology.* 2000;43:559-561.

Yuh WTC, Nguyen HD, Gao F, et al. Brain parenchymal infection in bone marrow transplantation patients. CT and MR findings. *AJR Am J Radiol.* 1994;162:425-430.

CHAPTER 10
Metabolic Disorders
Robert J. Young, Sofia S. Haque, and John K. Lyo

■ INTRODUCTION

Metabolic diseases of the brain represent a diverse group of diseases caused by inherited (inborn) and acquired (radiation, toxic) errors in metabolism. Many metabolic diseases consist of otherwise heterogeneous groups of disorders with varied pathophysiologies that interrupt critical metabolic pathways in different ways but with the common end result of abnormal accumulation or insufficient production of a critical brain compound.

Imaging of metabolic disorders often has high sensitivity but poor specificity. The end stage of most metabolic diseases is diffuse atrophy, enlarged ventricles, and abnormal white matter. This is true for both the leukodystrophies, which primarily involve the white matter, and the poliodystrophies, which primarily involve the gray matter. The greatest potential for differential accuracy and a positive impact on patient therapy lies in early imaging of these diseases, when distinctive patterns may be identified. Despite frequent limitations in establishing a definite diagnosis, imaging has a critical role in the triage, diagnosis, prognosis, and management of these patients. The diseases may be grouped according to the common biochemical defect (Table 10-1).

Although this categorization is accurate, it is impractical from an imaging approach due to the high variability and overlapping abnormalities of many diseases. In order to provide a practical radiographic framework from which a reasonable differential diagnosis may be formed, this chapter organizes the metabolic disorders into groups based on the most distinctive radiologic abnormality: white matter disease, cortical gray matter disease, and deep gray matter disease. These are followed by a discussion of magnetic resonance (MR) diffusion and MR spectroscopy. When a disorder displays multiple manifestations and may fall into more than one category, the disorder may be mentioned in different sections with the emphasis on the most characteristic imaging feature(s). As with the rest of this book, the purpose of this chapter is not to provide an extensive review but rather to suggest a systemic approach for radiologic interpretation. The classic or most common manifestations are discussed with the focus on the inherited metabolic disorders; the acquired metabolic and toxic metabolic disorders are briefly presented for comparison purposes.

■ PART I: WHITE MATTER DISEASE

Bilaterally symmetric white matter signal abnormalities suggest hereditary leukoencephalopathy, the primary white matter diseases. On imaging, white matter disease typically is seen as hypodense lesions on computed tomographic (CT) scan and as T1 hypointense and T2 hyperintense lesions on magnetic resonance imaging (MRI). These abnormalities may be symmetric or

Table 10-1 Inherited Metabolic Disorders

Mitochondrial disorders	• Mitochondrial myopathy, encephalopathy, lactic acidosis, and stroke-like episodes (MELAS) • Myoclonic epilepsy with ragged red fibers (MERRF) • Subacute necrotizing encephalomyelopathy (Leigh) • Kearns-Sayre syndrome (KSS) • Trichopoliodystrophy (Menkes syndrome) • Progressive cerebral poliodystrophy (Alpers syndrome) • Neurogenic weakness, ataxia, and retinitis pigmentosa (NARP) • Hearing loss, ataxia, myoclonus (HLAM) • Leber hereditary optic neuropathy (LHON) • Mitochondrial myopathy, neuropathy, and gastrointestinal encephalomyopathy (MNGIE)
Lysosomal storage disorders	• Mucopolysaccharidosis • GM_2 gangliosidosis • Metachromatic leukodystrophy (MLD) • Globoid cell leukodystrophy (Krabbe disease)
Peroxisomal disorders	• Zellweger disease • Adrenoleukodystrophy/adrenomyeloneuropathy
Organic acidemias and amino acidurias	• Glutaric acidemia • Proprionic acidemia • Canavan disease (spongiform degeneration of the brain, von Bogaert-Bertrand disease) • Maple syrup urine disease (MSUD) • Urea cycle disorders (UCD) • Methylmalonic acidemia (MMA) • Alexander disease • Phenylketonuria (PKU)
Other	• van der Knaap leukoencephalopathy • Neurodegeneration with brain iron accumulation (NBIA)/Hallervorden-Spatz syndrome (HSS) • Huntington disease • Wilson disease • Pelizaeus-Merzbacher disease

Table 10-2 Leukodystrophies Categorized by White Matter Abnormality

Hypomyelination
Dysmyelination
Delayed myelination
	• Pelizaeus-Merzbacher disease (PMD)
	• Mitochondrial disorders
	• Amino acidurias
	   Phenylketonuria (PKU)
	   Maple syrup urine disease (MSUD)
	   Methylmalonic acidemia (MMA)
	   Nonketotic hyperglycinemia (NKH)
	   Hydroxymethylglutaryl-coenzyme A (HMG-CoA) lyase deficiency
	• Organic acidopathies
	   Glutaric acidemia
	   Proprionic acidemia

Demyelination
Primary
Secondary
	• Globoid cell leukodystrophy (Krabbe disease)
	• Metachromatic leukodystrophy
	• Adrenoleukodystrophy / Adrenomyeloneuropathy
	• Cerebrohepatorenal syndrome (Zellweger disease)
	• Alexander disease
	• Lysosomal storage disorders
	   GM₂ gangliosidosis
	   Niemann-Pick disease
	   Fabry disease
	• Mucopolysaccharidosis
	• Sjoögren-Larsson syndrome
	• Cerebrotendinous xanthomatosis
	• Canavan disease

Vacuolating myelinopathies	• Megaloencephalic leukoencephalopathy with subcortical cysts (van der Knaap syndrome) • Leukoencephalopathy with vanishing white matter (LVWM)

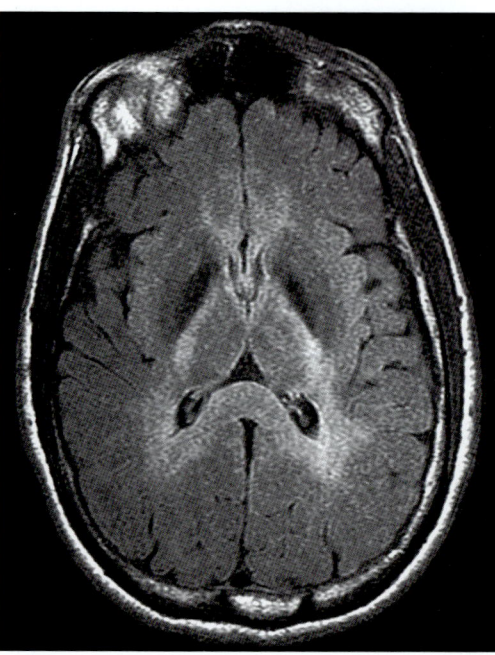

Figure 10-1 Adrenoleukodystrophy. Axial fluid-attenuated inversion recovery image showing symmetric regions of hyperintensity in the peritrigonal white matter, splenium of the corpus callosum, and along the corticospinal tracts in the posterior limbs of the internal capsules, with typical central and posterior distribution of disease.

geographic, patchy or confluent, and may be associated with swelling or volume loss. The wide range of biochemical disturbances includes peroxisomal disorders, lysosomal storage disorders, organic acidurias, and aminoacidemias. The three main pathophysiologic mechanisms affecting myelin are (1) deficient or abnormal myelin formation, (2) loss or destruction of previously normal myelin, and (3) vacuolation with rarefaction and replacement of myelin by cerebrospinal fluid (CSF) (Table 10-2).

The imaging changes reflect increased water content within the white matter tracts due to destruction or malformation of the myelin sheaths around the axons running in the white matter or due to edema related to abnormal water balance between the white matter and the extracellular spaces. A similar appearance can be caused by abnormal cellular infiltration (with or without demyelination and axonal loss) from processes such as inflammation due to infection or autoimmune disease, gliosis related to chronic insult to the white matter from radiation, trauma, or medication, or infiltrating neoplasms.

Distinguishing the heritable leukoencephalopathies from each other is difficult due to the broad overlap in the distribution of white matter signal abnormality and enhancement characteristics, and they are indistinguishable in the late stages due to diffuse symmetric white matter signal abnormalities and volume loss. Thus, early imaging offers the best possibility for detection of patterns that favor one or a few diagnoses, and imaging is generally *suggestive* (and aids in narrowing down clinical and laboratory tests for confirmation) rather than *diagnostic*.

Central White Matter Disorders

Is There Symmetric Peritrigonal Involvement Crossing the Posterior Corpus Callosum?

X-linked adrenoleukodystrophy is part of a spectrum of diseases that include adrenomyeloneuropathy and adrenoleukomyeloneuropathy. Adrenoleukodystrophy commonly presents with bilateral symmetric low attenuation of the peritrigonal white matter and the posterior corpus callosum, corticospinal tracts, and optic tracts. On MRI, corresponding areas of T2 hyperintensity with early sparing of the subcortical U fibers are seen (Figure 10-1). Centrifugal disease progression later involves the subcortical white matter. Three discrete zones of central gliosis, intermediate active demyelination with enhancement, and peripheral leading edge of active demyelination without enhancement have been described. Administration of steroids may cause the leading edge of enhancement to disappear. The nonenhancing abnormality peripheral to the enhancing margins may represent early demyelination that has not yet developed an inflammatory response. Decreased fractional anisotropy (FA) and increased mean diffusivity by diffusion tensor imaging (DTI) may be a more sensitive marker for demyelination. The nonenhancing signal abnormality central to the rim of enhancement

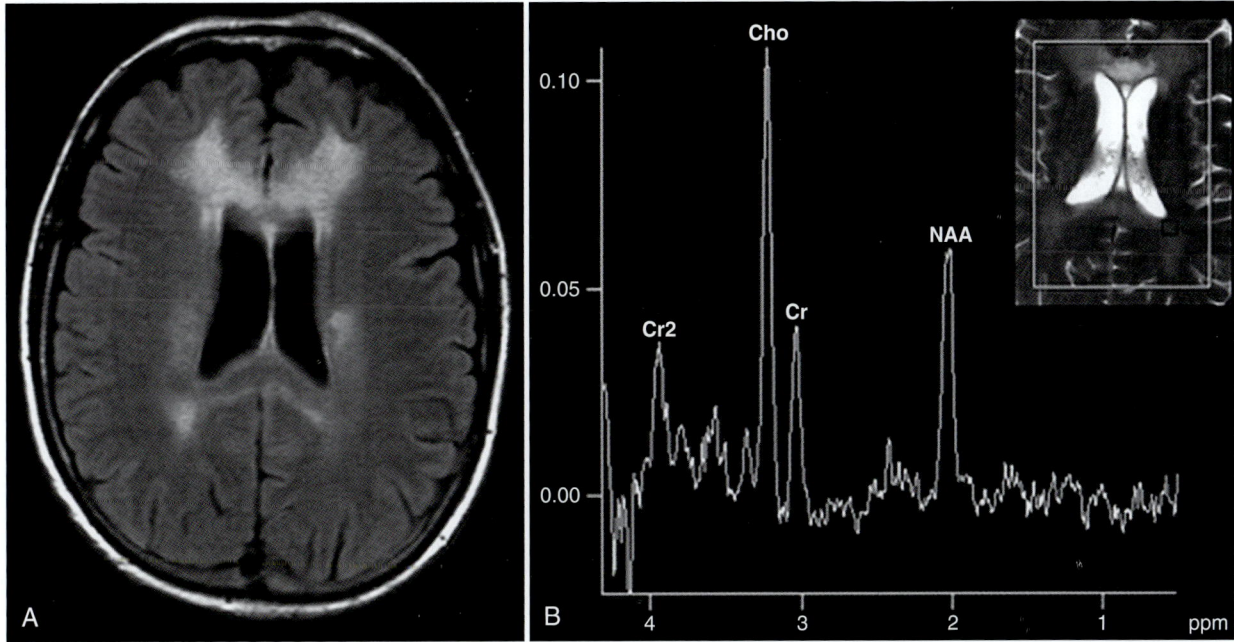

Figure 10-2 Adrenomyeloneuropathy. **A:** Fluid-attenuated inversion recovery image showing symmetric regions of hyperintensity in the hemispheric white matter with mild frontal lobe predominance and involvement of the corpus callosum. **B:** Spectroscopy of the posterior periventricular white matter reveals decreased N-acetylaspartate and increased choline, which are nonspecific but consistent with the demyelinating diseases.

may represent gliosis and scarring from burned out disease. Less frequently, the disease process begins in the frontal lobes and progresses posteriorly to resemble Alexander disease (Figure 10-2 and Box 10-1).

Is There Focal Involvement of Bilateral Caudothalamic Grooves?

Zellweger syndrome (cerebrohepatorenal syndrome) shows profound diffuse hypomyelination with diffuse white matter T2 signal hyperintensity and CT low attenuation. Small germinolytic cysts in the caudothalamic grooves and subependyma of the lateral ventricles are visible on fluid-attenuated inversion recovery images (also visible by ultrasound) (Figure 10-3). Abnormal signal in the basal ganglia can be seen related to hyperbilirubinemia from the related liver disease and can confuse the picture. Zellweger syndrome can be distinguished from the other leukodystrophies by the presence of disorganized cortical gyri, pachygyria, and other neuronal migration disorders. Optic nerve atrophy may be seen. Enhancement is not typical for Zellweger disease but can be seen with the related processes of neonatal adrenoleukodystrophy and infantile Refsum disease. This may be due to the earlier and more severe course of Zellweger with death before the inflammatory component becomes apparent (Box 10-2).

Is There Symmetric Anterior and Posterior Distribution?

Metachromatic leukodystrophy shows symmetric confluent areas of T2 hyperintensity in the anterior and posterior periventricular and peritrigonal white matter in a confluent butterfly pattern, which may also involve the cerebellar white matter. There is early

> **BOX 10-1 X-Linked Adrenoleukodystrophy (Spectrum: Adrenomyeloneuropathy, Adrenoleukomyeloneuropathy)**
>
> - X-linked mutations in ABCD1 gene
> - ABCD1 is a peroxisomal transporter for very long chain fatty acids, which are degraded within the peroxisome
> - Accumulation of undegraded very long chain fatty acids
> - Both males and females have noninflammatory axonal loss; heterozygotes females are resistant to the inflammatory demyelinating disease
> - Many clinical forms exist, including those without neurologic involvement, such as Addison disease
> - 31%–50%; childhood cerebral adrenoleukodystrophy (CCALD) onset at 3–10 years with "bronzed" skin, behavioral and learning problems, and gait, hearing, and vision disturbances, with rapid progression to dementia and death
> - 40%–46%; adrenomyeloneuropathy onset at 30 years with a chronic course that does not benefit from bone marrow transplantation (as opposed to CCALD)

sparing of the subcortical U fibers. There is also early sparing of the perivascular white matter, leading to radial stripes of spared white matter extending laterally from the edges of the lateral ventricles reminiscent of a "tigroid" appearance on T2-weighted sequences (a nonspecific finding also noted with Pelizaeus-Merzbacher disease) (Figure 10-4). Late disease demonstrates widespread white matter T2 hyperintense demyelination involving both deep and peripheral

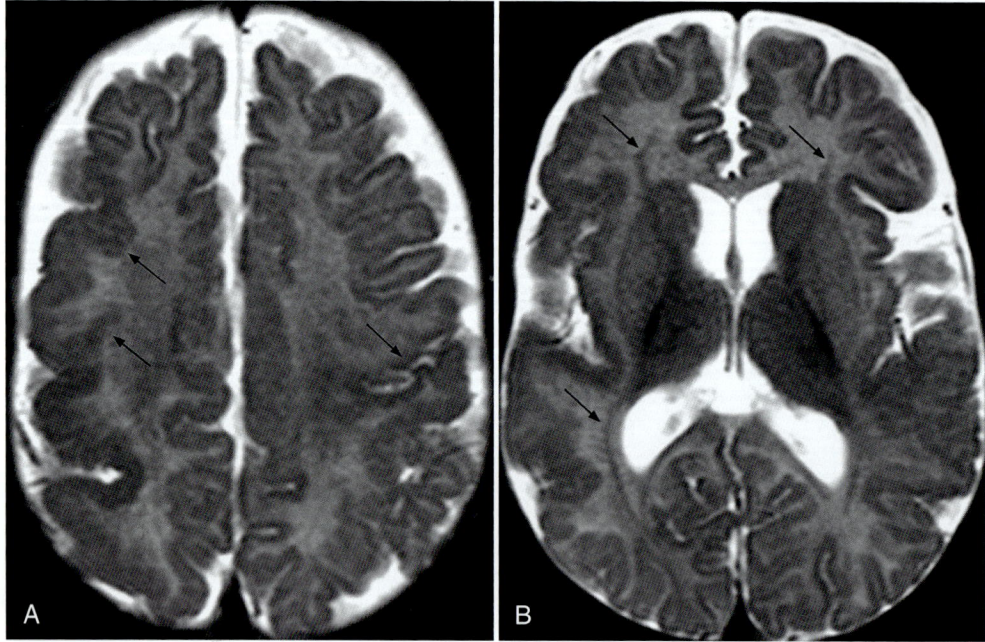

Figure 10-3 Zellweger syndrome. A, B: Axial T2-weighted images showing microgyria in the right frontal and parietal cortex and left rolandic cortex (arrows, A). Bilateral symmetrical laminar heterotopia is seen as a thin line of gray matter between the ventricle and the cortex in the frontal and parietal lobes (arrows, B). (From Huybrechts SJ, Van Veldhoven PP, Hoffman I, et al. Identification of a novel PEX14 mutation in Zellweger syndrome. J Med Genet 2008;45:376-383.)

BOX 10-2 Zellweger Syndrome (Cerebro-hepatorenal Syndrome) and Other Peroxisomal Disorders

- Spectrum of autosomal recessive mutations in one of several genes for peroxin proteins necessary for peroxisome assembly
- Mutation leads to near-complete absence of peroxisomes within cells
- Present at birth, with craniofacial dysmorphism, high forehead, ocular anomalies, hepatomegaly, severe hypotonia, and seizures
- Polymicrogyria and pachygyria with occasional abnormal clefting
- Diffuse hypomyelination may be caused by accumulation of abnormal compounds in brain, such as very long chain fatty acids and pipecolic acid, or by lack of sufficient myelin precursors
- Controversy as to whether Zellweger syndrome is distinct from infantile Refsum disease and neonatal adrenoleukodystrophy (NALD) or whether Zellweger is the most severe early-onset form of a common process

---

white matter, including the subcortical U fibers with associated cerebral atrophy. The corpus callosum, internal capsules, and descending corticospinal tracts can also be involved. There is no abnormal enhancement, perhaps due to a lack of an inflammatory component to the demyelination/dysmyelination, although cranial nerve enhancement on MRI has been reported. The lack of enhancement allows separation from X-linked adrenoleukodystrophy, which also commonly involves the splenium and peritrigonal white matter. Occasionally, T2 hypointense changes are seen in the thalamus, posterior limb of the internal capsule, and cerebellum (Box 10-3).

Is There Early Predilection for the Posterior White Matter?

Phenylketonuria demonstrates primarily supratentorial diffuse white matter T2 hyperintensity involving the posterior white matter with initial sparing of the subcortical white matter. The T2 signal abnormality often spares the frontal lobes or eventually may involve them as the disease worsens. The abnormal signal is thought to reflect abnormally high phenylalanine levels and may resolve with adequate dietary control. Involvement of the brainstem and cerebellum is less common but may occur in the setting of more severe supratentorial abnormalities. Restricted diffusion has been reported within the areas of signal abnormality and may be related to acute decompensation or very elevated serum phenylalanine concentrations. Enhancement is rare because there is no inflammatory component. There may be late volume loss related to white matter atrophy (Box 10-4).

Is There Early Predilection for the Anterior White Matter?

Alexander disease is a progressive nonfamilial demyelinating leukodystrophy characterized by increased astrocytic eosinophilic Rosenthal fibers and increased glial fibrillary acid protein. The rapidly fatal neonatal form presents with early megalencephaly and disproportionate frontal lobe disease. Contrast enhancement may occur at the margins of the symmetric bifrontal

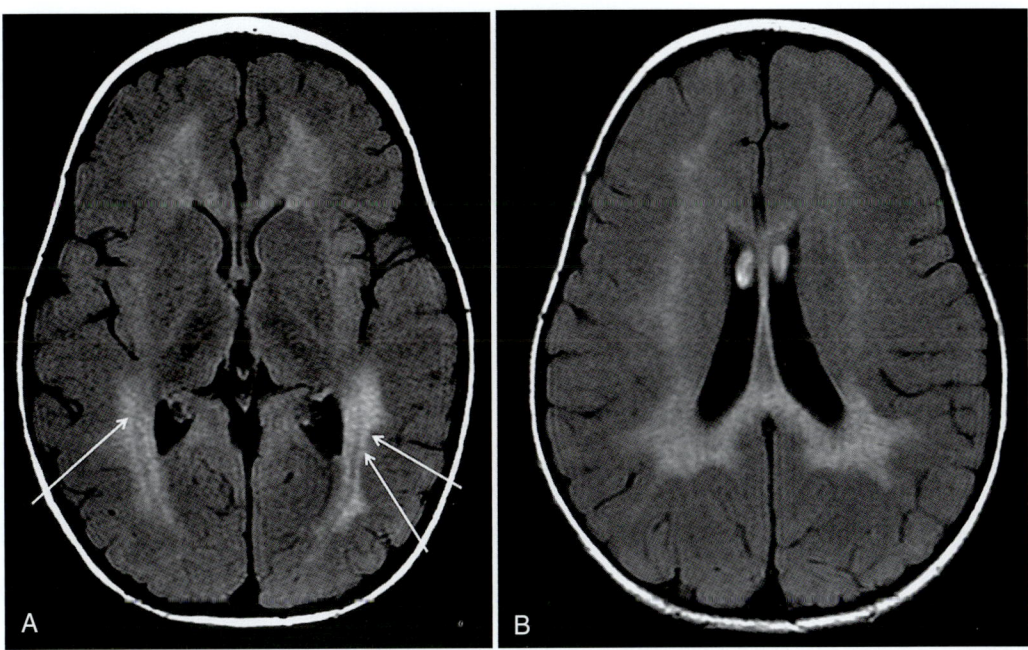

Figure 10-4 Metachromatic leukodystrophy. **A, B:** Fluid-attenuated inversion recovery images showing symmetric hyperintense regions in the periventricular white matter and corpus callosum that has not yet involved the subcortical U fibers. Sparing of the perivascular white matter creates a tigroid pattern of radiating linear hypointensities *(arrows,* **A**), which when seen end-on in the higher white matter can have a spotted leopard skin pattern (not shown). (Case courtesy of Azad Ghassemi, MD, and Nicholas D'Ambrosio, MD, New York Presbyterian Hospital / Weill Cornell Medical College, New York, NY.)

BOX 10-3   Metachromatic Leukodystrophy

- Autosomal recessive mutations in lysosomal enzyme arylsulfatase A (ARSA), which hydrolyzes intracellular sulfatides, or mutation of ARSA cofactor saposin B
- Accumulation of undegraded sulfatides in oligodendrocytes and Schwann cells causing demyelination of brain and spinal cord white matter and peripheral nerves
- Late infantile, juvenile, and adult forms
- Infantile form shows most severe and rapidly fatal disease
- Late infantile form is the most common, presenting at 2 years and progressing to death within 4 years

---

BOX 10-4   Phenylketonuria

- Autosomal recessive mutations of phenylalanine hydroxylase, an enzyme that allows conversion of excess amino acid phenylalanine into tyrosine
- Defective enzyme leads to accumulation of toxic phenylalanine compounds that damage the developing brain and can cause mental and growth retardation, eczema, epilepsy, "mousy" odor of urine and skin, and hypopigmentation
- Damage to brain may result from delayed myelination or malformed myelination with spongiotic changes, although mental retardation also may be due in part to reduced neurotransmitter production as a result of decreased tyrosine production
- Treatment involves dietary restriction of phenylalanine

---

regions of T2 hyperintensity and then progresses posteriorly to the parietal lobes and internal and external capsules. The subcortical U fibers typically are involved. In the late stages of the disease, cysts may develop. The more mild juvenile and adult forms do not show macrocephaly because the head has already formed. The adult form is characterized by areas of T2 hyperintensity and late atrophy of the medulla oblongata and upper spinal cord (Figure 10-5). The basal ganglia and thalami may also be involved. Hemispheric white matter disease and patchy enhancement may be seen in patients younger than 40 years (Box 10-5).

Are the Thalami and Basal Ganglia Also Too Dense?

Globoid cell leukodystrophy (Krabbe disease) can be separated from other leukodystrophies by early transient faint hyperdensity within the thalami, basal ganglia, corona radiata, and cerebellar dentate nuclei on CT scan of unknown etiology. Hyperdensity limited to the thalami may be seen with GM_2 gangliosidosis. Patchy hypodense changes occur in the deep and periventricular white matter with early sparing of the subcortical white matter. MRI shows corresponding areas of T2 hyperintensity that also involve the cerebellar white matter, cerebellar nuclei, corticospinal tracts, and posterior limbs of the internal capsules. The cerebellar white matter and deep gray matter changes only occur in early-onset disease before 2 years. Parietal periventricular white matter T2 signal abnormality and corpus callosal involvement are seen over time along with late T2 hyperintensity of the thalami (Figure 10-6). Adult-onset disease may present with fewer areas of signal abnormality, and there have been reports of normal

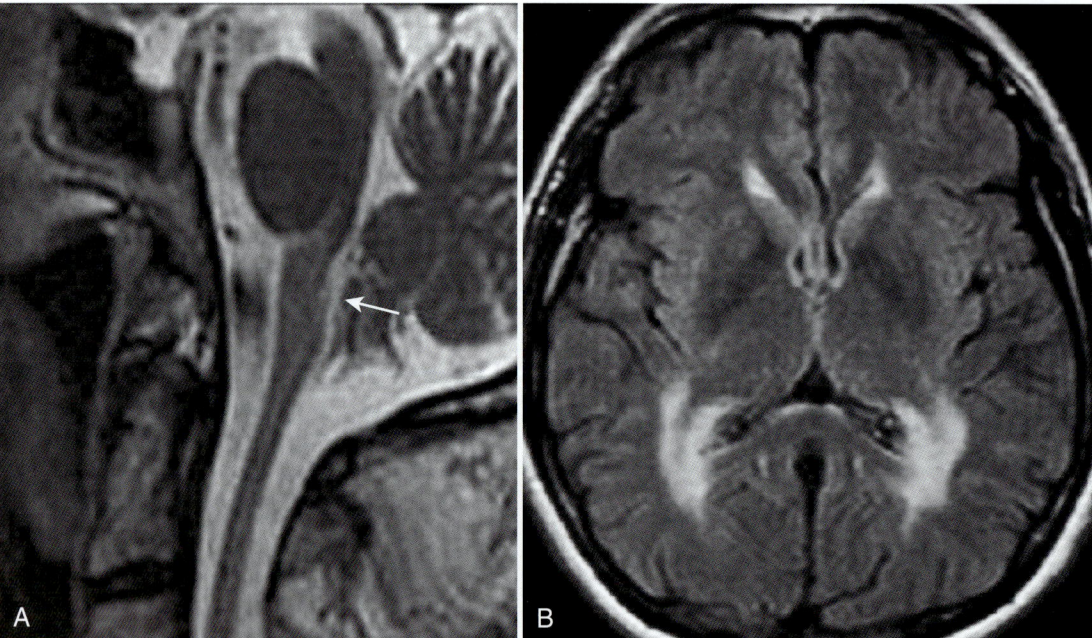

Figure 10-5 Adult-onset Alexander disease. **A:** Sagittal T2-weighted image showing atrophy and signal abnormalities in the medulla oblongata *(arrow)*. The hyperintensity fades away in the upper cervical cord, whereas the entire spinal cord is also atrophic. **B:** Fluid-attenuated inversion recovery image in another patient showing increased signal intensity of the periventricular white matter, which is more extensive in the posterior regions. (From Pareyson D, Fancellu R, Mariotti C, et al. Adult-onset Alexander disease: a series of eleven unrelated cases with review of the literature." Brain 2008;131:2321-2331.)

BOX 10-5   Alexander Disease (Fibrinoid Leukodystrophy)

- Mutation of glial fibrillary acid protein on chromosome 17q21
- Pathologic features are increased astrocytic eosinophilic Rosenthal fibers in subependymal, subpial, and perivascular regions
- Glial fibrillary acid protein increases
- Periventricular rim of high signal intensity T1, low signal intensity T2

MRI scans or initial T2 hyperintensity limited to the bilateral corticospinal tracts and posterior corpus callosum. Bilateral isolated corticospinal tract abnormalities are also seen in amyotrophic lateral sclerosis. The globoid cells of Krabbe disease can cause enlargement of the optic nerves and enhancement of cranial nerves (Box 10-6).

The thalami and basal ganglia may show hyperintense abnormalities in the peripheral white matter leukodystrophies, as in Alexander disease and Canavan disease.

Are There Cystic Lesions within the Involved White Matter?

The diagnosis of Lowe syndrome usually is made based on clinical findings at birth; thus this disease does not typically present an imaging or diagnostic quandary. There is nonenhancing central white matter T2 signal hyperintensity that spares the subcortical U fibers. Multiple cystic or punctate CSF signal lesions can be found within the symmetric and patchy white matter lesions (Figure 10-7 and Box 10-7).

Megaloencephalic leukoencephalopathy (MLC) with subcortical cysts is a slowly progressive disease that presents with early diffuse brain swelling in infancy. The white matter changes follow a centripetal course, with severe peripheral changes characterized by early large subcortical cysts, particularly in the frontal parietal and temporal lobes. The subcortical cysts and white matter lesions show facilitated diffusion with high apparent diffusion coefficient (ADC) as well as decreased FA at DTI. The cortical and deep gray matter structures are spared (Box 10-8).

The central cystic changes of Lowe syndrome and the peripheral cystic changes of MLC should be differentiated from the diffuse cribriform dilated perivascular spaces of the mucopolysaccharidoses. The cystic destruction in advanced Alexander disease and Leber hereditary optic neuropathy has strong frontal lobe predominance.

Peripheral White Matter Disorders

Is There Early Subcortical White Matter Disease?

Leukodystrophies with early subcortical white matter involvement include Alexander disease, Canavan disease, and galactosemia. The subcortical U fibers may be abnormal in Cockayne syndrome, but their involvement usually occurs later.

Canavan disease is a spongiform or vacuolating myelinopathy that shows diffuse demyelination that classically shows subcortical U-fiber white matter T2 hyperintense changes and symmetric involvement of the globi pallidi and thalami. The white matter disease has a centripetal progression pattern that extends into the central white matter as well as the internal and external

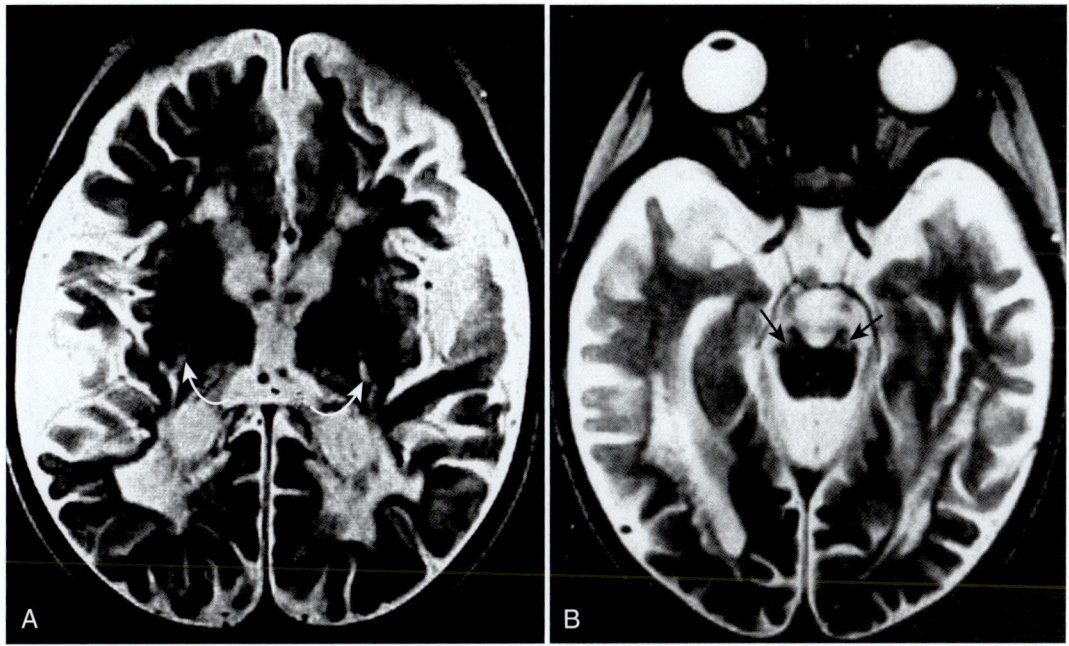

Figure 10-6 Late-infantile Krabbe disease. **A, B:** Axial T2-weighted images through the basal ganglia showing involvement of the occipital white matter and posterior limbs of the internal capsules *(curved arrows,* **A**). The thalamus and globus pallidus show symmetric decreased signal. The midbrain reveals small cerebral peduncles and increased signal along the course of the corticospinal tract *(arrows,* **B**). (From Zafeiriou DI, Michelakaki EM, Anastasiou AL, Gombakis NP, Kontopoulos EE. Serial MRI and neurophysiological studies in late-infantile Krabbe disease. Pediatr Neurol 1996;15:240-244.)

> **BOX 10-6 Krabbe Disease (Globoid Cell Leukodystrophy)**
>
> - Autosomal recessive mutation of galactosylceramide β-galactosidase (GALC) at chromosomal location 14q24
> - GALC deficiency leads to cytotoxic accumulation of cerebrosides within oligodendrocytes and Schwann cells causing demyelination of central nervous system and spinal cord white matter and peripheral nerves
> - Clinical subtypes (infantile, late infantile, juvenile, adult) categorized by age of onset, with infantile form most common
> - Later-onset forms may be due to less severe reductions in GALC activity, and the disease may be incidentally diagnosed in midlife due to presence of gait unsteadiness, paraparesis, or hyperreflexia

capsules (Figure 10-8). This demyelinating process is not accompanied by abnormal enhancement. Late disease may show tiny cysts in the subcortical U-fiber layer. MR spectroscopy shows a dramatic increase in N-acetylaspartate (NAA) that contrasts with the nearly universal decrease in almost all other white matter diseases (Box 10-9).

Galactosemia shows areas of T2 hyperintensity in the cerebral peripheral white matter with delayed myelination and diffuse atrophy (Box 10-10).

Is Macrocephaly Present?

Subcortical white matter disease and macrocephaly are seen in the infantile forms of Canavan disease, Alexander disease, and MLC. Canavan disease has a unique elevation in NAA, whereas MLC typically develops prominent subcortical cysts.

Are the Subcortical U Fibers and Bilateral Optic Nerves Involved?

Bilateral optic nerve involvement is typical for Leber hereditary optic neuropathy, a maternally inherited mitochondrial disorder. Patients present with severe acute or subacute bilateral visual loss in early adulthood. Although the disease usually is isolated to the optic nerves, some patients have Leber hereditary optic neuropathy plus diseases with widespread involvement of the central nervous system (CNS). They include multiple sclerosis-like demyelinating disease with otherwise indistinguishable lesions of the brain and spinal cord, Leigh-like encephalopathy with lesions of the brainstem, and dystonia disease with striatal necrosis in children. Patients may also demonstrate striking symmetric cystic destruction in the frontal lobes involving the subcortical U fibers and in the anterior corpus callosum (Figure 10-9). The frontal lobe lesions with cyst formation may mimic Alexander disease (also shows early subcortical U-fiber involvement) and MLC (reveals early sparing of subcortical U fibers), both of which cause macrocephaly in the infantile form (Box 10-11).

Nonspecific, Diffuse, Other

Is There a "Tigroid" Pattern of the Perivascular White Matter?

The tigroid pattern is formed by linear T2 hypointense stripes of spared perivascular white matter that extend from the ventricles in a radial pattern. This pattern is seen in metachromatic leukodystrophy, Pelizaeus-Merzbacher disease, and trichothiodystrophy. The tigroid

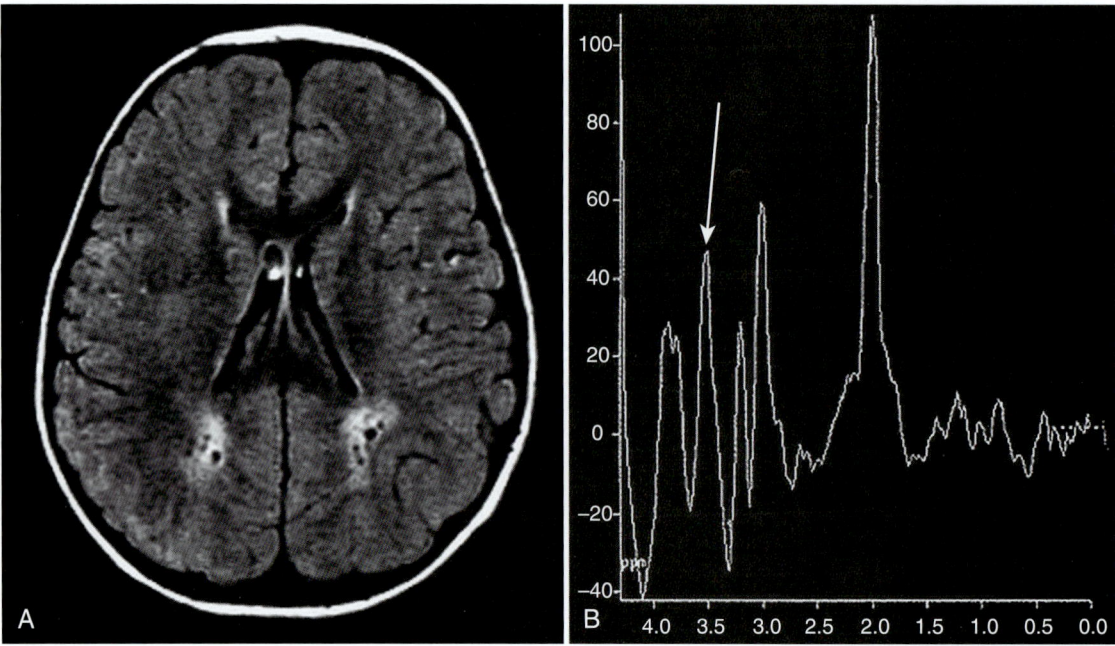

Figure 10-7 Lowe syndrome. **A:** Fluid-attenuated inversion recovery image revealing periatrial hyperintensities with multiple small, cyst-like structures. **B:** Spectrum from the left periatrial region showing the peak of myoinositol (at 3.56 ppm) is greater *(arrow)* than that of nearby choline (at 3.22 ppm). (From Sener RN. Lowe syndrome: proton MR spectroscopy, and diffusion MR imaging. J Neuroradiol 2004; 31:238-240.)

BOX 10-7 Lowe Syndrome (Oculocerebrorenal Syndrome [OCRL])

- X-linked recessive mutations of OCRL1 on chromosome Xq26
- OCRL1 encodes a Golgi body protein that modulates cellular trafficking and cytoskeleton remodeling
- High death rate in first months of life with failure to thrive, electrolyte imbalances, seizures, and recurrent pneumonias
- Present at birth with cataracts, hypotonia, absent deep tendon reflexes, and typical facies

BOX 10-8 Megaloencephalic Leukoencephalopathy with Subcortical Cysts (van der Knaap disease)

- Autosomal recessive
- Myelin splitting and intramyelinic vacuolization
- >60 mutations in MLC1 gene on chromosome 22q13.33
- Slow clinical progression despite marked radiographic abnormalities

---

pattern may be caused by sparing of myelin in the perivascular areas in the setting of diffuse white matter abnormality (Figure 10-4).

Is There Diffuse Hypomyelination?

Pelizaeus-Merzbacher disease shows diffuse hypomyelination of the central and peripheral white matter that resembles the appearance of a newborn brain. Some myelination may occur and then disappear with disease progression. The most severe form is the "connatal" or infantile form, which presents at birth without any evidence of myelination (Figure 10-10). There is no abnormal enhancement or evidence of white matter destruction. Late in the disease, there may be diffuse white matter atrophy (Box 10-12).

Is There Severe Atrophy of the Superior Cerebellar Peduncles?

Myoclonus epilepsy with ragged red fibers (MERRF) may present with severe atrophy that is limited to the superior cerebellar peduncles, which by DTI can also demonstrate decreased FA (Figure 10-11). The structural abnormalities are otherwise usually mild despite severe clinical disabilities. They include mild nonspecific atrophy of the cerebrum, cerebellum, and brainstem and areas of T2 hyperintensity in the hemispheric white matter, striatum, and brainstem (Box 10-13).

Is There Diffuse Cerebral, Cerebellar, and Brainstem Disease?

Maple syrup urine disease demonstrates diffuse white matter hypodensity that is more marked in the cerebellum and brainstem than in the cerebral hemispheres. This edema may be seen on transfontanelle ultrasound as diffuse white matter echogenicity. Early on, maple syrup urine disease can also present with a normal CT scan. MRI shows T2 hyperintense changes in the deep cerebellar white matter and dorsal brainstem, cerebral peduncles, posterior limbs of the internal capsule and corticospinal tracts (to the cortex), and, to a lesser extent, the supratentorial white matter and occasionally globus pallidi (Figure 10-12). Some of this signal abnormality may be related to cerebral edema from hyponatremia

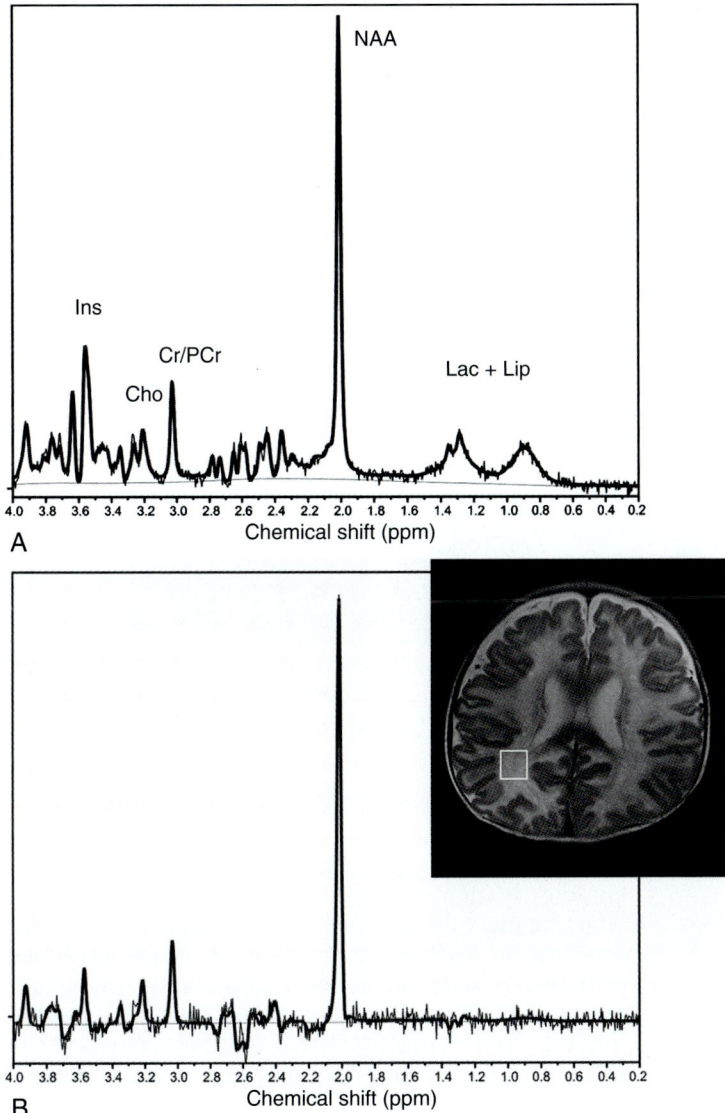

Figure 10-8 Canavan disease. Short **(A)** and long **(B)** TE spectra showing diffuse white matter changes and a nearly pathognomonic increase in *N*-acetylaspartate, which is nearly double the normal values from age-matched controls and even higher than the value seen in adults. (From Dezortova M, Hajek M. ^{1}H MR spectroscopy in pediatrics. Eur J Radiol 2008;67:240-249.)

BOX 10-9 Canavan Disease (Spongiform Leukoencephalopathy, Canavan–van Bogaert-Bertrand disease)

- Autosomal recessive
- Increased *N*-acetylaspartate due to deficiency of aspartoacylase on chromosome 17p
- Infantile form >> congenital and juvenile forms

BOX 10-10 Galactosemia

- Autosomal recessive disorder
- Kinase, transferase, or epimerase deficiency; most common is galactose-1-phosphate-uridyl transferase deficiency
- Treatment is dietary restriction of galactose

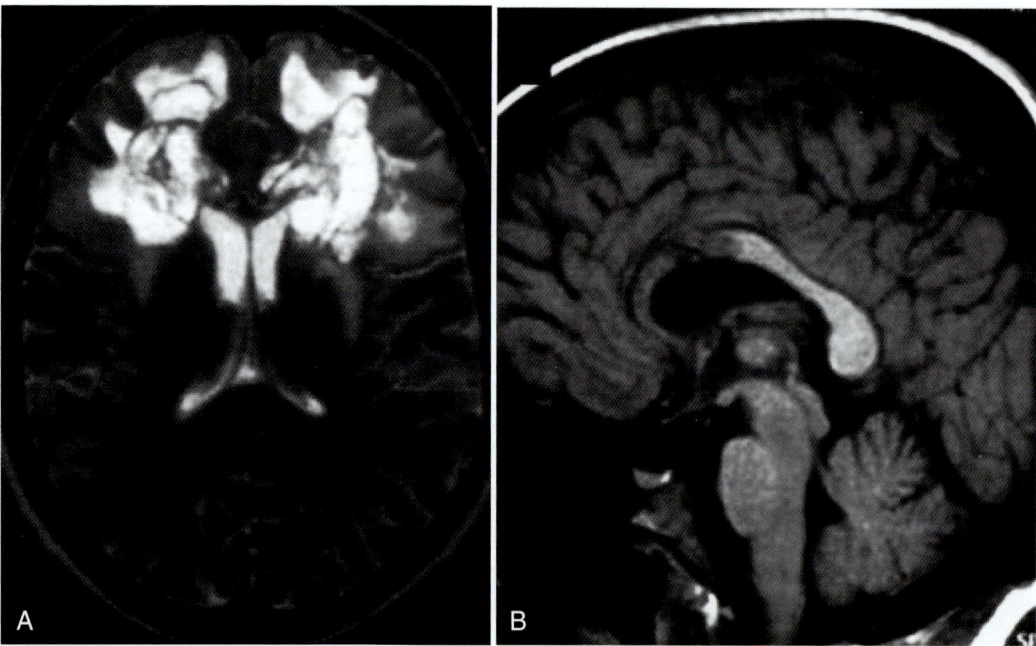

Figure 10-9 Leber hereditary optic neuropathy. Axial T2-weighted (A) and sagittal T1-weighted images (B) showing destructive cystic lesions in the frontal lobe deep and subcortical white matter. The genu and the rostral third of the corpus callosum are severely involved. (From Kovacs GG, Hoftberger R, Majtenyi K, et al. Neuropathology of white matter disease in Leber's hereditary optic neuropathy. Brain 2005;128:35-41.)

> **BOX 10-11 Leber Hereditary Optic Neuropathy**
>
> - Most common mitochondrial disorder to affect vision (acute or subacute)
> - >30 point mutations in mitochondrial DNA (11,778 >> 3460 > 14,484)
> - Males >> females; 40% in children
> - Bilateral optic nerve atrophy with degeneration of retinal ganglion cells and optic nerve axons

and may resolve with therapy or progression to subacute stage. Diffusion imaging shows restricted diffusion within the areas of T2 signal abnormality acutely, particularly the ventral lateral thalami, posterior limbs of the internal capsules, and globus pallidi. Contrast enhancement is not present because there is no inflammatory component (Box 10-14).

Central pontine myelinolysis is an acquired disorder that classically demonstrates abnormal T2 hyperintensity within the central pons that spares the peripheral brainstem and corticospinal tracts (Figure 10-13). This entity is more accurately referred to as *osmotic demyelination syndrome* due to the common involvement of extrapontine structures, including the basal ganglia, cerebral white matter (including subcortical U fibers), cerebellar peduncles, and cortex. Imaging abnormalities may lag behind clinical symptoms; restricted diffusion may occur prior to T2 hyperintense lesions.

Other

Nonspecific white matter patterns (diffuse, unilateral, bilateral, asymmetric) can be seen with nonketotic hyperglycinemia, the urea cycle disorders, and virtually any end-stage white matter disease. Nonketotic hyperglycemia is a hereditary amino acidopathy characterized by glycine accumulation. Patients present in early infancy with diffuse volume loss, abnormal white matter, thinned corpus callosum, and delayed myelination. The urea cycle disorders include ornithine carbamyl transferase deficiency, carbamyl phosphate synthetase deficiency, arginosuccinic aciduria, citrullinemia, and hyperargininemia. These disorders of increased ammonemia manifest with diffuse cerebral edema that involves the cortex and white matter, including the subcortical U fibers that develops into diffuse white matter lesions and marked atrophy.

Chemotherapy and radiation therapy often show early central white matter changes, although the subcortical U fibers may also be involved with diffuse toxic effects. The destruction of intrinsically normal myelin usually is asymmetric, with T2 hyperintense lesions that do not show significant mass effect or enhancement (Figure 10-14).

Are Dilated Perivascular Spaces Present?

Mucopolysaccharidosis is the only metabolic disorder to have dilated perivascular spaces in a symmetric cribriform pattern, although this may be seen in other nonmetabolic disorders. The dilated perivascular spaces may involve the periventricular white matter, thalami, basal ganglia, corpus callosum, and brainstem (Figure 10-15). They are thought to result from the macroscopic accumulation of glycosaminoglycans, although they also may reflect defective CSF resorption as part of communicating hydrocephalus. Other abnormalities of impaired CSF resorption include enlarged subarachnoid spaces, arachnoid cysts, and mega cisterna magna. Brain abnormalities include diffuse atrophy and areas of T2 hyperintensity in the periventricular white

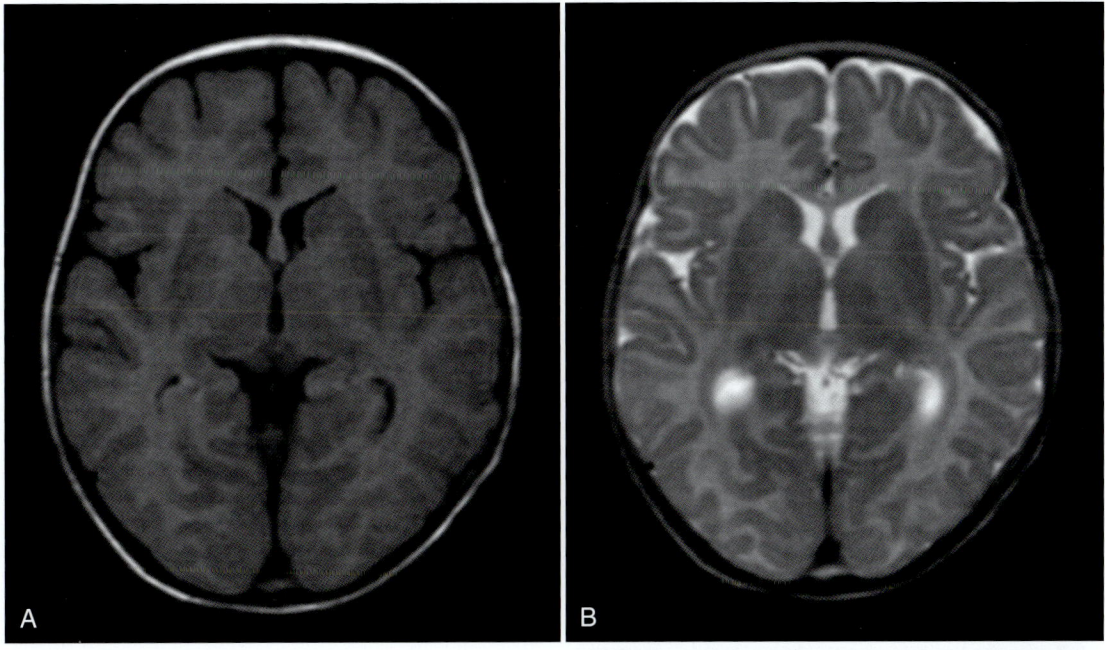

Figure 10-10 Pelizaeus-Merzbacher disease. Axial T1-weighted (A) and T2-weighted (B) images showing diffuse hypomyelination with abnormal T2 hyperintensity of the cerebral white matter. (Case courtesy of Yvonne W. Lui, MD, Montefiore Medical Center, New York, NY.)

BOX 10-12   Pelizaeus-Merzbacher Disease

- X-linked recessive disorder of proteolipid protein 1 (PLP1) gene on chromosome Xq22
- Pelizaeus-Merzbacher disease and spastic paraplegia 2 (SPG2) share PLP1 gene defects along a spectrum, with SPG2 showing milder and later onset symptoms
- PLP1 proteolipid protein makes up 50% of protein mass of myelin in oligodendrocytes
- Defective folding or transport of PLP to cell surface results in PLP accumulation that leads to oligodendrocyte and axonal cell death

---

matter, which along with the hydrocephalus correlate with disease duration and severity (Figure 10-16 and Box 10-15).

■ PART II: CORTICAL GRAY MATTER DISEASE

Poliodystrophies or disorders of the cortical gray matter often manifest with marked cortical atrophy and sulcal widening. Disorders include Alpers syndrome, Menkes syndrome, and neuronal ceroid lipofuscinosis (NCL). Variable white matter lesions and atrophy are often present.

Alpers syndrome usually affects infants and very young children with progressive neurologic disorders, including refractory epilepsy and severe liver disease. Older children and teenagers may have juvenile Alpers syndrome, which has a more protracted clinical course. The brain shows necrotizing lesions with severe neuronal loss and gliosis, decreased white matter volume, and delayed myelination. Marked cortical thinning is most conspicuous in the posterior temporal, occipital, and frontal lobes (Figure 10-17 and Box 10-16).

Is the White Matter More T2 Bright than the Gray Matter?

Although white matter lesions and atrophy are variably present in all the poliodystrophies, the white matter disease may be the most severe in NCL. Infantile NCL, which is the most severe form of NCL, causes extreme cortical atrophy and marked white matter T2 hyperintensity that becomes higher than that of gray matter. The progressive cortical atrophy is most marked in the cerebellum and frontal lobes. The white matter changes are thought to reflect myelin loss, wallerian degeneration, and gliosis after neuronal death. These changes occur rapidly during the first 4 years of life in parallel with clinical and histopathologic progression. The thalamus shows T2 hypointensity in infantile NCL and variant subtype (not classic) late infantile NCL. Late infantile NCL shows extensive T2 hyperintense lesions in the hemispheric white matter including the internal capsule. Whole-brain ADC measurements reveal facilitated diffusion (increasing ADC values) in patients with late infantile NCL that correlates with disease severity and duration; ADC values normally decrease with increasing age due to normal myelination (Box 10-17).

■ PART III: DEEP GRAY MATTER DISEASE

The combination of deep gray matter disease and peripheral white matter disease in a child or young adult strongly suggests the diagnosis of a mitochondrial disorder. Mitochondrial disorders represent a spectrum of clinically similar diseases that involve mutations in mitochondrial or nuclear deoxyribonucleic acid (DNA). Mitochondrial DNA has a maternal inheritance pattern. Mutations in mitochondrial DNA result in marked phenotypic heterogeneity due to heteroplasmy, in which variable amounts

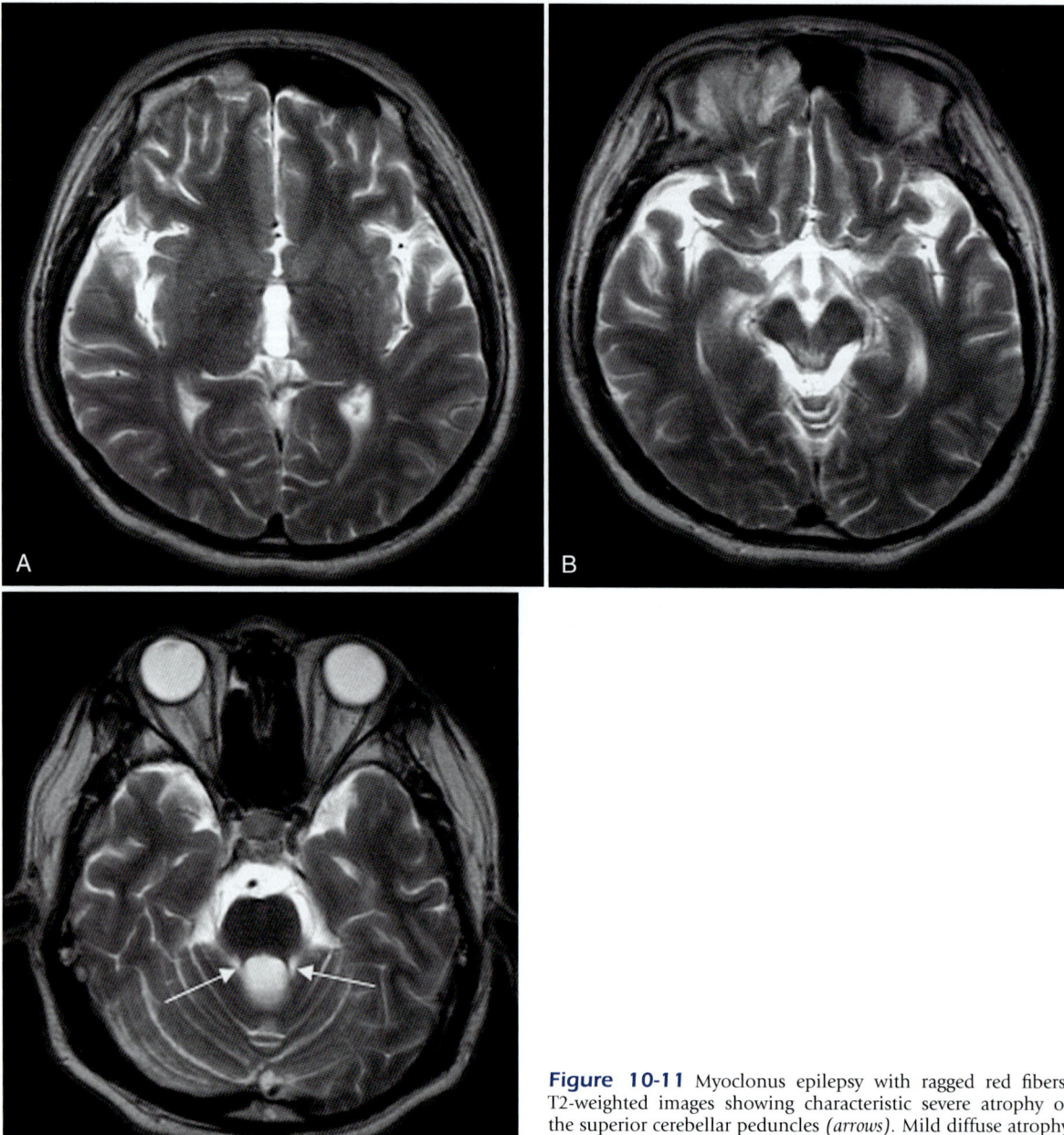

Figure 10-11 Myoclonus epilepsy with ragged red fibers. T2-weighted images showing characteristic severe atrophy of the superior cerebellar peduncles *(arrows)*. Mild diffuse atrophy and symmetric areas of hyperintensity are present in the medial thalami and periaqueductal gray matter.

BOX 10-13 Myoclonus Epilepsy with Ragged Red Fibers (MERRF)

- Myoclonus epilepsy, cerebellar ataxia, myopathy, and hearing loss
- A8344G >> A3243G mitochondrial DNA mutations
- A8344G is associated with slower, less severe disease than A3243G
- No cerebral lactic acidosis and no stroke-like episodes (unlike MERRF)
- Radionuclide single-photon emission computed tomography shows decreased, potentially reversible perfusion, particularly in the parietal occipital lobes (normal perfusion in most other mitochondrial disorders)
- Diffusion tensor imaging reveals decreased fractional anisotropy in the abnormal areas of the brain and spinal cord, although fiber tracking may be preserved

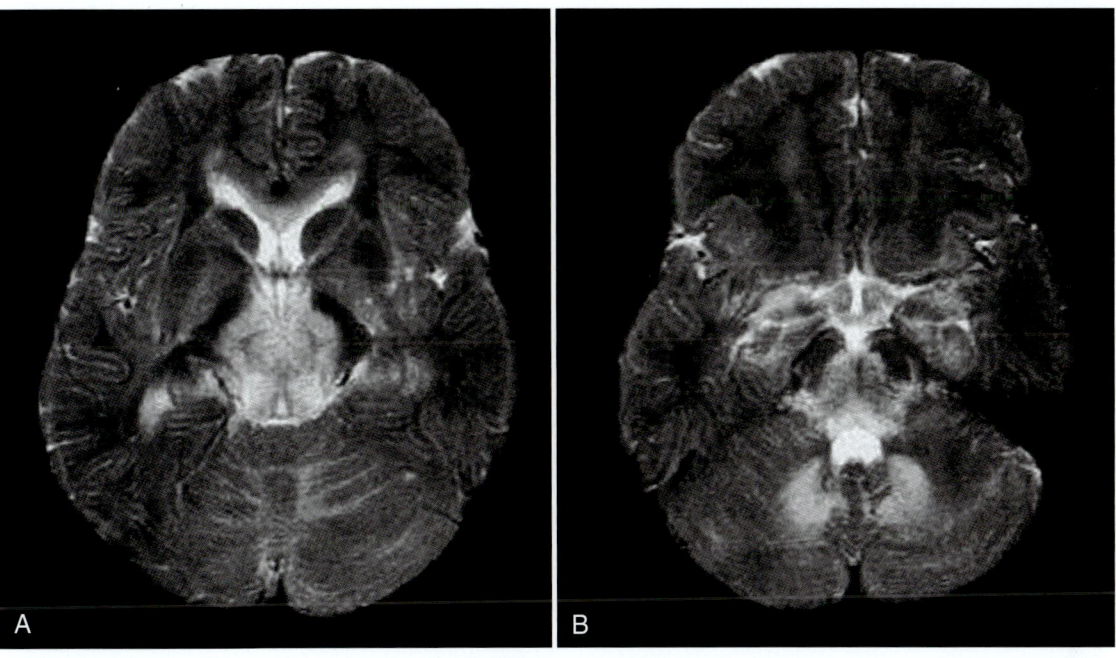

Figure 10-12 Maple syrup urine disease. Axial T2-weighted images showing diffuse hyperintense T2 signal involving the supratentorial white matter, basal ganglia, mesencephalon, and cerebellum. (From Schönberger S, Schweiger B, Schwahn B, Schwarz M, Wendel U. Dysmyelination in the brain of adolescents and young adults with maple syrup urine disease. Mol Genet Metab 2004;82:69-75.)

BOX 10-14   Maple Syrup Urine Disease (MSUD)

- Multiallelic autosomal recessive disorder of the mitochondrial enzymatic complex
- Neurotoxic accumulation of branched-chain amino acids (BCAA) and their ketoacid metabolite forms
- Excess BCAA in urine gives urine a maple syrup smell
- Five clinical phenotypes: classic, intermediate, intermittent, thiamin-responsive, and dihydrolipoamide dehydrogenase (E3) deficient
- Classic form has the most severe BCAA defect (<2% enzymatic activity) and presents within the first week of life
- Treatment involves restriction of dietary BCAA and/or oral thiamine

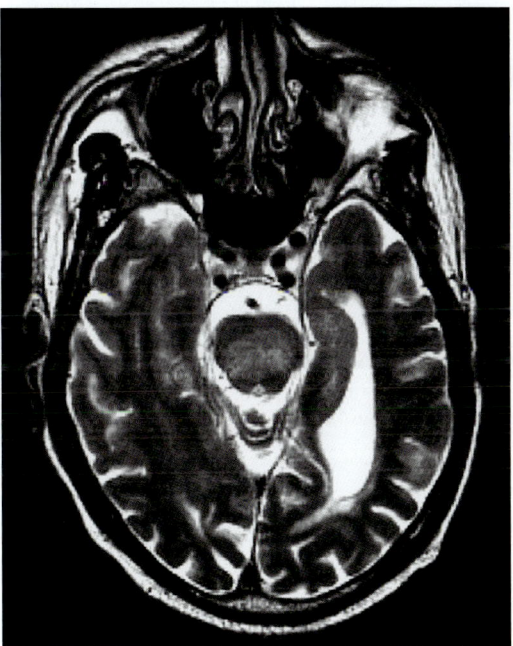

Figure 10-13 Central pontine myelinolysis. Axial T2-weighted image showing central hyperintensity and swelling that spares the peripheral brainstem.

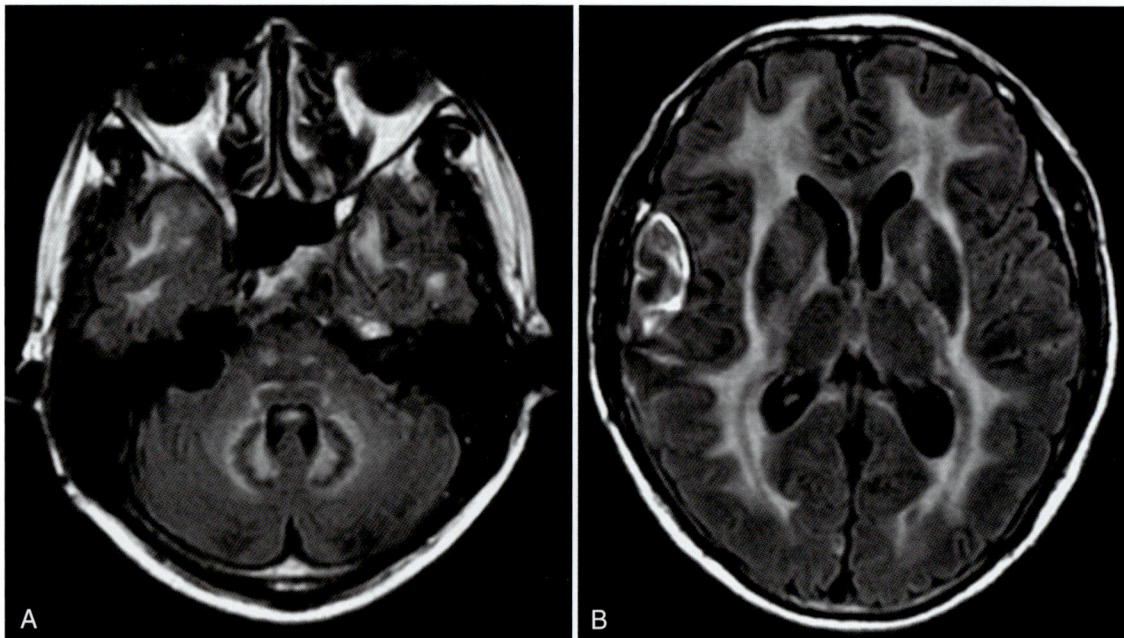

Figure 10-14 Methotrexate-based chemotherapy– and radiation therapy–induced necrotizing encephalopathy in a patient with treated brain and leptomeningeal metastases from non–small cell lung carcinoma. **A, B:** Fluid-attenuated inversion recovery images showing diffuse areas of hyperintensity involving the cerebral white matter, basal ganglia, cerebellum, and brainstem. Susceptibility artifact over the right sylvian region is due to an Ommaya reservoir (not shown).

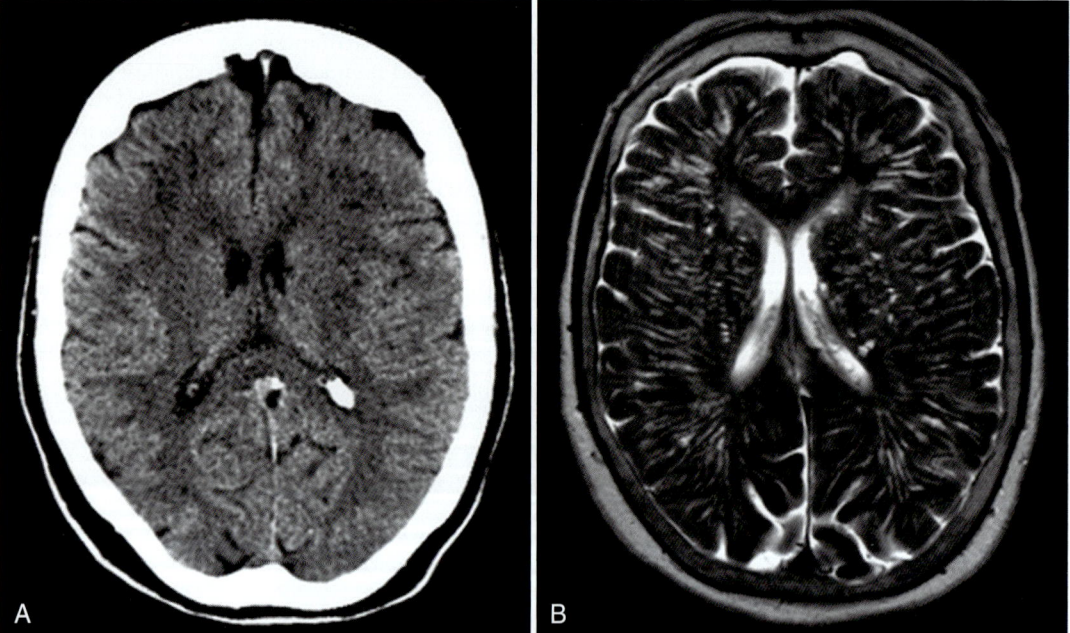

Figure 10-15 Mucopolysaccharidosis type IH (Hurler syndrome). Computed tomography **(A)** and T2-weighted images **(B)** showing cribriform dilated perivascular spaces in the hemispheric white matter as well as small cysts in the basal ganglia.

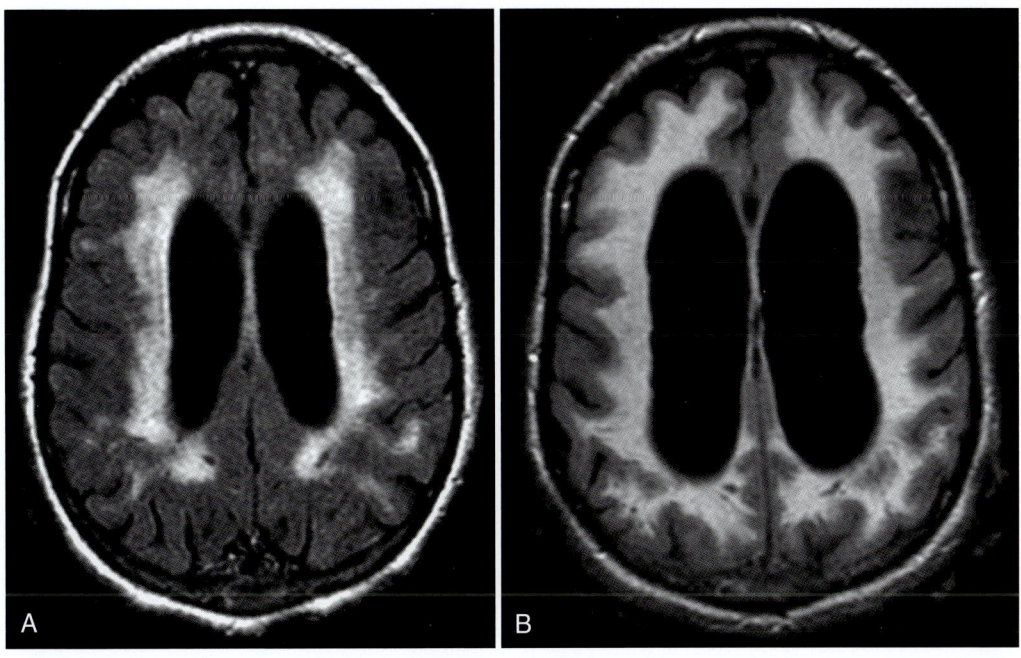

Figure 10-16 Mucopolysaccharidosis type IIA (Hunter syndrome). Axial fluid-attenuated inversion recovery images. **A:** Initial image showing cerebral atrophy, communicating hydrocephalus, and symmetric areas of hemispheric white matter hyperintensity, which all progressed after 1 year (**B**). (Case courtesy of Vinh Nguyen, MD, Long Island Jewish Medical Center, New Hyde Park, NY.)

BOX 10-15   Mucopolysaccharidosis (MPS)

- Heterogeneous group of lysosomal storage disorders
- Accumulation of incompletely degraded glycosaminoglycans in multiple organs
- Autosomal recessive, except for MPS II (X-linked recessive)
- Seven discrete MPS disorders, caused by 11 lysosomal enzyme deficiencies
- α-L-Iduronidase deficiency on chromosome 4p16.3 shared by severe MPS IH (Hurler syndrome), intermediate MPS IHS (Hurler-Scheie), and mild MPS IS (Scheie)
- MPS IH Hurler syndrome is the prototype MPS disorder
- Severe MPS with mental retardation: MPS IH (Hurler), MPS IIA (Hunter), MPS III (Sanfilippo), MPS VII
- MPS IV (Morquio) spares the central nervous system

---

of mutant and normal copies are present in each cell through the process of replicative segregation. Ragged red fibers may be found in many of these disorders, although only one incorporates this descriptive terminology into its name (myoclonic epilepsy associated with ragged red fibers) (Table 10-3). Mitochondrial encephalopathies often involve the globus pallidus, which may be more susceptible to injury due to the relatively high baseline metabolism of the pallidal neurons.

The white matter is commonly abnormal, with areas of T2 hyperintensity that may spontaneously resolve and subsequently recur. These changes are thought to reflect either mitochondrial cerebral angiopathy–induced ischemia or mitochondrial impairment–induced direct neuronal death. White matter disease occurs in Leigh syndrome; Kearns-Sayre syndrome (KSS); mitochondrial myopathy, encephalopathy, lactic acidosis, and stroke (MELAS); MERRF; mitochondrial neurogastrointestinal encephalopathy; and Leber hereditary optic neuropathy. The abnormal white matter may include small cyst-like lesions and involvement of the cerebral and cerebellar white matter. This should be contrasted from the leukoencephalopathies, which primarily involve the deep cerebral white matter with relatively less involvement of the deep gray nuclei.

Disorders of the deep gray matter may be separated by primary (or mixed) involvement of the individual components of the basal ganglia (caudate, putamen, corpus striatum [caudate and putamen], globus pallidus) and of the thalamus.

Caudate Nucleus

Are the Caudate Nuclei Atrophic?

Marked disproportionate atrophy of the caudate nuclei is the imaging hallmark of Huntington disease. Severe neuronal loss may also involve the putamen and less so the globus pallidus (Figure 10-18). The caudate nucleus atrophy results in ex vacuo dilatation of the frontal horns, which assume a boxcar-like configuration, and increased bicaudate ratio (minimum intercaudate distance divided by brain width, measured on an axial image at level of third ventricle). Early disease shows areas of T2 hyperintensity in the caudate heads and putamina prior to the atrophy. The striatum may also show areas of T2 hypointensity due to iron deposition. Advanced Huntington disease has generalized involvement of the brain with diffuse cerebral atrophy that often begins in the frontal lobes and has posterior progression (Box 10-18).

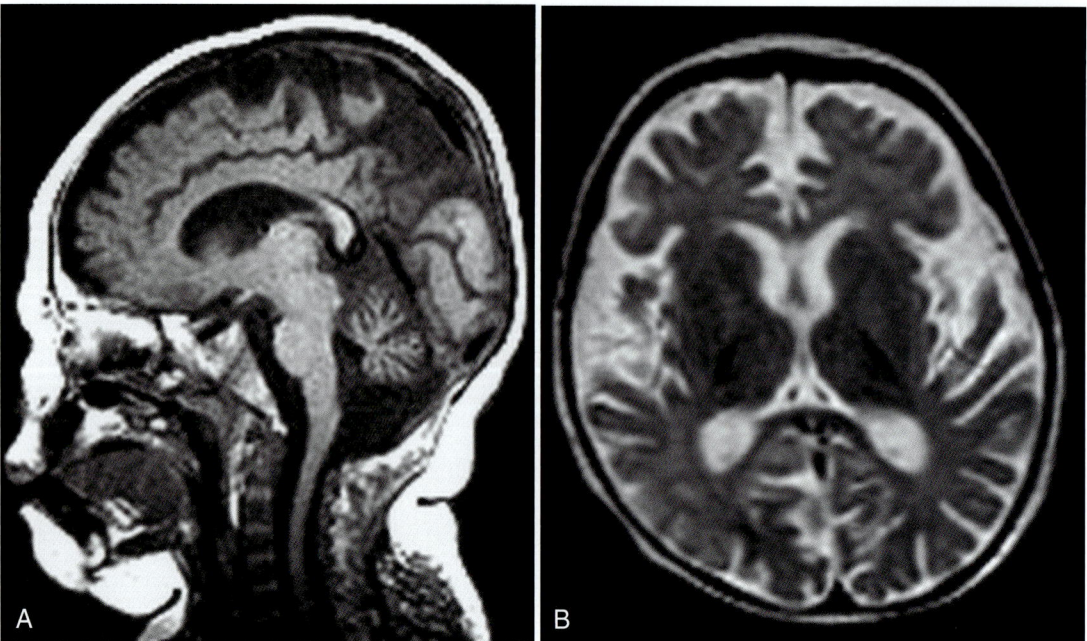

Figure 10-17 Alpers syndrome. **A:** Sagittal T1-weighted image showing diffuse atrophy. **B:** Axial T2-weighted image showing hyperintense lesions in the white matter. (Case courtesy of Sasan Karimi, MD, Memorial Sloan-Kettering Cancer Center, New York, NY.)

BOX 10-16 Progressive Cerebral Poliodystrophy (Alpers, Alpers-Huttenlocher Syndrome)

- Progressive neuronal degeneration of childhood with liver disease
- Autosomal recessive hepatocerebral disorder
- Heterogeneous group of similar clinical and metabolic disorders
- Spongiform atrophy of cortex (particularly occipital lobes), basal ganglia, and thalami

Trichopoliodystrophy (Menkes, Menkes kinky hair disease)
- X-linked recessive mitochondrial disorder that only affects male infants
- Decreased copper absorption results in poor cytochrome oxidase activity
- Secondarily abnormal mitochondria
- *Kinky hair* term arises from the coarse, stiff, and frayed hair ends
- Rapidly progressive atrophy with ventriculomegaly and cortical thinning
- Cortical shrinking and subsequent stretching of the subdural vessels may contribute to bilateral subdural hematomas, which should not be mistaken for non-accidental trauma

---

BOX 10-17 Neuronal Ceroid Lipofuscinosis (NCL)

- Heterogeneous group of genetically distinct progressive diseases
- Abnormal intracellular lipid pigment (lipofuscin) accumulation in lysosomes of different cells, including neurons, lymphocytes, vascular endothelium, and muscle
- Four major types (>20 different types described):
  1. Infantile NCL (Santavuori-Haltia disease)
  2. Late infantile NCL (Jansky-Bielschowsky disease)
  3. Juvenile NCL (Batten or Spielmeyer-Vogt-Sjögren-Batten disease)
  4. Adult NCL (Kufs or Parry disease)
- Juvenile NCL is the most common type (Batten occasionally used to refer to all NCLs)
- Childhood NCLs are autosomal recessive (infantile, late infantile, juvenile)
- Adult NCLs are autosomal recessive (Kufs) or dominant (Parry)
- More mild and slowly progressive than childhood forms
- Weill Cornell late infantile NCL scale incorporates quantitative magnetic resonance imaging criteria (apparent diffusion coefficient values, ventricular volumes) to monitor disease

Table 10-3 Ragged Red Fibers

- Muscle biopsy using the modified Gomori trichome stain
- Appearance caused by increased abnormal mitochondria, lack of cytochrome c oxidase, and mitochondrial DNA deletions
- Morphologic characteristic of mitochondrial encephalomyopathies
- Myoclonus epilepsy with ragged red fibers
- Mitochondrial myopathy, encephalopathy, lactic acidosis, and stroke
- Kearns-Sayre syndrome/chronic progressive external ophthalmoplegia
- Menkes syndrome

BOX 10-18 Huntington Disease

- Autosomal dominant, complete penetrance
- Classic adult form presents at 35–45 years and is fatal within 20 years
- Less common juvenile form in 1%–6% that presents before age 20 years with Parkinson like movements and rigidity rather than choreoathetoid movements
- Huntington disease gene on chromosome 4p16.3
- Repeat expansion of CAG (cytosine-adenosine-guanosine) trinucleotide; earlier age of onset and more rapidly progressive disease occur with increased repeats
- Toxic accumulation of mutant Huntington protein
- Impaired energy metabolism primarily affects the medium spiny GABAergic neurons in the striatum and less so the mesencephalon and cortex

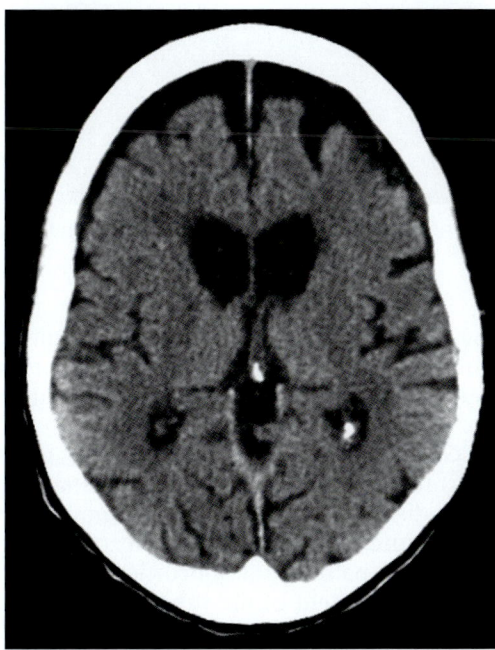

Figure 10-18 Huntington disease. Axial computed tomographic image showing severe caudate nucleus atrophy and subsequent ex vacuo, boxcar-like configuration of the frontal horns of the lateral ventricles. Widening of the frontal extraaxial cerebrospinal fluid spaces is present. Diffuse cerebral atrophy often begins in the frontal lobes and progresses posteriorly. (Case courtesy of Yvonne W. Lui, MD, Montefiore Medical Center, New York, NY.)

Corpus Striatum (Caudate Nucleus and Putamen)

Are the Putamina Too Bright?

Wilson disease shows symmetric regions of T2 hyperintensity or mixed signal intensity in the putamina and globi pallidi, caudate nuclei, and thalami (Figure 10-19). The putamina often show peripheral, laminar rims of T2 hyperintensity. The hyperintense areas reflect the portal–systemic encephalopathic effects of Wilson disease, whereas the hypointense areas represent copper deposition. The excess copper does not cause CT hyperdensity. These structures show restricted diffusion in the acute phase. Midbrain abnormalities may give the giant panda sign, which consists of tegmentum hyperintensity and superior colliculus hypointensity with sparing of the red nucleus and the lateral portions of the pars reticulata of the substantia nigra. Linear hyperintensities may involve the dentatorubrothalamic, pontocerebellar, and corticospinal tracts. Patchy cortical and subcortical lesions may occur, particularly in the frontal lobes. Generalized brain atrophy, particularly midbrain atrophy, usually is present (Box 10-19).

Isolated hyperintensity of the corpus striatum may be seen in a variety of metabolic diseases, such as Leigh syndrome and MELAS, as well as other acquired metabolic diseases, including thiamine deficiency and infections such as CNS aspergillosis (Figure 10-20). However, Leigh syndrome will classically show brainstem and cerebellar disease.

The putamen and thalamus are preferentially involved by severe hypoxic–ischemic encephalopathy, which may be due to increased activity of excitatory glutamatergic pathways. The globus pallidus may be protected in those situations by inhibitory neuronal activity, although the relatively high baseline activity of the pallidal neurons may make them more vulnerable to subacute oxidative stresses, such as the mitochondrial encephalopathies and kernicterus.

Are the Brainstem and Spinal Cord Also Abnormal?

Leigh syndrome shows hyperintense putamina in nearly all cases, with classic involvement of the basal ganglia, brainstem, and spinal cord. Symmetric gray and white matter T2 hyperintense lesions may also involve the caudate nuclei, globi pallidi, midbrain tegmentum, periaqueductal gray matter, pons, cerebral peduncles, and posterior column spinal cord (Figure 10-21). The basal ganglia is usually the site of initial involvement. The upper brainstem lesions are often transient and in parallel to reversible respiratory distress, whereas the lower brainstem lesions are usually present at the time of near-fatal respiratory failure. The lesions may resolve after several months, or they may progress to cavitary gliosis. Mild or absent basal ganglia lesions with bilateral subthalamic nuclei and brainstem lesions may suggest cytochrome c oxidase (COX) deficiency and underlying SURF1 gene mutations. The white matter is spared in Leigh syndrome,

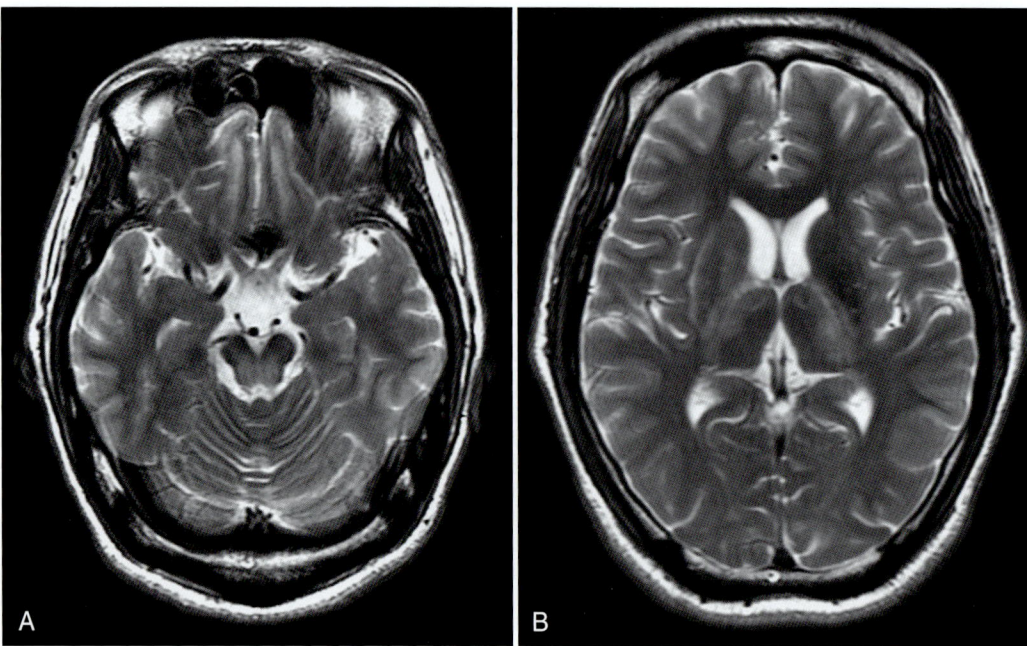

Figure 10-19 Wilson disease. T2-weighted images showing symmetric areas of hyperintensity in the putamina, thalami, and midbrain. (Case courtesy of Yvonne W. Lui, MD, Montefiore Medical Center, New York, NY.)

BOX 10-19 Hepatolenticular Degeneration (Wilson Disease)

- Autosomal recessive
- Deficient ceruloplasmin (serum transport protein for copper) due to ATP7B mutation on chromosome 13q14.3-q21.1

---

in contrast to the diffuse white matter and brainstem involvement of maple syrup urine disease (Box 10-20).

Is the Cortex Also Abnormal?
Creutzfeldt-Jakob disease is a rapidly progressive, fatal, potentially transmissible spongiform encephalopathy caused by prion infection. Both deep and superficial gray matter structures, including the caudate nuclei, putamina, thalami, and cerebral cortex, show T2 hyperintensity and diffusion restriction (Figure 10-22). Symmetric hyperintensity of the dorsomedial and pulvinar thalamic nuclei (hockey-stick sign) is characteristic for new variant Creutzfeldt-Jakob disease. The globi pallidi are usually spared.

Globus Pallidus

Are the Globi Pallidi Too Dark?
The metal deposition diseases typically cause symmetric areas of T2 hypointensity in the globi pallidi, among other structures. Neurodegeneration with brain iron deposition (NBIA) may show an eye-of-the-tiger appearance due to focal anterior medial hyperintensity in the otherwise hypointense globi pallidi (see below). Wilson disease is accompanied by laminar hyperintensity of the putamina. Hypothyroidism in children (endemic neurologic cretinism) may also show hypointensity of the globi pallidi and substantia nigra. Chronic hemochromatosis may show globus pallidus hypointensity.

Are the Globi Pallidi Too Bright?
KSS and chronic progressive external ophthalmoplegia are related diseases that involve both gray and white matter structures. Patients classically present with abnormal globi pallidi and subcortical white matter; the typical involvement of the subcortical U fibers and sparing of the central or periventricular white matter are important features distinguishing KSS from the leukodystrophies. Areas of T2 hyperintensity may be seen in the other basal ganglia structures, thalamus, brainstem tegmentum, and cerebellar white matter (Figure 10-23). Diffuse atrophy is the most common imaging finding, with good correlation between the severity of cerebellar atrophy and cerebellar signs and symptoms but poor correlation between cerebral and brainstem atrophy. Increased lactate in the abnormal white matter supports the mitochondrial respiratory chain insufficiency theory (Box 10-21).

Cockayne syndrome is an inherited disorder of DNA repair that shows dense calcifications of the basal ganglia (particularly the globus pallidus and putamen) and dentate nuclei in the cerebellum. The basal ganglia and dentate nuclei calcifications present with hyperintense areas on T1 and hypointense areas on T2-weighted images. The basal ganglia calcifications should be distinguished from mild physiologic calcifications that occur with normal aging and other causes such as infection. Patchy areas of T2 hyperintensity are also seen in the periventricular white matter, usually with late involvement of the subcortical U fibers, and in the thalami. The diffuse white matter changes tend to spare the corpus callosum (Box 10-22).

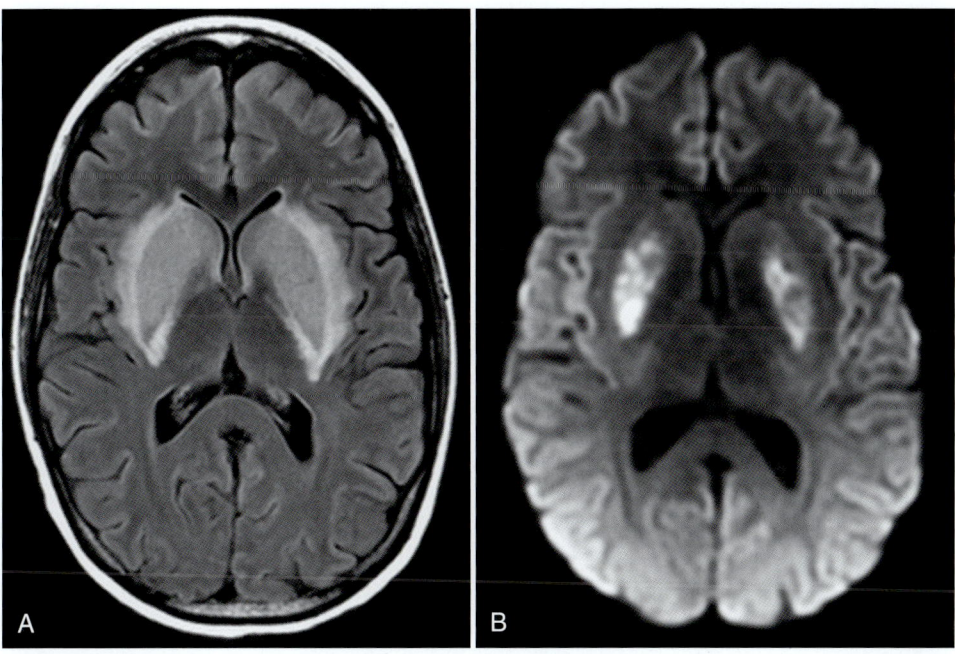

Figure 10-20 Thiamine deficiency. **A:** Fluid-attenuated inversion recovery image revealing symmetric hyperintensity and swelling of the basal ganglia. **B:** Diffusion-weighted image showing diffusion restriction in the globi pallidi and putamina.

The globus pallidus is often involved by the leukodystrophies, usually in conjunction or following the white matter lesions. Canavan disease may present with symmetric areas of T2 hyperintensity in the globi pallidi that precede the typical peripheral white matter changes.

Kernicterus or bilirubin encephalopathy in infants presents with areas of T2 hyperintensity in the globi pallidi, subthalamic nuclei, and hippocampi (Figure 10-24). A similar appearance may be found in hepatic encephalopathy and hyperalimentation (due to manganese in total parenteral nutrition). Similar appearances may be caused by methylmalonic acidemia, propionic acidemia, creatine deficiency, carbon monoxide poisoning, toxic including chemotherapeutic insults, and hypoglycemia. The toxic and ischemic exposures may often be distinguished based on the clinical scenario.

Are the Globi Pallidi Too Dark and Too Bright?

The eye-of-the-tiger sign is formed by focal anterior medial T2 hyperintensity and surrounding T2 hypointensity in the globus pallidus. The low signal intensity is due to iron deposition, whereas the central high signal intensity is due to loose tissue with axonal vacuolization. This sign is characteristic for the pantothenate kinase-associated neurodegeneration (PKAN) form of NBIA, which was formerly known as Hallervorden-Spatz syndrome (Figure 10-25). Early isolated T2 hyperintensity of the globi pallidi may also be found. PKAN patients have prevalent but late radiographic evidence of substantia nigra pars reticulata iron deposition and less marked cerebral and cerebellar atrophy than non-PKAN patients. No specific imaging features have been described for mutation-negative patients (Box 10-23).

Thalamus

Are the Thalami Too Dense/Dark?

Both Krabbe disease and GM_2 gangliosidosis (Tay-Sachs disease, Sandhoff disease) share the appearance of symmetric hyperdense thalami on CT scan. The hyperdensity and corresponding MR T1 hyperintensity and T2 hypointensity result from abnormal calcium deposition. Krabbe disease reveals hyperdensity of other structures and more extensive white matter changes that include the corpus callosum.

The hyperdense thalami of GM_2 gangliosidosis occur only in the infantile form. The diffuse patchy and confluent T2 hyperintense hemispheric white matter lesions tend to spare the internal capsule. The T2 hyperintense lesions demonstrate centripetal progression and may involve the basal ganglia, cerebellum, and brainstem. Severe cerebellar atrophy is characteristic for juvenile GM_2 gangliosidosis, which may also show mild preceding cerebral atrophy, callosal thinning, and white matter lesions (Figure 10-26). Adult GM_2 gangliosidosis may present with only progressive cerebellar atrophy and otherwise normal-appearing supratentorial structures (Box 10-24).

The metal deposition disorders, such as NBIA (Hallervorden-Spatz), may also cause T2 hypointensity of the thalamus, along with hypointensity of the basal ganglia and brainstem. Infantile NCL and variant subtype late infantile NCL may show T2 hypointensity of the thalamus, but as part of the poliodystrophies they are characterized by marked global gray matter loss and cortical atrophy.

Are the Thalami Too Bright?

Various diseases may result in T2 hyperintensity of the thalami, including the leukodystrophies (Canavan disease) and poliodystrophies (Alpers syndrome). Hyperintensity is not as useful a diagnostic sign as hypointensity.

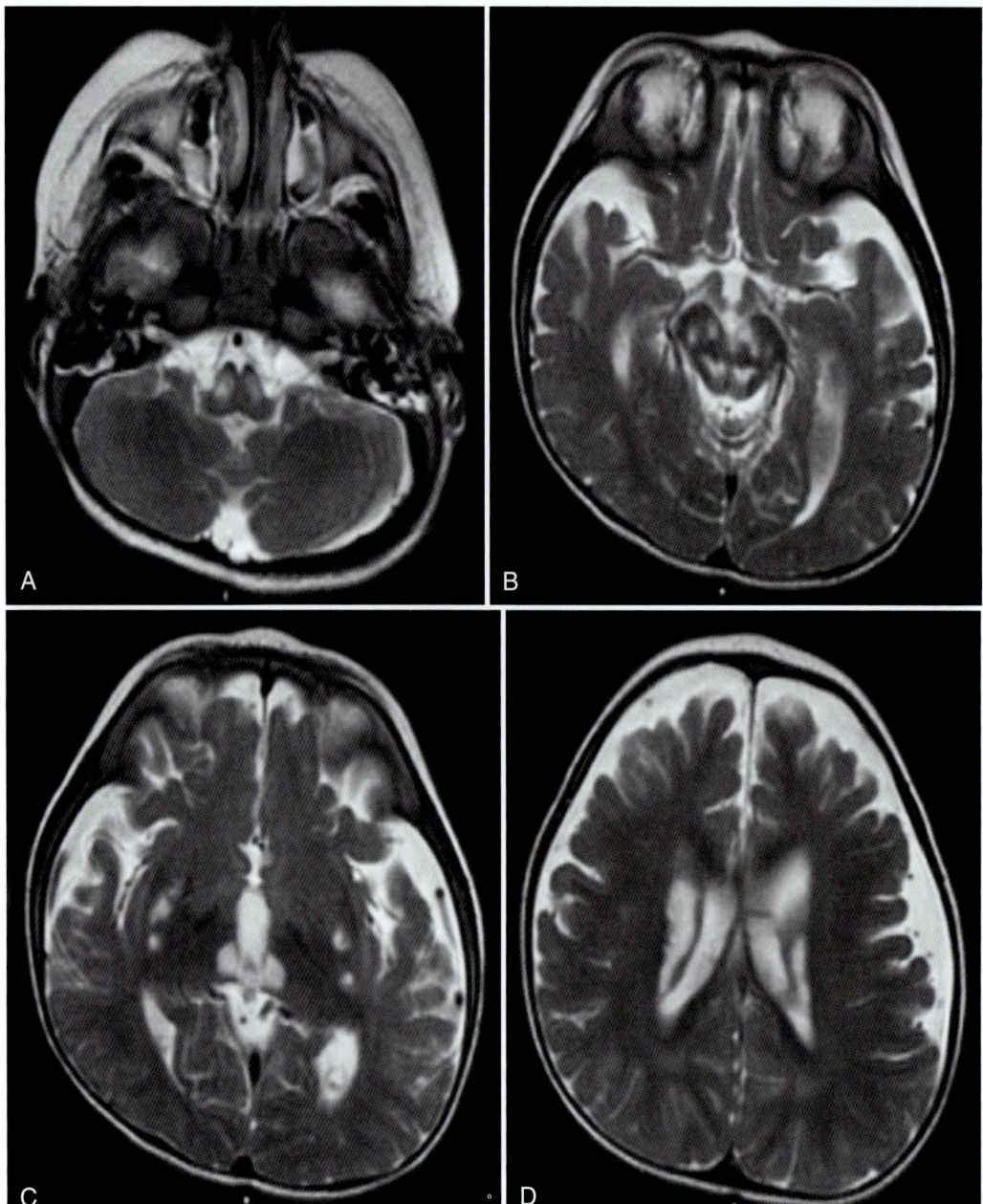

Figure 10-21 Infantile-type Leigh disease. T2-weighted images showing symmetric areas of hyperintensity in the basal ganglia, thalami, midbrain, and medulla. Abnormalities in the midbrain include the cerebral peduncles and periaqueductal gray matter. (Case courtesy of Vinh Nguyen, MD, Long Island Jewish Medical Center, New Hyde Park, NY.)

BOX 10-20 Subacute Necrotizing Encephalomyelopathy (Leigh Disease, Leigh Syndrome)

- Autosomal recessive >> X-linked or mitochondrial DNA (maternal)
- Multiple mitochondrial DNA mutations and enzyme defects, including pyruvate dehydrogenase complex deficiency and cytochrome c oxidase deficiency
- Leigh disease refers to patients with classic pathologic findings
- Leigh syndrome refers to related genetic and biochemical disorders with similar clinical features
- Infantile type presents before age 2 years with hypotonia, failure to thrive, nystagmus, and respiratory failure
- Less common juvenile and adult types present with more mild progressive neurologic problems, mental deterioration, and seizures

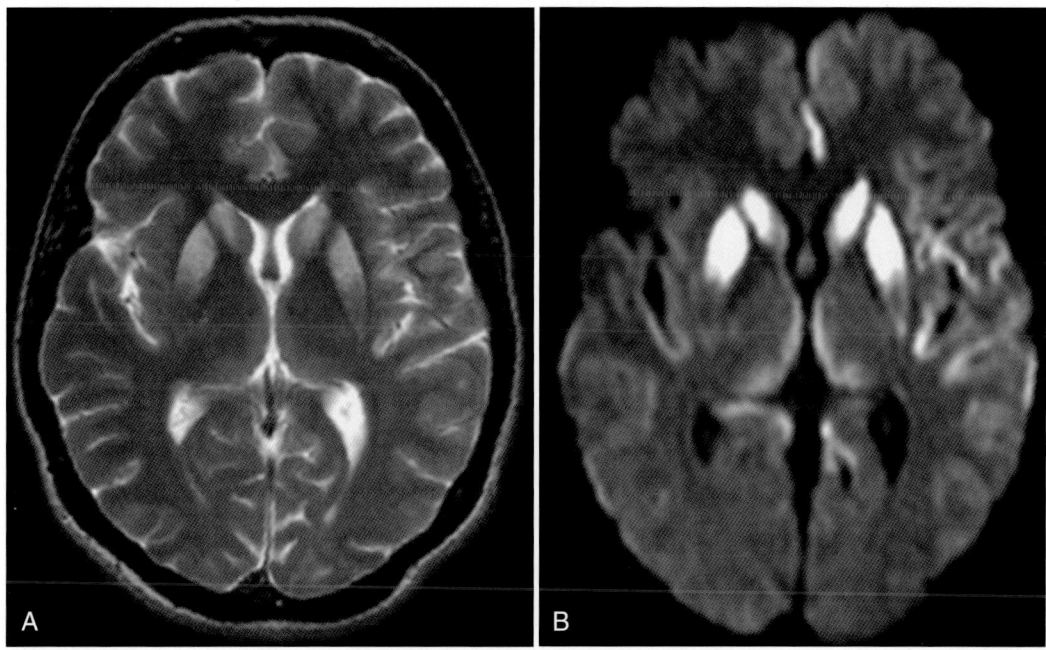

Figure 10-22 Creutzfeldt-Jakob disease. T2 (**A**) and diffusion-weighted images (**B**) showing marked hyperintense regions in the caudate nuclei, putamina, thalami, and bilateral cortices. Dorsomedial and pulvinar thalamic nuclei lesions yield the hockey-stick sign.

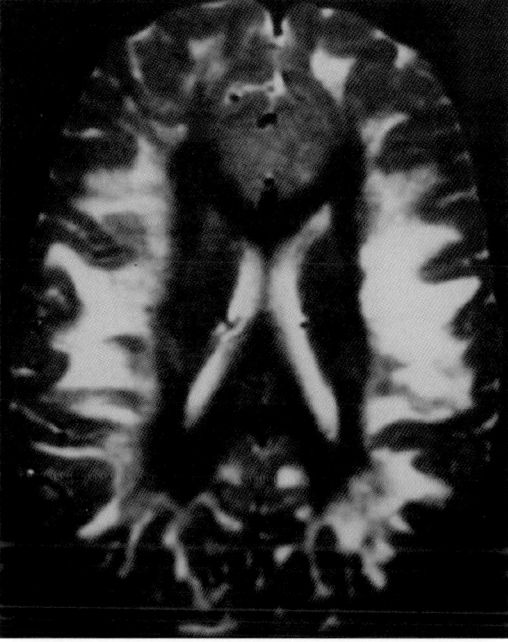

Figure 10-23 Kearns-Sayre syndrome. Axial T2-weighted image demonstrating diffuse high signal intensity regions within the corona radiata and subcortical white matter. (From Lerman-Sagie T, Leshinsky-Silver E, Watemberg N, Luckman Y, Lev D. White matter involvement in mitochondrial diseases. Mol Genet Metab 2005;84:127-136.)

BOX 10-21 Kearns-Sayre Syndrome (KSS) and Chronic Progressive external Ophthalmoplegia (CPEO)

- Pearson syndrome (hypocellular anemia and pancreatic exocrine deficiency) in infants may progress to Kearns-Sayre syndrome by school age
- KSS presents in the teenage years with progressive external ophthalmoplegia and pigmentary retinal degeneration, cardiac blockade, cerebellar signs, and sensorineural hearing loss
- KSS shares many clinical and imaging features with CPEO
- Diffuse spongiform encephalopathy of the white matter and less so the deep gray matter, brainstem, and spinal cord (spongiform degeneration may also occur in Leigh syndrome and Canavan disease)

BOX 10-22 Cockayne Syndrome

- Autosomal recessive
- Disorder of DNA repair (like ataxia-telangiectasia, Fanconi anemia)
- Characteristic facies
- Ultraviolet hypersensitivity, microcephaly, retinitis pigmentosa, cachexia

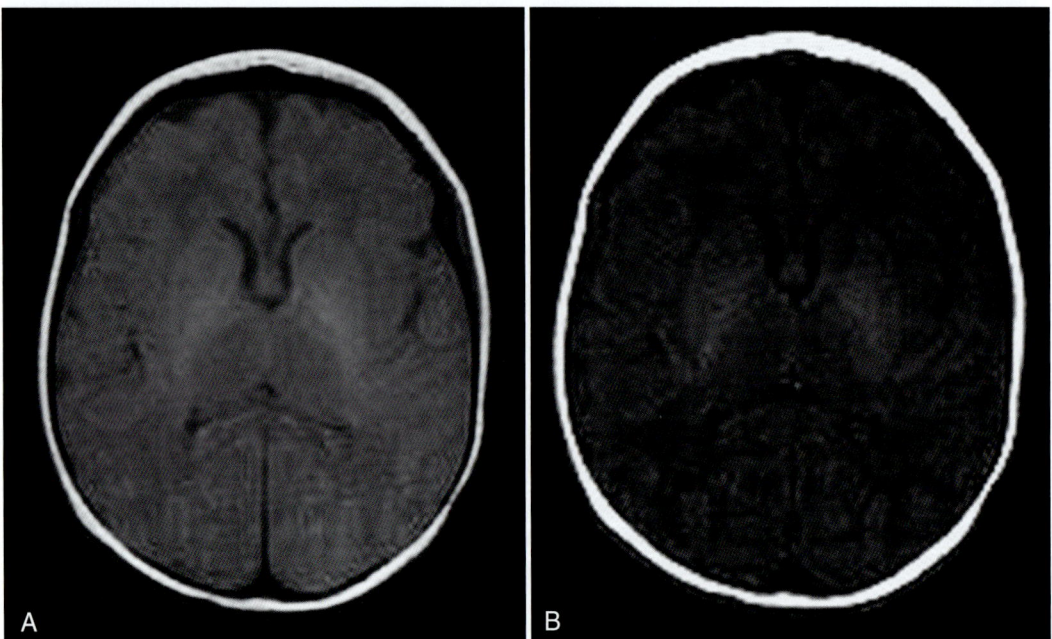

Figure 10-24 Infant with kernicterus. T1-weighted (A) and fluid-attenuated inversion recovery images (B) demonstrating symmetric regions of hyperintensity of the globi pallidi.

■ PART IV: DIFFUSION

Diffusion-weighted images (DWI) can often separate T2 hyperintense lesions into those due to vasogenic edema (facilitated diffusion) or cytotoxic edema (restricted diffusion). Facilitated diffusion is hyperintense on DWI and on ADC maps. Restricted diffusion is hyperintense on DWI and hypointense on ADC. DTI includes directional information about water diffusion, which is commonly measured as FA. The DTI metric mean diffusivity is analogous to ADC. The demyelinating leukoencephalopathies cause increased mean diffusivity and decreased FA on DTI, which may be more sensitive than conventional imaging. The diffusion findings are summarized here and are also discussed under the individual diseases.

Does the Lesion Show Facilitated Diffusion?

MELAS classically shows cortical and subcortical lesions with T2 hyperintensity and facilitated diffusion despite clinical evidence suggestive for acute infarction (Figure 10-27). The facilitated diffusion supports the defective neuronal metabolism hypothesis, in which the mitochondrial dysfunction causes anaerobic metabolism and neuronal death from acidosis. Less commonly, MELAS lesions may show restricted diffusion due to failed energy metabolism according to the vascular hypothesis, where metabolic damage to the endothelium causes small-vessel occlusion and neuronal death. Chronic MELAS reveals worsening cerebral atrophy with areas of cortical laminar necrosis and cortical and subcortical gliosis. Other diseases with facilitated diffusion include Zellweger syndrome, adrenoleukodystrophy,

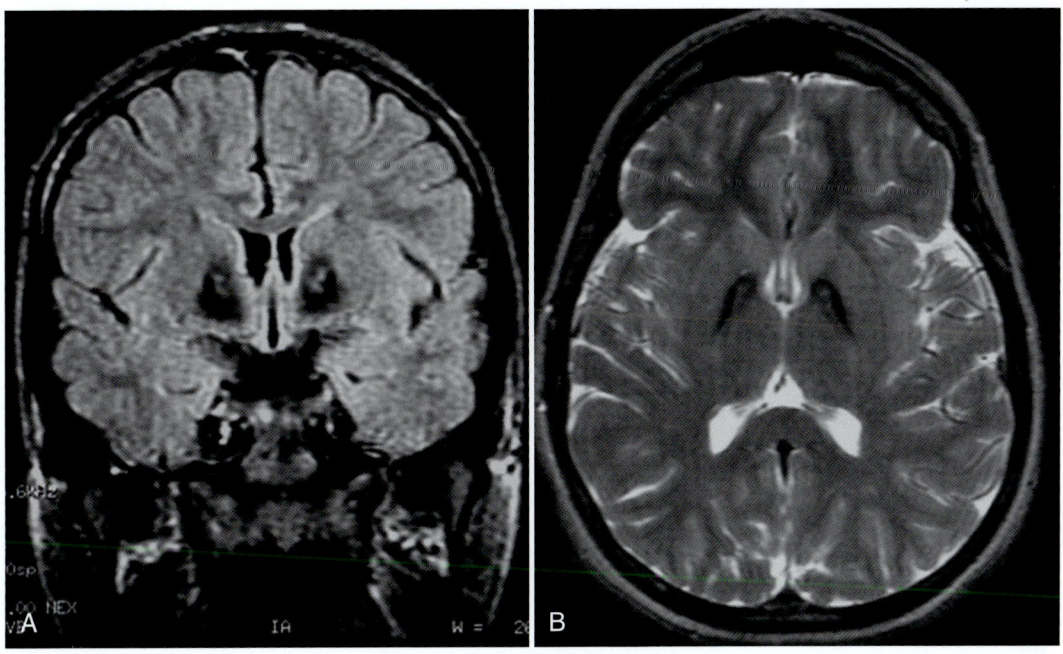

Figure 10-25 Pantothenate kinase-associated neurodegeneration, formerly known as Hallervorden-Spatz syndrome. Coronal fluid-attenuated inversion recovery (**A**) and axial T2-weighted images (**B**) showing classic hypointensity in the globus pallidus with anterior medial hyperintensity, the eye-of-the-tiger sign.

BOX 10-23 Neurodegeneration with Brain Iron Accumulation (NBIA)/Pantothenate Kinase-Associated Neurodegeneration (PKAN)/Hallervorden-Spatz Syndrome

- NBIA is the preferred umbrella term for autosomal recessive disorders characterized by abnormal brain iron accumulation, dystonia, and parkinsonism
- NBIA includes Hallervorden-Spatz syndrome, pantothenate kinase 2 (PANK2) deficiency, hereditary aceruloplasminemia, and neuroferritinopathy
- Classic rapidly progressive disease presents before age 10 years with dystonia and upper motor neuron signs and symptoms and intervening plateaus of stability
- Atypical disease presents at age 13 years with dystonia, psychiatric and speech disturbances, and slow disease progression
- All classic disease and one third of atypical disease have a PANK2 mutation on chromosome 20p13, which is responsible for coenzyme A biosynthesis
- PANK2 deficiency leads to accumulation of cystine-containing neurotoxins that result in edema, destruction, and iron accumulation in normally iron-rich parts of the brain

---

Krabbe disease, mucopolysaccharidosis, Lowe syndrome, Alexander disease, and van der Knaap disease. Facilitated diffusion in the leukoencephalopathies usually reflects slow progression with low-grade demyelination, tissue loss, and increased extracellular space (Box 10-25).

Does the Lesion Show Restricted Diffusion?
This finding is classic for infarction, particularly when it involves both gray and white matter in a vascular territory. Diffusion restriction may also be seen in metachromatic leukodystrophy, maple syrup urine disease, Canavan disease, phenylketonuria, Wilson disease, Cockayne syndrome, and glutaric aciduria type 1. The restricted diffusion may represent more acute ischemic, demyelinating, or vacuolating myelinopathy changes that mimic the cytotoxic edema diffusion pattern. The pattern of the diffusion restriction may vary depending upon the acuity of the lesion.

Mixed vasogenic and cytotoxic lesions may be seen in some diseases, such as MELAS. Other diseases such as Pelizaeus-Merzbacher disease may have normal diffusion imaging.

■ PART V: SPECTROSCOPY

The specificity of conventional MRI may be improved by proton MR spectroscopy, which allows in vivo semi-quantitative measurement of brain metabolites. In addition to helping to narrow the differential possibilities, spectroscopy has an important role during management of these patients to follow disease progression or treatment effects. Quantitative imaging biomarkers

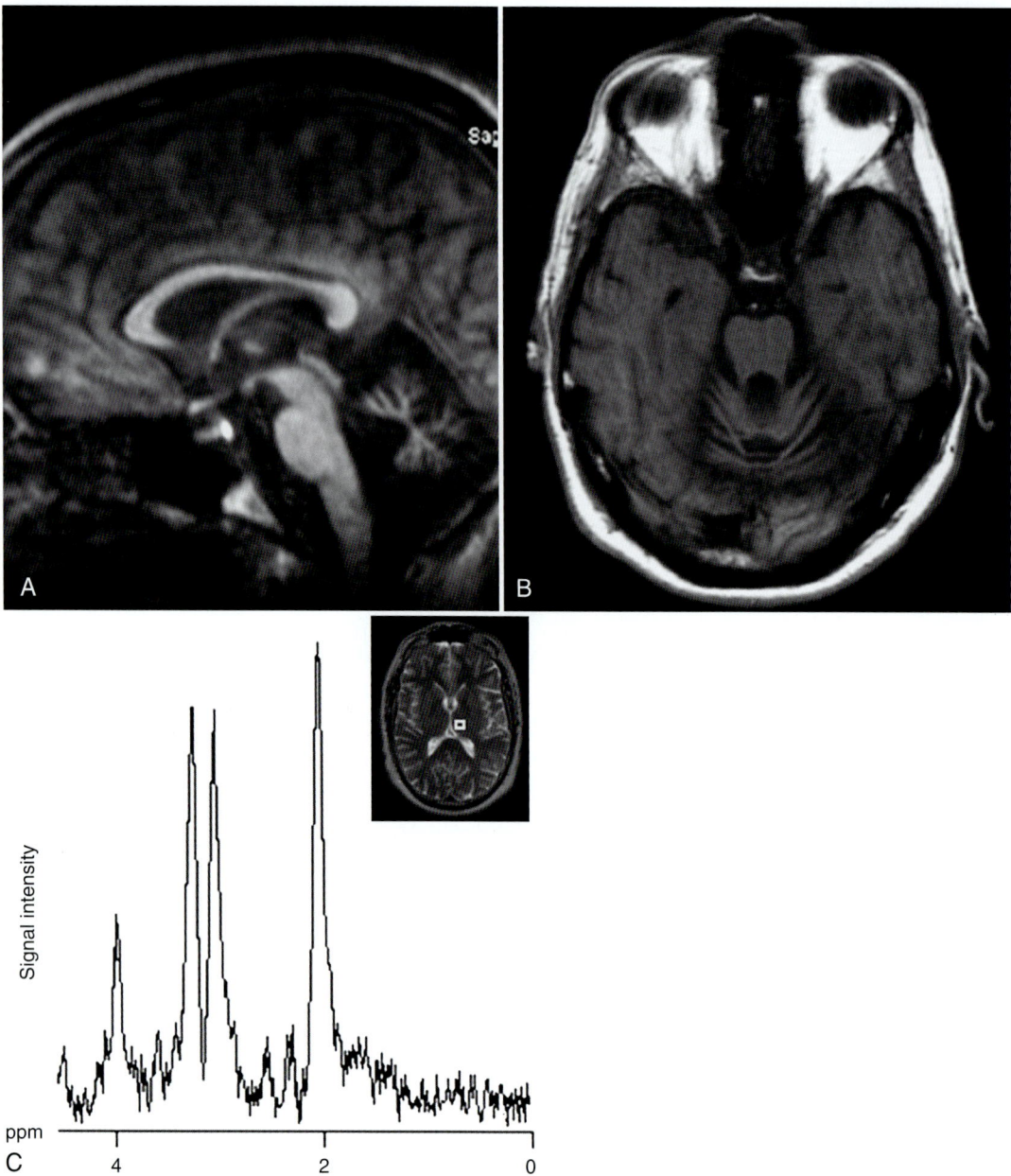

Figure 10-26 Adult form of GM_2 gangliosidosis B (Tay-Sachs disease) in a 47-year-old man. Sagittal **(A)** and axial T1-weighted images **(B)** showing isolated cerebellar atrophy, which may be the only abnormality seen on conventional images. (Courtesy Yvonne W. Lui, MD, Montefiore Medical Center, New York, NY.) **C:** Spectroscopy through the thalamus in another Tay-Sachs patient showing decreased N-acetylaspartate despite normal-appearing supratentorial gray and white matter structures.

BOX 10-24 GM_2 Gangliosidosis (Tay-Sachs Disease, Sandhoff Disease)

- Heterogeneous group of lysosomal storage disorders
- Autosomal recessive
- Defective sphingolipid metabolism causes abnormal accumulation of gangliosidoses
- Types B and O have discrete infantile, juvenile, and adult clinical forms
    - Earlier age of onset correlated with more rapid disease progression
    - Chronic adult form with neuropsychiatric disturbances that may mimic schizophrenia
- Type B (Tay-Sachs disease) caused by hexosaminidase A deficiency on chromosome 15q23-q24
- Type O (Sandhoff disease) caused by hexosaminidase A and B deficiency on chromosome 5q13; is less common but clinically indistinguishable
- Type AB is rare and has only an infantile form characterized by GM_2 activator deficiency on chromosome 5

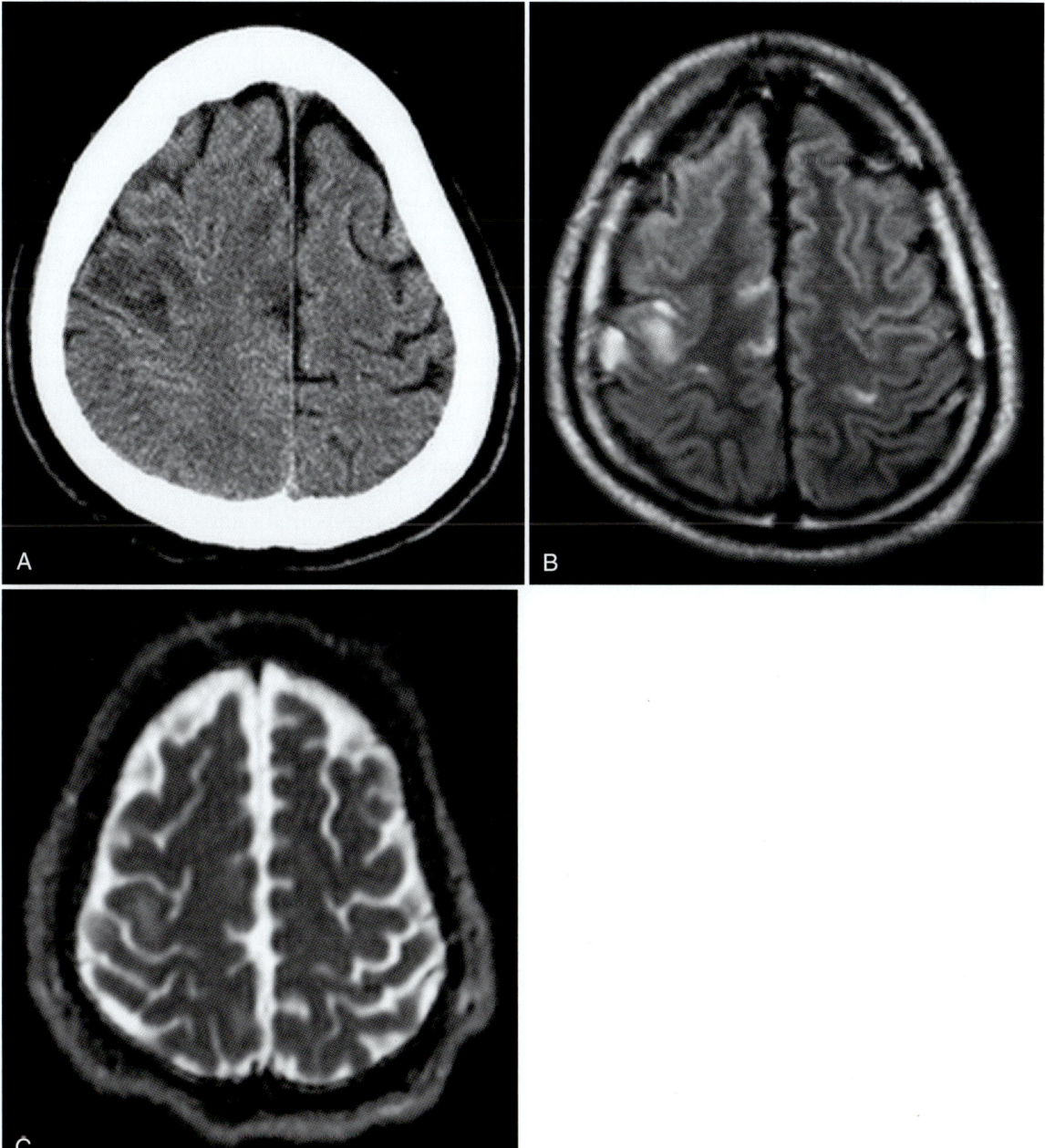

Figure 10-27 Mitochondrial myopathy, encephalopathy, lactic acidosis, and stroke (MELAS). Computed tomography **(A)**, fluid-attenuated inversion recovery **(B)**, and apparent diffusion coefficient (ADC) images **(C)** showing multiple bilateral cortical and subcortical stroke-like lesions in a nonvascular distribution in the frontal and parietal lobes. The typical facilitated diffusion (high ADC signal) reflects vasogenic edema, compared to the restricted diffusion and cytotoxic edema of acute infarction.

BOX 10-25   Mitochondrial Myopathy, Encephalopathy, Lactic Acidosis, and Stroke-Like Episodes (MELAS)

- Most common inherited mitochondrial abnormality
- Primary neuronal oxidative metabolic disturbance
- A3243G >> A8344G mitochondrial DNA mutations
    - Same mutation also causes mitochondrial epilepsy with ragged red fibers and chronic progressive external ophthalmoplegia
- Stroke-like episodes before age 40 years, seizures, dementia, and lactic acidosis
- Usually presents with gray and white matter lesions
- Fluctuating stroke-like events in the cortical gray matter and subcortical white matter in a nonvascular distribution, particularly in the temporal parietal and occipital lobes
- May have isolated or symmetric involvement of the basal ganglia (similar to Leigh syndrome)

Table 10-4 Common Compounds Resolved by Clinical Magnetic Resonance Spectroscopy

Major Compounds	Parts per Million (ppm)
Myoinositol (mI)	3.56
Choline (Cho)	3.22
Creatine (Cr)	3.03
Glutamine/glutamate (Glx)	2.2–2.4
N-acetylaspartate (NAA)	2.02
Lactate (Lac)	1.33

using conventional and spectroscopic MRI will be important tools for novel genetic and stem cell therapies approaching clinical trials.

The common metabolites demonstrated on routine clinical MR spectroscopy are summarized in Table 10-4. NAA is a marker of neuronal density and viability that is decreased in most disease processes. Creatine (Cr) and creatine phosphate are markers of cellular energetics and may be decreased due to higher metabolic demand and energy consumption. Choline (Cho) is a membrane turnover marker consisting of phosphorylcholine and glycerophosphorylcholine, which may be increased by accelerated membrane synthesis and myelination or breakdown. Lactate, which is normally not resolved, is elevated by anaerobic glycosis. Lipid is increased by cellular breakdown and necrosis. Glutamate is an excitatory neurotransmitter, γ-aminobutyric acid (GABA) precursor, and intermediate of amino acid metabolism. Myoinositol (mI) is found in glial cells and may be increased by myelin breakdown products, glial proliferation, and gliosis.

The leukodystrophies present three main spectroscopic metabolic patterns, which correlate with the underlying pathophysiologic mechanism:
1. The hypomyelination disorders show normal or near-normal spectra indicating relatively preserved membrane turnover and axonal density in the white matter despite deficient deposition of myelin. For example, Pelizaeus-Merzbacher syndrome may show relatively normal spectra despite extensive white matter disease.
2. The demyelination disorders are characterized by increases in Cho, Cho/NAA, and Cho/Cr, and decreases in NAA. Cho increases are due to membrane turnover, accumulation of myelin breakdown products, and presence of inflammatory cells. NAA decreases result from loss of neuronal cells.
3. The vacuolization disorders show overall decreases in Cho, Cr, and NAA due to rarefaction, cystic degeneration, and neuronal and axonal loss. MLC is an example.

Is NAA Increased?

An increase in NAA is pathognomonic for Canavan disease because virtually all other diseases result in nonspecific decreases in NAA (Figure 10-8). Canavan disease is caused by deficiency of the aspartoacyclase enzyme, which causes the abnormal neurotoxic accumulation of NAA in the brain and urine. Alexander disease, which can also present with macrocephaly and have early subcortical U-fiber involvement, is among the innumerable diseases that show decreased NAA.

Is NAA Decreased?

The combination of decreased NAA and increased Cho is the most common and therefore least specific spectroscopic pattern. Decreases in NAA reflect neuronal loss and increases in Cho demyelination and inflammation. This may be seen in both malignant (neoplastic) and nonneoplastic diseases. In addition to the demyelinating leukodystrophies, other metabolic disorders that may display this pattern include NCL, NBIA/PKAN2, MERRF, MELAS, Huntington, mucopolysaccharidosis, adrenoleukodystrophy, and GM_2 gangliosidosis (Figure 10-2). MERRF and MELAS often show decreased NAA/Cr and NAA/Cho. Adrenoleukodystrophy may show spectroscopic abnormalities even in areas that appear normal on T2-weighted and FA maps. GM_2 gangliosidosis may also reveal decreases in NAA in the normal-appearing gray and white matter structures (Figure 10-26).

Decreased NAA and decreased Cr may be seen in the PKAN form of NBIA. Spectroscopy in these patients is complicated by the high iron concentration, which may broaden the calculated metabolite signals and alter the baseline values.

Is Lactate Present?

The mitochondrial disorders often present with lactic acidemia, variable encephalopathy, and myopathy. They include Leigh syndrome, MERRF, MELAS, pyruvate dehydrogenase complex deficiency, and respiratory chain complex enzyme deficiency. Increases in lactate are also common to many extramitochondrial neurodegenerative disorders, as a result of increased reliance on the glycolytic pathway due to abnormal oxidative phosphorylation.

Leigh syndrome shows increased lactate in the basal ganglia, brainstem, and occipital cortex. This CNS lactate elevation may occur in the setting of normal peripheral lactate. These lesions will also have increased Cho, thought to reflect demyelinating changes even in the normal-appearing white matter. Increased lactate and Cho and decreased NAA, although not particularly specific, may help distinguish Leigh syndrome from similar-appearing basal ganglia disorders, such as maple syrup urine disease and Wilson disease. Finding lactate in normal-appearing brain in both Leigh syndrome and MELAS can help distinguish these disorders from other mitochondrial disorders such as KSS.

Acute MELAS lesions will have increased lactate and Cho and decreased NAA. These changes return to baseline parallel with improved symptoms. Less marked abnormalities can be found even in patients without focal signal abnormalities on MRI. Increased CSF lactate in the lateral ventricle has been correlated with the degree of chronic neurologic impairment. Lactate may decrease with resolving symptoms.

Increased lactate may also be seen in maple syrup urine disease, methylmalonic acidemia, glutaric acidemia type II.

Is Myoinositol Increased?

Infantile NCL shows an early and persistent increase in mI, even after 4 years when there is a uniform decrease in all main metabolites. Early increases in mI, Cho, and glutamine/glutamate (Glx) may reflect glial proliferation, demyelination, and gliosis, and decreases in NAA neuronal loss and/or damage. Spectroscopy of the thalamus is thought to have better correlation with disease severity than spectroscopy of the white matter or cortex. Lactate and lipids may be observed at 4 years.

GM_2 gangliosidosis (Tay-Sachs disease, Sandhoff disease) show increased mI reflecting gliosis due to toxic accumulation of GM_2 gangliosides.

Alexander disease reveals a prominent increase in mI due to intense gliosis. This is accompanied by decreased NAA, increased Cho, and increased lactate, with abnormalities more obvious in the frontal lobes that correlate with the usual anteroposterior progression of disease.

Metachromatic leukodystrophy demonstrate an increase in mI due to the increase of phosphatidylinositol in myelin, particularly in patients with severe disease.

Lowe syndrome has increased mI that may be due to gliosis and possibly abnormal accumulation of phosphatidylinositol 4,5-biphosphate (Figure 10-7).

NBIA may show an increase in mI in the deep cerebral white matter.

Is Glx Increased?

Huntington disease may show increases in mI and Glx in the striatum from glutamate excitotoxicity. The striatum may also demonstrate asymmetric increases in lactate, left greater than right, due to asymmetric basal ganglia activity during motor performance in right-handed subjects. Increased lactate in the occipital and frontal lobes may represent similar defective oxidative phosphorylation. The decreased NAA and increased lactate in the striatum correlate with symptom duration and increased CAG repeat length. Cr may be a more sensitive marker in juvenile and presymptomatic Huntington disease. Spectroscopy in preclinical mutation carriers is usually normal.

Proprionic acidemia, an organic acidemia due to an inborn error of propionyl coenzyme A (CoA) carboxylase, causes increased Glx in the basal ganglia. This is thought to reflect hyperammonemia and increased excitotoxic damage. Patients may also show decreases in NAA and mI, and increases in lactate.

Is There an Extra Peak?

At 7.36 ppm, a specific peak of brain phenylalanine concentration may be seen in phenylketonuria.

At 5.25 ppm and 4.57 ppm, doublets corresponding to galactitol are found in galactosemia.

At 3.7 ppm, a broad peak may be caused by the accumulated glycosaminoglycans of some forms of the mucopolysaccharidoses. Spectroscopy may otherwise show decreased NAA, decreased NAA/Cr, and increased Cho/Cr. Patients with cognitive impairment have higher mI/Cr levels than those without cognitive impairment.

At 3.56 ppm, nonketotic hyperglycemia shows an abnormal peak that may be separated from the normal mI peak by long echo spectroscopy.

At 2.42 ppm, a 3-hydroxy-isovalerate and/or 3-hydroxy-3-methylglutarate specific peak may be seen in hydroxymethylglutaryl (HMG)-CoA lyase deficiency.

At 0.9 to 1.0 ppm, a specific peak may be found during decompensation of maple syrup urine disease.

■ CONCLUSION

The metabolic diseases represent a diverse group of inherited and acquired disorders, which are variably classified according to the genetic, phenotypic, histopathologic, or biochemical defect. Despite often nonspecific, overlapping clinical, laboratory, and radiographic appearances, many disorders have distinctive features that can be used to suggest a specific diagnosis or at least narrow the differential possibilities to direct additional testing. Advanced imaging techniques, such as MR diffusion and spectroscopy, offer additional tools to improve the sensitivity and characterization of the metabolic diseases. MR spectroscopy in particular adds valuable information through the in vivo measurement and tracking of specific brain metabolites to aid the diagnosis, prognosis, and management of these patients.

Suggested Readings

A novel gene containing a trinucleotide repeat that is expanded and unstable on Huntington's disease chromosomes. The Huntington's Disease Collaborative Research Group. *Cell.* Mar 26 1993;72(6):971-983.

Adachi M, Kawanami T, Ohshima F, Hosoya T. MR findings of cerebral white matter in Cockayne syndrome. *Magn Reson Med Sci.* Apr 2006;5(1):41-45.

Arii J, Tanabe Y. Leigh syndrome: serial MR imaging and clinical follow-up. *AJNR Am J Neuroradiol.* Sep 2000;21(8):1502-1509.

Austin J, McAfee D, Armstrong D, O'Rourke M, Shearer L, Bachhawat B. Abnormal sulphatase activities in two human diseases (metachromatic leucodystrophy and gargoylism). *Biochem J.* Nov 1964;93(2):15C-17C.

Austin JH. Metachromatic form of diffuse cerebral sclerosis. III. Significance of sulfatide and other lipid abnormalities in white matter and kidney. *Neurology.* May 1960;10:470-483.

Autti T, Raininko R, Santavuori P, Vanhanen SL, Poutanen VP, Haltia M. MRI of neuronal ceroid lipofuscinosis. II. Postmortem MRI and histopathological study of the brain in 16 cases of neuronal ceroid lipofuscinosis of juvenile or late infantile type. *Neuroradiology.* May 1997;39(5):371-377.

Aydin K, Bakir B, Tatli B, Terzibasioglu E, Ozmen M. Proton MR spectroscopy in three children with Tay-Sachs disease. *Pediatr Radiol.* Nov 2005;35(11):1081-1085.

Bajaj NP, Waldman A, Orrell R, Wood NW, Bhatia KP. Familial adult onset of Krabbe's disease resembling hereditary spastic paraplegia with normal neuroimaging. *J Neurol Neurosurg Psychiatry.* May 2002;72(5):635-638.

Barkovich AJ, Good WV, Koch TK, Berg BO. Mitochondrial disorders: analysis of their clinical and imaging characteristics. *AJNR Am J Neuroradiol.* Sep-Oct 1993;14(5):1119-1137.

Barkovich AJ, Peck WW. MR of Zellweger syndrome. *AJNR Am J Neuroradiol.* Jun-Jul 1997;18(6):1163-1170.

Beglinger LJ, Nopoulos PC, Jorge RE, et al. White matter volume and cognitive dysfunction in early Huntington's disease. *Cogn Behav Neurol.* Jun 2005;18(2):102-107.

Bergman AJ, Van der Knaap MS, Smeitink JA, et al. Magnetic resonance imaging and spectroscopy of the brain in propionic acidemia: clinical and biochemical considerations. *Pediatr Res.* 1996;40(3):404-409.

Bernal OG, Lenn N. Multiple cranial nerve enhancement in early infantile Krabbe's disease. *Neurology.* Jun 27 2000;54(12):2348-2349.

Berry GT, Hunter JV, Wang Z, et al. In vivo evidence of brain galactitol accumulation in an infant with galactosemia and encephalopathy. *J Pediatr.* Feb 2001;138(2):260-262.

Bizzi A, Castelli G, Bugiani M, et al. Classification of childhood white matter disorders using proton MR spectroscopic imaging. *AJNR Am J Neuroradiol.* Aug 2008;29(7):1270-1275.

Boor PK, de Groot K, Waisfisz Q, et al. MLC1: a novel protein in distal astroglial processes. *J Neuropathol Exp Neurol.* May 2005;64(5):412-419.

Brockmann K, Dechent P, Meins M, et al. Cerebral proton magnetic resonance spectroscopy in infantile Alexander disease. *J Neurol.* 2003;250(3):300-306.

Brockmann K, Finsterbusch J, Terwey B, Frahm J, Hanefeld F. Megalencephalic leukoencephalopathy with subcortical cysts in an adult: quantitative proton MR spectroscopy and diffusion tensor MRI. *Neuroradiology.* Mar 2003;45(3):137-142.

Castillo M, Kwock L, Green C. MELAS syndrome: imaging and proton MR spectroscopic findings. *AJNR Am J Neuroradiol.* Feb 1995;16(2):233-239.

Choksi V, Hoeffner E, Karaarslan E, Yalcinkaya C, Cakirer S. Infantile Refsum disease: case report. *AJNR Am J Neuroradiol.* Nov-Dec 2003;24(10):2082-2084.

Chu BC, Terae S, Takahashi C, et al. MRI of the brain in the Kearns-Sayre syndrome: report of four cases and a review. *Neuroradiology.* Oct 1999;41(10):759-764.

Chuang DT, Chuang JL, Wynn RM. Lessons from genetic disorders of branched-chain amino acid metabolism. *J Nutr.* Jan 2006;136(suppl 1):243S-249S.

Demaerel P, Wilms G, Verdru P, Carton H, Baert AL. MR findings in globoid cell leucodystrophy. *Neuroradiology.* 1990;32(6):520-522.

Dezortova M, Hajek M. ^{1}H MR spectroscopy in pediatrics. *Eur J Radiol.* 2008;67(2):240-249.

Ducreux D, Nasser G, Lacroix C, Adams D, Lasjaunias P. MR diffusion tensor imaging, fiber tracking, and single-voxel spectroscopy findings in an unusual MELAS case. *AJNR Am J Neuroradiol.* August 1, 2005;26(7):1840-1844.

Dyke JP, Voss HU, Sondhi D, et al. Assessing disease severity in late infantile neuronal ceroid lipofuscinosis using quantitative MR diffusion-weighted imaging. *AJNR Am J Neuroradiol.* August 1, 2007;28(7):1232-1236.

Eichler FS, Itoh R, Barker PB, et al. Proton MR spectroscopy and diffusion tensor brain MR imaging in X-linked adrenoleukodystrophy: initial experience. *Radiology.* Oct 2002;225(1):245-252.

Engelbrecht V, Scherer A, Rassek M, Witsack HJ, Modder U. Diffusion-weighted MR imaging in the brain in children: findings in the normal brain and in the brain with white matter diseases. *Radiology.* Feb 2002;222(2):410-418.

Fabrizi GM, Cardaioli E, Grieco GS, et al. The A to G transition at nt 3243 of the mitochondrial tRNALeu(UUR) may cause an MERRF syndrome. *J Neurol Neurosurg Psychiatry.* Jul 1996;61(1):47-51.

Faerber EN, Poussaint TY. Magnetic resonance of metabolic and degenerative diseases in children. *Top Magn Reson Imaging.* Feb 2002;13(1):3-21.

Farina L, Pareyson D, Minati L, et al. Can MR imaging diagnose adult-onset Alexander disease? *AJNR Am J Neuroradiol.* Jun 2008;29(6):1190-1196.

Flanigan KM, Johns DR. Association of the 11778 mitochondrial DNA mutation and demyelinating disease. *Neurology.* Dec 1993;43(12):2720-2722.

Gabrielli O, Polonara G, Regnicolo L, et al. Correlation between cerebral MRI abnormalities and mental retardation in patients with mucopolysaccharidoses. *Am J Med Genet A.* 2004;125A(3):224-231.

Garbern J, Cambi F, Shy M, Kamholz J. The molecular pathogenesis of Pelizaeus-Merzbacher disease. *Arch Neurol.* Oct 1999;56(10):1210-1214.

Gelal F, Calli C, Apaydin M, Erdem G. van der Knaap's leukoencephalopathy: report of five new cases with emphasis on diffusion-weighted MRI findings. *Neuroradiology.* Jul 2002;44(7):625-630.

Grodd W, Krageloh-Mann I, Klose U, Sauter R. Metabolic and destructive brain disorders in children: findings with localized proton MR spectroscopy. *Radiology.* 1991;181(1):173-181.

Halliday GM, McRitchie DA, Macdonald V, Double KL, Trent RJ, McCusker E. Regional specificity of brain atrophy in Huntington's disease. *Exp Neurol.* Dec 1998;154(2):663-672.

Harris RA, Joshi M, Jeoung NH. Mechanisms responsible for regulation of branched-chain amino acid catabolism. *Biochem Biophys Res Commun.* Jan 9 2004;313(2):391-396.

Hayflick SJ, Hartman M, Coryell J, Gitschier J, Rowley H. Brain MRI in neurodegeneration with brain iron accumulation with and without PANK2 mutations. *AJNR Am J Neuroradiol.* Jun-Jul 2006;27(6):1230-1233.

Hayflick SJ, Westaway SK, Levinson B, et al. Genetic, clinical, and radiographic delineation of Hallervorden-Spatz syndrome. *N Engl J Med.* Jan 2 2003;348(1):33-40.

Henseler M, Klein A, Reber M, Vanier MT, Landrieu P, Sandhoff K. Analysis of a splice-site mutation in the sap-precursor gene of a patient with metachromatic leukodystrophy. *Am J Hum Genet.* Jan 1996;58(1):65-74.

Huang CC, Kuo HC, Chu CC, Liou CW, Ma YS, Wei YH. Clinical phenotype, prognosis and mitochondrial DNA mutation load in mitochondrial encephalomyopathies. *J Biomed Sci.* 2002;9(6 Pt 1):527-533.

Inglese M, Nusbaum AO, Pastores GM, Gianutsos J, Kolodny EH, Gonen O. MR imaging and proton spectroscopy of neuronal injury in late-onset GM_2 gangliosidosis. *AJNR Am J Neuroradiol.* Sep 2005;26(8):2037-2042.

Ito S, Shirai W, Asahina M, Hattori T. Clinical and brain MR imaging features focusing on the brain stem and cerebellum in patients with myoclonic epilepsy with ragged-red fibers due to mitochondrial A8344G mutation. *AJNR Am J Neuroradiol.* Feb 2008;29(2):392-395.

Jenkins BG, Koroshetz WJ, Beal MF, Rosen BR. Evidence for impairment of energy metabolism in vivo in Huntington's disease using localized ^{1}H NMR spectroscopy. *Neurology.* Dec 1993;43(12):2689-2695.

Johnston MV, Hoon Jr AH. Possible mechanisms in infants for selective basal ganglia damage from asphyxia, kernicterus, or mitochondrial encephalopathies. *J Child Neurol.* Sep 2000;15(9):588-591.

Jones BV, Barron TF, Towfighi J. Optic nerve enlargement in Krabbe's disease. *AJNR Am J Neuroradiol.* Aug 1999;20(7):1228-1231.

Kaback MM, Howell RR. Infantile metachromatic leukodystrophy. *N Engl J Med.* Jun 11 1970;282(24):1336-1340.

Kamada K, Takeuchi F, Houkin K, et al. Reversible brain dysfunction in MELAS: MEG, and (1)H MRS analysis. *J Neurol Neurosurg Psychiatry.* May 2001;70(5):675-678.

Kang PB, Hunter JV, Kaye EM. Lactic acid elevation in extramitochondrial childhood neurodegenerative diseases. *J Child Neurol.* 2001;16(9):657-660.

Kaufmann P, Shungu DC, Sano MC, et al. Cerebral lactic acidosis correlates with neurological impairment in MELAS. *Neurology.* April 27, 2004;62(8):1297-1302.

Kim TS, Kim IO, Kim WS, et al. MR of childhood metachromatic leukodystrophy. *AJNR Am J Neuroradiol.* Apr 1997;18(4):733-738.

Kovacs GG, Hoftberger R, Majtenyi K, et al. Neuropathology of white matter disease in Leber's hereditary optic neuropathy. *Brain.* 2005;128(1):35-41.

Kreis R, Pietz J, Penzien J, Herschkowitz N, Boesch C. Identification and quantitation of phenylalanine in the brain of patients with phenylketonuria by means of localized in vivo ^{1}H magnetic-resonance spectroscopy. *J Magn Reson B.* 1995;107(3):242-251.

Krivit W, Shapiro E, Kennedy W, et al. Treatment of late infantile metachromatic leukodystrophy by bone marrow transplantation. *N Engl J Med.* Jan 4 1990;322(1):28-32.

Kwan E, Drace J, Enzmann D. Specific CT findings in Krabbe disease. *AJR Am J Roentgenol.* Sep 1984;143(3):665-670.

Lerman-Sagie T, Leshinsky-Silver E, Watemberg N, Luckman Y, Lev D. White matter involvement in mitochondrial diseases. *Mol Genet Metab.* 2005;84(2):127-136.

Loes DJ, Peters C, Krivit W. Globoid cell leukodystrophy: distinguishing early-onset from late-onset disease using a brain MR imaging scoring method. *AJNR Am J Neuroradiol.* February 1, 1999;20(2):316-323.

Lucotte G, Turpin JC, Riess O, et al. Confidence intervals for predicted age of onset, given the size of (CAG)n repeat, in Huntington's disease. *Hum Genet.* Feb 1995;95(2):231-232.

MacQueen GM, Rosebush PI, Mazurek MF. *Neuropsychiatric Aspects of the Adult Variant of Tay-Sachs Disease. J Neuropsychiatry Clin Neurosci.* February 1, 1998;10(1):10-19.

Maegawa GH, Stockley T, Tropak M, et al. The natural history of juvenile or subacute GM_2 gangliosidosis: 21 new cases and literature review of 134 previously reported. *Pediatrics.* Nov 2006;118(5):e1550-1562.

Maia Jr AC, da Rocha AJ, da Silva CJ, Rosemberg S. Multiple cranial nerve enhancement: a new MR imaging finding in metachromatic leukodystrophy. *AJNR Am J Neuroradiol.* Jun-Jul 2007;28(6):999.

Man PY, Turnbull DM, Chinnery PF. Leber hereditary optic neuropathy. *J Med Genet.* Mar 2002;39(3):162-169.

Martin JJ, Leroy JG, Ceuterick C, Libert J, Dodinval P, Martin L. Fetal Krabbe leukodystrophy. A morphologic study of two cases. *Acta Neuropathol.* 1981;53(2):87-91.

Matheus MG, Castillo M, Smith JK, Armao D, Towle D, Muenzer J. Brain MRI findings in patients with mucopolysaccharidosis types I and II and mild clinical presentation. *Neuroradiology.* Aug 2004;46(8):666-672.

Mehndiratta MM, Agarwal P, Tatke M, Krishnamurthy M. Neurological mitochondrial cytopathies. *Neurol India.* Jun 2002;50(2):162-167.

Moller HE, Kurlemann G, Putzler M, Wiedermann D, Hilbich T, Fiedler B. Magnetic resonance spectroscopy in patients with MELAS. *J Neurol Sci.* Mar 15 2005;229-230:131-139.

Morton DH, Strauss KA, Robinson DL, Puffenberger EG, Kelley RI. Diagnosis and treatment of maple syrup disease: a study of 36 patients. *Pediatrics.* Jun 2002;109(6):999-1008.

Moser H, Dubey P, Fatemi A. Progress in X-linked adrenoleukodystrophy. *Curr Opin Neurol.* Jun 2004;17(3):263-269.

Moser HW, Loes DJ, Melhem ER, et al. X-Linked adrenoleukodystrophy: overview and prognosis as a function of age and brain magnetic resonance imaging abnormality. A study involving 372 patients. *Neuropediatrics.* Oct 2000;31(5):227-239.

Moser HW. Adrenoleukodystrophy: phenotype, genetics, pathogenesis and therapy. *Brain.* Aug 1997;120(Pt 8):1485-1508.

Narahara K, Takahashi Y, Murakami M, et al. Terminal 22q deletion associated with a partial deficiency of arylsulphatase A. *J Med Genet.* Jun 1992;29(6):432-433.

Novotny Jr EJ, Avison MJ, Herschkowitz N, et al. In vivo measurement of phenylalanine in human brain by proton nuclear magnetic resonance spectroscopy. *Pediatr Res.* 1995;37(2):244-249.

Oppenheim C, Galanaud D, Samson Y, et al. Can diffusion weighted magnetic resonance imaging help differentiate stroke from stroke-like events in MELAS? *J Neurol Neurosurg Psychiatry.* August 1, 2000;69(2):248-250.

Otaduy MCG, Leite CC, Lacerda MTC, et al. Proton MR Spectroscopy and Imaging of a Galactosemic Patient before and after Dietary Treatment. *AJNR Am J Neuroradiol.* January 1, 2006;27(1):204-207.

Page RA, Davie CA, MacManus D, et al. Clinical correlation of brain MRI and MRS abnormalities in patients with Wilson disease. *Neurology.* Aug 24 2004;63(4):638-643.

Parmar H, Sitoh YY, Ho L. Maple syrup urine disease: diffusion-weighted and diffusion-tensor magnetic resonance imaging findings. *J Comput Assist Tomogr*. Jan-Feb 2004;28(1):93-97.

Parry-Jones AR, Mitchell JD, Gunarwardena WJ, Shaunak S. Leber's hereditary optic neuropathy associated with multiple sclerosis: Harding's syndrome. *Pract Neurol*. 2008;8(2):118-121.

Paulsen JS, Magnotta VA, Mikos AE, et al. Brain structure in preclinical Huntington's disease. *Biol Psychiatry*. Jan 1 2006;59(1):57-63.

Pavlakis SG, Phillips PC, DiMauro S, De Vivo DC, Rowland LP. Mitochondrial myopathy, encephalopathy, lactic acidosis, and strokelike episodes: a distinctive clinical syndrome. *Ann Neurol*. Oct 1984;16(4):481-488.

Reynolds Jr NC, Prost RW, Mark LP. Heterogeneity in 1H-MRS profiles of presymptomatic and early manifest Huntington's disease. *Brain Res*. Jan 7 2005;1031(1):82-89.

Rossi A, Biancheri R, Bruno C, et al. Leigh Syndrome with COX deficiency and SURF1 gene mutations: MR imaging findings. *AJNR Am J Neuroradiol*. Jun-Jul 2003;24(6):1188-1191.

Sartor H, Loose R, Tucha O, Klein HE, Lange KW. MELAS: a neuropsychological and radiological follow-up study. Mitochondrial encephalomyopathy, lactic acidosis and stroke. *Acta Neurol Scand*. Nov 2002;106(5):309-313.

Savoiardo M, Halliday WC, Nardocci N, et al. Hallervorden-Spatz disease: MR and pathologic findings. *AJNR Am J Neuroradiol*. Jan-Feb 1993;14(1):155-162.

Schapiro M, Cecil KM, Doescher J, Kiefer AM, Jones BV. MR imaging and spectroscopy in juvenile Huntington disease. *Pediatr Radiol*. Aug 2004;34(8):640-643.

Schneider JF, Boltshauser E, Neuhaus TJ, Rauscher C, Martin E. MRI and proton spectroscopy in Lowe syndrome. *Neuropediatrics*. Feb 2001;32(1):45-48.

Schneider JF, Il'yasov KA, Boltshauser E, Hennig J, Martin E. Diffusion tensor imaging in cases of adrenoleukodystrophy: preliminary experience as a marker for early demyelination? *AJNR Am J Neuroradiol*. May 2003;24(5):819-824.

Schönberger S, Schweiger B, Schwahn B, Schwarz M, Wendel U. Dysmyelination in the brain of adolescents and young adults with maple syrup urine disease. *Mol Genet Metab*. 2004;82(1):69-75.

Seitz D, Grodd W, Schwab A, Seeger U, Klose U, Nagele T. MR imaging and localized proton MR spectroscopy in late infantile neuronal ceroid lipofuscinosis. *AJNR Am J Neuroradiol*. August 1, 1998;19(7):1373-1377.

Semnic R, Svetel M, Dragasevic N, et al. Magnetic resonance imaging morphometry of the midbrain in patients with Wilson disease. *J Comput Assist Tomogr*. Nov-Dec 2005;29(6):880-883.

Sener RN. Canavan disease: diffusion magnetic resonance imaging findings. *J Comput Assist Tomogr*. Jan-Feb 2003;27(1):30-33.

Sener RN. Diffusion magnetic resonance imaging patterns in metabolic and toxic brain disorders. *Acta Radiol*. Aug 2004;45(5):561-570.

Sener RN. Diffusion MRI findings in Wilson's disease. *Comput Med Imaging Graph*. 2003;27(1):17-21.

Sener RN. Lowe syndrome: proton MR spectroscopy, and diffusion MR imaging. *J Neuroradiol*. Jun 2004;31(3):238-240.

Sener RN. Metachromatic leukodystrophy. Diffusion MR imaging and proton MR spectroscopy. *Acta Radiol*. Jul 2003;44(4):440-443.

Sener RN. Pantothenate kinase-associated neurodegeneration: MR imaging, proton MR spectroscopy, and diffusion MR imaging findings. *AJNR Am J Neuroradiol*. Sep 2003;24(8):1690-1693.

Sener RN. Pelizaeus-Merzbacher disease: diffusion MR imaging and proton MR spectroscopy findings. *J Neuroradiol*. Mar 2004;31(2):138-141.

Seto T, Kono K, Morimoto K, et al. Brain magnetic resonance imaging in 23 patients with mucopolysaccharidoses and the effect of bone marrow transplantation. *Ann Neurol*. Jul 2001;50(1):79-92.

Sijens PE, Smit GPA, Rödiger LA, et al. MR spectroscopy of the brain in Leigh syndrome. *Brain Dev*. 2008;30(9):579-583.

Sparaco M, Simonati A, Cavallaro T, et al. MELAS: clinical phenotype and morphological brain abnormalities. *Acta Neuropathol*. Sep 2003;106(3):202-212.

Takanashi J, Sugita K, Osaka H, Ishii M, Niimi H. Proton MR spectroscopy in Pelizaeus-Merzbacher disease. *AJNR Am J Neuroradiol*. 1997;18(3):533-535.

Taylor-Robinson SD, Weeks RA, Bryant DJ, et al. Proton magnetic resonance spectroscopy in Huntington's disease: evidence in favour of the glutamate excitotoxic theory. *Mov Disord*. Mar 1996;11(2):167-173.

Teijido O, Martinez A, Pusch M, et al. Localization and functional analyses of the MLC1 protein involved in megalencephalic leukoencephalopathy with subcortical cysts. *Hum Mol Genet*. 2004;13(21):2581-2594.

van der Knaap MS, Bakker HD, Valk J. MR imaging and proton spectroscopy in 3-hydroxy-3-methylglutaryl coenzyme A lyase deficiency. *AJNR Am J Neuroradiol*. 1998;19(2):378-382.

van der Knaap MS, Naidu S, Breiter SN, et al. Alexander disease: diagnosis with MR imaging. *AJNR Am J Neuroradiol*. Mar 2001;22(3):541-552.

van Oostrom JC, Sijens PE, Roos RA, Leenders KL. 1H magnetic resonance spectroscopy in preclinical Huntington disease. *Brain Res*. Sep 7 2007;1168:67-71.

Vanhanen SL, Puranen J, Autti T, et al. Neuroradiological findings (MRS, MRI, SPECT) in infantile neuronal ceroid-lipofuscinosis (infantile CLN1) at different stages of the disease. *Neuropediatrics*. Feb 2004;35(1):27-35.

Vanhanen SL, Raininko R, Autti T, Santavuori P. MRI evaluation of the brain in infantile neuronal ceroid-lipofuscinosis. Part 2: MRI findings in 21 patients. *J Child Neurol*. Nov 1995;10(6):444-450.

Vedolin L, Schwartz IV, Komlos M, et al. Brain MRI in mucopolysaccharidosis: effect of aging and correlation with biochemical findings. *Neurology*. Aug 28 2007;69(9):917-924.

Vedolin L, Schwartz IV, Komlos M, et al. Correlation of MR imaging and MR spectroscopy findings with cognitive impairment in mucopolysaccharidosis II. *AJNR Am J Neuroradiol*. Jun-Jul 2007;28(6):1029-1033.

Vonsattel JP, DiFiglia M. Huntington disease. *J Neuropathol Exp Neurol*. May 1998;57(5):369-384.

Wang C, Melberg A, Weis J, Mansson JE, Raininko R. The earliest MR imaging and proton MR spectroscopy abnormalities in adult-onset Krabbe disease. *Acta Neurol Scand*. Oct 2007;116(4):268-272.

Wang XY, Noguchi K, Takashima S, Hayashi N, Ogawa S, Seto H. Serial diffusion-weighted imaging in a patient with MELAS and presumed cytotoxic oedema. *Neuroradiology*. Sep 2003;45(9):640-643.

Wang ZJ, Berry GT, Dreha SF, Zhao H, Segal S, Zimmerman RA. Proton magnetic resonance spectroscopy of brain metabolites in galactosemia. *Ann Neurol*. Aug 2001;50(2):266-269.

Watanabe Y, Hashikawa K, Moriwaki H, et al. SPECT Findings in Mitochondrial Encephalomyopathy. *J Nucl Med*. June 1, 1998;39(6):961-964.

Wenger DA, Rafi MA, Luzi P. Molecular genetics of Krabbe disease (globoid cell leukodystrophy): diagnostic and clinical implications. *Hum Mutat*. 1997;10(4):268-279.

Woodward KJ. The molecular and cellular defects underlying Pelizaeus-Merzbacher disease. *Expert Rev Mol Med*. 2008;10:e14.

Worgall S, Kekatpure MV, Heier L, et al. Neurological deterioration in late infantile neuronal ceroid lipofuscinosis. *Neurology*. August 7, 2007;69(6):521-535.

Wray SH, Provenzale JM, Johns DR, Thulborn KR. MR of the brain in mitochondrial myopathy. *AJNR Am J Neuroradiol*. May 1, 1995;16(5):1167-1173.

Yalcinkaya C, Dincer A, Gunduz E, Ficicioglu C, Kocer N, Aydin A. MRI and MRS in HMG-CoA lyase deficiency. *Pediatr Neurol*. 1999;20(5):375-380.

Yoneda M, Maeda M, Kimura H, Fujii A, Katayama K, Kuriyama M. Vasogenic edema on MELAS: A serial study with diffusion-weighted MR imaging. *Neurology*. December 1, 1999;53(9):2182-2184.

Yuksel A, Yalcinkaya C, Islak C, Gunduz E, Seven M. Neuroimaging findings of four patients with Sandhoff disease. *Pediatr Neurol*. Aug 1999;21(2):562-565.

Zafeiriou DI, Michelakaki EM, Anastasiou AL, Gombakis NP, Kontopoulos EE. Serial MRI and neurophysiological studies in late-infantile Krabbe disease. *Pediatr Neurol*. 1996;15(3):240-244.

Tumor

Marco Essig

CHAPTER 11

■ INTRODUCTION

The goals and requirements for brain tumor imaging are multiplex and involve making a diagnosis and a differential diagnosis, and accurate lesion grading is needed for tumor description. Imaging is also involved in the decision-making process for therapy and later for precise planning of surgical or radiotherapeutic interventions. After therapy, neuroimaging techniques have been shown to be mandatory for monitoring of disease and possible therapy-related side effects.

Because of the high tissue contrast and the noninvasive nature of the method, magnetic resonance imaging (MRI) is accepted as the most sensitive method for characterizing brain tumors. Ruling out a brain tumor in patients with unspecific neurologic symptoms is one of the most common indications for neuroimaging using MRI. In the past years it has become generally recognized that MRI would be the imaging study of choice in the evaluation of intracranial tumors if availability and cost were not issues.

The classification of brain tumors still is controversial and includes classification by location or by histology. The most common classification is that of the World Health Organization (WHO), which is summarized in the WHO Blue Book series (latest edition 2007).

Brain tumors are categorized into primary versus secondary tumors based on the origin tissue and intraaxial versus extraaxial tumors based on origin of growth. The most common primary intraaxial tumors are neuroepithelial tumors, which include astrocytomas, oligodendrogliomas, mixed gliomas, and other neuronal–glial tumors. Glioblastoma multiforme is the most common brain tumor. Meningiomas are the most common primary extraaxial tumors, accounting for about 20% of all brain tumors. In adults, secondary metastatic brain lesions from systemic cancer far outnumber primary tumors.

■ KEY QUESTIONS FOR PROBLEM SOLVING IN BRAIN TUMOR IMAGING

For the radiologic imaging of cerebral lesions, a few key questions have to be answered in order to solve problems in brain tumor imaging.
1. Is a lesion present?
2. Is the lesion a tumor?
3. Are any complications present that need an immediate intervention?
4. What is the most likely differential diagnosis?

The first question can be easily addressed by using an appropriate brain tumor imaging protocol in MRI and should include the following sequences (Table 11-1):

Unenhanced T1-weighted spin-echo (SE) or fast SE sequences are used to rule out intralesional bleeding and to visualize, for example, melanin, which is frequently found in metastases from malignant melanoma (Figure 11-1).

T2-weighted fast SE sequences and fluid-attenuated inversion recovery (FLAIR) are used to display the margins of a tumor and its surrounding edema or a direct tumor infiltration. In the past years, FLAIR has mainly replaced proton density weighted sequences. In uncooperative patients, motion-insensitive acquisition techniques should be used (Figure 11-2).

Contrast enhancement studies are mandatory in the assessment of patients with cerebral tumors. The standard dose used for MRI of the central nervous system is 0.1 mmol per kilogram of body weight, although numerous studies have shown that lesion detection may be improved by use of higher doses and dedicated sequences. Contrast-enhanced MRI helps in distinguishing tumors from other pathologic processes and enables optimal characterization of tumor response to therapy, such as change in size, morphology, and degree of contrast material enhancement (Figure 11-3).

The sequences after contrast administration should include at least two planes of T1-weighted sequences and, if possible, a volumetric sequence (e.g., three-dimensional gradient-recalled echo) to allow for reconstruction in different planes and volumetric assessment of the lesions.

In the past few years, a number of advanced, nonenhanced, and contrast-enhanced MRI techniques have been developed that provide new insights into the pathophysiology of brain tumors, mainly gliomas. They include MR spectroscopy (MRS), perfusion MRI, dynamic contrast-enhanced MRI, and diffusion tensor MRI. These techniques may help to answer the second question: Is the lesion a tumor?

If the presence of a tumor is determined, the best possible differential diagnosis should be given. In addition to the actual radiologic appearance of the tumor, including the characterization obtained with different modalities (e.g., MRI, computed tomography [CT], and positron emission tomography), the following parameters that help with the differential diagnosis should be considered (Table 11-2 and Figure 11-4):
■ Age of the patient (most important in pediatric patients)
■ Relevant clinical history
■ Previous available imaging studies and/or clinical and radiologic follow-up

Table 11-1 Proposed MRI Protocol for Brain Tumor Imaging Including Advance Techniques

Sequence	TR Range (ms)	TE Range (ms)	Orientation	Acquisition Time (min)
T1 SE	500–700	10–12	Tra/Cor	2–4
T2 FSE	3,000–5,000	80–100	Tra/Cor	2–4
FLAIR	9,000–9,500	100–110	Tra/Cor	3–5
Administration of 0.1 mmol Gadolinium Contrast Agent per Kilogram of Body Weight				
T1 SE	500–700	10–12	Tra/Cor	2–4
T1 3D GRE	8–15	5–7	Isotropic	3–5
Alternative Sequences				
DWI/DTI	2,900	90	Tra	1.30
PWI	1,400	32	Tra	1.40
MRS	Variable	Variable		Up to 12
T1 Dynamic MRI (DCE-MRI)	2.03	0.95	Tra	3–5

3D GRE, Three-dimensional gradient-recalled echo; *Cor,* coronal; *DTI,* diffusion tensor imaging; *DWI,* diffusion-weighted imaging; *FLAIR,* fluid-attenuated inversion recovery; *FSE,* fast spin echo; *MRS,* magnetic resonance spectroscopy; *PWI,* perfusion-weighted imaging; *SE,* spin echo; *Tra,* transverse.

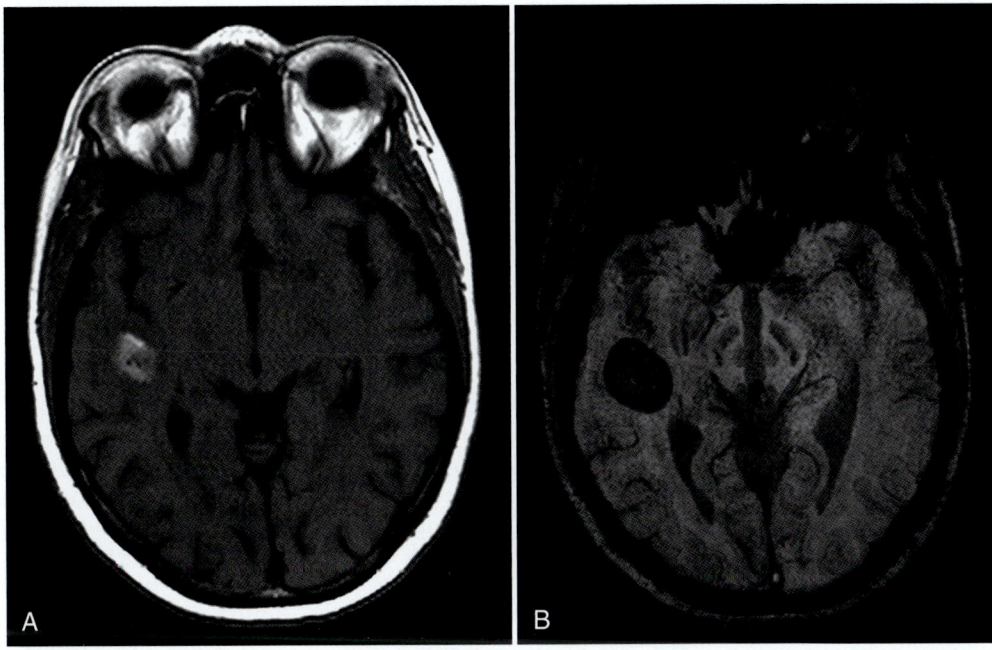

Figure 11-1 **A:** Unenhanced T1 spin echo on a 3-T system in a patient with melanoma. The cerebral lesion presented with increased signal intensity representing melanin or blood products (methemoglobin) in the metastatic lesion. **B:** On susceptibility-weighted magnetic resonance imaging, both melanin and blood products may cause susceptibility artifacts, which clearly present the size and origin of the lesion.

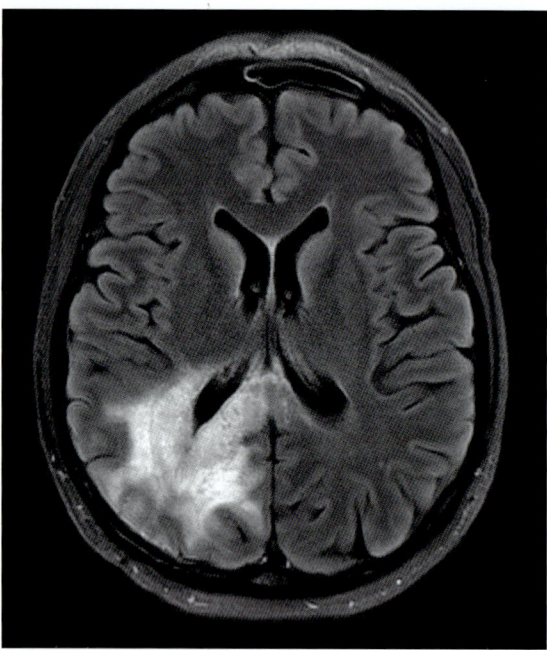

Figure 11-2 BLADE FLAIR acquisition for therapy planning in an uncooperative patient with oligoastrocytoma grade III. Note the few artifacts using the BLADE technique. The tumor tissue appears bright on T2 and BLADE FLAIR with infiltration of the cortical U fibers, the cortical gray matter, and the corpus callosum. Infiltration of cortical and periventricular tissue is best seen on FLAIR images.

■ PRACTICAL ASPECTS OF MRI IN BRAIN TUMORS

Using a standard MRI protocol for cerebral neoplasms as provided in Table 11-1 allows high-resolution imaging and characterization of lesions. Most tumors present low intensity on T1-weighted images and high intensity on T2-weighted images (Figure 11-5).

More recently, FLAIR imaging, a T2-weighted sequence with suppression of the signal intensity of cerebrospinal fluid (CSF) or any fluid with the T1 of CSF, has become a part of most brain imaging protocols. Initially used for imaging white matter changes, FLAIR has become a standard sequence in brain tumor imaging protocols. It can be particularly useful in proving the cystic content of a lesion or in the delineation of tumor from CSF containing areas, for example, the ventricles, surgical defects, or cystic tumor parts. A lesion that is exactly isointense to CSF on T1-weighted, T2-weighted, and FLAIR images can confidently be stated as being cystic, a pattern followed by arachnoid cysts and cysts associated with extraaxial masses (Figure 11-6).

In patients with cerebral gliomas, FLAIR was found to be superior to conventional imaging in tumor delineation and in the differentiation between tumor and edema. Due to the suppression of the CSF signal and a reduced gray-to-white matter contrast on the FLAIR images, periventricular, cortical, and callosal lesions could be better detected and delineated. Unfortunately for the radiologist, tumor cysts and cystic necrosis within neoplasms often contain blood products or have a high protein content that does not allow for optimal suppression of the cystic fluid on FLAIR imaging. Therefore, these regions are hyperintense to normal CSF on FLAIR, with increasing signal parallel to increasing protein content. Fluid debris intensity levels are a pathognomonic sign of cystic tissue and often are quite striking and frequent in cases of cystic tumors.

Hemorrhage is uniquely depicted by MRI because of the paramagnetic properties of many of the blood products. The appearance of those products depends on their age and amount. On MRI, old hemorrhage is easily distinguished from other fluid (e.g., CSF) because of the paramagnetic properties of methemoglobin, a marker of subacute to chronic intracranial hemorrhage. However, the tendency of certain primary intracranial neoplasms to bleed (e.g., glioblastoma, ependymoma, oligodendroglioma) and metastases (e.g., melanoma, lung carcinoma, renal cell carcinoma, choriocarcinoma) can be of great importance for the differential diagnosis and increases the sensitivity (Figures 11-1 and 11-4).

Although it is important to discover hemorrhage, it also is critical to define its etiology. CT is of limited value for this purpose. The signal intensity pattern of intratumoral hemorrhage differs from that of benign intracranial hematoma. Signal intensity presents as heterogeneous in tumor bleeds but is more homogeneous in parenchymal hemorrhage. The appearance of blood also is different between the entities. Blood may not evolve as rapidly if it is within tumor tissue, presenting different stages of blood, in comparison with the fast evolution of benign hematomas. Some tumors contain tissue that may mimic a hematoma. The most important tumors are metastases from melanoma. The melanin pigments substantially shorten the T1 relaxation time, and the tumors appear hyperintense on unenhanced T1 sequences. The effect on T2 relaxation is small, and no signal changes are seen in most cases. However, melanoma metastases are commonly both hemorrhagic and melanotic, so imaging is less specific in many subjects.

Calcifications can be depicted only if they are extensive or with the use of susceptibility weighted MRI sequences. Rim-shaped calcifications, as in cystic lesions, may mimic chronic hemorrhage in the hemosiderin stage (Figure 11-7).

The enhancement seen in brain tumors is based on a disrupted blood–brain barrier (BBB), which can be compromised by neovascularization and direct tumoral damage. Because nonneoplastic astrocytes are required to induce BBB features of cerebral endothelial cells, it is conceivable that malignant variants of these cells have lost this ability due to dedifferentiation. Alternatively, glioma cells might actively degrade previously intact BBB tight junctions. Although the integrity of the barrier within the tumor often is compromised, the alteration in permeability is variable and dependent on the tumor type and size. Moreover, it is extremely heterogeneous in a given lesion. Although the BBB frequently is leaky in the center of malignant brain tumors, the well-vascularized, actively proliferating edge of the tumor, in the brain adjacent to tumor

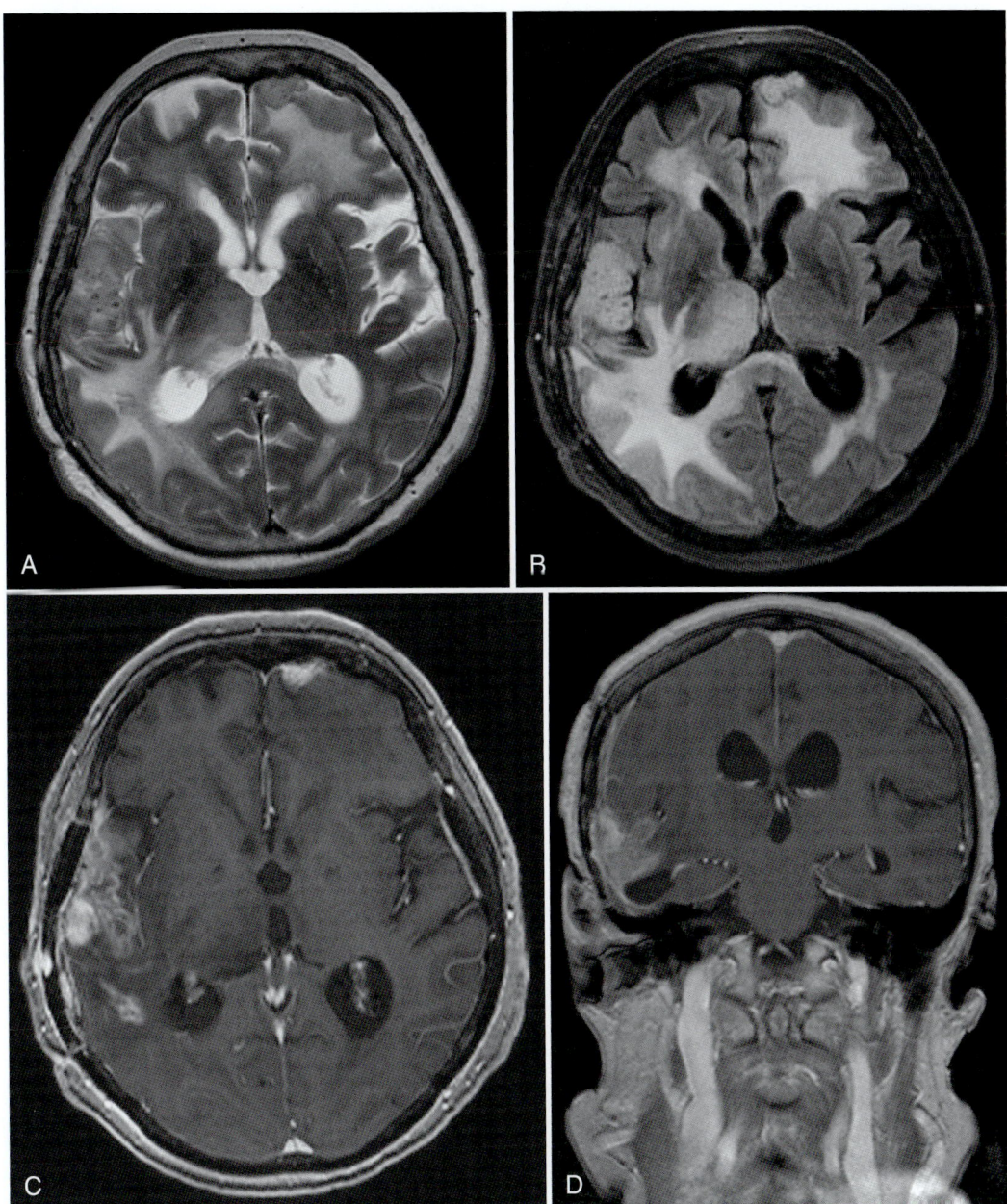

Figure 11-3 Contrast-enhanced (0.1 mmol per kilogram of body weight) magnetic resonance imaging of a patient with recurrent malignant glioma (World Health Organization grade IV). T2-weighted **(A)** and FLAIR **(B)** images showing a large area of T2 hyperintensity with small foci of lower signal representing the high cellular density tumor areas. **C, D:** These tumor areas show pronounced contrast media enhancement with the typical pattern of high-grade gliomas. The frontal lesion can be considered tumor spread via the meninges or a second malignant tumor change in a large area of suspected low-grade tumor tissue.

area, has been shown to have variable and complex barrier integrity (Figure 11-8).

In secondary metastatic intraaxial tumors and extraaxial tumors, the vessels are different from normal cerebral vasculature and have no or strongly disturbed BBB. Those entities normally have a strong enhancement pattern, presenting the whole tumor as an enhancing mass (Figure 11-9).

Because brain edema is also thought to be due to breakdown of the BBB, a correlation between the degree of enhancement and the volume of the peritumoral edema could be expected. Holodny et al studied this correlation in malignant gliomas representative of primary intraaxial tumors and meningiomas representative of extraaxial tumors. In their study, no correlation was found for meningiomas, which proved that the meningioma vessels have no BBB or no effect on the BBB in the surrounding brain tissue. A strong correlation was found for malignant gliomas, which offers evidence that the BBB defect is directly related to both the degree of lesion enhancement and the amount of edema, and that the two interfere with each other. The interference may influence both conventional contrast-enhanced MRI as well as some of the flow-dependent functional imaging techniques.

Problem Solving: Common Intraaxial Tumors

The most common intraaxial lesions to be differentiated are the following:
- Astrocytic tumors
- Lymphomas
- Metastases
- Abscesses
- Tumefactive demyelinating lesions

The main problem to be solved is the differentiation between primary and secondary tumors, the grading of primary intraaxial tumors, and the therapeutically important difference between gliomas and lymphomas.

A common problem with intraaxial tumors is that cerebral metastases can mimic cerebral tumors with isointense to hypointense signal on T1-weighted imaging and hyperintensity on T2-weighted imaging. Intensive

Table 11-2 Key Imaging Characteristics for Differential Diagnosis/Problem Solving

Location of lesion	Supratentorial versus infratentorial
	Intraaxial versus extraaxial location
	Single lesion versus multiple lesions
Associated findings	Edema and/or tumor infiltration
	Mass effect
Signal characteristics of lesions that are helpful in the differential diagnosis	
High signal on unenhanced T1	Metastases of melanoma (Figure 11-1)
	Subacute bleeding/hemorrhage, e.g., in oligodendroglioma (Figure 11-4)
Signal on T2	High = low cellularity
	Low = high cellularity
Low signal on both T1 and T2	Calcifications

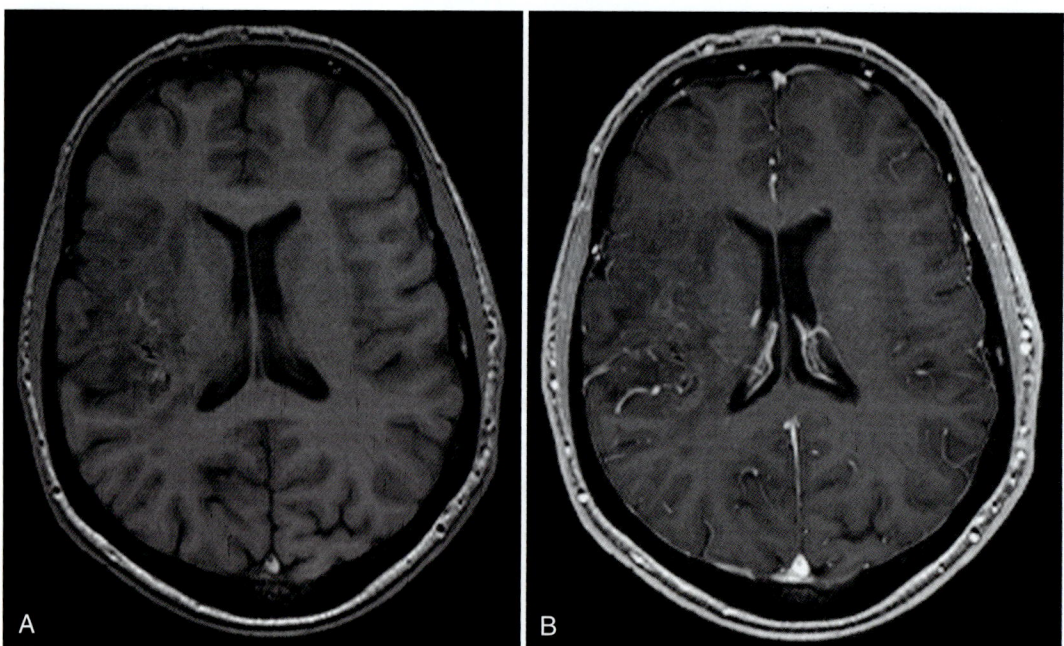

Figure 11-4 A: Magnetic resonance image of a patient with a grade II oligodendroglioma showing the typical patterns of streaky high signal on unenhanced T1 representing blood products. B: After contrast media, only subtle signs of enhancement could be detected.

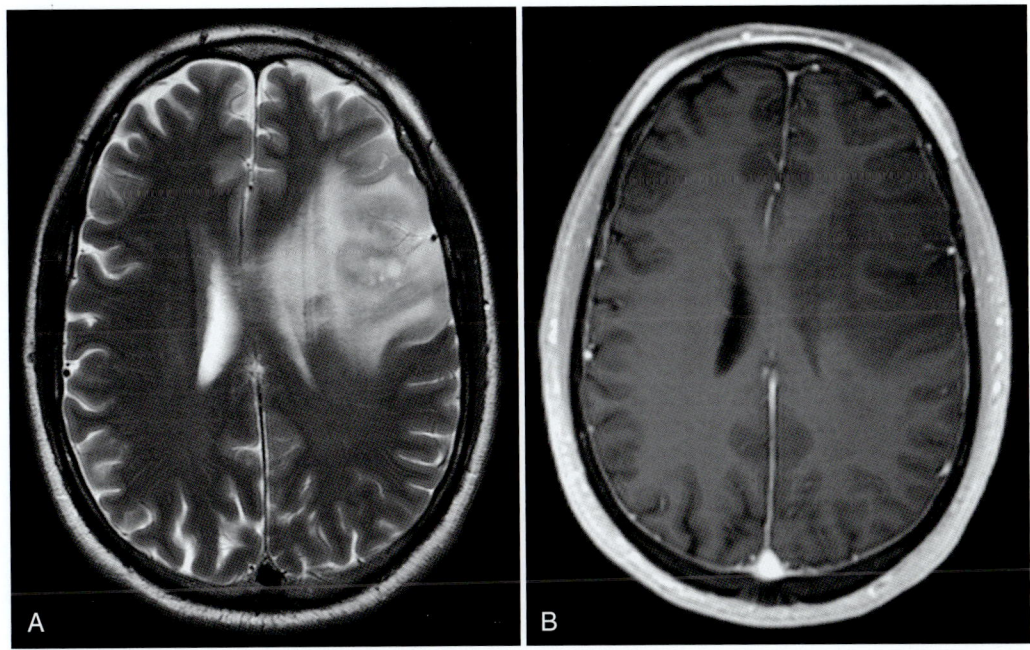

Figure 11-5 T2-weighted (A) and T1-weighted (B) images of a patient with low-grade astrocytoma showing the typical signal changes of cerebral tumors with high intensity on T2. In this case, infiltration into the corpus callosum and low signal on T1 are clearly seen.

edema is present in large lesions but frequently is absent in small metastatic lesions.

Astrocytic tumors account for up to 80% of glial neoplasms and refer to diffuse infiltrating tumors originating from glial cells. The tumor border on both imaging and histology is ill defined with an infiltration that primarily does not obey the anatomic cerebral structures. The tumors often distort the structures with the appearance of cysts.

Under the recent WHO classification of primary intracranial tumors, grade I to grade IV tumors can be differentiated.

Grade I or pilocytic tumors are normally present in children and young adults. The main problem is the differentiation between low-grade (grade II) and high-grade or malignant gliomas (grades III–IV). Based on imaging and enhancement characteristics, this differentiation is not possible in about 20% to 30% of cases. In these cases, a more sophisticated imaging strategy that includes MRS and perfusion MRI is required (Figure 11-10).

For enhancing lesions, gliomas and lymphomas often cannot be differentiated, especially if the lesions present with a butterfly appearance.

Besides the clinical history (e.g., immunocompromise), functional imaging tools may help in the differential diagnostic process. Whereas astrocytomas often present with high values of perfusion and a high ratio of choline to N-acetylaspartate (NAA) (Figure 11-11), lymphomas normally present with substantially lower perfusion values. The extent of edema is normally less than observed in gliomas or metastases. The enhancement is intensive (Figure 11-12), and detection of a strong enhancement along the perivascular spaces is typical for lymphomas, with sarcoidosis the only differential diagnosis.

Problem Solving: Differentiating Recurrent Tumor from Therapeutic-Induced Changes

The differentiation of recurrent tumor from therapeutic-induced changes is another common problem in brain tumor imaging.

After radiation or chemotherapy, BBB breakdown can occur and mimic tumor recurrence. Differentiation between these two entities often is not possible using standard MRI techniques. MRS has been shown to be useful in identifying tumoral tissue by the presence of choline and, in high-grade tumors, lactate. Choline, which is a marker of membrane turnover, is normally not present in necrosis (Figure 11-13).

Problem Solving: Common Extraaxial Tumors

Extraaxial masses arise from tissue at the surface of the brain and include lesions that arise from the ventricles or ependyma (Figure 11-14). They tend to displace the brain structures and may cause a CSF cleft. They preserve the normal cerebral structures and the gray–white matter junctions (Figure 11-14).

The main extraaxial lesions are meningiomas, choroids plexus tumors, tumors of the sella, and cerebral nerve sheath tumors. Metastases can originate from extraaxial tissue.

Common problems with extraaxial tumors are differentiation between meningiomas and nerve sheath tumors (e.g., schwannomas) and differentiation of cystic lesions. Clinically, the description of the mass effect in extraaxial lesions and the influence of neuronal functions are of importance.

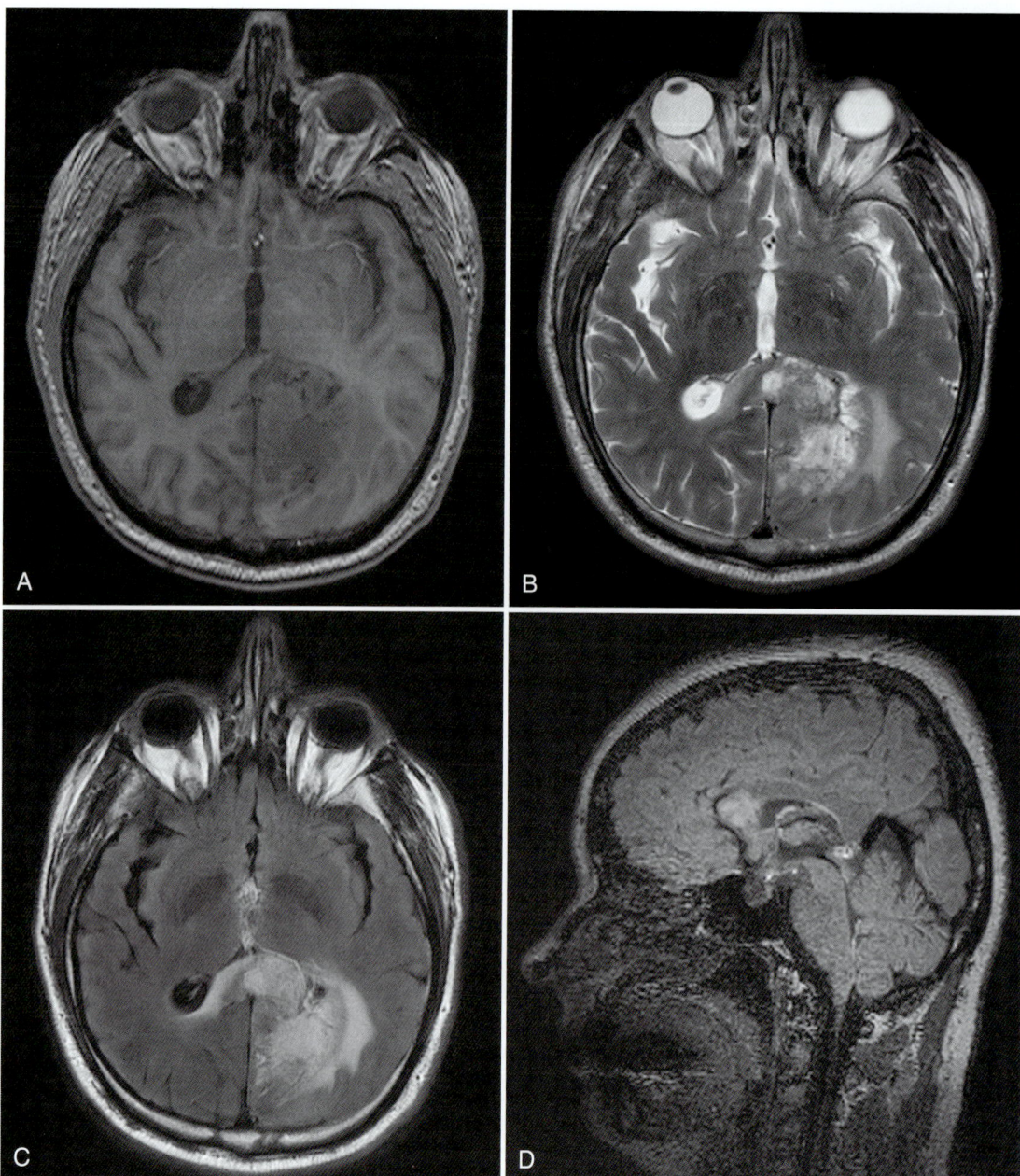

Figure 11-6 Magnetic resonance imaging of a patient with anaplastic (grade III) astrocytoma. On unenhanced T1-weighted (**A**) and T2-weighted (**B**) images, one can speculate about an infiltration of the corpus callosum. However, the best visualization of the infiltration can be achieved by using FLAIR acquisition. Due to the high signal-to-noise ratio and the suppression of cerebrospinal fluid, the tumor tissue can be nicely seen (**C**). In another case (**D**), infiltration in the genu of the corpus callosum can be appreciated.

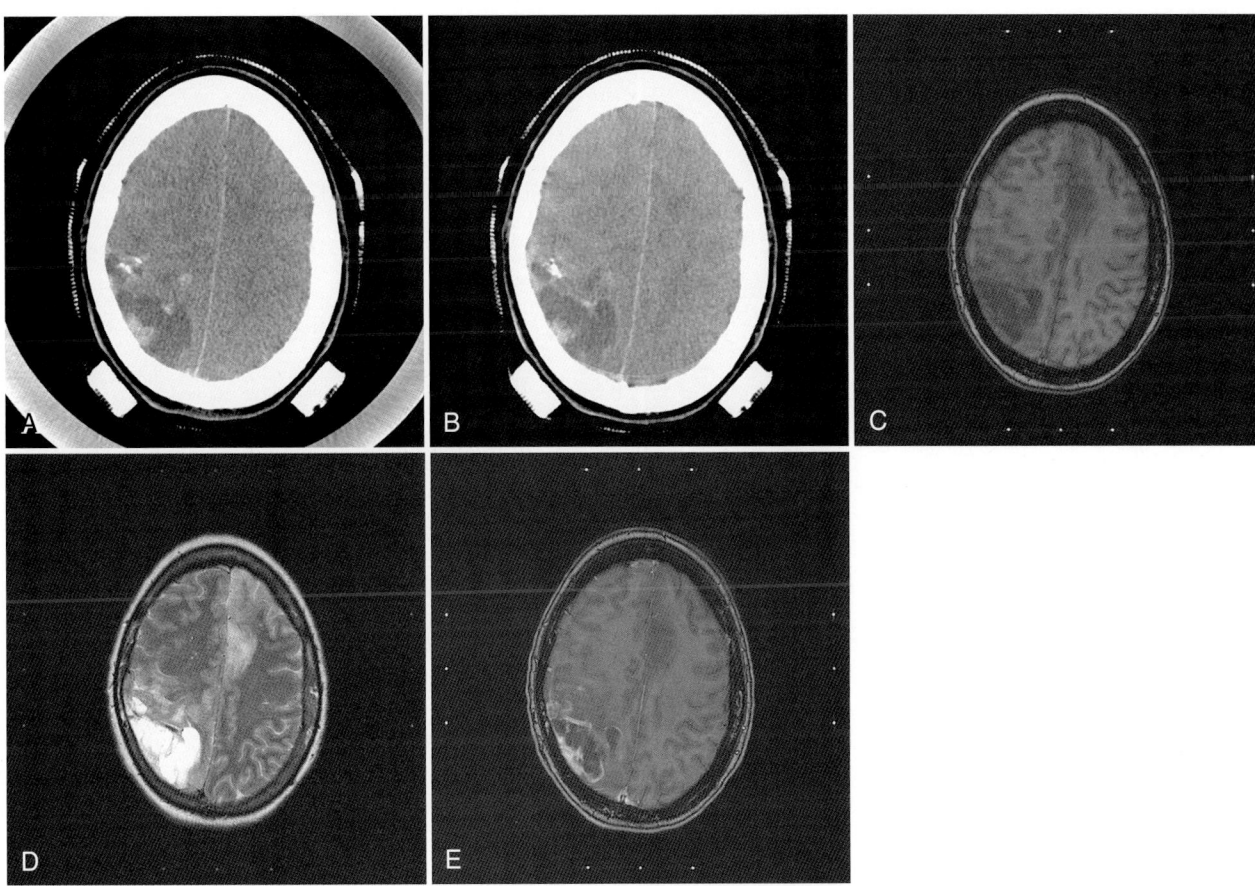

Figure 11-7 Computed tomography (CT) **(A, B)** and magnetic resonance imaging **(C–E)** in a patient with multiple cerebral lesions. CT shows a large cystic lesion in the right parietal lobe with calcifications and faint enhancement. T1 unenhanced spin echo (SE) showed a faint high signal indicating blood byproducts and areas of low signal that are also present on T2-weighted fast SE sequences. The latter are seen in concordance to the calcifications on CT. The solid-appearing left frontal lesion shows no enhancement and no calcification. Enhancement was visible only in the right-sided lesion. The signal characteristics combined with knowledge of calcification favor the diagnosis of an oligodendroglioma, which was confirmed at histology.

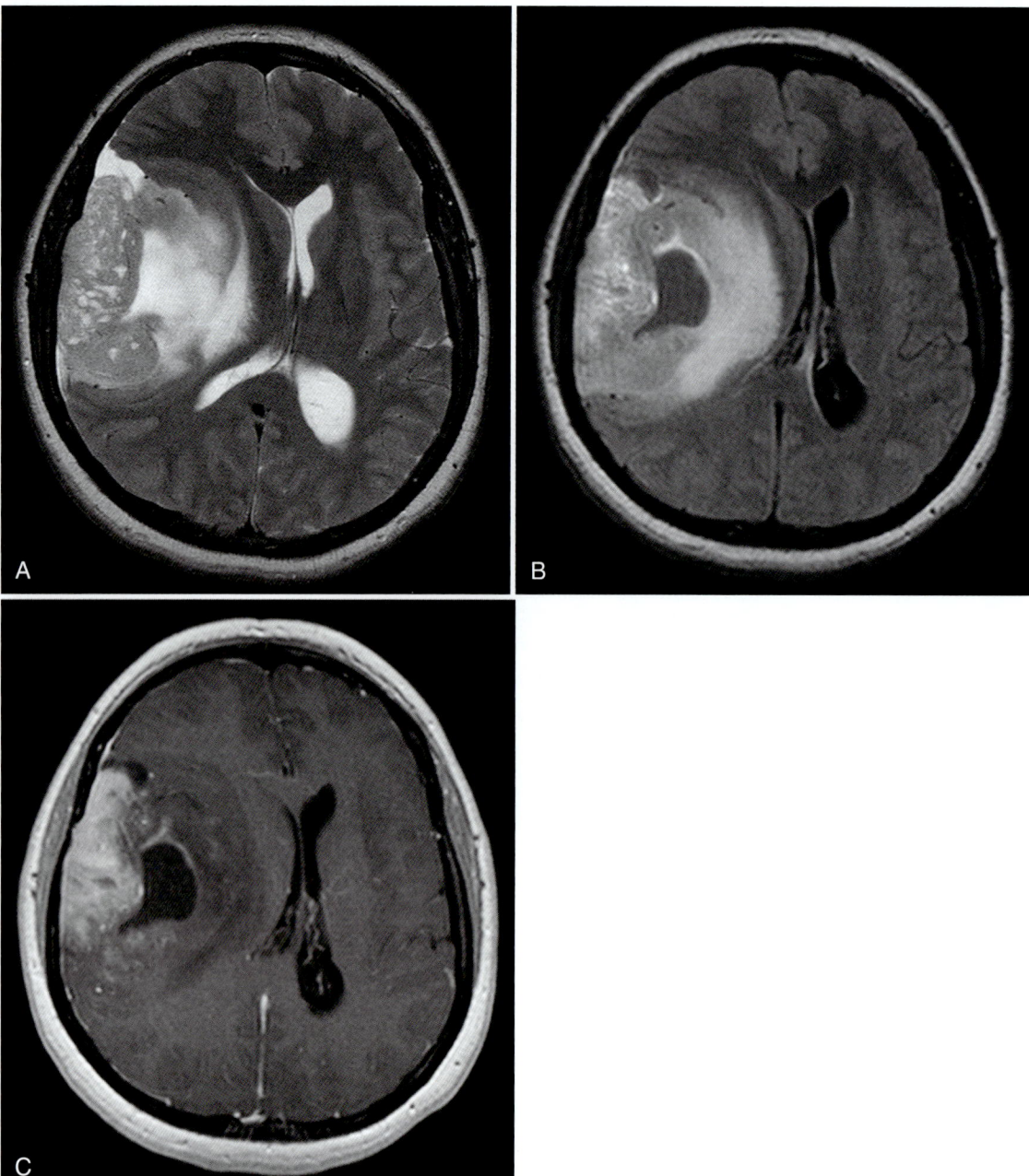

Figure 11-8 Typical enhancement pattern in a patient with malignant glioma. The more solid parts appear darker in T2 (**A**) and FLAIR (**B**) and present with a strong enhancement (**C**). The surrounding lower tumor grade tissue still has an intact blood–brain barrier.

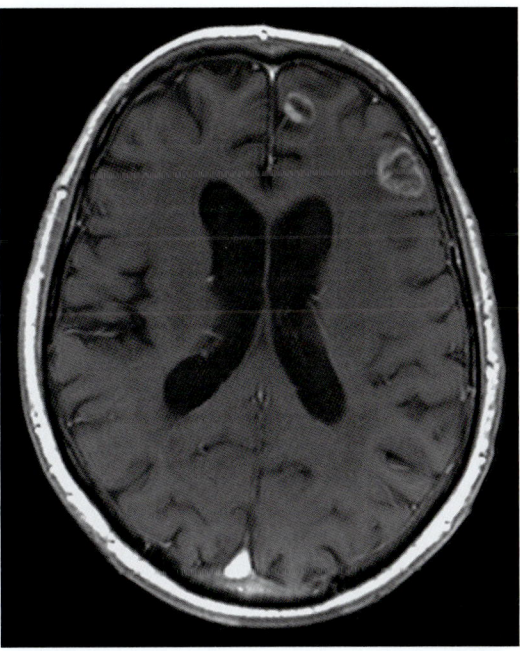

Figure 11-9 Typical rim-shaped enhancement in a patient with metastatic disease. Metastases can show any type of enhancement; however, the most common is the rim shape with substantial surrounding edema.

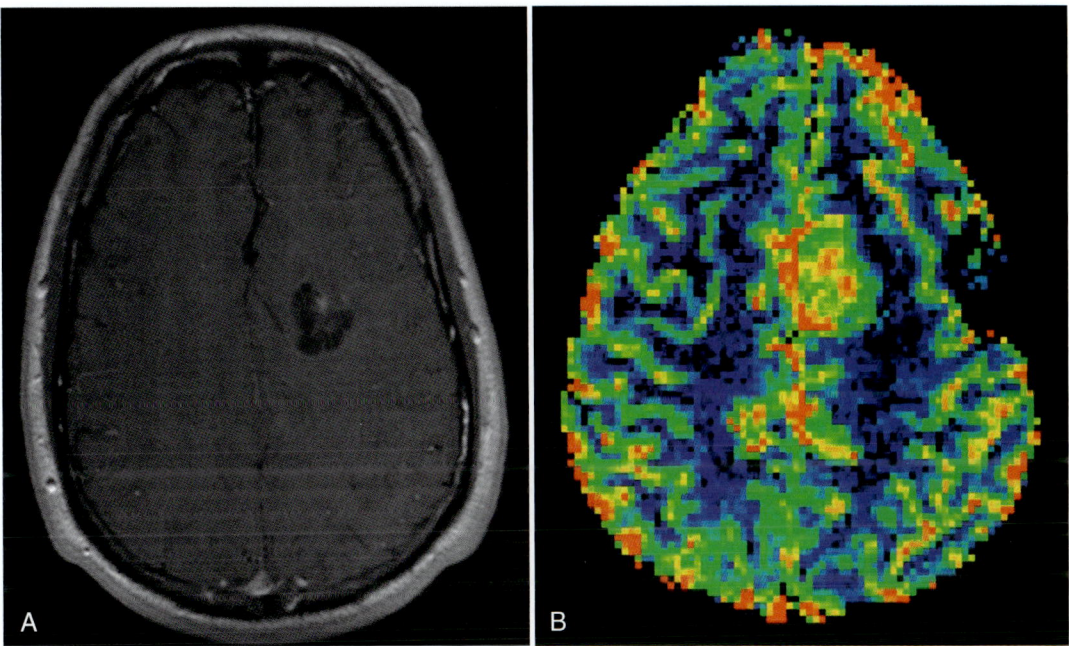

Figure 11-10 Perfusion magnetic resonance imaging (MRI) of lesions with unknown histology. **A:** The lesions showed hyperintensity on T2, a focus of enhancement not easily differentiated from a vascular structure. **B:** Perfusion MRI, displayed is the regional cerebral blood flow map, demonstrating a lesion with high perfusion, which can be classified as a high-grade glioma. Histology confirmed a grade IV astrocytoma or glioblastoma multiforme.

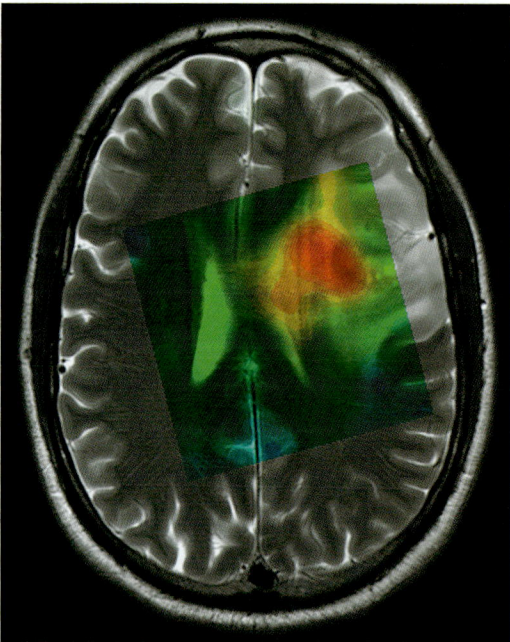

Figure 11-11 Choline to *N*-acetylaspartate (NAA) ratio color coded from magnetic resonance CSI data. Note the hot spot in *red* in the center of the tumor representing a ratio of high choline and low NAA, which is typical for a high-grade astrocytic tumor.

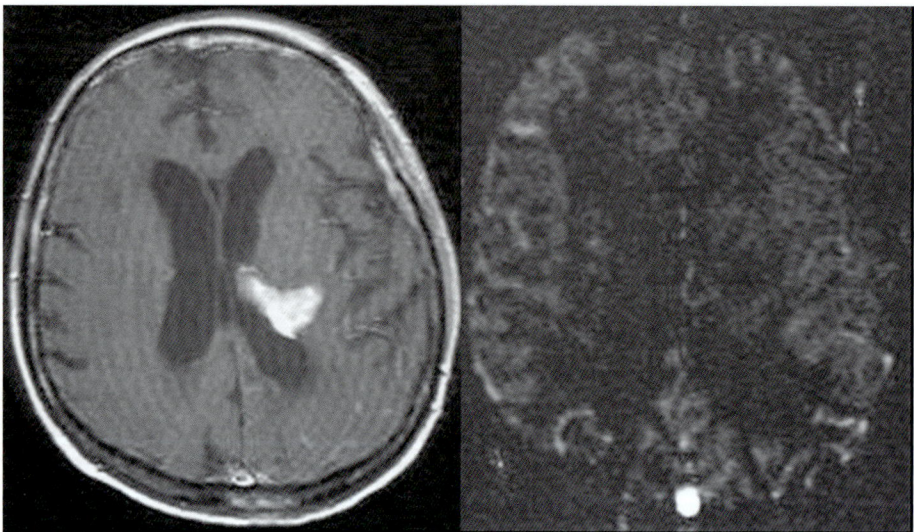

Figure 11-12 Contrast-enhanced T1 and arterial spin labeling perfusion magnetic resonance imaging in a patient with cerebral lymphoma. Although the tumor presents with avid contrast enhancement, the perfusion values are low, which allows differentiation from the normally highly perfused primary intraaxial tumors and central nervous system lymphoma.

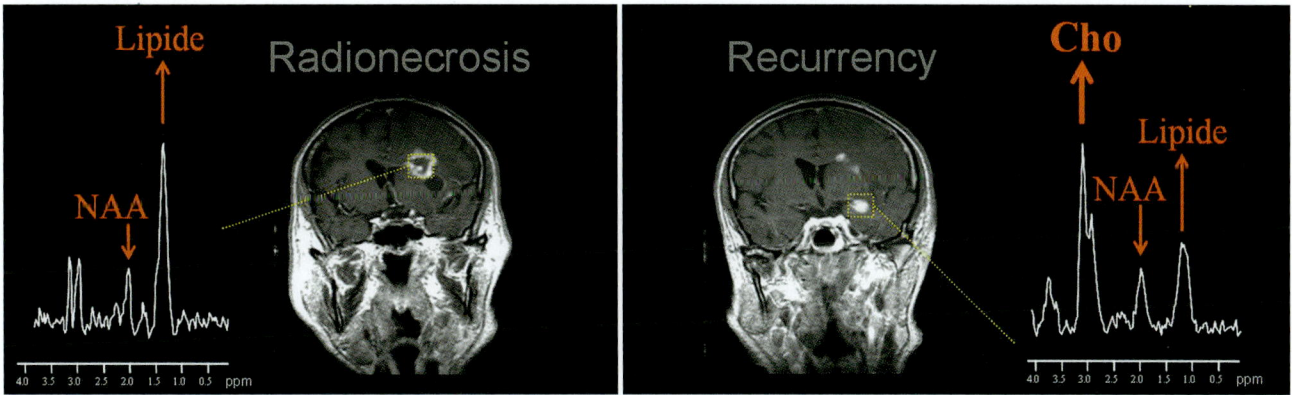

Figure 11-13 Tumor necrosis and recurrent tumor in the same patient after radiation therapy of an anaplastic (grade III) astrocytoma. The patient presented 9 months after radiation with multiple new enhancing, partially cystic lesions, all suspicious for tumor progression. Magnetic resonance spectroscopy was used for further differentiation. The lesion adjacent to the lateral ventricle showed no choline and was histologically proven radionecrosis, whereas the lesion on the left temporal lobe presented a typical tumor spectrum and was confirmed as recurrent tumor. *Cho*, Choline; *NAA*, N-acetylaspartate.

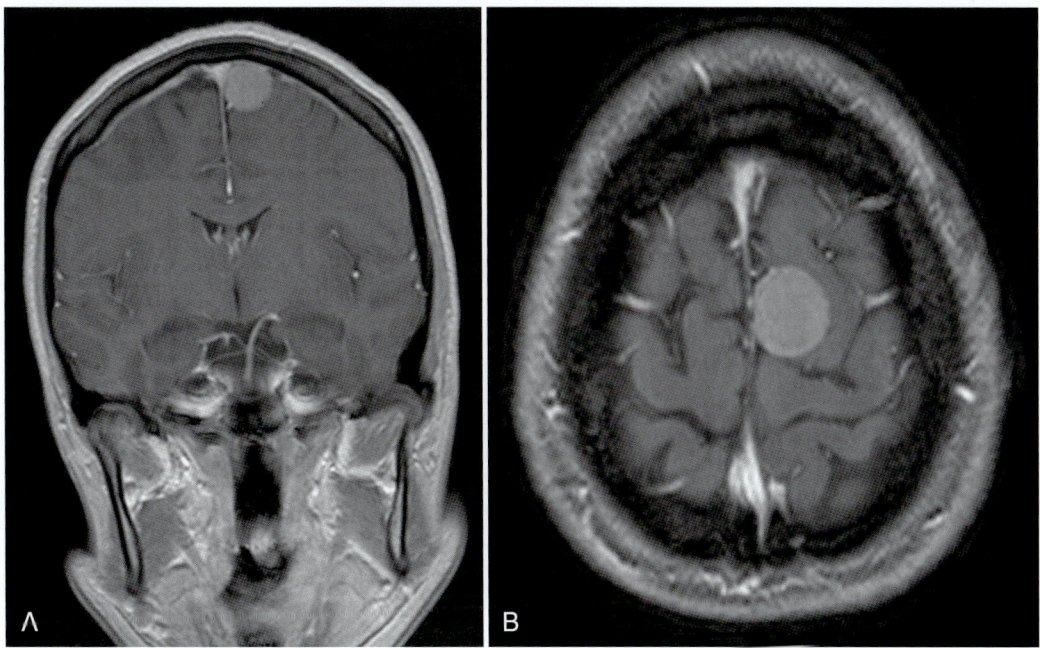

Figure 11-14 Typical magnetic resonance image of a supratentorial extraaxial lesion that can clearly be identified radiologically as a meningeoma. Extraaxial location with slight displacement of the adjacent cerebral tissue and homogeneous enhancement.

Meningiomas versus Schwannomas

Compared to schwannomas, meningiomas tend to show calcifications, especially if they are large, have a periosteal bony reaction/exostosis, and have broader contact with the skull with a typical dural tail sign in the majority of cases (Figure 11-15).

A common problem that is easy to solve is the differentiation between arachnoidal cysts and epidermoid cysts (Figure 11-16). Although the differential diagnosis is difficult based on CT alone, MRI with diffusion-weighted imaging sequences is the key diagnostic step. Arachnoid cysts contain CSF with normal protein content and therefore have identical signal as the ventricles in all sequences, including FLAIR (Figure 11-16).

Epidermoid cysts usually are located at the skull base and may have CSF-like signal in conventional imaging sequences. However, in most cases they appear hyperintense on FLAIR. The surface may be irregular and can show calcification on CT. The diagnostic key is use of diffusion-weighted imaging sequences in which the lesion appears very bright due to restricted diffusion (Figure 11-17).

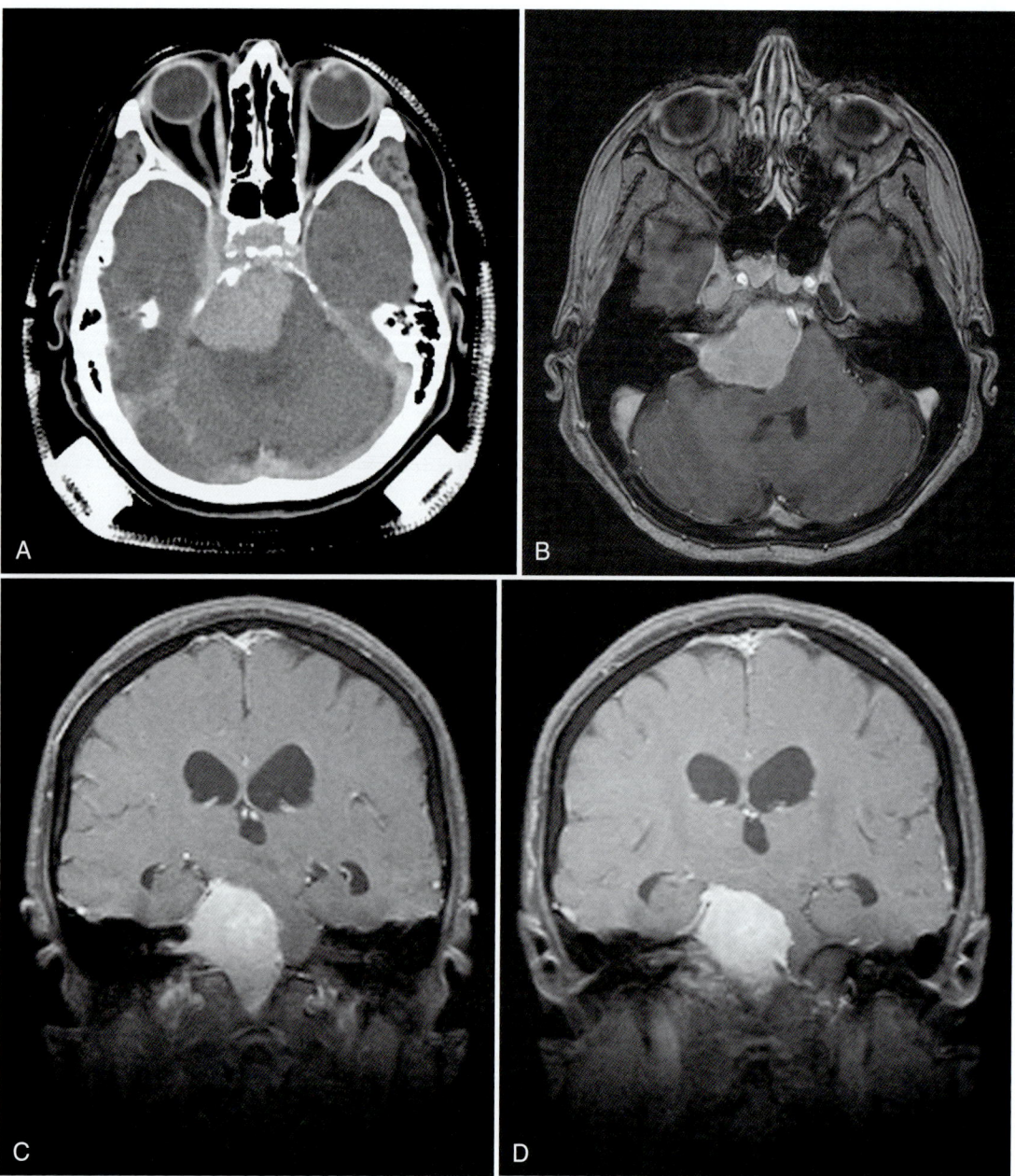

Figure 11-15 Skull base lesion in computed tomography (A) and axial magnetic resonance imaging (B) showing some bone reaction and strong contrast enhancement extending into the inner auditory canal (C). The diagnosis of meningioma is based on the dural tail sign, which is most obvious in the coronal orientation (C, D).

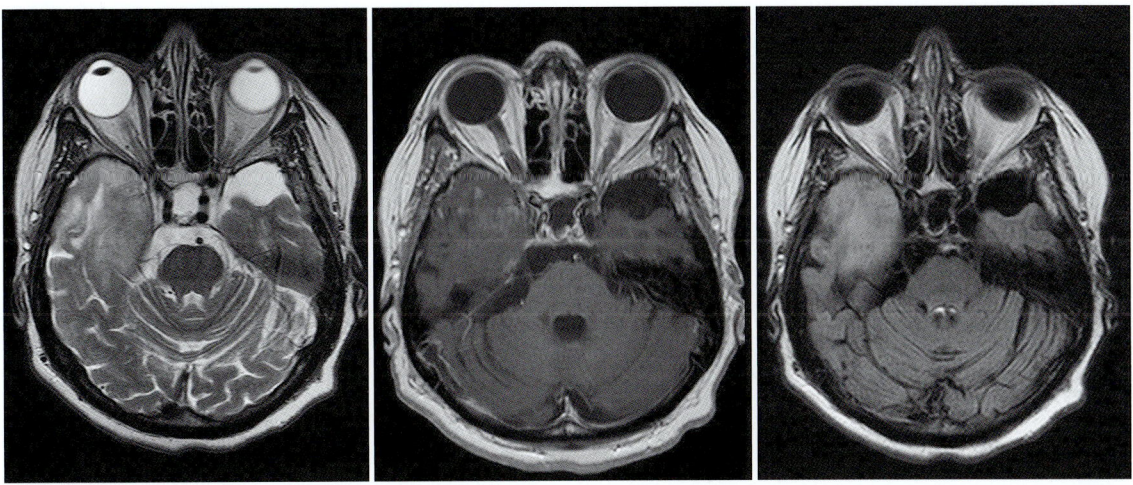

Figure 11-16 Uncomplicated arachnoid cyst of the temporal lobe as an incidental findings in a young volunteer. Note the cerebrospinal fluid (CSF)-like signal in all sequences. A pitfall, which can be a helpful sign in the presence of CSF, is pulsation artifact within the cyst on FLAIR imaging.

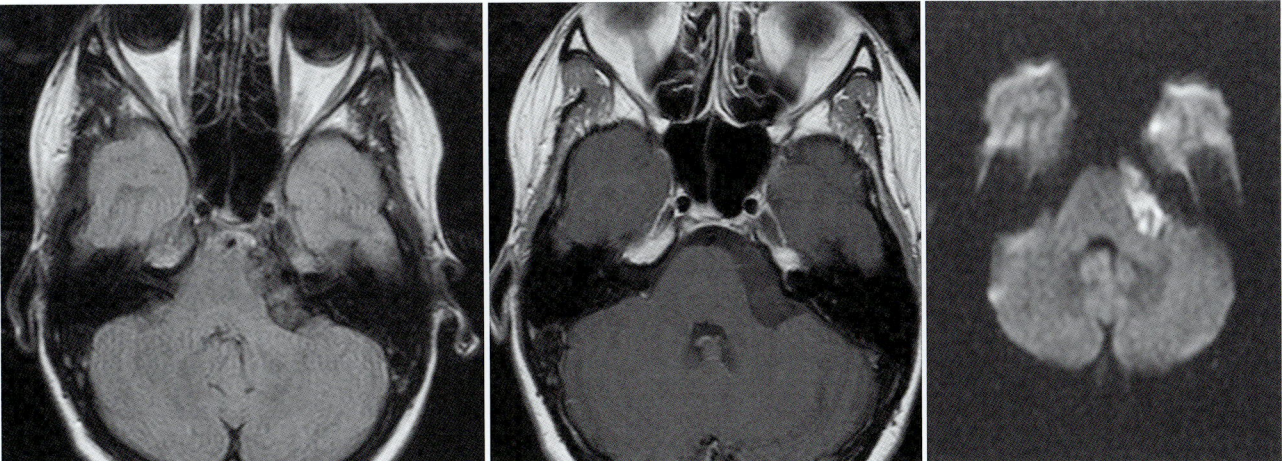

Figure 11-17 Epidermoid cyst in typical location and high signal on diffusion-weighted imaging sequences. This helps to differentiate the lesion from an arachnoid cyst (see Figure 11-16). Note the intermediate signal on FLAIR imaging.

Suggested Readings

Behin A, Hoang-Xuan K, Carpentier AF, Delattre JY. Primary brain tumours in adults. *Lancet*. 2003;361:323-331.

Bisese J. MRI of cranial metastasis. *Semin Ultrasound CT MR*. 1992;13:473-483.

Brant-Zawadzki M, Norman D, Newton TH, et al. Magnetic resonance of the brain: the optimal screening technique. *Radiology*. 1984;152(1):71-77.

Byrne TN. Imaging of gliomas. *Semin Oncol*. 1994;21:162-171.

Cenacchi G, Giangaspero F. Emerging tumor entities and variants of CNS neoplasms. *J Neuropathol Exp Neurol*. 2004;63:185-192.

De Coene B, Hajnal JV, Gatehouse P, et al. MR of the brain using fluid-attenuated inversion recovery (FLAIR) pulse sequences. *Am J Neuroradiol*. 1992;13:1555-1564.

Earnest 4th F, Kelly PJ, Scheithauer BW, et al. Cerebral astrocytomas: histopathologic correlation of MR and CT contrast enhancement with stereotactic biopsy. *Radiology*. 1988;166:823-827.

Erickson BJ, Campeau NG, Schreiner SA, Buckner JC, O'Neill BP, O'Fallon JR. Triple-dose contrast/magnetization transfer suppressed imaging of "non-enhancing" brain gliomas. *J Neurooncol*. 2002;60:25-29.

Essig M, Hawighorst H, Schoenberg SO, et al. Fast fluid-attenuated inversion-recovery (FLAIR) MR imaging in the assessment of intraaxial brain tumors. *J Magn Reson Imag*. 1998;8:789-798.

Essig M, Reichenbach JR, Schad LR, Schoenberg SO, Debus J, Kaiser WA. High resolution MR venography of cerebral arteriovenous malformations. *Magn Reson Imaging*. 1999;17:1417-1425.

Essig M, Schoenberg SO, Hawighorst H, et al. Cerebral gliomas and metastases: Assessment with contrast enhanced fast fluid-attenuated inversion-recovery MR imaging. *Radiology*. 1999;210:551-557.

Fidler IJ, Yano S, Zhang RD, Fujimaki T, Bucana CD. The seed and soil hypothesis: Vascularization and brain metastases. *Lancet Oncol*. 2002;3:53-57.

Forsting M, Albert FK, Kunze S, Adams HP, Zenner D, Sartor K. Extirpation of glioblastomas: MR and CT follow-up of residual tumor and regrowth patterns. *Am J Neuroradiol*. 1993;14:77-87.

Groothuis DR. The blood-brain and blood tumor barriers: a review of strategies for increasing drug delivery. *Neuro Oncol*. 2000;2:45-59.

Holodny AJ, Nusbaum AO, Festa S, Pronin IN, Lee HJ, Kalnin AJ. Correlation between the degree of contrast enhancement and volume of peritumoral edema in meningiomas and malignant gliomas. *Neuroradiology*. 1999;41:820-825.

Jeyapalan S, Batchelor T. Diagnostic evaluation of neurologic metastases. *Cancer Invest*. 2000;18:381-394.

Kido G, Wright JL, Merchant RE. Acute effects of human recombinant tumor necrosis factor-alpha on the cerebral vasculature of the rat in both normal brain and in an experimental glioma model. *J Neurooncol*. 1991;10:95-109.

Kleihues P, Burger PC, Scheithauer BW. The new WHO classification of brain tumours. *Brain Pathology*. 1993;3:255-268.

Kleihues P, Ohgeki H. Primary and secondary glioblastomas: from concept to clinical diagnosis. *Neuro Oncol*. 2001;52:181-188.

Koeller KR, Smirniotopoulos JG, Jones RV. Primary central nervous system lymphoma: Radiologogic-pathologic correlation. *Radiographics*. 2007;17:1497-1526.

Levin VA, Leibel SA, Gutin PH. Neoplasms of the central nervous system. In: DeVita VTJr, Hellman S, Rosenberg SA, eds. *Cancer: Principles and Practice of Oncology*. 6th ed. Philadelphia, Pa: Lippincott Williams & Wilkins; 2001:2100-2160.

Longstretz WE, Dennis LK, McGuire VM, et al. Epidemiology of intracranial meningioma. *Cancer*. 1993;72:639-664.

Lopes MBS, VandenBerg SR, Scheithauer BW. The World Health Organization classification of nervous system tumors in experimental neuro-oncology. In: Levine AJ, Schmidek HH, eds. *Molecular Genetics of Nervous System Tumors*. New York: Wiley-Liss; 1993:1-36.

Muroff LR, Runge VM. The use of MR contrast in neoplastic disease of the brain. *Top Magn Reson Imaging*. 1995;7(3):137-157.

Patchell RA. Brain metastases. *Neurol Clin*. 1991;9:817-827.

Pronin IN, Holodny AI, Petrainkin AV. MRI of high-grade glial tumors: correlation between the degree of contrast enhancement and the volume of surrounding edema. *Neuroradiology*. 1997;39:348-350.

Rydberg JN, Hammond CA, Grimm RC, et al. Initial clinical experience in MR imaging of the brain with a fast fluid-attenuated inversion-recovery pulse sequence. *Radiology*. 1994;193:173-180.

Schneider G, Kirchin MA, Pirovano G, et al. Gadobenate dimeglumine-enhanced magnetic resonance imaging of intracranial metastases: effect of dose on lesion detection and delineation. *J Magn Reson Imaging*. 2001;14:525-539.

Schneider SW, Ludwig T, Tatenhorst L, Braune S, Oberleithner H, Senner V, Paulus W. Glioblastoma cells release factors that disrupt blood-brain barrier features. *Acta Neuropathol*. 2004;107:272-276.

Stieber VW. Low-grade gliomas. *Curr Treat Options Oncol*. 2001;2:495-506.

Thomas B, Somasundaram S, Thamburaj KE, et al. Clinical applications of susceptibility weighted MR imaging of the brain—a pictoral review. *Neuroradiology*. 2008;29:9-17.

Tsuchiya K, Mizutani Y, Hachiya J. Preliminary evaluation of fluid-attenuated inversion-recovery MR in the diagnosis of intracranial tumors. *Am J Neuroradiol*. 1996;17:1081-1086.

van den Bent MJ. Management of metastatic (parenchymal, leptomeningeal, and epidural) lesions. *Curr Opin Oncol*. 2004:309-313.

Walker AE, Robins M, Weinfled FD. Epidemiology of brain tumors: the national survey of intracranioa neoplasms. *Neurology*. 1985;35:219-226.

Wintersperger BJ, Runge VM, Biswas J, et al. Brain magnetic resonance imaging at 3 Tesla using BLADE compared with standard rectilinear data sampling. *Invest Radiol*. 2006;41:586-592.

World Health Organization. Classification of brain tumors. Zürich. WHO. 1990-2007.

CHAPTER **12**

Brain Trauma

Alessandro Cianfoni and Cesare Colosimo

■ HEAD TRAUMA

Who Needs to Be Imaged? When to Best Image? What Are the Most Optimal Imaging Techniques?

Traumatic injuries of the brain and spinal cord are a leading cause of death and permanent disability among individuals younger than 50 years, accounting for 15% to 20% of deaths in the age group comprising individuals aged 5 to 35 years. Clinical management of the head-injured patient begins with assessment of the degree of patient risk according to the symptoms of intracranial injury. This assessment then can be used as a guide to further treatment.

What Are the Indications for Imaging in Head Trauma?

Debate continues in the medical literature about which patients with head trauma need to be imaged in the emergency situation. Various authors note indications for imaging of the head in patients who sustained head trauma. The indications are listed in Table 12-1 and include Glasgow Coma Scale (GCS) score <15; clinical signs of basal skull fracture or depressed skull fracture; all penetrating head injuries; anisocoria or fixed and dilated pupils; neurologic deficit, including focal motor paralysis, cranial nerve deficit, and abnormal Babinski reflex; loss of consciousness for more than 5 minutes; and antegrade amnesia.

The role of computed tomography (CT) in severely head-injured patients is well documented. The indications for CT in patients with minor head injury are less clear than for those with severe head injury.

What Are the Indications for Imaging in Minor Head Trauma?

Minor head injury usually is defined as a blunt injury to the head, after which the patient may briefly lose consciousness, may have short posttraumatic amnesia, but have a normal mental status at presentation (GCS score = 15). In patients with mild traumatic brain injury who present to the hospital with GCS = 15, the estimated prevalence of intracranial CT scan abnormalities is as high as 5%. Approximately 0.1% to 1% of all patients with mild traumatic brain injury present to the emergency room require neurosurgical intervention. Miller et al. determined that four simple clinical variables—severe headache, nausea, vomiting (more than one episode), and skull depression on physical examination—can be used to define which patients with head trauma and GCS score = 15 require a head CT scan. Although there is strong evidence that clinical factors can predict imaging abnormalities and the need for intervention in adults, there is no such evidence for mild traumatic brain injury in children. Given the difficulty in assessment of these patients, the threshold for performing CT is lower. Other risk groups include elderly people, intoxicated individuals, and patients with a coagulopathy (history of bleeding, clotting disorder, current treatment with anticoagulants). These concepts are summarized on Table 12-2. It is safe to state that, whenever in doubt, head imaging should be obtained, even in patients with mild head injury.

What Are the Most Optimal Imaging Techniques and Protocols in Head Trauma?

CT scanning is the primary imaging technique for acute brain injury. It provides rapid information and is part of a general trauma workup in emergency situations.

Head CT should be performed in sequential axial, rather than helical, mode to avoid artifacts that might affect the quality of the images for brain parenchyma evaluation. Noncontrast CT is fast and accurate for the detection of intracranial hemorrhage, mass effect and edema (including brain herniation), skull fractures, displaced bone fragments, foreign bodies, and intracranial air. CT scan with intravenous contrast usually is unnecessary. Furthermore, contrast infusion imaging may obscure some pathology in the acute setting, most notably subarachnoid hemorrhage. In severely head-injured patients, CT should be performed as soon as possible to assess the possible need for surgical intervention and for intracranial pressure (ICP) management. In the following hours and days, critically injured patients can be monitored within the scanner with relative ease. Most trauma centers now use multidetector computed

Table 12-1 Indications for Head Computed Tomographic Imaging in Patients with Head Trauma

Glasgow Coma Scale <15
Loss of consciousness >5 minutes
Antegrade amnesia
Penetrating head injury
Clinical signs of skull base fracture
Clinical evidence of depressed skull fracture
Anisocoria or fixed dilated pupils
Neurologic deficit (central nervous system, cranial nerves)

tomography (MDCT). This technology provides isotropic datasets that can be used for high-resolution three-dimensional (3D) postprocessing to better show fractures of the skull vault, maxillofacial region, and even the petrous bones and skull base. In patients with craniocerebral trauma, CT images of the head are best viewed in three window/level (W/L) settings as follows (Figure 12-1): brain parenchyma setting (W 80–120 Hounsfield units [HU], L 30–50 HU); bone setting to identify skull fractures (W 2,000–4,000 HU, L 500 HU); and intermediate setting for detection of thin layer of subdural or epidural blood against the dense calvarium (W 150–300 HU, L 50–100 HU).

In order to promptly diagnose patients with blunt vascular injury who are at risk for major strokes, some authors suggest the routine use of computed tomographic angiography (CTA) to simultaneously examine the cervical spine and cervical arterial system during assessment of acute multitrauma patients.

For the detection of subacute and delayed sequelae of head trauma, magnetic resonance imaging (MRI) is more sensitive than CT for evaluating the full extent of brain injury and has the ability to identify posttraumatic encephalomalacia, reactive gliosis, and hemosiderin deposits. MRI also is useful in cases with unexplained findings on CT scanning or when CT cannot explain the current clinical findings, such as patients with a focal neurologic deficit or prolonged period of unconsciousness. MRI is superior to CT in visualizing posterior fossa or brainstem lesions and in delineating vascular or diffuse axonal injuries. The most useful MR pulse sequences for head trauma imaging are the spin-echo (SE) T1-weighted image (T1-WI), fluid-attenuated inversion recovery (FLAIR) image, T2-weighted image (T2-WI), gradient-recalled echo (GRE) T2*-WI, and, in the acute or early subacute stage, the diffusion-weighted image (DWI).

What Is the Role of Skull Plain X-Ray Films in Problem Solving?

Plain films represent a valid technique for diagnosing skull vault fractures. However, skull fractures can occur without associated loss of consciousness; conversely, severe intracranial pathology can be present even in the absence of a fractured skull. Therefore, the diagnostic yield of plain films is low because of the poor correlation between skull fractures and intracranial injury. Plain x-ray films of the skull contribute little or no additional information in the clinical management of the acute head trauma patient. In most major trauma centers, plain x-ray films of the skull have been supplanted by CT scanning.

ACUTE ADMISSION IMAGING

Head

What Is the Role of Imaging in the Acute Phase?

Acute head trauma imaging, obtained as soon as possible after resuscitation, is directed at evaluating diffuse and focal lesions, identifying lesions that need urgent surgical intervention, and assessing the mass effect caused by the primary lesions and by the early development of brain edema.

Table 12-2 Indications for Head Computed Tomographic Imaging in Mild Head Trauma (Glasgow Coma Scale=15)

Severe headache
Nausea and vomiting (>1 episode)
Clinical suspicion of depressed skull fracture or large scalp hematoma obscuring clinical examination
Children, especially <2 years (keep radiation dose as low as possible)
Elderly patients
Intoxicated patients
Coagulopathic or anticoagulated patients

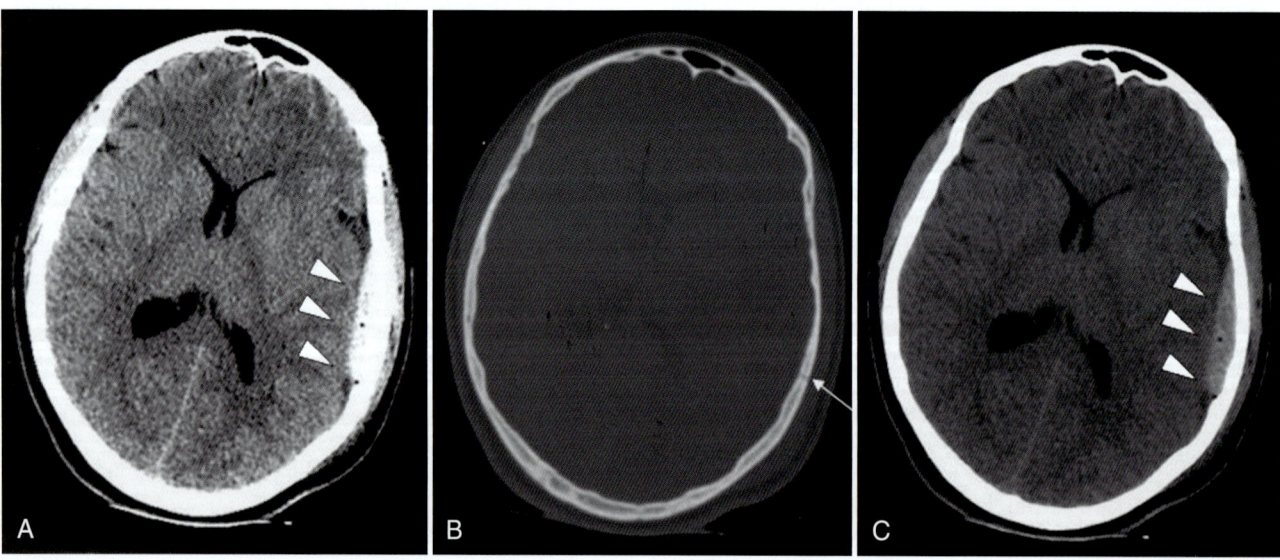

Figure 12-1 Window settings for noncontrast head computed tomography (CT) in trauma. Head CT images should be evaluated with brain parenchyma window settings **(A)** to appreciate good gray–white matter contrast, sensitive to intraaxial blood and edema; with bone window settings **(B)** to visualize skull fractures *(arrow)*; and with intermediate window settings **(C)** to enhance visualization of small extraaxial blood collection adjacent to the inner surface of the calvarium. Note better visualization of this small epidural hematoma *(arrowheads)* in C than in A.

Which Are the Possible Traumatic Lesions to Look for in the Acute Stage?
Problem Solving: Are There Primary Versus Secondary Lesions?

Head trauma can cause primary and secondary lesions (Table 12-3). Primary lesions are directly and immediately caused by the impact, the penetrating injury, or the deceleration forces. Secondary injuries are determined by the ensuing rise of ICP, edema, brain herniation, vascular damage and compression, embolism, hypotension, and hypoxia.

Primary Lesions
Skull Fractures

Skull fractures are often present in severe craniocerebral trauma. However, about 20% of patients with fatal head injuries do not have a skull fracture, so the absence of a skull fracture does not necessarily predict better clinical status. On the other hand, fractures can also be associated with mild clinical conditions. The diagnosis of a skull fracture requires visualization of the CT images with a bone window setting and can be further aided by 3D surface-shaded volume-rendering images (Figure 12-2). Skull fractures can be linear, complex, or comminute. Depending on their location, they can cause vascular lacerations resulting in arterial or venous epidural hematomas (EDHs) that have to be actively searched using various window settings and possibly multiplanar reformatting. An important feature of a fracture to define is whether it is depressed (Figure 12-2). A depressed skull fracture is important clinically because it may cause injury of the brain parenchyma, may be associated with penetration of the brain by foreign bodies, and may compress the brain parenchyma. As a rule of thumb, if the depression of the fracture's margins is equal or greater than the calvarium thickness, surgery to reduce the fracture is considered. Special attention should be directed to the extension of the fracture line to the skull base because of the possible risks of cerebrospinal fluid (CSF) fistula and vascular damage. The presence of pneumocephalus implies that the fracture may be connected to a penetrating injury, the paranasal sinuses, or mastoid air cells and represents a risk factor for CSF fistula and intracranial infection. In penetrating injuries, a detailed description of the size and location of intracranial bony fragments and foreign bodies might be helpful to the neurosurgeon.

Table 12-3 Primary and Secondary Brain Traumatic Lesions

Primary Lesions	Secondary Lesions
Skull fracture	Brain swelling (hyperemia and edema)
Epidural hematoma	
Subdural hematoma	Brain herniation
Subarachnoid and intraventricular hemorrhage	Vascular complications
	Cerebrospinal fluid fistula and pneumocephalus
Cortical contusion	
Brain hematoma	
Diffuse axonal injury	
Brainstem contusion	

Problem Solving: Is There an Extraaxial Collection? How to Differentiate Between Different Types of Extraaxial Collections?
Epidural Hematoma

An EDH is an extracerebral collection of blood within the epidural space, which is the potential space between the inner table of the skull and the firmly adherent outer layer of the dura mater. An EDH can be of arterial (90%) or venous (10%) origin. Arterial EDH is typically found at the coup site and is associated with a skull fracture, most commonly of the squamosal portion of the temporal bone (Figure 12-3), due to injury of one or more branches of the meningeal arteries. Arterial EDH tends to enlarge. Hyperacute EDH can appear heterogeneous on CT, with areas of high density representing clotted blood and hypointense lucent swirls indicating blood that has not yet clotted (Figure 12-3). These features indicate the greatest potential for rapid enlargement. As the EDH matures, hyperdensity distribution becomes more homogeneous. Venous EDH is due to injury to the sphenoparietal sinus, transverse sinus, or superior sagittal sinus and is typically found along the anterior wall of the middle cranial fossa, at the vertex, or against the occipital bone along the transverse sinus (Figure 12-4). The venous EDH seldom enlarges because of the containing force of the dural adhesion to the inner table of the calvarium.

CT is the preferred imaging technique because of its rapid accessibility and because it shows both the hemorrhage and the causative skull fracture. Due to the attachment of the dura to the calvarium, EDH has a typical focal biconvex configuration that may cross dural folds, such as falx and tentorium, but not sutures, where the dura is even more firmly anchored. A vertex EDH may not be seen on axial CT images unless it has a significant mass effect or it is imaged on reformatted coronal or sagittal images.

Subdural Hematoma

A subdural hematoma (SDH) is an extracerebral collection of blood within the subdural space, which is the virtual space between the dura mater and the arachnoid membrane. It is due to tearing of bridging veins (Figure 12-5) as they pierce the outer arachnoid membrane. There is no consistent relationship with skull fractures. SDH does cross suture lines but is limited by falx and tentorium. Most SDHs are ipsilateral to the site of trauma, but approximately one third occur contralateral to the site of injury. SDHs are also seen within the interhemispheric fissure, along the falx, and along the tentorium. Due to the absence of attachment between the dura mater and the outer arachnoid membrane, SDH is seen, differently from EDH, as a crescent-shaped fluid collection lying between the brain and the inner skull table (Figure 12-5). Due to the anatomy of the subdural space, a considerable volume of blood can be seen as a relatively thin SDH and still cause significant mass effect on the brain. On CT the density of an SDH depends on the interval between the last major episode of bleeding and the time of examination. Acute SDH is seen as a dense, crescent-shaped collection. Mixed density of an acute SDH might indicate very recent or active bleeding that

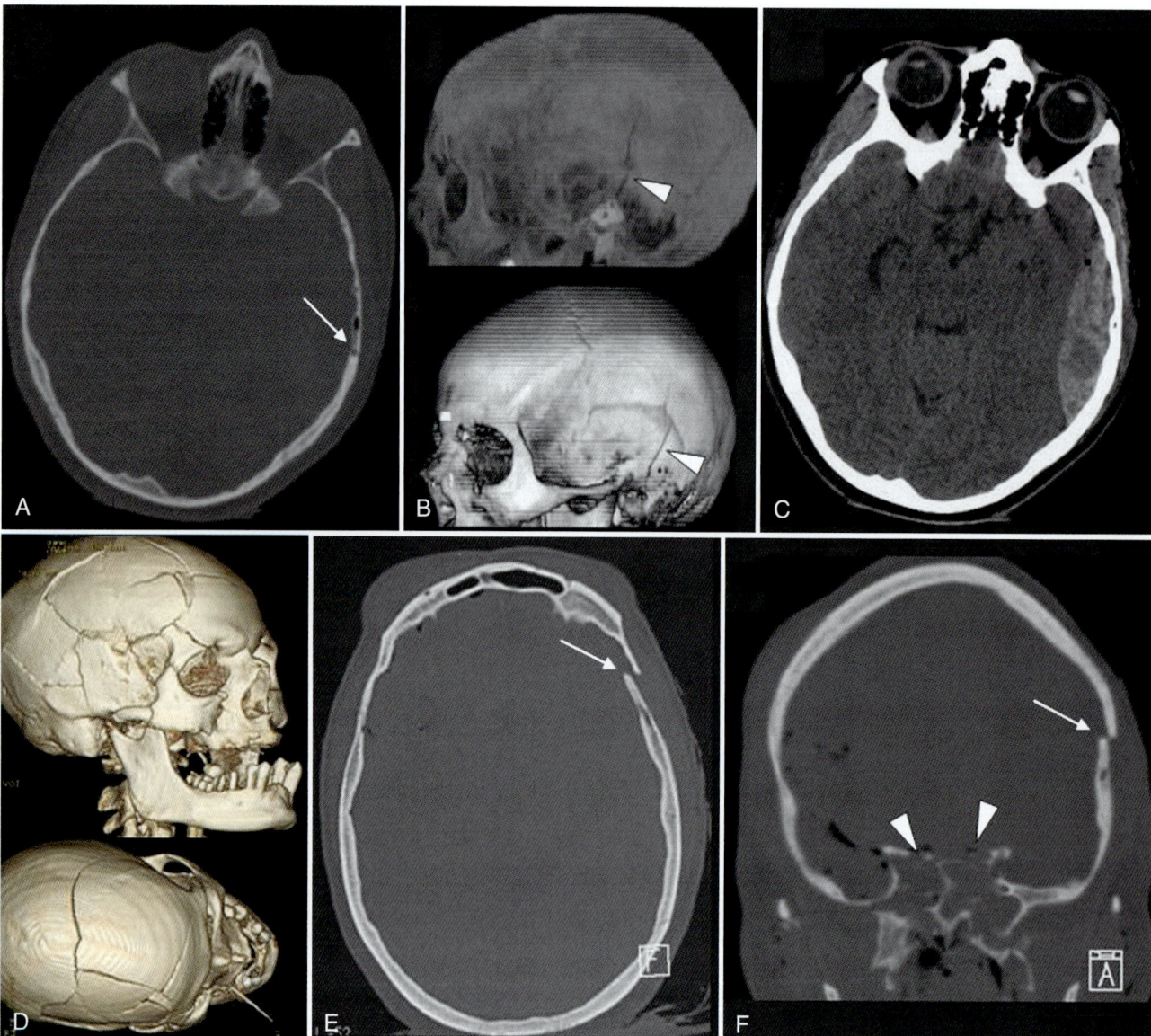

Figure 12-2 Computed tomography of skull fractures. **A–C:** Linear lucency, consistent with a fracture, of the left temporal squama (*arrow* in **A**), better appreciated in its entire course on three-dimensional volume-rendering reformatted images (*arrowheads* in **B**). **C:** This fracture is associated with an epidural hematoma visible with intermediate windowing. **D:** Three-dimensional views are especially useful in case of complex and comminuted fractures, as in this case. **E, F:** Multiple skull and skull base fractures. Depressed fractures (*arrow* in **E** and **F**) might represent a surgical indication, whereas fractures causing pneumocephalus, such as these ethmoid plate comminuted fractures (*arrowheads* in **F**), are a risk factor for cerebrospinal fluid fistula and intracranial infection.

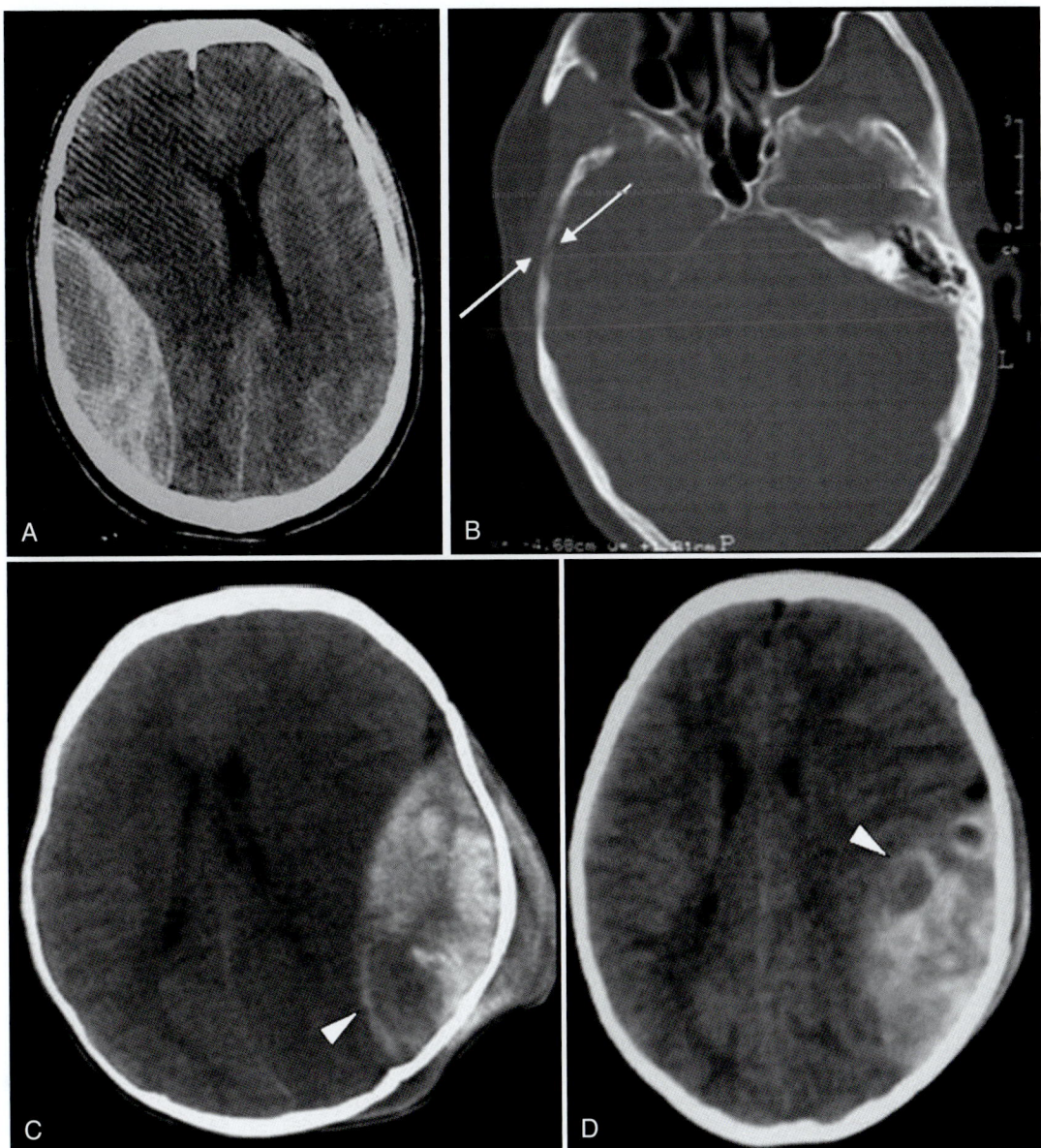

Figure 12-3 **A, B:** Large acute epidural hematoma causing mass effect and subfalcine herniation is associated with a fracture of the right temporal squama *(arrows* in **B)**, likely involving a branch of the middle meningeal artery. **C, D:** Two different acute epidural hematomas characterized by heterogeneous density. The hypodense areas *(arrowheads)* are represented by hyperacute and nonclotted components, suggesting active bleeding and rapid growth potential.

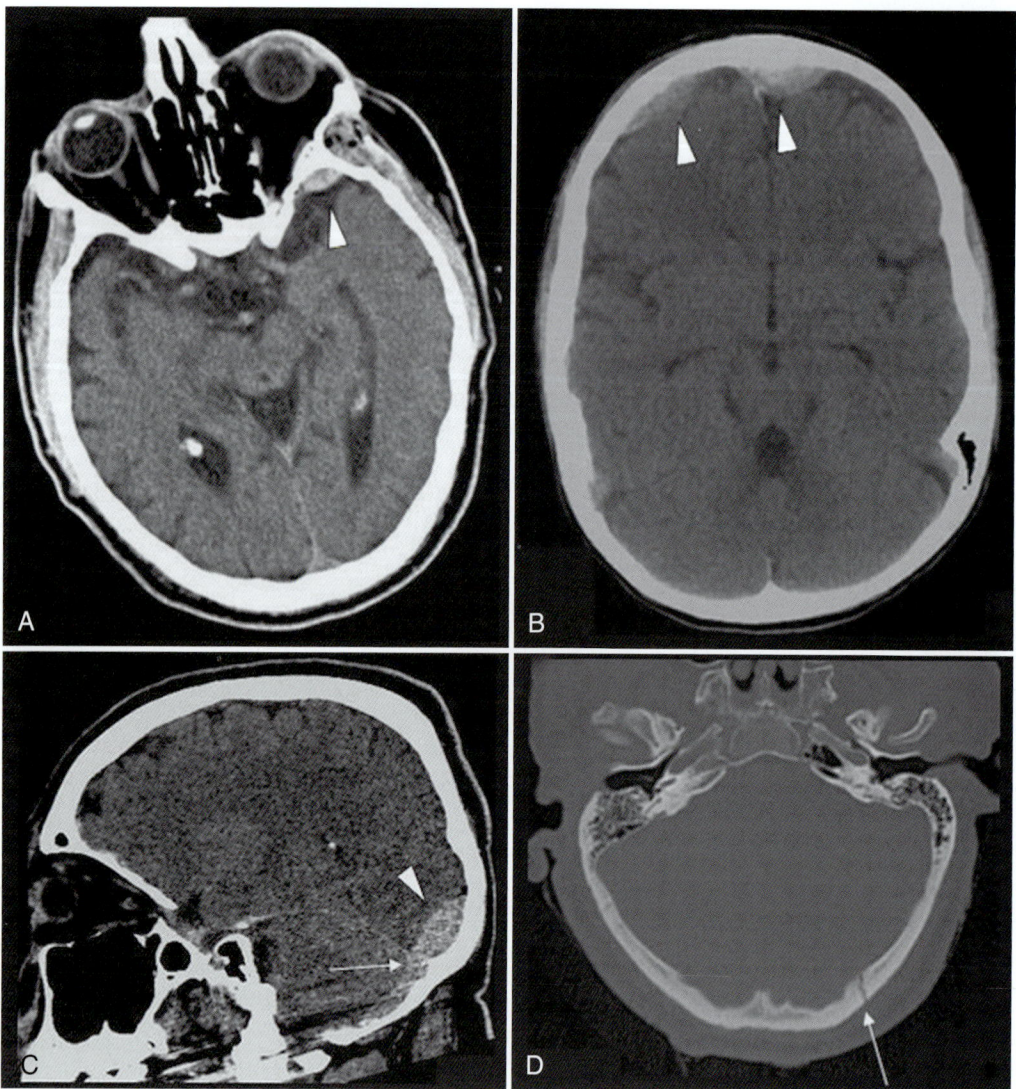

Figure 12-4 Venous epidural hematomas usually are self-limited and commonly are found in the anterior portion of the middle cranial fossa (*arrowhead* in **A**), adjacent to the superior sagittal sinus (*arrowheads* in **B**) or the transverse sinuses. *Hematoma* is indicated by *arrowhead* in **C**. Transverse sinus is indicated by *arrow* in **C**. These hematomas can be associated with skull fractures involving the dural sinuses (*arrow* in **D**).

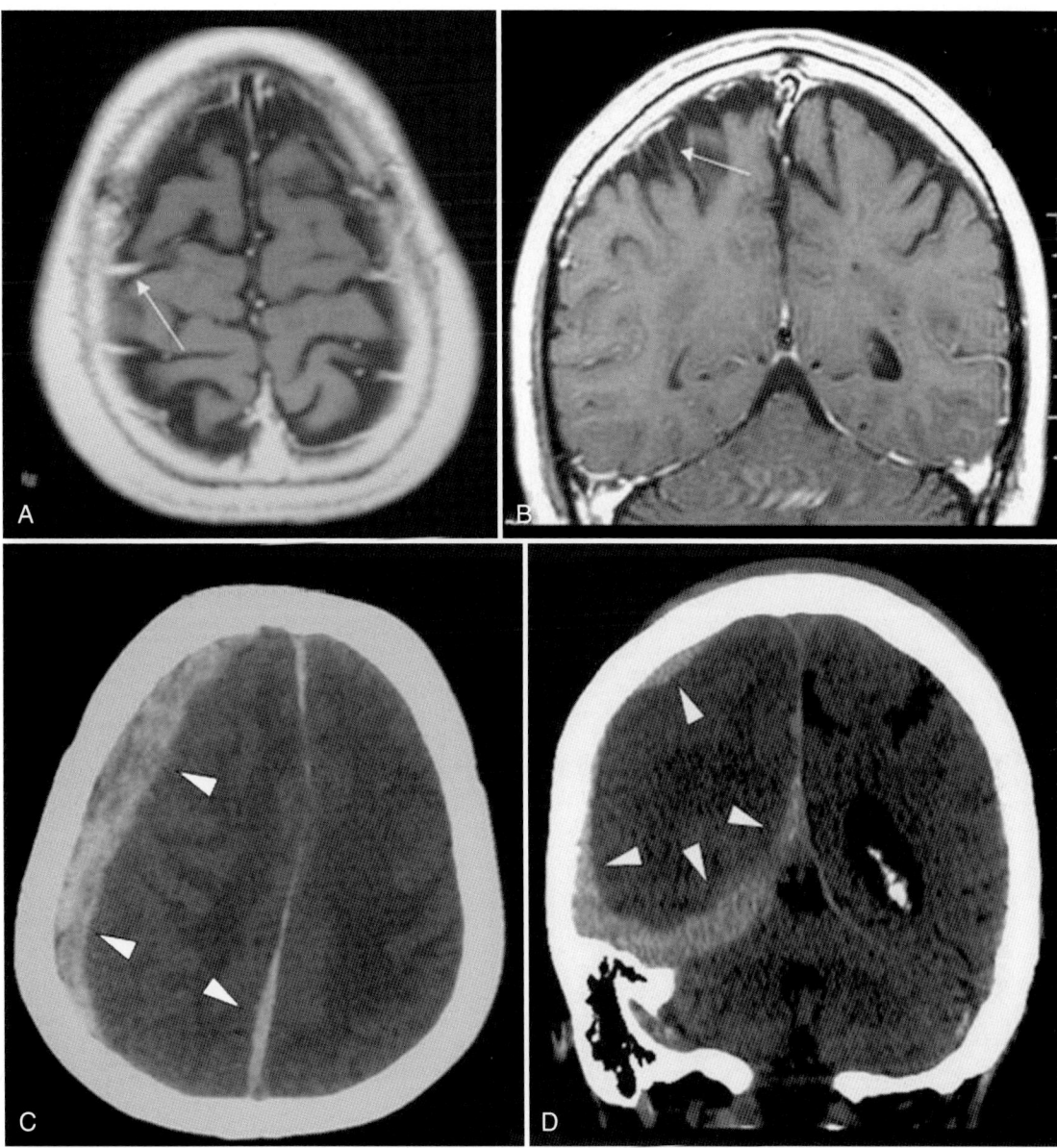

Figure 12-5 Bridging veins and subdural hematomas. Bridging veins drain the brain surfaces, traverse the subarachnoid space, pierce the arachnoid, and connect to larger venous collector draining into the dural sinuses. They are best visualized in their subarachnoid course on postcontrast T1-weighted images *(arrow* in **A** and **B)**. Tearing of bridging veins causes subdural hematomas, which are characterized by their crescent shape. Subdural hematomas are not limited by sutures, can extend along the whole calvarium, falx and, tentorium *(arrowheads* in **C** and **D)**, but are limited by dural reflection, so they cannot pass midline.

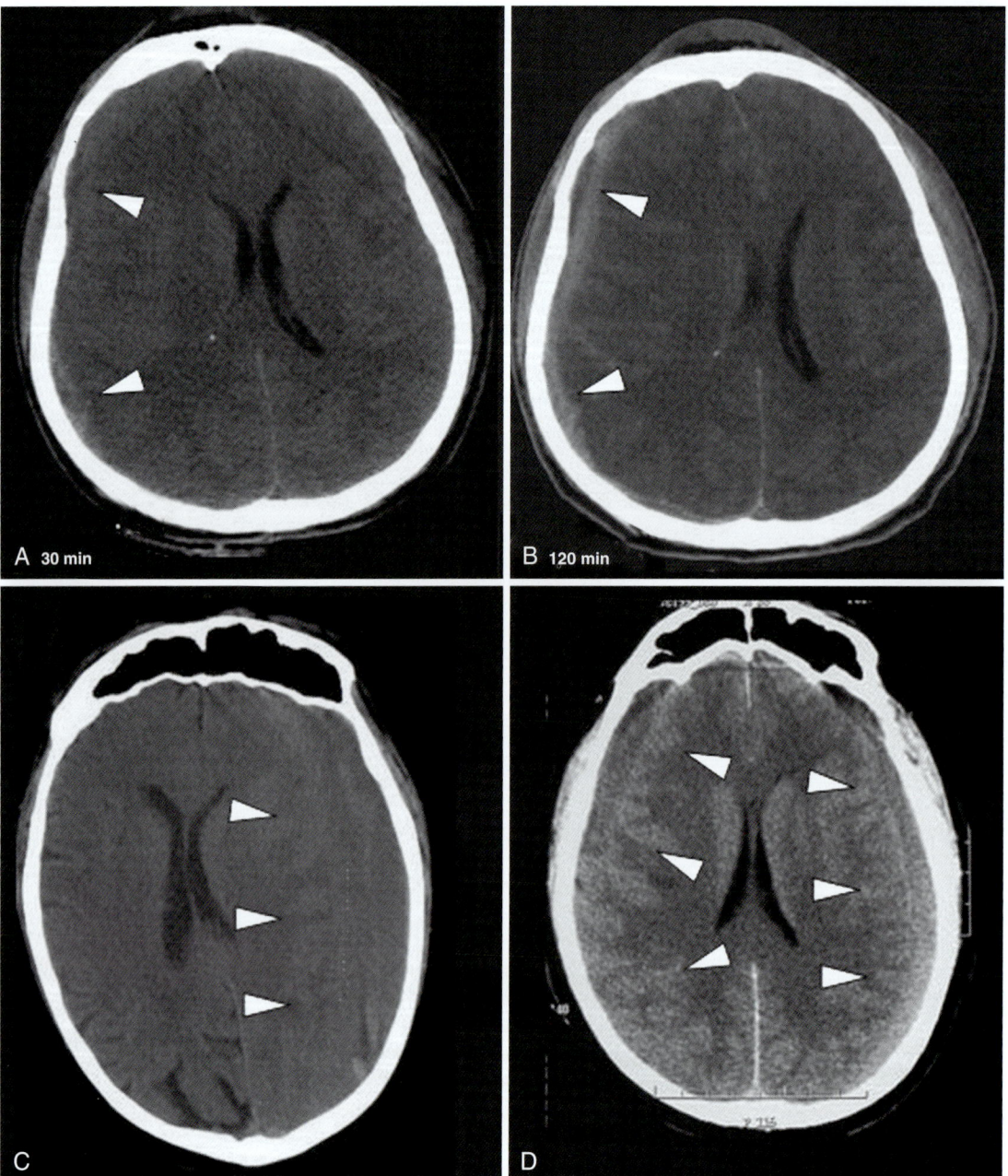

Figure 12-6 Isodensity and rebleeding in subdural hematomas. **A:** Hyperacute subdural blood collection, imaged before clot formation, appears isodense to the brain (*arrowheads*) and therefore may be overlooked, although careful attention should be posed to indirect signs such as mass effect on the ventricles and inward displacement of the cortical gyri. **B:** Follow-up scan obtained 90 minutes later clearly shows shift to hyperdensity of the subdural hematoma (*arrowheads*). **C:** Large isodense subdural hematoma (*red dotted line*) along its inner margins is clearly revealed by inward displacement of the gray–white matter junction (*arrowheads*). **D:** Bilateral isodense subdural collections displace symmetrically the gray–white matter junction inward (*arrowheads*).

is at high risk for rapid enlargement. Hyperacute SDH, before blood clotting, and subacute SDH can be nearly isodense with the adjacent cerebral cortex and difficult to differentiate from normal brain tissue. Acute SDH also can appear isodense to gray matter if the hemoglobin concentration is less than 10 to 11 g/dl. Asymmetry of the subarachnoid spaces and inner displacement of the cortex may reveal the presence of the isodense blood collection (Figure 12-6). Bilateral isodense SDHs should not be difficult to detect if attention is given to identifying the displacement of gray matter with effacement of cortical sulci and compressed ventricles (Figure 12-6). A mixed density pattern or a hemorrhagic sedimentation level may also indicate rebleeding into a preexisting chronic SDH (Figure 12-6). MRI is superior to CT in identifying the relative age of the various blood breakdown products of a layered, multicompartmental SDH.

Subarachnoid and Intraventricular Hemorrhage

Traumatic subarachnoid hemorrhage (SAH) is common. The most common cause of SAH is head trauma. It can be caused by direct injury to the pial vessels,

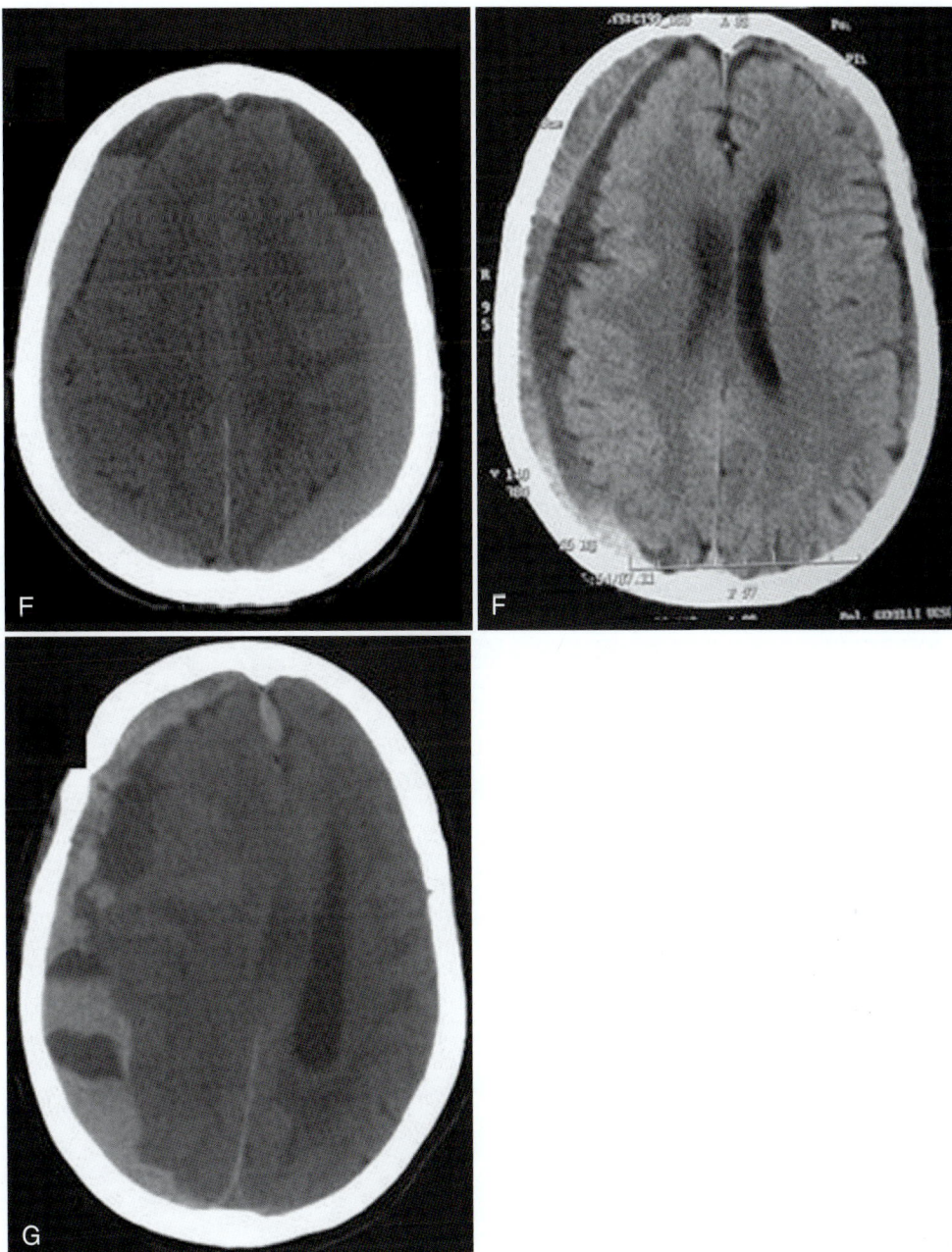

Figure 12-6, cont'd E–G: Different examples of rebleeding phenomena occurring in chronic subdural hematomas as revealed by layers and fluid–fluid levels of different densities, suggesting coexistence of blood products of different ages.

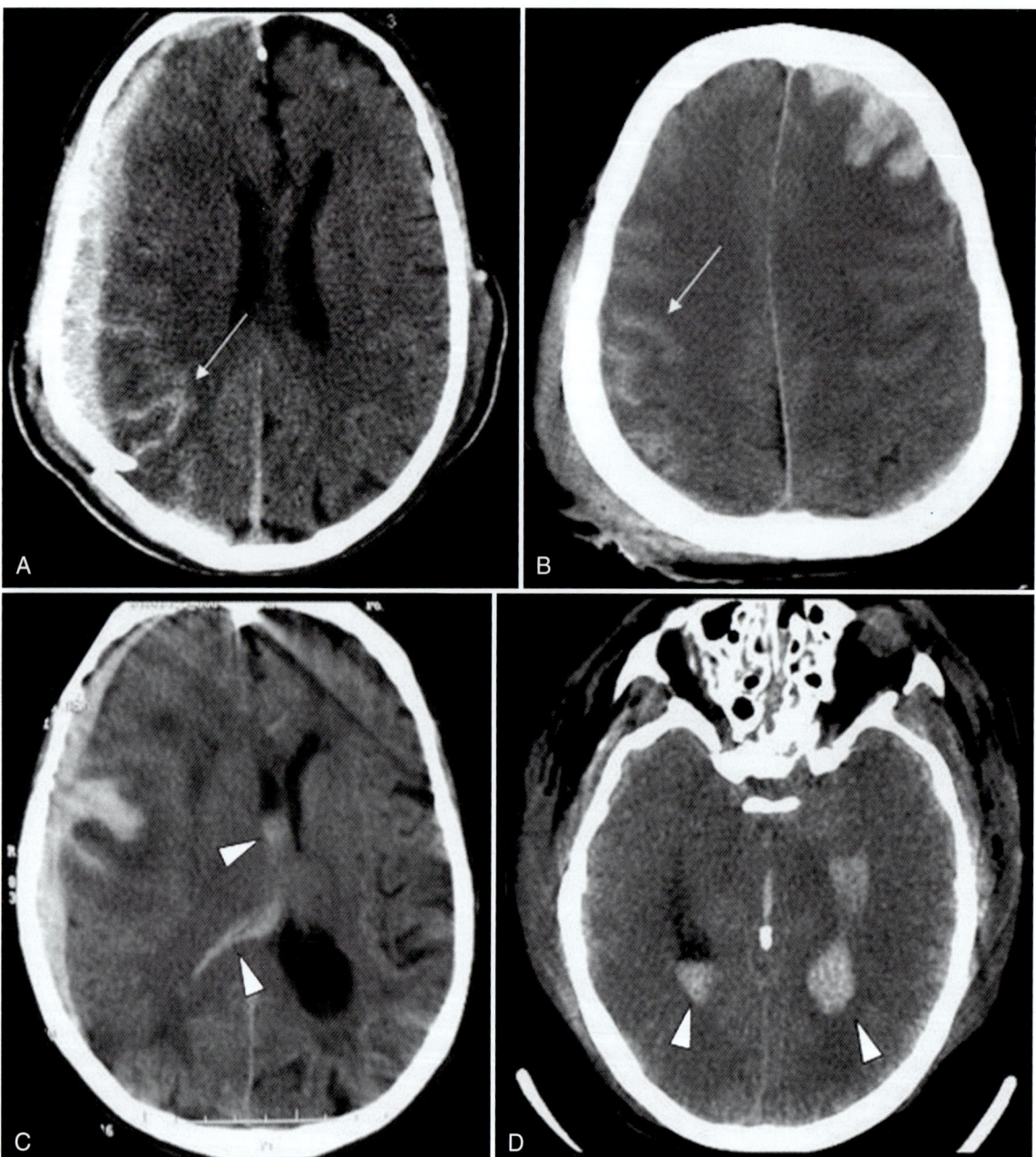

Figure 12-7 Subarachnoid and intraventricular hemorrhage. Traumatic subarachnoid hemorrhage is usually more focal than what is seen in aneurysm ruptures. Traumatic subarachnoid hemorrhage is seen in a parietal location (**A**, *arrow*) adjacent to a subdural hematoma and depressed fracture, and in a frontal location (**B**, *arrow*), overlying the site of a contusion, with scalp hematoma. Intraventricular hemorrhage can fill the ventricles, clot, and float attached to ventricular walls (*arrowheads* in **C**) or layer in a dependent position, usually in the ventricular trigones (*arrowheads* in **D**).

hemorrhagic cortical contusion, or extension of intraventricular hemorrhage (IVH) into the subarachnoid space. Traumatic SAH is an adverse, independent, prognostic factor in worsening outcomes. On a nonenhanced CT scan, acute SAH appears as linear high-density fluid collections within the superficial sulci and CSF cisterns. Compared to SAH related to an aneurysm, traumatic SAH is often focal, overlying the site of cortical bruising, or subjacent to an SDH (Figure 12-7). Diffuse spread throughout all the subarachnoid spaces is less common. Nevertheless, if the history of trauma is unclear and SAH is present, angiography should be used to identify a ruptured aneurysm. Traumatic SAH usually resolves over the following days.

As many as 25% of patients with severe head injury have IVH. Traumatic IVH occurs as a result of the tearing of subependymal veins, rupture of an intracerebral hemorrhage into the adjacent ventricle, or reflux of SAH into the ventricular system. On CT, look for a horizontally layered blood–CSF level in the dependent portions of the lateral ventricles (occipital horns, if the patient is supine) (Figure 12-7).

The detection of acute blood into the CSF (ventricles and subarachnoid spaces) with MRI is more complicated.

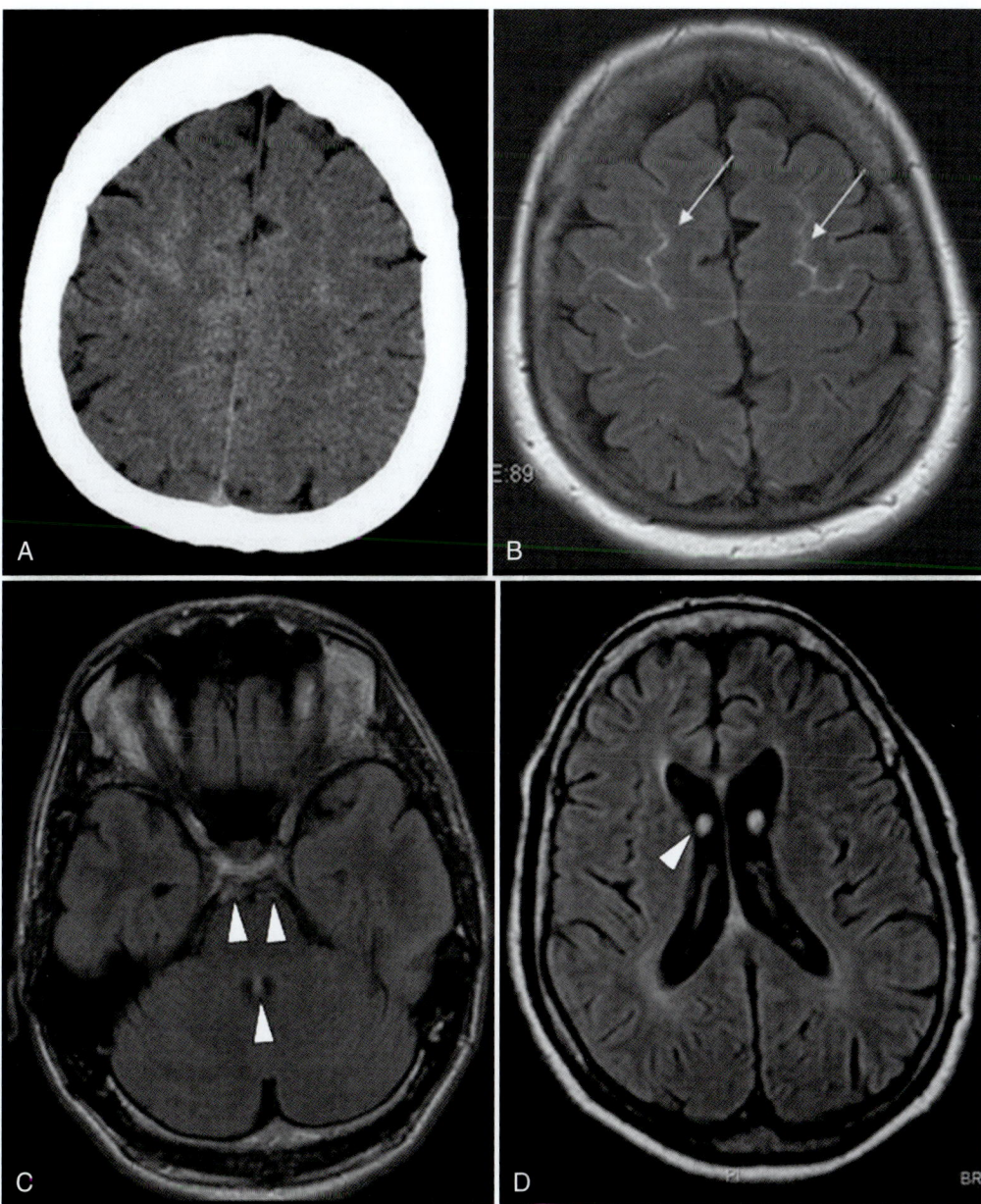

Figure 12-8 Magnetic resonance imaging for detection of subarachnoid hemorrhage. Acute subarachnoid hemorrhage, seen as cerebrospinal fluid (CSF) hyperdensity along the frontal sulci on computed tomography (A) is clearly revealed as high signal on FLAIR T2-weighted image (*arrows* in B). The extreme sensitivity of FLAIR imaging for detecting subtle changes in protein concentration of CSF is counterbalanced by its poor specificity. Infectious and neoplastic meningeal disease, as well as hyperoxygenation (frequent in patients ventilated with high concentrations of O_2 under general anesthesia) may cause similar CSF hyperintensity. Commonly observed hyperintense CSF pulsatility artifacts further decrease FLAIR specificity in the basal and prepontine cisterns and in the ventricles (*arrowheads* in C and D).

The higher oxygen tension (pO_2) in the CSF slows the transformation of oxyhemoglobin to paramagnetic breakdown products such as deoxyhemoglobin and methemoglobin. Traditional T1-W or T2-W SE or fast SE sequences have not been able to detect SAH reliably. Fast FLAIR sequences show traumatic SAH on MR with a sensitivity that is as good as, or even better than, CT. SAH produces dramatic hyperintensity in the normally hypointense CSF on FLAIR due to the sensitivity of this pulse sequence to the high protein content of the blood (Figure 12-8). Nevertheless, FLAIR specificity fro SAH is particularly low. High CSF signal can be observed that are due to other causes of increased protein concentration in the CSF, such as meningeal infection or tumor, and when CSF has high oxygen concentrations (as in patients ventilated with oxygen). The presence of high-signal CSF pulsatility artifacts on FLAIR further limits its specificity in identifying hemorrhage in the prepontine cistern, in the frontal horns of the lateral ventricles, in the III and IV ventricles (Figure 12-8).

Cortical Contusions, Cerebral Hematomas, Diffuse Axonal Injuries, Brainstem Injuries

Cerebral primary injuries occur due to impact of the cerebral parenchyma against the inner calvarium and to shear–strain forces caused by rotational acceleration

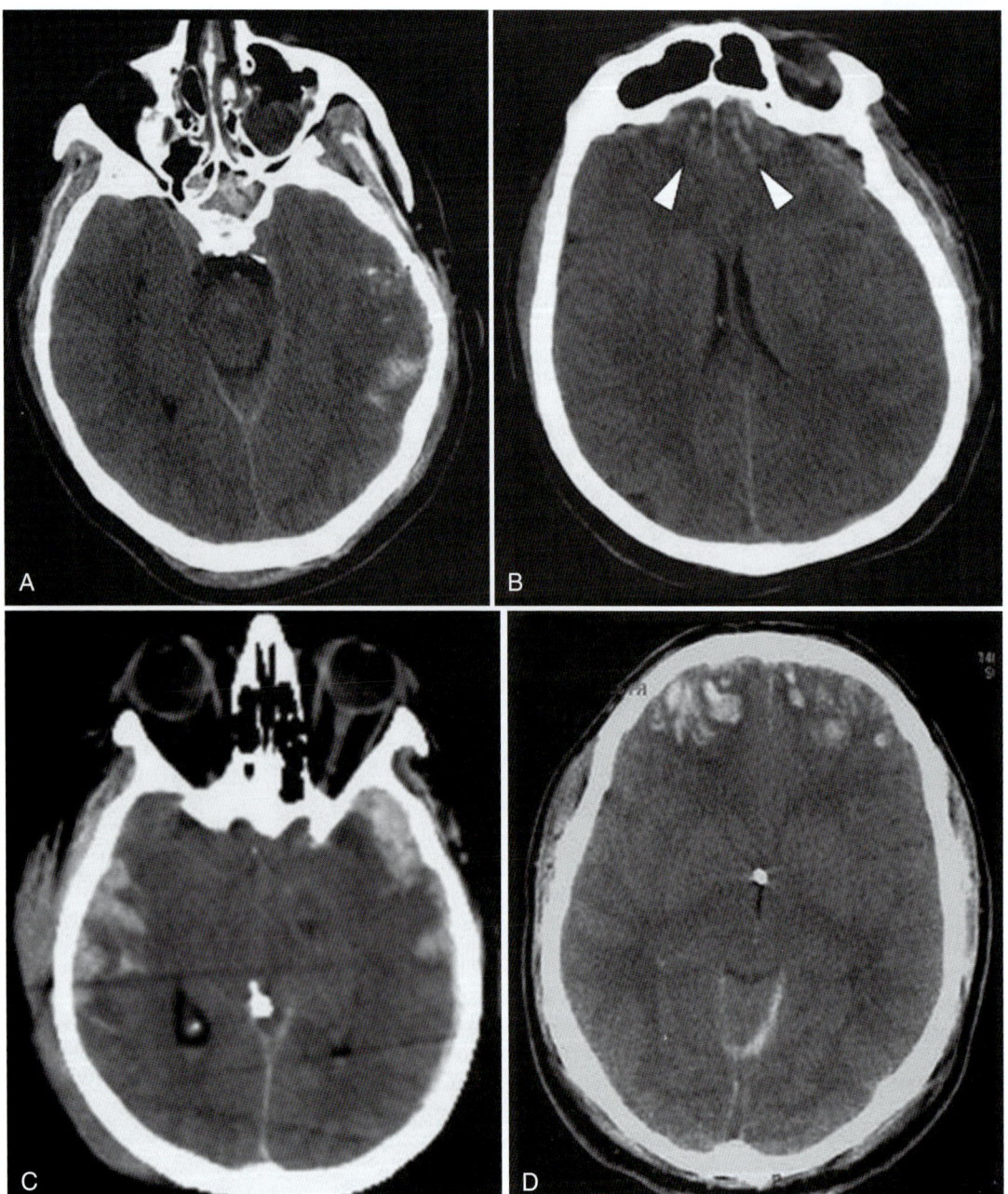

Figure 12-9 Different examples of cerebral contusions are seen as superficial cortical and subcortical small punctuate but sometimes larger and confluent edematous and hemorrhagic injuries. Predilections sites are the frontal and temporal lobes, especially in areas in contact with uneven bone surfaces, such as the ethmoid cribiform plate (*arrowheads* in **B**) and the petrous ridges.

of the head. Brain injuries consist of cortical contusions and intracerebral hematomas, diffuse axonal injury (DAI), and brainstem injury. They can present with different levels of clinical severity.

Cortical Contusion and Intracerebral Hematomas. Cerebral contusions are small, punctuate, often multiple, superficial parenchymal injuries with hemorrhage and variable amounts of surrounding vasogenic edema, resulting from coup or contrecoup mechanisms. Hemorrhagic cerebral contusions are most often encountered supratentorially. Sites of predilection include the anterior and inferior frontal lobes and the anterior and inferior temporal lobes, due to the rough surfaces of the adjacent cribrous ethmoid plate and the petrous ridges. Contusions occur much less frequently in the cerebellar hemispheres, which are protected by the smooth inner surface of the thick occipital bone. On CT, acute brain contusions are recognized as patchy, ill-defined cortical and subcortical low-density lesions (edema, nonhemorrhagic contusion) containing small, hyperdense, punctate foci of petechial hemorrhage (hemorrhagic contusion), more often in the frontal and temporal lobes (Figure 12-9).

Associated SAH is a common finding. In acceleration or deceleration brain injuries, a specific lesion pattern is often encountered, the so-called *coup–contrecoup*

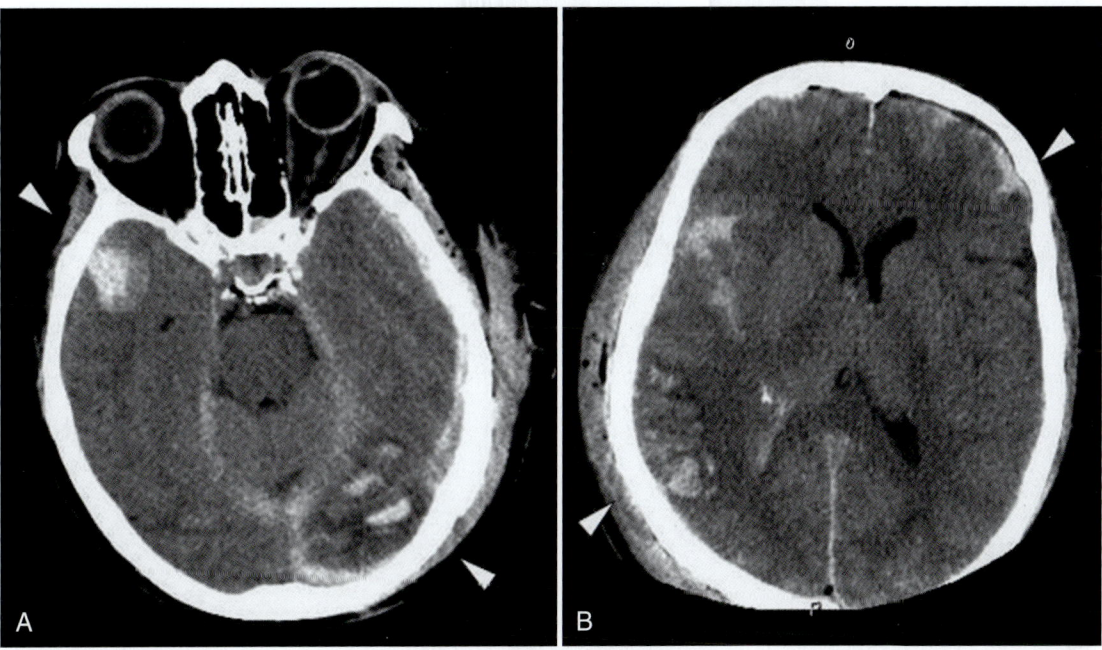

Figure 12-10 Two examples of coup–contrecoup injury revealing hemorrhagic brain contusions in opposite location across an ideal vector of acceleration–deceleration impact type of injury mechanism. **A:** Left occipital injury is opposed to a right temporal pole contusion (*arrowheads*). **B:** Right parietal lesion connects along an ideal line with the left frontal contusion. The primary site of impact is usually revealed by the soft tissue scalp hematoma.

injury. The intraparenchymal *coup injury* occurs at the site of primary impact, which is identified by the associated scalp injuries or skull fractures, whereas the *contrecoup injury* arises on the opposite side (Figure 12-10). Hemorrhagic cerebral contusions are more common and tend be larger on the contrecoup side, although both coup and contrecoup injuries can be hemorrhagic. A severe impact on the stationary head (e.g., a blow with a blunt object) results in skull fractures but generally does not cause contrecoup contusions. This is because, in these cases, the head does not accelerate or decelerate, and there is no brain lag.

The term *cerebral hematoma* refers to a well-circumscribed larger parenchymal hemorrhage. Cerebral hematomas tend to be found in the deeper parts of the brain. Delayed development of a posttraumatic intracerebral hemorrhage is not uncommon and should be suspected when the patient's neurologic condition is worsening. In the acute phase, hematomas may show little or no surrounding edema. However, as the hematoma matures and clot retraction occurs, the hematoma becomes surrounded by a hypodense rim of edema. Hemorrhagic sedimentation levels may develop (Figure 12-11). Cerebral hematomas can spontaneously decompress into the ventricles, thereby causing IVH.

Diffuse Axonal Injury. The brain can suffer severe damage by shearing injuries caused by acceleration, deceleration, or rotational forces. DAI represents approximately 48% of all primary lesions in head trauma and is one of the most common causes of poor clinical outcome. Clinically, DAI is characterized, in the acute phase, by impairment or complete loss of consciousness from the moment of impact.

Depending on rotation or deceleration of adjacent brain tissues of different density and rigidity, DAI may occur in white matter or subcortical gray matter. Most injuries occur in gray matter–white matter junction areas of the frontal and temporal lobes or in the internal capsules. The corpus callosum or brainstem seldom sustain injury without associated lesions in the lobar white matter. Callosal injuries occur more commonly in the posterior body and the splenium of the corpus callosum. In brainstem injuries, the posterior lateral quadrant of the midbrain and upper brainstem are most commonly involved. Shearing injuries in the cerebellum are infrequent. Despite the clinical severity, only 10% of patients with DAI demonstrate significant abnormalities on CT scan. CT may identify punctate hemorrhages in the acute setting or may reveal multiple, small, focal low-density lesions in the white matter (Figure 12-12). However, CT underestimates DAI lesions because nonhemorrhagic lesions are difficult to identify. Therefore, when a patient's neurologic or psychiatric status is worse than predicted from the CT findings, MRI must be performed (Figure 12-13). MRI is far more sensitive for detecting DAI lesions. FLAIR sequences are useful for the detection of nonhemorrhagic lesions. Gradient echo $T2^*$-weighted images are used to detect the susceptibility effects of paramagnetic blood degradation products. Evidence indicates that DWI is valuable in closed head injury because it identifies additional shearing injuries that are not visible on T2/FLAIR or $T2^*$ sequences. Decreased apparent diffusion coefficient values can be found in DAI and indicate restricted diffusion.

Brainstem Injury. Acute posttraumatic primary brainstem injury usually involves the dorsolateral aspect of the upper midbrain, as a result of a contusion, as the

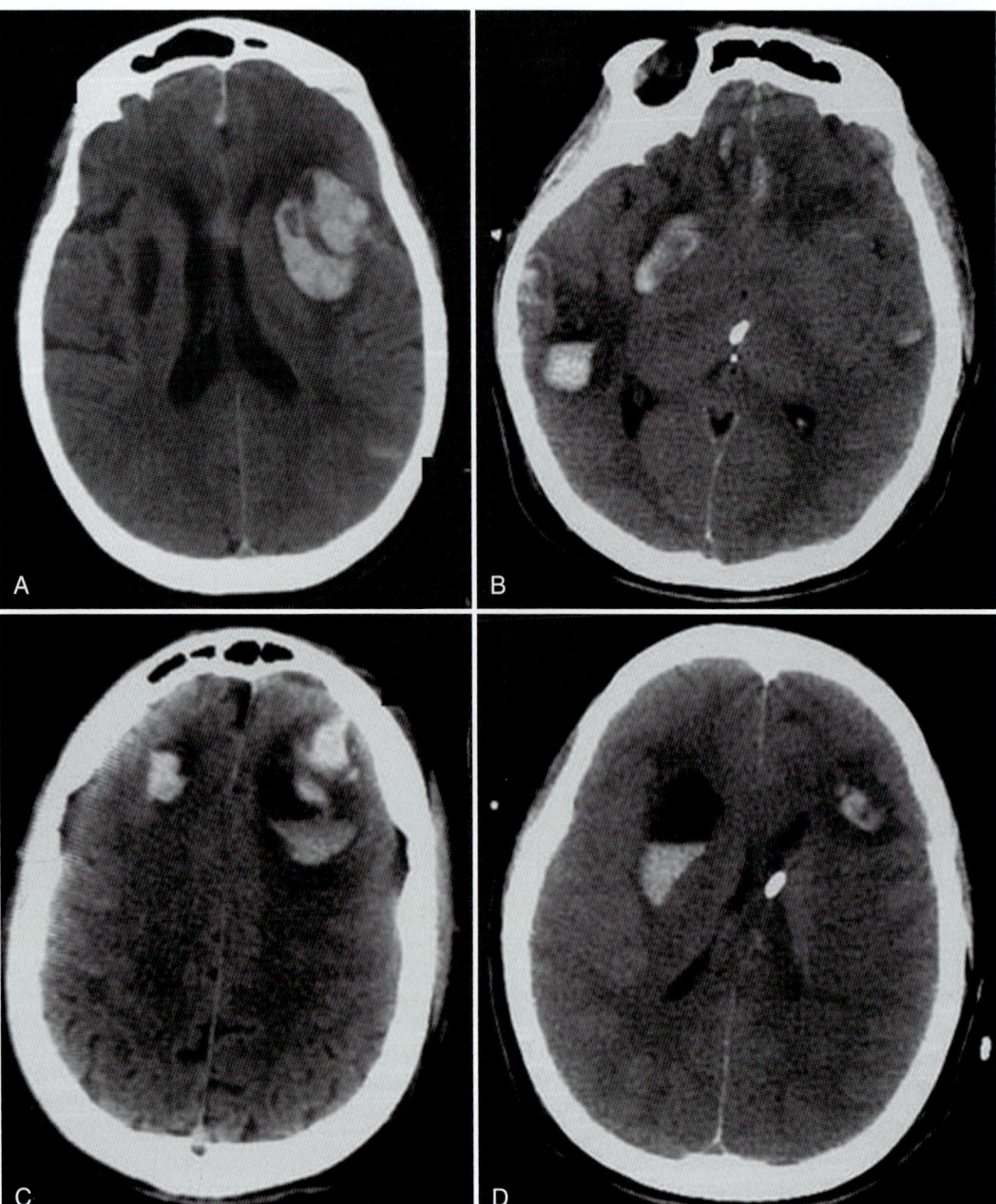

Figure 12-11 Four different cases of traumatic cerebral hematomas. These hematomas are generally located deep in the brain and might not be present on the admission study but develop in the early subacute phase. The amount of surrounding vasogenic edema and mass effect is variable, and commonly blood–fluid levels are present.

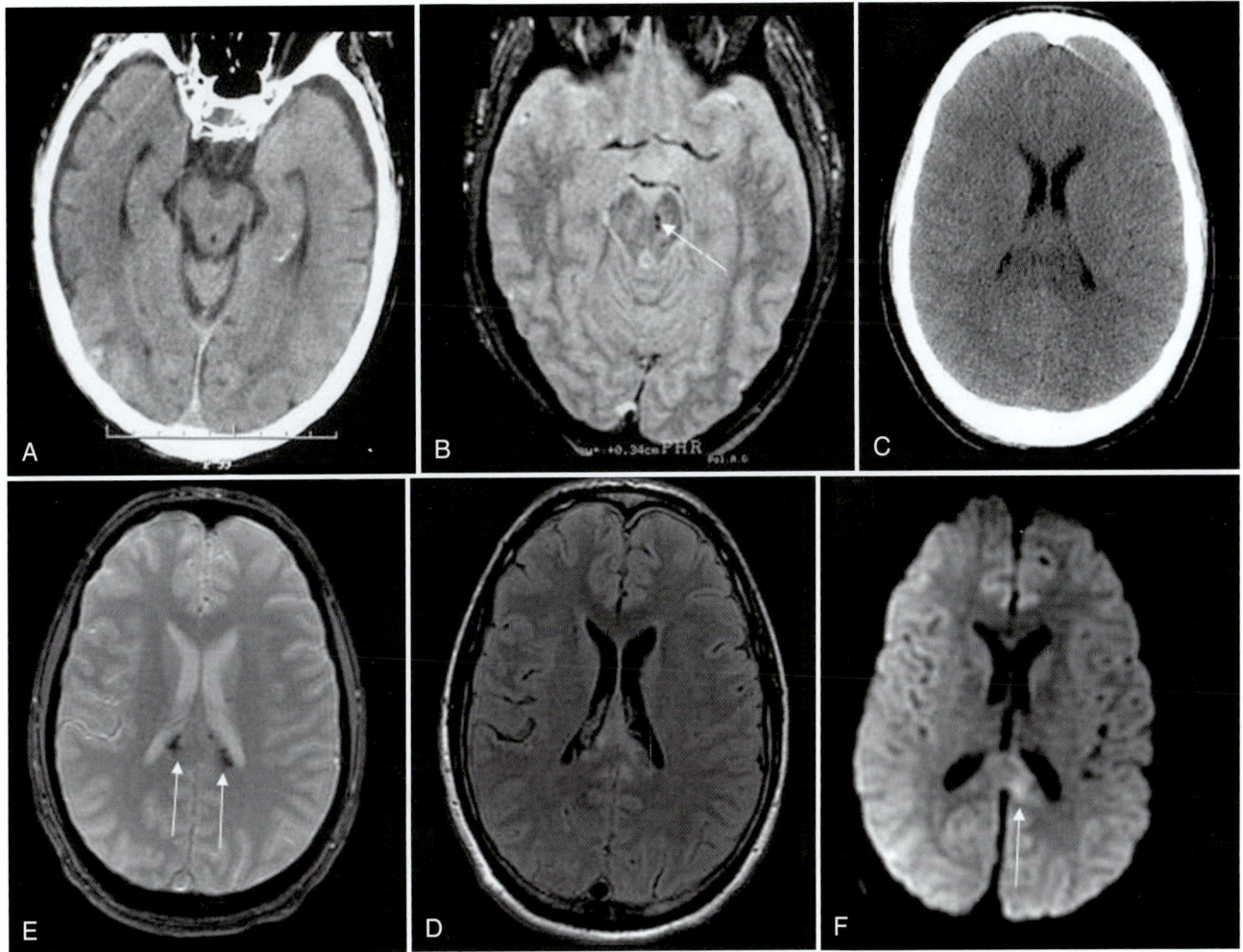

Figure 12-13 Diffuse axonal injuries (DAIs) on magnetic resonance imaging (MRI). MRI, with its multiparametric capabilities and inherent great sensitivity for brain signal abnormalities, is superior to computed tomography (CT) for the diagnosis and full estimation of shearing injuries. Whenever the clinical picture is not completely explained by CT findings, a subtle but eloquent shearing injury should be suspected and MRI should be performed. **A, B:** Patient who suffered severe acceleration–deceleration head impact and presented with otherwise unexplained right hemiparesis. CT cut through the midbrain (**A**) is nonconclusive, whereas gradient-recalled echo (GRE) T2* MRI reveals a small hemorrhagic DAI in the left cerebral peduncle (*arrow* in **B**). **C–F:** Another severe craniocerebral trauma patient in a coma but with no obvious hemorrhagic lesions on CT examination (**C**), whose MRI shows diffuse shearing injuries of the splenium of the corpus callosum, hemorrhagic on GRE T2* image (**D**), high T2 signal on FLAIR (**E**), and restricted diffusion on diffusion-weighted imaging b1000 (**F**).

gradually herniate through the tentorial incisura and the foramen magnum.

Brain Herniations

Severe brain swelling and intraaxial and extraaxial hemorrhage cause mass effect and may lead to displacement of brain tissue. The intracranial dural reflections, the falx and the tentorium, are the boundaries of the intracranial compartments and limit the amount of compensatory shift and displacement, which develop in response to general or localized increased ICP. When the pressure in one of the dural compartments increases beyond the physiologic compensatory mechanisms, a pressure gradient ensues. This leads to brain herniation, which is a displacement of brain, CSF, and blood vessels, from one cranial compartment to another, along the free margins of the dural reflections, following the pressure gradient direction (Figure 12-15).

What Are the Different Types of Brain Herniations?

1. *Subfalcine herniation:* Brain hemispheres can shift from side to side under the falx, with the risk of compression of the anterior cerebral artery (ACA) against the rigid falx, possibly resulting in ACA infarcts, and distortion of the ventricular foramina of Monro, possibly resulting in ventricular entrapment and hydrocephalus.
2. *Transtentorial descending herniation (uncal herniation):* Brain hemispheres can shift downward so that the mesial temporal lobe "slips" medially and inferiorly along the free margin of the tentorium. The herniated temporal lobe can compress the ipsilateral oculomotor nerve and cerebral peduncle, causing ipsilateral mydriasis and contralateral hemiparesis, or can push the contralateral cerebral peduncle against the adjacent tentorium, causing ipsilateral

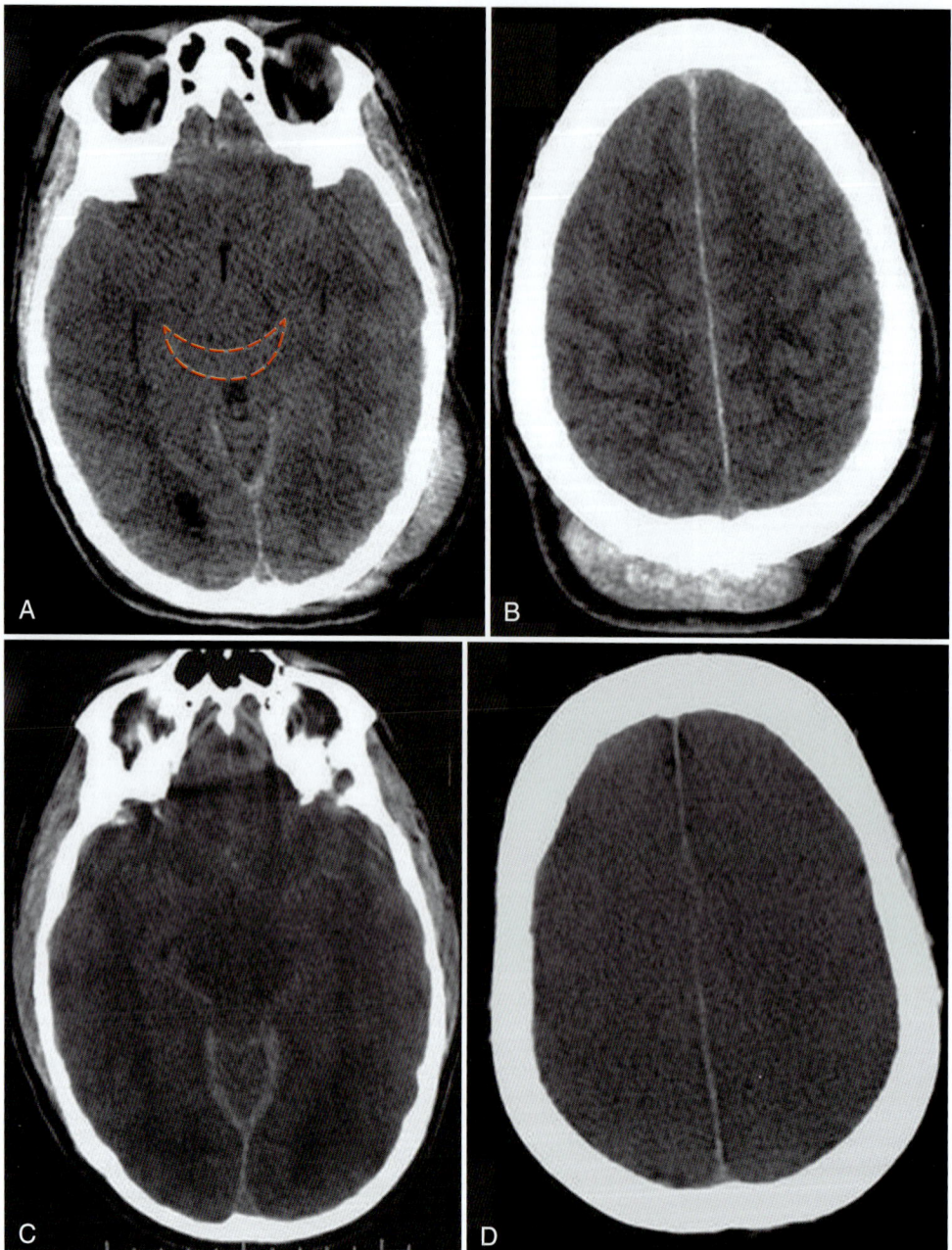

Figure 12-14 Posttraumatic brain swelling: hyperemia and cerebral edema. **A, B:** Diffuse brain swelling revealed by effacement of the cerebrospinal fluid (CSF) spaces in the sulci along the vault (**B**) and of the cisterns at the base of the brain (**A**). Disappearance of the perimesencephalic cistern, the so-called smile, represented here by the red dotted line crescent in **A**, is a very important sign of brain swelling and impending descending transtentorial herniation. Note that the natural density difference at the gray–white matter junction is preserved, so this is defined as swelling in hyperemic state rather than brain edema. **C, D:** Diffuse and severe brain swelling (note effacement of CSF spaces at base and along vault) is accompanied by homogeneous parenchymal hypodensity (blood-containing structures, such as dural sinuses and large vessels, and the tentorium appear hyperdense compared to brain) and gray–white matter junction visibility loss. This is defined as brain swelling and diffuse cerebral edema, a prognostically much worse condition than hyperemia.

mydriasis and ipsilateral hemiparesis, the so-called *Kernohan notch syndrome* or false-localizing sign. The posterior cerebral and superior cerebellar arteries can be compressed along their course lateral to the midbrain, possibly resulting in infarcts in their respective territories.

3. *Central herniation:* In response to generalized and severe increased pressure in the supratentorial compartment, the diencephalon can shift downward through the tentorial hiatus. As a result, the brainstem is compressed and pushed downward and the arterial and venous pontine perforators can be stretched, possibly resulting in devastating pontine hemorrhage, also known as *Duret hemorrhage*.

4. *Transtentorial ascending herniation:* Mass effect in the posterior fossa can push the superior vermis and cerebellar hemispheres in the supratentorial compartment through the tentorial hiatus.

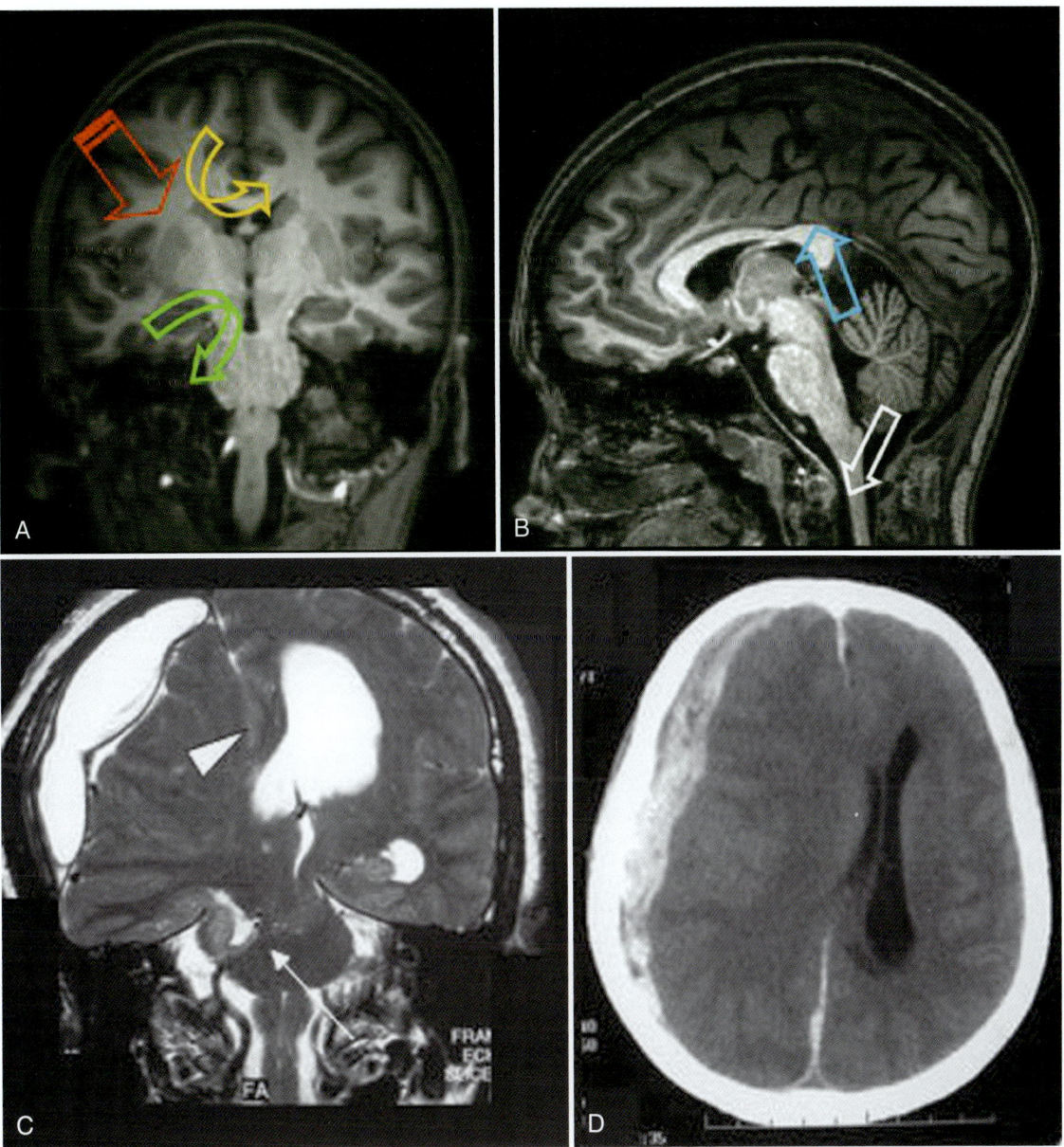

Figure 12-15 Brain herniations. **A:** Expected effects of a pressure increase in the supratentorial compartment, creating a pressure gradient directed downward *(red arrow)*. The brain shifts contralaterally below the falx, featuring a subfalcine herniation *(yellow arrow)*, and caudally across the free margin of the tentorium, featuring a transtentorial descending or uncal herniation *(green arrow)*. **B:** Increased mass effect in the posterior fossa causes the cerebellum to herniate upward through the tentorial hiatus *(blue arrow)* and downward through the foramen magnum *(white arrow)*, featuring ascending transtentorial and tonsillar herniation, respectively. **C:** Coronal plane display of a large subdural hematoma compressing the right cerebral hemisphere, resulting in subfalcine herniation *(arrowhead)* and transtentorial herniation *(arrow)* that impinges on the brainstem.

5. *Tonsillar herniation:* Mass effect in the posterior fossa can push the inferior vermis and cerebellar tonsils in the spinal canal through the foramen magnum, possibly compressing the lower medulla, the vertebral arteries, and the posterior inferior cerebellar arteries.
6. *Herniation through the craniectomy:* To prevent brain herniation in the acute trauma setting, a craniectomy, often bilateral, is commonly performed to relieve intracranial hypertension. The swollen brain then herniates through the craniectomy defect without compressing other intracranial nervous or vascular structures. The craniectomy should be wide so that no additional brain compression occurs against the bony margins. Some neurosurgeons also perform duraplasty, a procedure that widens the dura at the level of the craniectomy, with apposition of an extra sheet of artificial dura.

Displacement of brain tissue across intracranial compartments causes compression on vital brain tissue and stretching and compression of cranial nerves and vessels, possibly resulting in profound neurologic deficits, ischemic infarcts, and perhaps even death. Early detection of brain herniation is of vital importance in clinical patient management. CT is able to identify all types of

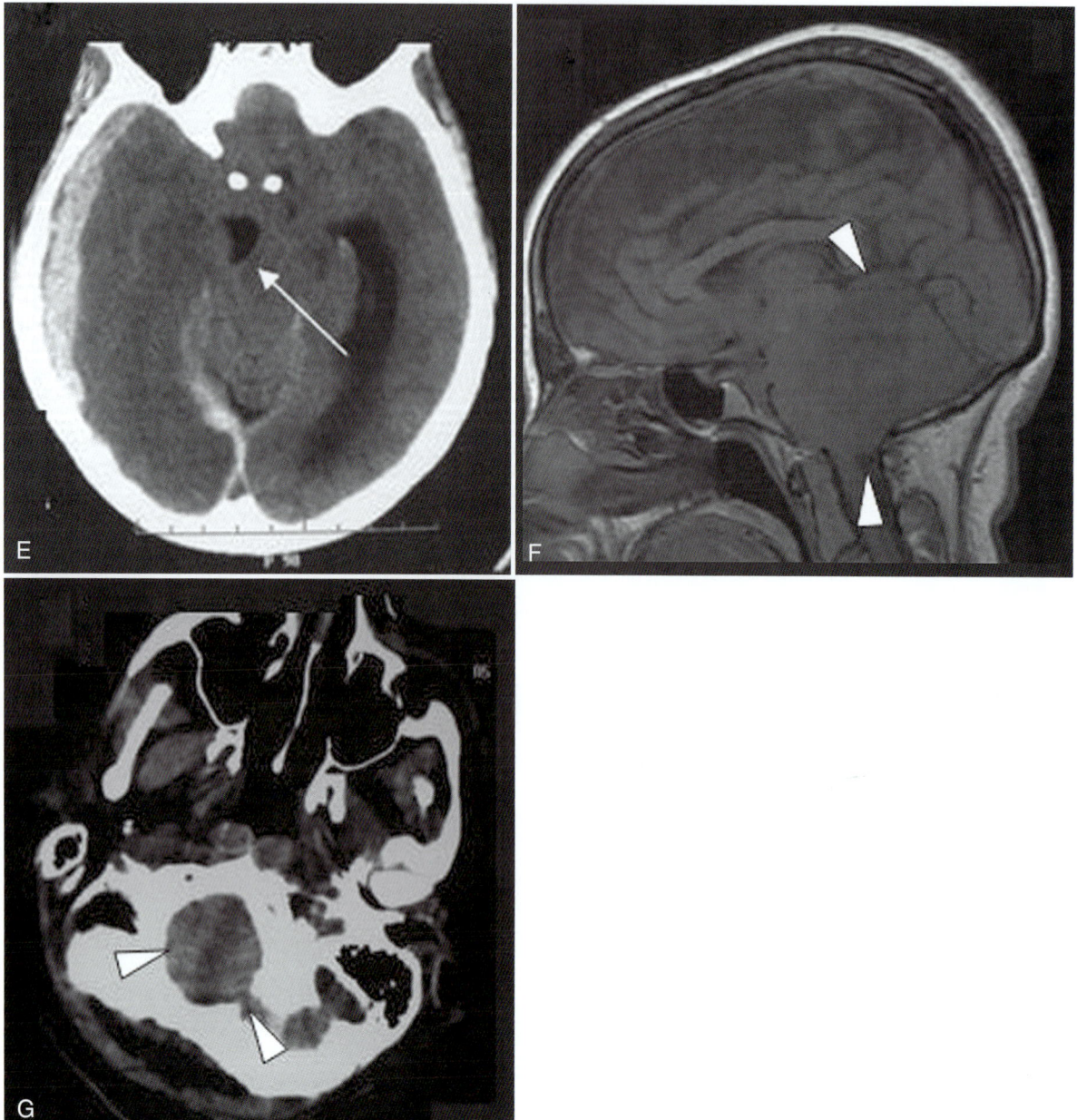

Figure 12-15, cont'd D, E: Axial plane appearance of a right subdural hematoma causing subfalcine (D) and uncal (E) herniation. The left lateral ventricle is entrapped and dilated. The *arrow* in E points to a medially displaced and dilated right temporal horn. F: Sagittal magnetic resonance image showing mass effect in the posterior fossa with upward and downward herniation (*arrowheads*). G: Axial plane computed tomography of a tonsillar herniation revealed by effacement of cerebrospinal fluid spaces around the inferior brainstem at the level of the foramen magnum (*arrowheads*).

brain herniations based on direct and indirect signs of displacement.

Vascular Complications

Posttraumatic ischemia and infarction are common complications in severe head injury, especially among patients with associated SDH, brain swelling/edema, and traumatic SAH. The most common cause of posttraumatic infarction is extrinsic compression of a blood vessel due to mechanical shift of the brain and herniation across the falx and/or tentorium (e.g., caused by EDH or SDH). The infarcts can occur on the same side or on the contralateral side of the herniation. Vasospasm can cause cerebral infarction in head injury patients, usually induced by SAH. Direct vessel injury can occur, possibly resulting in arterial dissection, laceration, formation of pseudoaneurysms, arteriovenous fistula, thrombosis, or distal embolization. Diagnosis of arterial lesions usually requires CTA, digital subtraction angiography, or MRI/MR angiography. Related ischemic lesions are rarely evident on the admission CT study but become evident on follow-up imaging studies (Figure 12-16). More rarely, cerebral fat microembolisms may occur in patients with long bones fractures.

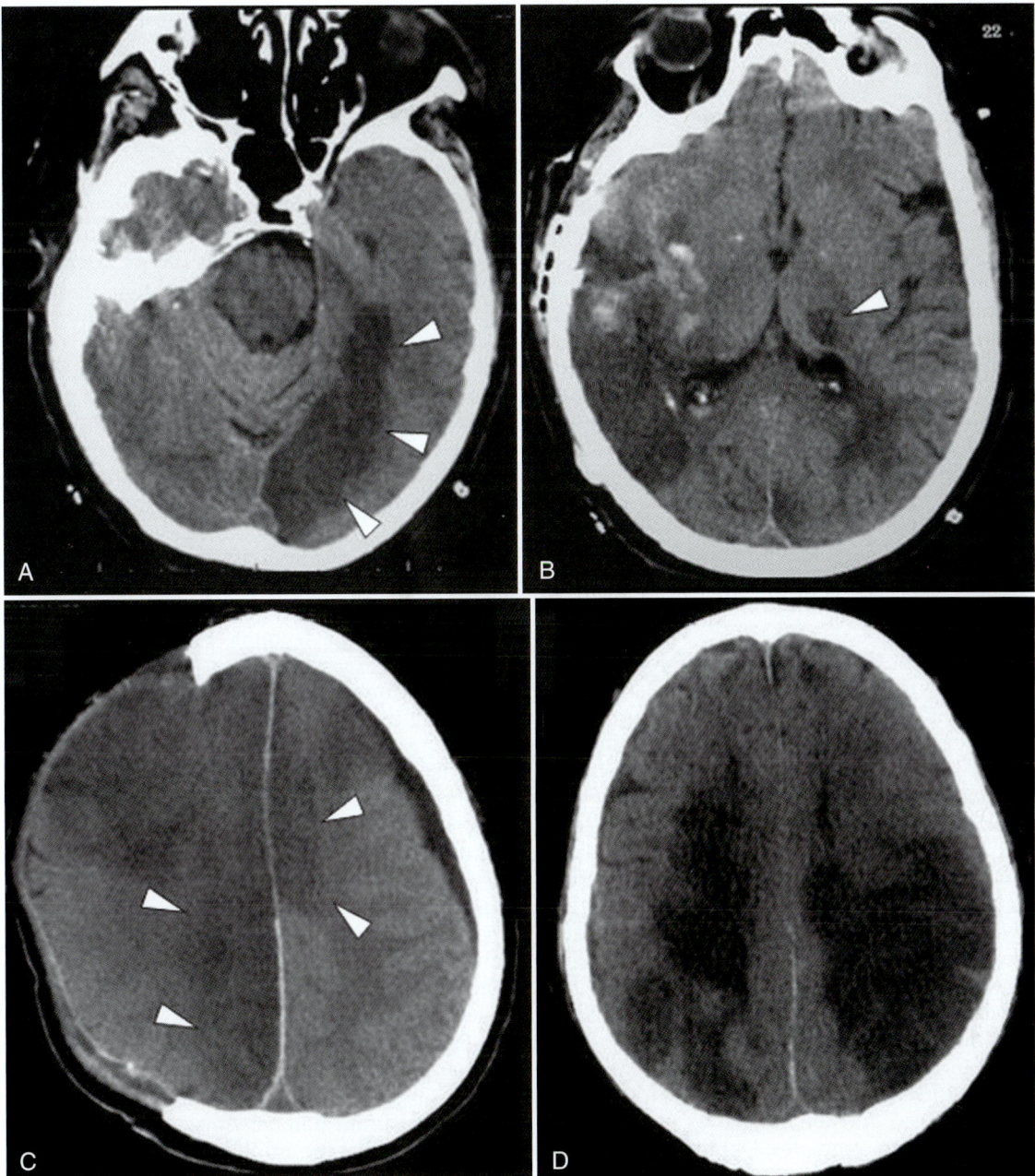

Figure 12-16 Posttraumatic ischemic vascular complications. **A, B:** Patient with head injury presented with right subdural hematoma and descending transtentorial brain herniation. After hematoma evacuation and brain decompression was performed, follow-up computed tomography (CT) reveals a left posterior cerebral artery (PCA) ischemic infarct involving the mesial temporooccipital lobe (*arrowheads* in **A**) and thalamus (*arrowhead* in **B**) due to herniation-related PCA compression. **C:** Patient with posttraumatic subfalcine herniation underwent decompressive craniectomy. Follow-up CT scan reveals bilateral anterior cerebral artery (ACA) ischemic infarcts (*arrowheads*) due to herniation-related compression of the ACAs against the falx. **D:** Follow-up CT images of patient who presented with severe traumatic subarachnoid hemorrhage showing multiple and bilateral large ischemic infarcts involving arterial and watershed territories. This distribution suggests vasospasm as the responsible injury mechanism.

On the venous side, dural venous sinus laceration is almost always associated with depressed skull fracture or penetrating wounds.

CSF Fistulae and Pneumocephalus

CSF fistulae and pneumocephalus can occur as secondary events if there is a skull fracture with an associated dural laceration. Posttraumatic CSF fistulae occur in up to 9% of patients with head injury. Most of these fistulae close spontaneously, whereas a persistent CSF leak carries significant risk for the development of meningitis. CSF fistulae are rarely addressed by acute imaging. Pneumocephalus is detected in the presence of a penetrating injury, a mastoid fracture extended to the tegmen tympani, or a fracture of the inner wall of the frontal sinuses and implies an increased risk of intracranial infection. Large pneumocephalus, as with any extraaxial collection, has mass effect and an irritating effect on the brain but usually undergoes spontaneous resorption. Noncontrast CT, visualized with bone window settings, optimally detects even very small pneumocephalus.

Which Lesions Require Immediate Surgical Intervention?

One of the most critical questions the radiologist needs to answer in the most timely manner is "Does this patient require an emergency surgical intervention?"

As a general rule, because the intracranial compartment is a rigid closed space capable of tolerating only limited increase in internal pressure, all conditions characterized by significant focal mass effect or potential for rapid evolving mass effect are candidates for surgical decompression. Such conditions are represented by large cerebral hematomas and large SDHs, with significant mass effect and brain herniation, and almost any EDH, even of small size, due to possible rapid growth. Significant brain swelling is amenable to decompressive craniectomy in order to prevent brain herniation and ischemic complications. A raise of ICP in the infratentorial compartment may represent a surgical emergency due to the limited compensatory spaces in the posterior fossa and the dangerous compression of the brainstem's vital structures. Depressed skull fractures usually need surgical reduction to relieve brain compression and prevent further neuronal damage. Ventricular shunting is performed in case of ventricular hemorrhage, massive SAH, or hydrocephalus due to ventricular incarceration. Finally, aggressive intensive care management of severe head trauma often requires the placement of a subdural or intraventricular catheter for invasive ICP monitoring.

SAH, cerebral contusions, and DAI, although possibly clinically relevant, are not lesions amenable to surgery.

What to Look for on the Admission CT Scan

"The Container"

Review of CT images with soft tissues and bone window settings allows identification of large scalp hematomas and skull fractures. In cases of linear fractures, differential must be made with sutures: sutures are bilateral and symmetrical and show sclerotic margins, whereas no sclerosis is seen along the borders of an acute fracture. The extent of a linear or a complex fracture can be better appreciated on panoramic 3D surface-shaded reformatted images, although this technique might underestimate or overlook thin fracture lines. Particular attention is needed for fractures in the temporoparietal area, where the large-caliber middle meningeal artery and its branches run along the inner calvarium, because of frequent association with EDH. In case of depressed fractures, inward displacement of the calvarium has to be measured and reported because of the possible coexistence of adjacent brain injuries. The craniocervical junction should be included in the CT evaluation and examined for fractures or dislocations. Skull base fractures must be actively searched for because of possible involvement of the bony carotid canal, cranial nerve foramina, tegmen tympani, middle ear ossicles, and otic capsules. Fracture of the posterior wall of the frontal sinuses must be ruled out in frontal impacts because of the infectious risks carried by direct communication between the sinonasal air spaces and the intracranial compartment. Presence of air bubbles in the intracranial compartment suggests a penetrating injury or a fracture of the tegmen tympani, ethmoid plate, or frontal sinuses, whereas air around the temporomandibular joints is a strong indicator of a mastoid fracture (Figure 12-17).

"The Extraaxial Compartment"

CT images are viewed with standard brain parenchyma and subdural (W 150–300 HU, L 50–100 HU) window settings in order to visualize the thinner layers of EDH or SDH against the inner margins of the calvarium. Be aware that thin extraaxial hematomas along the inferior portion of the occipital squama, along the petrous ridge and along the floor of the anterior cranial fossa, hence the ones that are parallel to the axial plane of the CT cuts, are easier to miss.

Particular attention must be directed to the mass effect caused by the extraaxial blood collection. Mass effect can be visible locally on the adjacent CSF spaces, sulci, and brain parenchyma, or remotely on the ventricular system, the midline brain structures, the basal cisterns, and the brainstem. EDHs, with their typical biconvex shape, especially those in the temporoparietal region, must be considered with particular attention and alarm because they are usually caused by an arterial bleed and can grow in size very rapidly, with possible devastating effects. The usually associated skull fracture should be visualized and reported.

SDHs on the other side, with their crescentic shape, are usually caused by a venous bleed and hold a lesser growth potential. However, due to their large surface of spread, they can occupy a large volume and cause significant mass effect and brain displacement, even when their thickness might seem not considerable.

Although acute extraaxial blood collections commonly appear hyperdense and grossly homogeneous at the time of admission imaging, inhomogeneity and nonlayered patchy isodense components within might represent very recent and nonclotted bleed or active and/or repetitive hemorrhage, with rapid growth potential.

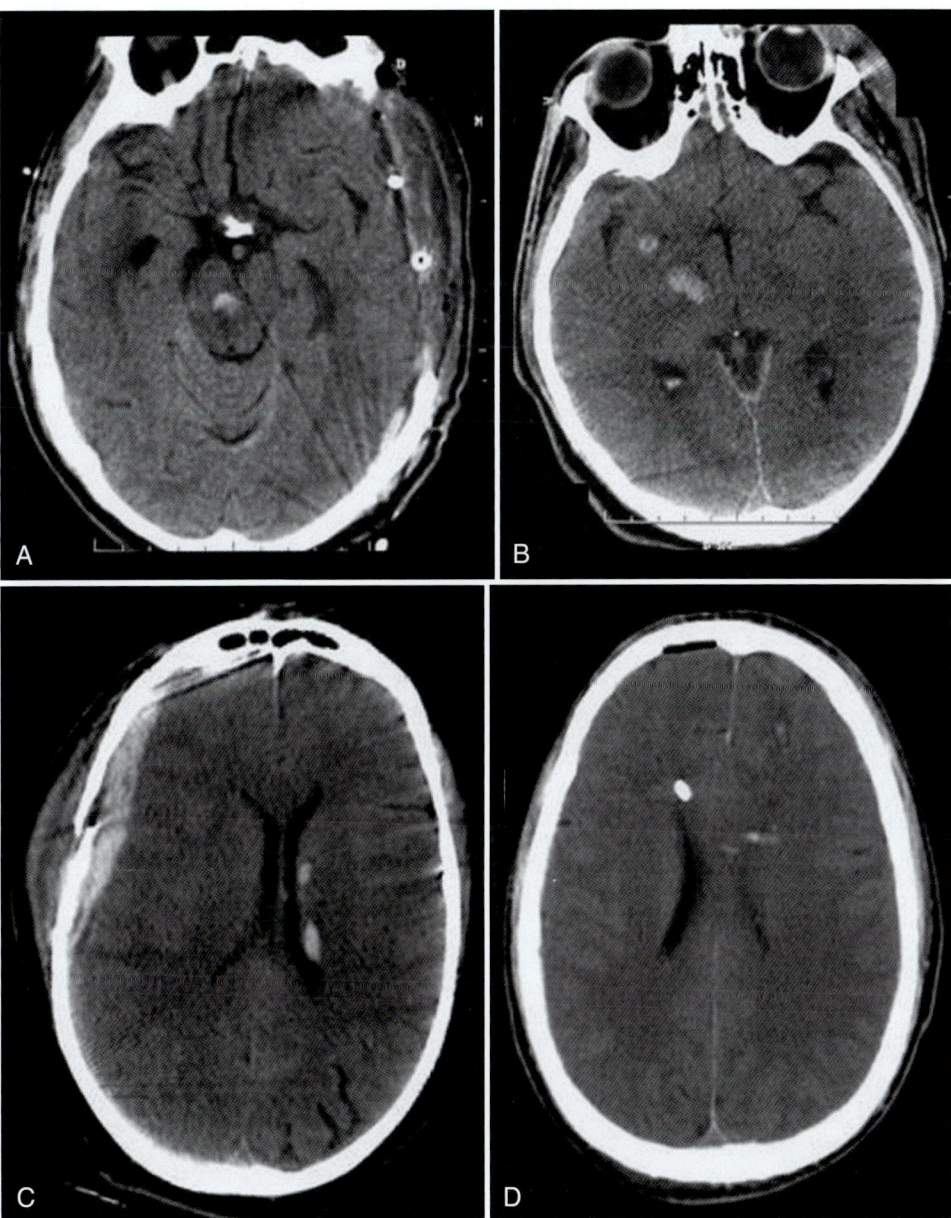

Figure 12-12 Diffuse axonal injuries (DAIs) on computed tomography (CT). **A–D:** Different cases showing the most common shearing injuries locations, such as the midbrain, basal regions of the brain (here also called *intermediate injuries*), deep white matter, corpus callosum, and subcortical white matter at gray–white matter junction. CT performs better at identifying hemorrhagic rather than nonhemorrhagic DAI and usually identifies them better in the early subacute stage rather than on admission scan.

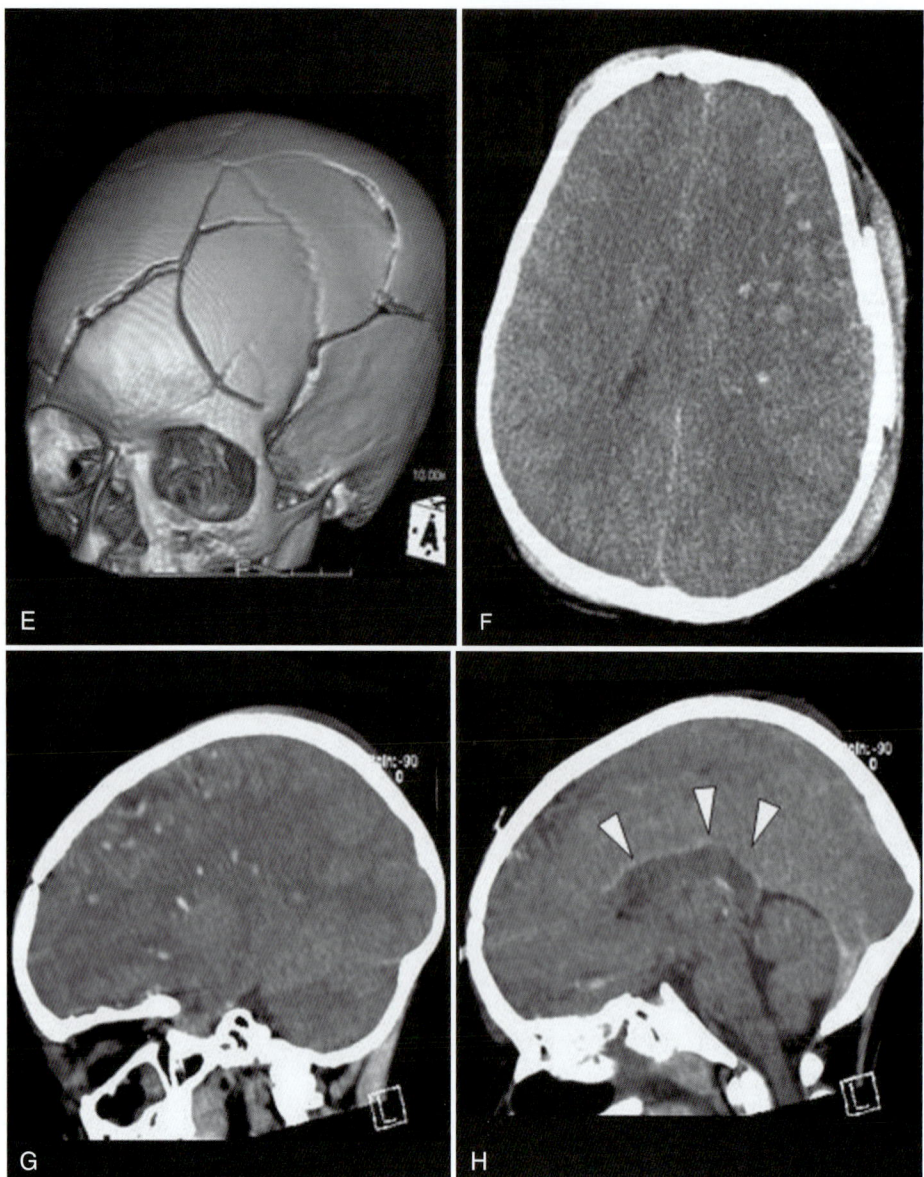

Figure 12-12, cont'd E–H: Different images from the same severe craniocerebral trauma showing multiple complex skull fractures, multiple punctuate hemorrhagic DAI in the deep and subcortical white matter, predominantly of the left hemisphere, and extensive, but more subtle, non-hemorrhagic shearing injuries of the corpus callosum (*arrowheads* in **H**). The corpus callosum appears irregularly swollen and hypodense, with bumpy contours, on the midline sagittal reformatted image (**H**).

brainstem hits the edge of the tentorium. Although this lesion can be highly significant with regard to clinical status and prognosis, admission CT will show a very low percentage of these lesions. In doubtful cases or in patients with unexplained clinical status, MRI might be necessary.

Secondary Lesions
The clinical outcome sometimes depends on the secondary effects of cranial trauma: brain swelling, brain herniations, vascular complications, CSF fistulae, and pneumocephalus.

Brain Swelling
Brain swelling with intracranial hypertension is a life-threatening, secondary, traumatic brain lesion. Clinically, an increase in ICP is indicated by bradycardia and hypertension. It starts immediately after injury and is caused by traumatic loss of vascular autoregulation with massive vasodilation. In the initial stage the brain swelling is caused by diffuse increase of the cerebral blood volume, called *hyperemia*.

What Are the Signs of Secondary Brain Swelling? Hyperemia is revealed on CT by diffuse CSF space effacement, preserved gray–white matter junction visibility, and grossly normal brain density (Figure 12-14). Hyperemia can progress to frank brain edema, usually after 24 to 48 hours, revealed as loss of gray–white matter junction visibility and diffuse brain parenchyma hypoattenuation (Figure 12-14). The large arterial vessels and the venous dural sinuses might appear relatively hyperdense compared to the brain parenchyma in this stage. If the ICP is not relieved, the brain will

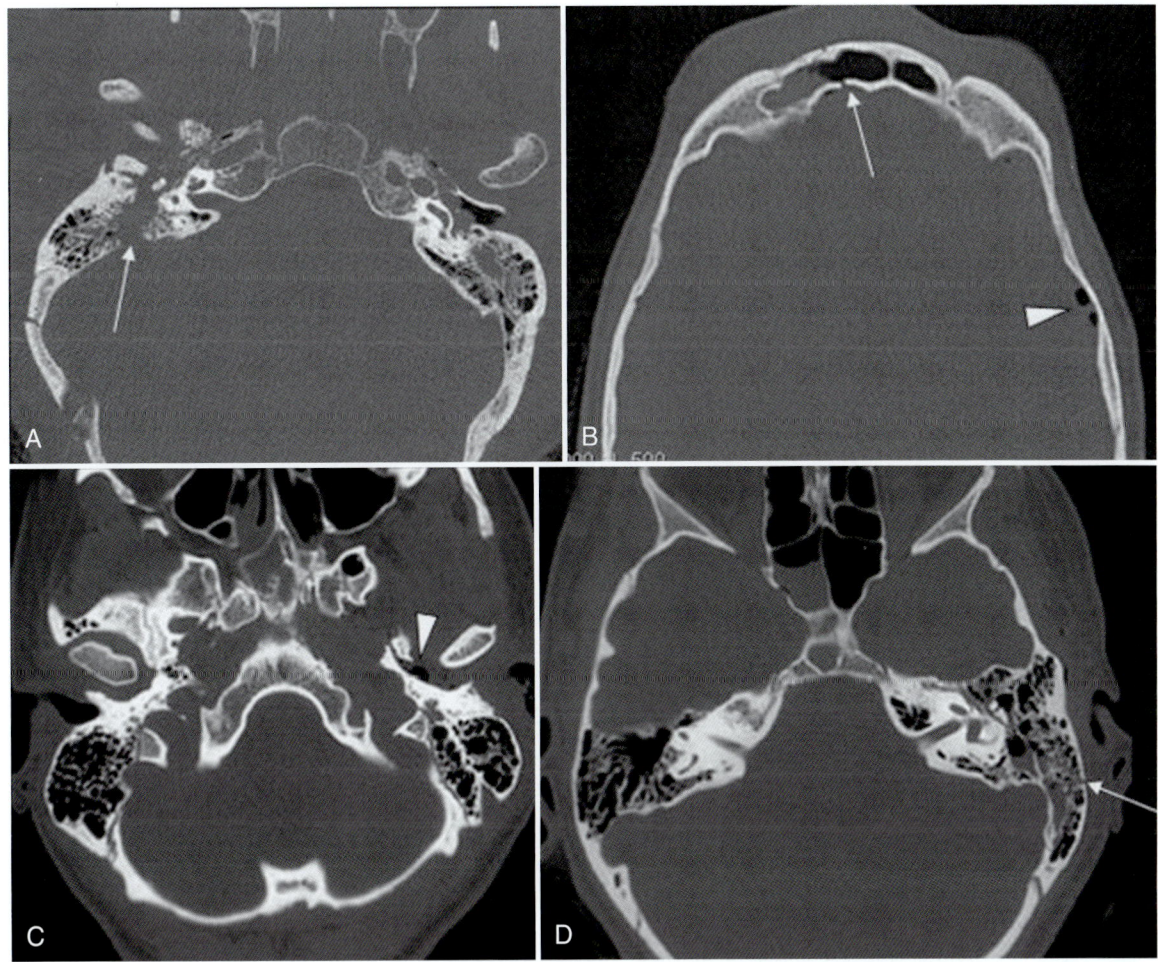

Figure 12-17 Head fractures of particular interest. **A:** Obvious right mastoid fracture (*arrow*) coursing through the middle ear. Integrity of the ossicular chain and carotid canal and the likely cerebrospinal fluid (CSF) fistula are of special concern in these fractures. Opacification of the contralateral mastoid and middle ear should raise the suspicion of a more subtle fracture of the left mastoid as well. **B:** Small linear fracture of the posterior wall of the frontal sinus (*arrow*) associated with pneumocephalus (*arrowhead*) is at risk for intracranial infection and CSF fistula. **C, D:** Air in the temporomandibular joint (*arrowhead* in **C**) is an indirect sign of a temporal bone/mastoid fracture, as confirmed in this case by fluid in the left mastoid and direct visualization of a thin fracture line (*arrow* in **D**).

Common pitfalls are represented by invisible thin extraaxial collections, due to improper window-settings (Figure 12-18), and by isodense EDHs and SDHs. Hyperacute bleed before clot retraction and low hemoglobin concentration (<10 g/dl) in anemic patients may cause the extraaxial hematoma to appear isodense to the brain parenchyma (Figure 12-18). Asymmetry of the CSF spaces, sulcal effacement, and inward displacement of the gray–white matter junction depict the presence and the location of the isodense extraaxial blood collection.

Finally, the density of the CSF spaces in the sulci must be examined to rule out SAH.

"The Content"
CT images are visualized with standard brain parenchyma window settings. At first glance, note the following:
- Obvious intraaxial hemorrhages need to be grossly measured in size, and the presence of vasogenic edema and mass effect must be evaluated, along with the presence of IVH.
- In the presence of IVH, early signs of developing hydrocephalus, such as mild dilatation of the temporal horns or convex margins of the third ventricle, with initial sulcal effacement, have to be ruled out.
- Signs of ICP have to be recognized.

Generalized increase of ICP, caused by hyperemia or brain edema, is revealed by diffuse and bilateral sulcal effacement, reduced ventricular size due to compression, and basal cistern effacement. In young patients with normally small ventricles and CSF spaces, it may be difficult to judge the width of the subarachnoid spaces along the convexities; therefore, it is advisable to evaluate the most cranial axial cuts, where CSF spaces in the parasagittal regions should always be visible in normal conditions (Figure 12-19). Another area to focus attention is certainly the basal cisterns, particularly the ambiens cistern, around the midbrain, called the *brain smile*, whose effacement indicates bilateral descending transtentorial herniation and severe intracranial hypertension (Figure 12-19). If signs of generalized increased ICP are observed, the next judgment required is the differential diagnosis between hyperemia (a more benign

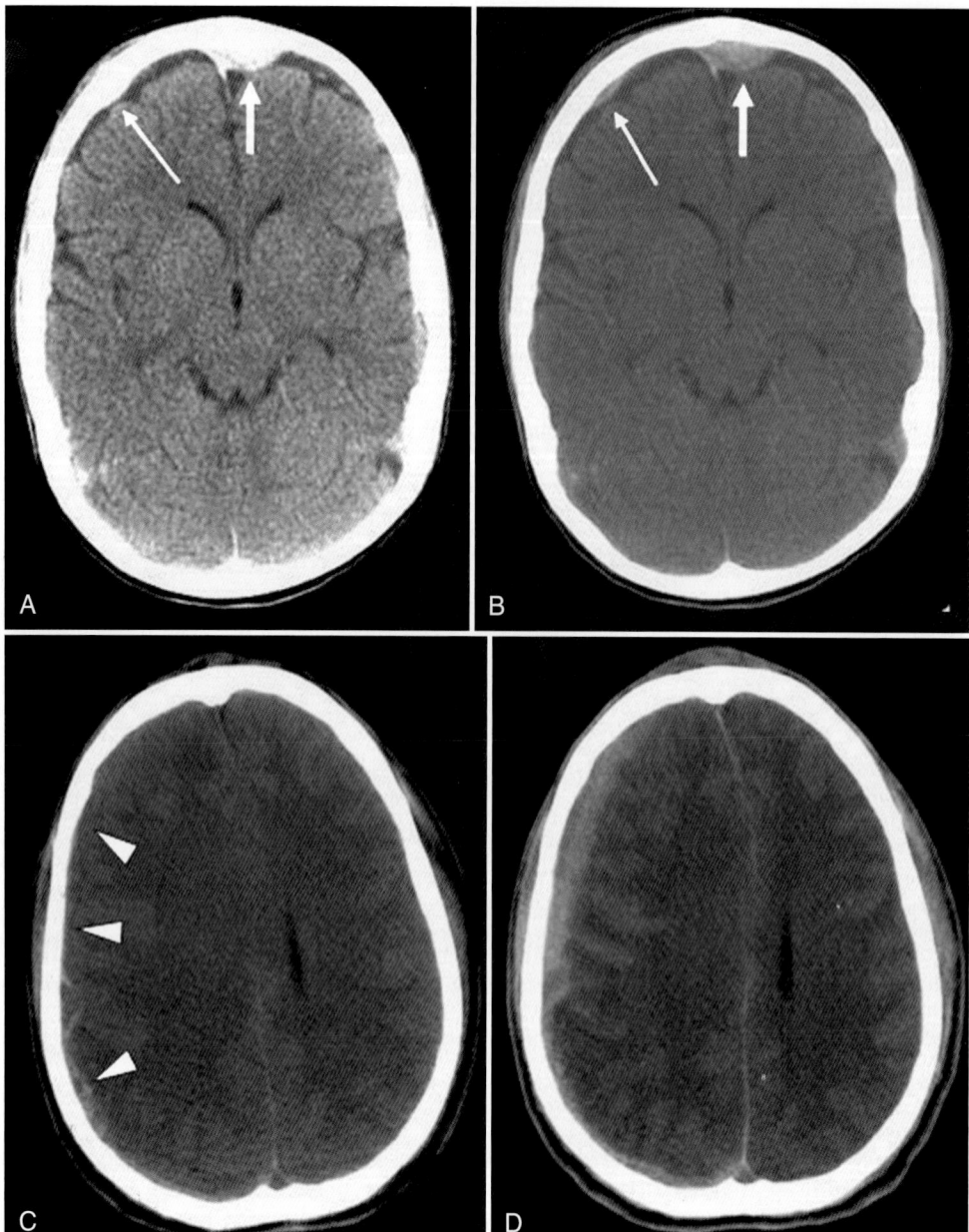

Figure 12-18 Common pitfalls in extraaxial collections. **A, B:** Improper window setting might underestimate or overlook small extraaxial hemorrhagic collections, such as these two small epidural hematomas (*thin* and *thick arrows*). **C, D:** Hyperacute bleeds, before clot retraction occurs, display isodensity with the gray matter, as in this subdural hematoma (SDH) (*arrowheads* in **C**). At follow-up few hours later, the SDH is much more obvious because of enlargement and increase in density (**D**).

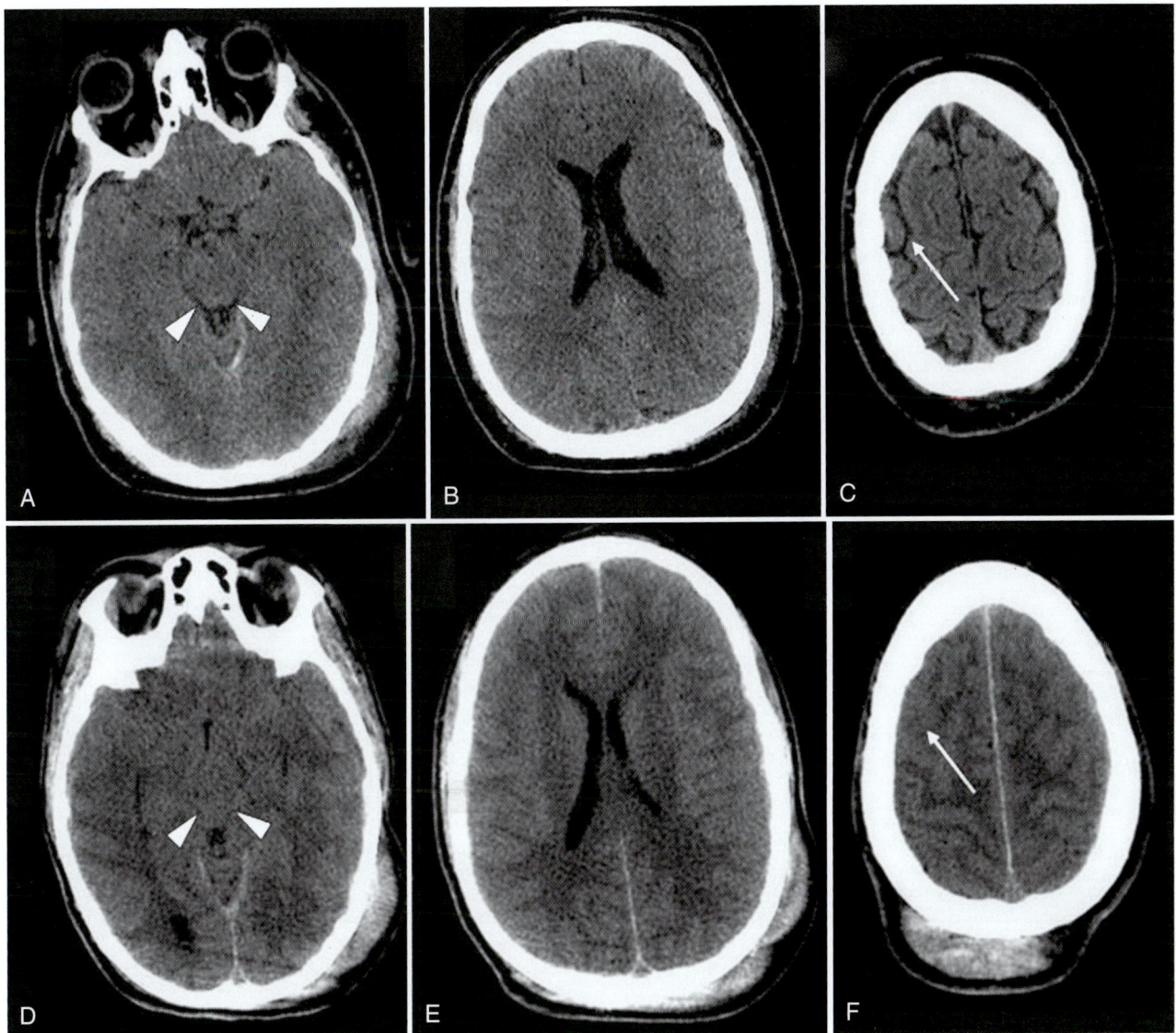

Figure 12-19 Cerebrospinal fluid (CSF) space effacement as a sign of intracranial hypertension. In normal healthy brains, CSF space width is highly variable. **A–C:** In a normal young individual, although sulci can be very tight along the convexities and in the sylvian fissures, they should always be visible around the midbrain (ambiens cistern, *arrowheads* in **A**) and at the level of the most upper cuts along the vault (*arrow* in **C**). **D–F:** Loss of visibility of the basal cisterns (*arrowheads* in **D**) and of the CSF spaces at the upper cuts along the vault (*arrow* in **F**) should raise concern for intracranial hypertension caused by enlarged ventricles or brain swelling.

and initial condition), and brain edema (a more severe and advanced pathologic condition). In hyperemia, gray–white matter junction visibility is preserved, and the brain has a normal density, whereas in brain edema, the brain is diffusely hypodense and gray–white matter junction visibility is lost. If the scan was acquired in helical rather than sequential mode, be aware that the gray–white matter junction might be poorly visible due to "dragging" artifacts (Figure 12-20).

Localized supratentorial increase of ICP, caused by intraaxial or extraaxial hemorrhage, can result in asymmetric sulcal effacement, ventricular compression, and subfalcine and uncal herniation. Obvious subfalcine brain herniation is readily appreciated by observing the asymmetry of the lateral ventricles and the position of the septum pellucidum and third ventricle in relation the midline. In case of subfalcine brain shift, because of the risk of vascular compression of the anterior cerebral arteries against the falx, search for early CT signs of ischemia in their respective vascular territories, in the superior frontal gyri, along the parasagittal areas. Uncal herniation is recognized by mesial displacement of the uncus and mesial temporal lobe, with asymmetry of the interpeduncular cistern, unilateral ambiens cistern effacement, and contralateral midbrain displacement. When an uncal herniation is diagnosed, due to the risk of posterior cerebral artery and superior cerebellar artery compression between the mesial temporal lobe and the midbrain, rule out early signs of ischemia in the thalamus and in the temporooccipital regions.

Increased ICP in the posterior fossa, caused by intraaxial or extraaxial hemorrhage, is indicated by effacement of the subarachnoid spaces around the cerebellum and

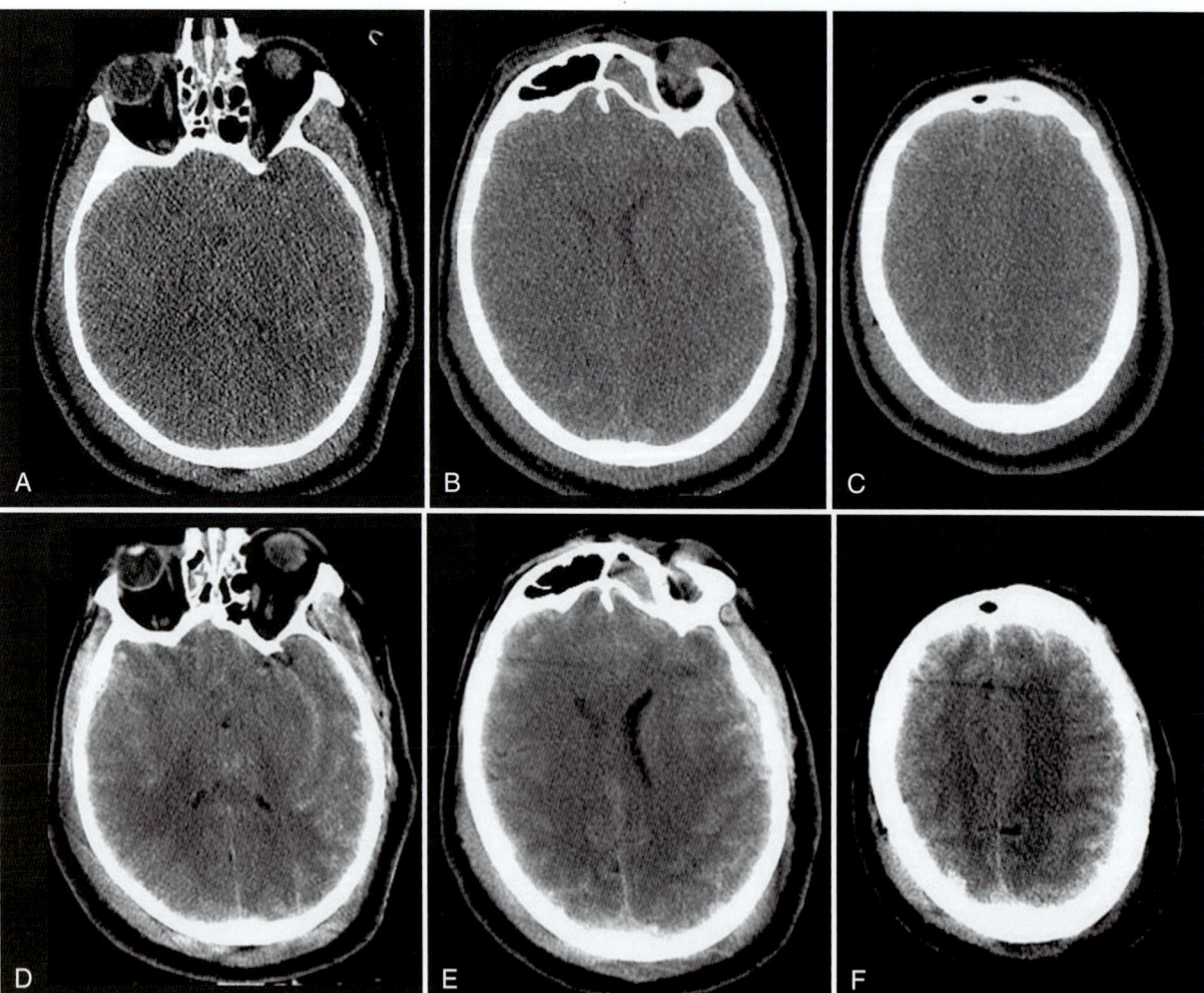

Figure 12-20 Dragging artifact of helical computed tomography (CT) acquisition. Ideally the brain CT should be acquired in sequential rather than helical mode due to the possible dragging artifact that may give the false appearance of gray–white matter junction effacement, possibly leading to a false diagnosis of brain edema. **A–C:** Images of the brain acquired in helical mode having an appearance of brain hypodensity and abnormal homogeneous density. **D–F:** Images obtained immediately after repeated scan in sequential mode shows brain swelling (but with preserved gray–white matter contrast) and diffuse subarachnoid hemorrhage.

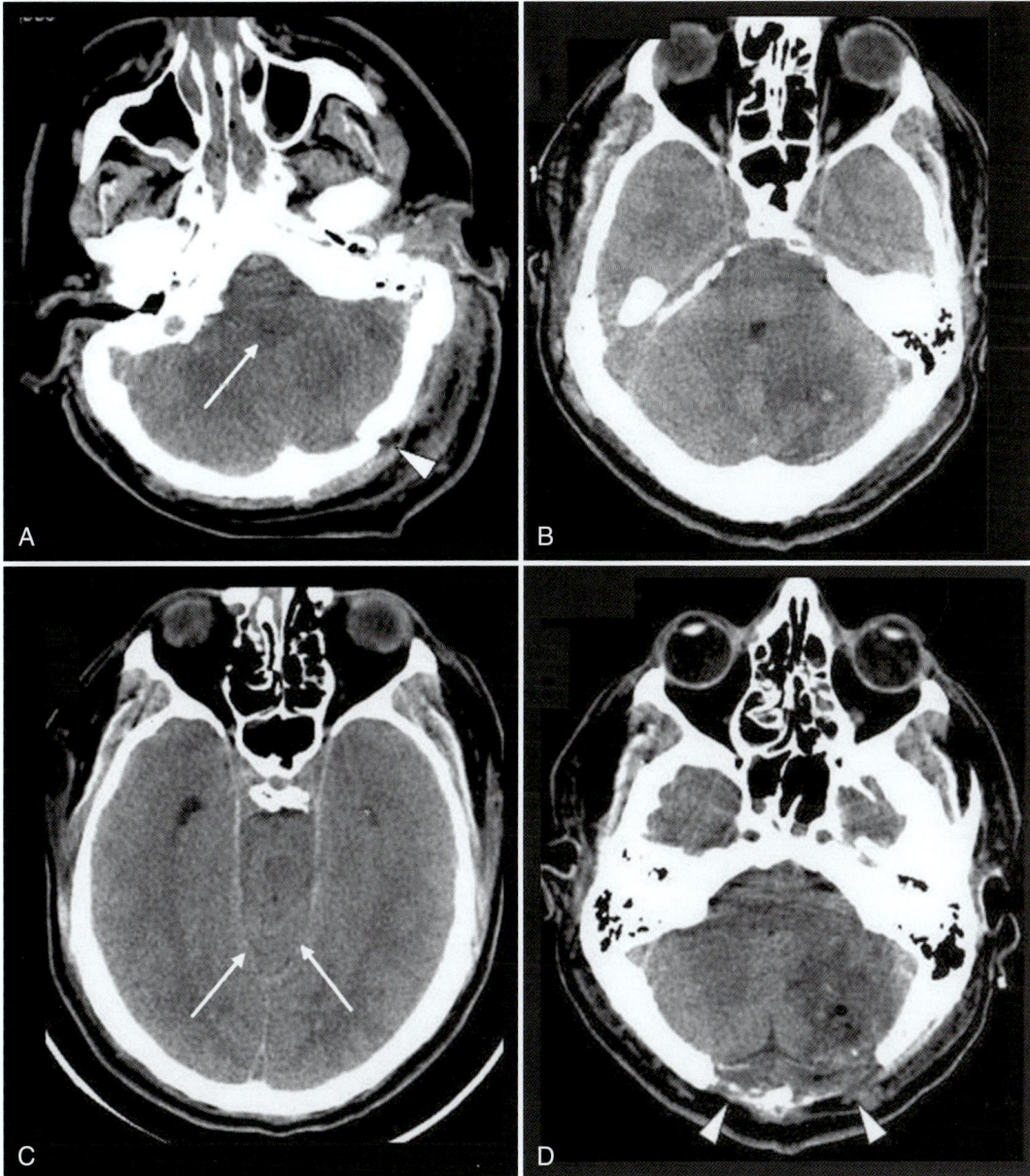

Figure 12-21 Increased intracranial pressure in the posterior fossa. **A–C:** Occipital fracture (*arrowhead* on **A**), accompanied by left cerebellar edematous and hemorrhagic contusion resulted in posterior fossa hypertension as demonstrated by fourth ventricle compression and effacement (*arrow* in **A**), effacement of the prepontine cistern, and ascending transtentorial herniation, as revealed by upward displacement of the superior vermis through the tentorial hiatus (*arrows* in **C**). These findings prompted an emergency decompressive craniectomy (*arrowheads* in **D**).

of the prepontine cistern, with compression or dislocation of the fourth ventricle. The inferior vermis and the tonsils herniate downward through the foramen magnum (tonsillar herniation), as revealed by effacement of the CSF spaces around the inferior medulla on the lower axial cuts or on reformatted sagittal images. The superior vermis herniates upward through the tentorial hiatus (ascending transtentorial herniation), filling the superior vermian and the pulvinar cisterns. Direct or indirect CT signs of increased ICP in the posterior fossa require thorough and rapid reporting, representing a possible indication to an emergency decompressive suboccipital craniectomy (Figure 12-21).

- Cortical contusions revealed by a variable combination of small hemorrhagic and edematous superficial lesions must be sought in the anterior temporal poles and in the basal and orbital portion of the frontal lobes, with particular attention to the undersurface of the gyri recti because they rub against the uneven surfaces of the ethmoidal plate at the moment of the impact (Figure 12-22). When it is important to clarify the mechanism of the head injury, whether it is due to a fall or to a blow, look for evidence of coup–contrecoup injury, which is present in acceleration–deceleration injuries but not in purely impact lesions.
- After the most immediate observations, the radiologist should actively and carefully search for the less evident DAI, which often is an underestimated lesion on the admission imaging and sometimes is responsible for otherwise unexplained severe clinical conditions.

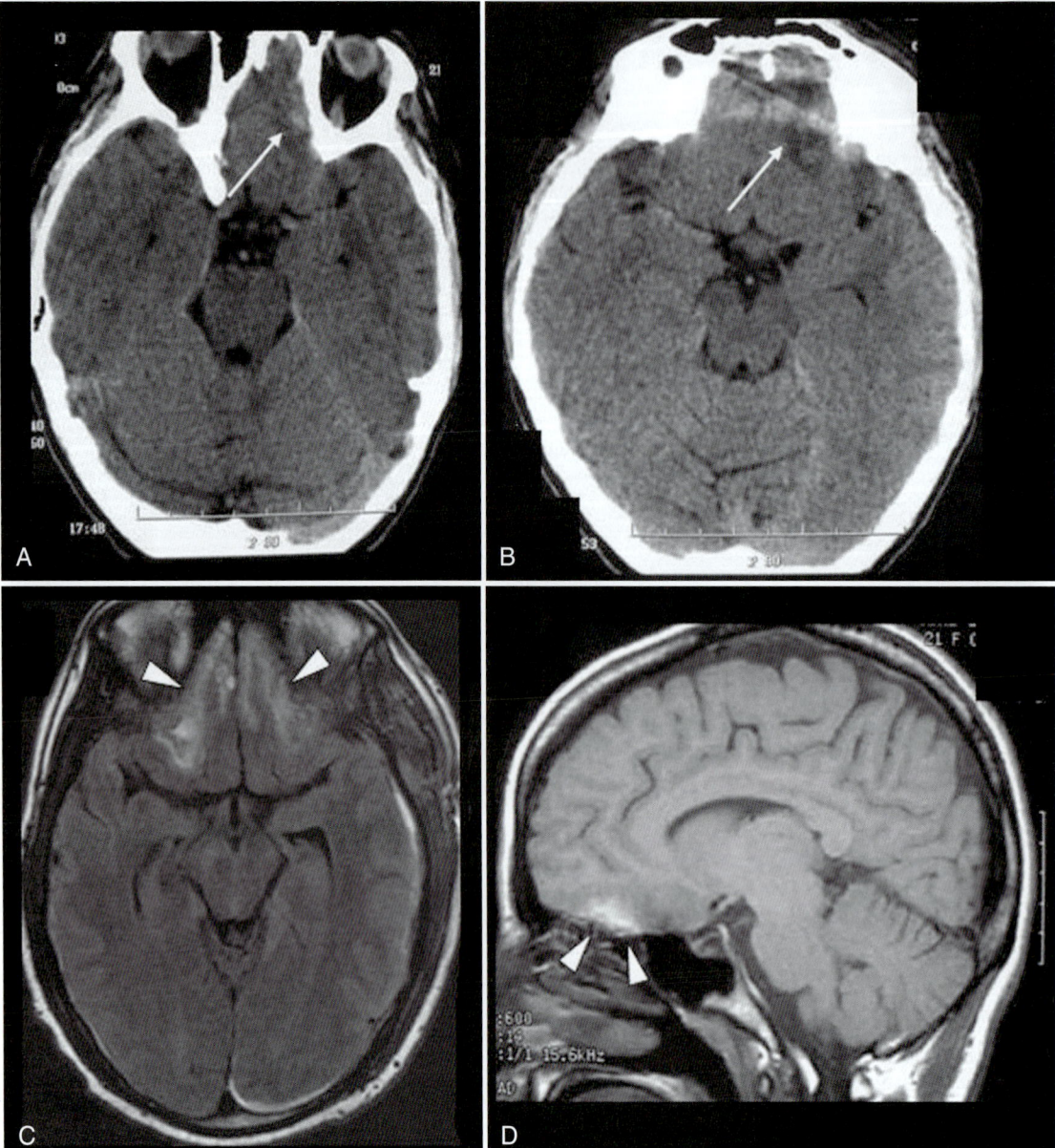

Figure 12-22 Hot spots for brain contusions. Subtle contusive injuries have to be searched for at the temporal poles and along the straight gyri (*arrows* and *arrowheads*) because they are in contact with and rub against the uneven bony surface of the ethmoid cribrous plate during head trauma.

Sites of focused attention to look for DAI are the subcortical white matter at the centri semiovale, the splenium of the corpus callosum, the internal capsules, and the dorsolateral portions of the brainstem.
- Axial cuts through the brainstem itself deserve a specific and thorough analysis to rule out hemorrhagic contusions, DAI, and, in case of descending transtentorial herniation, usually in a later phase, so-called Duret hemorrhage (see section: Subacute Head Imaging: Early Follow-Up and Management).
- If diagnostic imaging is performed at admission to rule out blunt vascular injuries, look for arterial caliber irregularities, such as dissection-related stenosis, beading, pseudoaneurysms, intimal flaps, and mural hematomas. A dilated superior ophthalmic vein in the orbit, with exophthalmus and variable edema in the orbital fat, might be indirect signs of a carotid–cavernous fistula (Figure 12-23).

Is There Any Facial and/or Orbital Trauma?

Facial fractures are often associated with brain traumatic injuries in severe craniofacial traumas. For most isolated facial fractures, plain film radiographs are generally considered a satisfactory screening imaging tool. However, the need for multiple and high technical value views, the increasingly widespread use of MDCT in busy emergency rooms, and the frequent association of facial trauma with intracranial injuries are making MDCT a more often used primary imaging method for diagnosing facial and orbital fractures. This preference for CT

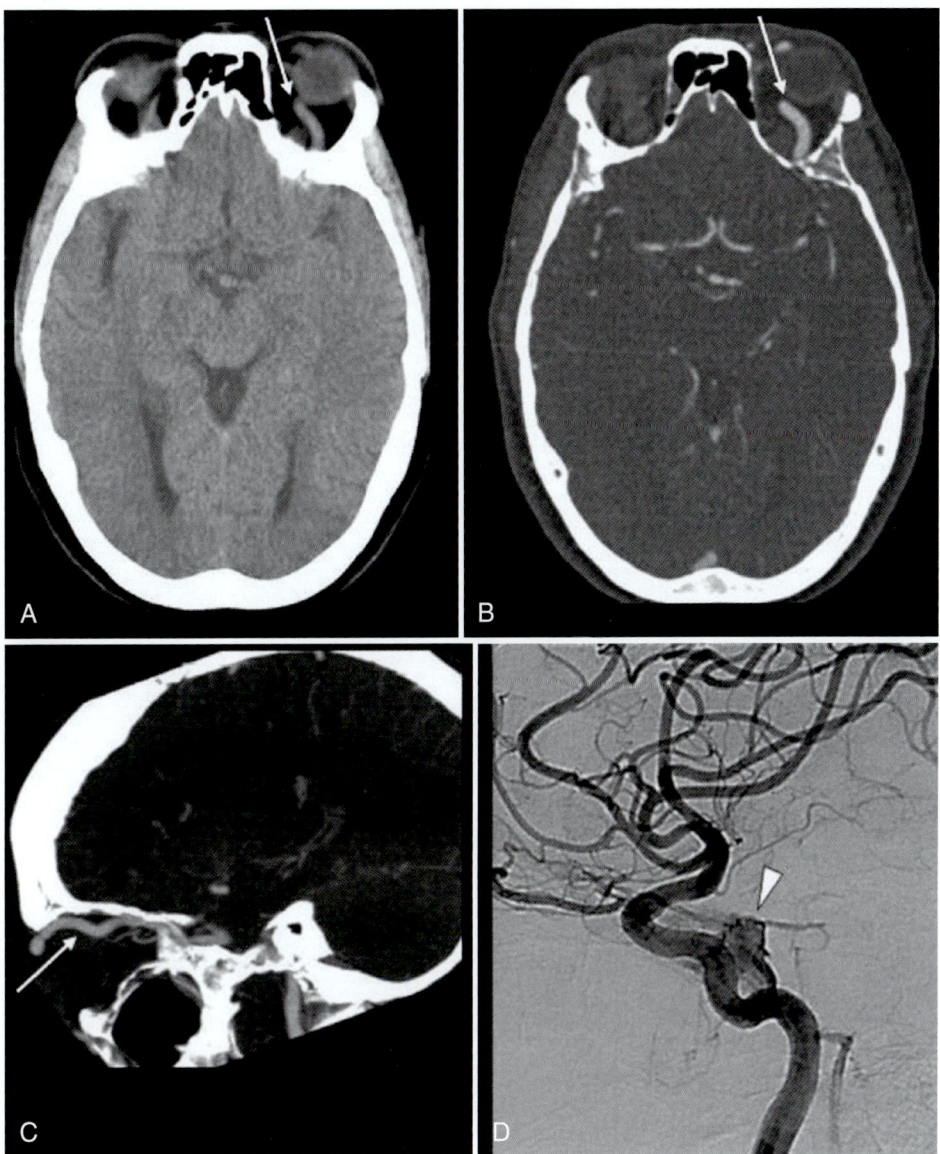

Figure 12-23 Carotid-cavernous fistula. Two months after head trauma, this patient presented with left proptosis, pulsatile eye pain, and an orbital bruit at auscultation. Noncontrast computed tomography showing an asymmetrically enlarged superior ophthalmic vein on the left side (*arrow* in **A**), confirmed by computed tomographic angiography (*arrow* in **B** and **C**). **D:** Carotid angiogram showing a carotid-cavernous fistula with opacification of the left cavernous sinus in the arterial phase (*arrowhead*).

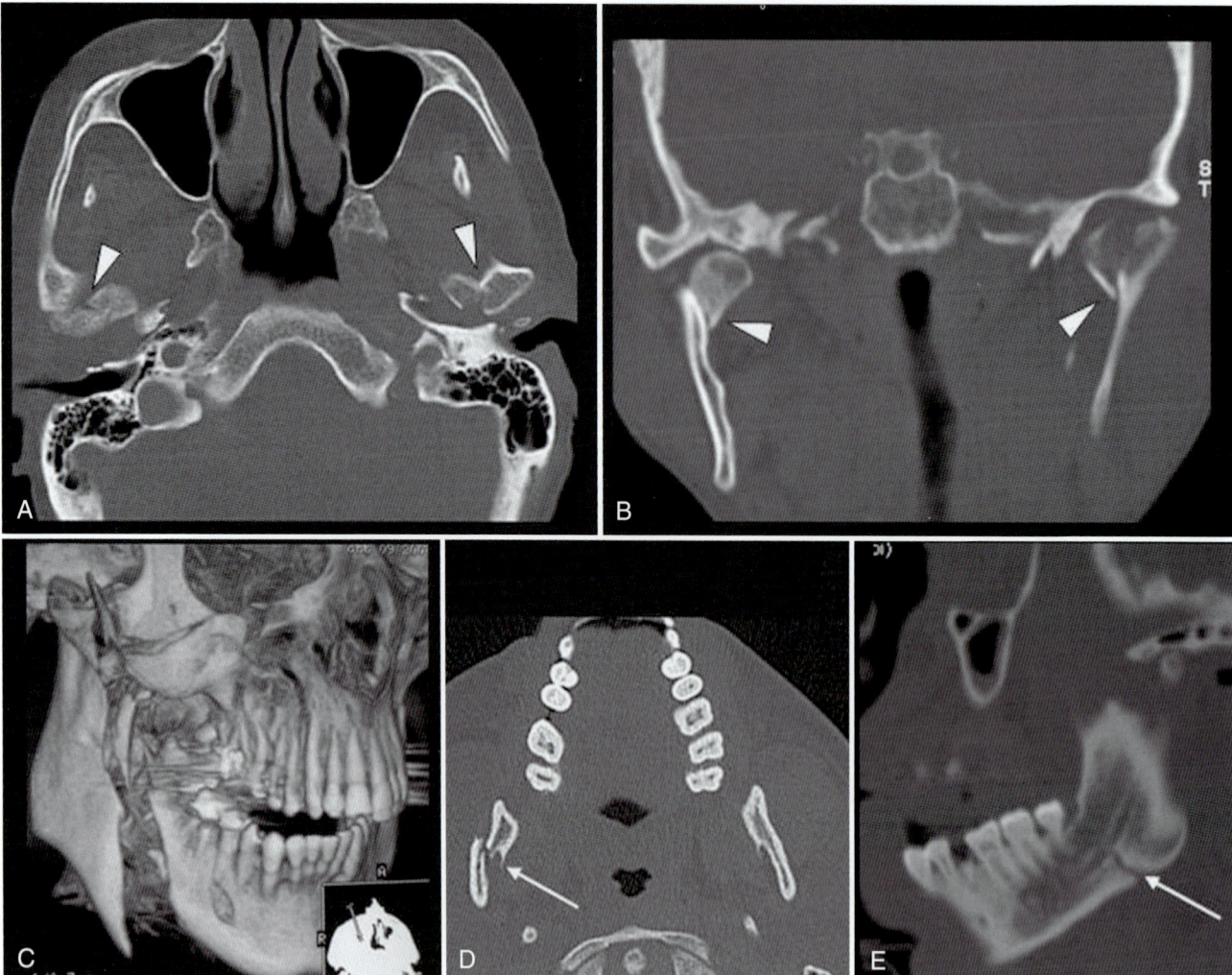

Figure 12-24 Mandibular fractures. **A, B:** Bilateral mandibular condylar fractures (*arrowheads* in **A** and **B**) carrying the risk of malunion and late degenerative OA of the temporomandibular joints. (Courtesy Dr. MV Spampinato, MUSC.) **C–E:** Three examples of mandibular fractures involving the mandibular inferior alveolar nerve foramen (*arrow* in **D** and **E**) at risk for associated nerve injury.

over radiography is unfortunately accompanied by a decreased level of confidence in interpreting face radiographs among radiologists, who are also pressured by the high risk of litigation. When MDCT is used, thin slice (0.5–2.0 mm) volumetric acquisition should be obtained, and the same datasets should be used to obtain coronal and sagittal reformatted images, to be viewed with bone and soft tissue window settings, as well as 3D volume-rendering surface-shaded reconstructions. MRI, ultrasound, color Doppler, and angiography are used to perform further and targeted assessment of soft tissue or vascular abnormalities, such as lesions of the optic globe, optic nerve, and cavernous sinus.

Although very accurate systems of classification for facial and orbital fractures exist, a thorough description is beyond the aim of this chapter. Clinical routine usually adopts a descriptive approach to diagnosing fractures of the facial bones, considering bone involvement, fracture morphology and extent, displacement of osseous fragments, and soft tissue involvement, with particular attention to "hot spots" or particular injuries with specific clinical relevance.

- *Mandible:* Attention should be directed to involvement of the articular condylar components and the mandibular nerve canal (Figure 12-24). The radiologist should be wary of the "flail" mandible, in which a parasymphyseal fracture occurs in conjunction with bilateral posterior fractures, allowing posterior displacement of the genioglossus muscle attachment and potential difficulty in keeping a patent airway in a patient who is lying supine. Complications include malunion, excessive mobility, infection, and temporomandibular joint ankylosis resulting from intracapsular fracture.
- *Ethmoid:* Air cell walls act as an energy dissipating crumple zone, resulting in complex fractures, often associated with CSF leaks if the dura mater is torn. Nasolacrimal duct involvement can lead to nasolacrimal sac mucocele.
- *Midface:* Although high-energy impact forces, such as those that occur in motor vehicle accidents, often result in complex fracture patterns with comminution and displacement, the classic and simplified classification of midface fractures by Le Fort

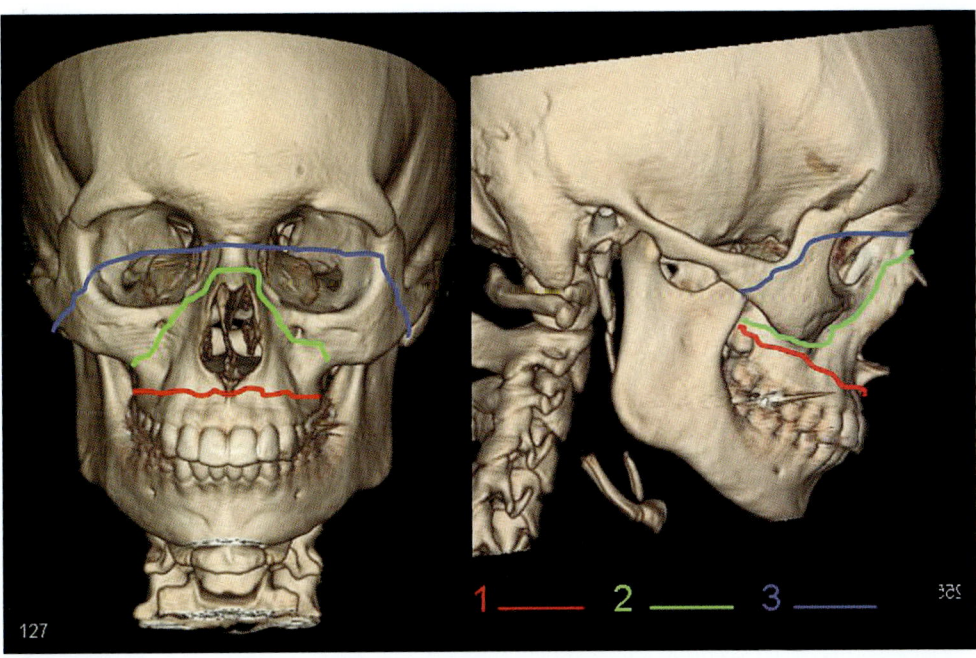

Figure 12-25 Le Fort midface fracture classification. Schematic representation of the classic Le Fort fracture classification system as it appears on anterior and lateral views. *Red line* indicates type I fractures, *green line* type II, and *blue line* type III. See text for details. (Modified from Le Fort classification of midface fractures.)

(Figure 12-25) is still used by surgeons and therefore is worthy of consideration. *Le Fort I:* horizontal fracture line above the hard palate, separating the caudal maxilla from the midface and coursing through the three walls of the maxillary sinuses, the nasal septum, and the pterygoid plates. *Le Fort II:* pyramidal fracture involving the nasoethmoidal region, the orbital floor, and the anterior and posterior (not the medial) walls of the maxillary sinuses. *Le Fort III:* more cranial fracture line involving medial and lateral orbit walls, the zygomatic arch, and the pterygoid plates; maxillary sinuses are spared.

- *Frontal sinus:* Fractures of frontal sinuses may lead to cosmetic deformity, CSF fistula, chronic meningitis, and mucocele. Points for the radiologist to note are whether the fracture of the anterior wall extends to the medial supraorbital rim or nasoethmoidal complex and whether there is persistent fluid in the sinus making damage to the nasofrontal recess more likely. In this situation, the surgeon may consider sinus obliteration to prevent chronic sinusitis or mucocele. Detection of a posterior wall fracture is often associated with intracranial injuries and requires a careful study for extension to the anterior skull base, intracranial air, and any displaced fragments that may lead the surgeon to consider sinus cranialization to prevent CSF leak and meningitis.
- *Orbits:* In patients with acute orbital trauma, visual acuity and extraocular muscle motility are the two most important ophthalmologic functions to be evaluated emergently. Assessment of these capabilities may be difficult due to the severity of the head injury, the extent of periorbital soft tissue edema, inadequate cooperation from alert patients, and reduced level of consciousness in obtunded individuals. CT has come to play a major role in the orbital examination of acute trauma patients.

The term *orbital blowout fracture* is used to describe a fracture resulting from a blow to the orbit by an object too large to enter the orbit. Fractures of the orbital floor (sparing the rim) and the medial wall are typical. These fractures can be accompanied by indirect signs, such as inferior and medial displacement of orbital soft tissue, respectively, in the maxillary sinus and in the ethmoid air cells, orbital fat edema, orbital emphysema, and fluid in the maxillary sinus. Diplopia may result from muscle injury or entrapment of the extraocular muscles, more often the inferior rectus, which usually represents a surgical emergency (Figure 12-26). A tension pneumoorbit may occasionally occur.

Roof of the orbit fractures are uncommon and are often associated with intracranial complications.

Intraocular injury is reported in 15% to 30% of patients with orbital fractures. Although CT may show features of globe disruption, lens dislocation, and vitreous hemorrhage, these abnormalities are often better demonstrated with ultrasound. When intraocular and intraconal causes of posttraumatic visual loss have been excluded, visual impairment is usually due to optic nerve injury, edema or ischemia, or perineural or retrobulbar hematoma. Compression of the optic nerve most frequently occurs within the intracanalicular segment. Any fracture of the orbital roof, lamina papyracea, and sphenoid bone body should prompt careful analysis of the optic canal.

Foreign bodies in the orbit may be intraocular or extraocular. Intraorbital displaced bone fragments can cause entrapment, nerve, and vascular injury and usually require surgical removal. Although radiopaque foreign bodies do not represent a diagnostic problem,

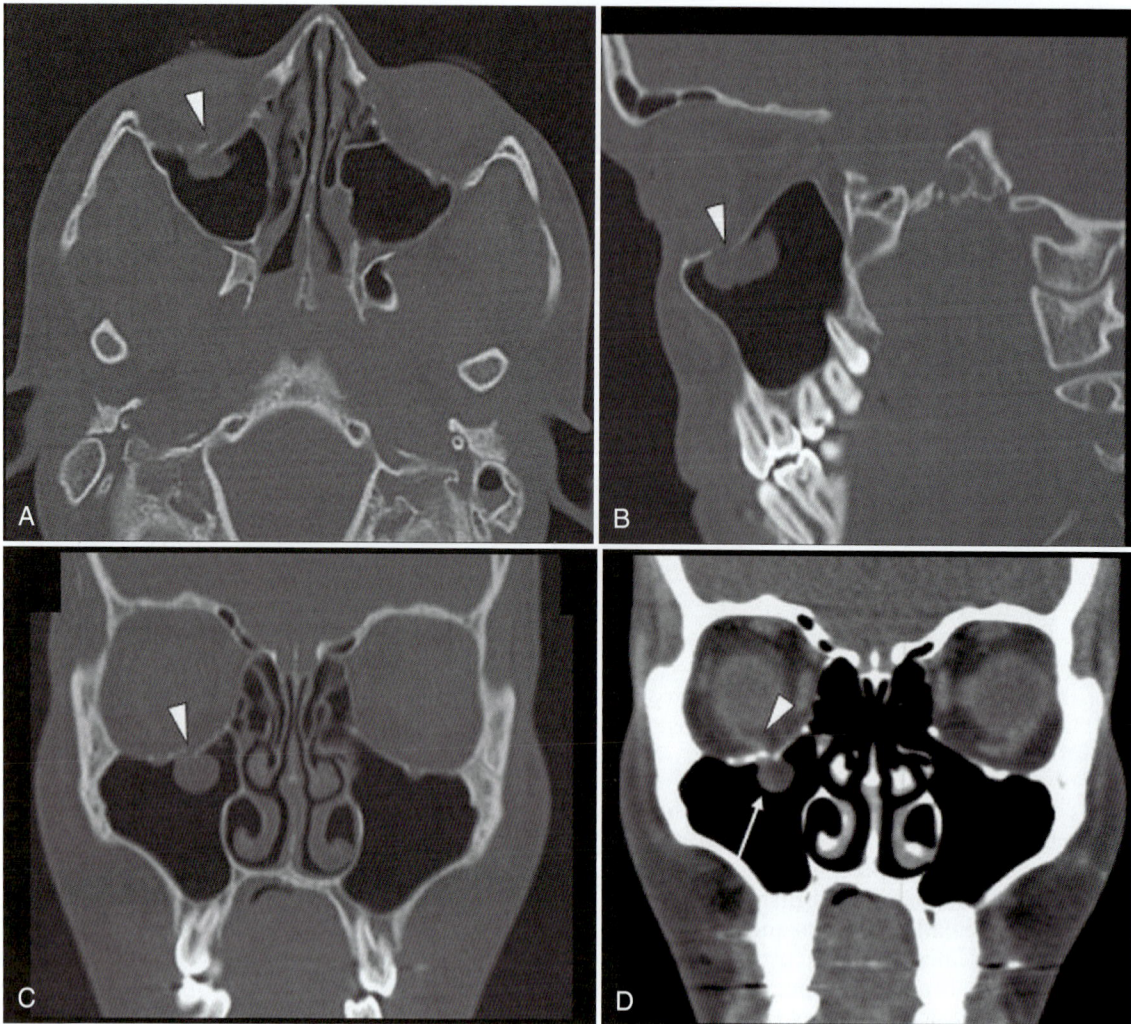

Figure 12-26 Orbital floor fracture and extraocular muscle entrapment. **A–D:** Fracture of the floor of the right orbit (*arrowheads* in **A–C**) complicated by herniation in the adjacent maxillary sinus of orbital soft tissues. **D:** Coronal image with soft tissue window settings showing distortion and inferior deviation of the inferior rectus (*arrowhead*) and mixed density of the herniated soft tissues, composed of fat and muscle (*arrow*). The patient presented with diplopia and upward gaze limitation due to the muscle entrapment, which required emergent surgical correction.

the radiologist should be aware that wooden fragments are markedly hypodense and may mimic locules of air if images are viewed with narrow window settings.

■ SUBACUTE HEAD IMAGING: EARLY FOLLOW-UP AND MANAGEMENT

What Is the Most Optimal Imaging Approach to Follow-up in Different Clinical Settings?

After acute head trauma admission imaging, further imaging is obtained in the following settings:
- Follow-up imaging in patients who have undergone surgical procedures
- Routine serial follow-up imaging
- Follow-up imaging focused toward a new clinical issue

Which Imaging Is Best?

In this phase when patients usually are monitored in an intensive care unit, the most rapid, accessible, cost-effective, satisfactory, and comparable imaging method remains CT. MRI in these patients is reserved for those cases whose clinical findings are not explained by the CT findings and is mainly aimed at detecting subtle brainstem injuries or better defining location and extent of DAI.

Postsurgical Imaging

The main classes of surgical procedures performed on acute head trauma patients are
- drainage of intraaxial and extraaxial hematomas
- decompressive craniectomies
- placement of intracranial catheters

After surgical drainage of intraaxial or extraaxial hematomas, the radiologist should note the type of surgical procedure that was performed. When comparing presurgical and postsurgical studies, it is important to note whether the drainage has been completely or partially

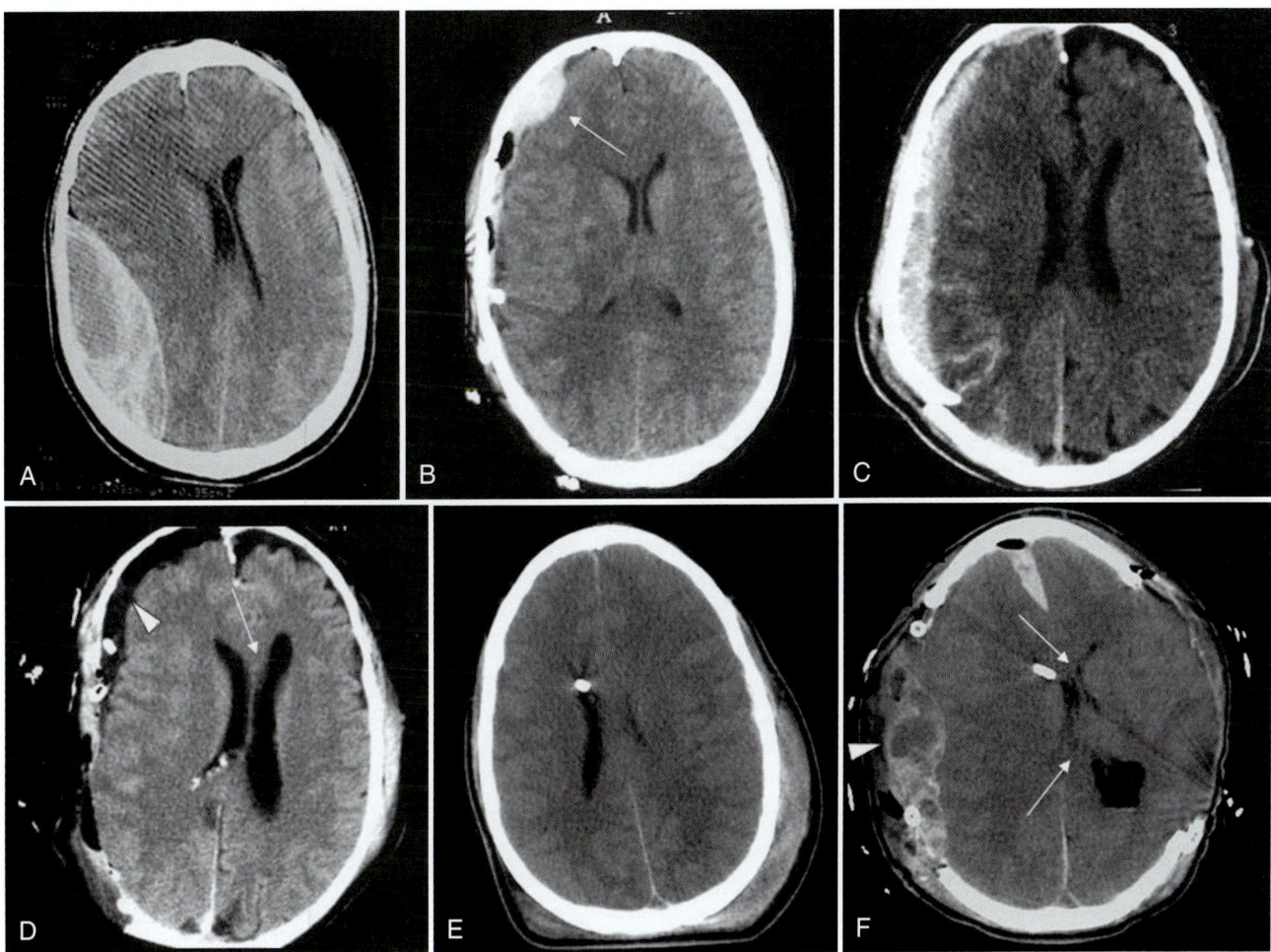

Figure 12-27 Postsurgical follow-up. **A, B:** Follow-up of surgical treatment of a large epidural hematoma. **B:** Decompression with resolution of midline shift and a new small epidural hematoma *(arrow)* at the anterior edge of the craniotomy that will require close radiologic follow-up because of its rapid growth potential. **C, D:** Craniectomy performed to decompress the right hemisphere from a subdural hematoma and a depressed skull fracture. The hematoma has been drained, but the midline shift persists and appears increased *(arrow* in **D**) partly due to parenchymal plasticity and especially due to a new cerebrospinal fluid subdural collection on the right side *(arrowhead* in **D**), with mass effect. **E, F:** Bilateral decompressive craniectomy performed to relieve intracranial pressure in this patient with hyperemic brain swelling (**E**). **F:** Postsurgical follow-up shows subfalcine herniation *(arrows)* due to the mass effect of a large heterogeneous epidural hematoma that developed at the site of the right craniectomy *(arrowhead)*.

successful and whether rebleeding has occurred, locally or remotely. The decompressive result of the drainage must be evaluated, looking at the signs of intracranial hypertension and brain herniation: Are the subarachnoid spaces reexpanded? Are the midline structures back in place? Are the cisterns around the midbrain patent? Has the ventricular incarceration resolved? Is there evolution of the lesions seen at admission?

Often a severe displacement of the brain tends to persist on the first follow-up studies after decompression due to brain parenchymal plasticity (Figure 12-27). In these cases, the place of the hematoma can be temporarily occupied by CSF. Sometimes a decompression is complicated by ex vacuo contralateral SDH or hygroma. After decompression, some hemorrhagic, edematous, and ischemic lesions appear more evident. Particular attention must be directed to the brainstem: During descending transtentorial herniation the brainstem is pushed downward and stretching of the perforating pontine arteries might cause the typical and severe hemorrhagic lesion in the ventral portion of the pons seen in association with uncal herniation, so-called *Duret hemorrhage* (Figure 12-28). After craniotomy, the dura is detached from the inner calvarium, and, despite the reanchoring surgical attempt, it is usually very difficult to discern the epidural from the subdural location of fluid or hemorrhagic extraaxial collections unless the dura itself is visible.

In case of brain swelling and often after hematoma drainage, a decompressive craniectomy is performed, usually in association with a duraplasty. On the postsurgical study it is important to evaluate the effect of the craniectomy on the pressure equilibria in the intracranial compartment. Have the brain, ventricles, and CSF spaces reexpanded? Are the cisterns around the midbrain patent? Are the craniectomy and the duraplasty wide enough to allow the brain to protrude freely through the craniectomy? Are extraaxial fluid or hemorrhagic collections limiting the degree of decompression? Has the decompression caused a contralateral SDH or hygroma?

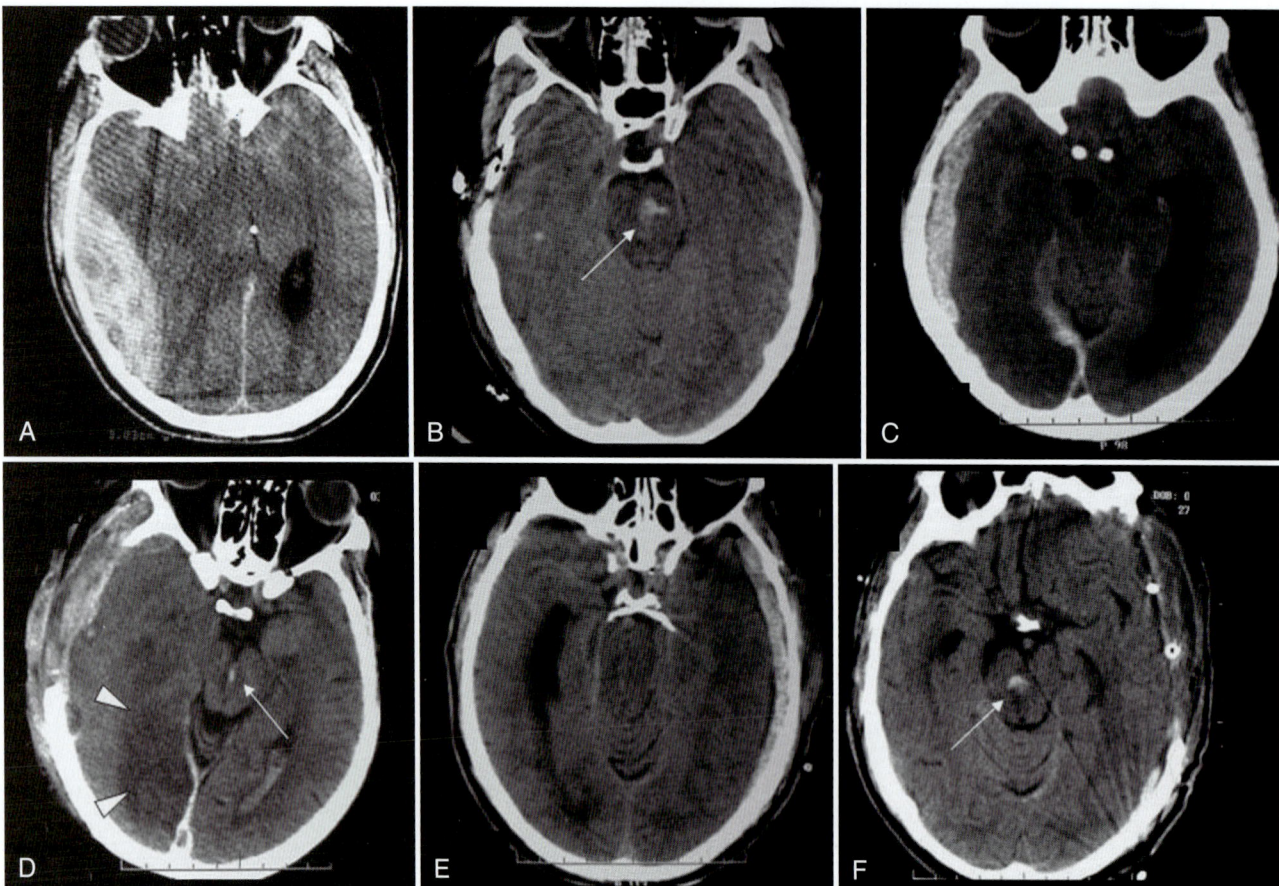

Figure 12-28 Duret hemorrhage, a specific type of brainstem hemorrhage that can be observed in patients who suffer descending transtentorial herniation (see text for details). It usually is better visualized in the subacute phase, at follow-up imaging, when the brain herniation has been decompressed. (A, B), (C, D), and (E, F) show three examples of patients with extraaxial hematoma and uncal herniation (A, C, E) who developed Duret brainstem hemorrhage (*arrows* in B, D, F), visible after surgical decompression. *Arrowheads* in D point to a posterior cerebral artery ischemic infarct caused by brain herniation.

Intracranial catheters can be inserted in the ventricles or in the subdural space for drainage and ICP monitoring. An intraparenchymal catheter can be used, usually in children, for ICP monitoring purposes. The role of radiologist is to verify the correct positioning of the catheters, their site of insertion, course, and distal tip position, and to report complications and visible effects on ventricular and subarachnoid spaces if a drainage is attempted.

Routine Serial Follow-up Imaging
- Why?
  To follow up the evolution of acute lesions and of delayed secondary lesions, to detect new lesions not present or not visible at the admission imaging, and to monitor indirectly the ICP in patients under sedation with no intracranial catheters.
- When?
  After admission imaging, a follow-up CT is usually obtained at 24 hours. Earlier follow-up at 12 hours is recommended if the admission imaging was performed less than 6 hours after the trauma or in presence of risk factors, such as anticoagulation, hypotension at admission, or posterior fossa lesions (Figure 12-29).
- What?

Interval Evolution of Primary Lesions
When hemorrhagic extraaxial collections are not surgically drained and a conservative approach is chosen, imaging follow-up is requested to evaluate signs of growth and increased mass effect of extraaxial hematomas. New evidence of mixed density or different density layering might indicate rebleeding. It is noteworthy that the mass effect caused by an enlarging EDH is usually greater than the mass effect caused by an SDH, due to the rapidity and the more focal nature of the compression, which does not allow the brain to adapt and conform to the mass.

In case of traumatic SAH, rebleeding is very rare. Most times at the follow-up imaging, a stable appearance or progressive resorption of the hyperdense blood in the subarachnoid space is observed.

Primary parenchymal lesions, such as cerebral hematomas, cerebral contusions, and DAI, are very likely to change appearance and size from the admission imaging through the follow-up studies. Rebleeding, increased edematous changes, hemorrhagic transformation of edematous lesions, confluence of lesions, and fluid–blood layering can be seen (Figure 12-30). Edema that is associated with intracerebral hemorrhagic contusions often increases dramatically

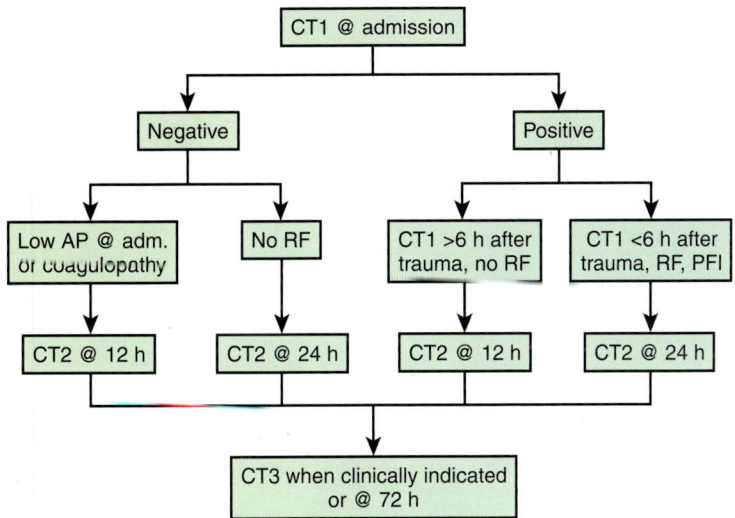

Figure 12-29 Recommended intervals of follow-up head imaging after admission imaging. AP, arterial pressure; adm, admission; RF, risk factors; PFI, posterior fossa injuries.

during the days following the acute event. It is not unusual for the initial CT scan to show no, or only limited, edema and for follow-up examination to reveal massive perilesional edema and associated mass effect. The majority of relevant CT changes develop within 48 hours after injury; therefore, serial imaging with early control CT scan is recommended. These modifications are due to the normal temporal evolution of the parenchymal lesions and to the general interval changes in the intracranial compartment. For example, it is not uncommon to better see DAI or to observe intracerebral hematomas enlarge after a craniectomy that has relieved intracranial hypertension.

Interval Evolution of Secondary Lesions
In the hours and days after the trauma, relevant intracranial changes, lesion evolution, and complications have to be expected.
Brain swelling initially due to hyperemia can gradually progress and evolve into brain edema. This shift is signaled by loss of visibility of the gray–white matter junction, diffuse parenchymal hypodensity, and progressive effacement of the CSF spaces in the basal region and along the convexities. As previously mentioned, brain swelling is usually accompanied by brain herniations. The most frequent type of brain herniation, the descending transtentorial herniation, is revealed by progressive effacement of ambiens cistern, the so-called disappearance of the "brain smile." The generalized parenchymal hypodensity is more striking when compared to the adjacent vascular structures, which appear hyperdense, and to the superior portion of the cerebellum. The cerebellar folia are more resistant than the cerebral hemispheres to the edematous changes, so axial CT cuts through the tentorial hiatus show the contrast between the normal cerebellar density and the hypodense temporal and occipital lobes, recognizable as the "dense cerebellum" sign (Figure 12-31).

Ischemic infarcts represent a frequent complication in severe head trauma. They are usually visible at follow-up imaging. Infarcts can occur very early after the trauma but be invisible at the time of admission imaging, or they can occur in the hours or days following the trauma. Ischemic infarctions are more frequently caused by arterial compression due to brain herniations. In case of subfalcine herniation, the expected infarcted areas are in the anterior cerebral artery territory, whereas in case of uncal herniation the expected infarcts involve the posterior thalamus, the temporooccipital lobes, and the superior cerebellum, along the distribution of the posterior cerebral and superior cerebellar arteries. Massive brain shift and swelling can result in compression of basically all major arteries of the circle of Willis, resulting in extremely extensive infarcts (Figure 12-32). Less frequent causes of ischemia are embolic phenomena from arterial dissection, vasospasm (if SAH is present), and excitotoxic injuries.

Special attention must be directed to ventricular size changes. Increased brain edema tends to reduce the size of the ventricles; on the other hand, hydrocephalus can occur. In a swollen brain, with effacement of the CSF spaces and reduced compensatory reserve, even a minimal increase in ventricular volume can cause a significant ICP rise and worsening clinical conditions. Therefore it is a special responsibility of the neuroradiologist to detect in serial scans the more subtle signs of developing hydrocephalus, such as a slight increase in size of the temporal horns or mild convexity of the walls of the third ventricle. In addition, brain herniation can cause ventricular entrapment, followed by monoventricular or compartmental hydrocephalus.

Dural tears can cause CSF fistulas, but more often they will result in subdural hygroma, typically crescentic in morphology, CSF-like in density, and with variable mass effect. Although the subdural hygroma can occur anywhere in the supratentorial and infratentorial

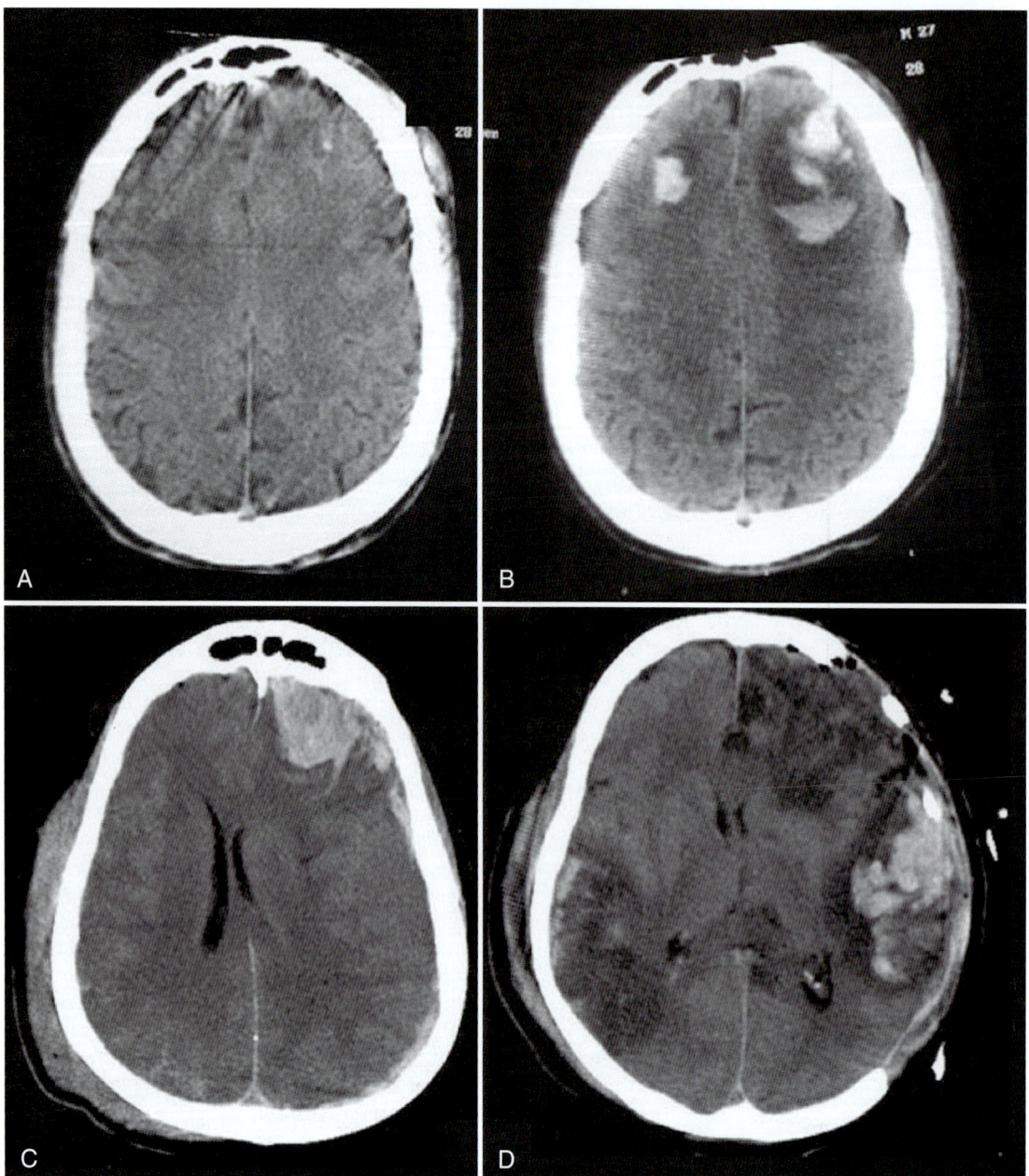

Figure 12-30 Evolution of primary lesions. Dramatic changes in appearance, number, and size of primary traumatic lesions seen at admission computed tomography are common occurrences. **A, B:** Small punctate hemorrhagic contusions in the frontal lobes (**A**) can develop into large brain hematomas a few hours later (**B**). **C, D:** After drainage of a frontal subdural hematoma (**C**), large edematous and hemorrhagic contusive lesions appear (**D**) in areas that showed no visible parenchymal lesions at the time of the admission scan.

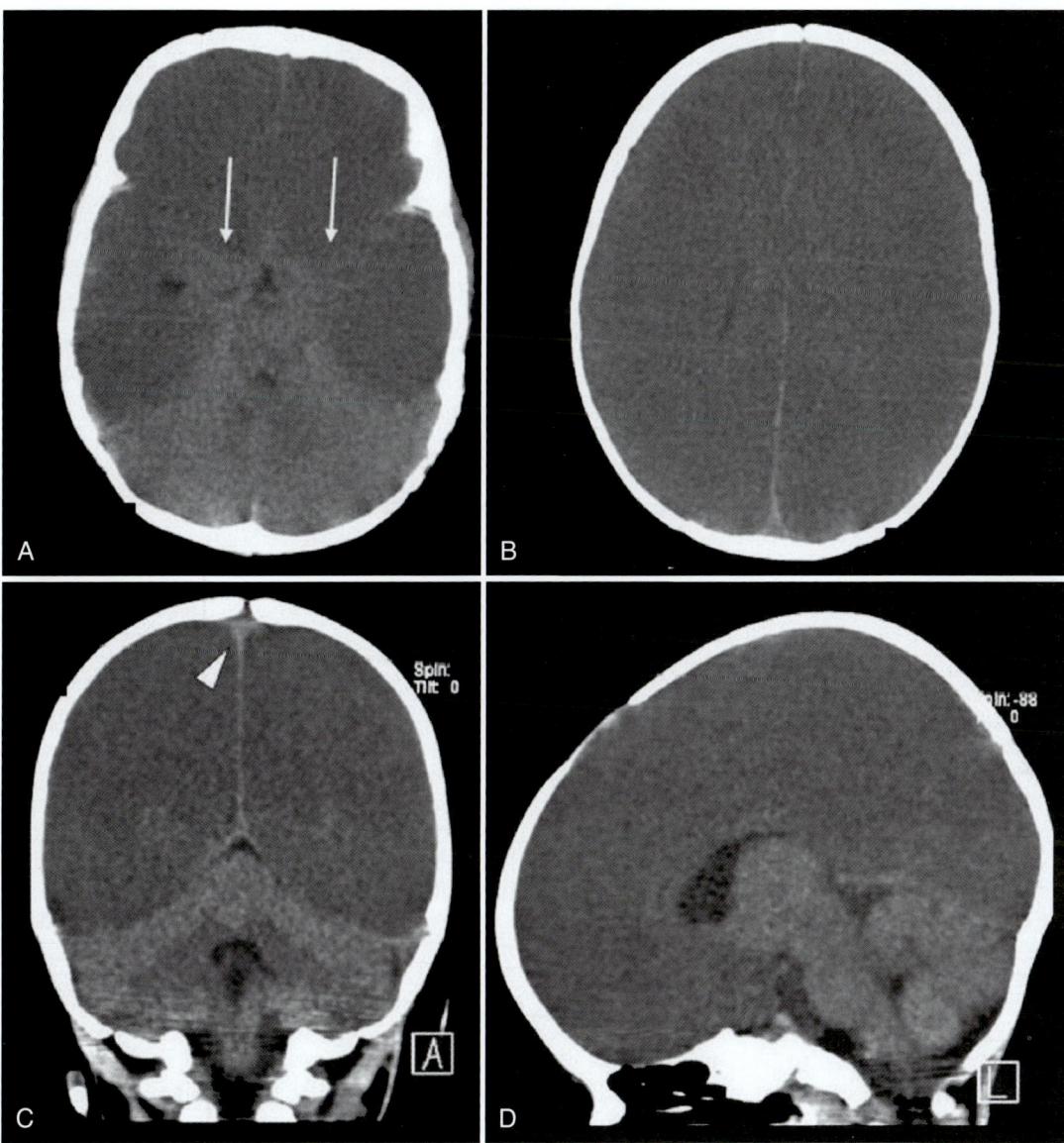

Figure 12-31 Brain edema and the "dense cerebellum sign." **A–D:** Multiplanar reformatted images of a noncontrast computed tomographic scan of a child with severe posttraumatic cerebral edema. The cerebral hemispheres are swollen and abnormally hypodense and homogeneous, with loss of gray–white matter contrast and sulcal effacement. The supratentorial hypodensity is striking compared to normal cerebellar density. The cerebellum is more resistant than the cerebral hemispheres to edematous changes. Blood-containing structures such as the middle cerebral arteries (*arrows* in **A**) and the venous sinuses (*arrowhead* in **C**) also appear relatively hyperdense to the brain.

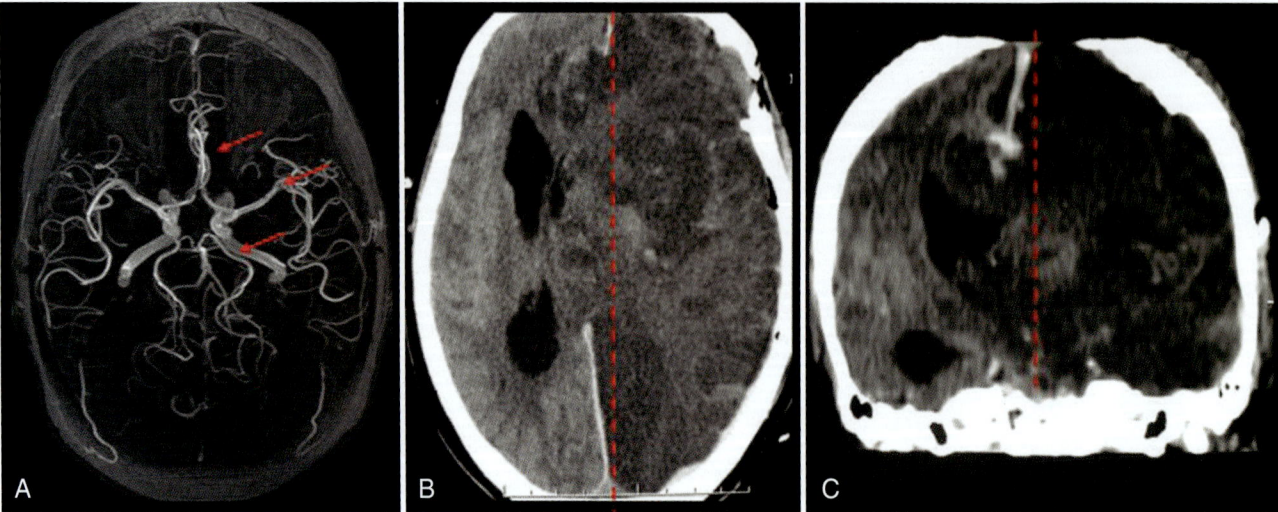

Figure 12-32 Complications of brain herniation. Massive brain shift can result in severe compression of all major intracranial arteries, possibly leading to extensive holohemispheric infarcts. **A:** Normal magnetic resonance angiogram of the circle of Willis. *Red arrows* point to the three major arteries branching off the anastomotic circle. In brain herniation, the anterior cerebral artery can be compressed against the falx by the displaced frontal lobe, the posterior cerebral artery can be compressed between the brainstem and the medial temporal lobe, and the middle cerebral artery can be distorted and compressed along its horizontal cisternal M1 segment. Massive subfalcine and descending transtentorial brain shift causes the ischemic infarct and in turn is further complicated by the ensuing brain edema **(B, C)**, revealed by the parenchymal hypodensity and swelling.

compartments, they are often located in the frontal region and can be bilateral (Figure 12-33). In patients with wide CSF spaces, the differential diagnosis between bilateral subdural hygromas and brain volume loss is usually obtained by detection of mass effect and displacement of the bridging veins toward the pial surface in the former and stretching of the veins in the latter (better seen on contrast CT or MR) (Figure 12-33).

New Lesions

New lesions that were not present or simply not visible at the acute admission imaging can appear on follow-up studies. New SDH or cerebral hematomas can present; DAI are usually much better evident hours after the trauma either because of the increase in vasogenic edema or because of their hemorrhagic transformation. Associated with uncal herniation, a delayed focal and very severe hemorrhagic lesion in the brainstem occurs and is revealed by CT or to better advantage by MR. This lesion, called *Duret hemorrhage* (Figure 12-28), is different from contusive lesions and brainstem DAI. Duret hemorrhage usually is located in a central or ventral location in the pons or midbrain, whereas contusions and DAI more frequently involve the dorsolateral portions of the brainstem. Duret hemorrhage probably is due to stretching and laceration of the perforating arterial branches of the basilar artery following downward displacement of the brainstem caused by descending transtentorial herniation.

ICP Monitoring

Serial subacute imaging can serve as a tool to explain unexpected ICP increases in patients with intracranial monitoring or to assess indirect evaluation of ICP in patients without invasive ICP monitoring. As explained earlier, lesions with mass effect, brain swelling, ventricular morphology and size, patency of CSF spaces along the convexities, in the basal cisterns, and in the posterior fossa, brain herniations, and their serial changes must be evaluated. Their final effect as a whole on the volume and pressure equilibrium of the intracranial compartment can serve as a tool to grossly assess signs of intracranial hypertension. Careful reporting of imaging findings, along with clinical data, can guide the invasive or conservative treatment.

Follow-up Imaging Focused toward a New Clinical Issue

Additional follow-up imaging can be obtained in the presence of new clinical issues, such as unexpected increased ICP >25 mmHg, anisocoria, focal neurologic signs, and seizures, to detect any treatable complication or evolution of primary or secondary lesions.

More advanced imaging, usually performed with MRI, is necessary when the clinical picture is not fully explained by CT findings. MRI is more sensitive than CT for the detection of thin SDHs or small cortical contusions, but it is mainly used in patients with unexplained comatose conditions to assess the presence and extent of DAI, especially with nonhemorrhagic lesions, that are distributed in particular locations, such as the corpus callosum and brainstem. Small Duret hemorrhages of the brainstem are also detected to better advantage by MRI.

■ CHRONIC IMAGING: TRAUMATIC SEQUELAE AND LATE COMPLICATIONS

Imaging at a long distance from the trauma may be necessary to evaluate the sequelae of head trauma and to investigate the presence of lesions responsible for

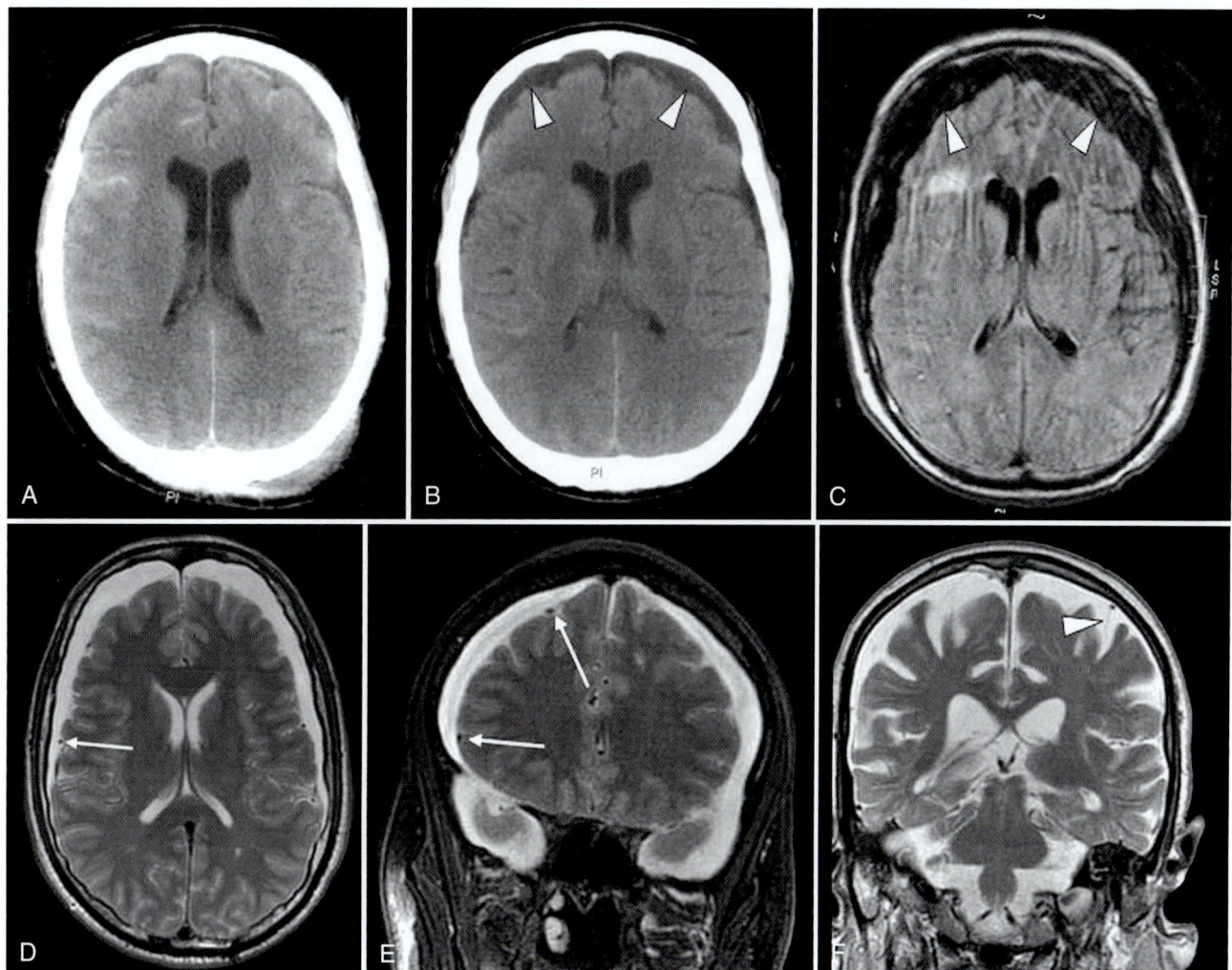

Figure 12-33 Subdural hygroma. **A–C:** Follow-up neuroimaging of a patient with head trauma, showing progressive enlargement of bilateral, extraaxial, subdural, frontal, and cerebrospinal fluid (CSF)-like density/signal fluid collections (*arrowheads* in **B** and **C**), causing progressive mass effect on the frontal lobes. **D–F:** Elements of differential diagnosis between subdural hygroma (**D**, **E**) and CSF space expansion due to brain volume loss (**F**). Hygromas tend to compress the brain, effacing the sulci, and displace the vessels inward, toward the pial surface (arrows in **D** and **E**), whereas in brain volume loss the CSF spaces and the sulci are widened, no mass effect is seen, and the vessels are seen stretched and coursing across the subarachnoid space (*arrowhead* in **F**).

permanent or newly developed clinical signs and symptoms. In other cases, imaging can be obtained for other reasons, and the signs of an old head trauma can represent incidental findings.

Patients who have suffered head trauma can present with permanent focal neurologic deficits, seizures, headaches, behavioral or cognitive problems, CSF rhinorrhea, anosmia, and hypoacusia.

CT and MR can serve as complementary imaging diagnostic tools in the chronic setting, with scanning techniques targeted to the diagnostic questions.

Although a general imaging assessment of the sequelae of head trauma is used to evaluate the correct repositioning of the craniectomy operculum, the resolution of extraaxial collections, the presence of gliotic or encephalomalacic changes, and volume loss and ventricular enlargement (Figure 12-34) in the presence of specific clinical conditions, more focused imaging studies are required to address the particular issues, as follows:.

- The patient has developed epilepsy.

    The culprit most likely is a cortical gliotic or encephalomalacic supratentorial lesion as a result of contusive or ischemic injury. MRI is the imaging method of choice to detect subtle cortical abnormalities. FLAIR T2-WI is the sequence of choice to detect subtle signal abnormalities of the brain parenchyma adjacent to the CSF, and GRE T2*-WI is very sensitive to foci of hemorrhage in the late stage due to the susceptibility effect and blooming artifacts created by hemosiderin deposits. The anterior and basal frontal regions, the temporal lobes, and the occipital poles deserve most of the attention. Hemorrhagic and nonhemorrhagic DAI sequelae are best assessed by FLAIR T2-WI and GRE T2*-WI.

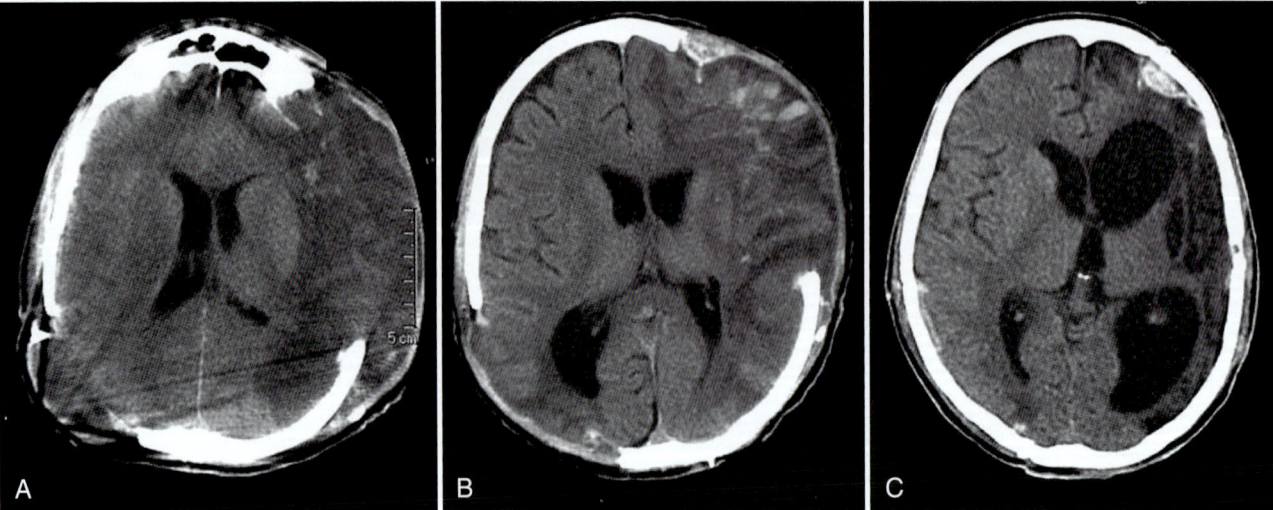

Figure 12-34 General late subacute head trauma imaging follow-up. **A–C:** Follow-up imaging of severe head trauma in a patient who underwent bilateral decompressive craniectomies (**A**). Brain edema gradually subsided (**B**), eventually allowing the repositioning of the craniectomy operculum (**C**). **C:** Final assessment of permanent encephalomalacic changes, brain volume loss, and compensatory ventricular enlargement.

- The patient has clear fluid rhinorrhea and positional headache.
  The working diagnosis is a CSF fistula caused by arachnoid and dural tear in communication with a bone defect in the region of the petrous ridges (mastoid and tegmen tympani), sella, ethmoid plate, or frontal sinuses. Targeted CT study, with bone algorithm, thin slice acquisition, and multiplanar reformatting, is able to show small bony defect along the inner surface of the skull, whereas MR with high resolution T2-WI or heavily T2-W cisternographic techniques shows the dural defect and herniation of CSF spaces and rules out encephaloceles (Figure 12-35). Sometimes the fistulous site is not found on conventional imaging, but CSF collection can be found in the mastoid cells, middle ear cavities, or ethmoid cells, indicating the possible site to address by surgical repair. A striking indirect sign of chronic CSF hypotension caused by the fistula is represented by generalized thickening and enhancement of the dura, better seen on fat-suppressed enhanced T1-WI, along with sagging of the brain on sagittal images and expansion of the venous dural sinuses and pituitary gland (Figure 12-35).
- The patient has lost the function of smell.
  Loss of smell, called *anosmia*, is a frequent condition after severe head trauma. It is caused by lesion of the thin olfactory nerve fibers that travel from the nasal mucosa through the cribrous ethmoid plate, to the olfactory bulbs, just below the gyri recti of the anterior frontal lobes, and can be sheared by acceleration–deceleration forces of the brain. MRI, with high-resolution coronal T2-WI or cisternographic sequences, can visualize the CSF space of the olfactory grooves along the ethmoid plate and show atrophy of the olfactory bulbs as a late sequela (Figure 12-36).
- Incidental findings.
  Some lesion patterns can be recognized as traumatic lesions, even when they are noted as incidental findings and when a history of past head trauma is not given. Typical old traumatic lesion patterns include cortical and subcortical amputation with gliosis, often bilateral, of the frontal rectus gyrus, supraorbital gyrus, and temporal poles. These structures are likely to suffer contusion and injury from rubbing against the uneven surfaces of the anterior and middle cranial fossae. Another very typical finding in the late stages after trauma is evidence of bilateral and symmetrical leukoencephalopathic changes in the anterior frontal subcortical and deep white matter, resembling the horns of a moose, called the "moose sign" (Figure 12-37). Such changes are often misdiagnosed as chronic ischemic lesions, but their distribution in the anterior and basal frontal lobes, across the vascular territories of the anterior and middle cerebral arteries and often accompanied by the lesions in the gyri recti, should orient toward the correct diagnosis.

■ PEDIATRIC HEAD TRAUMA

How to Problem Solve and Approach the Peculiarities?

The head, skull, and brain present different characteristics in children and adults, so the pathophysiology of pediatric head trauma and consequently its imaging have a few peculiarities that are important to know.

Labor and Delivery Head Trauma

Labor and delivery, even when uneventful, is a form of physiologic trauma that can cause minor head injuries, most often with no clinical consequences. These minor and benign traumatic injuries need to be differentiated from the more serious injuries related to complications that occurred during labor and delivery, such as hypoxic–ischemic damage.

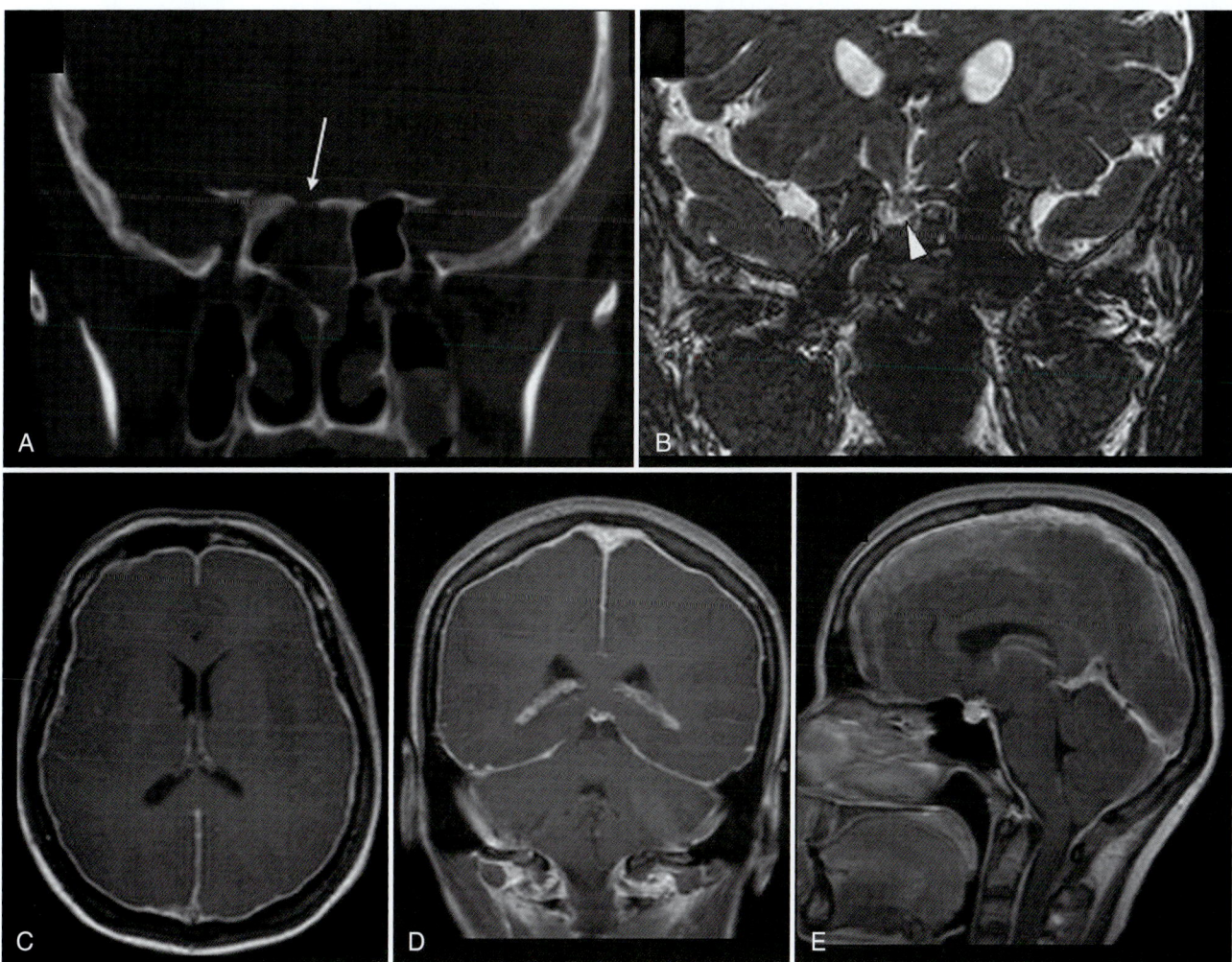

Figure 12-35 Posttraumatic cerebrospinal fluid (CSF) fistula. **A:** In a patient with CSF rhinorrhea after head trauma, thin coronal head computed tomography cuts with bone window settings shows a bony defect in the ethmoid plate *(arrow)* and obliteration of the adjacent sphenoid sinus, suggesting CSF leak. **B:** In preoperative planning, magnetic resonance imaging with cisternographic thin partitions is required to further characterize the fistula, here complicated by herniation of the dura, arachnoid space, and part of the right straight gyrus *(arrowhead)*, configuring a posttraumatic meningoencephalocele. **C–E:** Gadolinium-enhanced magnetic resonance imaging in another patient with CSF fistula showing indirect signs of chronic intracranial hypotension, characterized by diffuse dural thickening and enhancement, venous dural sinus expansion, pituitary gland enlargement, and sagging of the brain across the tentorium and foramen magnum.

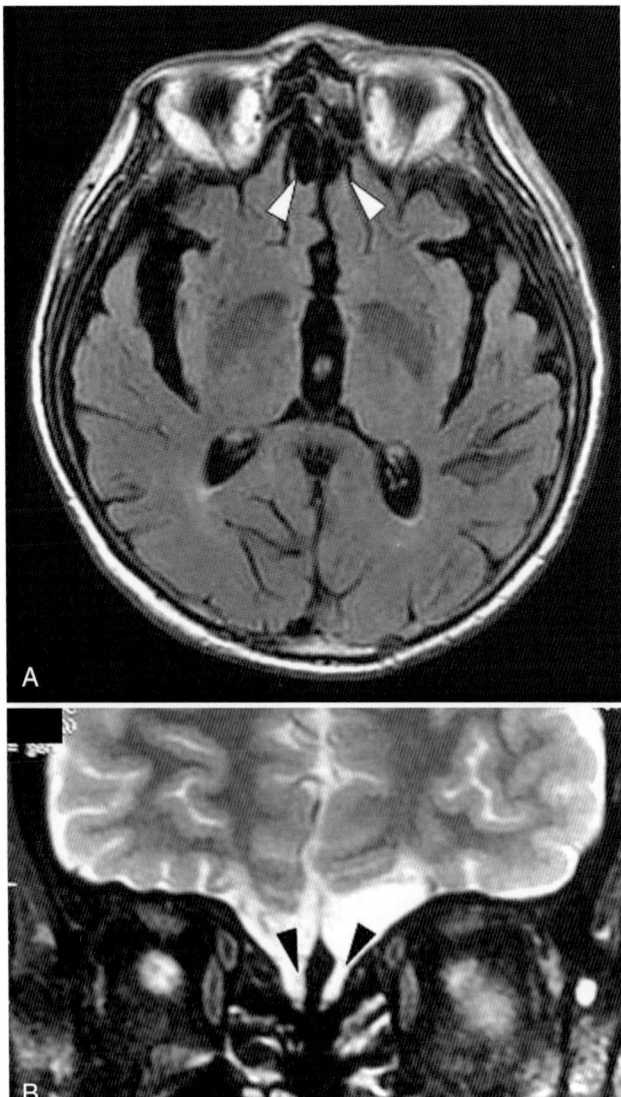

Figure 12-36 Posttraumatic anosmia in a patient with posttraumatic loss of smell. Magnetic resonance imaging showing encephalomalacia of the straight gyri (*white arrowheads* in **A**) and coronal T2-weighted image demonstrating atrophy of the olfactory bulbs revealed by cerebrospinal fluid signal and absence of normal olfactory bulbs in the olfactory grooves (*black arrowheads* in **B**).

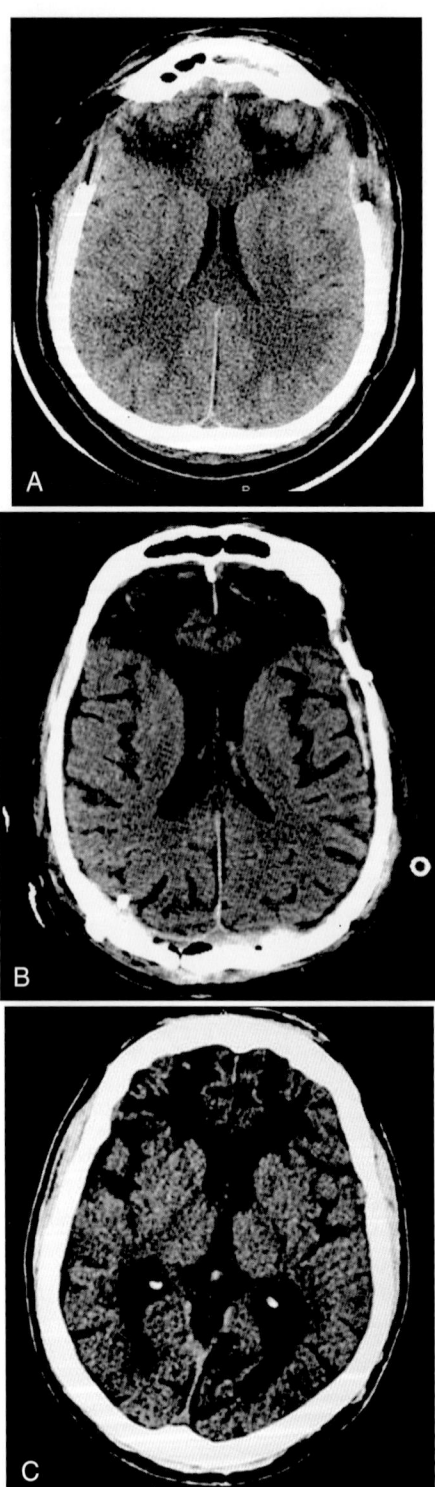

Figure 12-37 Posttraumatic bifrontal leukoencephalopathy (the "moose sign"). Different examples of bilateral frontal subcortical white matter gliotic changes, a typical posttraumatic contusive sequela, resembling the horns of a moose. This can be an incidental finding, often misdiagnosed as ischemic lesions, but prior head trauma should be inquired for when obtaining the patient's history.

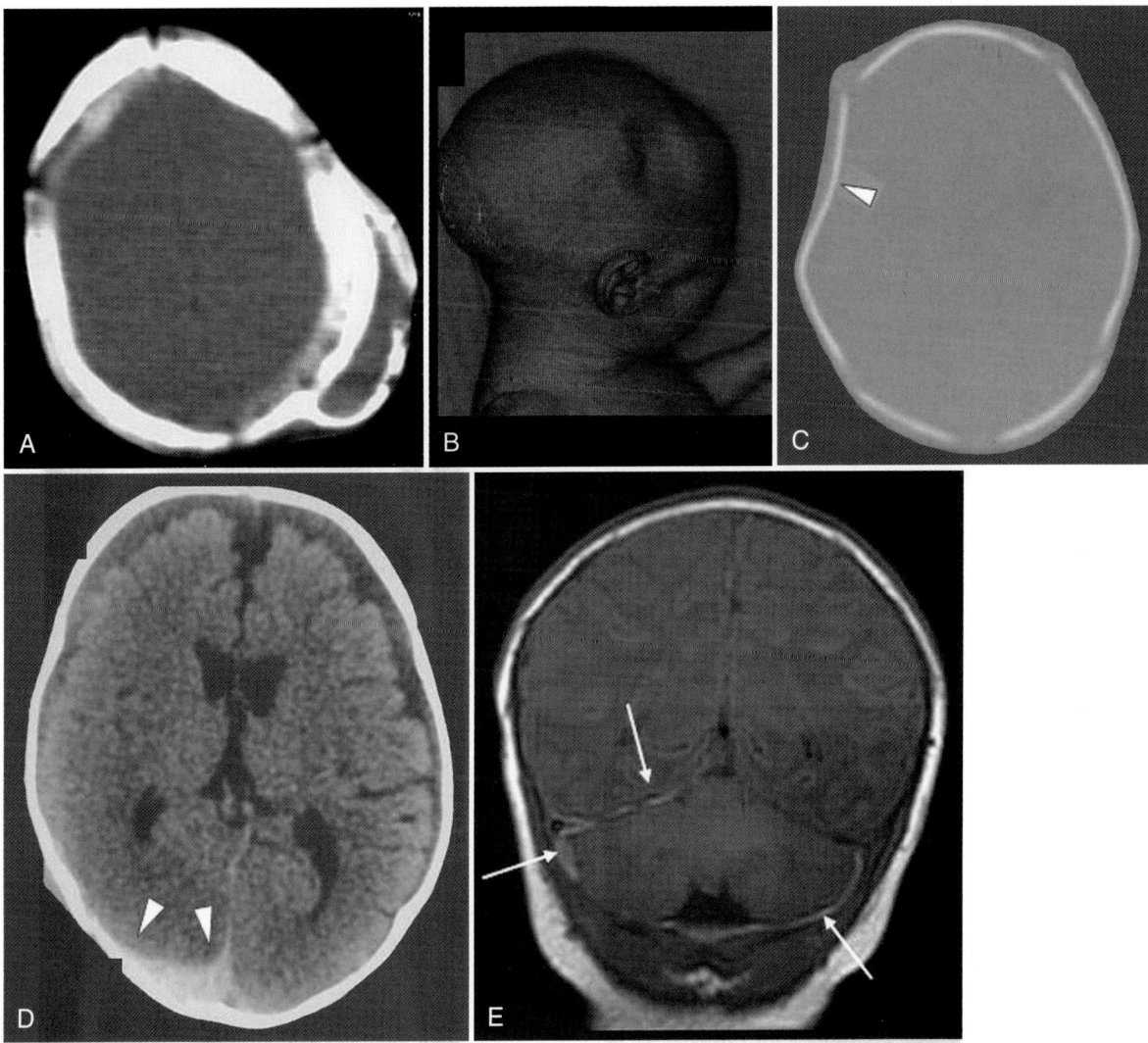

Figure 12-38 Delivery-related head trauma. **A:** Cephalohematoma in the typical subperiosteal location, expanding the periosteum, confined by sutures. **B, C:** Depressed skull fracture, with the feature of a deformation rather than a true fracture (*arrowhead* on **C**), due to the calvarium plasticity in newborns (Courtesy Dr. F. Velardi, Rome, Italy.) **D, E:** Typical asymptomatic incidental small subdural hematomas at the falcotentorial junction (*arrowheads* in **D**) and in the posterior fossa (*arrows* in **E**) can be considered part of the physiologic trauma of delivery.

Head injuries seen in neonates just after delivery (Figure 12-38) can be classified as follows:
- *Extracranial hemorrhages:* These range from the most superficial, so-called *caput succedaneum*, which is hemorrhagic thickening of the superficial scalp soft tissues, mobile at palpation, for which imaging is not required; to *subgaleal hematoma*, which is located deep to the galea capitis, superficial to the skull, mobile at palpation; and finally *cephalohematoma*, which is a subperiosteal hematoma that remodels the periosteum, is hard and nonmobile at palpation, stops at the sutures, and can be seen in association with fractures and intracranial injuries.
- *Fractures:* These can be result from uterine contractions or compression against the pelvic ring bones during delivery. The skull fractures can be linear or depressed, sometimes with the appearance of a focal impression and deformation rather than a true bony fracture. Overlapping displaced sutures can also be seen, and they usually spontaneously resolve.
- *Intracranial extraaxial hemorrhages:* The most common intracranial extraaxial hemorrhages are SDHs. Very often these SDHs are small and are seen as incidental findings at the junction of falx and tentorium, with no significant mass effect. In these cases the radiologic report should state that such an SDH can be considered a relatively normal finding, related to the physiologic trauma of delivery. SAH is rare in neonates, more frequently observed in preterm babies.
- *Intraaxial injuries:* Cortical contusions, although rare, can be seen in association with SDHs and fractures.

Postnatal Pediatric Head Trauma

Which Factors Account for the Peculiarities of Pediatric Head Trauma?
- Clinical assessment of children is difficult. The history often is unreliable, and a history of loss of consciousness can be impossible to establish. For these reasons, clinicians should have a low threshold for

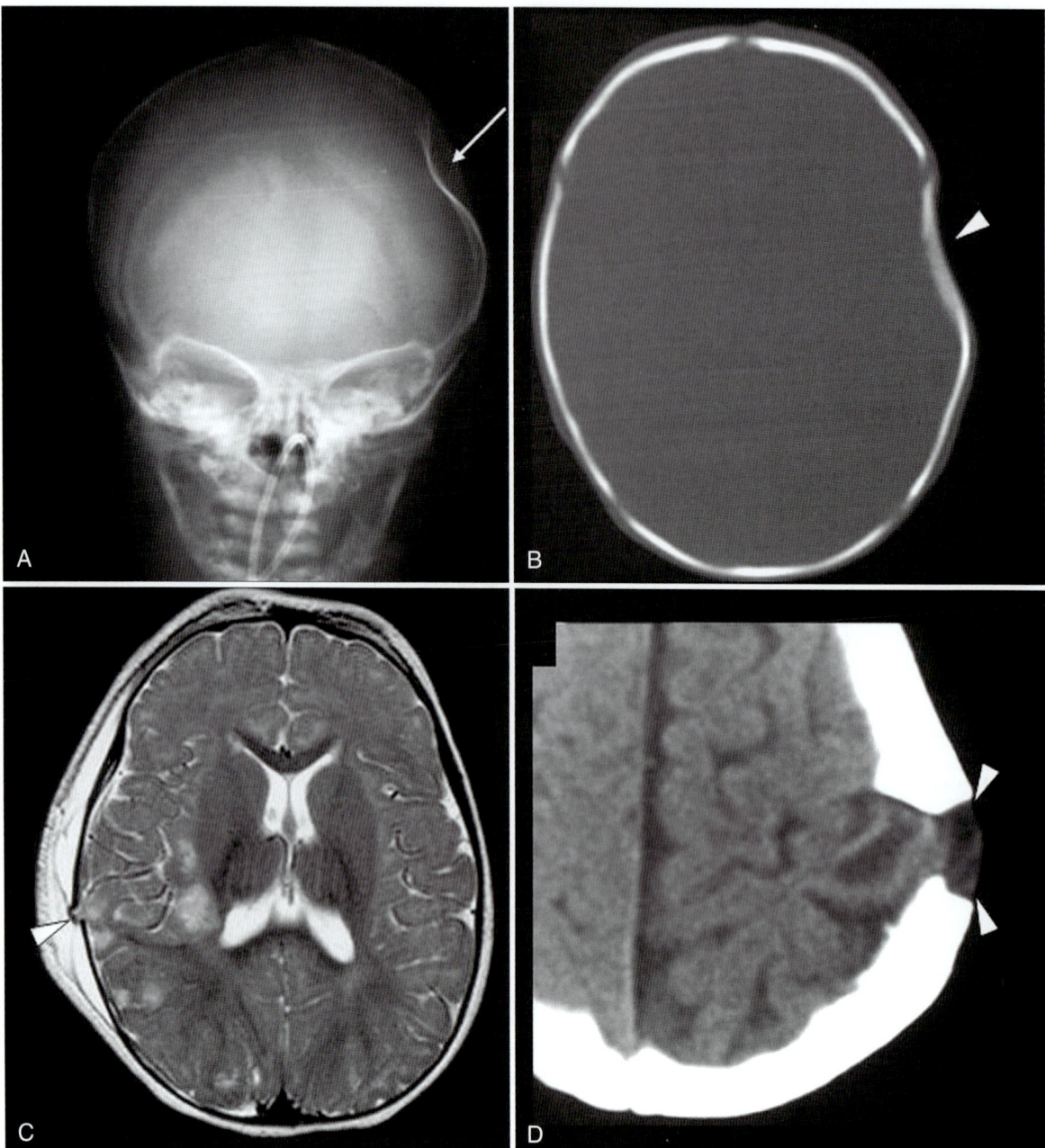

Figure 12-39 Pediatric skull fracture peculiarities. **A, B:** "Ping-pong fracture" resulting from direct impact on the calvarium. There are no fracture lines but inward focal depression of the deformable skull (*arrow* in **A**, *arrowhead* in **B**). **C, D:** Two different stages of growing fractures. **C:** Small outpouching of arachnoid and cerebrospinal fluid (CSF) through a small fracture line (*arrowhead*). **D:** CSF pulsatility can expand the fracture line and result in larger herniation of intracranial structures through the bony defect (*arrowhead*). (Courtesy Dr. A. Rossi, Genoa, Italy).

ordering neuroimaging studies in children. In particular, age less than 2 years is itself a risk factor that should prompt head imaging after significant head trauma. Every effort should be made to minimize radiation dose during CT imaging of the head and cervical spine while ensuring that image quality and coverage are sufficient to achieve an adequate diagnostic study.

- In children, the ratio of head to body weight is higher than in adults (about 10%) and neck muscles are relatively weak, which account for the potential for more violent head impact and higher acceleration/deceleration forces applied to the head.

- The pediatric skull has plasticity and deformability, which account for EDHs and brain contusions that occur in the absence of skull fractures, the peculiar appearance of the so-called *ping-pong fracture* (Figure 12-39), a depressed fracture with the appearance of a squished table-tennis ball, and the increased risk of dural lacerations. In children younger than 3 years fractures can evolve into "growing fractures" (Figure 12-39). These fractures show progressive enlargement of the fracture defect, usually greater than 3 to 4 mm, due to meningeal interposition and CSF pulsatility, possibly leading to meningoceles and encephaloceles of variable size.

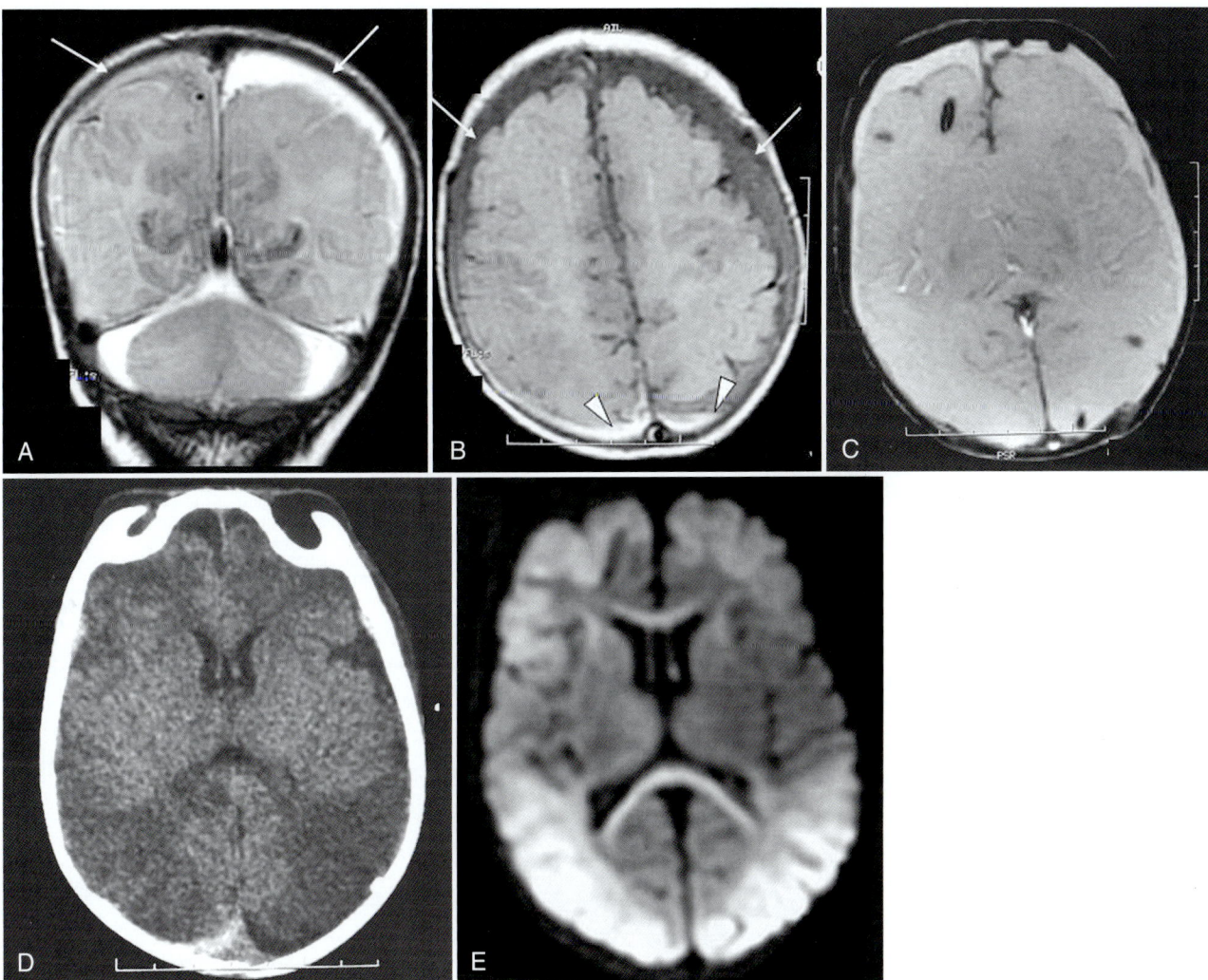

Figure 12-40 A–E: Neuroimaging of child abuse. Bilateral subdural hematomas *(arrows on* **A** and **B**), with different magnetic resonance signals suggesting different ages. Blood–fluid levels in the dependent regions *(arrowheads* on **B**) suggest rebleeding phenomena, along with pericerebellar hygromas, and hemorrhagic axonal injuries "blooming" on gradient-recalled echo T2* (**C**). Bilateral excitotoxic injuries in a nonvascular distribution, visible on computed tomography (**D**) and diffusion-weighted imaging (**E**), are almost pathognomonic of shaken baby injuries until proven otherwise.

- The brain parenchyma is soft and poorly myelinated so delamination injuries can occur in acceleration/deceleration traumas.
- The CSF spaces are wide, which accounts for the incidence of SDHs due to rupture of bridging veins. Moreover, the presence of unfused sutures and fontanelles allows intracranial hemorrhages to reach considerable volumes before clinical signs are seen, so the clinical evolution of intracranial hemorrhages in children is often characterized by lucid intervals and sudden deterioration.
- Immature autoregulation and increased vasoreactivity make hyperemia and brain swelling more frequent subacute complications of head trauma in children, usually 24 to 48 hours after the primary event.
- The developing brain is particularly susceptible to apoptotic neuronal death following traumatic injury, which accounts for the not rarely observed rapid and extensive encephalomalacic evolution of initially smaller traumatic brain injuries. The presence of a lactate (Lac) peak on MR spectroscopy has proved to be an early bad prognostic indicator in children with a normal-appearing brain on MRI acquired in the acute or early subacute phase after head trauma.

Nonaccidental Head Trauma: Child Abuse

In infants and young children, the possibility of nonaccidental injury should always be kept in mind. The radiologist plays an important role in accurately identifying nonaccidental cranial trauma and is in the front line for suggesting the possibility of child abuse.

Child abuse should be suspected in presence of disproportion between the neuroradiologic findings (Figure 12-40) and the referred clinical history. Skull x-ray films, as part of a series of plain x-ray films (skeletal survey), retain a role in detecting nonaccidental head injuries in children. CT is able to detect skull fractures and typical bilateral SDHs, often parasagittal, often of different ages, with signs of rebleeding. MRI with FLAIR images is much more sensitive for small SDHs and is accurate in detecting rebleeding of different ages, whereas DWI is extremely sensitive for detecting the usually associated acute parenchymal injuries, especially in shaken babies, represented by contusions, DAI, and hypoxic–ischemic and excitotoxic injuries. If the red flag of a suspected child abuse has been raised, MRI, including fast FLAIR and DWI, should be performed as soon as possible (on the day of admission). DWI is the most sensitive and specific method of confirming a shaking injury.

In chronic phases, brain volume loss due to diffuse atrophy and SDHs of different ages can be seen.

Associated evidence of long bone fractures and retinal hemorrhages reinforce the diagnosis of child abuse.

Suggested Readings

Brandstack N, Kurki T, Tenovuo O, Isoniemi H. MR imaging of head trauma: visibility of contusions and other intraparenchymal injuries in early and late stage. *Brain Inj.* 2006 Apr;20(4):409-416.

Cihangiroglu M, Ramsey RG, Dohrmann GJ. Brain injury: analysis of imaging modalities. *Neurol Res.* 2002 Jan;24(1):7-18:Review.

Connor SEJ, Chaudhary N. Imaging of maxillofacial and skull base trauma. *Imaging.* 2007;19:71-82.

Demaerel P, Casteels I, Wilms G. Cranial imaging in child abuse. *Eur Radiol.* 2002 Apr;12(4):849-857.

Gallagher CN, Hutchinson PJ, Pickard JD. Neuroimaging in trauma. *Curr Opin Neurol.* 2007 Aug;20(4):403-409.

Grossman RI, Yousem DM. Head trauma. In: Grossman RI, Yousem DM, eds. *Neuroradiology: the Requisites.* 2nd ed. Philadelphia: Mosby; 2003:243-272.

Holm L, Cassidy JD, Carroll LJ, Borg J. Neurotrauma Task Force on Mild Traumatic Brain Injury of the WHO Collaborating Centre. Summary of the WHO Collaborating Centre for Neurotrauma Task Force on Mild Traumatic Brain Injury. *J Rehabil Med.* 2005 May;37(3):137-141.

Lee HJ, Jilani M, Frohman L, Baker S. CT of orbital trauma. *Emerg Radiol.* 2004 Feb;10(4):168-172.

Lobato RD, Gomez PA, Alday R, et al. Sequential computerized tomography changes and related final outcome in severe head injury patients. *Acta Neurochir (Wien).* 1997;139(5):385-391.

Nortje J, Menon DK. Traumatic brain injury: physiology, mechanisms, and outcome. *Curr Opin Neurol.* 2004 Dec;17(6):711-718:Review.

Parizel PM, Ceulemans B, Laridon A, Ozsarlak O, Van Goethem JW, Jorens PG. Cortical hypoxic-ischemic brain damage in shaken-baby (shaken impact) syndrome: value of diffusion-weighted MRI. *Pediatr Radiol.* 2003 Dec;33(12):868-871.

Parizel PM, Makkat S, Jorens PG, et al. Brainstem hemorrhage in descending transtentorial herniation (Duret hemorrhage). *Intensive Care Med.* 2002 Jan;28(1):85-88.

Parizel PM, Ozsarlak Van Goethem JW, et al. Imaging findings in diffuse axonal injury after closed head trauma. *Eur Radiol.* 1998;8(6):960-965.

Parizel PM, Van Goethem JW, Ozsarlak O, Maes M, Phillips CD. New developments in the neuroradiological diagnosis of craniocerebral trauma. *Eur Radiol.* 2005 Mar;15(3):569-581:Review.

Poussaint TY, Moeller KK. Imaging of pediatric head trauma. *Neuroimaging Clin N Am..* 2002 May;12(2):271-294:ix. Review.

Sklar EM. What more can MR imaging teach us about brain injury? *AJNR Am J Neuroradiol.* 2000 May;21(5):808-809.

Sliker CW, Mirvis SE. Imaging of blunt cerebrovascular injuries. *Eur J Radiol.* 2007 Oct;64(1):3-14.

Smits M, Dippel DW, de Haan GG, et al. Minor head injury: guidelines for the use of CT—a multicenter validation study. *Radiology.* 2007 Dec;245(3): 831-838.

Vincent JL, Berré J. Primer on medical management of severe brain injury. *Crit Care Med.* 2005 Jun;33(6):1392-1399:Review.

CHAPTER 13

Imaging of Spine Trauma

Alessandro Cianfoni and Cesare Colosimo

■ SPINE TRAUMA

Imaging: Why, Who, and How? (Computed Tomography: When, Why, and How; Magnetic Resonance Imaging; When, Why, and How; Computed Tomographic Angiography)

Why Imaging?
Spinal injuries are common sequelae of high-energy acute traumas. The role of imaging is to establish the radiologic diagnosis, classify it, determine the stability and instability, evaluate the integrity of neural elements, and provide further radiologic evaluation when appropriate. Given that spinal injuries can cause spinal cord injury and major permanent disability, there is no controversy regarding the need for accurate and emergent imaging assessment of the traumatized spine.

Who Needs Imaging?
It is important to judge the appropriate use of imaging in patients referred for spine imaging after trauma. A set of clinical and/or amnestic criteria can be very useful in identifying patients who have an extremely low probability of injury and who consequently have no need for imaging studies and those who are at high risk for having spinal injuries and therefore must undergo a thorough imaging evaluation of the spine.

Any trauma patient who is unconscious or intoxicated in the emergency department, and therefore is not easily evaluated, needs spinal imaging to rule out significant and possibly unstable spinal lesions. More controversial debate exists about the selection criteria for imaging in trauma patients who are fully alert. Most studies have focused on cervical spine trauma, and the conclusions of those studies are routinely extrapolated to the thoracolumbar spine injuries in the clinical practice. In alert (Glasgow Coma Scale score = 15) and stable patients, the Canadian C-Spine Rule study established an accurate set of criteria to triage trauma patients who are at low risk and therefore do not need spinal imaging (Table 13-1).

How to Image: Which Imaging Techniques and Protocols Are Best?
Problem Solving with Plain Film Radiography
In general, when plain film radiography is used for the initial assessment, most institutions perform a minimum of three views: anteroposterior (AP), lateral, and open-mouth odontoid necessary for C-spine clearance. AP and lateral plain radiographs should be taken without change of the patient's position. If the cervicothoracic junction is not clearly visualized, additional swimmer's view or supine oblique views may be obtained. Additional flexion–extension radiographs are of questionable use in the acute phase due to poor feasibility, technical reproducibility, and sensitivity and the theoretical risk of causing additional spinal cord injury. (In rare cases, flexion–extension can be useful for excluding delayed instability 2 to 4 weeks after trauma.) On the lateral view, attention should be directed toward assessing the integrity of the vertebral bodies and of four parallel longitudinal lines (Figure 13-1): a line joining the anterior margins of the vertebral bodies (anterior spinal line), the posterior margin of the vertebral bodies (posterior spinal line), the interapophyseal line along the posterior margin of the lateral masses, and the spinolaminar line joining the junction of the laminae with the anterior margin of spinous processes. On the AP view, a line along the tips of spinous processes should be running straight downward (Figure 13-1). In cervical and upper thoracic spine fractures, abnormal widening of prevertebral or paravertebral soft tissue structures is significant. In the case of a patient who shows an abnormal positioning of head and/or spine, repositioning for imaging is contraindicated until it is proven that the reason for the abnormal position is not a life-threatening/painful pathology.

Problem Solving with Multidetector Computed Tomography
Until a few years ago, plain film radiography was the initial imaging procedure in the evaluation of the spine in trauma patients. However, plain radiographs have proved to have intrinsic low to medium sensitivity for traumatic spinal injuries and suffer from additional technical limits in acute and immobilized patients. Some authors advocate the use of conventional radiographs, as a sole modality, only in low-risk patients and direct use of multidetector computed tomography (MDCT) in high-risk patients. Many other authors now recognize MDCT as the preferred initial imaging procedure in acute (blunt) spinal trauma patients who need imaging. MDCT is accurate and fast, and it can be performed simultaneously with head, thoracic, and/or abdominal computed tomography (CT), even using the same raw data, in the polytraumatized patient, thereby reducing patient manipulation. Complex lesions can be

more clearly depicted using the reformatting and three-dimensional (3D) capabilities of MDCT. It is important to note that the axial CT images alone may miss fracture lines that run parallel to the scans, compression fractures, and subtle subluxations. Therefore, the whole diagnostic potential of MDCT should be used to advantage (Figure 13-2), routinely obtaining multiplanar reformatted thin section views for bone and soft tissues and possibly 3D volume-rendering images as well, which are especially useful at the craniocervical and atlantooccipital junctions. Evidence-based research has established that MDCT improves patient outcome and saves money in comparison to plain film. Our institution includes oblique reconstructions for the facet joints as well as the routine sagittal and coronal reconstructions of the C-spine.

Problem Solving with CT Angiography

Because blunt vascular injuries of the neck arterial vessels associated with cervical spinal trauma are more frequent than believed and can have devastating consequences with cerebral embolism and infarction when undiagnosed, we suggest obtaining the cervical spine MDCT study just after injection of contrast agent bolus used for other purposes in polytraumatized patients in order to obtain simultaneous evaluation of the bony spinal structures, and a CT angiogram of the neck to rule out arterial dissection of the carotid and vertebral arteries.

Problem Solving with Magnetic Resonance Imaging

Magnetic resonance imaging (MRI) can demonstrate the presence, location, and extent of spinal cord lesions, ligament and muscular injuries, disc herniation, epidural hematomas (EDHs), and bone marrow edema. MRI should not be used as a primary screening tool in spinal trauma, but it certainly should play a prominent role in the thorough assessment of severe spinal trauma to evaluate instability possibly caused by soft tissues injury and in any case of suggested spinal cord or nerve root compromise. A quick assessment of the

Table 13-1 Canadian C-spine Rule: Criteria to Triage Low-Risk Patients with Spinal Trauma Who Do Not Need Imaging

A. Absence of high risk factors, including the following:

Age 65 years or older
Dangerous mechanism (fall from elevation of 5 feet/five stairs or more; axial load to the head)
>100 km/h MVA, rollover or ejection MVA
Motorized recreational vehicle, bicycle collision
Paresthesias in extremities

B. Presence of low-risk factors, including the following:

Simple rear-end MVA (excluding pushed into oncoming traffic, hit by bus or large truck, rollover, hit by high-speed vehicle)
Sitting position at admission
Ambulatory at any time since trauma
Delayed onset of neck pain
No midline C-spine tenderness

C. Able to actively rotate neck 45 degrees bilaterally

Patients who satisfy all of the A, B, C criteria are triaged as low risk and do not need C-spine imaging.

Modified from Stiell IG, Wells GA, Vandemheen KL, et al. The Canadian C-spine rule for radiography in alert and stable trauma patients. JAMA. 2001;286(15):1841-1848.
MVA, Motor vehicle accident.

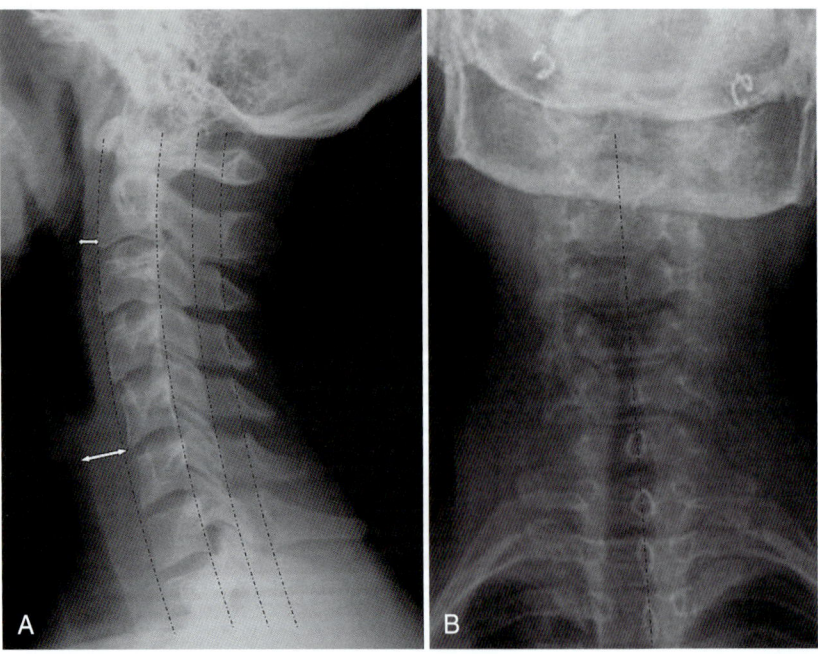

Figure 13-1 Assessment of C-spine radiographs in trauma. **A:** On this normal examination, the lateolateral view shows four uninterrupted parallel longitudinal lines *(black dotted lines)*. The line's stepoff suggests dislocation. Thickness of the prevertebral soft tissues is <6 mm at C2 *(short white arrow)* and <22 mm at C5 *(long white arrow)*. Increased thickness suggests hematoma due to rupture of the anterior longitudinal ligament. **B:** Anteroposterior view showing alignment of the spinous processes *(black dotted line)*. Misalignment suggests rotatory dislocation, such as unilateral facet luxation.

spine can be obtained by a set of T1-weighted and fat-suppressed T2-weighted or short tau inversion recovery (STIR) sagittal images to detect alignment abnormalities, bone marrow edema (believed to be a sign of osseous trabecular microfractures), ligamentous injuries, acute disc lesions and herniations, central canal compromise, cord contusions, compression, or transection. The addition of a sagittal gradient-recalled echo (GRE) T2*-weighted sequence, which is sensitive to susceptibility effects, allows the prognostically relevant distinction between hemorrhagic and nonhemorrhagic cord contusions.

Problem Solving with CT Myelography

CT myelography can only partially replace MRI in detecting central canal compromise and spinal cord compression. In cases where MRI is unavailable, CT offers no information on the cord parenchyma. CT myelography also can have a role, after acute trauma management, in rare cases of dural sac tears or unclear nerve root problems.

Acute Spinal Trauma Imaging

What Is the Role of Acute Spinal Trauma Imaging in Problem Solving?

The role of acute spinal trauma imaging is to assess the spinal injury, to direct appropriate management, and to predict neurologic outcome. The risk of mis(under)diagnosis is extremely high because of the possible life-long devastating sequelae. Awareness of the strengths and limitations of plain radiography, MDCT, and MRI in the diagnosis of spinal injuries is fundamental, and most often a multimodal imaging is required for best practice.

One single concept is worth keeping in mind when imaging the acute spinal trauma: *stability versus instability.*

Stability is the capacity of the spine to limit segmental motion so as to not risk damage to the neural structures. Stability is provided by intact bony and ligamentous structures. The implication of clinical instability is the risk of delayed neurologic injury and the need for surgical intervention to stabilize the spine.

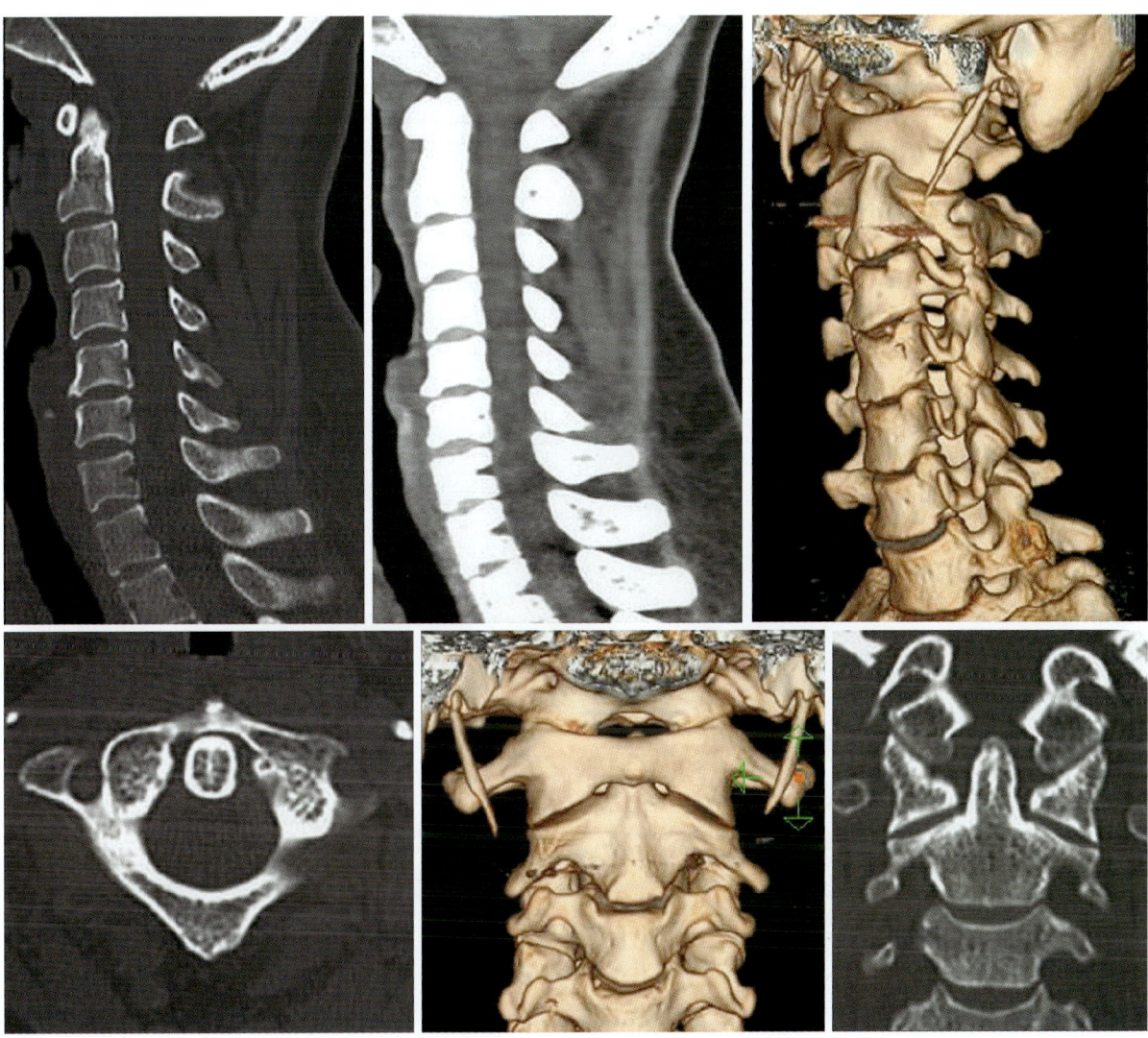

Figure 13-2 Multidetector computed angiography (MDCT) of the C-spine. In the spine trauma setting, the full diagnostic potential of MDCT should be exploited, obtaining thin axial cuts and multiplanar two-dimensional reformats, viewed with bone and soft tissue windows, as well as multiple three-dimensional views, especially useful at the craniovertebral and C1–C2 junctions.

Despite numerous and complex classification systems, Denis' concept of stability based on the three columns still holds valid. In the lower cervical segment of C3–C7 and in the thoracolumbar spine, support is provided by three columns (Figure 13-3).

The anterior column consists of the anterior vertebral bodies, the anterior annulus fibrosus, and the anterior longitudinal ligament. The middle column consisted of the posterior vertebral bodies, posterior longitudinal ligament, and posterior annulus fibrosus. The posterior column includes the posterior bony elements, the ligamenta flava, and the posterior ligaments. A spinal lesion is considered unstable if it involves the middle column, which is considered the most crucial for spinal stability. Middle column lesions are most often associated with lesions of the adjacent anterior or posterior column, so lesions involving two or more columns are considered unstable. With the more widespread use of MR in acute spinal trauma, it is not too uncommon to encounter extensive ligamentous lesions on STIR images, in absence of bony fractures. In these cases, although no rigid rules are given, a little flexibility in thinking is required. Ligamentous disruption involving all three columns at one level certainly is considered as an unstable lesion. However, most spinal surgeons do not feel quite comfortable fusing a spine with only two-column soft tissue injury and will ask for further dynamic imaging such as flexion-extension x-ray films to assess stability.

The Important Problem-Solving Questions

Imaging a traumatized spine implies answering a set of important questions regarding the status of the spinal supporting structures (bony elements, ligaments, and discs) and the content (spinal cord, nerve roots, cerebrospinal [CSF] spaces, meninges, vessels).

Which Lesions Are Present? What Is the Mechanism of Injury? Is There Instability?

Traumatic spinal lesions are represented by fractures, dislocations, ligamentous disruption, disc injury, acute disc herniations, and EDHs, often combined.

Fractures and dislocations usually occur based on a single predominant mechanism of injury. The six major mechanisms of injuries are (1) hyperflexion, (2) simultaneous hyperflexion and rotation, (3) hyperextension, (4) simultaneous hyperextension and rotation, (5) vertical compression, and (6) lateral flexion. The injuries in each class have characteristic radiologic abnormalities, which are more or less specific for that group.

- Hyperflexion implies distraction of posterior elements and compression of the anterior columns. It can result in compression fractures, which involve the anterior column and therefore are stable, or burst fractures, which involve the anterior and middle columns and therefore are considered unstable. Hyperflexion causing significant distraction of the posterior elements results in severe instability, with anterior luxation, facet dislocation, and flexion teardrop fractures.
- Hyperextension involves distraction of the anterior column and compression/rotation/translation of the middle and posterior columns.
- The addition of rotational forces to both hyperflexion and hyperextension results in more complex patterns of injury.

With minor modifications due to anatomic and biomechanical differences, the same principles apply to all the spine segments in the lower C-spine and thoracolumbar

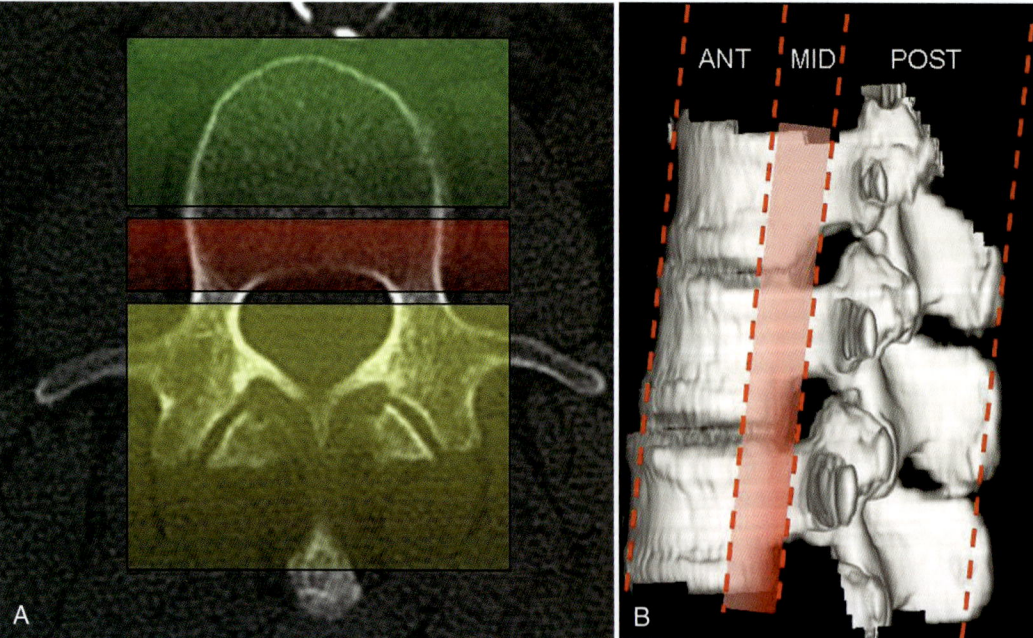

Figure 13-3 Denis' three-column stability concept. Delineation of the three columns over axial (**A**) and three-dimensional lateral views (**B**) of lumbar vertebrae. The middle column *(red)* plays a crucial role in the stability of the spine from C3 to L5. Fractures of the middle column are rarely isolated and usually are associated with anterior or posterior column fractures, featuring unstable lesions.

spine. The craniovertebral junction (CVJ) has specific peculiarity and therefore is treated separately.

Craniovertebral Junction (C0–C2)
The CVJ is a specialized structure with peculiar anatomy that results in patterns of injuries specific to this region. The CVJ is formed by the atlantooccipital and atlantoaxial joints, and it is well adapted to provide a remarkable range of motion, with most of neck rotation occurring at the C1–C2 articulation. The CVJ is the most frequently injured spine segment in children, but because of the relatively large spinal canal diameter at this level, neurologic deficits occur only in the most severe dislocations.

Atlantooccipital Dislocations (C0–C1) (Figure 13-4)
Look for increased basion–dens tip distance (>12 mm), increased Powers ratio, occipital condylar fractures, misalignment of atlas and occipital condyles on reformatted coronal CT images, prevertebral soft tissue hematoma at C2, edema in the alar ligaments on sagittal or coronal STIR MRI, and disruption of the tectorial membrane on sagittal T2-weighted MRI.

Atlantoaxial Dislocation (C1–C2) (Figure 13-5)
Caused by severe hyperextension, implies ligamentous disruption, especially of the transverse ligament of the dens, resulting in widened distance between the anterior arch of C1 and the dens (>3 mm in adults). STIR images show extensive soft tissues injuries. The odontoid tip can be fractured.

Atlantoaxial Rotation (C1–C2) (Figure 13-6)
The atlas loses articular congruence with the lateral articular masses of C2, there is asymmetric articular distance at C1–C2, the odontoid is in an asymmetric position with respect to the anterior arch of C1, and the C1 spinous process is rotated. The luxated joints are locked, so the patient presents with traumatic torticollis, and the asymmetry of joints, dens, and spinous process does not correct with head rotation. Normal patients scanned with the head tilted even mildly on one side can show a significant degree of mobility at this joint on CT. Such articular excursion should not be diagnosed as an injury. Trying to position patients in the scanner with head and shoulder straight and aligned, multiplanar reformatting, and, when needed, a repeat scan with contralateral head rotation can prevent overdiagnoses.

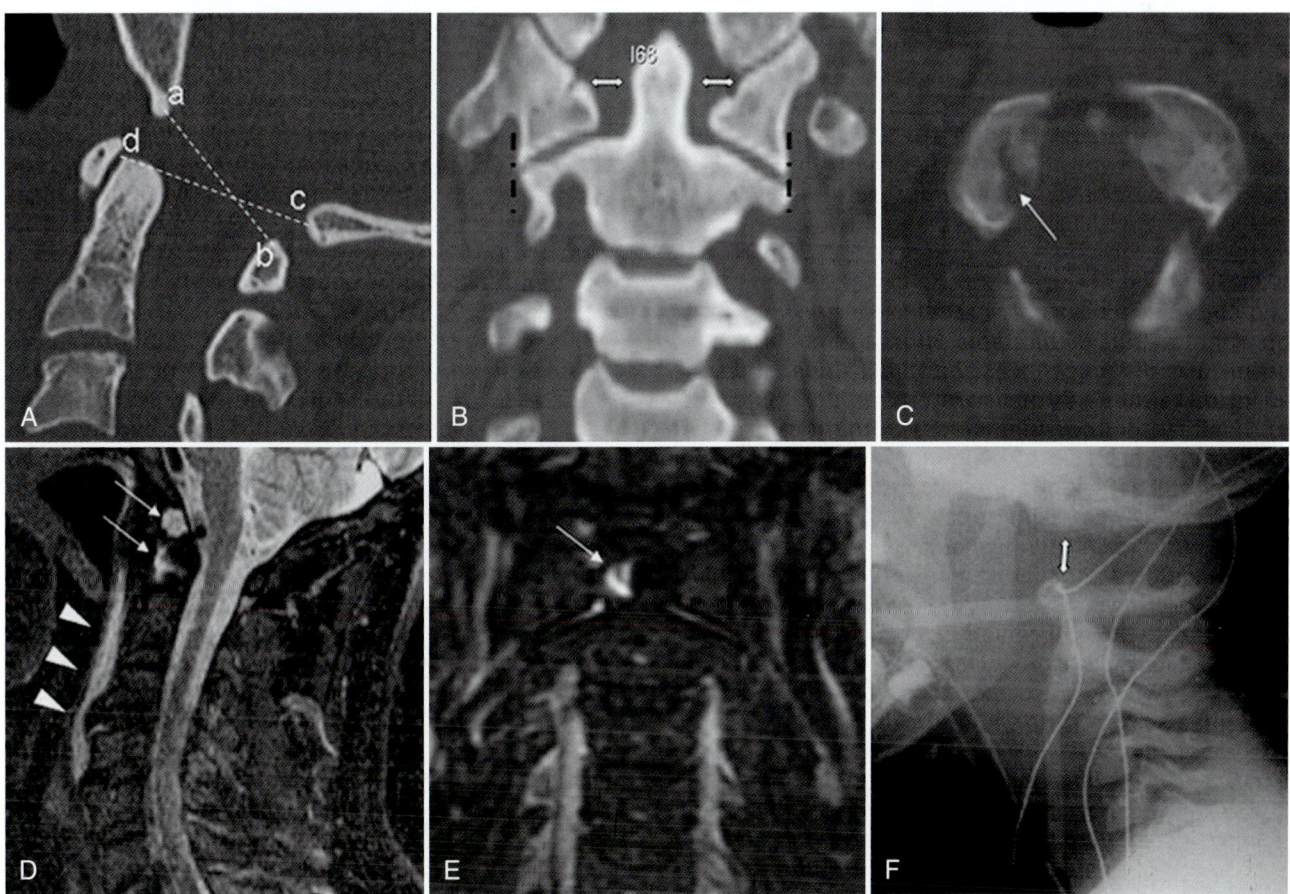

Figure 13-4 Hot spots for assessment of atlantooccipital dislocations. **A:** On the sagittal view, basion–dens tip distance should not exceed 12 mm, and Powers ratio (ab/cd) should not exceed 1. **B:** Coronal view showing the distance between the dens and the C1 lateral masses (double arrows) and the articular alignment between C1 and C2 lateral masses (black dotted lines). **C:** Attention should be directed to note condylar fractures (white arrow). **D, E:** Magnetic resonance imaging fat-suppressed T2-weighted images showing ligamentous injuries revealed by high signal in the predental space and along the alar ligaments (white arrows) and along the anterior longitudinal ligament in the prevertebral soft tissues (arrowheads). **F:** Laterolateral radiograph of a complete atlantooccipital dislocation revealed by loss of articulation at the craniovertebral junction (double arrow). (Courtesy of Dr. A. Leone, Rome, Italy.)

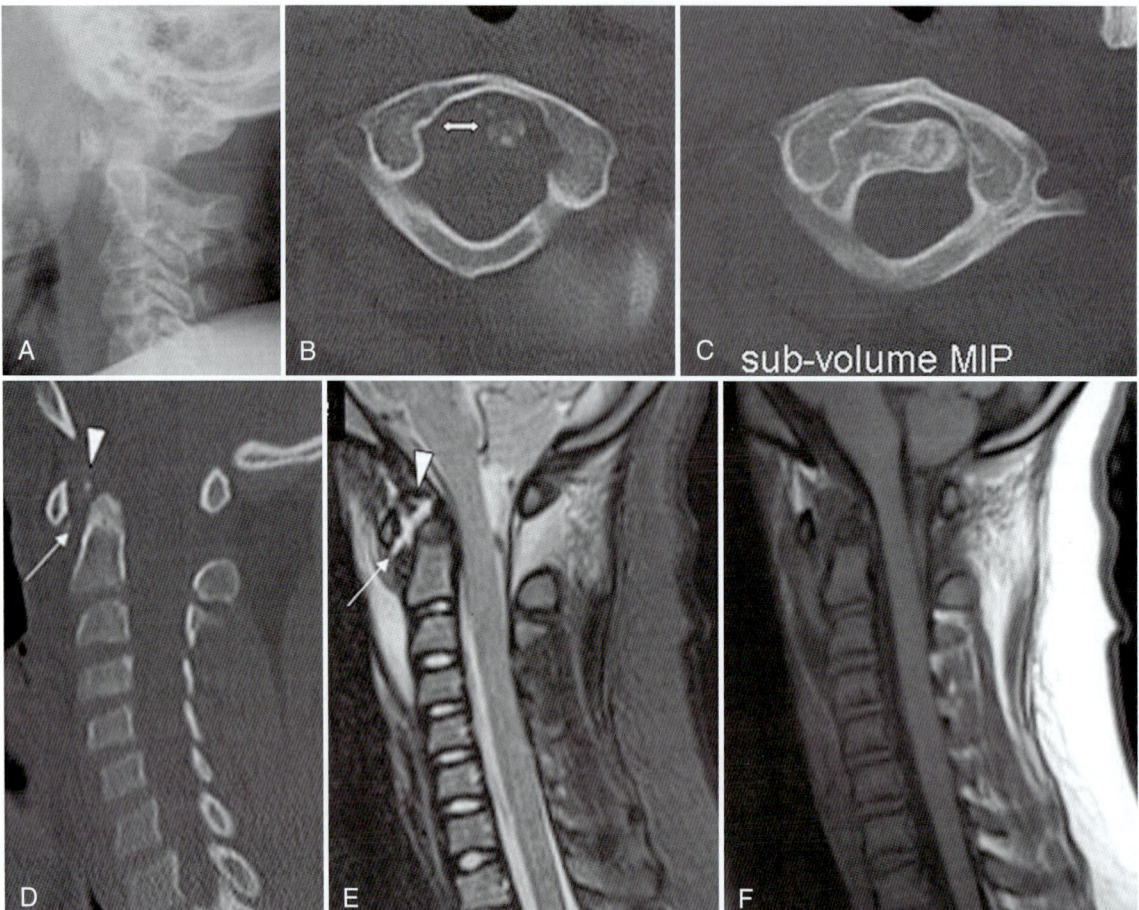

Figure 13-5 Atlantoaxial dislocation. As a result of severe extension injury, there is fracture of the odontoid tip *(arrowheads* in **D** and **E**) and rupture of the transverse ligament of the dens, revealed on plain films and computed tomography by increased anteroposterior distance between the arch of C1 and the dens *(arrow* in **D**) and by asymmetric lateral C1–C2 dislocation *(double arrow* in **B**). The full degree of C1–C2 dislocation is best appreciated on the subvolume axial maximal intensity projection (MIP) superimposing the C1–C2 junction **(C)**. Magnetic resonance imaging shows high T2 signal on the STIR image at the atlantoaxial joint *(arrow* in **E**), accompanied by prevertebral hematoma, extending from the clivus to C7, suggesting rupture of the anterior longitudinal ligament, and high T2 signal in the interspinous ligaments at C1–C2, indicating further soft tissue injury.

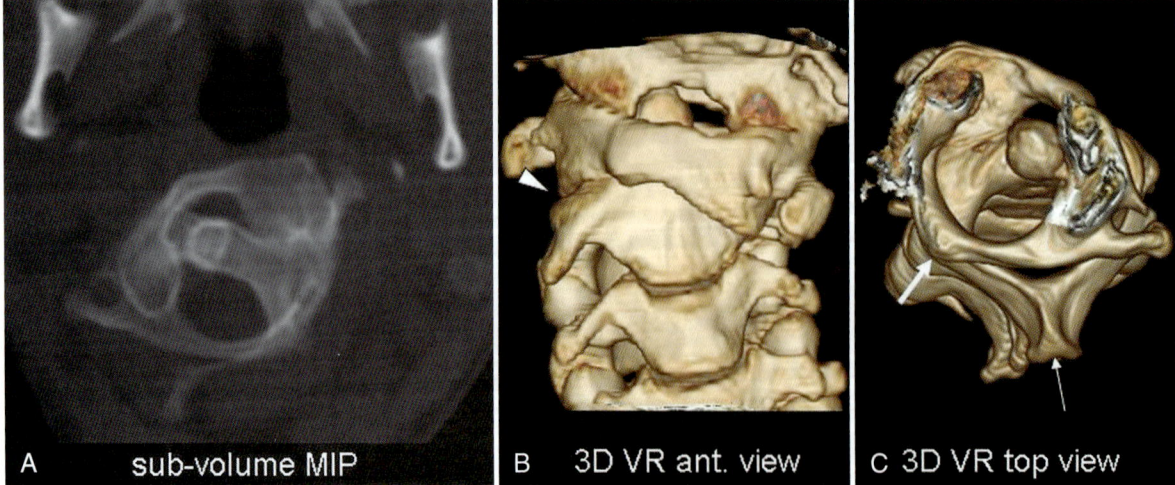

Figure 13-6 Atlantoaxial rotatory luxation. Axial subvolume maximal intensity projection (MIP) **(A)** and three-dimensional (3D) VR views **(B, C)** of the C1–C2 junction clearly showing rotatory luxation at C1–C2, with increased predental distance and loss of articular congruence between the C1 and C2 lateral masses *(arrowhead* in **B**). There is striking misalignment of the C1 and C2 spinous processes *(arrows* in **C**).

C1 Fractures

A burst fracture (Jefferson fracture) is the result of axial loading with bilateral outward displacement of the lateral masses of C1. This injury can be diagnosed by recognizing the fractures in both the anterior and posterior arches of C1 and on coronal images by the increased distance between the lateral masses of C1 (Figure 13-7). Separation of the lateral masses from the dens greater than 7 mm implies atlantoaxial instability due to tearing of the transverse ligament. An isolated fracture of the posterior arch of C1 may result from hyperextension with impaction of the posterior arch of C1 between the occiput and C2. This injury is distinguished from C1 burst fracture by involvement of only the posterior arch. An isolated fracture of the anterior arch of C1 is less common. It also results from hyperextension with avulsion of the attachment of the anterior spinal ligament. The small avulsed bone fragment is visible ventral to the anterior arch of C1.

C2 Fractures

C2 fractures can involve the dens, the body, the pars interarticularis, and the posterior arch. Dens fractures are frequently observed in elderly patients and are classified according to a scheme proposed by Anderson and D'Alonzo (Figure 13-8). They are commonly classified into *type I*, rare, involving the dens tip, to be differentiated from an os odontoideum; *type II*, most common, consisting of a fracture through the base of the dens at its junction with the body of C2, unstable, with a high incidence of nonunion if not surgically fused; and *type III*, involving the upper body of C2. The body of C2 can also be involved in burst fractures resulting from hyperflexion or axial loading forces. Traumatic spondylolysis of C2 (hangman's fracture) is caused by hyperextension with resultant bilateral fractures of the pars interarticularis (C2 vertebra is only cervical vertebra with a true pars interarticularis); there is anterior displacement of the anterior portion of C2 to C3 (Figure 13-9). This fracture is often associated with spinal cord injury.

What to Look for on CVJ Acute Trauma Imaging?

- On axial thin CT sections: Look for obvious fracture lines of the occipital condyles, the atlas arches, the C2 vertebral body, and the posterior elements. Check the midline position of the spinous process of C1 and the central position of the odontoid to the anterior arch of C1.
- On sagittal reformatted CT images: Look for the basion–odontoid distance, the Powers ratio, the C0–C1 joints, the integrity of the dens and the C2 pars interarticularis, and the distance between dens and C1 anterior arch. On soft tissue window images, rule out gross prevertebral hematomas and central canal compromise.
- On coronal reformatted CT images: Look for occipital condyle fractures, splaying of C1 lateral masses, uncovering of C2 lateral masses by exaggerated and locked atlas rotation, and correct midline position of the dens.
- On MRI: STIR or fat-suppressed fast spin-echo (FSE) T2-weighted images are useful for detecting soft tissue edema suggesting ligamentous disruption and prevertebral hematomas along the anterior longitudinal ligament. Assess the bulbomedullary junction and the cervical spinal cord for extrinsic compression and cord injuries with T2- and T2*- weighted images. Although any severe cervical spine trauma harbors the risk of vertebral and carotid artery dissection even without evidence of fractures or direct arterial injury, when a

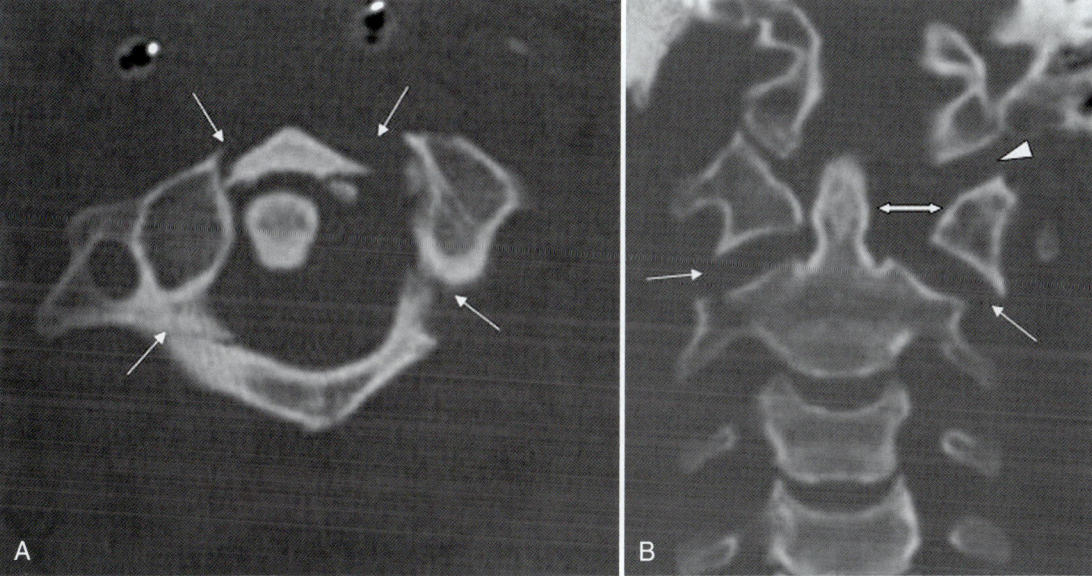

Figure 13-7 C1 burst fracture (Jefferson fracture). **A:** Axial computed tomographic image through C1 showing bilateral fractures of the anterior and posterior arches of the C1 ring *(white arrows)*. **B:** Coronal reformatted two-dimensional view showing increased distance between the C2 dens and the left C1 lateral mass *(double pointed arrow)*, suggesting unstable transverse ligament rupture, increased distance between the occipital condyle and the C1 lateral mass on the left *(arrowhead)*, and loss of articular congruence at the C1–C2 lateral masses *(arrows)*. There is also a right C2 lateral mass fracture.

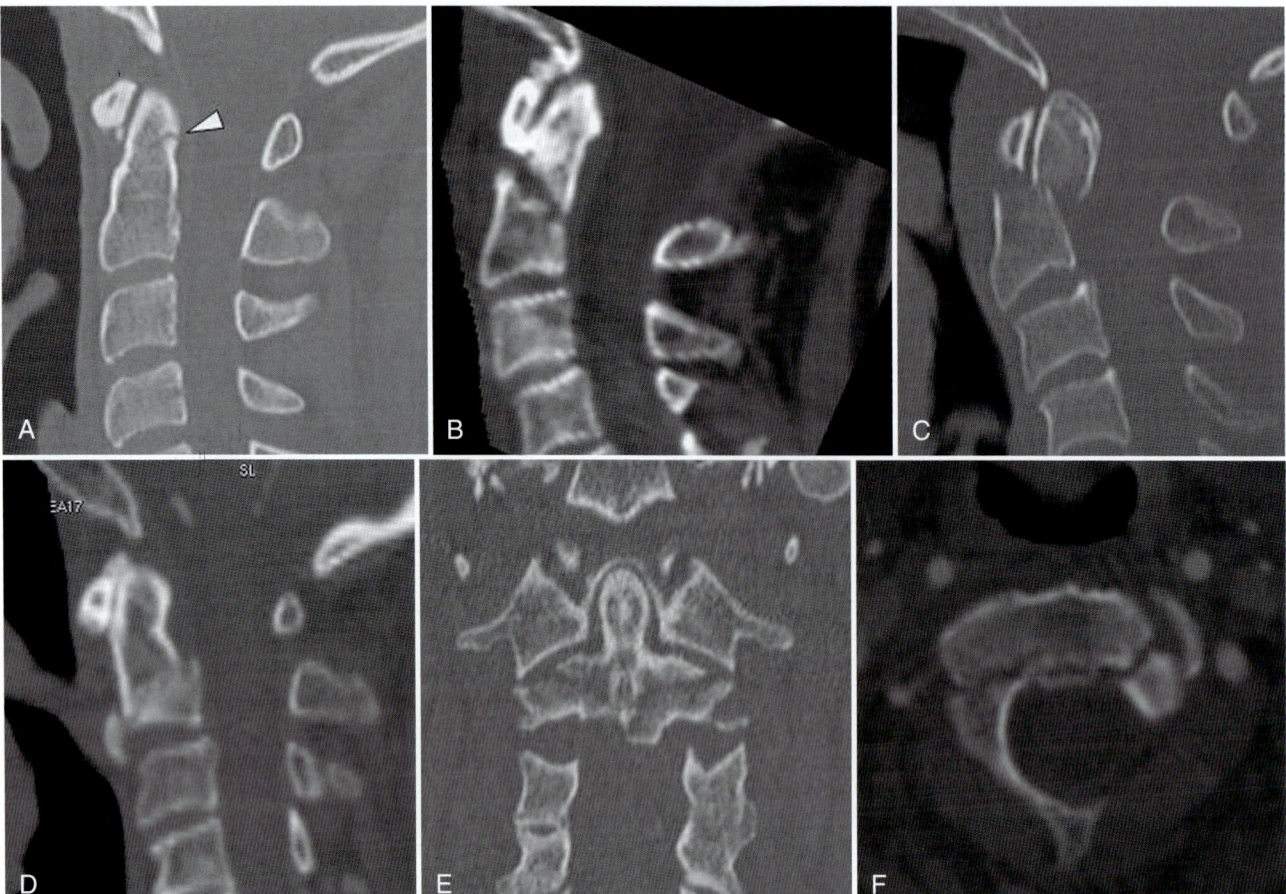

Figure 13-8 Odontoid fractures following the scheme proposed by Anderson and D'Alonzo. **A:** Thin fracture line of the dens tip *(arrowhead)* featuring a nondisplaced type 1 fracture. **B:** Aligned type 2 fracture. **C:** Displaced type 2 fracture. Both **B** and **C** involve the base of the dens. **D–F:** Multiplanar views of a type 3 odontoid fracture coursing through the body of C2.

fracture is seen involving the vertebral artery transverse foramen, arterial dissection absolutely needs to be ruled out with vascular imaging (CT angiography or MR angiography and fat-suppressed axial T1- weighted imaging, or digital subtraction angiography) (Figure 13-10).

Lower C-Spine (C3–C7) and Thoracolumbar Spine

Hyperflexion Injuries. These injuries, which are especially common in divers, are characterized by abnormal widening between adjacent posterior elements, variable degree of kyphotic angulation at the level of injury, and wedge-shaped deformity of the vertebral body. They include wedge fractures, disruption of the posterior ligaments (interspinous ligaments, facet capsules, and posterior longitudinal ligament), bilateral facet joint dislocations, and teardrop fractures. The different combination of these elementary lesions depends on the magnitude of the lesional forces and determines the severity and the stability of the injury.

- Wedge-shaped fracture is caused by impaction fracture of the superior end plate, with integrity of the inferior end plate and height loss of the anterior column. If height loss is less than 50%, the wedge fracture is considered stable; if height loss is greater than 50%, it usually is associated with posterior ligamentous injury and facet dislocation. A simple wedge fracture involves only the anterior column, whereas a complex fracture involves the middle column and can have a retropulsed posterior vertebral wall (Figure 13-11).
- Posterior ligament disruption is best shown by MRI on STIR and fat-suppressed FSE T2- weighted images as ill-defined high T2 signal or fluid collection in the ligaments between the spinous processes, adjacent to facet joints, along the posterior margins of the vertebral bodies.
- Facet dislocation requires greater forces, especially in the thoracolumbar region, and consists of anterior luxation of the inferior articular process of the upper vertebra above and in front of the superior articular process of the lower vertebra. It is associated with facet capsules, posterior longitudinal ligament, annulus fibrosus, and interlaminar and interspinous ligament disruption. On axial images it is revealed by the "naked facet" sign, whereas reformatted sagittal images give the impression that the facets of the upper vertebra have jumped over the inferior ones, which remain uncovered. The jumped facet can encroach on the articular pillar ("perched facet") or be lodged in the neural foramen ("locked facet"). Despite their denomination, when bilateral, these injuries are unstable (Figure 13-12).

Chapter 13 Imaging of Spine Trauma 481

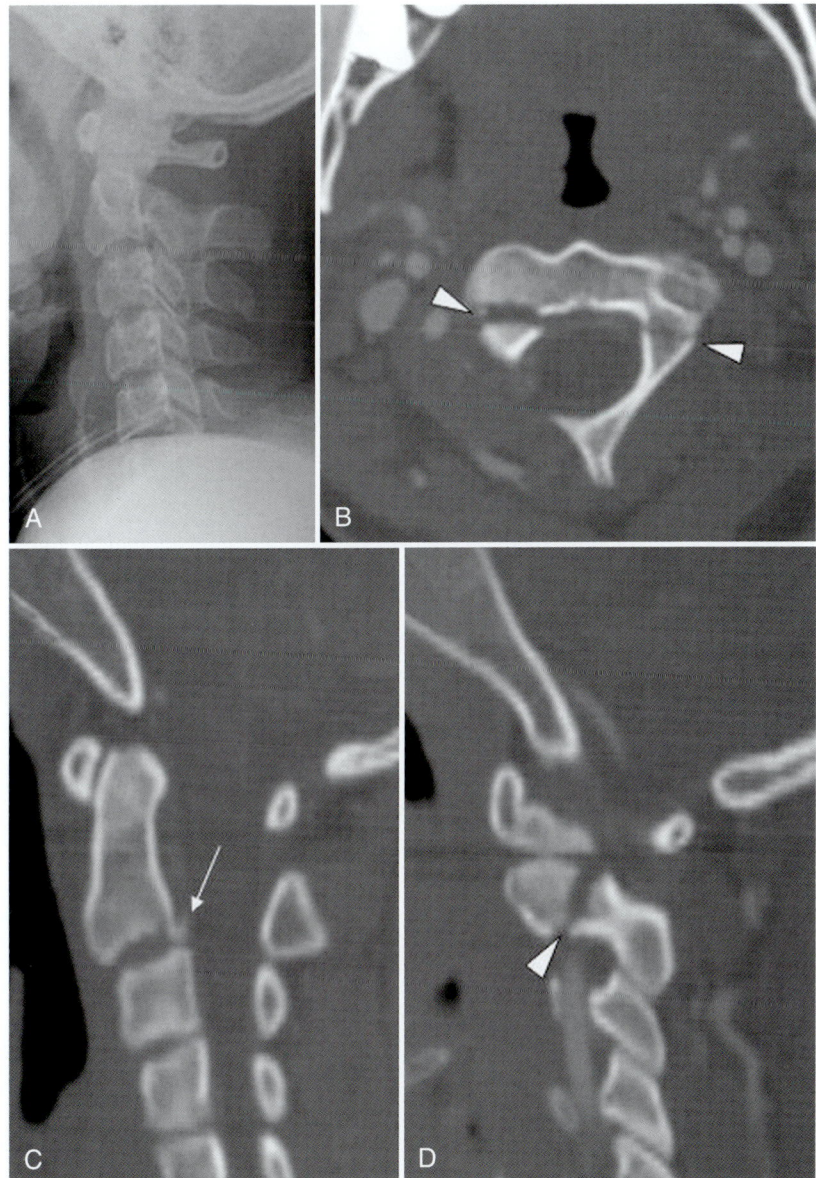

Figure 13-9 Traumatic C2 spondylolysis (hangman's fracture). This fracture involves the C2 pars interarticularis bilaterally *(arrowheads* in B and D) and causes mild C2–C3 anterolisthesis *(arrow* in C). Due to the frequent compromise of the C2 vertebral artery foramen, computed tomographic angiogram is recommended for these fractures. Laterolateral plain film (A) fails to clearly identify this extremely important finding.

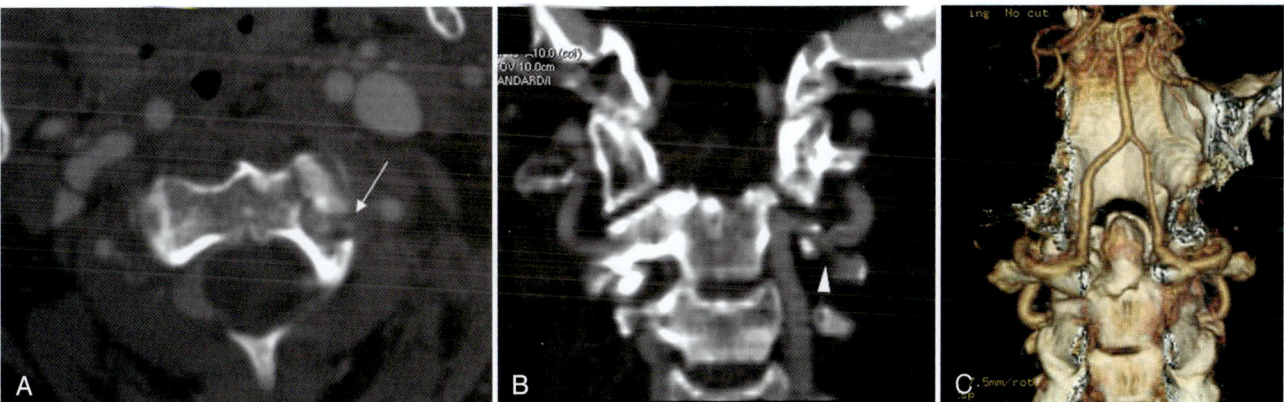

Figure 13-10 Neck computed tomographic angiogram (CTA) in cervical spinal trauma. In this type 2 odontoid fracture associated with a comminuted left C2 lateral mass fracture, CTA shows compression and narrowing of the left vertebral artery in its bony foramen *(arrow* in A and *arrowhead* in B), with preserved patency (C) and no clear signs of vertebral dissection.

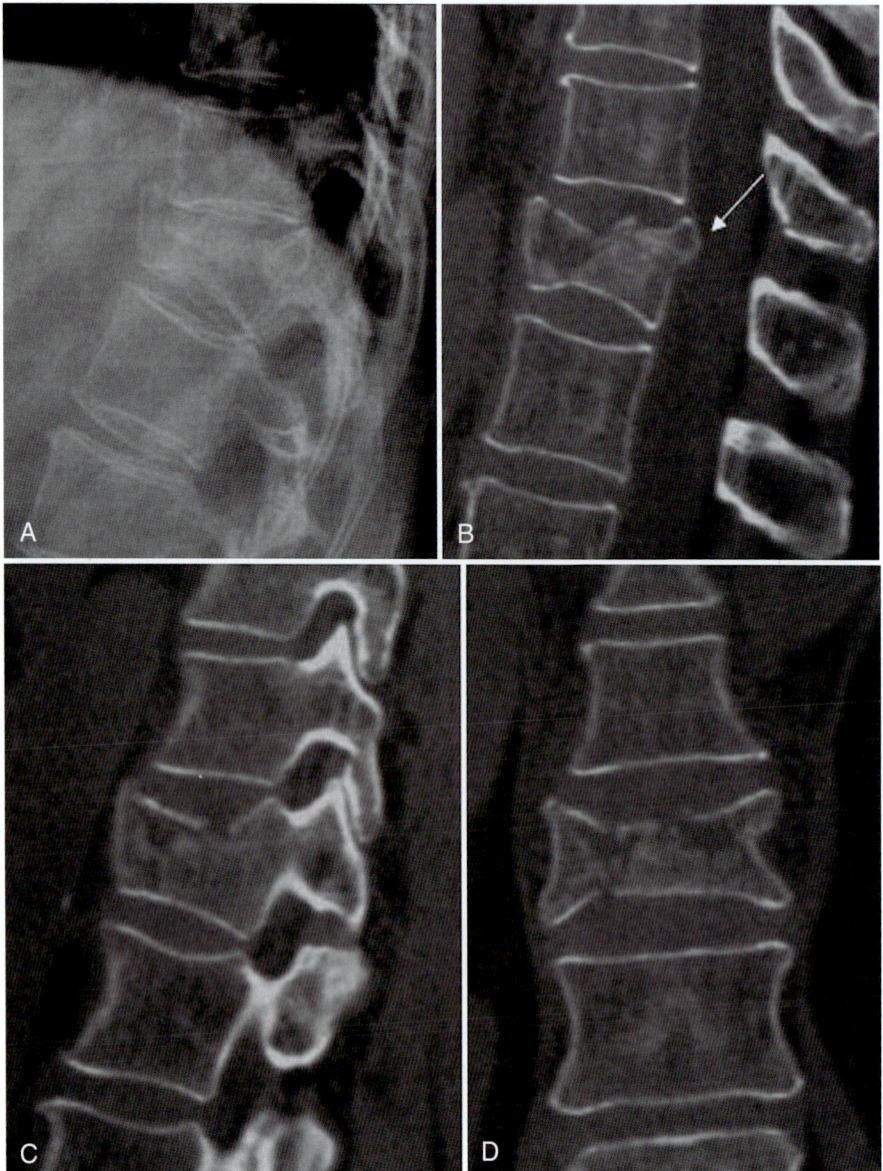

Figure 13-11 Wedge fractures. Traumatic injuries are often more complex than their classification systems. **A–D:** Wedge fracture of the T-spine with anterior vertebral body height loss of about 50% and middle column involvement in the form of a retropulsed fragment *(arrow* in **B)** indenting the central canal and possibly compressing the spinal cord.

- Teardrop fracture consists of a large triangular fracture fragment arising from the anteroinferior margin of the upper vertebral body, associated with posterior ligament complex disruption. Flexion teardrop fractures are the result of greater magnitude forces and usually are complicated by middle column fractures and retropulsion of bony fragments into the spinal canal (Figure 13-13).

What Are the Typical Variants of Hyperflexion Injuries that Occur at Different Levels?

Clay shoveler's fractures is a stable fracture of the spinous process seen in the cervical spine or at the cervicothoracic junction.

Chance fracture is an unstable fracture that occurs nearly exclusively at the thoracolumbar junction. It is thought to be the result of distractive forces generated when the spine is flexed about a fulcrum point, such as a car lap seatbelt, and is defined as a horizontally oriented fracture that passes through the spinous process, laminae, and vertebral body. A horizontal disruption involving the intervertebral disc or posterior ligaments, rather than the vertebral body or posterior bony elements, is considered a variation of the Chance fracture (Figure 13-14).

Hyperextension Injuries

Extension injury of the cervical and thoracolumbar spine results in backward rotation or translation of the vertebra in the sagittal plane. It often results from an anterior impact on the mandible, face, or forehead, or from sudden deceleration. They are less frequent than flexion fractures. These injuries may result in either hyperextension dislocation or hyperextension teardrop

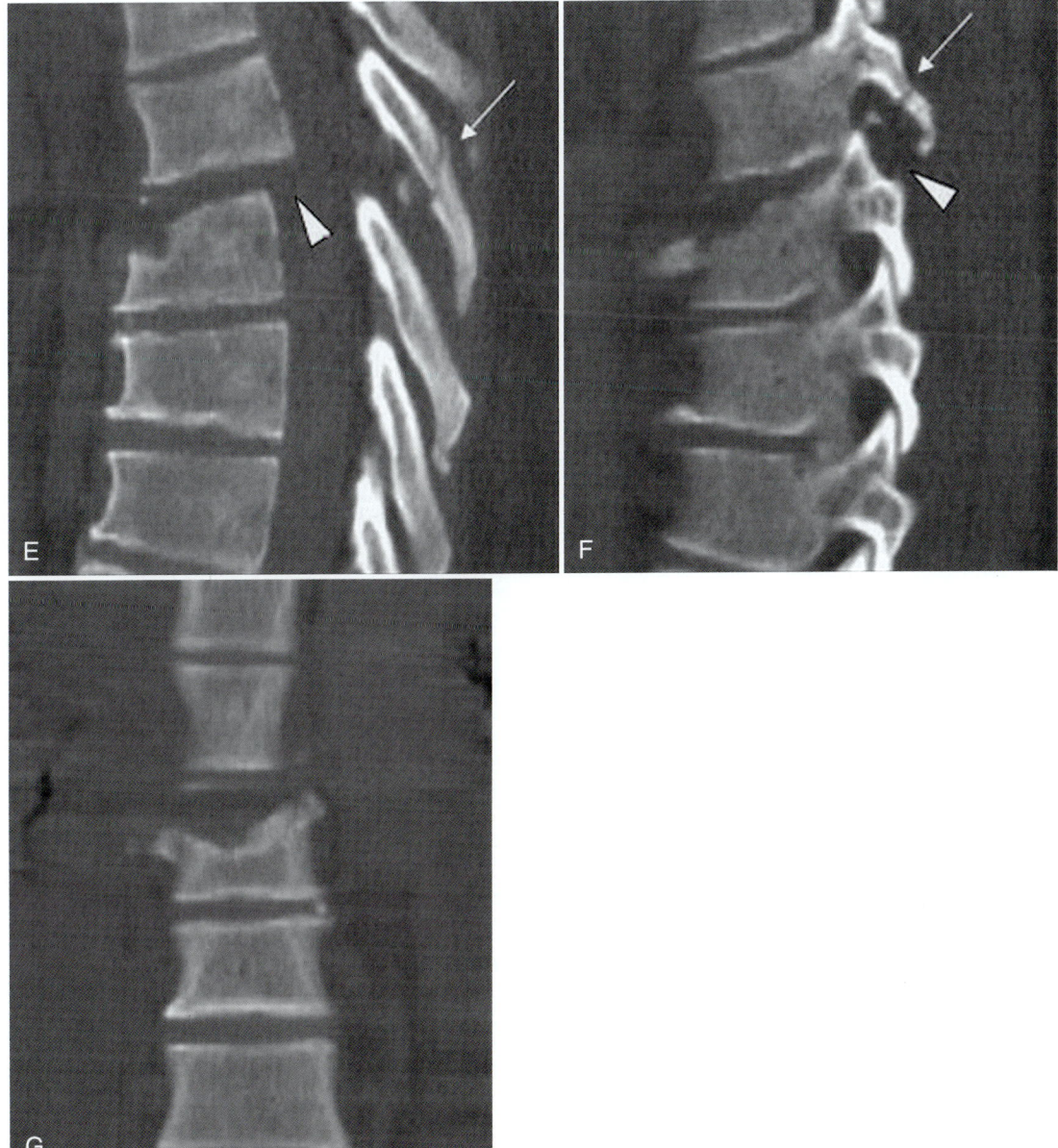

Figure 13-11, cont'd E–G: Another T-spine wedge fracture with anterior vertebral body height loss less than 50% but with complex middle column posterior longitudinal ligament disruption and retrolisthesis *(arrowhead* in **E)**, posterior column fractures *(arrows* in **E** and **F)**, and ligamentous injury with facet capsule disruption *(arrowhead* in **F)**.

fracture, almost invariably associated with intervertebral disc disruption.

Hyperextension dislocation is a disruption of the ligaments between adjacent vertebrae, including the anterior longitudinal ligament, annulus fibrosus, and facet capsular ligaments. Because there may be no fracture, the only clue on radiographs and CT may be thickening of the prevertebral soft tissues, which is better seen on MRI. This injury is frequently associated with severe spinal cord contusion, especially in patients with preexisting degenerative changes and central canal stenosis. Hyperextension dislocation injury is often accompanied by an avulsion fracture of the anteroinferior margin of the affected vertebral body, caused by traction of the annulus fibrosus. This has an almost horizontally oriented fracture line.

Hyperextension teardrop fracture is an avulsion fracture of the anteroinferior margin of the vertebral body caused by excessive stress on the anterior longitudinal ligament. The fracture fragment can be distinguished from the avulsion fracture of hyperextension dislocation by the obliquity of the fracture line (approximately 45 degrees from vertical) and the relatively greater height of the fragment. In contrast to hyperflexion teardrop fractures, hyperextension teardrop fractures show no evidence of posterior ligament disruption.

Vertical Compression Injuries

Axial loading injury of the cervical and thoracolumbar spine results from an impact to the top of the head when the spine is straight and vertical compressive forces are transmitted through the intervertebral disc with radial

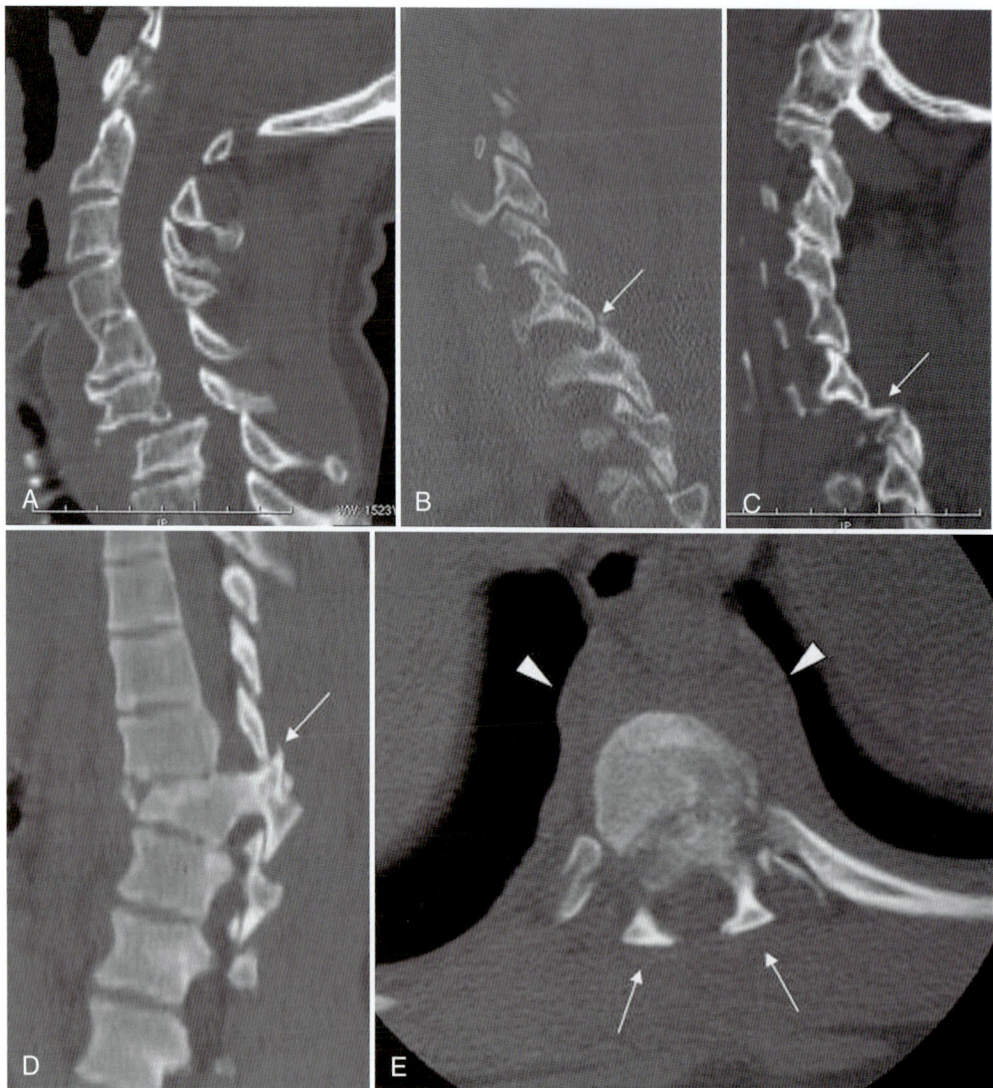

Figure 13-12 Facet dislocation. **A, B:** C6–C7 facet dislocation causing severe anterior spondylolisthesis, canal narrowing, and very likely spinal cord compression. There is evident discontinuity of the anterior and posterior spinal and spinolaminar lines on the midline sagittal image **(A)** suggesting extensive three-column ligamentous injury, whereas the off-midline sagittal image **(B)** shows the "jumped facet" *(arrow)* that encroaches over the articular pillar, featuring the so-called perched facet. **C:** Another example of facet dislocation associated with a facet fracture *(arrow)*. **D, E:** Thoracic facet dislocation example where the jumped facet is completely dislodged and locked in the neuroforamen *(arrow in D)*, whereas the axial image shows the "naked facet" sign *(arrows in E)* and the prevertebral hematoma *(arrowheads in E)*. This facet dislocation is associated with a wedge fracture as well.

outward forces generated in the vertebral body. Typical representative example is the burst fracture in the lower cervical and thoracolumbar spine. Burst fractures consist of a vertically oriented fracture of the vertebral body with lateral dispersion of the fracture fragments (Figure 13-15). The posterior wall of the vertebral body is disrupted, which does not occur with wedge fractures, and the distance between the pedicles is widened. Usually, there are associated fractures in the posterior elements. Burst fractures are either stable or unstable. The encroachment of the spinal canal may lead to cord injuries in up to 50% of cases.

Other Mechanisms

Less common mechanisms of injury may lead to recognized fracture patterns. A combination of flexion and rotational forces can result in a unilateral facet dislocation. Lateral force vectors may lead to isolated fractures of the uncinate processes, lateral wedge, and lateral burst fractures. Combined extension and rotation forces may result in pillar or pediculaminar fractures.

Disc Injuries

Disc disruption is demonstrated by MRI T2-weighted images as increased T2 signal in the intervertebral space, more often as a rim lesion near the anterior vertebral rim. If the posterior annulus is also disrupted, an acute traumatic disc herniation, characterized by high T2 signal and mass effect on the spinal cord, may occur (Figure 13-16). Disc injury is caused by distraction and shearing in sudden extension, in which case both the posterior disc and the facets are compressed, causing disc contusion or herniation, facet hemarthroses, or fractures of articular processes. Traumatic disc lesions also occur after flexion injuries.

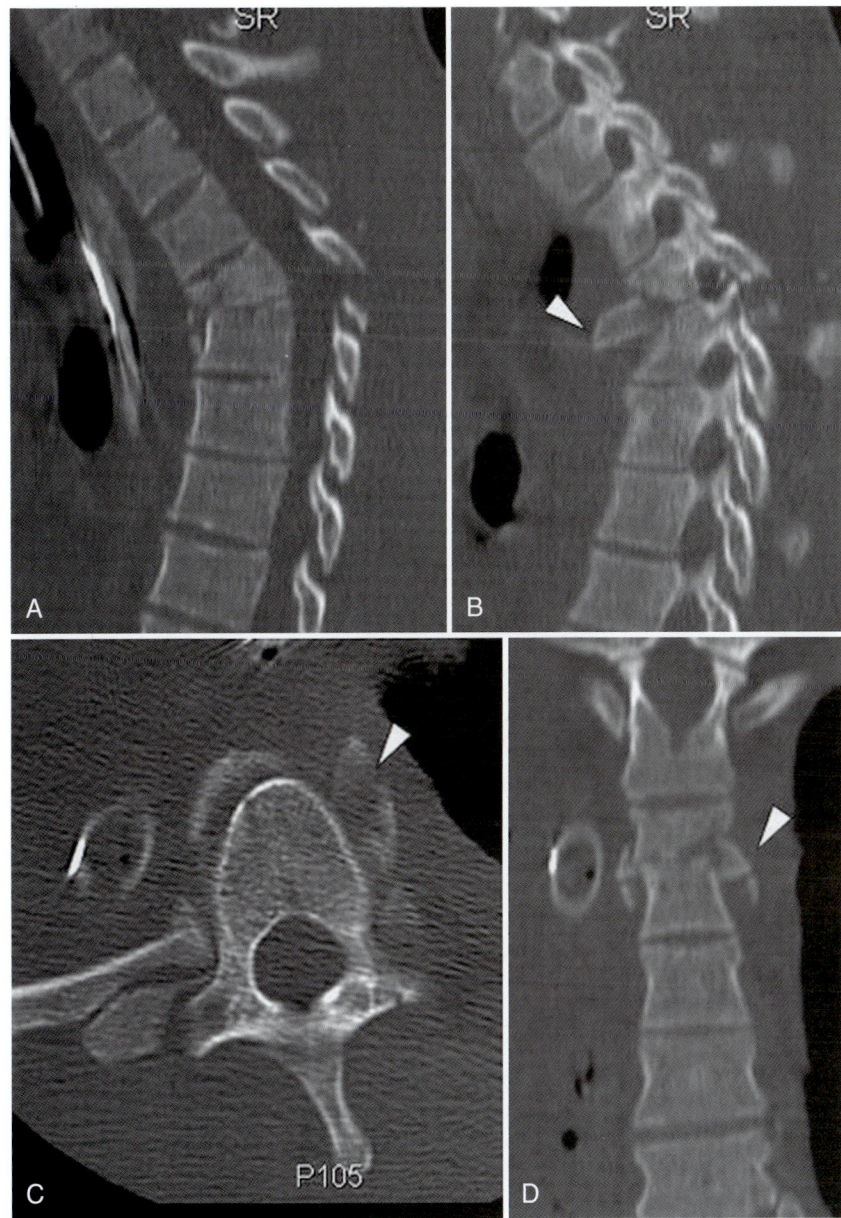

Figure 13-13 Flexion teardrop fracture. Hyperflexion forces of great magnitude caused a wedge deformity and a fracture of a large triangular portion of the anteroinferior portion of the vertebral body *(arrowheads)*. There is also evidence of disruption of the posterior ligamentous complex with facet subluxation. This degree of kyphotic deformity caused a spinal cord injury.

Ligamentous Injuries
Ligamentous injuries can occur even in absence of detectable fractures. They are suspected on MRI by direct visualization of a gap or by an increased signal in the ligament or the surrounding structures on STIR images or fat-suppressed FSE T2-weighted images, which might represent edema or acute hemorrhage (Figure 13-17). However, the sensitivity of MRI in detecting ligamentous injuries is relatively low.

Bone Contusions/Microfractures
Bone marrow edema, suggesting bone bruises or microfractures, usually is revealed by MRI in patients with significant spinal trauma as focal areas of abnormal high signal on STIR or fat-suppressed T2-weighted images against the dark background of normal bone marrow. At times the pattern of bone marrow edema further clarifies the injury mechanism or leads to a retrospective identification of subtle fractures originally missed on CT (Figure 13-17).

Whiplash Injuries
Whiplash is one of the most common mechanisms of injury to the cervical spine and cord. The term *whiplash* describes the manner in which a head is moved suddenly to produce a sprain in the neck.

Whiplash has become a popular term commonly used to refer to a syndrome following a neck sprain. Evidence suggests that whiplash injuries are real and are manifested by symptoms consistent with the anatomic lesion sustained and that they are a potential cause of significant impairment. The diagnosis of a

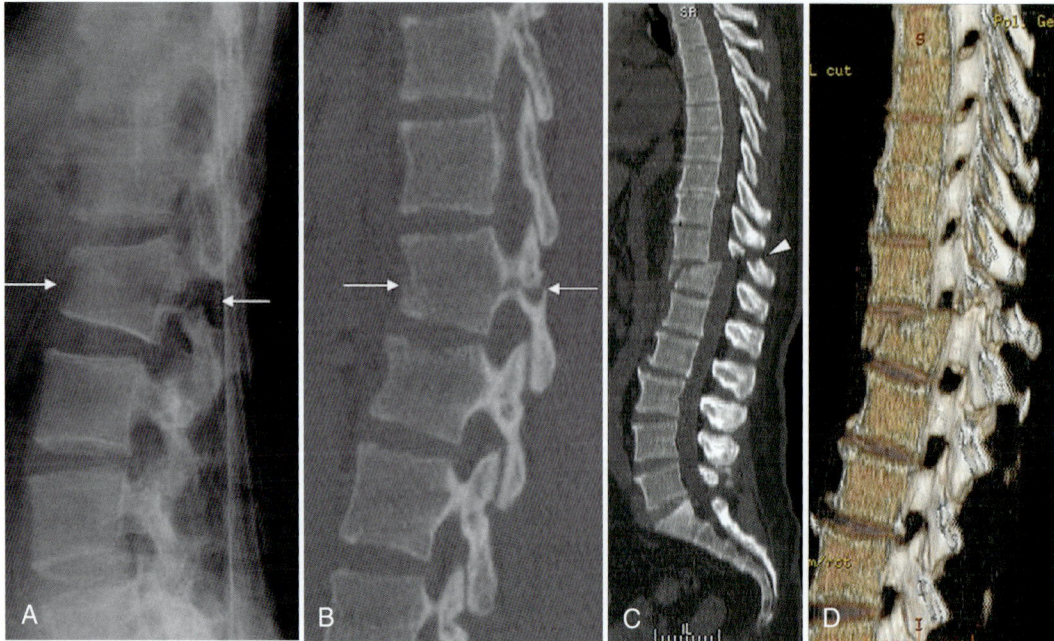

Figure 13-14 Chance fracture. A, B: Horizontally oriented fracture at the thoracolumbar junction coursing in the axial plane through the posterior and anterior bony elements (arrows). (Courtesy Drs. Z. Rumboldt and D. Nissman, Charleston, SC.) C, D: Variant of Chance fracture, with the horizontally oriented fracture traversing the posterior bony elements (arrowhead in C) and the disc space, disrupting the ligamentous structures, and causing anterior listhesis, central canal narrowing, and very likely spinal cord injury. The sagittal images clearly suggest that this type of injury occur with hyperflexion at the site of a fulcrum, as occurs with use of a pelvic seatbelt.

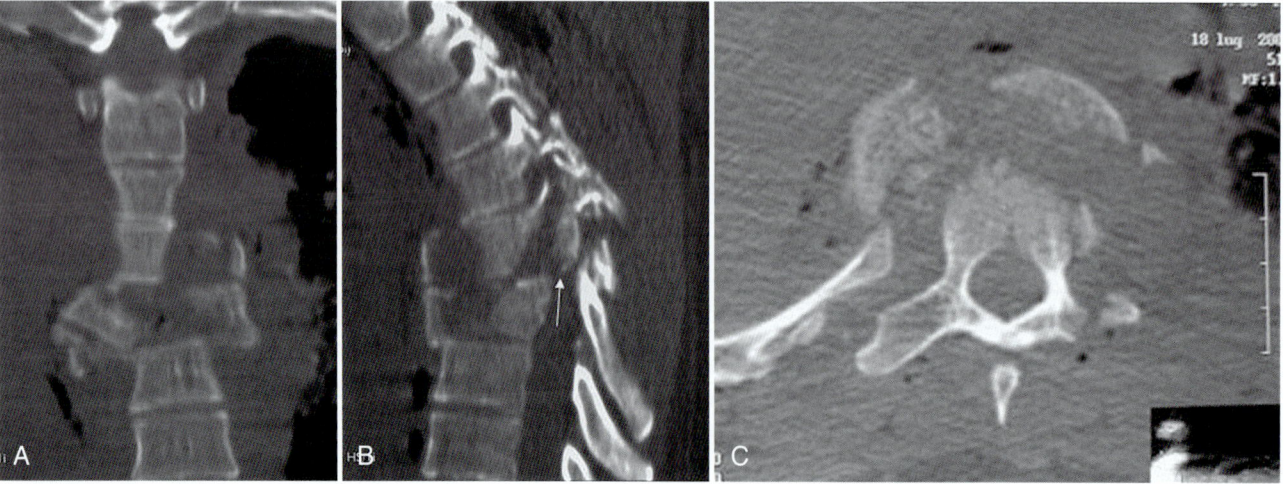

Figure 13-15 Burst fracture. Multiplanar computed tomographic views showing the striking outward displacement of multiple vertebral fracture fragments due to vertical compression force. There is a large retropulsed bone fragment occupying the central canal (arrow in B) and voluminous soft tissue hematoma in the perivertebral space. (Courtesy of Dr. A. Leone, Rome, Italy.)

whiplash injury is determined by the history provided, the mechanism of injury, the symptoms, and the physical findings on examination. Patients usually report nonradicular upper extremity pain, neck pain, headache, paresthesia, vertigo, and fatigue. The role of medical imaging in the evaluation of whiplash injuries remains to be determined. One of the key problems in imaging whiplash-injured patients is the lack of knowledge of the underlying pathology of the trauma. Recent studies suggest that a whiplash injury is not a hyperextension/hyperflexion injury but a combined axial loading and rotation resulting in anterior discal distraction and posterior facet compression lesions. Therefore, some research is focused on detecting disc–endplate lesions, facet capsule disruption, or facet microfractures.

What About the Spinal Content (Spinal Cord and Nerve Roots)?

The discussion on the possible mechanisms and the appearance of trauma of the spinal column is finalized to rule out injury or risk of injury of what really matters: the content of the spinal supporting structures, consisting of the neural structures, spinal cord, and nerve roots.

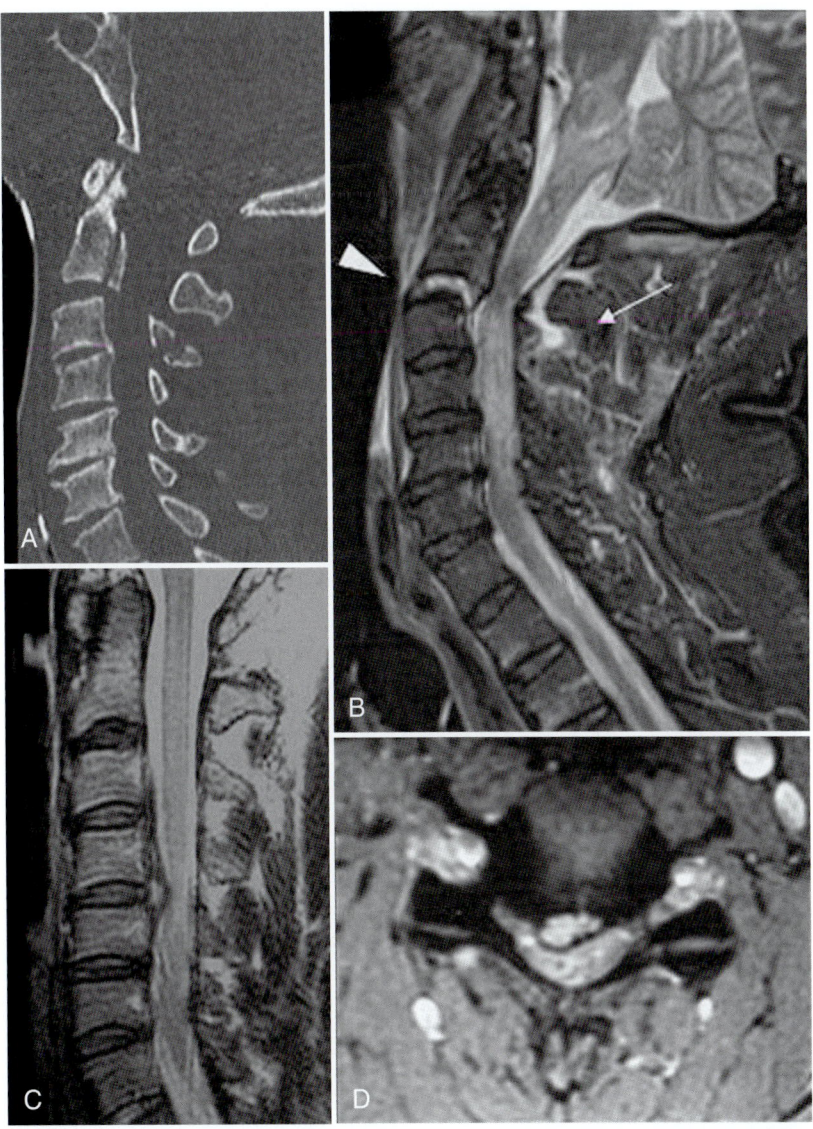

Figure 13-16 Traumatic disc injuries. A, B: Hyperextension injury characterized by multiple vertebral fractures on computed tomography and soft tissue injuries on magnetic resonance imaging, such as ligamenta flava and interspinous ligament disruption *(arrow* in **B)** and high T2 signal in the C2–C3 disc *(arrowhead* in **B)**, with retrolisthesis and cord compression. Anterior longitudinal ligament injury is suggested by the retropharyngeal hematoma, but the posterior longitudinal ligament is stretched but not torn, and is visualized as a thin black line at the posterior disc margin on **B**; no disc herniation is seen. C, D: Large T2-hyperintense C4–C5 disc extrusion compressing the spinal cord following a rear-end motor vehicle collision. High T2 signal of the disc fragment indicates a high water content of this extrusion, probably coming directly and acutely off the nucleus pulposus.

How Can the Neural Structures Be Injured?
The spinal cord and the nerve roots can be traumatically injured by transection, compression, contusion, stretching, and, much more rarely, by direct vascular compromise.

What Do Traumatic Spinal Cord Lesions Look Like?
MRI is the imaging method of choice for demonstrating acute intramedullary abnormalities in traumatized patients, such as medullary transection, contusion, and hemorrhage (Figure 13-18). Contusion of the cord is best seen on T2-weighted images as a high-signal lesion within the cord, with variable mass effect due to swelling. T1-weighted images show little or no signal abnormality. When hemorrhagic cord contusion is present, the prognosis is much more unfavorable. In these cases, bleeding within the cord may cause signal loss on T2*-weighted images. Adding a sagittal GRE T2*-weighted sequence to the imaging protocol is helpful in assessing more reliably the prognosis of spinal cord injuries. The spinal cord edema caused by contusion usually is focal, at the site of the injury, but in most severe injuries edema and swelling can extend to upper and lower adjacent levels. In follow-up studies the edema can gradually resolve, usually accompanied by improvement of clinical conditions, or it can evolve in a progressive ascending myelopathy, presenting as an enlarged cord with high signal on T2-weighted imaging several segments superior to the original injury site. In the subacute phase, the spinal cord lesion can also show abnormal enhancement after contrast injection.

In some cases the swollen and enlarged cord appears compressed in a central canal that would otherwise be

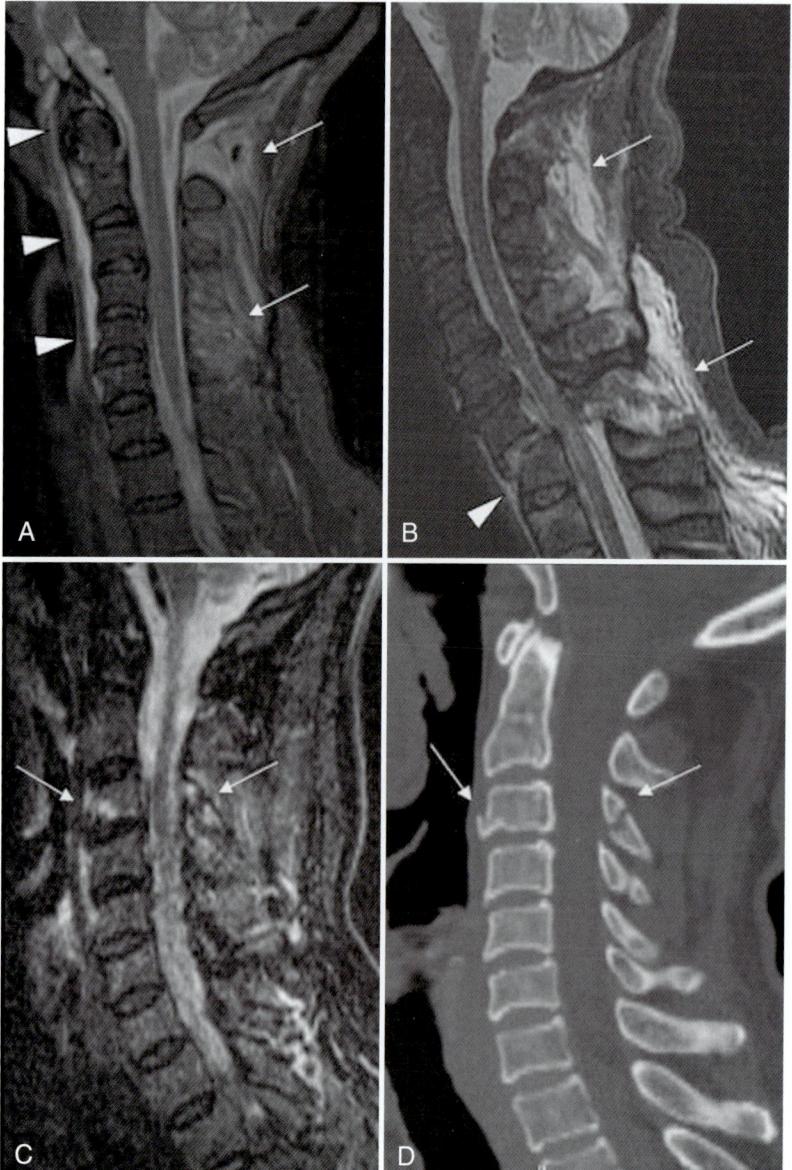

Figure 13-17 Soft tissue injury and bone bruise. **A:** Sagittal STIR image of patient with no C-spine fractures on computed tomography showing extensive soft tissue injuries, with high signal in the prevertebral/retropharyngeal space *(arrowheads)*, suggesting anterior longitudinal ligament (ALL) lesion with hemorrhage or edema, and along the interspinous and supraspinous ligaments *(arrows)*, suggesting ligamentous disruption. **B:** Another case of C-spine trauma where dislocation and disc injury at C7–T1 is associated with ALL injury *(arrowhead)* and striking posterior ligamentous complex injury *(arrows)*. **C, D:** High T2 signal is noted on STIR sagittal image in the bone marrow of the C3 vertebral body and spinous process *(arrows* in **C**), so-called bone bruising, in correspondence with subtle fractures as seen on computed tomography *(arrows* in **D**).

of normal width. Nevertheless, surgical decompression in such instances should be considered given the risk of further spinal cord damage caused by secondary compromise of the cord vascular supply.

What is SCIWORA?

The acronym SCIWORA stands for "spinal cord injury without radiographic abnormalities." It is a type of spinal cord injury that occurs in the absence of fractures or dislocations. The lesion is usually due to contusion or cord stretching and is more commonly seen in infants and young children as a consequence of their vertebral column elasticity and vulnerability to deforming forces, and in elderly patients with preexisting spinal narrowing (Figure 13-19). SCIWORA can present clinically in acute fashion as the so-called *central spinal cord syndrome* or acute traumatic central cord syndrome, a reversible or partially reversible paralysis affecting the arms more than the legs, bladder dysfunction, and variable sensory loss. This syndrome correlates with microscopic features of white matter injury revealed by loss of axons in the lateral corticospinal tracts. SCIWORA can also present with delayed onset of neurologic symptoms, up to 4 days after injury.

Do Epidural and Subdural Hematomas Occur in the Spine As Well?

The answer is yes, although subdural hematomas of the spine are exceptionally rare. EDHs, on the other hand, occur quite frequently in the presence of vertebral

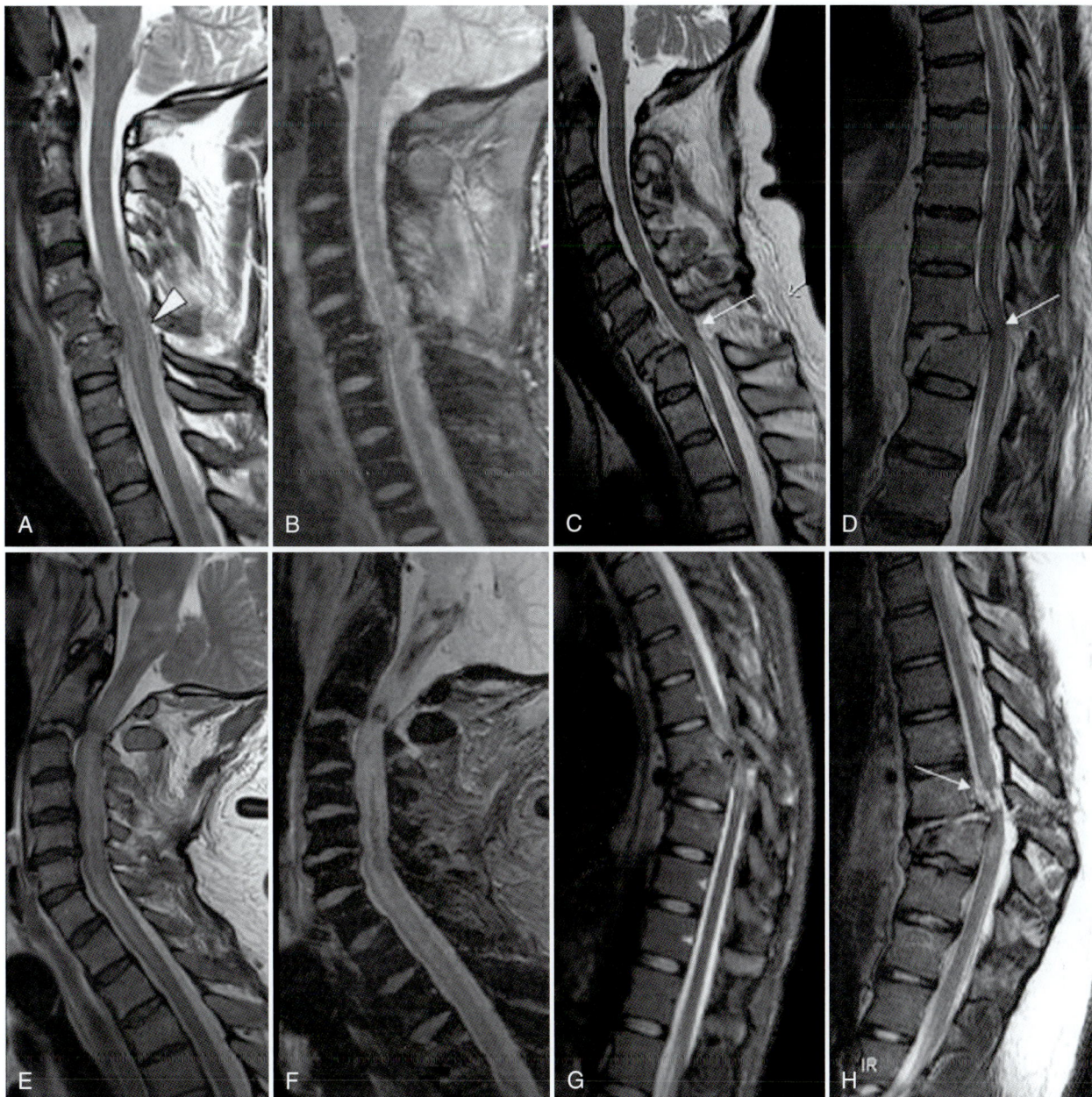

Figure 13-18 Spinal cord injuries. **A, B:** Spinal cord nonhemorrhagic contusion due to C5–C6 osteophyte and disc extrusion, with spinal cord swelling and faint and ill-defined high T2 signal. The cord is encroached, but there is no true cord compression. The posterior subarachnoid space is patent *(arrowhead* in **A**). Gradient-recalled echo (GRE)-T2* image, which is sensitive to blood products, does not show any cord hemorrhage. **C, D:** Cord contusion with different degree of cord compression. In both cases there is vertebral dislocation narrowing the central canal and distorting the spinal cord, which also shows high T2 signal, consistent with compressive myelopathic edema *(arrows* in **C** and **D**). **E, F:** Following cord contusion, the cord shows abnormal high T2 signal **(E)**, is swollen, and appears compressed due to the effacement of the subarachnoid spaces, but there is no true central canal narrowing. **F:** GRE T2*-weighted image showing extensive hemorrhage within the cord, visible as low signal, which makes the prognosis more dismal. **G, H:** Two examples of very severe cord injury, with extreme compression **(G)** and complete cord transection **(H)**, indicated by the cerebrospinal fluid–filled gap along the cord *(arrow* in **H**).

fractures, but usually they are of venous origin. MRI is the imaging method of choice to demonstrate EDH, although it also should be actively ruled out on the admission CT scan images viewed with a soft tissue windowing setting. The epidural collection on MRI (Figure 13-20) usually is isointense to hyperintense on T1-weighted images and hyperintense to hypointense on T2-weighted images. It does not enhance after contrast administration and its signal does not suppress; therefore, it is more evident on fat-suppressed sequences. Because the dura mater is not firmly attached to the walls of the bony canal as it is to the calvarium, the typical biconvex shape of an intracranial EDH is not observed in the spine, and the EDH can extend circumferentially around the dural sac, possibly causing severe compression of the neural structures. On good-quality sagittal or axial T2-weighted images, a thin dark line representing the dura is usually appreciable between the hemorrhagic collection and the CSF.

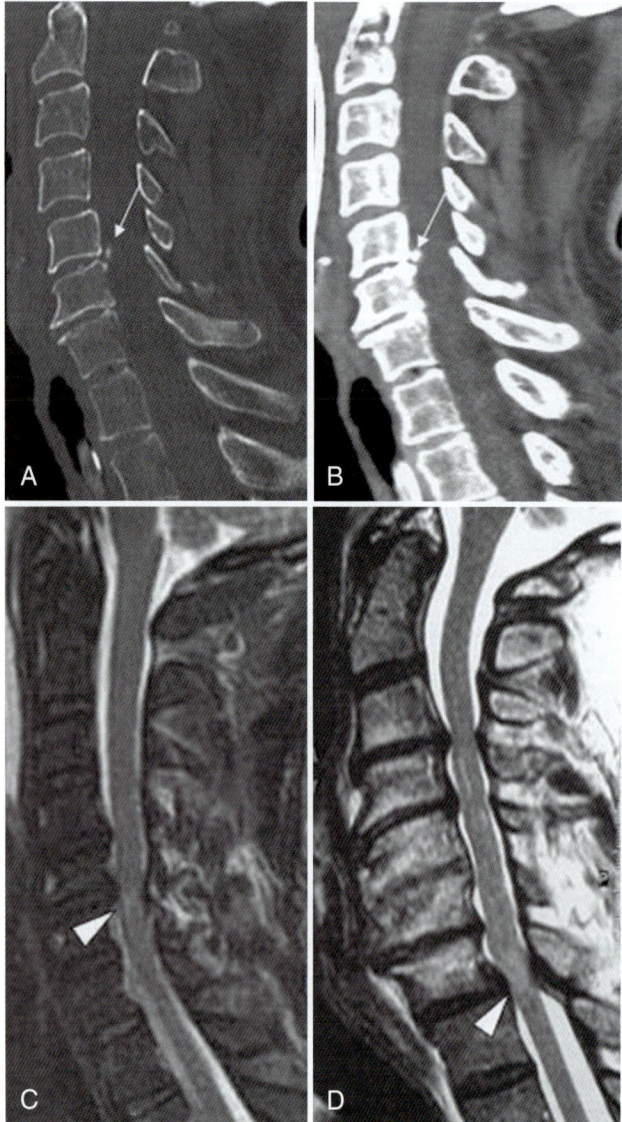

Figure 13-19 SCIWORA (spinal cord injury without radiographic abnormalities). Preexisting degenerative conditions, such as disc–osteophyte complexes, disc herniations, and central canal stenosis, may cause spinal cord injury with minor spinal trauma, even in the absence of evident acute traumatic fractures or dislocations. **A, B:** Partially calcified posterior disc–osteophyte complex (*arrows* in **A** and **B**) is a quite common and apparently benign degenerative finding, but it can represent a risk factor for SCIWORA in the trauma setting. **C, D:** Two cases of spinal cord contusion (*arrowheads* in **C** and **D**) with no radiographic evidence of fracture or dislocation in trauma patients with preexisting congenital (**C**) or degenerative (**D**) spinal stenosis.

How to Identify Nerve Root Avulsions, Particularly If There Is a Clinical Problem?

Nerve root avulsion from the cord can occur at the cervical level and usually occurs in conjunction with brachial plexus injuries due to traction forces on the arm or the shoulder. Nerve root avulsion is often associated with nerve root sleeve disruption. The best imaging technique to demonstrate nerve root avulsion is MRI with 3D acquisition producing strongly T2-weighted thin sections, so-called *MR myelography sequences* such as 3D-CISS (constructive interference in steady state)/3D-FIESTA (fast imaging employing steady-state acquisition), or alternative CT myelography. On these images the normal nerve filaments are directly visualized, whereas the avulsed filaments are either absent or detached from the spinal cord. Indirect signs of nerve root avulsion also can be observed on less sophisticated axial T2-weighted MRI, such as contralateral displacement of the spinal cord in the central canal due to traction from the intact nerve roots, and the appearance of traumatic meningoceles and focal extradural pooling of CSF, often in the foramen or in the paraspinal soft tissues, caused by nerve root sleeve disruption (Figure 13-21). Brachial plexus injuries are best imaged in the coronal plane through fat-suppressed or STIR T2-weighted images. These injuries are usually imaged in the subacute phase, and it is not uncommon to see abnormal contrast enhancement of the avulsed nerve roots or of the injured brachial plexus elements (Figure 13-22).

What to Look for on Acute Spinal Trauma Imaging

- Obtain multiplanar reformatted thin CT sections of the spine.
- Check different views for CVJ, general spinal alignment, vertebral body height, central canal width, facet joints, fractures, with particular attention to integrity of walls of posterior vertebral bodies, and retropulsed bone fragments.
- Use soft tissue window settings to look for soft tissue density masses in the central canal, such as traumatic disc herniations and EDH, which may cause or worsen the associated spinal cord injury, and in the prevertebral space, such as prevertebral hematomas.
- If a fracture or dislocation is present, estimate the central canal compromise and the possible related injury to the spinal cord, as well as the presence of possible vascular injuries, especially in cervical spine fractures involving the foramen transversarium, which constitutes the bony canal for the vertebral arteries.
- If a facet dislocation is present, assess facet fractures that could interfere with attempts at reduction. Try to identify a lesion pattern that suggests a specific mechanism of injury.
- Judge stability versus instability of the different spine lesions.
- Be aware that degenerative changes, such as posterior osteophytes and central canal stenosis, increase the likelihood of serious spinal cord injuries even with minor spine trauma.
- If neurologic symptoms or signs are present, an emergent MRI study is warranted to assess spinal cord lesions or compression.
- If a spinal cord lesion is present, a severe compression needs to be differentiated from a complete transection. Although the prognosis is sometimes equally grim, compression of a nontransected spinal cord poses an indication for emergent decompressive surgery.
- Detect signs of bleeding in the spinal cord, which worsens the prognosis of spinal cord injuries.
- On axial T2-weighted images of the cervical spine, do not miss indirect signs of nerve root avulsion, such as traumatic meningoceles and off-center contralateral position of the spinal cord in the canal.

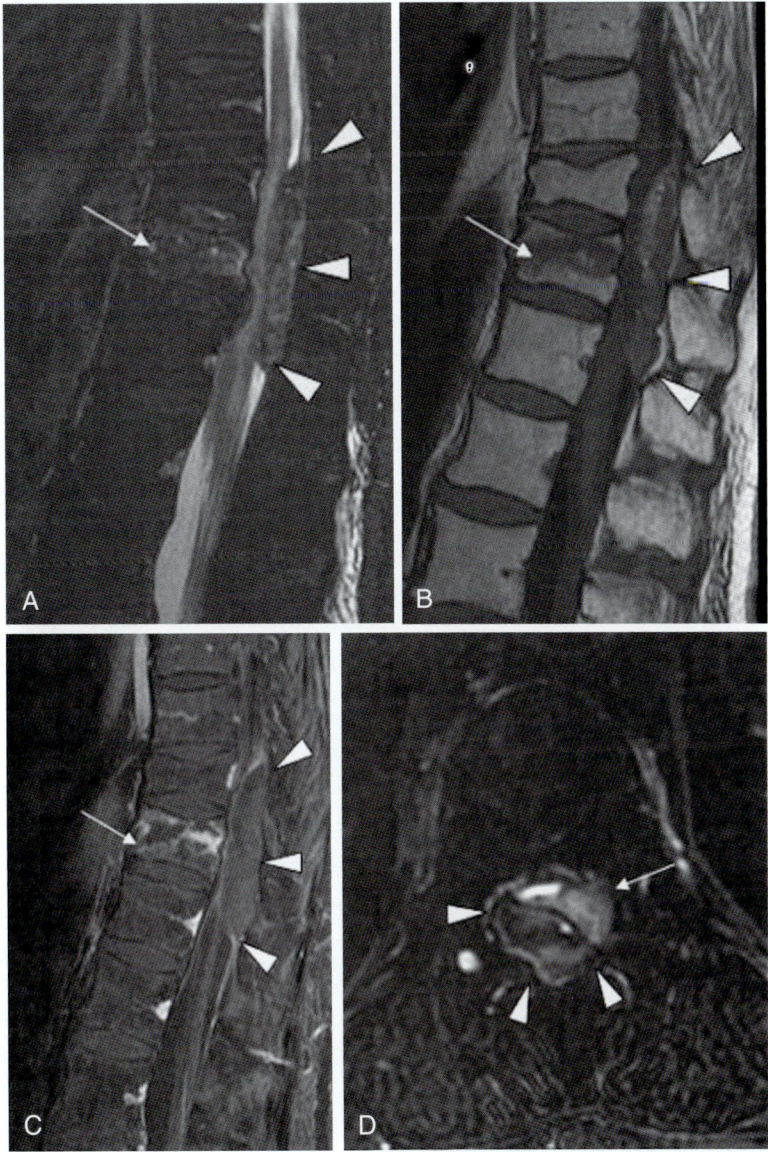

Figure 13-20 Epidural hematoma. Fat-suppressed T2-weighted (**A**), nonenhanced T1-weighted (**B**), gadolinium-enhanced fat-suppressed T1-weighted sagittal image (**C**), and fat-suppressed T2-weighted axial image (**D**) showing an acute traumatic compression fracture of T11 vertebral body *(arrows* in **A–C**), complicated with an epidural hematoma *(arrowheads* in **A–D**) occupying the right posterior half of the central canal and compressing the spinal cord *(arrow* in **D**). The hematoma is of heterogeneous high and low T2 signal, isointense to hyperintense on T1, and shows no enhancement after contrast. The cord appears displaced and compressed, and displays high T2 signal consistent with edema. On the axial image (**D**), the inward displaced dura is visible as a thin dark line between the hematoma and the spinal cord.

Traumatic disc herniations and EDHs are shown on MRI to better advantage and are important findings, often representing surgical indications.

Use MRI to assess soft tissue injuries, thereby increasing the accuracy of assessment of stable versus unstable spinal lesions.

On T2-weighted sagittal images, check for hyperintense signal in the discs, which could reveal traumatic disc injuries.

On STIR images, look for high-signal injuries of the ligaments for prevertebral and paravertebral hematomas and for bone marrow edema. Bone marrow edema, also called *bone bruise,* is a sign of trabecular microfractures, useful in further clarifying the injury mechanism and sometimes helpful in retrospectively diagnosing subtle fractures originally missed on CT.

What Are the Possible Pitfalls in Spinal Trauma Imaging?
- Subtle patient movements during MDCT scanning, such as breathing, shaking, or coughing, can originate false images of fracture or dislocation when reformatted on different planes (Figure 13-23). Looking at the skin contours and double checking the axial source images help avoid wrong diagnosis and, in the worst case scenario, unnecessary interventions.
- MR T2-weighted sagittal images are usually the most informative of spinal cord status. High T2 signal in the spinal cord is worrisome for cord lesions, edema,

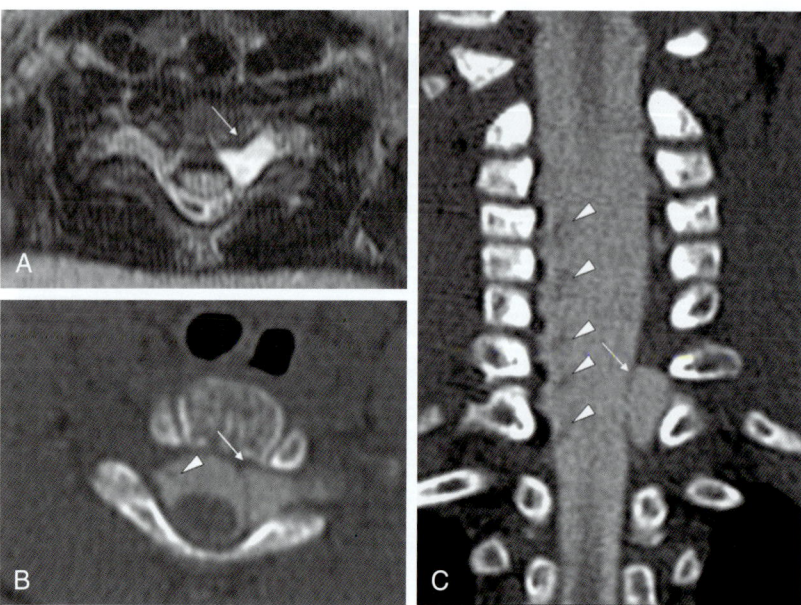

Figure 13-21 Cervical nerve root avulsion due to delivery trauma. T2-weighted axial image (**A**) and computed tomographic myelogram (**B**) reveal an extradural foraminal cerebrospinal fluid collection, representing a traumatic pseudomeningocele *(arrows on **A**, **B** and **C**)* following root sleeve laceration. The dural margins are clearly visible. The intradural nerve roots are not visualized ipsilaterally but are individually visualized contralaterally *(arrowheads on **B** and **C**)*. Note the slightly off-center and rotated position of the spinal cord (**B**) due to asymmetric traction by the intact nerve roots toward the normal side. (Courtesy Dr. Z. Rumboldt, Charleston, SC.)

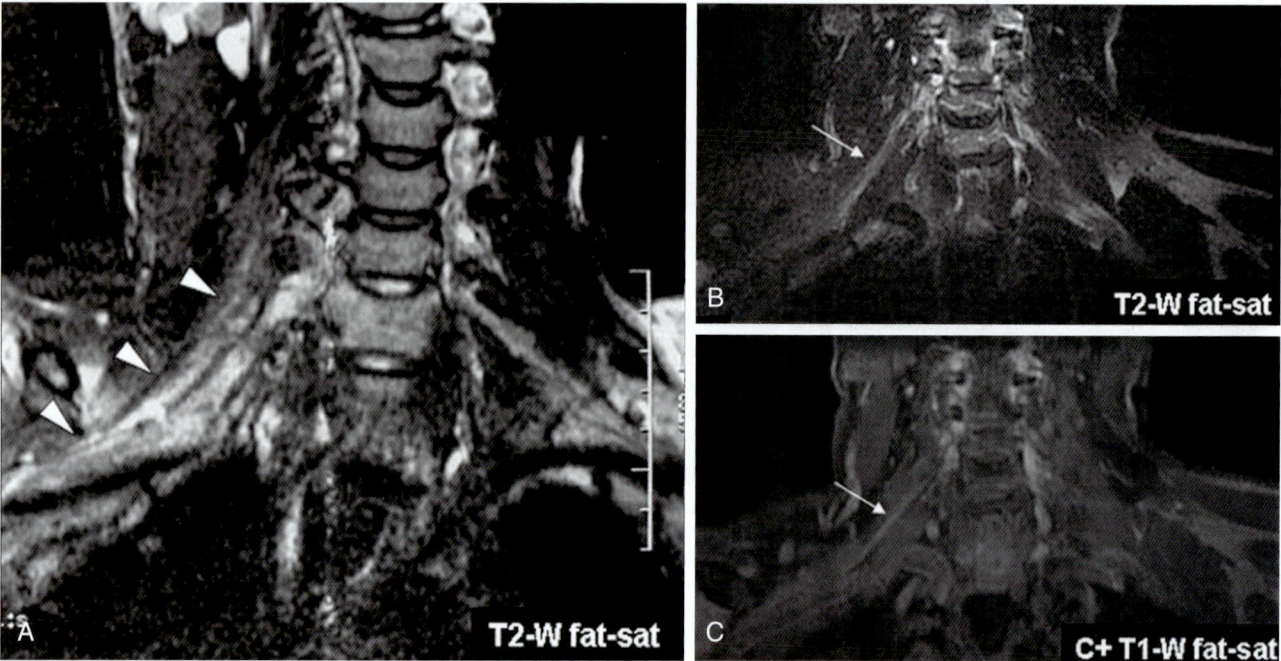

Figure 13-22 Brachial plexus traumatic injuries. **A:** T2-weighted fat-saturated coronal image showing striking swelling and high T2 signal of the right brachial plexus *(arrowheads)* in a patient with traumatic distraction injury of the right shoulder and monoplegia of the right upper limb. **B, C:** More subtle case showing mild asymmetric T2 hyperintensity of the right upper trunk *(arrow in **B**)*. In such cases, the diagnosis is reinforced by evidence of contrast enhancement in the same region on postcontrast fat-saturated T1-weighted images *(arrow in **C**)*.

or syrinx. A common artifact, called *truncation artifact*, gives the false appearance of subtle linear T2 hyperintensities along the spinal cord, mimicking pathology. The technical solution to this artifact is to increase the frequency matrix of the pulse sequence, usually achieved at no extra scan time cost. Moreover, any signal abnormality in the spinal cord needs to be confirmed on another imaging plane, usually the axial plane.

- Fat-suppressed T2-weighted images used to assess soft tissues injuries of the spine can suffer from uneven and inhomogeneous fat suppression, especially in patients with metallic instrumentation, thereby failing to completely suppress the high signal from fat

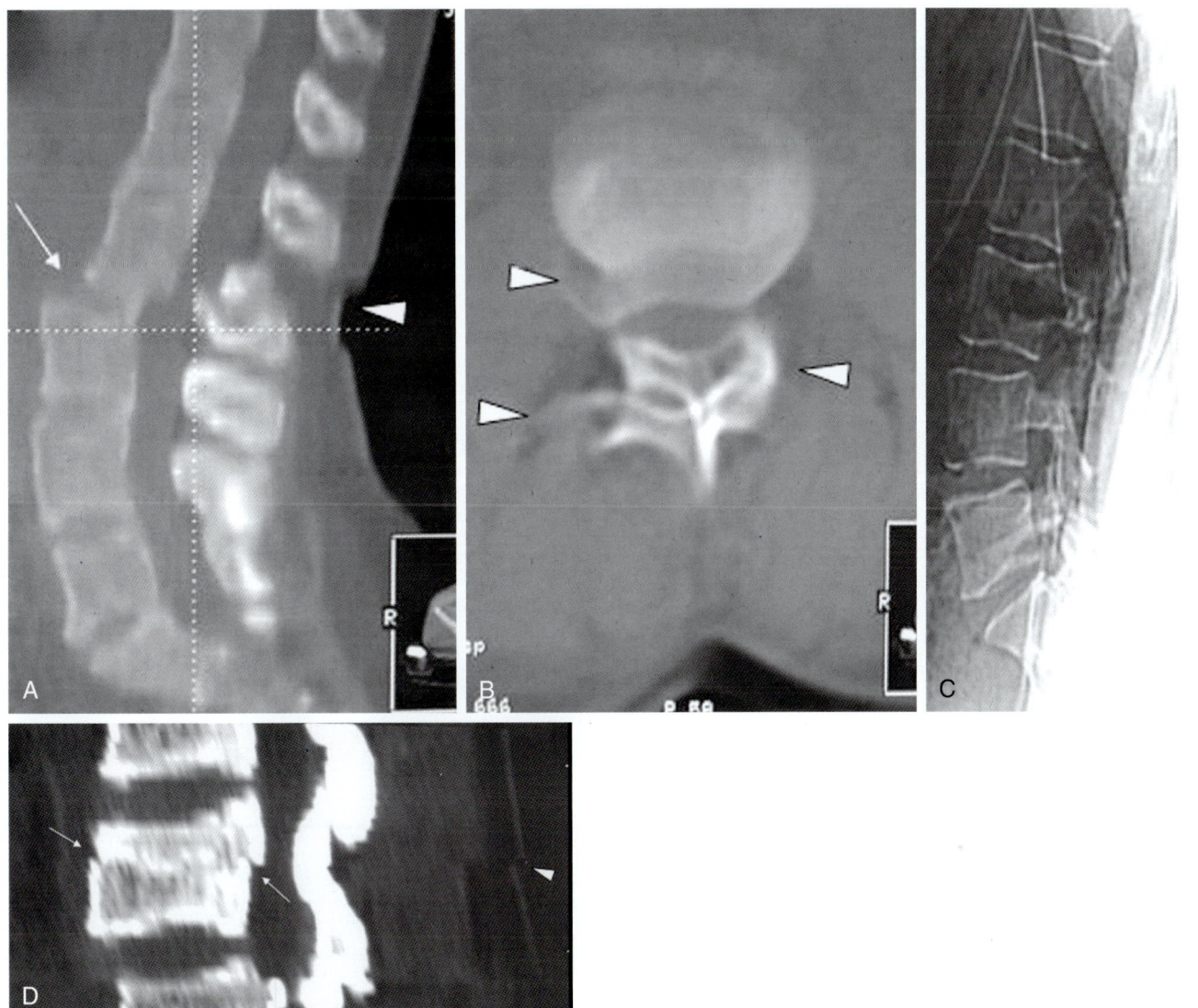

Figure 13-23 Multidetector computed tomography (CT) pitfalls in spinal trauma imaging. **A:** Sagittal reformatted CT view showing L2–L3 dislocation *(arrow)*, but the stepoff of the skin contour line *(arrowhead)* suggests it might be an artifact caused by minimal patient motion during the volumetric CT acquisition. This is confirmed by looking at the axial image at the L2–L3 level **(B)**, showing motion *(arrowheads)*, and at the scout view **(C)**, displaying normal alignment. **D:** Similar case in which motion during scan acquisition created a fake "bony fracture" *(arrows)*, which is confirmed by focal discontinuity of the skin contour line *(arrowhead)*.

adjacent to muscles and ligaments. This could be erroneously interpreted as soft tissue edema and injury. STIR images, although more noisy and of worse quality than FSE T2-weighted images, guarantee more homogeneous fat signal nulling and are more specific in identifying soft tissue injuries. Newer fat suppression techniques, such as two- and three-point Dixon and adiabatic inversion recovery methods, which are being implemented, will provide superior fat suppression compared to traditional chemical suppression techniques.

What Are the Delayed Findings in Spinal Trauma Imaging?

After spinal trauma and related interventions, follow-up imaging is usually performed with plain films radiography or CT to confirm realignment and correct positioning of hardware implants and to detect signs of instability. Instability can be diagnosed in the presence of abnormal intersegmental motility of the spine elements during flexion–extension maneuvers or in the presence of lucent bone resorption around the screws of metallic fixation devices. In case of instability, at the same level, MR STIR images can show high bone marrow signal as well.

After a spinal cord injury, the spinal cord abnormality is expected to evolve in the late chronic phase into a focal area of myelomalacia, characterized by CSF-like T1 and T2 signal and cord thinning due to atrophic volume loss (Figure 13-24). In this phase following spinal cord injury, MRI often reveals further hyperintense signal on T2-weighted imaging in the white matter tracts above (dorsal columns) and below (lateral columns) the injury level. This finding is believed to represent wallerian degeneration.

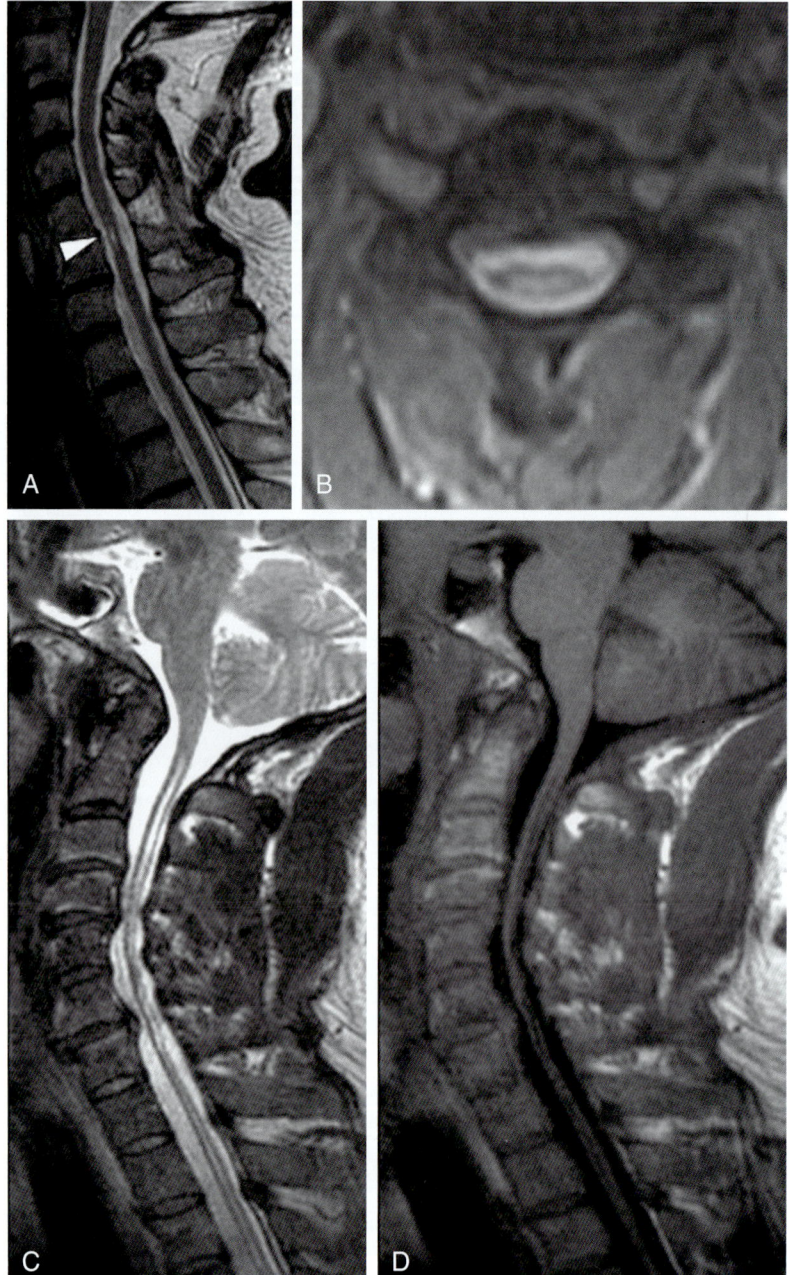

Figure 13-24 Spinal cord injury in the chronic phase. **A, B:** Months after a spinal cord contusion, there is focal thinning and volume loss of the spinal cord and a central small myelomalacic area in the spinal cord displaying well-defined high T2 cerebrospinal fluid–like signal *(arrowhead in A)*. **C, D:** Another case months after a severe cervical spinal cord injury showing diffuse spinal cord volume loss and extensive central high T2, low T1 signal in the cord. In the absence of cord expansion this more likely is myelomalacia than syrinx.

The neurologic deficit after trauma is supposed to remain stable; therefore, further MRI follow-up is needed in the presence of unexpected worsening of the clinical conditions to rule out the late sequelae of spinal cord injury, including progressive syrinx or intramedullary cysts, arachnoiditis with adhesions and tethering (Figure 13-25), hardware failure, or new compression.

Suggested Readings

Anderson LD, D'Alonzo RT. Fractures of the odontoid process of the axis. *J Bone Joint Surg Am.*. 1974 Dec;56(8):1663-1674.

Besman A, Kaban J, Jacobs L, Jacobs LM. False-negative plain cervical spine x-rays in blunt trauma. *Am Surg.* 2003 Nov;69(11):1010-1014.

Blackmore CC. Evidence-based imaging evaluation of the cervical spine in trauma. *Neuroimaging Clin N Am.*. 2003 May;13(2):283-291.

Denis F. Spinal instability as defined by the three-column spine concept in acute spinal trauma. *Clin Orthop Relat Res.* 1984 Oct(189):65-76.

Geck MJ, Yoo S, Wang JC. Assessment of cervical ligamentous injury in trauma patients using MRI. *J Spinal Disord.* 2001 Oct;14(5):371-377.

Grossman RI, Yousem DM. Non-degenerative diseases of the spine. In: Grossman RI, Yousem DM, eds. *Neuroradiology: the Requisites.* 2nd ed. Philadelphia: Mosby; 2003:837-849.

Hanson JA, Blackmore CC, Mann FA, Wilson AJ. Cervical spine injury: a clinical decision rule to identify high-risk patients for helical CT screening. *AJR Am J Roentgenol.* 2000 Mar;174(3):713-717.

Imhof H, Fuchsjäger M. Traumatic injuries: imaging of spinal injuries. *Eur Radiol.* 2002 Jun;12(6):1262-1272.

Mann FA, Cohen WA, Linnau KF, Hallam DK, Blackmore CC. Evidence-based approach to using CT in spinal trauma. *Eur J Radiol.* 2003 Oct;48(1):39-48.

Ross JS, Brant-Zawadzki M, Moore KR, Crim J, Chen MZ, Katzman GL. Trauma. In: Ross JS, ed. *Diagnostic Imaging: Spine.* Salt Lake City: Amyrsis; 2004.

Rumboldt Z, Castillo M, Smith K. The spine. In: Lee JKT, Sagel SS, Stanley RJ, Heiken JP, eds. *Computed body tomography with MRI correlation.* 4th ed. Philadelphia: Lippincott Williams & Wilkins; 2006:1669-1683.

Stiell IG, Wells GA, Vandemheen KL, et al. The Canadian C-spine rule for radiography in alert and stable trauma patients. *JAMA.* 2001 Oct 17;286(15):1841-1848.

Takhtani D, Melhem ER. MR imaging in cervical spine trauma. *Magn Reson Imaging Clin N Am.* 2000 Aug;8(3):615-634.

Van Geothem JW, Biltjes IG, van den Hauwe L, Parizel PM, De Schepper AM. Whiplash injuries: is there a role for imaging? *Eur J Radiol.* 1996 Mar;22(1):30-37.

Van Goethem JW, Maes M, Ozsarlak O, van den Hauwe L, Parizel PM. Imaging in spinal trauma. *Eur Radiol.* 2005 Mar;15(3):582-590.

Wilmink JT. MR imaging of the spine: trauma and degenerative disease. *Eur Radiol.* 1999;9(7):1259-1266.

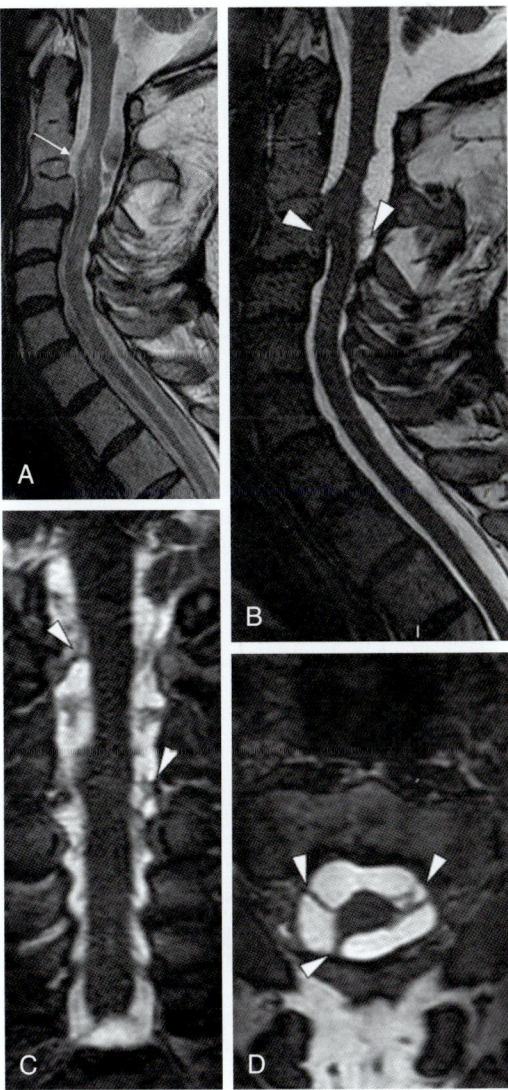

Figure 13-25 Posttraumatic arachnoiditis. Several months after suffering a spinal cord injury, this patient noted new onset of further progressive neurologic deficit. Magnetic resonance imaging with sagittal T2-weighted **(A)** and multiplanar reformatted images from a three-dimensional constructive interference in steady state myelographic sequence **(B–D)** showing irregular and multifocal C-spine tethering with thick irregular septations in the subarachnoid space *(arrowheads)* representing arachnoid adhesions. At C2–C3, the site of most severe cord tethering, there is spinal cord high T2 signal, possibly representing edema or gliosis *(arrow)*.

CHAPTER 14
Imaging of Congenital Brain Abnormalities

Andrea Rossi

■ INTRODUCTION

Brain malformations are extremely polymorphous, and individual cases very often escape rigid categorization. Moreover, several malformations are frequently associated with one another in individual patients, and many are comprised within complex multiorgan syndromes. Classifications schemes are continuously challenged by new advances in the understanding of the pathologies they attempt to describe. This has especially been the case with brain malformations. Knowledge of the basic molecular and genetic processes that direct normal brain development and, when deranged, result in congenital abnormalities has literally boomed in the past decade. For this reason, we are now witnessing a delicate transition from a purely morphologic to a molecular genetic approach. At present, both perspectives probably are equally unsatisfactory because the molecular and genetic background is well known for a few entities but is still unavailable for many others. Causes of malformations can be divided into four groups: chromosomal abnormalities, single gene mutations, environmental agents, and unknown; unfortunately, the last category is the largest. Therefore, neuroradiologic classifications are still mostly based on morphology or on a combination of morphologic and biochemical data.

■ ANOMALIES OF THE CORPUS CALLOSUM AND TELENCEPHALIC COMMISSURES

The corpus callosum, hippocampal commissure, and anterior commissure form the midline telencephalic commissural plate. The corpus callosum is the largest commissure in the brain. It is anatomically divided in five portions from anterior to posterior: the rostrum, genu, body, isthmus, and splenium. The hippocampal commissure connects the posterior pillars of the fornix and lies along the inferior aspect of the callosal isthmus and splenium, so the term *callosohippocampal commissure* has been introduced to illustrate such continuity. The anterior commissure crosses the midline at the superior end of the lamina terminalis. Embryologically, the telencephalic commissures derive from the lamina reuniens, a dorsal thickening of the embryonic lamina terminalis. The concept that callosal development starts from the posterior portion of the genu and proceeds bidirectionally toward the splenium and rostrum has been questioned by Raybaud and Girard, who introduced a new classification of the abnormalities traditionally known as "agenesis and hypoplasia of the corpus callosum," a simplified version of which is presented here. Patients with commissural abnormalities are often impaired intellectually and neurologically (about 90% of cases), a fact that should be considered when such anomalies are discovered antenatally.

Commissural Agenesis

Commissural agenesis is categorized in three subsets: complete commissural agenesis, callosohippocampal agenesis, and isolated callosal agenesis. The most frequent among the three is callosohippocampal agenesis, in which the anterior commissure is preserved. Commissural agenesis is characterized by a host of magnetic resonance imaging (MRI) features (Figure 14-1), first and foremost the absent visualization of the corpus callosum in midsagittal scans. Developing axons fail to cross the midline and remain in their native hemisphere, forming the so-called *Probst bundles*. These run along the medial walls of the lateral ventricles, characteristically resulting in crescent-shaped frontal horns in coronal sections. Because the cingulum (forming the white matter core of the cingulate gyrus) is consistently absent, the cingulate gyrus does not fold, the callosomarginal sulcus does not form, and the mesial cortical sulci show a radial arrangement. Moreover, absence of the cingulum produces thinning of the parahippocampal convolutions, leading to dilatation of the temporal horns and rudimentary hippocampal infolding. Hypoplasia of occipital associative bundles causes colpocephaly, an ex vacuo dilatation of the trigones of the lateral ventricle. A large amount of genetic syndromes may be associated with commissural abnormalities. Among these, the Aicardi syndrome is a dominant X-linked entity characterized by a variable association of asymmetric infantile spasms, commissural agenesis, and chorioretinal lacunae, found in infant girls. Choroid plexus papillomas may also be associated.

Commissural Hypoplasia

Commissural hypoplasia is divided into three categories: partial posterior commissural agenesis, diffuse commissural hypoplasia, and segmental callosal hypoplasia.

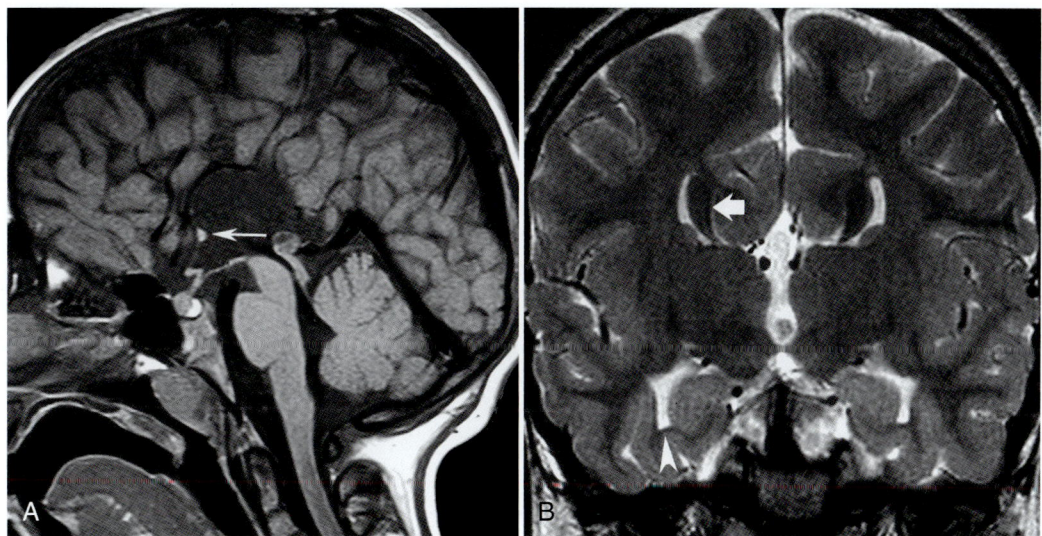

Figure 14-1 Callosohippocampal agenesis in a 7-year-old girl. **A:** Sagittal T1-weighted image showing complete absence of the corpus callosum and the hippocampal commissure. The anterior commissure is present *(arrow)*. The roof of the third ventricle bulges upward slightly. The normal appearance of the cingulate gyrus is not found. **B:** Coronal T2-weighted image confirming no interhemispheric commissure. The medial cortex is rolled-in over the thalami. The lateral ventricles are away from each other, closed medially by the primordial septal leaves that contain the longitudinal bundles of Probst *(arrow)*. The temporal horns have an abnormal appearance, extending below the hippocampus into the parahippocampal gyrus *(arrowhead)*, presumably because of the lack of cingulum. This lack of cingulum could also explain the loss of the normal pattern of the cingulate gyrus.

Partial posterior commissural agenesis is characterized by partial agenesis of the posterior portion of the corpus callosum. The extent of the agenetic portion may be variable, with only part of the genu (corresponding to the portion of the corpus callosum that forms first) present in the most severe cases. It is predictable based on the traditional theory of bidirectional development of the corpus callosum. *Diffuse commissural hypoplasia*, characterized by diffuse thinning of the three commissures, could be related to errors occurring later during commissural plate development, resulting in a lesser amount of fibers crossing the commissures. *Segmental callosal hypoplasia*, in which an intermediate portion of the corpus callosum is thinned, must be differentiated from secondary callosal destruction.

Associated Findings

Interhemispheric Cysts
Cerebrospinal fluid (CSF)–filled cavities associated with commissural abnormalities belong to two main categories: *diencephalic pseudocysts*, representing superior bulging of the tela choroidea of the third ventricle, and *interhemispheric cysts* (Figure 14-2, A), which are independent from the ventricles and may in turn be intraparenchymal, subarachnoid, arachnoid, or even intradural. True interhemispheric cysts suggest that commissural development may influence, and in turn be influenced by, development of the meninx primitiva.

Lipomas
The deep interhemispheric fissure is a common location for intracranial lipomas (so-called *lipomas of the corpus callosum*). Commissural plate abnormalities are almost invariably associated (Figure 14-2, B).

■ HOLOPROSENCEPHALIES AND RELATED ENTITIES

Holoprosencephaly
Holoprosencephaly (HPE) is a complex developmental anomaly of the brain and skull, characterized by hypoplasia of the most rostral portions of the neural tube resulting in noncleaved cerebral hemispheres and absence of midline structures such as the rhinencephalon, corpus callosum, and septum pellucidum. Both genetic factors (either chromosomal aberrations or single-gene mutations) and extrinsic teratogens (including maternal diabetes mellitus) may be involved in the pathogenesis. Currently, nine human HPE genes are known, and more likely will be discovered in the future; therefore, it probably is incorrect to think of a gene "for" HPE. Rather, it is the action of a gene(s) with the environment of the developing embryo that determines the outcome. HPE is classically divided into alobar, semilobar, and lobar types according to the severity of the malformation. However, a precise boundary among the three groups does not exist, and intermediate cases may be identified.

Alobar HPE
Midline structures such as the falx cerebri, superior sagittal sinus, interhemispheric fissure, septum pellucidum, corpus callosum, third ventricle, pituitary gland, and olfactory bulbs are absent. The thalami are fused and abut a rudimentary ventricle that freely communicates with a large cyst, the dorsal sac, that extends upward to the calvarium. Facial abnormalities ranging from cyclopia to ethmocephaly are commonly associated. The diagnosis usually is made antenatally by ultrasound. Neonates usually are stillborn and therefore are rarely imaged by MRI.

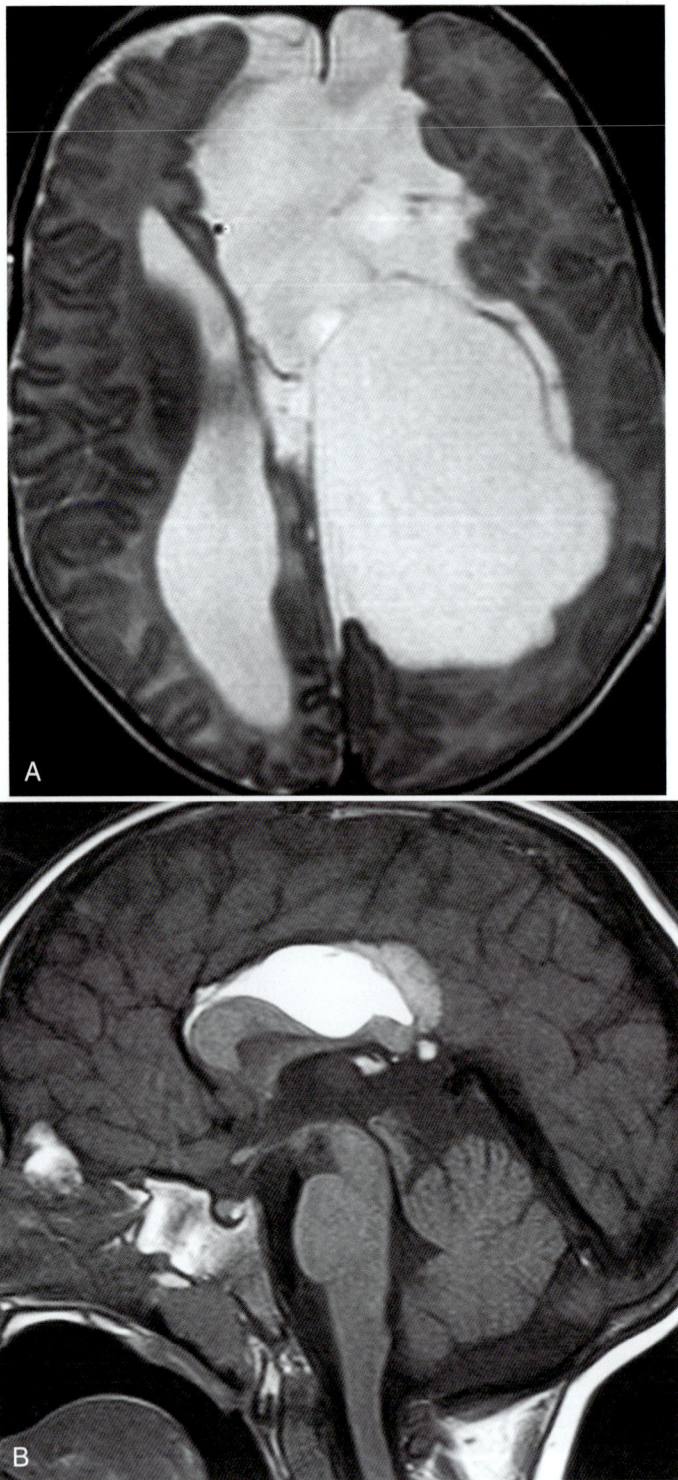

Figure 14-2 Callosohippocampal agenesis and associated anomalies. **A:** Axial T2-weighted image of a 2-month-old girl showing multiple interhemispheric cavities. The right lateral ventricle is enlarged, whereas the left lateral ventricle is difficult to identify. The cortex of the medial aspect of the left cerebral hemisphere is dysplastic, with subcortical heterotopia. **B:** Sagittal T1-weighted image of a 3-year-old boy showing tubulonodular lipoma overlying a dysplastic corpus callosum. (From Tortori-Donati P, Rossi A, Biancheri R. Brain malformations. In: Tortori-Donati P (ed) Pediatric Neuroradiology. Berlin: Springer, 2005:71-198.).

Semilobar HPE

The brain is less dysmorphic. Rudimentary lateral ventricles are present, and the cortex is more developed. The thalami may be partially separated, and a rudimentary third ventricle may be seen. The interhemispheric fissure and the falx cerebri are partially developed posteriorly, whereas the frontal lobes and basal ganglia are not separated (Figure 14-3). The corpus callosum is absent in the fused regions, whereas a commissure ("pseudosplenium") is visible where the two cerebral hemispheres are separated. Affected patients are usually afflicted by severe psychomotor delay.

Lobar HPE

Lobar HPE is the mildest form, usually found in asymptomatic or mildly retarded individuals. The lateral ventricles are formed. The frontal lobes may be partially fused in some cases and separated in others, but the septum pellucidum is constantly absent. The mildest forms show only the absence of the septum pellucidum and therefore require differentiation from septooptic dysplasia, in which optic nerves are hypoplastic. The differentiation from the semilobar variant is sometimes difficult by MRI due to the large amount of intermediate forms. The degree of anterior extension of the corpus callosum in midsagittal planes may be used as a gross indicator of the severity of the malformation.

Syntelencephaly (Middle Interhemispheric HPE)

This rare abnormality is characterized by failure of cleavage of the posterior frontal and parietal regions of the brain despite separation of the rostrobasal forebrain, with presence of an interhemispheric fissure anteriorly (Figure 14-4). The nervous tissue that bridges the midline may be represented by a heterotopic nodule or cortical dysplasia. Patients are usually severely retarded developmentally, although normal intelligence was reported in one case.

Septooptic Dysplasia

It is characterized by the association of hypoplastic optic nerves and absent septum pellucidum. The clinical presentation is related to the association with either schizencephaly (presenting with seizures) or hypothalamic and pituitary hypoplasia (presenting with pituitary insufficiency). The diagnosis of septooptic dysplasia is based on ophthalmoscopy, which shows hypoplastic optic discs, and a MRI picture of small optic nerves and chiasm and absent septum pellucidum. The association with schizencephaly ("septooptic dysplasia plus") must be accurately scrutinized.

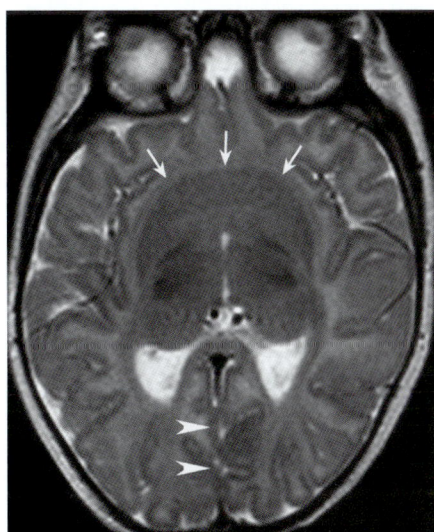

Figure 14-3 Semilobar holoprosencephaly in a 5-month-old girl. Axial T2-weighted image showing incomplete cleavage of the frontal lobes and basal ganglia (*arrows*). The interhemispheric fissure is formed posteriorly (*arrowheads*), consistent with normal cleavage of the posterior region of the brain. Correspondingly, the trigones of the lateral ventricles, albeit rudimentary, are formed, whereas the frontal horns show agenesis.

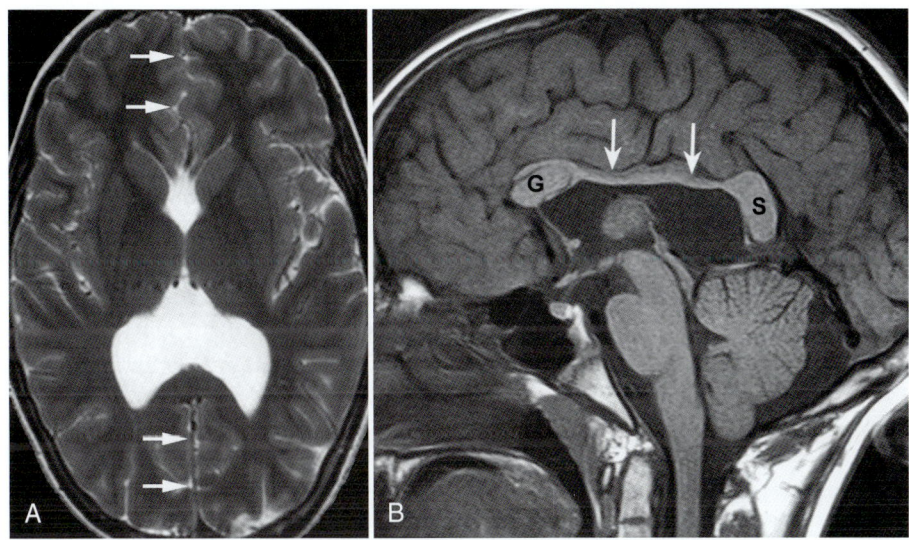

Figure 14-4 Syntelencephaly in a mildly hypotonic 14-year-old boy with normal intelligence. **A:** Axial T2-weighted image showing rudimentary lateral ventricles but septum pellucidum is absent; however, normally developed interhemispheric fissure both anteriorly and posteriorly (*arrows*) does not suggest holoprosencephaly at first glance. **B:** Sagittal T1-weighted image showing partial intermediate dysgenesis of the corpus callosum. A thin cortical bridge (*arrows*) overlies the markedly thinned callosal body. G, Genu; S, splenium. (From Tortori-Donati P, Rossi A, Biancheri R. Brain malformations. In: Tortori-Donati P (ed) Pediatric Neuroradiology. Berlin: Springer, 2005:71-198.)

The frontal horns show a square-like shape due to the absence of the septum pellucidum, a feature in common with lobar HPE.

MALFORMATIONS OF THE CEREBRAL CORTEX

Embryology and Classification

The complex events leading to the formation of the cerebral cortex may be simplified in three main steps: *proliferation*, *migration*, and *organization*. Proliferation begins during the seventh gestational week, when cells in the subependymal layer of the walls of the lateral ventricles form the germinal matrix. During the following week, neurons generated by intense mitotic activity in the germinal matrix begin to migrate radially toward the surface of the brain; such migration follows a track laid by specialized radial glial fibers. When migration in the cortex of the human fetus stops is not clear. However, distal processes of the radial glia disappear by 20 to 28 weeks of gestation, suggesting no or little migration on glial guides at this stage. Organization of the cortex to the eventual six-layer configuration occurs next and is completed by the seventh lunar month. The current classification categorizes cortical malformations into defects of proliferation, migration, and organization. Only the main entities are described here.

Hemimegalencephaly

Hemimegalencephaly results from a disorder in neuronal and glial proliferation in the germinal matrix. It may be isolated or occur in patients with neurocutaneous syndromes. MRI shows enlargement of a whole hemisphere (Figure 14-5). The cortex is affected by diffuse migration anomalies, whereas the white matter is gliotic and dysmyelinated. The ipsilateral ventricle is frequently dilated, and the frontal horn is stretched. The homolateral cerebellar hemisphere is usually enlarged as well. Affected newborns suffer from untreatable epilepsy, so hemispherectomy is often necessary. However, because hemispherectomy is contraindicated if the contralateral hemisphere has cortical malformations, assessment of the contralateral hemisphere is crucial.

Focal Cortical Dysplasia

Focal cortical dysplasia (FCD) affects children with partial, intractable epilepsy. It presently is categorized into three grades. Grade I (or architectural) and grade II (or cytoarchitectural) are often found in association with hippocampal sclerosis (dual pathology). They are characterized by a hypoplastic appearance of one temporal lobe with loss of gray–white matter demarcation. Grade III FCD corresponds to the so-called Taylor-type FCD, which in turn is categorized into two subgroups based on the presence or absence of balloon cells (i.e., large cells with abundant eosinophilic cytoplasm, showing intermediate features between neuronal and glial elements). Such classification is valuable because it correlates with epilepsy surgery outcome. In fact, an inverse correlation between histologic grade and percentage of seizure-free patients after 1 year of follow-up has been found. Patients usually suffer from partial intractable epilepsy. Because the histologic abnormality, which is reflected in corresponding MRI features (see below), involves not only the cortex but the whole thickness of the cerebral mantle (i.e., from the ventricular to the pial surface), Taylor-type FCD has also been called *focal transmantle dysplasia*. On MRI, Taylor-type FCD shows a triad of focal cortical thickening with enlargement of the affected gyri, blurred gray–white matter interface, and a funnel-shaped high T2/fluid-attenuated inversion recovery signal intensity in the subcortical white matter that tapers toward the lateral ventricle (Figure 14-6).

The Lissencephaly Spectrum

The term *lissencephaly* refers to a complete lack of sulcation of the cortical plate and therefore should be considered synonymous with agyria, whereas pachygyria indicates few, broad gyri with shallow sulci. However, there is a wide spectrum of intermediate features in which variably combined areas of agyria and pachygyria coexist. Several forms of lissencephaly have been identified, the most relevant of which are briefly discussed here.

Classical lissencephaly can be caused by abnormalities of either the LIS1 gene on chromosome 17 or the DCX gene on chromosome X (i.e., X-linked lissencephaly). Patients are usually severely affected with intractable epilepsy and profound psychomotor delay. Histologically, there is a four-layered cortex with a thick sparse cell layer interposed between the external and internal cellular layers. On MRI (Figure 14-7), the cortical surface is flat and the sylvian cisterns are broad and vertically oriented; therefore, the brain has a figure-of-eight shape in axial sections. The cortex is

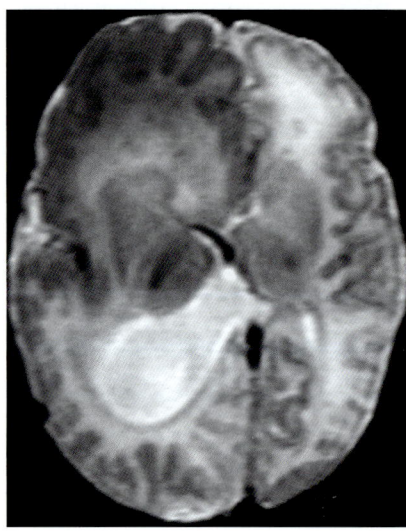

Figure 14-5 Hemimegalencephaly in a newborn. Axial T2-weighted image showing general increase in size of right cerebral hemisphere with cortical thickening. Relative hypointensity of the frontal white matter is consistent with hypermyelination. Notice marked dilatation of the lateral ventricle.

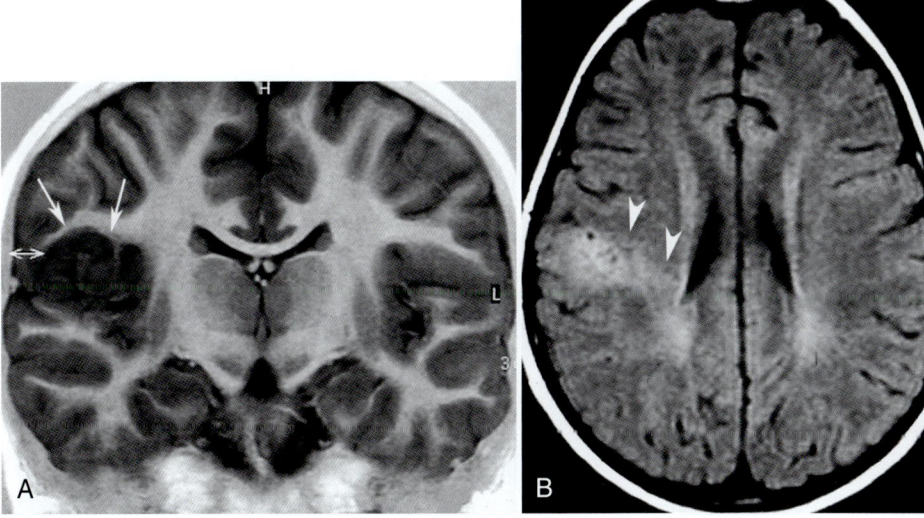

Figure 14-6 Taylor-type focal cortical dysplasia in a 5-year-old boy. On magnetic resonance imaging, Taylor-type focal cortical dysplasia shows a triad of focal cortical thickening with enlargement of the affected gyri, blurred gray–white matter interface, and funnel-shaped high T2/fluid-attenuated inversion recovery (FLAIR) signal intensity in the subcortical white matter that tapers toward the lateral ventricle. **A:** Coronal inversion recovery image showing focal cortical thickening in the right frontal lobe *(arrows)*. **B:** Axial FLAIR image showing hyperintensity that tapers toward the lateral ventricle *(arrowheads)*.

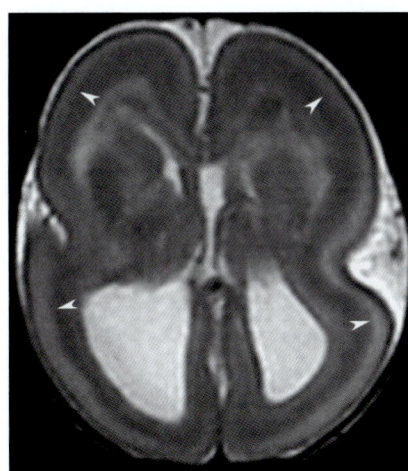

Figure 14-7 Classic lissencephaly in a 3-month-old boy. Axial T2-weighted image showing the brain has a figure-of-eight appearance due to shallow, vertically oriented sylvian fissures. The brain surface is entirely smooth. Thickness of the cortical plate is much greater than that of white matter. The sparse cells layer, separating the thin outer cortical layer from the thick layer of arrested neurons, is clearly recognizable as a hyperintense stripe *(arrowheads)*.

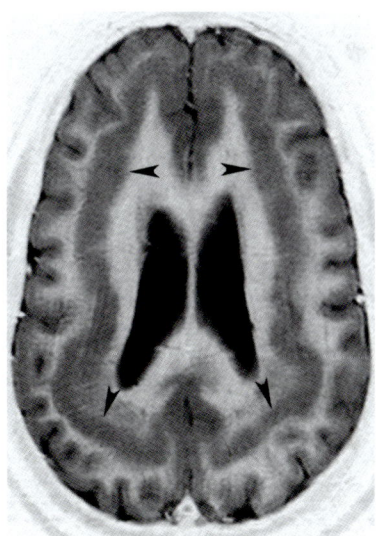

Figure 14-8 Subcortical band heterotopia in a 13-year-old girl. Axial inversion recovery image showing thick layer of heterotopic neurons *(arrowheads)* located deep to a grossly normal-appearing cortex and extending continuously along both hemispheres bilaterally. The band is separated from the cortex by a layer of myelinated white matter. Note that the convolutions are somewhat coarse, and the gyral pattern probably is simplified.

thickened, and the hyperintense sparse cells layer is usually visualized. A variable degree of sulcation can be present in individual patients. LIS1 gene mutation is characterized by a combination of posterior agyria and anterior pachygyria, whereas the opposite pattern (i.e., anterior agyria and posterior pachygyria) is found in DCX mutations.

Subcortical band heterotopia is found in female carriers of the DCX mutation. In this entity, the majority of radial glial fibers are damaged, manifesting with bilateral, thick layers of arrested neurons located approximately halfway between the ventricles and the cortical plate, resembling a doubling of the cortex (Figure 14-8).

Cobblestone lissencephaly is usually found in children with Fukuyama congenital muscular dystrophy, Walker-Warburg syndrome, and muscle-eye-brain disease. There is a more anarchic disorganization of the cortex, with zones of typical lissencephaly interspersed among areas of polymicrogyria. Cortical lamination is absent, and subcortical heterotopia may be found. On MRI (Figure 14-9), the cortex is thinner than in classic lissencephaly, and there may be concurrent hypomyelination of the white matter. Brainstem hypoplasia and cerebellar malformations are commonly associated.

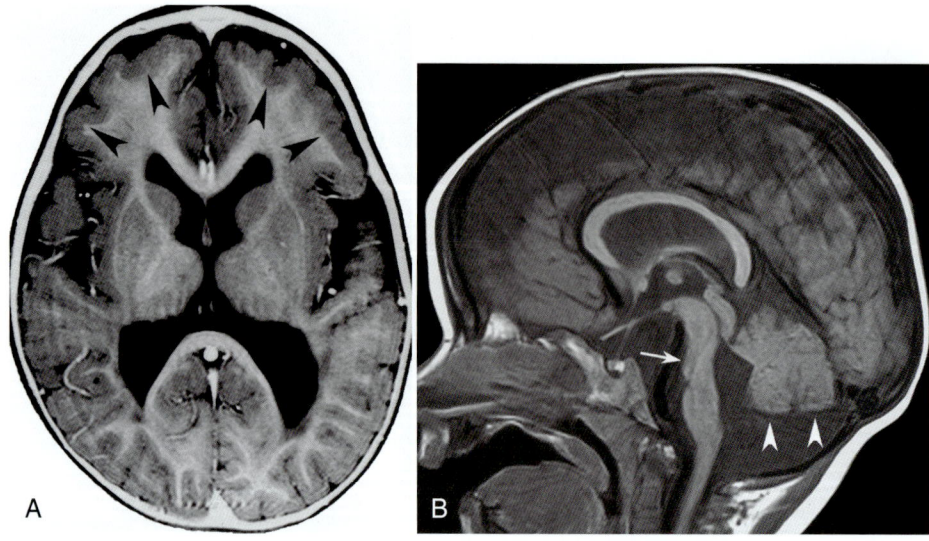

Figure 14-9 Cobblestone lissencephaly in a 3-year-old girl with muscle-eye-brain disease. **A:** Axial inversion recovery image showing thickened cortical ribbon with coarse gyration involving both frontal lobes *(arrowheads)*. **B:** Sagittal T1-weighted image showing hypoplasia of the pons *(arrow)* and inferior vermis *(arrowheads)*.

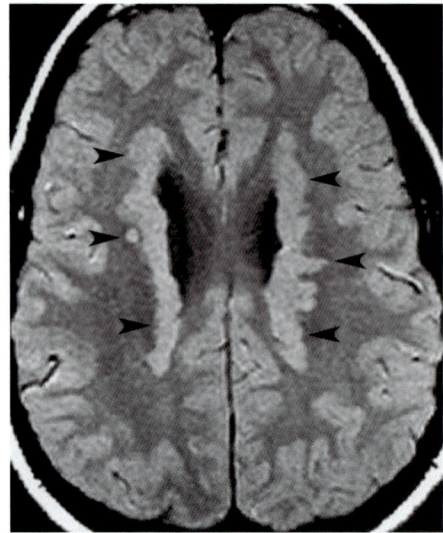

Figure 14-10 X-linked bilateral periventricular nodular heterotopia in a 16-year-old girl who had her first seizure at age 14 years. Axial fluid-attenuated inversion recovery image showing bilateral subependymal nodules that are isointense with gray matter *(arrowheads)*. (Courtesy Dr R. Guerrini, Florence, Italy.)

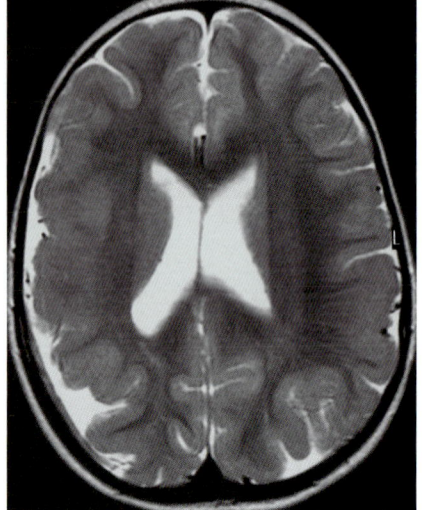

Figure 14-11 Polymicrogyria in a 2-year-old girl with congenital left hemiplegia. Axial T2-weighted image showing the right cerebral hemisphere is smaller than the left and the cortical mantle is apparently thickened, resulting from fusion of multiple adjacent small gyri. The cortical surface is flattened.

Subependymal Heterotopia

Damage of radial glial fibers may arrest neuronal migration at anomalous sites, where neurons conglomerate in a disorganized fashion. Patients almost always present with a seizure disorder. Gray matter heterotopia may be subependymal, subcortical, or meningeal. Among these, subependymal heterotopia is by far more common. The heterotopic nodules are isointense with normal gray matter in all MRI sequences. Focal nodules are found in sporadic cases. Diffuse heterotopia bordering the walls of the lateral ventricles is more likely to be X-linked due to defects of the FLN1 gene (Figure 14-10).

Polymicrogyria

Polymicrogyria is the most frequent cause of partial epilepsy in pediatric patients, although unilateral polymicrogyria may present with congenital hemiparesis. Either genetic or acquired factors, including vascular events or congenital infection, can be implicated in the pathogenesis. Polymicrogyria may be unilateral or bilateral, resulting in various appearances depending on the extent of hemispheric involvement. Macroscopically, there is excessive infolding of the cortex with thin, numerous microconvolutions separated by narrow and often obliterated sulci. On MRI (Figure 14-11), polymicrogyria appears as an area of increased cortical

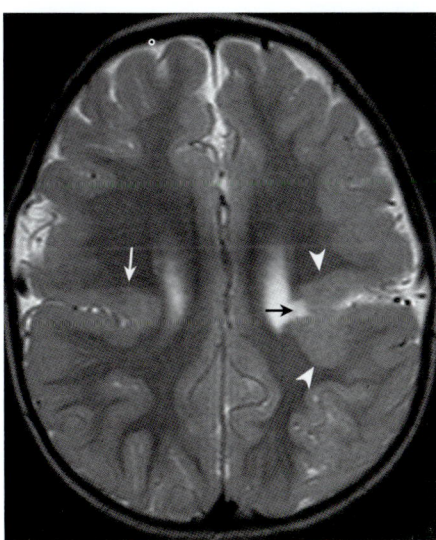

Figure 14-12 Schizencephaly in a 3-year-old girl. Axial T2-weighted image showing deep fissure involving the entire thickness of the right cerebral hemisphere. The deep portion of the cleft is fused, with a dimple along the ventricular wall *(black arrow)*. Polymicrogyric cortex surrounds both lips of the fissure *(arrowheads)*. Polymicrogyria also involves the contralateral hemisphere, with deep infolding *(white arrow)*. Large drainage veins into the dilated cerebrospinal fluid spaces are visible on both sides.

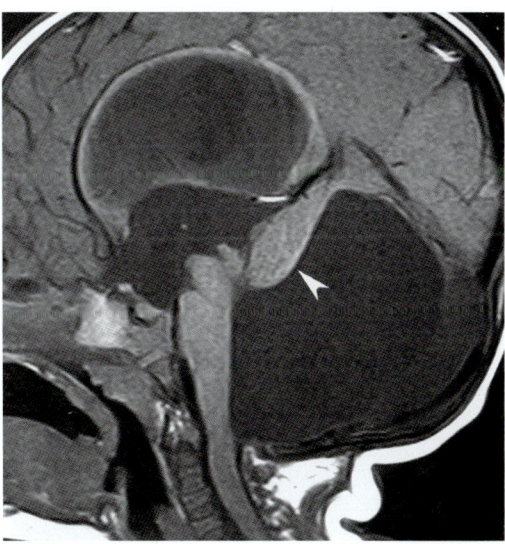

Figure 14-13 Dandy-Walker malformation in a 20 month old girl. The posterior fossa is enlarged and filled with a huge cerebrospinal fluid cavity, corresponding to an enlarged fourth ventricle. The vermis is hypoplastic with verticalization (i.e., counterclockwise rotation of the vermis) *(arrow)* and elevated tentorial insertion/torcula. Associated hydrocephalus is evident.

thickness with an irregular gray–white matter junction, whereas the cortical surface may be flat or extend inward, producing a cortical infolding around an abnormally oriented sulcus. Anomalous venous drainage is common in dysplastic cortical areas, and large veins may often be seen within the abnormal sulci.

Schizencephaly

Schizencephaly is characterized by a cleft extending through the whole hemisphere, from the ependymal lining of the lateral ventricle to the pia covering the brain. The cleft may be unilateral or bilateral and is constantly lined by polymicrogyric cortex. The walls of the cleft may be widely separated by intervening CSF *(open lips)* or abut one another *(closed lips)*. In the latter case, the cleft may not be easily visible, although a dimple may be seen in the wall of the lateral ventricle where the cleft communicates (Figure 14-12). Presence of dysplastic cortex lining the cleft is of primary importance to differentiate schizencephaly from porencephalic cavities.

■ MALFORMATIONS OF THE CEREBELLUM

Embryology

By gestational day 28 to 37, the thin roof of the rhombencephalon (future fourth ventricle) is formed by an ependymal membrane coated by pia mater. The plica choroidea, a precursor of the future choroid plexus, divides the rhombencephalic roof into the *anterior membranous area* (AMA) lying cephalad and the *posterior membranous area* (PMA) lying caudad. The edges of the AMA thicken progressively by cellular proliferation, forming the *rhombic lips*. These paired structures approach each other until they eventually fuse in the midline to form the vermis. The intervening AMA progressively involutes until its remnants are incorporated in the choroid plexus. Meanwhile, the PMA shows a transient posterior finger-like expansion, the *Blake pouch*, which disappears as the foramen of Magendie opens. Cerebellar malformations derive from an imbalance between the formation of the rhombic lips and of the choroid plexuses on one side and the involution of the AMA and PMA on the other side. A further categorization individuates *cystic malformations*, in which a collection resulting from active expansion of CSF spaces is found within the posterior cranial fossa, and *noncystic malformations*, which are usually dominated by vermian dysgenesis.

Dandy-Walker Malformation

The definition of Dandy-Walker malformation classically includes partial or complete vermian agenesis associated with hypoplastic cerebellar hemispheres, cystic dilatation of the fourth ventricle, and expansion of the posterior fossa associated with high insertion of the tentorium, torcular Herophili, and transverse sinuses (Figure 14-13). Vermian hypoplasia may be more or less severe; however, the hypoplastic superior vermis is constantly rotated in a counterclockwise fashion and often lies posterior to the quadrigeminal plate. Cerebellar hemispheres are also hypoplastic and abut the petrous ridges. The posterior fossa is occupied by a large cyst that corresponds to a dilated fourth ventricle. Hydrocephalus develops in up to 80% of untreated cases. In some cases, key features of Dandy-Walker malformation (e.g., rotated, hypoplastic vermis and cystic dilatation of the fourth ventricle) may be found in patients with a normal-sized posterior fossa. The term *Dandy-Walker variant* was used to describe these minor forms. However, there presently is no consensus regarding the

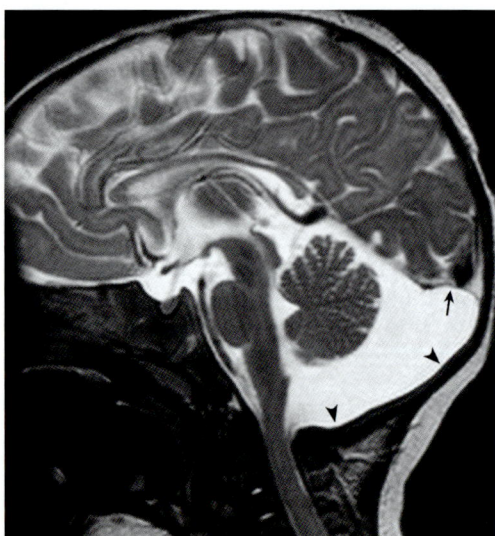

Figure 14-14 Mega cisterna magna in a 2-month-old boy. Sagittal T2-weighted image showing the subarachnoid spaces of the posterior fossa are enlarged, with scalloping of the occipital squama *(arrowheads)*. Note there is no hydrocephalus. Both the vermis and brainstem are normally formed. Posteriorly, the mega cisterna magna insinuates itself into a small fenestration of the tentorial insertion *(arrow)*.

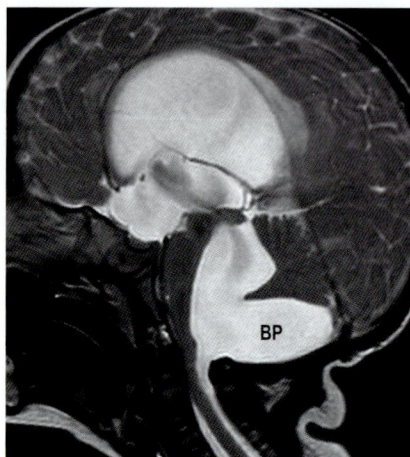

Figure 14-15 Persistent Blake pouch in a 6-month-old boy. Sagittal T2-weighted image showing tetraventricular hydrocephalus. The fourth ventricle is markedly enlarged and communicates with a large infravermian cystic formation representing persistence of the Blake pouch *(BP)*. The cerebellar vermis is normally formed and not rotated, although its inferior surface is compressed. Posterior fossa size is normal.

exact significance of this term. Probably, Dandy-Walker malformation and Dandy-Walker variant represent two ends of the spectrum of AMA anomalies, with the main difference being the degree of dilatation of the fourth ventricle and, therefore, of the posterior fossa.

Mega Cisterna Magna

This abnormality is characterized by dilatation of the cisterna magna with free communication with both the fourth ventricle and the adjacent subarachnoid spaces (Figure 14-14). The vermis, cerebellar hemispheres, and fourth ventricle are normal. Hydrocephalus is never associated, and the anomaly is constantly clinically silent but usually is encountered during MRI for other indications.

Persistent Blake Pouch

Persistent Blake pouch is characterized by a retrocerebellar CSF collection that, in itself, is similar to a mega cisterna magna. However, persistence of the Blake pouch is characterized by failed permeabilization of the Magendie foramen, resulting in tetraventricular hydrocephalus (Figure 14-15). Shunting of the retrocerebellar pouch restores normal CSF outflow so that both the hydrocephalus and the pouch are resolved.

Molar Tooth Malformation

Molar tooth malformation consists of the following triad: (1) dysgenesis of the isthmic portion of the brainstem with elongation and thinning of the pontomesencephalic junction and elongation of the interpeduncular fossa; (2) thickened superior cerebellar peduncles that project straight back, coursing perpendicular to the brainstem; and (3) hypoplasia of the vermis. This malformation typically is found in patients with Joubert syndrome, who present clinically in the neonatal age with hyperpneic–apneic spells, ataxia, nystagmus, and developmental delay. Other entities in the so-called *cerebello-oculo-renal syndrome spectrum* (including Arima, Senior-Loken, and Coach syndromes) may display a similar malformation. On MRI (Figure 14-16), the vermis is completely or partially absent, with only the anterior lobules visible. The fourth ventricle is high riding with an umbrella shape on axial images. The superior cerebellar peduncles are elongated, thickened, and project straight back, running parallel with each other.

■ CHIARI MALFORMATIONS

Chiari I

Chiari I malformation is characterized by bilateral or, less frequently, unilateral ectopia of the cerebellar tonsils into the foramen magnum by greater than 5 mm (Figure 14-17). The posterior fossa is usually normal or slightly smaller than normal, and the vermis is normally shaped and located. Associated hydrocephalus and hydromyelia are frequent and may be secondary to restricted CSF flow at level of the crowded foramen magnum. In rare cases, the medulla oblongata is elongated sagittally and shows a prominent obex *(myelencephalic variant)*. Affected patients may be asymptomatic or may complain of headache, torticollis, cervical pain, and cranial nerve palsies. Cine MRI studies of CSF flow are useful for selecting candidates for decompression surgery and for evaluating the results.

Chiari II

There is a consistent association between myelomeningoceles and Chiari II malformation, a complex congenital anomaly of the hindbrain characterized

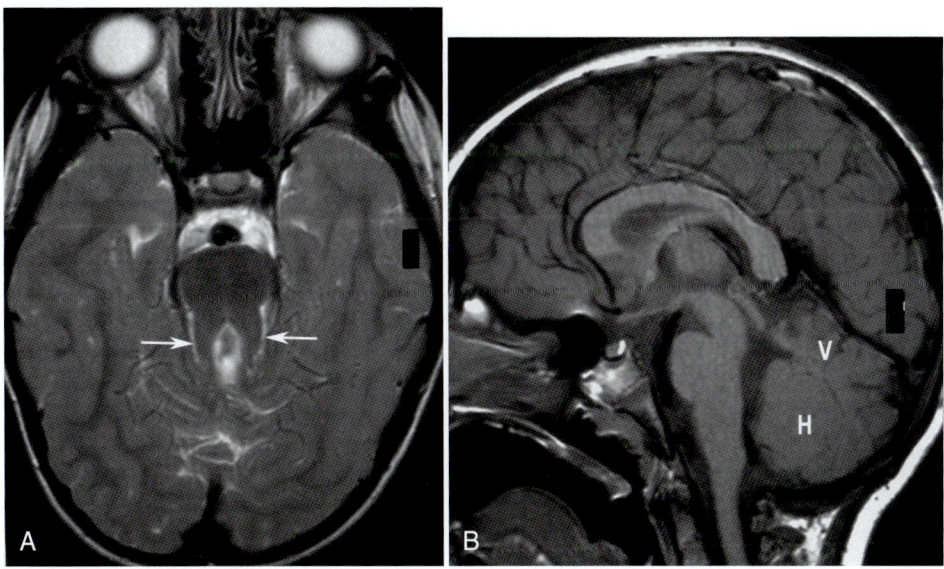

Figure 14-16 Molar tooth malformation in a 4-year-old girl. **A:** Axial T2-weighted image showing thickening of the superior cerebellar peduncles *(arrows)* resulting in a molar tooth appearance of the midbrain. Note abnormal foliation of the superior vermis. **B:** Sagittal T1-weighted image showing marked hypoplasia of the cerebellar vermis *(V)*. The hemispheres *(H)* abut one another on the midline.

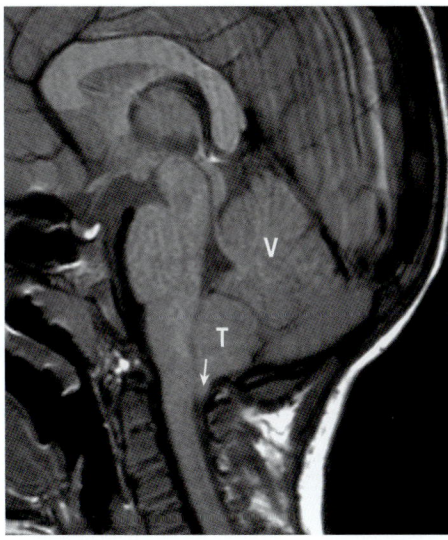

Figure 14-17 Chiari I malformation in a 6-year-old boy. Sagittal T1-weighted image showing the cerebellar tonsils *(T)* herniating into the foramen magnum by more than 5 mm *(arrow)*. Note that the vermis *(V)* is not herniated; instead, it is raised by the underlying tonsils.

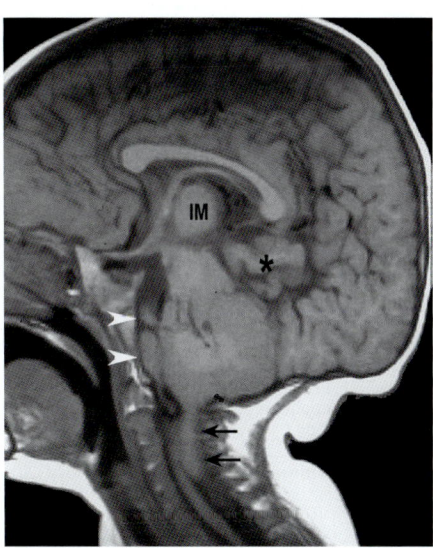

Figure 14-18 Chiari II malformation following ventriculoperitoneal shunting in a 2-year-old boy who had previously undergone myelomeningocele surgery. The posterior fossa is markedly small and crowded. The vermis herniates through the foramen magnum *(arrows)*, whereas the cerebellum engulfs the brainstem *(arrowheads)*. The fourth ventricle is effaced. Additional signs include crowding of the occipital convolutions (i.e., stenogyria), an "accessory lobe" *(asterisk)* due to medialization of the posterior temporal lobe, and a thickened interthalamic mass *(IM)*.

by caudal displacement of the vermis, brainstem, and fourth ventricle. However, the severity of the hindbrain malformation may be variable, so patients with a nearly normal-sized posterior fossa may sometimes be found. Therefore, subtle minimal features of Chiari II malformation should be actively sought in all newborns with open spinal dysraphisms. CSF leaks through the spinal defect into the amniotic sac result in chronic CSF hypotension within the developing neural tube, insufficient dilatation of the rhombencephalic vesicle (future fourth ventricle), and lack of induction of the perineural mesenchyma of the posterior cranial fossa. Therefore, both the cerebellum and the brainstem are eventually forced to develop within a smaller than normal posterior fossa (Figure 14-18) and consequently herniate through both the tentorial groove and the foramen magnum. The inferior vermis herniates into the foramen magnum and wraps around the posterior surface of the cord (cerebellar peg). The medulla is stretched downward into the foramen magnum while the cervical cord is anchored by the dentate ligaments, resulting in the cervicomedullary kink, best seen on sagittal views. Hydrocephalus is a consistent finding in newborns within 48 to 72 hours of repair of the spinal dysraphism.

Chiari III

This rare abnormality is characterized by herniation of the cerebellum into an occipitocervical cephalocele, associated with other typical features of Chiari II malformation.

Suggested Readings

Aicardi J. Aicardi syndrome. In: Guerrini R, et al. ed. *Dysplasias of cerebral cortex and epilepsy.* Philadelphia: Lippincott-Raven; 1996:211-216.
Barkovich AJ. Imaging of the cobblestone lissencephalies. *AJNR Am J Neuroradiol.* 1996;17:615-618.
Barkovich AJ, Fram EK, Norman D. Septo-optic dysplasia: MR imaging. *Radiology.* 1989;171:189-192.
Barkovich AJ, Gressens P, Evrard P. Formation, maturation, and disorders of brain neocortex. *AJNR Am J Neuroradiol.* 1992;13:423-446.
Barkovich AJ, Hevner R, Guerrini R. Syndromes of bilateral symmetrical polymicrogyria. *AJNR Am J Neuroradiol.* 1999;20:1814-1821.
Barkovich AJ, Jackson Jr DE, Boyer RS. Band heterotopias: a newly recognized neuronal migration anomaly. *Radiology.* 1989;171:455-458.
Barkovich AJ, Kjos BO. Schizencephaly: correlation of clinical findings with MR characteristics. *AJNR Am J Neuroradiol.* 1992;13:85-94.
Barkovich AJ, Kuzniecky RI. Gray matter heterotopia. *Neurology.* 2000;55: 1603-1608.
Barkovich AJ, Kuzniecky RI, Bollen AW, Grant PE. Focal transmantle dysplasia: a specific malformation of cortical development. *Neurology.* 1997;49: 1148-1152.
Barkovich AJ, Kuzniecky RI, Jackson GD, et al. A developmental and genetic classification for malformations of cortical development. *Neurology.* 2005;65:1873-1887.
Bhadelia RA, Bogdan AR, Wolpert SM, et al. Cerebrospinal fluid flow waveforms: analysis in patients with Chiari I malformation by means of gated phase-contrast MR imaging velocity measurements. *Radiology.* 1995;196:195-202.
Biancheri R, Rossi A, Tortori-Donati P, et al. Middle interhemispheric variant of holoprosencephaly: a very mild clinical case. *Neurology.* 2004;63:2194-2196.
Castillo M, Quencer RM, Dominguez R. Chiari III malformation: imaging features. *AJNR Am J Neuroradiol.* 1992;13:107-113.
Colombo N, Tassi L, Galli C, et al. Focal cortical dysplasias: MR imaging, histopathologic, and clinical correlations in surgically treated patients with epilepsy. *AJNR Am J Neuroradiol.* 2003;24:724-733.
Di Rocco C. Surgical treatment of hemimegalencephaly. In: Guerrini R, et al. ed. *Dysplasias of Cerebral Cortex and Epilepsy.* Philadelphia: Lippincott-Raven; 1996:295-304..
Dobyns WB, Truwit CL, Ross ME, et al. Differences in the gyral pattern distinguish chromosome 17-linked and X-linked lissencephaly. *Neurology.* 1999;53:270-277.
Kash F, Brown G, Smirniotopoulos JA, et al. Intracranial lipomas. Pathology and imaging spectrum. *Int J Neuroradiol.* 1996;2:109-116.
Kollias SS, Ball Jr WS, Prenger EC. Cystic malformations of the posterior fossa: differential diagnosis clarified through embryologic analysis. *Radiographics.* 1993;13:1211-1231.
Maria BL, Boltshauser E, Palmer SC, Tran TX. Clinical features and revised diagnostic criteria in Joubert syndrome. *J Child Neurol.* 1999;14:583-591.
McLone DG, Knepper PA. The cause of Chiari II malformation: a unified theory. *Pediatr Neurosci.* 1989;15:1-12.
Milhorat TH, Chou MW, Trinidad EM, et al. Chiari I malformation redefined: clinical and radiological findings for 364 symptomatic patients. *Neurosurgery.* 1999;44:1005-1017.
Miller SP, Shevell MI, Patenaude Y, et al. Septo-optic dysplasia plus: a spectrum of malformations of cortical development. *Neurology.* 2000;54:1701-1703.
Naidich TP, McLone DG, Fulling F. The Chiari II malformation. Part IV. The hindbrain deformity. *Neuroradiology.* 1983;25:179-197.
Norman MG, McGillivray BC, Kalousek DK, Hill A, Poskitt KJ. *Congenital Malformations of the Brain. Pathological, Embryological, Clinical, Radiological and Genetic Aspects.* New York: Oxford University Press; 1995.
Patel S, Barkovich AJ. Analysis and classification of cerebellar malformations. *AJNR Am J Neuroradiol.* 2002;23:1074-1087.
Pilz DT, Matsumoto N, Minnerath S, et al. LIS1 and XLIS (DCX) mutations cause most classical lissencephaly, but different patterns of malformation. *Hum Mol Genet.* 1998;7:2029-2037.
Quisling RG, Barkovich AJ, Maria BL. Magnetic resonance features and classification of central nervous system malformations in Joubert syndrome. *J Child Neurol.* 1999;14:628-635.
Raybaud C, Girard N. Étude anatomique par IRM des agénésies et dysplasies commissurales télencéphaliques (agénesies du corps calleux et anomalies apparentées). Corrélations cliniques et interprétation morphogénétique. *Neurochirurgie.* 1998;44(suppl 1):38-60.
Raybaud C, Girard N. Malformations of the telencephalic commissures. Callosal agenesis and related disorders. In: Tortori-Donati P, ed. *Pediatric Neuroradiology.* Berlin: Springer; 2005:41-70.
Roessler E, Muenke M. The molecular genetics of holoprosencephaly: a model of brain development for the next century. *Childs Nerv Syst.* 1999;15:646-651.
Sarnat HB. Molecular genetic classification of central nervous system malformations. *J Child Neurol.* 2000;15:675-687.
Sarnat HB, Flores-Sarnat L. A new classification of malformations of the nervous system: an integration of morphological and molecular genetic criteria as patterns of genetic expression. *Eur J Paediatr Neurol.* 2001;5:57-64.
Satran D, Pierpont ME, Dobyns WB. Cerebello-oculo-renal syndromes including Arima, Senior-Löken and COACH syndromes: more than just variants of Joubert syndrome. *Am J Med Genet.* 1999;86:459-469.
Sheen VL, Dixon PH, Fox JW, et al. Mutations in the X-linked filamin 1 gene cause periventricular nodular heterotopia in males as well as in females. *Hum Mol Genet.* 2001;10:1775-1783.
Simon EM, Hevner RF, Pinter JD, et al. The middle interhemispheric variant of holoprosencephaly. *AJNR Am J Neuroradiol.* 2002;23:151-156.
Tassi L, Colombo N, Garbelli R, et al. Focal cortical dysplasia: neuropathological subtypes, EEG, neuroimaging and surgical outcome. *Brain.* 2002;125:1719-1732.
Tortori-Donati P, Fondelli MP, Rossi A, Carini S. Cystic malformations of the posterior cranial fossa originating from a defect of the posterior membranous area. Mega cisterna magna and persisting Blake's pouch: two separate entities. *Childs Nerv Syst.* 1996;12:303-308.
Tortori-Donati P, Rossi A, Biancheri R. Brain malformations. In: Tortori-Donati P, ed. *Pediatric Neuroradiology.* Berlin: Springer; 2005: 71-198.
van der Knaap MS, Valk J. Classification of congenital abnormalities of the CNS. *AJNR Am J Neuroradiol.* 1988;9:315-326.

CHAPTER **15**

Epilepsy

Pascal Bou-Haidar, Saulo Lacerda, and Meng Law

■ INTRODUCTION

Seizures are caused by abnormal and excessive discharges from the cortical neurons. Epilepsy is a general term used for a group of chronic neurologic disorders manifesting as spontaneous, recurrent seizures. The mean prevalence of epilepsy is estimated at 0.52% in Europe, 0.68% in the United States, and peaks up to 1.5% in developing countries.

The epilepsies are broadly classified into generalized and focal groups. Partial or focal seizures start from a localized unilateral area of the cerebrum versus simultaneously from both hemispheres in generalized seizures. In one fourth of patients who suffer from partial seizures, the condition is not adequately controlled with anticonvulsive medication. This is the group of patients who are potential candidates and could profit from surgical epilepsy treatment. The success rate for such surgery is greatest when a structural lesion related to the epilepsy can be identified. This lesion usually points to the epileptogenic zone. Resection of the epileptogenic zone is needed to stop the recurrence of seizures. Hence the primary goal of imaging epilepsy patients is detecting these lesions and determining their spatial relationship to eloquent cortical areas. Table 15-1 lists definitions of the zones and lesions of the cortex.

■ ROLE OF MAGNETIC RESONANCE IMAGING IN EPILEPSY WORKUP

Magnetic resonance imaging (MRI) plays a central role in the evaluation of patients with epilepsy. Computed tomographic (CT) imaging still is useful in emergency settings for screening patients with new onset of seizure and for ruling out surgical emergencies such as acute intracranial hemorrhage.

MRI is a versatile diagnostic tool in the evaluation of patients with epilepsy due to its inherent excellent soft tissue contrast and high spatial resolution. MRI protocols should be optimized and selected based on their ability to assess epileptogenic lesions such as cortical dysplasia, gray matter heterotopia, and hippocampal sclerosis. In 60% of patients with partial seizures and focal brain lesions, the lesion is located in the temporal or frontal lobe.

■ MRI PROTOCOL

The core imaging protocol is different for new-onset versus recurrent seizures.

New-onset seizures:
- Routine brain with contrast
- Axial gradient-recalled echo (GRE) T2*
- Diffusion weighted images

Recurrent seizures:
- Noncontrast MRI study
- Coronal T2, fluid-attenuated inversion recovery (FLAIR)
- Coronal three-dimensional (3D) volume T1 (1.5 mm) whole-brain GRE

Seizure protocol (Figure 15-1, *A* and *B*):
- Magnetization-prepared rapid acquisition of gradient echo (MPRAGE), whole-brain sagittal T1
- Coronal, axial T1
- Coronal T2 (512 × 512 matrix)
- Coronal FLAIR
- Axial GRE
- Diffusion MRI
- Postcontrast axial T1
- [1]H Magnetic resonance spectroscopy and dynamic susceptibility contrast MRI

The standard imaging protocol for evaluation of epilepsy at the Mount Sinai Medical Centre is given in Table 15-2.

Excellent alignment is particularly important for evaluating the hippocampus. The hippocampus is best visualized along its long axis (~35% to the orbitomeatal line) and orthogonal to this line. The axial plane, which is along the line joining the base of the splenium of the corpus callosum to the inferoposterior border of the frontal lobe, is determined on a sagittal scout image (Figure 15-2).

■ LOCATIONS FOR TYPES OF CLINICAL PRESENTATION: CLUES TO LOCATION

The clinical symptoms and particular auras in partial seizure often serve as useful clues to possible focal regions of the brain from which seizures are generated (Table 15-3).

Limbic System Anatomy

The noncortical areas that are part of the limbic system include the following (Figure 15-3):
- Amygdala
- Septal nuclei
- Basal ganglia
- Thalamus
- Hypothalamus

Table 15-1	Zones and Lesions of the Cortex
Epileptogenic zone	Region of cortex indispensible for generation of seizures By definition, total removal is necessary and sufficient for seizure freedom
Irritative zone	Region of cortex that generates interictal epileptiform discharges on EEG or MEG
Seizure-onset zone	Region of cortex where the clinical seizure originates
Epileptogenic lesion	Structural lesion that is causally related to the epilepsy
Ictal symptomatogenic zone	Region of cortex that generates the initial seizure symptoms
Functional deficit	Region of cortex that in the interictal period is functionally abnormal as indicated by neurologic examination, neuropsychological testing, and functional imaging or nonepileptiform EEG or MEG abnormalities
Eloquent cortex	Region of cortex that is indispensible for defined cortical functions

EEG, Electroencephalography; *MEG*, magnetoencephalography.

- Limbic midbrain
- Olfactory system

Extensive texts discuss the limbic system in detail; however, for our purpose, one important circuit (of Papez) and hippocampal formation are briefly discussed here because they are important for understanding changes in temporal lobe epilepsy.

Papez Circuit

In 1937, Papez postulated a classic neuronal circuit representing one of the anatomic substrates of memory and emotion. It is important for understanding the pathologic findings in mesial temporal sclerosis (MTS), discussed later. The Papez circuit starts in the cingulated cortex, which projects to the parahippocampal gyrus via the cingulated bundle and then to the hippocampus via the entorhinal cortex. The fornix connects the hippocampus with the mamillary body and via the mamillothalamic tract project to the anterior thalamic nucleus. The thalamocingulate fibers complete the Papez circuit by connecting back to the cingulated gyrus. More recent work has expanded the circuitry to encompass the remainder of the complex limbic system and includes structures such as the amygdala, prefrontal cortex, and other parts of the hypothalamus.

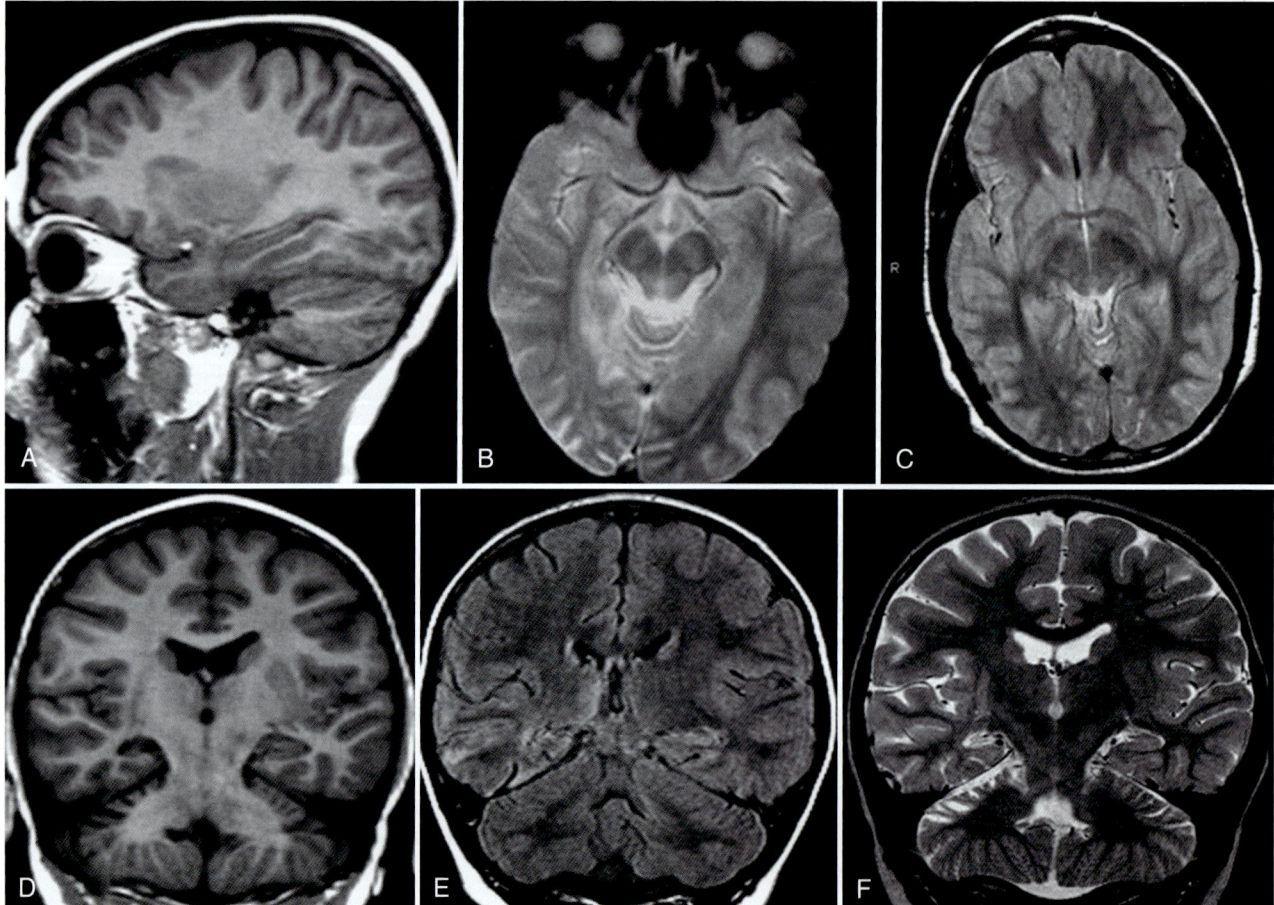

Figure 15-1 Magnetic resonance imaging protocol, sample sequences. **A:** Sagittal T1-weighted imaging **B:** Axial diffusion-weighted imaging and apparent diffusion coefficient. **C:** Axial T2-weighted imaging. **D:** Coronal T1-weighted imaging. **E:** Coronal fluid-attenuated inversion recovery. **F:** Coronal T2-weighted imaging.

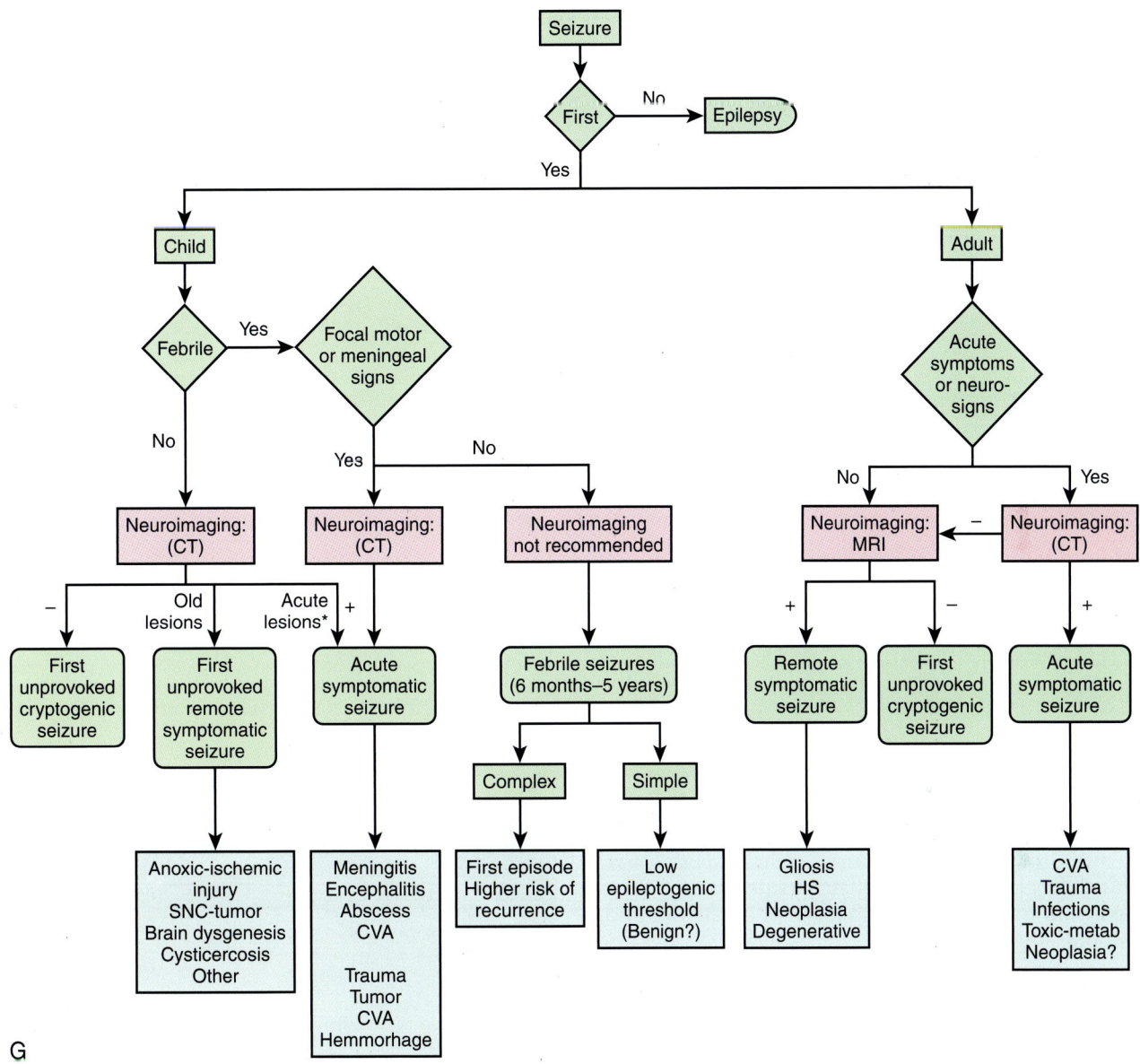

Figure 15-1, cont'd G: New-onset seizure flowchart. *CVA,* Cerebrovascular accident; HS, hippocampal sclerosis.

Table 15-2 Standard Imaging Protocol for Evaluation of Epilepsy at the Mount Sinai Medical Centre

Sequence	Sagittal T1 FLAIR	Axial T2 Propeller	Coronal Oblique 3D SPGR	Coronal Oblique XETA T2 FLAIR	3D SWAN*	Axial DWI	Axial T2 FLAIR
FOV	220	210	210	240	240	240	220
Matrix	288 × 192	320 × 256	512 × 192	256 × 256	320 × 192	96 × 128	288 × 256
Scan (%)	100	100	100	90	80	100	100
TI	785	—	—	—	—	—	—
TR	1839	4800		6250	MIN	7625	9500
TE	24	91.2	MIN	MIN	55	MIN	135.1
FA			35		30		
Slice thickness (mm)	5	5	2.5	2.0	3.0	5.0	5.0
Interslice gap (mm)	2.5	0	0	0	0	0	0
No. of slices	17	30	32	60	50	30	30
NSA	2	1.5	1	1	1	1	1
Acquisition time/min	1:35	2:30	1:10	3:48	4:03	1:09	2:51

*An alternative sequence to 3D SWAN is a coronal gradient-recalled echo sequence.
3D, Three-dimensional; DWI, diffusion-weighted imaging; FA, flip angle; FLAIR, fluid-attenuated inversion recovery; FOV, field of view; NSA, number of signal averages; SPGR, spoiled gradient-recalled; SWAN, T2 star-weighted angiography; XETA, extended echo-train acquisition.

Temporal Lobe Anatomy

The fusiform gyrus is also known as the *occipitotemporal gyrus*. It lies lateral to the collateral sulcus and is separated from the interior temporal gyrus by the occipitotemporal sulcus.

Internal Architecture of the Hippocampus

The hippocampal formation includes older cortical regions, all consisting of fewer than six layers deep in the most medial aspect of the temporal lobe (Figure 15-4). The term includes the following:
- Hippocampus proper or cornus ammonis (CA), which is divided into four regions (CA1 to CA4) and has a three-layered cortical area
- Dentate gyrus, which also has three layers
- Subiculum, a transitional cortical area of three to five layers that becomes continuous with the parahippocampal gyrus and is the origin of the majority of forniceal fibers

■ COMMON EPILEPTOGENIC LESIONS

Mesial Temporal Sclerosis

The most common candidates for surgical treatment of epilepsy are patients with intractable temporal lobe epilepsy. MST is one of the most common causes of epilepsy in the adolescent and young adult populations, and surgical therapy offers cures of approximately 90%. Patients

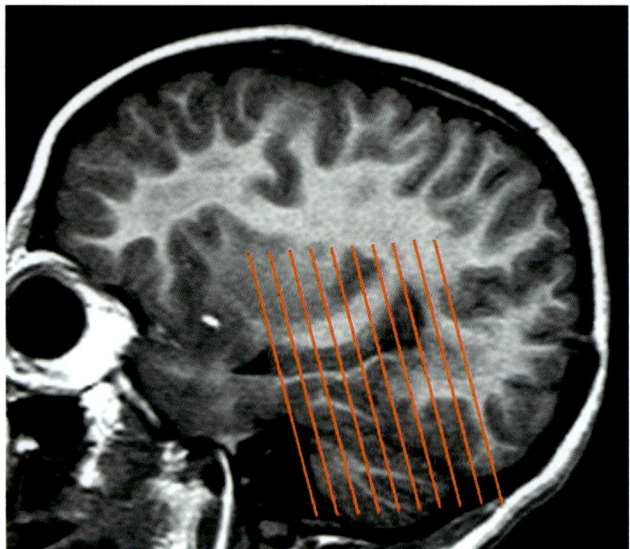

Figure 15-2 Magnetic resonance imaging technique used to plan coronal sections perpendicular to the long axis of the hippocampus (*red lines*).

may have a remote history of a cortical insult, such as head trauma, complicated febrile seizures, or infection in the first decade of life. Histologic findings include hippocampal atrophy with neuronal loss in the dentate, CA1 (Sommer sector), and CA3/CA4 regions with gliosis (Figure 15-5). Given the connections to other neuronal structures via the Papez circuit, it is not uncommon to find that extrahippocampal abnormalities also occur in patients with MTS. Findings include atrophy of the fornix, mamillary body, anterior thalamic nucleus, cingulated gyrus, and parahippocampus. Secondary effects include dilatation of the temporal horn (Figures 15-6 and 15-7). Atrophy of the contralateral cerebellum is also described as crossed cerebellar diaschisis.

Other proposed pathogenic processes involved include excitotoxins, particularly glutamate and aspartate.

Diagnosis
The combination of clinical, electroencephalographic, and MRI imaging features is usually sufficient for diagnosis. Three MRI criteria are required for diagnosis of MTS:
1. Atrophy
2. Signal change (high signal on T2-weighted and FLAIR imaging seen most often)
3. Derangement of anatomy (loss of digitations of dentate is useful sign)

Table 15-3 Clinical Presentation and Aura Based on Suspected CNS Location

Aura and/or Clinical Presentation	Suspected CNS Location
Focal motor seizure, jacksonian seizure, Todd paralysis	Primary motor cortex (precentral gyrus)
Involuntary turning during seizure (aversive movement)	Motor cortex anterior to precentral gyrus
Somatosensory seizures	Primary sensory cortex (postcentral gyrus)
Bilateral tonic postures	Supplementary motor area
Gelastic seizures	Hypothalamic region
Altered affect, crying	Frontal gyrus, anterior cingulated gyrus
Auditory auras	Region of Heschl gyrus
Seizure with olfactory or gustatory symptoms	Mesial temporal lobe
Vertigo	Insular or parietal cortex

CNS, Central nervous system.

Associated findings include the following:
- Dilated temporal horn
- Atrophy of fornix and mamillary body
- Increased signal in amygdala
- Increased signal in anterior temporal cortex
- ^{1}H MR spectroscopy in MTS

Proton spectroscopy has demonstrated abnormalities of N-acetylaspartate (NAA), a mitochondrial neuronal compound, creatine, and choline in patients with temporal lobe epilepsy. The abnormalities typically consist of reduced NAA signal and increased choline, creatine, and myoinositol signals. These MR spectroscopy findings are consistent with the histopathologic characteristics of reduced neuron cell counts with neuronal dysfunction and increased glial cellularity. Spectroscopy can show reduced NAA peak in asymmetric MTS and has a lateralizing sensitivity of approximately 80% (Figure 15-8).

Single-Photon Emission Computed Tomography
Single-photon emission computed tomography (SPECT) scans show the distribution of blood flow in the brain at the time of the injection of a radiotracer, which is injected ictally or interictally. If the radiotracer is injected ictally, focally increased uptake is identified in the affected temporal lobe (hot focus). If the radiotracer is injected interictally, the affected temporal lobe demonstrates decreased uptake compared with that of the rest of the brain (cold focus) (Figure 15-9). The advantage of SPECT is that it can used to demonstrate cerebral blood flow during seizure activity.

OTHER PATHOLOGIC PROCESSES AND CAUSES OF EPILEPSY

Apart from hippocampal/MTS, other causes of epilepsy to be considered include the following:
- Cerebral neoplasms
- Vascular malformations
- Developmental anomalies
- Gliosis (including posttraumatic, postsurgical causes)
- Infectious/inflammatory

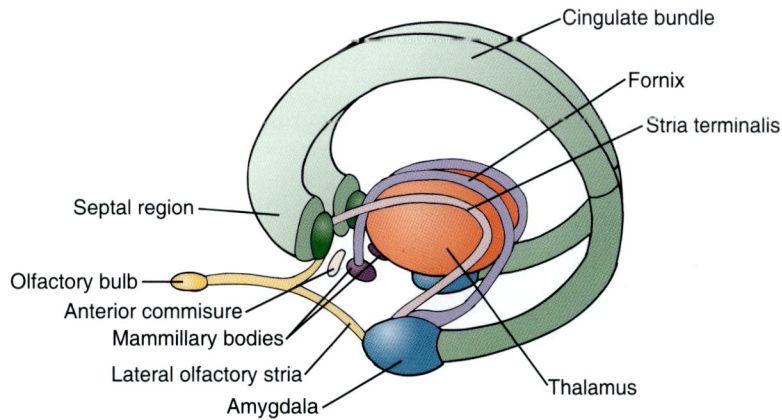

Figure 15-3 Schematic limbic system anatomy.

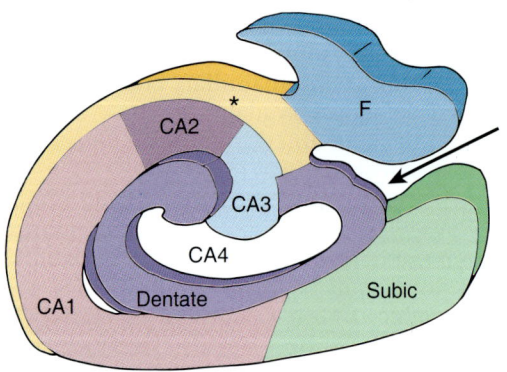

Figure 15-4 Schematic diagram of internal architecture of the hippocampus. Arrow indicates hippocampal fissure. *, alveus; *CA1-CA4*, Cornus ammonis; *F*, fimbria; *Subic*, subiculum.

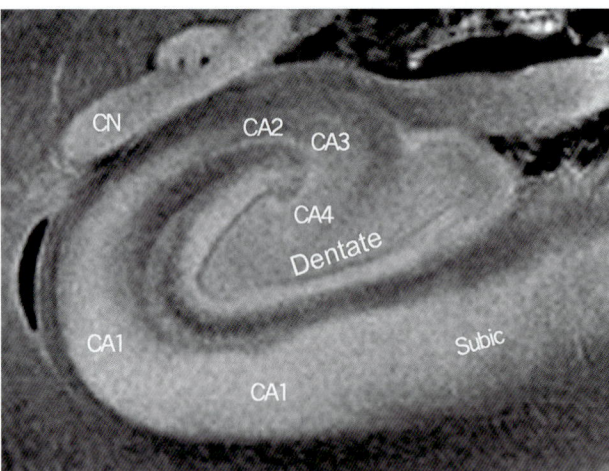

Figure 15-5 Microanatomy of the hippocampus. Microscopic magnetic resonance imaging at 9.4 T. Neurons in CA1 (Sommer sector) are most sensitive to ischemia. *CA1–CA4*, Cornus ammonis; *CN*, caudate nucleus; *Subic*, subiculum. (From Fatterpekar GM, Delman BN, Boonn WW, et al. MR microscopy of normal human brain. Magn Reson Imaging Clin N Am 2003;11(4):641-653.)

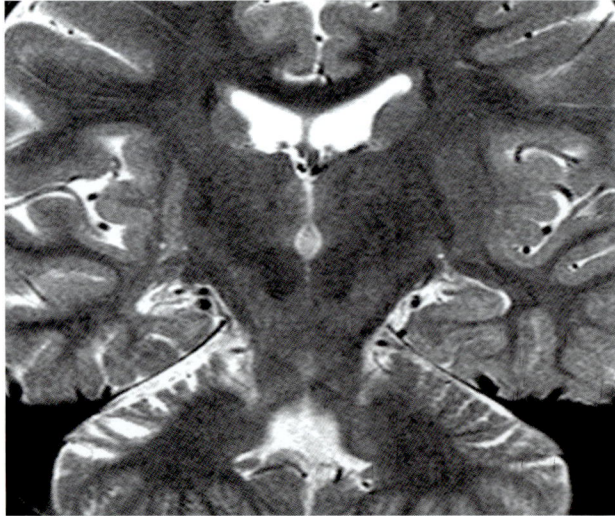

Figure 15-6 Mesial temporal sclerosis. Note right-sided derangement of hippocampal anatomy, volume loss, and increased T2-weighted signal. Compare to normal left side.

Cerebral Neoplasms

Neoplasms represent 2% to 4% of the epileptogenic causes in the general epilepsy population. The occurrence of epileptic seizures in patients suffering from primary brain tumors, as well as in patients with cerebral metastases, varies depending on the tumor entity. Slow-growing lesions are associated with a higher incidence of seizures than rapidly growing lesions. In patients with brain metastasis, melanoma is associated with the highest likelihood of seizures (Figure 15-10). Lung cancer, breast, and gastrointestinal tumor primaries are also associated with a high frequency of seizures.

In the pediatric population, epilepsy-associated tumors are more frequently located in the cortex of the temporal lobes. They are not usually associated with mass effect or vasogenic edema.

Common epilepsy associated primary brain tumors include gangliogliomas, dysembryoplastic neuroepithelial tumors (DNETs), pilocytic astrocytomas, pleomorphic xanthoastrocytomas, and World Health Organization (WHO) grade II astrocytomas (Figure 15-11).

Gangliogliomas

Gangliogliomas are slowly growing, well-differentiated neuroepithelial tumors composed of a mixture of neoplastic ganglion and glial cells. They are the most common mixed neuronal–glial tumor. They are often partially cystic, often cortically based masses presenting in children and young adults with temporal lobe epilepsy (Figure 15-12). They are usually located in the temporal lobes but can occur throughout the cerebrum. They are commonly associated with cortical dysplasia, and calcification is often present. Little mass effect or vasogenic edema is seen. Gangliomas demonstrate variable enhancement pattern and rarely can have malignant degeneration attributable to its glial component.

Dysembryoplastic Neuroepithelial Tumors

DNETs are classically seen as a wedge-shaped, well-defined intracortical partially cystic and nodular lesions. They present in young patients with a longstanding history of partial seizures most commonly located in the temporal lobe, hippocampus, and/or amygdala. Convex lesions tend to cause inner table scalloping. They have very slow or no growth potential and are unlikely to recur following resection. Enhancement is a rare and unusual feature (Figure 15-13).

Pilocytic Astrocytomas

This is the most common primary brain tumor in children and is the prototypic WHO grade I neoplasm most frequently located in the posterior fossa. Although more than two thirds of all patients demonstrate the classic imaging manifestation of a cystic mass with an enhancing mural nodule, approximately 17% of cases can be predominantly solid masses with minimal to no cyst-like component. Hence these tumors can be difficult to differentiate from DNETs and gangliogliomas, especially when they occur in supratentorial locations and present as partial seizures.

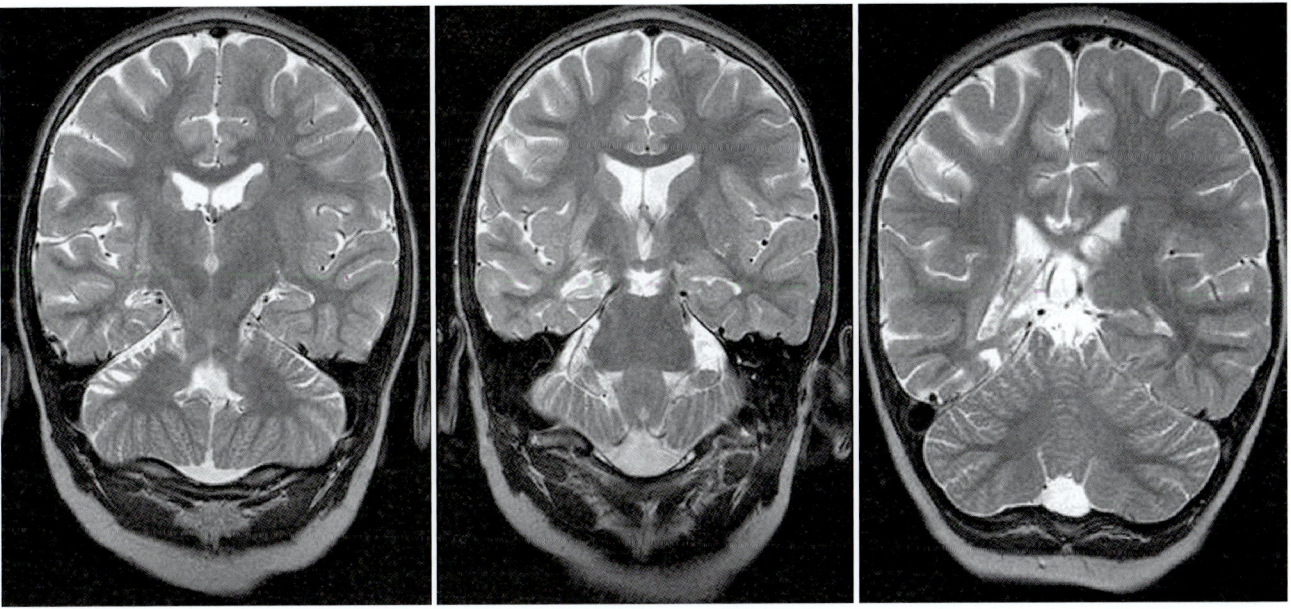

Figure 15-7 Mammillary body atrophy on the right side in a patient with mesial temporal sclerosis. Other associated findings include dilated temporal horn, atrophy of fornix, increased signal in amygdala, and increased signal in anterior temporal cortex.

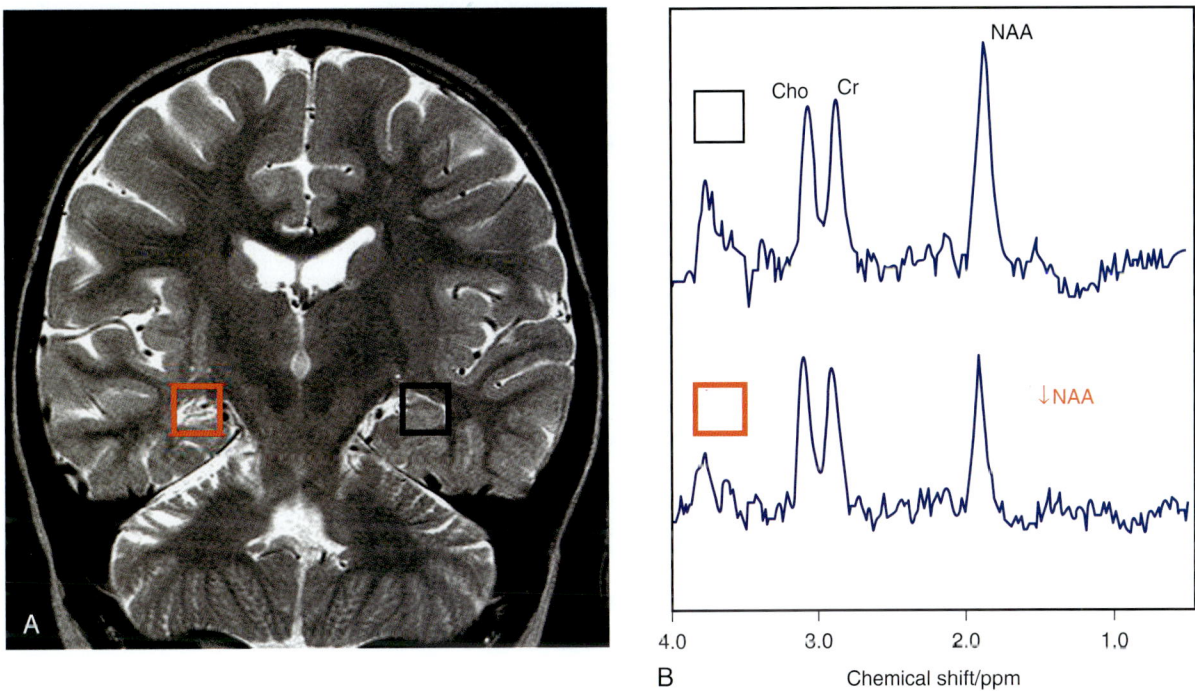

Figure 15-8 Magnetic resonance spectroscopy for detecting laterality in mesial temporal sclerosis (MTS). **A:** Coronal T2-weighted imaging through mesial temporal lobes with single-voxel spectroscopy over each hippocampal formation. **B:** Corresponding ¹H spectroscopy demonstrating reduced N-acetylaspartate (NAA) peak in asymmetric MTS. Spectroscopy has a lateralizing sensitivity of approximately 80%. *Cho,* Choline; *Cr,* creatine.

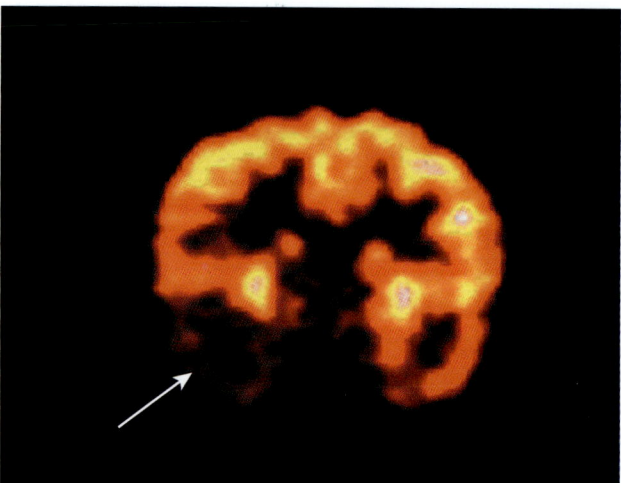

Figure 15-9 Single-photon emission computed tomography (SPECT) imaging in a patient with mesial temporal sclerosis performed interictally demonstrating hypoperfusion of the right temporal lobe. SPECT scans show the distribution of blood flow in the brain at the time of injection of a radiotracer, which is injected ictally or interictally. If the radiotracer is injected ictally, focally increased uptake is identified in the affected temporal lobe (hot focus). If the radiotracer is injected interictally, the affected temporal lobe demonstrates decreased uptake compared with that of the rest of the brain (cold focus).

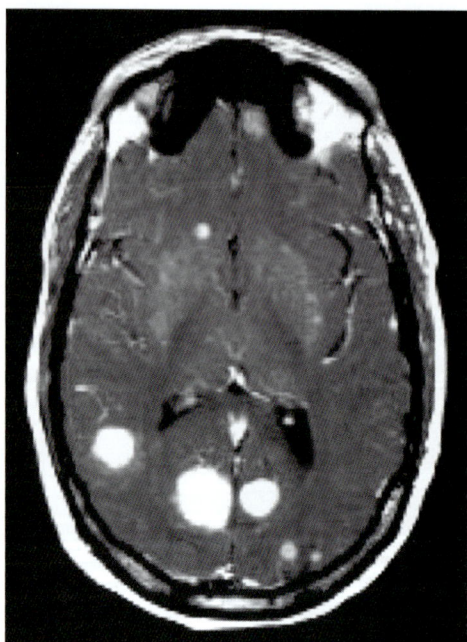

Figure 15-10 Cerebral metastasis. In patients with brain metastasis, melanoma is associated with the highest likelihood of seizures.

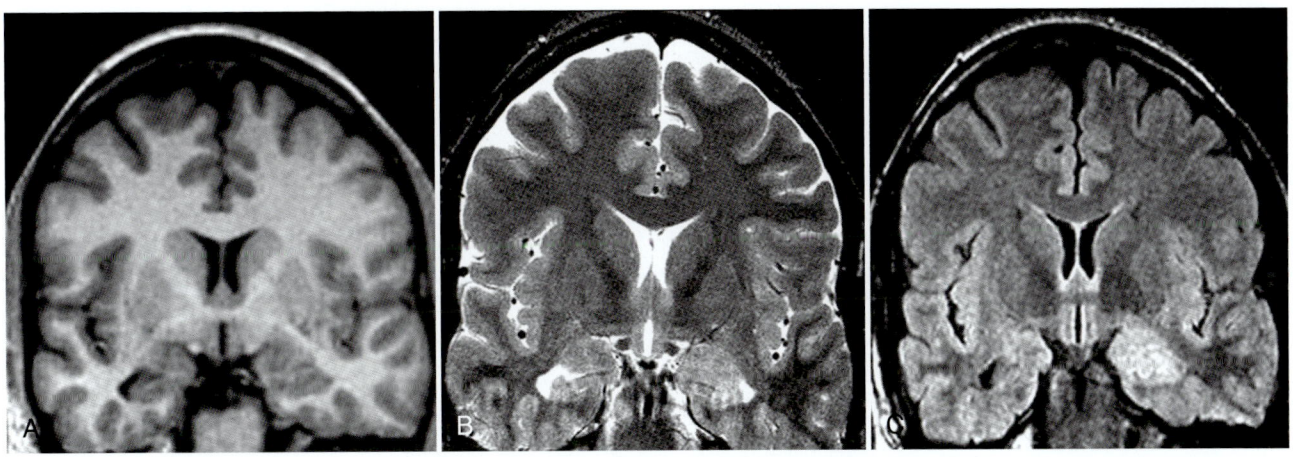

Figure 15-11 Low-grade glioma in left medial temporal lobe. Coronal T1-weighted image **(A)** demonstrates a mass in the left mesial temporal cortex of intermediate to low signal. T2-weighted image **(B)** and fluid-attenuated inversion recovery image **(C)** shows hyperintense signal involving the mass with no surrounding vasogenic edema and little mass effect. Differential diagnosis includes ganglioglioma, dysembryoplastic neuroepithelial tumor, low-grade astrocytoma, and pleomorphic xanthoastrocytoma.

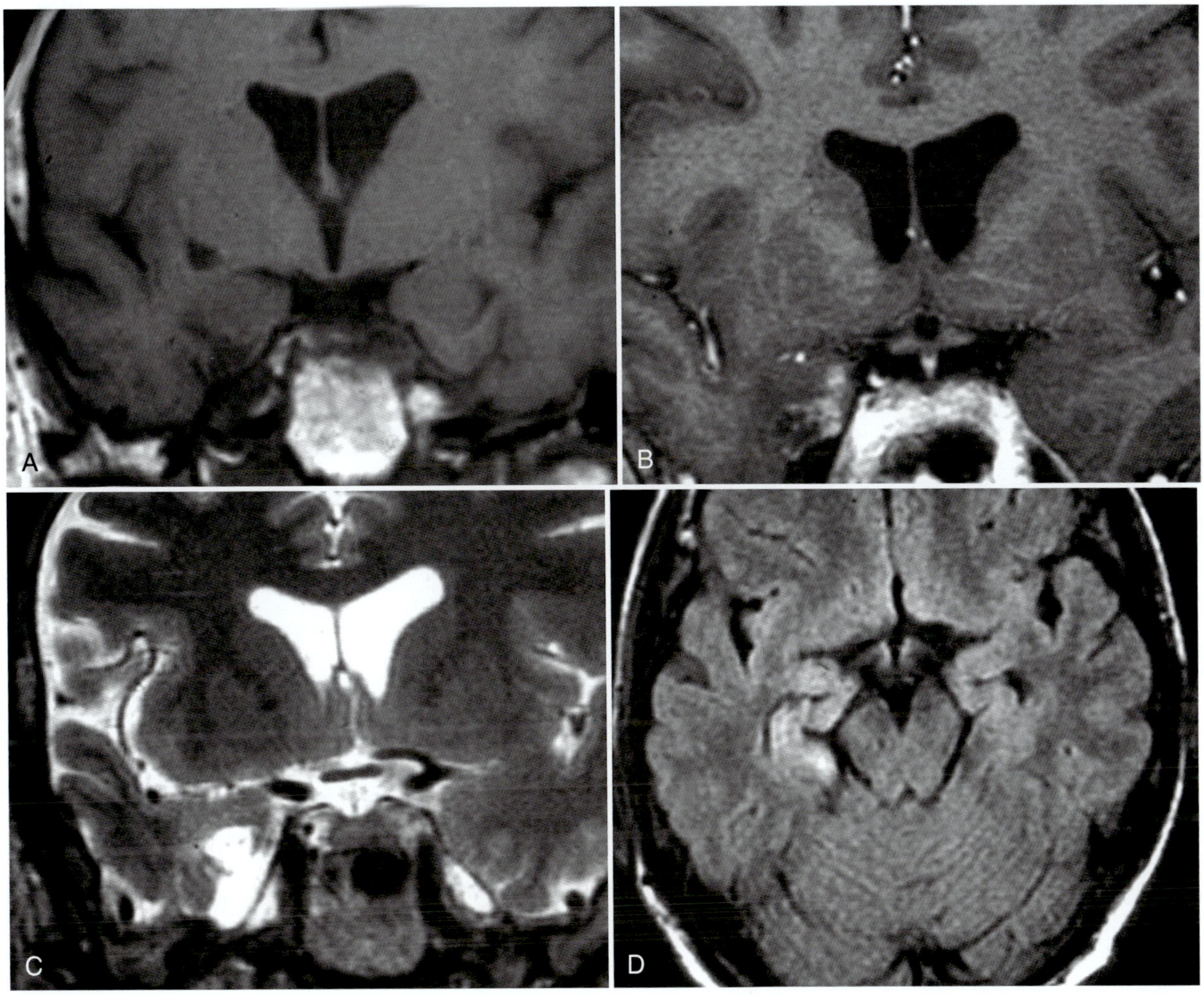

Figure 15-12 Proven case of ganglioglioma in right medial temporal lobe in an 18-year-old male patient. **A:** Coronal T1-weighted image following contrast demonstrating subtle lobulated rim enhancement in the same region. **B:** Coronal fluid-attenuated inversion recovery (FLAIR) image showing hyperintensity outlining a slightly lobulated cortical mass and marked hyperintensity on T2-weighted **(C)** and FLAIR **(D)** images.

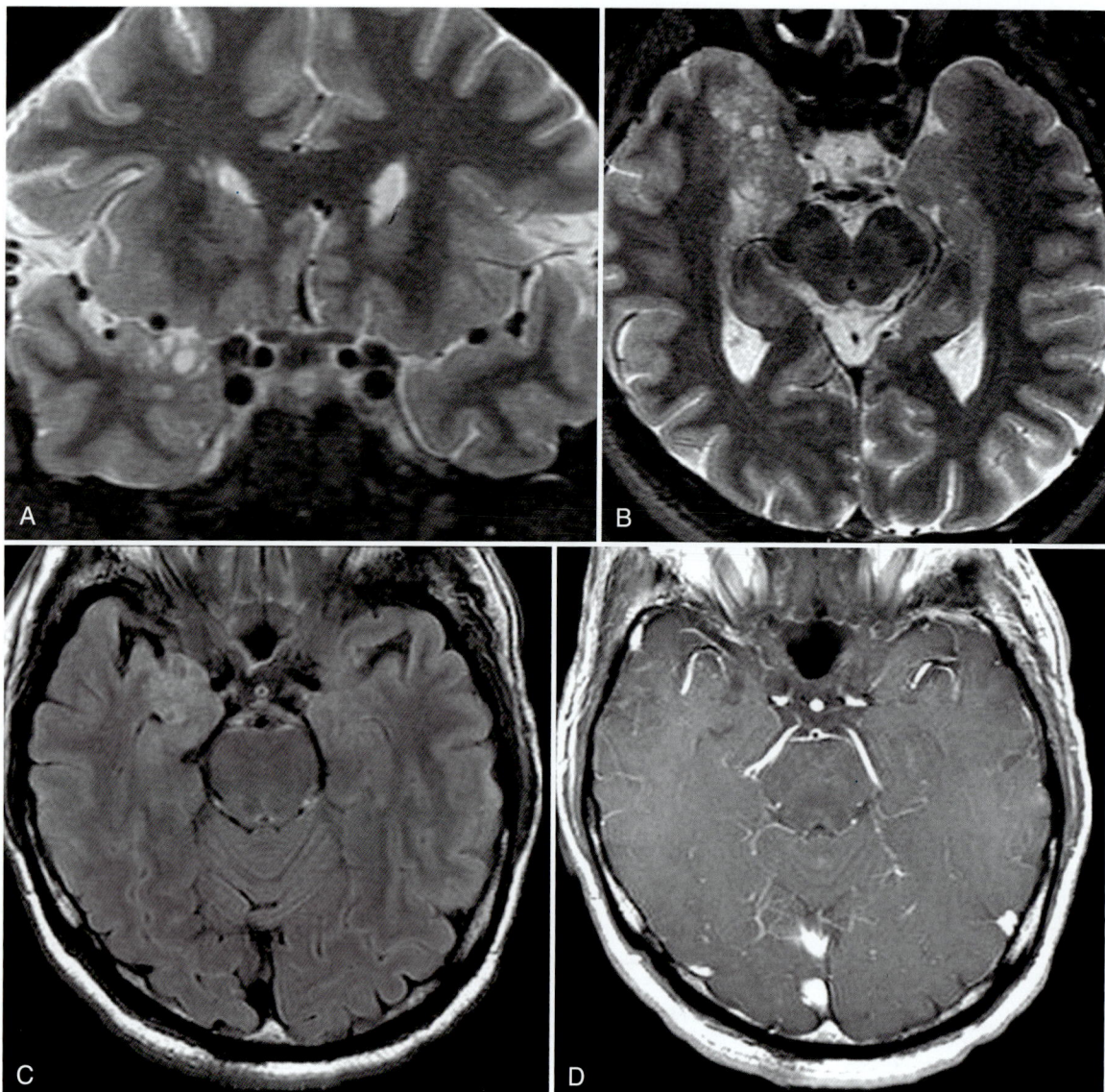

Figure 15-13 Patient in late teens with typical dysembryoplastic neuroepithelial tumor in right temporal lobe. **A, B:** Coronal and axial T2-weighted magnetic resonance images showing a multicystic (bubbly) lesion extending from the mesial right temporal cortex and temporal pole into the subcortical white matter. **C:** Axial fluid-attenuated inversion recovery image demonstrating the lesion is hyperintense. **D:** No significant enhancement is seen after contrast.

Sturge-Weber Syndrome

Sturge-Weber syndrome is usually a sporadic congenital neurocutaneous syndrome in which fetal cortical veins fail to develop normally with ipsilateral facial angioma in the distribution of ophthalmic branch of the trigeminal nerve. This condition does not usually present a diagnostic challenge because of its stark clinical and imaging features. Patients can present with variable neurologic symptoms, including intractable seizures and hemiparesis.

Imaging features are the result of progressive venous and chronic venous ischemia. Classic tramtrack calcification is often diagnostic on CT. MRI can demonstrate pial angiomatosis, unilateral atrophy, hyperintense cortical signal from gliosis, cortical signal loss to calcification, leptomeningeal enhancement, and ipsilateral engorged and enhancing choroid plexus (Figure 15-16).

Malformations of Cortical Development

Developmental malformations constitute 10% to 50% of pediatric epilepsy cases and 4% to 25% of adult cases.

Malformations of cortical development can be classified into four categories:

1. Malformations due to abnormal neuronal and glial proliferation or apoptosis
2. Malformations due to abnormal neuronal migration
3. Malformations due to abnormal cortical organization
4. Malformation of cortical development not otherwise classified

Focal cortical dysplasia (FCD) is a distinct subtype of malformation of cortical development. The findings in FCD can be very subtle and sometimes can only be appreciated microscopically. Epilepsy secondary to FCD is thought to be difficult to treat by medication because they have high intrinsic epileptogenicity. It is the most common cause of intractable epilepsy in children, accounting for the vast majority of surgically treated cases in children younger than 3 years. Linear subcortical T2 hyperintensity extending to the ventricle and associated with cortical thickening is associated with a particular subtype of FCD containing "balloon cells," first described by Taylor et al (type IIB FCD). It is also the most common operated FCD (Figure 15-17). Other findings include blurring of the gray–white matter junction, focal cortical thickening, and gray matter T2 hyperintensity (Figure 15-18).

Malformations due to abnormal neuronal migration are rarely operated on for seizure control. They include the heterotopias, such as band type (Figure 15-19), subependymal type (Figure 15-20), lissencephalies (Figure 15-21), and schizencephalies (Figure 15-22). Holoprosencephaly is a congenital brain malformation wherein the forebrain fails to normally bifurcate of which there are four types: alobar, with complete failure of separation; semilobar, the intermediate form; lobar, the least severe form; and middle interhemispheric variant (MIH), also know as *syntelencephaly* (Figure 15-23).

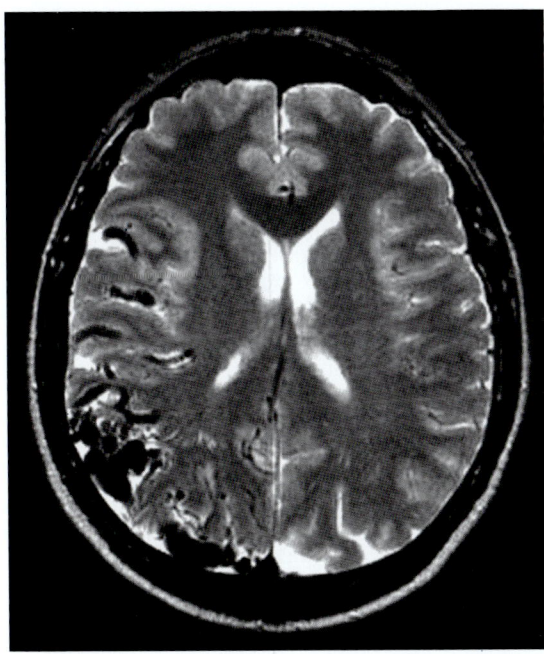

Figure 15-14 Pial/parenchymal arterio venous malformation. Axial T2-weighted image showing a large right parietooccipital parenchymal arteriovenous malformation characterized by large serpentine flow voids. There is no mass effect and the adjacent cortex is atrophic, "accommodating" the malformation.

Pleomorphic Xanthoastrocytomas

Like DNETs and gangliogliomas, pleomorphic xanthoastrocytomas, a benign subtype of astrocytoma, are found almost exclusively in young adults and most frequently in the temporal lobes. They are WHO grade II neoplasms and represent less than 1% of all astrocytomas. A supratentorial cortical mass with an adjacent enhancing dural tail should raise suspicion of pleomorphic xanthoastrocytoma. Involvement of the leptomeninges is a feature of this tumor. The deep margin of the tumor may show infiltration of the brain parenchyma.

Vascular Malformations

Arteriovenous malformations (Figure 15-14) and cavernous hemangiomas are the most frequent vascular malformations causing seizure in epilepsy patients.

Cavernous Hemangiomas/Cavernomas

Cavernomas are more frequently associated with seizures, particularly partial seizures, than are arteriovenous malformations. Cavernomas are mulberry-like vascular lesions consisting of ectatic endothelium-lined channels. Imaging with gradient and susceptibility-weighted imaging have made cavernomas even more conspicuous as focal "blooming" low-signal lesions that may also have "popcorn" high signal contrast on T2-weighted images (Figure 15-15). Cavernoma-related epileptogenicity is thought to be due to chronic, clinically silent, microhemorrhaging. Epileptic seizures that are linked to cavernomas are often medically refractory.

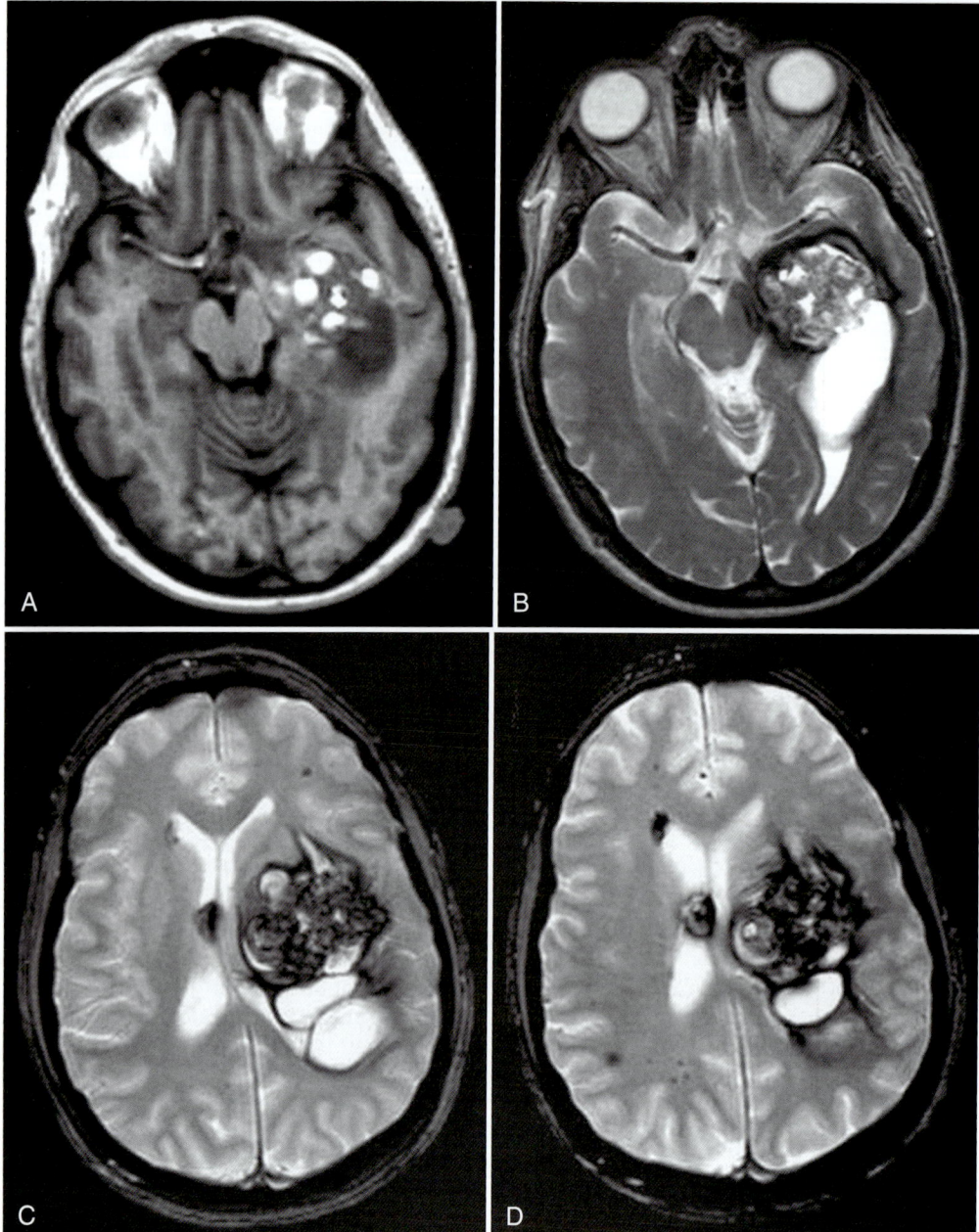

Figure 15-15 Cavernous malformation. **A:** Axial T1-weighted image demonstrating a large lobulated left temporal mass with multiple hyperintense internal regions. **B:** Axial T2-weighted image showing a rim of low signal involving the same lesion. **C, D:** Unusually large cavernous malformation in left hemisphere and multiple other smaller lesions revealed by gradient imaging seen in the right hemisphere.

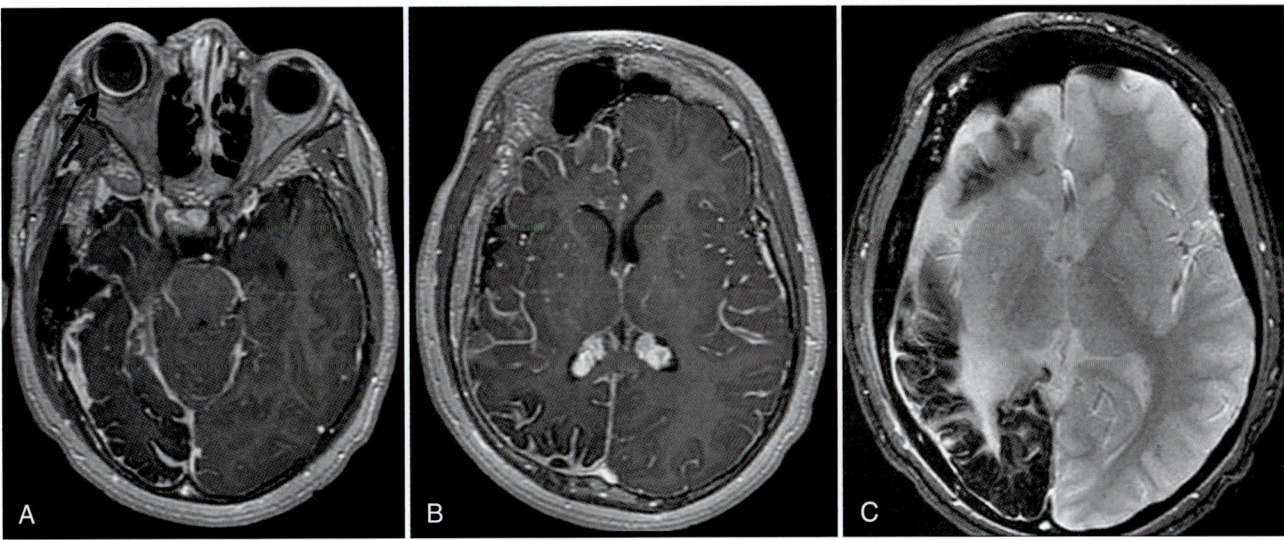

Figure 15-16 Severe case of right-sided Sturge-Weber syndrome in an 11-year-old male patient with choroidal angioma. **A, B:** Contrast-enhanced axial T1 magnetic resonance image showing choroidal angioma *(arrow)*, periorbital enhancement, and enhancement of the enlarged ipsilateral greater wing of sphenoid. **C:** Axial T2* gradient-recalled echo showing striking cortical susceptibility from chronic hemosiderin deposition. Note ipsilateral hemispheric volume loss.

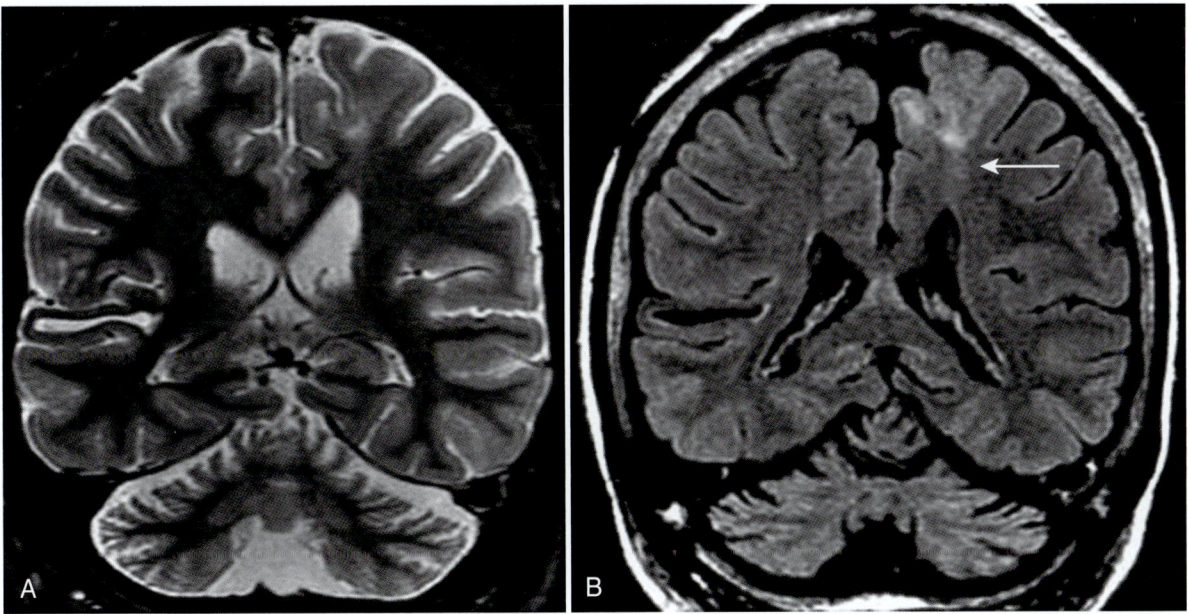

Figure 15-17 Type II focal cortical dysplasia in a 43-year-old female patient. Coronal T2-weighted **(A)** and coronal fluid-attenuated inversion recovery **(B)** magnetic resonance images showing focal cortical thickening of the gray matter in the left frontal region with linear subcortical hyperintensity extending to the ventricle *(arrow)*.

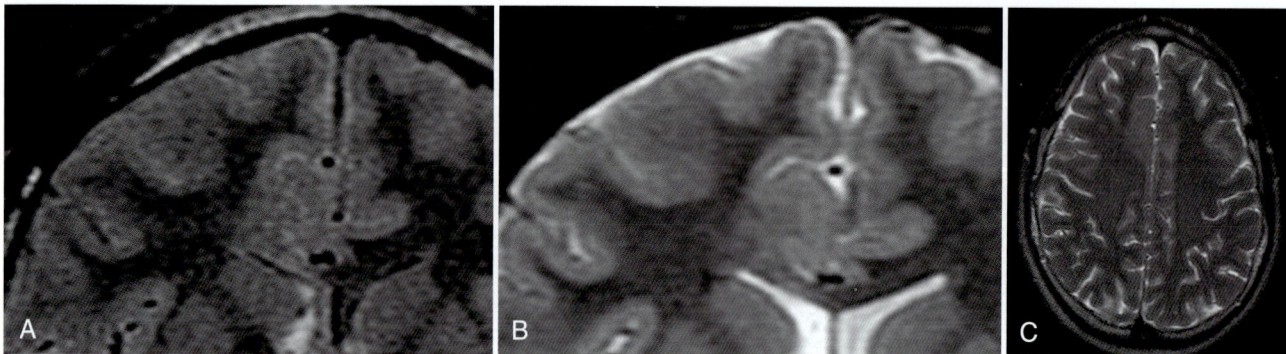

Figure 15-18 Type I focal cortical dysplasia in the region of the anterior right cingulate gyrus. Magnified coronal fluid-attenuated inversion recovery (**A**) and T2-weighted (**B**) magnetic resonance images showing a subtle hyperintense area in the subcortical white matter of the anterior right cingulate gyrus and subjacent corpus callosum. **C:** Axial T2-weighted image demonstrating the subtle finding and blurring of the gray–white matter junction compared to the normal contralateral side.

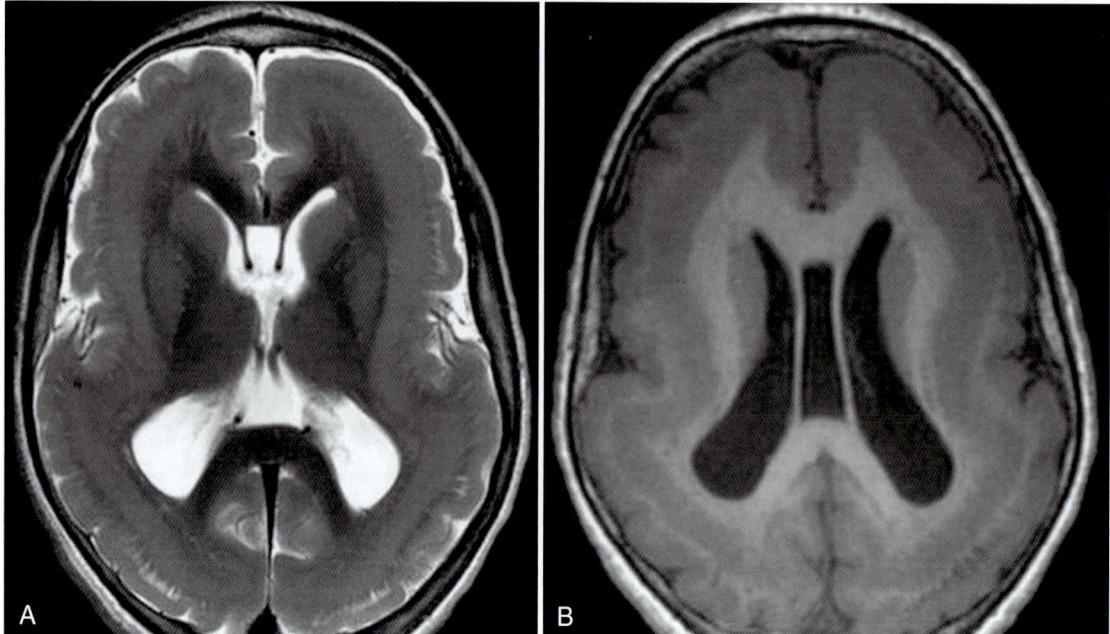

Figure 15-19 Band heterotopia, double cortex in an infant. **A:** Axial T2-weighted image. **B:** Axial T1-weighted image. Global simplification of the cortical gyration and bilateral thick subcortical heterotopic gray matter bands are seen. Note shallow sylvian fissures and incidental cavum septi pellucidi with cavum vergae.

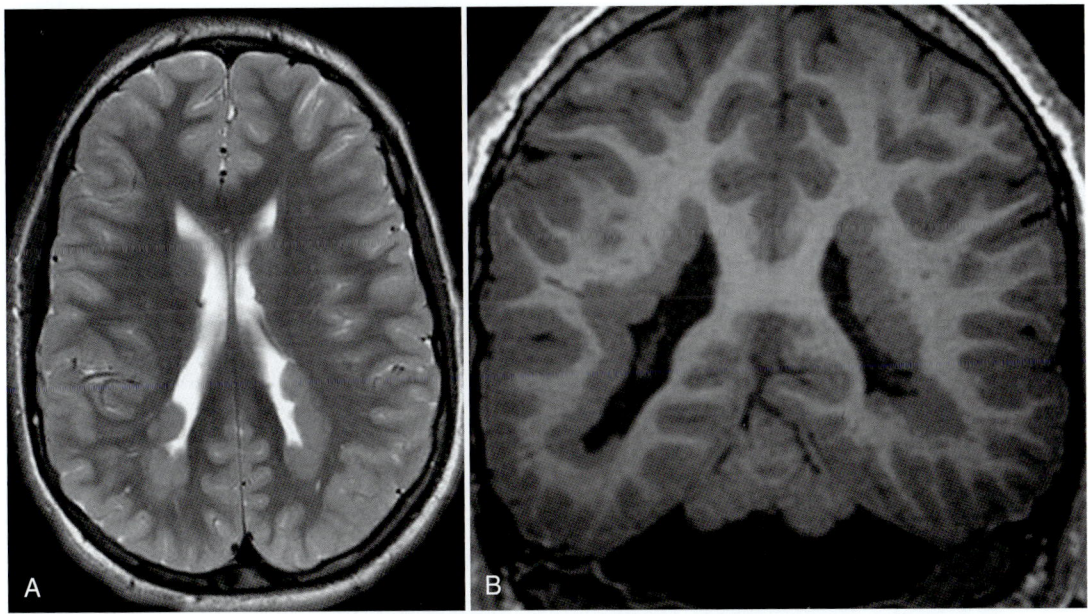

Figure 15-20 Nodular subependymal heterotopic gray matter in a 13-year-old male patient. **A:** Axial T2-weighted image showing bilateral subependymal heterotopia lining the arium of the lateral ventricles. **B:** Coronal T1-weighted image showing extensive bilateral subependymal heterotopia of the left frontal gray matter cortex is thin with shallow sulci. Polymicrogyria is also demonstrated in the right parietal and temporal regions.

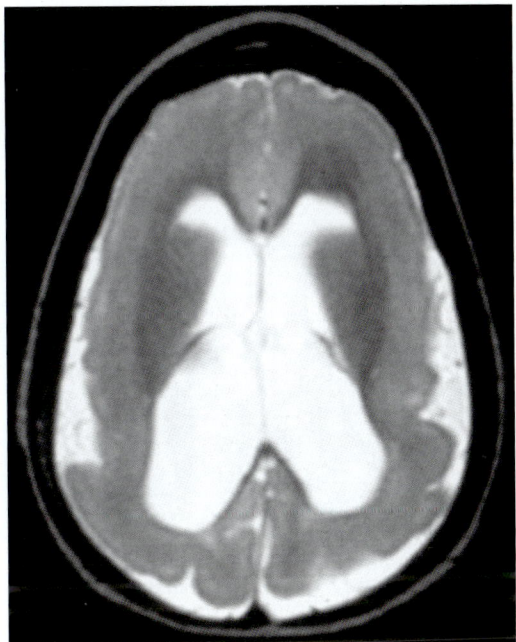

Figure 15-21 Axial T2-weighted image showing classic type 1 lissencephaly resulting in a smooth brain surface, shallow sylvian fissures, and arrested neuronal migration.

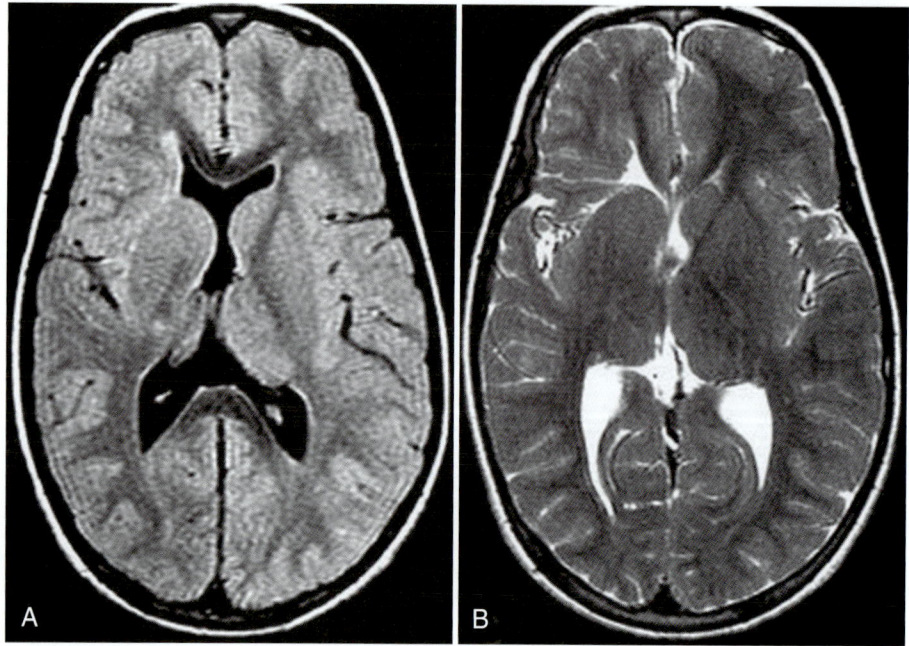

Figure 15-22 Closed-lip schizencephaly extending to the right frontal horn. Axial fluid-attenuated inversion recovery (A) and axial T2-weighted (B) images revealing a "nipple-shaped" outpouching of cerebrospinal fluid from the right frontal horn extending to the subpial surface of the brain. This tract is lined with gray matter.

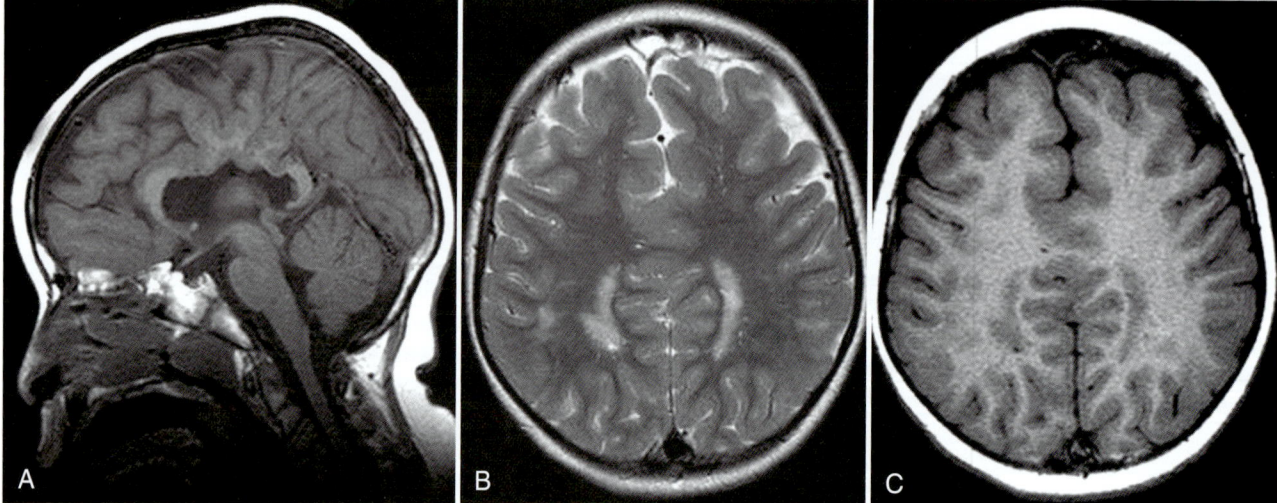

Figure 15-23 Middle interhemispheric variant of holoprosencephaly (syntelencephaly) in a 5-year-old male patient. A: Sagittal T1-weighted image revealing the absence of the body of the callosum in the region of noncleaved parenchyma. Axial T2-weighted (B) and axial T1-weighted (C) images showing abnormal communication across the midline with a bridge of gray and white matter.

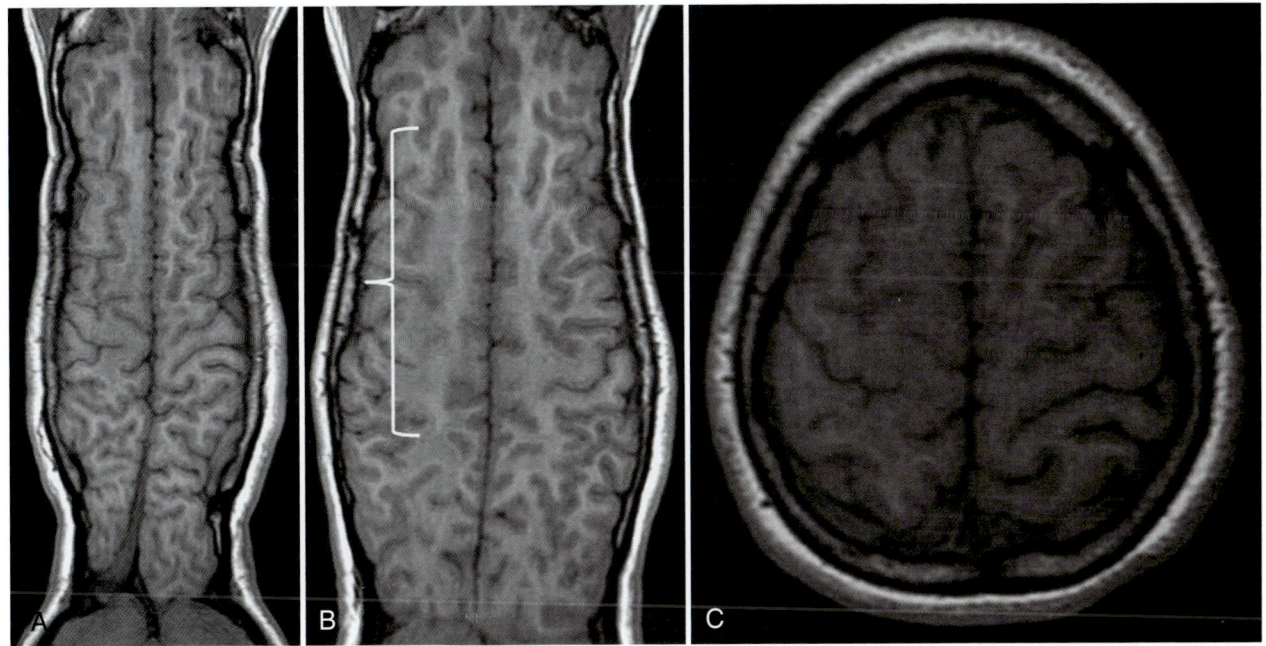

Figure 15-24 Utility of curved multiplanar reconstruction for assessment of cortical dysplasia. **A, B:** High-resolution three-dimensional T1-weighted image dataset can be reconstructed and "rolled out" to aid in the screening of cortical dysplasia *(white bracket)*, which involves almost the entire right high frontoparietal convexity. **C:** Original axial T1-weighted image of the same region for comparison showing the abnormality is less conspicuous to the reader.

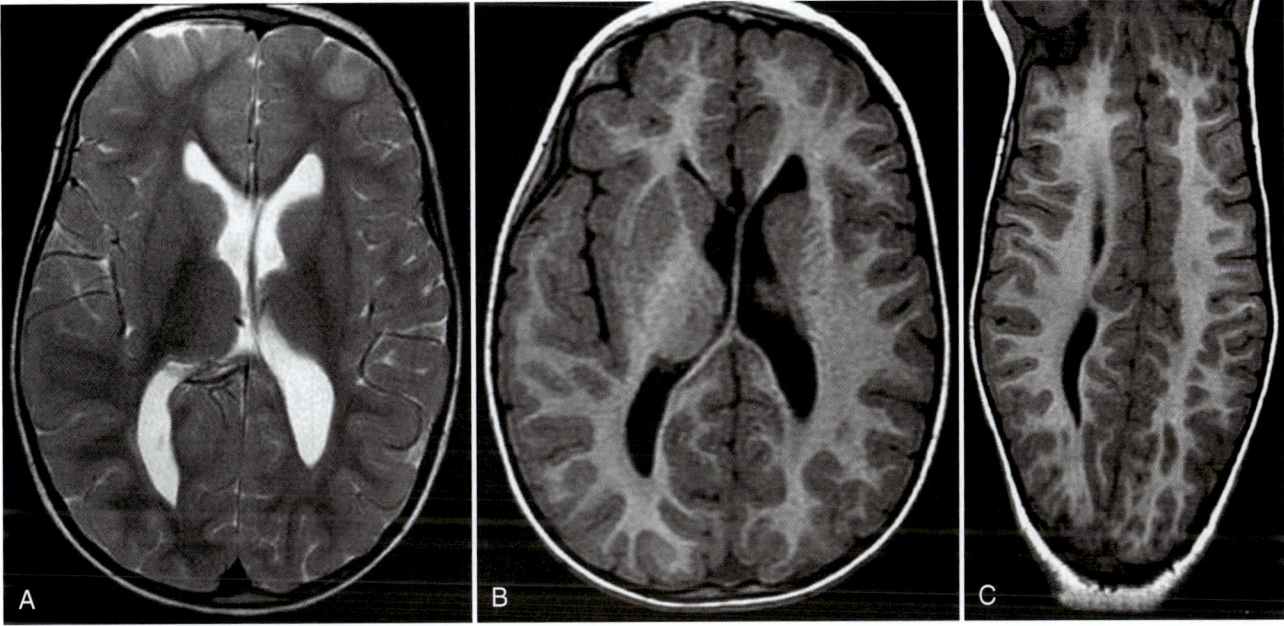

Figure 15-25 Subtle case of hemimegalencephaly. Axial T2-weighted **(A)** and axial T1-weighted **(B)** images revealing asymmetrically enlarged right lateral ventricle and subtle midline shift to the left. **C:** Curved multiplanar reconstruction of the same patient demonstrates subtle "bulky" right hemispheric white matter.

Curved reconstructions of the cortical surface from a high-resolution 3D T1-weighted MR sequence can aid in detecting subtle dysplasias (Figure 15-24) and subtle cases of hemimegalencephaly (Figure 15-25).

Microcephaly in itself can be associated with epilepsy and often is secondary to maternal toxin exposure, such as smoking or alcohol ingestion during early gestation (Figure 15-26).

Tuberous Sclerosis

Tuberous sclerosis is a multisystemic autosomal dominant disorder involving primarily the central nervous system (CNS), the skin, and the kidneys. Neurologic features include infantile spasms, intractable epilepsy, and cognitive disability. In the brain, the characteristic features are cortical tubers, subependymal nodules, and giant cell astrocytomas. Cortical tubers are more directly

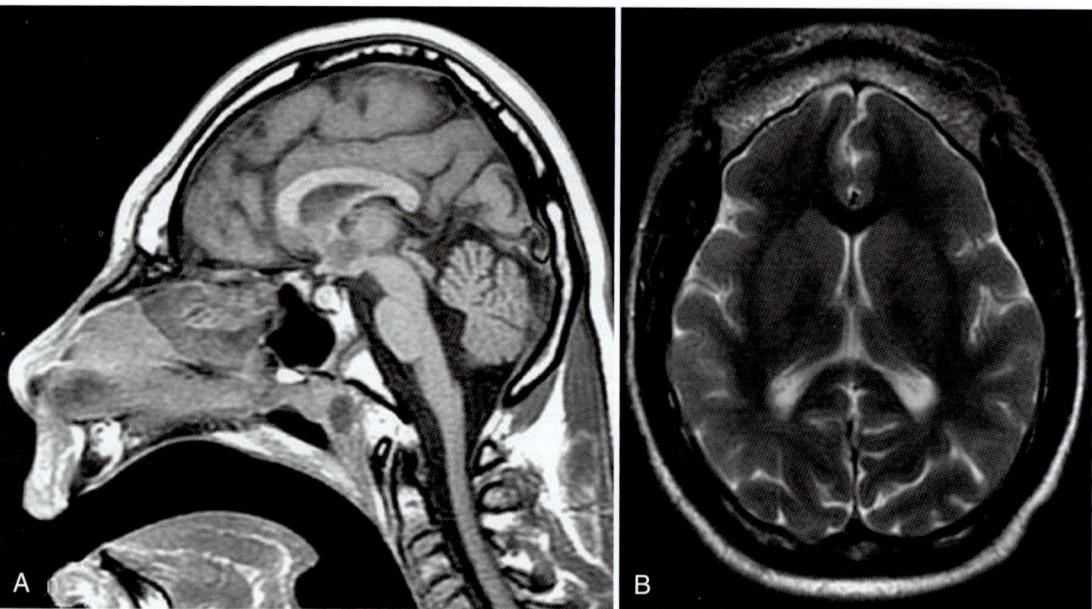

Figure 15-26 Microcephaly. **A:** Sagittal T1-weighted image demonstrating marked decrease in cranial to facial proportions and a conical head shape. **B:** Axial T2-weighted image demonstrating simplification of cortical gyri and a thickened calvarium.

related to epileptogenesis. The junction between gray and white matter in the cortical and subcortical tubers is indistinct. Pathologic changes are similar to those seen in FCD. Cortical tubers are usually well visualized by MRI as enlarged gyri with atypical shape and abnormal signal intensity, mainly involving the subcortical white matter (Figure 15-27). Patients with tuberous sclerosis must be carefully investigated in order to determine whether a single epileptogenic area exists because its surgical removal can yield good seizure control. Two genetic loci for tuberous sclerosis, on chr 9q34 and 16p13.3, form a gene complex product that controls mammalian target of rapamycin (mTOR) signaling, and early trials have shown that mTOR inhibitors such as rapamycin could play a dominant roll in the treatment of tuberous sclerosis in the future.

Gliosis

Gliosis is the end result of various focal and diffuse CNS injuries. Acute cerebral vascular events are a common cause of epilepsy in the elderly. Approximately 4% of patients with an acute stroke will have at least one seizure in the early or late period, and half of these patients will develop epilepsy (Figure 15-28). Hemosiderin and gliosis are known to be involved in seizure generation and propagation. Therefore, any processes that result in gliosis and hemosiderin deposition can lead to epilepsy. Causes include operative factor, closed head injury, diffuse axonal injury, hypoxic–ischemic injury, infarctions, and lobar hemorrhage.

Hypoxic–ischemic brain injury sustained in the perinatal period is a major cause of subsequent chronic disability including seizures. MRI features often reveal symmetric lesions within the basal ganglia and thalami with abnormal signal intensity in the intervening posterior limb of internal capsule. Injury to the cortex and subcortical white matter is most commonly seen around the central sulcus, the interhemispheric fissure and the insula. The greatest cortical damage involves the depth of the sulcal spaces while sparing the apex of the convolutions and resulting in a mushroom gyric or ulegyric pattern.

Posttraumatic epilepsy and seizures are common in children experiencing traumatic brain injury and predict a worse functional outcome. They have an incidence of about 10% in series of severe head injuries (Figure 15-29). Recurring late seizures (relatively remote from the initial event) make up the clinical syndrome of posttraumatic epilepsy. Susceptibility-weighted imaging is a high-spatial-resolution, 3D GRE MR technique with phase postprocessing that accentuates the paramagnetic properties of blood products. It is particularly useful and sensitive for detecting extravascular blood products, as in the setting of diffuse axonal injury, posttraumatic epilepsy, and vascular malformations.

Infection and Inflammatory Causes

Seizures can be the earliest clinical sign of a CNS infection, particularly herpes simplex encephalitis (herpes simplex virus [HSV]) in the elderly population. Tuberculous meningitis or cerebritis and suppurative CNS infections are among the most common causes of seizures worldwide, particularly in developing countries (Figure 15-30). The seizure may be related to the acute inflammatory response early in the infectious process and may be due to gliotic changes in the chronic phase.

Herpes Simplex Encephalitis

HSV type 1 encephalitis is the most common cause of fatal sporadic encephalitis. It can present with variable neurologic symptoms, ranging from altered mental status and focal deficits to focal and generalized seizures. MRI typically demonstrates hyperintensity in the medial

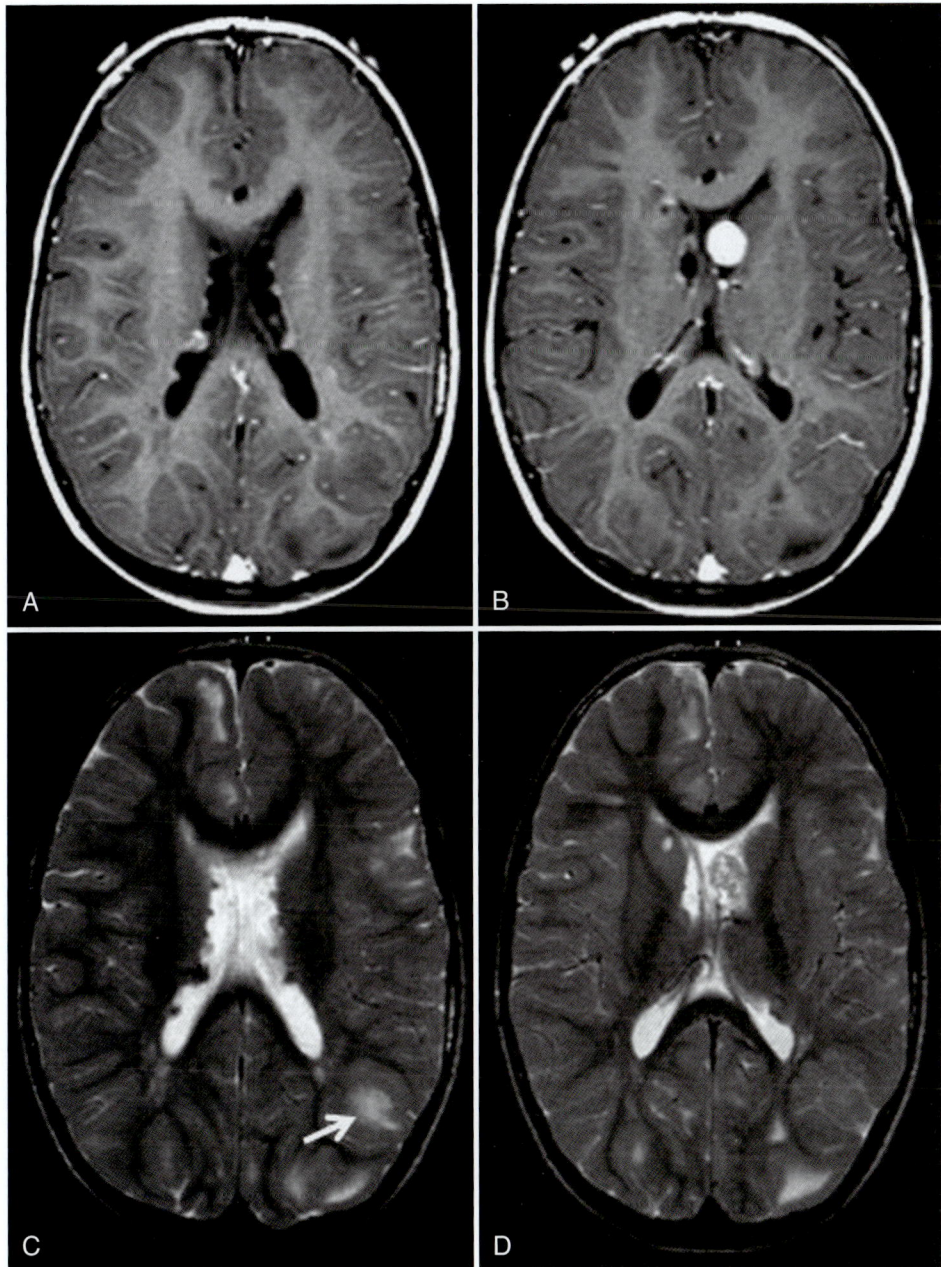

Figure 15-27 Tuberous sclerosis. **A, B:** Axial postcontrast T1-weighted images. **C, D:** Axial T2-weighted images. Multiple cortical, subcortical, and subependymal tubers are seen. The subcortical tubers are best appreciated on the T2-weighted image *(arrow* in **C**). A giant cell astrocytoma is demonstrated adjacent to the left foramen of Monro (**C, D**).

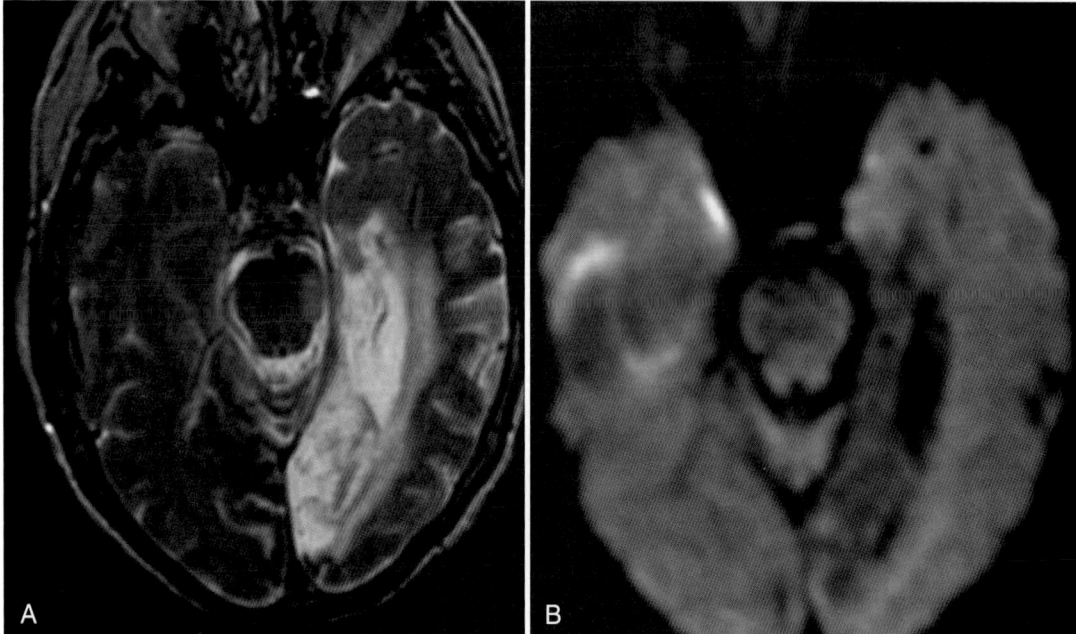

Figure 15-28 Chronic infarction. Seizures may be an early or late complication of cerebral infarcts or hemorrhages. **A:** Axial T2-weighted image demonstrating hyperintense signal and cerebral volume loss in the left posterior cerebral artery distribution. **B:** Diffusion-weighted image showing no evidence of restriction. Overall, approximately 4% of patients with an acute stroke will have at least one seizure in the early or late period, and half of them will develop epilepsy.

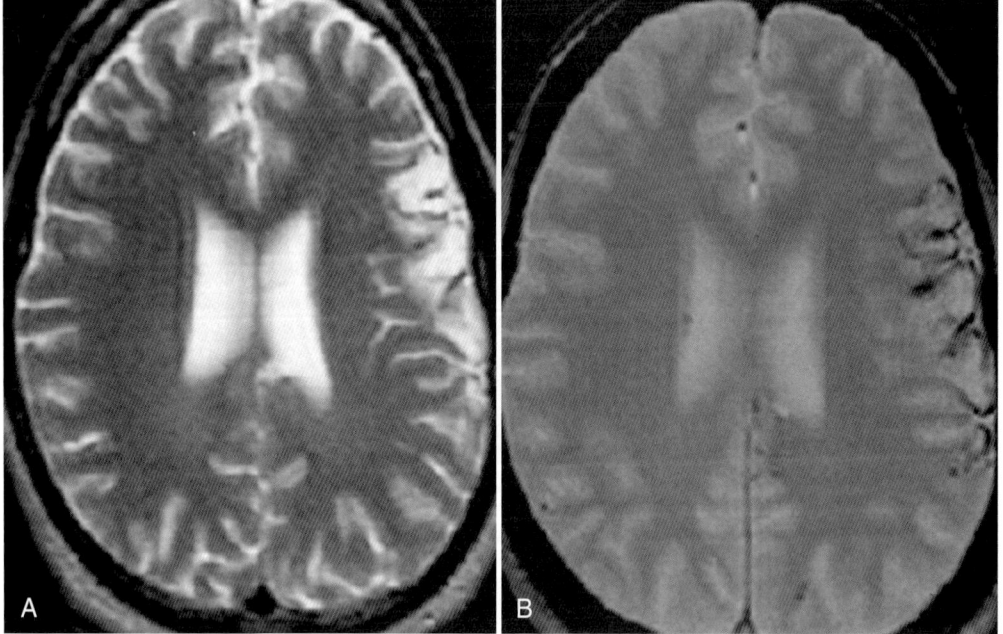

Figure 15-29 Gliosis secondary to trauma. **A:** Axial T2-weighted image showing cortical atrophy and gliosis in the left frontal convexity. **B:** Gradient imaging revealing old blood product in this region of volume loss.

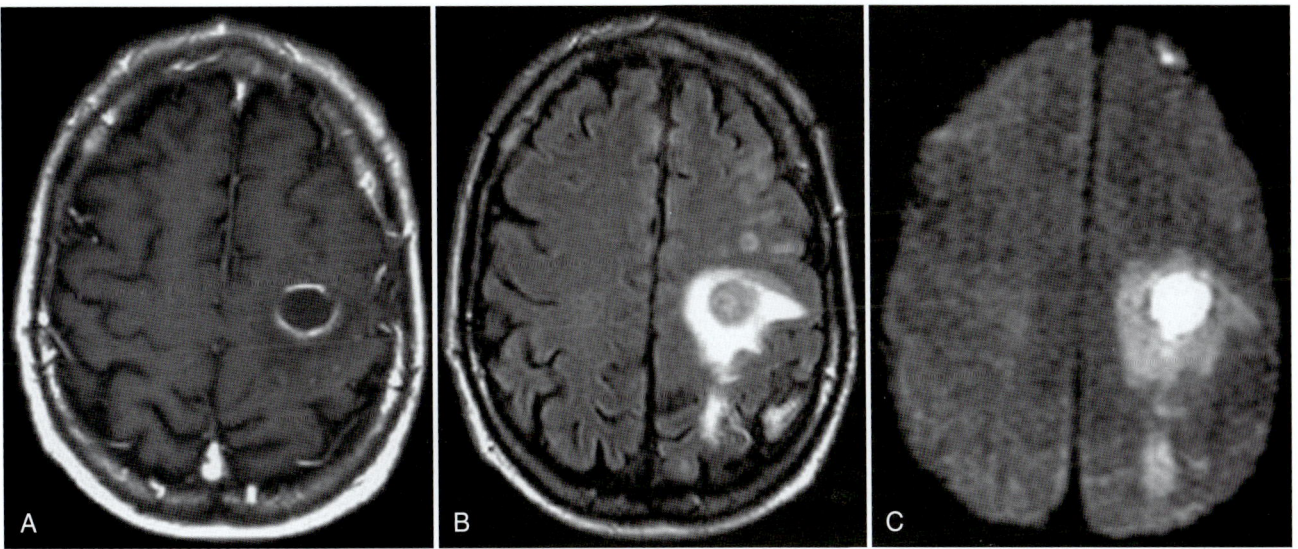

Figure 15-30 Cerebral abscess. **A:** Contrast enhanced T1-weighted image showing a smooth ring enhancing the left frontal lobe mass with extensive vasogenic edema. **B:** Axial fluid-attenuated inversion recovery image. **C:** Diffusion restriction is a relatively consistent finding in pyogenic cerebral abscess.

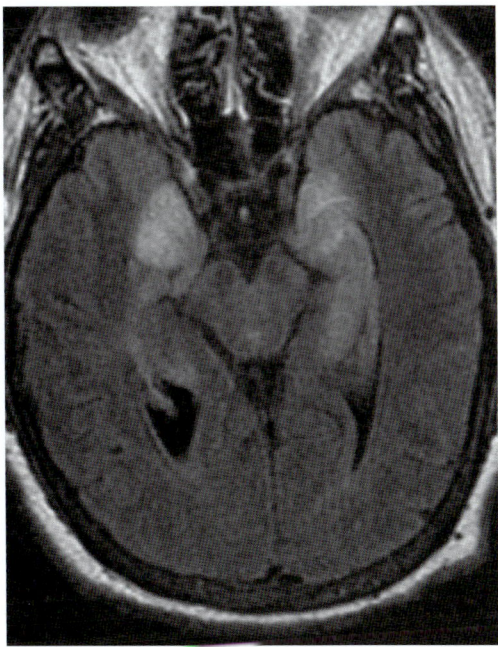

Figure 15-31 Herpes encephalitis. Abnormal high signal intensity on fluid-attenuated inversion recovery imaging is seen bilaterally in the medial temporal lobes, particularly in the uncus and rhinencephalon regions.

temporal, inferior frontal, and cingulate gyrus in a bilateral and asymmetric pattern (Figure 15-31). Late acute and subacute cases can often demonstrate hemorrhage as well as restricted diffusion in the involved portion of the limbic system. Basal ganglia are usually spared, although the cerebral convexity can be involved (Figure 15-32).

Limbic Encephalitis

Limbic encephalitis is thought to be a paraneoplastic syndrome manifesting with neurologic effects associated with extra-CNS tumors. The neurologic disorder and partial seizures may develop before the cancer becomes clinically, overt and the patient may be referred to the neurologist as the primary physician. This paraneoplastic syndrome is caused by autoimmune processes triggered by the cancer and directed against antigens common to both the cancer and the nervous system (onconeural antigens such as anti-HU or anti-Yo in small cell lung and ovarian cancers, respectively) (Figure 15-33). MRI often presents on T2-weighted imaging with hyperintensity in the mesial temporal lobes and limbic system that closely mimics HSV encephalitis but has a different

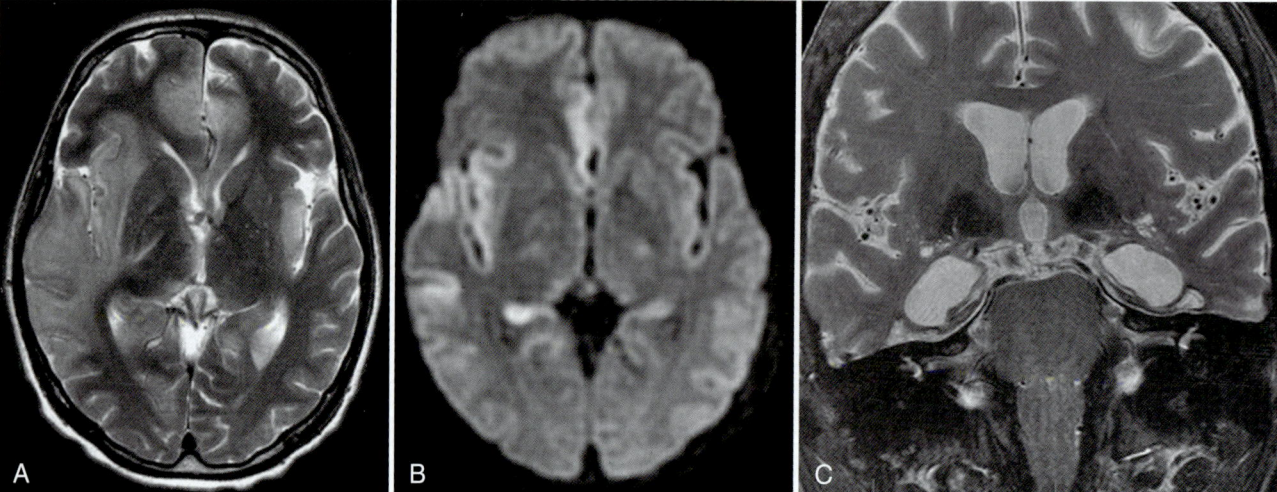

Figure 15-32 Herpes simplex encephalitis type 1 in a middle-aged female. **A:** Axial T2-weighted image demonstrating abnormal hyperintensity in the temporal and insular cortex that is bilaterally greater on the right, sparing the lentiform nucleus. **B:** Diffusion-weighted image showing cortical restrictions in the right insular, temporal opercula, and cingulate gyrus. **C:** Axial T1-weighted image with contrast showing striking cortical enhancement in the right temporal lobe and insular but also subtly on the left side. Enhancing lesions are also seen in the cingulate gyri.

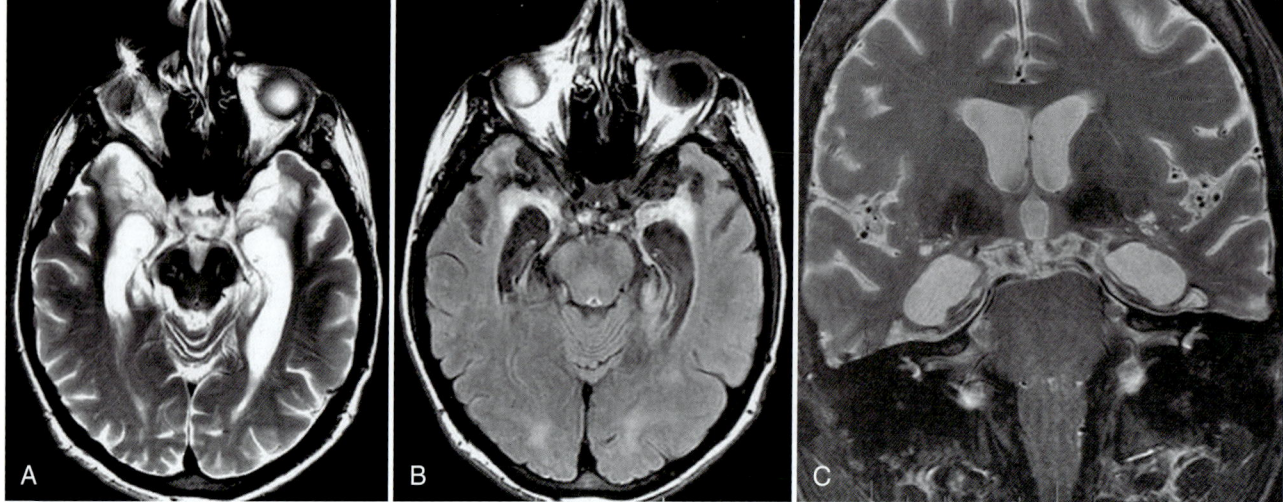

Figure 15-33 Subacute limbic encephalitis and *N*-methyl-D-aspartate receptor antibodies in a 46-year-old male patient with lung cancer. Axial T2-weighted (**A**) and axial fluid-attenuated inversion recovery (**B**) magnetic resonance images demonstrating striking atrophy in the temporal lobes and hyperintense signal in the white matter. **C:** Coronal T2-weighted image best demonstrates the expanded temporal horns reflecting the subacute nature of the presentation.

clinical course due to its subacute or chronic presentation (Figure 15-34). Unlike HSV encephalitis, hemorrhage is not seen in limbic encephalitis.

Rasmussen Encephalitis

A chronic encephalitis called *Rasmussen encephalitis* can be seen in children and young adults as progressive unilateral cortical atrophy, with enlargement of the ventricular system seen over time. It is one of the causes of Dyke-Davidoff-Masson syndrome (Figure 15-35). Degeneration of the corticopontocerebellar fibers can also result in contralateral cerebellar diaschisis. The condition is of uncertain etiology, although autoimmune and prior viral infections are postulated, and in many cases the condition is preceded by an inflammatory episode. Focal swelling of gyri can be seen early during the course of the disorder.

■ PITFALLS IN IMAGING

There are several common pitfalls to be aware of in order to avoid overdiagnosing or underdiagnosing imaging findings suggestive of focal lesions.

If head rotation is present, assessment of hippocampal symmetry must be performed by comparing compatible coronal hippocampal sections in the setting of MTS. Nonrotation can be quickly confirmed by noting if the cochlea and internal auditory meatus bilaterally are in the same coronal image (Figure 15-36). Another potential pitfall in assessing patients for MTS is the

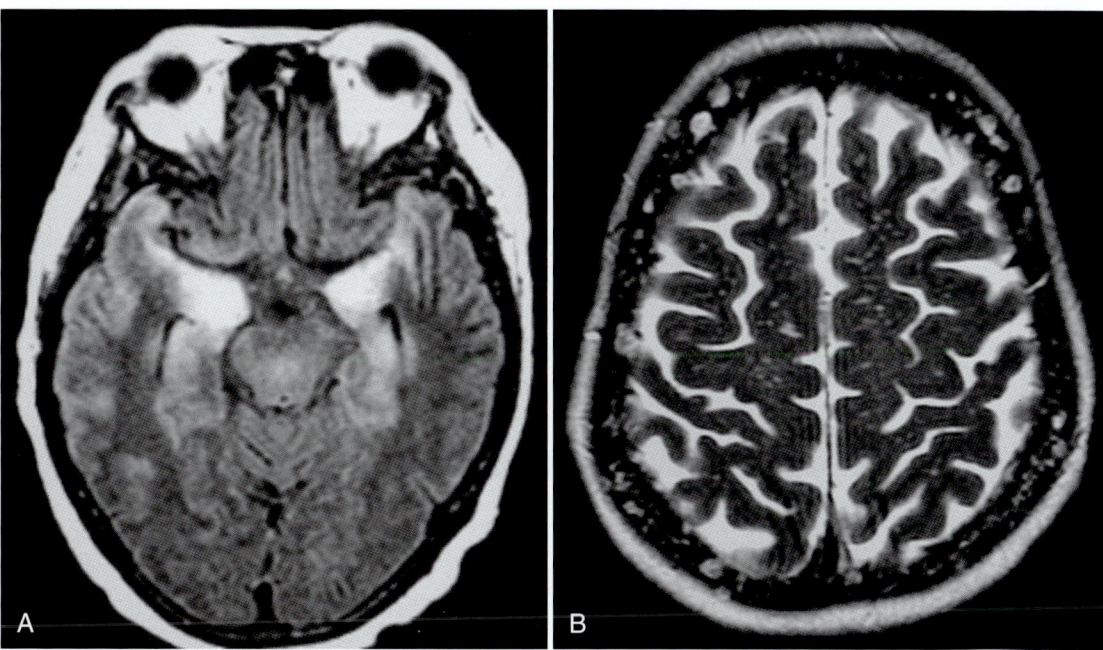

Figure 15-34 Limbic encephalitis in a patient with multiple myeloma. **A:** Axial fluid-attenuated inversion recovery image showing high signal intensity in both medial temporal lobes. **B:** Axial T2-weighted image demonstrating several multiple myeloma skull lesions.

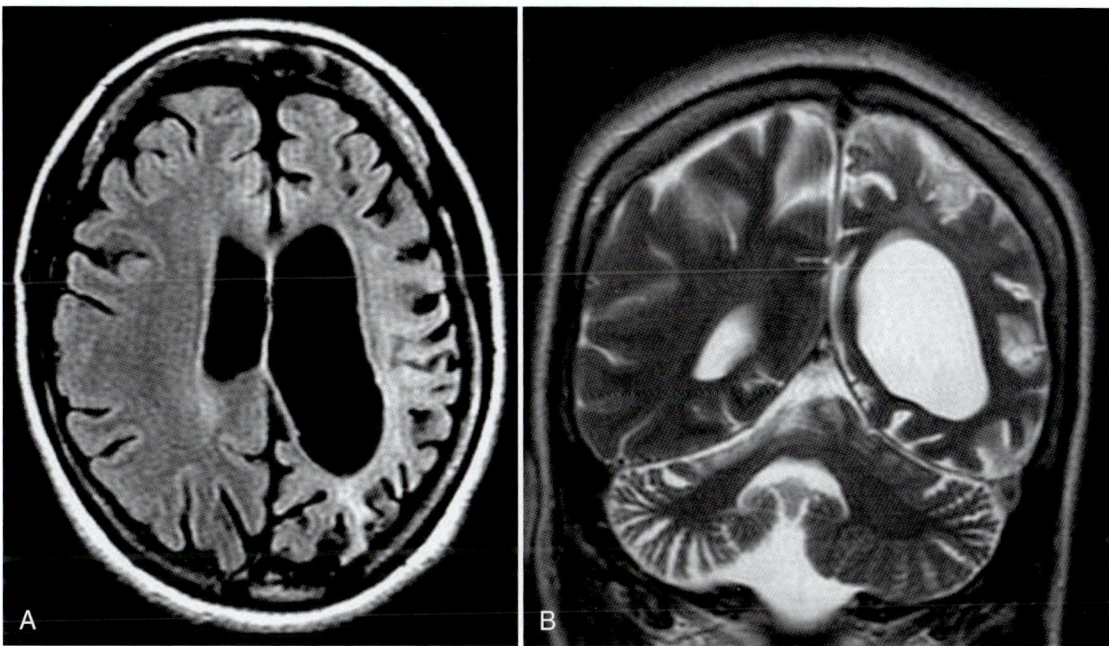

Figure 15-35 Rasmussen encephalitis in a 20-year-old female patient with a history of refractory epilepsy. **A:** Axial fluid-attenuated inversion recovery magnetic resonance image showing marked enlargement of the left hemispheric sulci and ipsilateral lateral ventricle. Increased signal is seen in the underlying white matter. **B:** Coronal T2-weighted image demonstrating crossed cerebellar diaschisis.

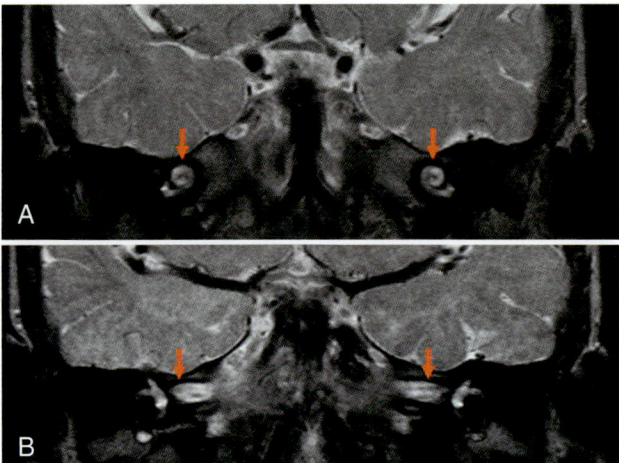

Figure 15-36 Confirmation of nonrotation of coronal images through the temporal lobe. Check that the cochlea (*arrows* in **A**) and internal auditory meatus (*arrows* in **B**) are in the same coronal image.

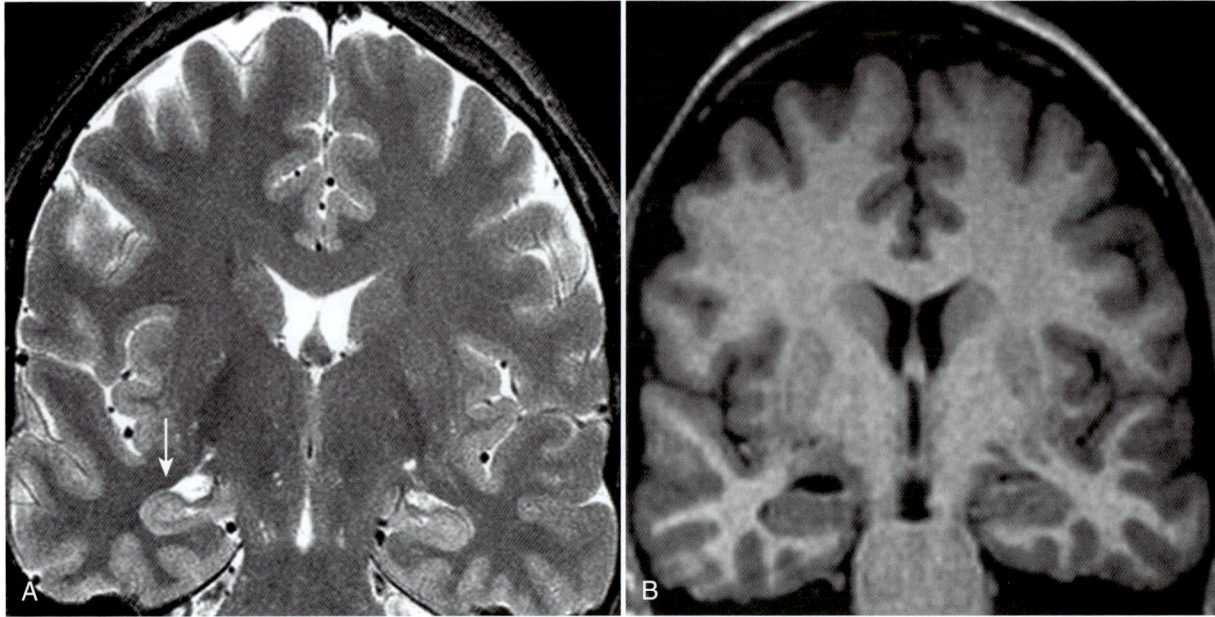

Figure 15-37 Asymmetric temporal horns. This is a potential pitfall in assessing patients for mesial temporal sclerosis. **A:** Coronal T2-weighted image showing asymmetry of the temporal horns due to a choroid fissure cyst, an incidental normal variant. Note the absence of increased signal in the hippocampus or derangement of its anatomy. **B:** Coronal T1-weighted image.

normal variant of asymmetry of the temporal horns (Figure 15-37).

Postictal changes can present as focal or multifocal hyperintense abnormalities of the cortex or hippocampus on long TR imaging and as restricted diffusion on diffusion-weighted imaging (Figure 15-38). Caution should be exercised in interpreting findings and recommending invasive studies for actively seizing patients. Transient lesions can be seen in the splenium of the corpus callosum. This particular lesion is thought to result from either frequent seizures or abrupt changes in antiepileptic drug concentrations that may cause cytotoxic edema in the splenium. Slight mass effect from cortical edema way be mistaken for a neoplastic lesion, and follow-up imaging is crucial to confirm this reversible imaging finding and support the diagnosis (Figure 15-39).

An important pitfall to avoid relates to dual pathology, which is defined as the coexistence of hippocampal sclerosis with another epileptogenic substrate. It is easy to focus on an obvious lesion and neglect assessment of the hippocampus. Coincidental hippocampal sclerosis is not infrequent, especially with developmental anomalies.

■ SUPPLEMENTARY AND COMPLEMENTARY TESTS

Subdural grid arrays are used when seizure activity cannot be located by ictal scalp recordings and when functional cortical mapping is required before surgery

Chapter 15 Epilepsy 531

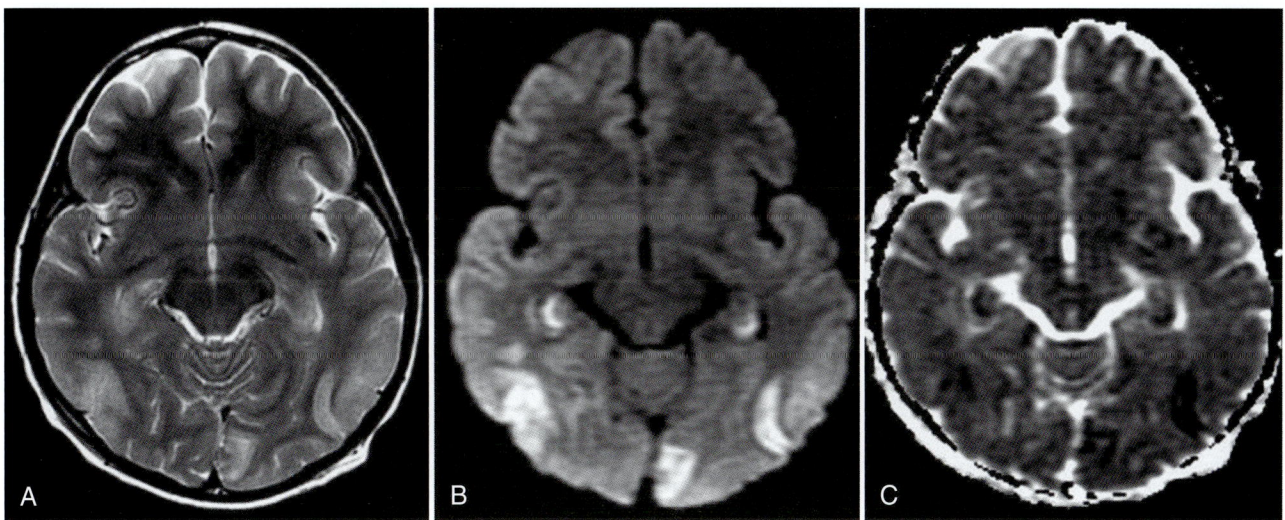

Figure 15-38 Status epilepticus in a 9-year-old male patient immediately prior to imaging. **A:** Axial T2-weighted image showing hyperintensity in the parietooccipital regions bilaterally in a cortical and subcortical distribution. There is sulcal effacement secondary to cortical edema. Diffusion-weighted image **(B)** and apparent diffusion coefficient image **(C)** demonstrate diffusion restriction in the affected areas.

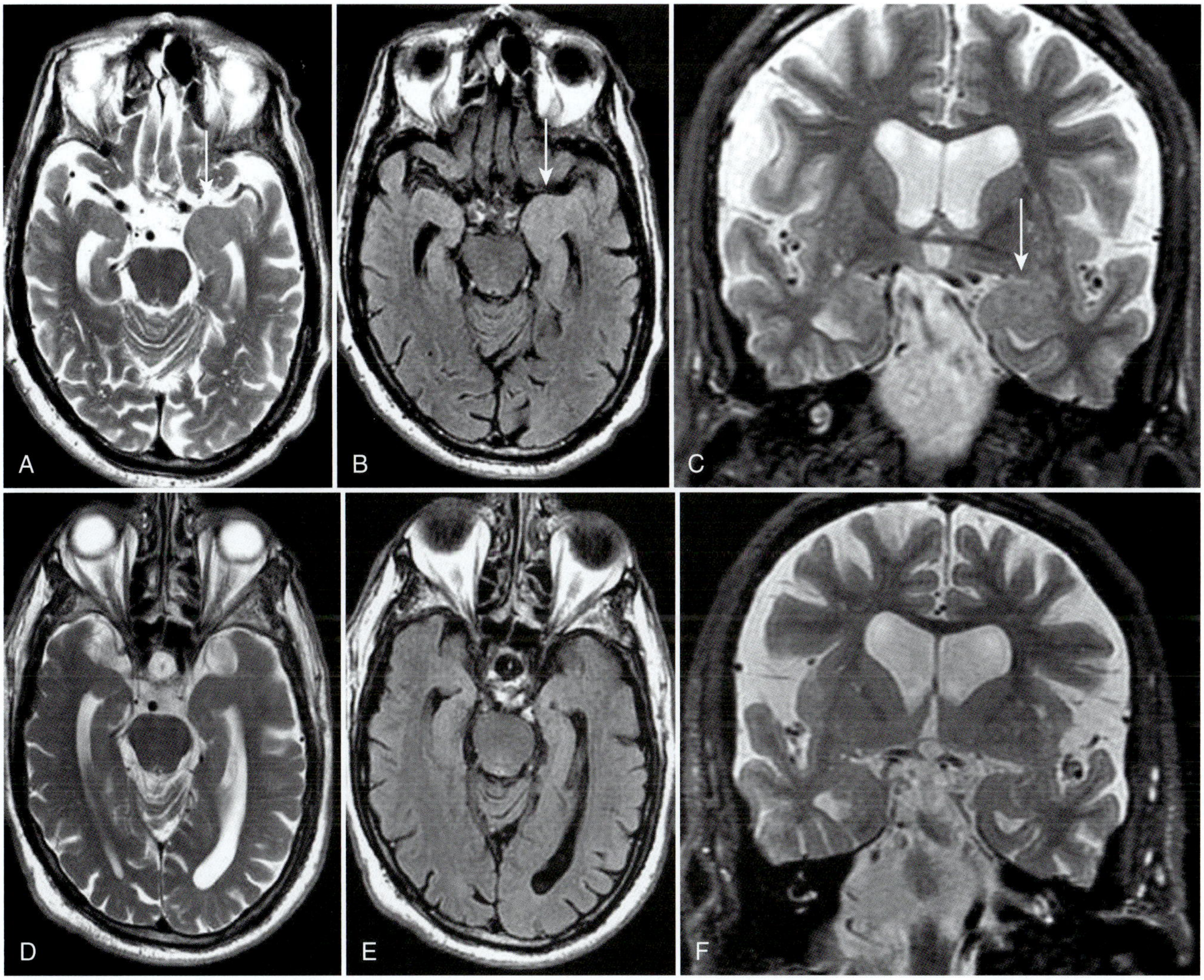

Figure 15-39 Postseizure edema in a 68-year-old patient. Axial T2-weighted **(A)**, axial fluid-attenuated inversion recovery **(B)**, and coronal T2-weighted **(C)** images show an asymmetrically enlarged left mesial temporal cortex and uncus from a 2006 study performed soon after an episode of seizure *(arrows)*. **D–F:** Magnetic resonance images from a follow-up study in 2008 reveal resolution of cortical edema.

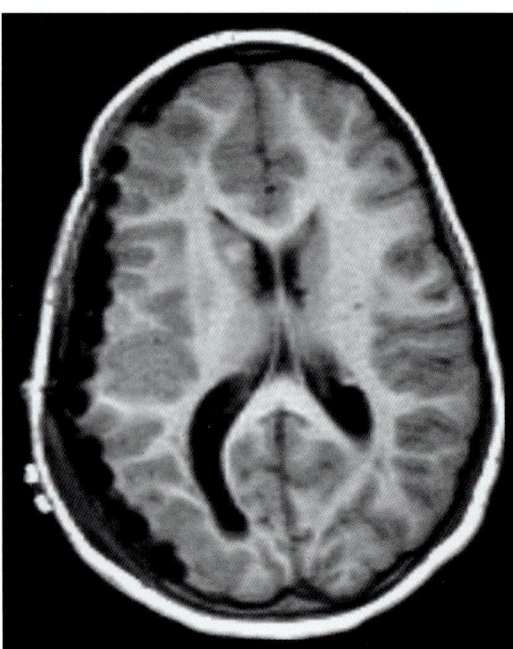

Figure 15-40 Subdural platinum grid electrodes in situ over the right cerebral hemisphere for identification of the seizure-onset zone and mapping of language and motor cortex.

(Figure 15-40). Advanced noninvasive neuroimaging techniques with multimodality imaging are increasingly being used, particularly in cases of pediatric epilepsy. These approaches include fluorodeoxyglucose-positron emission tomography (FDG-PET), magnetoencephalography, diffusion tensor imaging, and magnetic source imaging in combination with conventional MRI. Techniques such as MR/FDG-PET fusion imaging allows the detection of many subtle abnormalities that may go undetected with conventional MRI. Furthermore, these techniques can guide surgical resection in patients with multiple lesions by selecting those with greatest epileptogenic activity. For example, MR/FDG-PET in patients with tuberous sclerosis who present with medically refractory epilepsy and multiple tubers can demonstrate tubers with epileptogenic activity, seen as regions of hypometabolic activity in the tubers during interictal imaging.

Suggested Readings

Bote RP, Blázquez-Llorca L, Fernández-Gil MA, Alonso-Nanclares L, Muñoz A, De Felipe J. Hippocampal sclerosis: histopathology substrate and magnetic resonance imaging. *Semin Ultrasound CT MR*. 2008;29(1):2-14.

Cepeda C, André VM, Levine MS, et al. Epileptogenesis in pediatric cortical dysplasia: the dysmature cerebral developmental hypothesis. *Epilepsy Behav*. 2006;9(2):219-235.

Chan S, Erickson JK, Yoon SS. Limbic system abnormalities associated with mesial temporal sclerosis: a model of chronic cerebral changes due to seizures. *Radiographics*. 1997;17(5):1095-1110.

Concha L, Gross DW, Beaulieu C. Diffusion tensor tractography of the limbic system. *AJNR Am J Neuroradiol*. 2005;26(9):2267-2274.

Duncan JS. Imaging and epilepsy. *Brain*. 1997;120(Pt 2):339-377.

El Kamar FG, Posner JB. Brain metastases. *Semin Neurol*. 2004;24(4):347-362.

Engel Jr J. Surgery for seizures. *N Engl J Med*. 1996;334(10):647-652.

Ferroli P, Casazza M, Marras C, Mendola C, Franzini A, Broggi G. Cerebral cavernomas and seizures: a retrospective study on 163 patients who underwent pure lesionectomy. *Neurol Sci*. 2006;26(6):390-394.

Hogan RE, Wang L, Bertrand ME, et al. Predictive value of hippocampal MR imaging-based high-dimensional mapping in mesial temporal epilepsy: preliminary findings. *AJNR Am J Neuroradiol*. 2006;27(10):2149-2154.

Maehara T. Neuroimaging of epilepsy. *Neuropathology*. 2007;27(6):585-593.

Ng YT, McGregor AL, Wheless JW. Magnetic resonance imaging detection of mesial temporal sclerosis in children. *Pediatr Neurol*. 2004;30(2):81-85.

Oikawa H, Sasaki M, Tamakawa Y, Kamei A. The circuit of Papez in mesial temporal sclerosis: MRI. *Neuroradiology*. 2001;43(3):205-210.

Ozturk A, Yousem DM, Mahmood A, El Sayed S. Prevalence of asymmetry of mamillary body and fornix size on MR imaging. *AJNR Am J Neuroradiol*. 2008;29(2):384-387.

Papez JW. A proposed mechanism of emotion. 1937. *J Neuropsychiatry Clin Neurosci*. 1995;7(1):103-112.

Rastogi S, Lee C, Salamon N. Neuroimaging in pediatric epilepsy: a multimodality approach. *Radiographics*. 2008;28(4):1079-1095.

Strzelczyk A, Reese JP, Dodel R, Hamer HM. Cost of epilepsy: a systematic review. *Pharmacoeconomics*. 2008;26(6):463-476.

Taylor DC, Falconer MA, Bruton CJ, Corsellis JA. Focal dysplasia of the cerebral cortex in epilepsy. *J Neurol Neurosurg Psychiatry*. 1971;34(4):369-387.

Urbach H. Imaging of the epilepsies. *Eur Radiol*. 2005;15(3):494-500.

Villemure JG, de Tribolet N. Epilepsy in patients with central nervous system tumors. *Curr Opin Neurol*. 1996;9(6):424-428.

Willmore LJ. Post-traumatic epilepsy: cellular mechanisms and implications for treatment. *Epilepsia*. 1990;3(Suppl 31):S67-S73.

CHAPTER 16
Neuroimaging of Pediatric Hypoxic–Ischemic Injury

Andre D. Furtado, Saulo Lacerda, and Thomas P. Naidich

■ WHY IMAGING?

Hypoxic–ischemic injury in preterm or full-term neonates is a major cause cerebral palsy, seizures, and cognitive disorders. Additionally, preterm neonates with periventricular leukomalacia also present spastic paraparesis. In older children, the incidence of ischemic stroke is higher than once suspected. Imaging should be performed when hypoxic-ischemic injury is suspected in infants, toddlers, or children.

■ WHO NEEDS IMAGING?

1. Very-low-birthweight preterm neonates. These neonates are at risk for neurodevelopmental disability. Intraventricular hemorrhage is a major cause of adverse outcome. Clinical manifestations of hypoxic-ischemic injury in preterm neonates include spastic paraplegia, cerebral palsy, seizures, and cognitive disorders.
2. Neonates with clinical hypoxic-ischemic encephalopathy (HIE). Neonatal encephalopathy is a syndrome of neurologic dysfunction including difficulty to initiate and maintain respiration, depression of tone and reflexes, subnormal level of consciousness, and seizures. Neonates with stage 2 or 3 encephalopathies are at risk to have cerebral injury and should be imaged (Table 16-1).
3. Any infant or child with new neurologic deficit. Imaging is indicated to any pediatric patient with new neurologic deficit, especially if stroke is suspected.

■ PROBLEM SOLVING: HOW TO IMAGE/WHICH IMAGING?

Cerebral ultrasound (US) can be useful for detection of periventricular leukoencephalomalacia (PVL) and germinal matrix hemorrhage (GMH). It is considered less sensitive than magnetic resonance (MR) for detection of white matter changes and is less sensitive than CT in the detection of small subependymal hemorrhage.

CT scanning is an alternative to magnetic resonance imaging (MRI) for excluding hemorrhage and has some prognostic information. CT should be performed with the low-dose protocol during the perinatal period, which results in a lower signal-to-noise ratio.

MRI is the best modality for diagnosis and prognosis of hypoxic–ischemic injury. T1, T2, gradient echo, and diffusion-weighted imaging (DWI) sequences provide most of the diagnostic information. Perfusion weighted imaging (PWI) can be helpful to define the penumbra ("area at risk") in children with focal ischemic stroke.

■ FETAL AND NEONATAL HYPOXIC–ISCHEMIC BRAIN INJURY

Imaging findings in hypoxic–ischemic brain injury are influenced by brain maturity of the newborn infant as well as severity and duration of insult. The gestational age is one of the most important factors when determining the pattern of the brain damage.

Hypoxic–Ischemic Injury in Preterm Neonates (<36 Weeks' Gestational Age)

In premature infants, the injury occurs mainly in the deep areas of the brain. The periventricular white matter is more susceptible to hypoxic–ischemic injury because it receives blood supply from terminal circulation between the superficial and deep branches of the middle cerebral artery. Diffuse noncystic white matter changes are one of the most common imaging findings.

When the insult occurs from 24 to 26 weeks of gestational age, irregularly enlarged ventricular trigones with minimal periventricular gliosis is most frequently seen. When the insult occurs from 28 to 32 weeks, the typical finding is variably dilated ventricles with more evident periventricular gliosis. Insults at 36 weeks characteristically result in cortical and subcortical atrophy with periventricular gliosis. Early diagnosis of severe hypoxic–ischemic injury is particularly important in the immediate postnatal period, when decisions about active life support must be made.

Cranial Sonography in Hypoxic–Ischemic Injury in Preterm Neonates

Initially, PVL presents as periventricular areas of increased echogenicity that may progress to cystic changes after 3 to 4 weeks. Preterm neonates may have mild periventricular increased echogenicity of uncertain significance (Figure 16-1); however, periventricular white matter as echogenic as the choroid plexus or asymmetric white matter hyperechogenicity should be considered abnormal (Figure 16-2). Cysts are identified as areas with echogenicity similar to that of cerebrospinal fluid (CSF). Of note, congenital periventricular cysts and frontal horn coarctation may simulate PVL (Figure 16-3). With more severe insult, the areas of echogenicity may extend into the subcortical white matter and develop into extensive periventricular and subcortical cystic lesions. To confirm the presence of a structural abnormality rather than an artifact, the periventricular hyperechogenicity and the cysts should be seen in both coronal and parasagittal planes.

Computed Tomography in Hypoxic–Ischemic Injury in Preterm Neonates

Although head computed tomography (CT) is very sensitive to subependymal hemorrhage, it provides little information during the early stages of PVL due to its limited differentiation of periventricular injury and normal myelinization. CT can demonstrate late findings of PVL with reduction in volume of the periventricular white matter, ventriculomegaly particularly with dilatation of the trigones, and irregular ventricular walls. CT should be avoided in neonates given the associated ionizing radiation exposure. A low-dose radiation protocol for neonates should always be applied.

MRI in Hypoxic–Ischemic Injury in Preterm Neonates

Maintenance of body temperature and oxygen saturation greater than 95% is critical during neonatal MR examination. MR-compatible incubators have been developed to provide a less stressful environment for extreme preterm neonates. Infants may be sedated with 50 or 75 mg/kg of chloral hydrate orally prior to the MR examination if not contraindicated. Heart rate and transcutaneous oxygen saturation should always be monitored during the scanning time and supplemental oxygen should be available if necessary. Dedicated head coils has made possible high resolution images of the neonatal brain in a reasonable scanning time.

MR findings in premature neonates with PVL include decreased signal intensity on T1-weighted images and increased signal intensity on T2-weighted images involving the periventricular white matter (Figure 16-4), which below a certain threshold is of unclear clinical relevance. Some neonates may progress to periventricular cysts (Figure 16-5). Cystic lesions are defined as areas with signal intensity identical to that of CSF in all sequences. In more severe cases, intraparenchymal hemorrhagic or cystic lesions may involve both periventricular and subcortical white matter. Of note, dilated perivascular spaces in the peritrigonal white matter may resemble cystic PVL, however, without atrophy (Figure 16-6).

Table 16-1 Clinical Stages of Neonatal Encephalopathy

Stage of Neonatal Encephalopathy	Clinical Criteria
1	<24 hours with hyperalertness Moro and stretch reflexes Sympathetic effects Normal electroencephalogram
2	Obtundation Hypotonia Decreased spontaneous movements
3	Stupor Flaccidity Seizures Suppressed brainstem and autonomic functions Electroencephalogram with isopotential or infrequent periodic discharges

Patients with grade 2 or 3 encephalopathy usually have a poor prognosis and should undergo imaging.

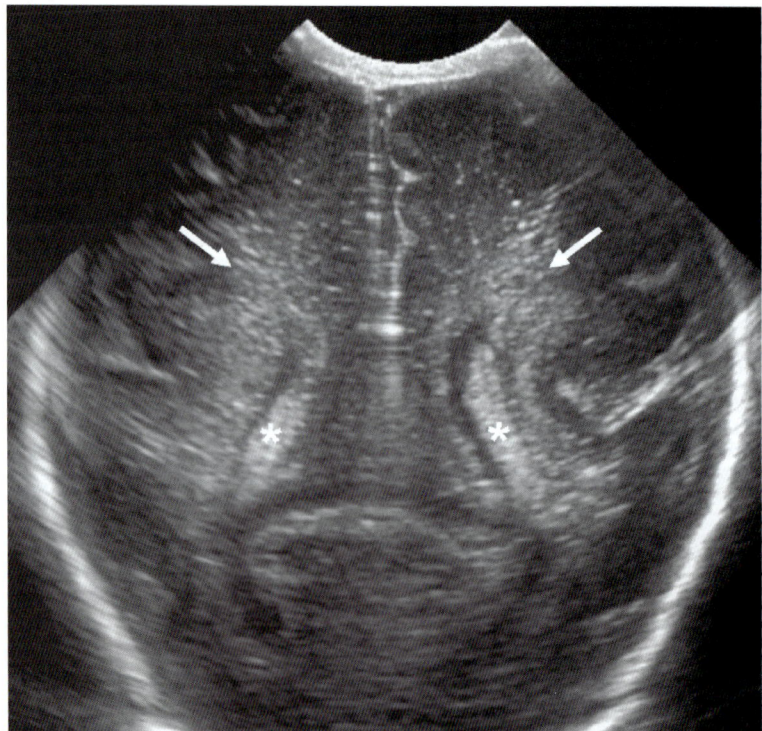

Figure 16-1 Normal periventricular echogenicity in a 5-day-old 30-week preterm neonate. Cranial US demonstrates normal periventricular white matter echogenicity (arrows) that are less echogenic than the choroid plexus (*).

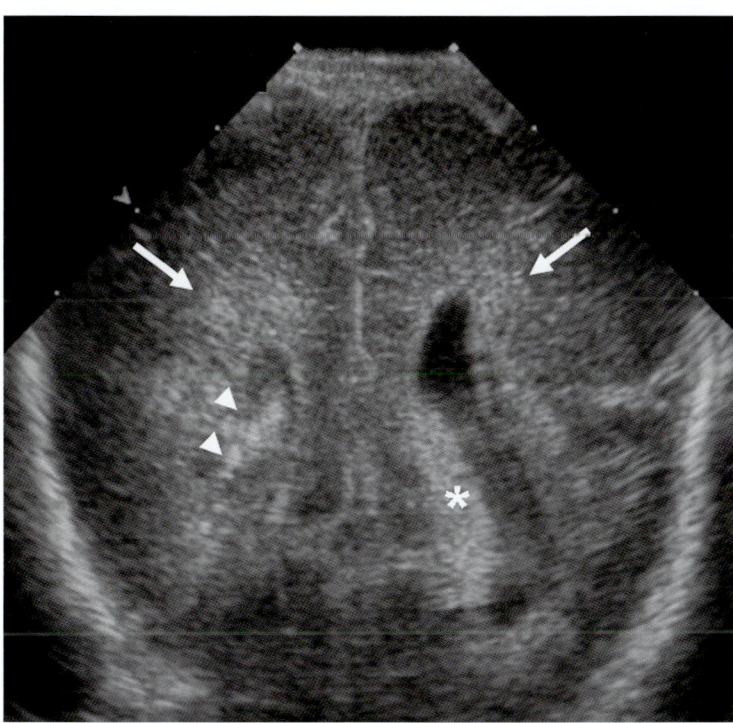

Figure 16-2 Periventricular leukoencephalomalacia in a 6-day-old 25-week preterm neonate. Cranial US demonstrates asymmetric periventricular white matter echogenicity *(arrows)*. The right periventricular white matter is as echogenic as the choroid plexus *(*)*. Note hyperechogenic foci in the right choroid plexus, suggestive of hemorrhage *(arrowheads)*.

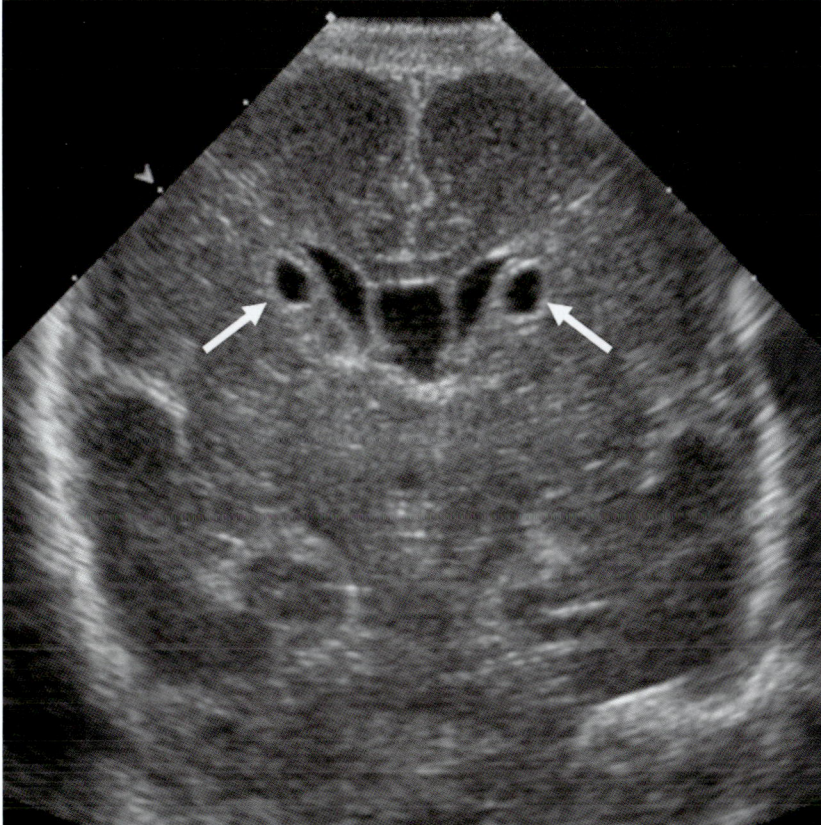

Figure 16-3 Congenital periventricular cysts in a 5-day-old 30-week preterm neonate. Cranial US demonstrates bilateral well-defined areas with echogenicity similar to that of cerebrospinal fluid in the periventricular white matter *(arrows)*. These congenital cysts typically occur below the level of the ventricular angles.

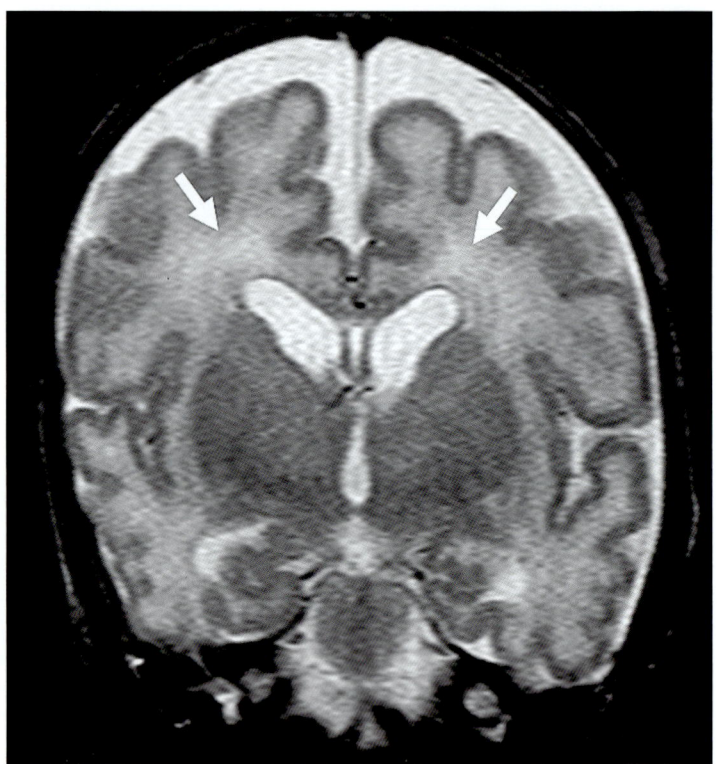

Figure 16-4 Periventricular increased signal intensity on coronal T2 (5610/159) image of a 37-day-old 28-week preterm neonate. This finding is of uncertain clinical significance.

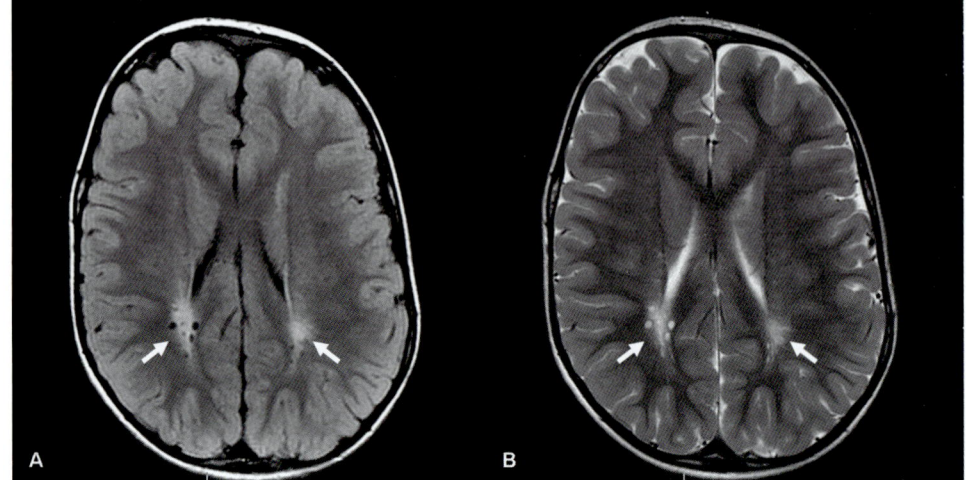

Figure 16-5 Periventricular leukoencephalomalacia in a 3-year-old 29-week preterm neonate. Axial T2 fluid-attenuated inversion recovery (10002/101.4) **(A)** and axial T2 (4700/111.6) **(B)** images show area of T2 hyperintensity and cyst formation in the periventricular white matter bilaterally (arrows).

MRS in PVL

It has been reported that a lactate peak may be seen in preterm infants and infants who are small for their gestational age, as well as in cases of head trauma, inborn errors of metabolism, or mitochondrial disease. It has also been reported that pentobarbital commonly used in neonates with HIE can lower lactate/choline and lactate/N-acetylaspartate (NAA) ratios in the basal ganglia of premature neonates. Therefore, it seems that the role of MRS in hypoxic–ischemic injury of preterm infants is still unclear.

DWI in PVL

The time of the hypoxic-ischemic event in PVL is usually not clear. It has been reported that reduced diffusion and abnormally decreased apparent diffusion coefficient (ADC) values may be evident from a few hours to almost 1 week after the insult. Because the ADC values change with time, pseudonormalization may occur if imaging is performed after 8 or 10 days. Elevated ADC values may not be apparent for two to three weeks. Therefore, lack of abnormality on DWI and normal ADC does not exclude PVL.

Germinal Matrix Hemorrhage

Germinal matrix is the subependymal region of neuronal precursors before their migration to the cortex. Premature and low-birthweight newborns are at risk for germinal matrix hemorrhage (GMH). Birth trauma and hypoxic–ischemic events are the most frequent causes of GMH. Clinically, intraventricular hemorrhage is

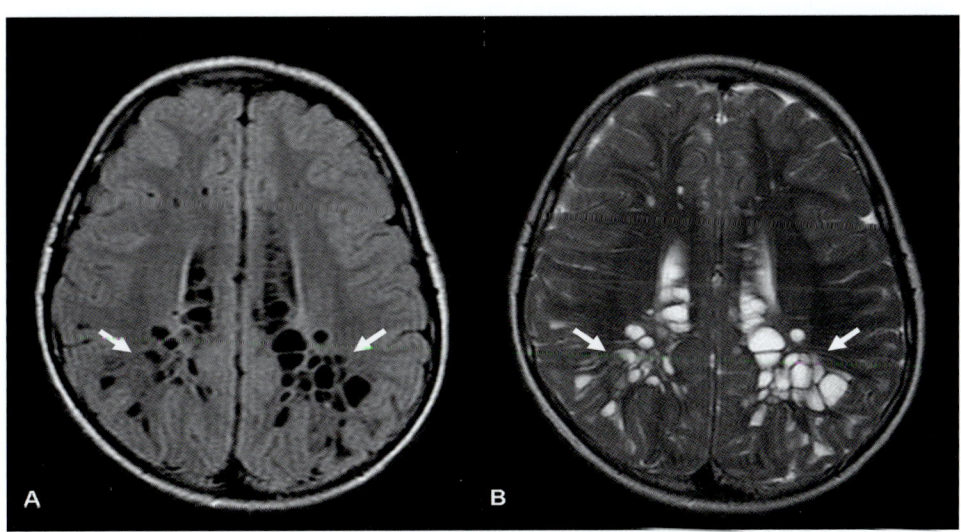

Figure 16-6 Enlarged perivascular spaces in an 8-year-old 27-week preterm neonate resembling periventricular leukomalacia. Axial T2 (4700/111.6) **(A)** and axial T2 fluid-attenuated inversion recovery (10002/101.4) **(B)** images show cluster of cyst formations in the parietal white matter bilaterally without evidence of gliosis of volume loss (arrows).

Table 16-2	Classification of Germinal Matrix Hemorrhage
Grade	**Definition**
I	Hemorrhage confined to germinal matrix
II	Hemorrhage extents to ventricles
III	Hemorrhage extents to ventricles with ventriculomegaly
IV	Hemorrhage into cerebral parenchyma

frequently associated with a drop in the hematocrit. The most used classification for GMH is listed in Table 16-2.

Grade 1 and 2 GMH are associated with a low mortality rate whereas grade 3 and 4 are associated with a poor neurodevelopment outcome and a high mortality rate. GMH typically occurs in the first seven days after birth with a peak on day 3. Early GMH has a higher mortality rate whereas late GMH has a more benign prognosis. Late GMH occurs in less than 5% of the cases and can be of minor severity or clinically silent.

US in GMH
US scans show unilateral or bilateral hyperechoic hemorrhagic material in the caudothalamic groove. Depending on the severity, this may extend into the lateral ventricles and cause hydrocephalus (Figures 16-7 and 16-8). Initially, decreased resistive index (RI) may be seen on Doppler US; however, sustained asphyxia with significant intracranial hemorrhage or diffuse cerebral edema may result in increased RI, which is indicative of a poor outcome.

CT in GMH
CT provides a rapid mode of cranial screening for a GMH hemorrhage in neonates without the need for sedation; however, it is the least sensitive modality for evaluation PVL and is disadvantaged due to the exposure to ionizing radiation. CT can be useful when suspicion for germinal matrix hemorrhage is high and US is equivocal, particularly if MR is contraindicated or not available.

MRI in GMH
GMH typically have increased signal intensity on T1-weighted images and decreased signal intensity on T2-weighted images, but signal intensity can vary. Gradient-recalled echo and susceptibility-weighted imaging may demonstrate blood products (ferritin/hemosiderin) deposition (Figure 16-9). DWI can be helpful as late acute or subacute blood clots may demonstrate reduced diffusibility. Neonates with acute large intraventricular hemorrhages may have fluid-fluid level in the lateral ventricle. Hydrocephalus and parenchymal atrophy can be seen as a complication of high grade GMH (Figure 16-10).

Cerebellar hemorrhage is usually under recognized in preterm neonates. It often occurs concomitantly with supratentorial hemorrhage and is associated with high mortality. US is particularly insensitive for cerebellar hemorrhage compared to MRI. Cerebellar hemorrhage may also be a manifestation of an associated blood disorder. Hemorrhagic foci without PVL are suggestive of blood disorder rather than a hypoxic–ischemic injury.

Profound Asphyxia in Full-Term Neonates (>36 Weeks' Gestational Age)

Profound asphyxia in full-term neonates is associated with injury to the thalami, basal ganglia, and brainstem. Full-term neonates may also have cortical and subcortical involvement and atrophy with more severe insults. Grade 2 or 3 encephalopathy in term infants are known to have a high incidence of neurologic damage and should undergo imaging.

Other findings from a difficult delivery such as caput succedaneum, cephalohematoma, subdural hematoma, or subarachnoid or intracranial hemorrhages may be present.

Transcranial US in Profound Asphyxia
Sagittal sonogram of a term neonate with hypoxic–ischemic encephalopathy shows hyperechogenicity in the basal ganglia and thalami (Figure 16-11). It may be transient or persistent and may progress to cavitation.

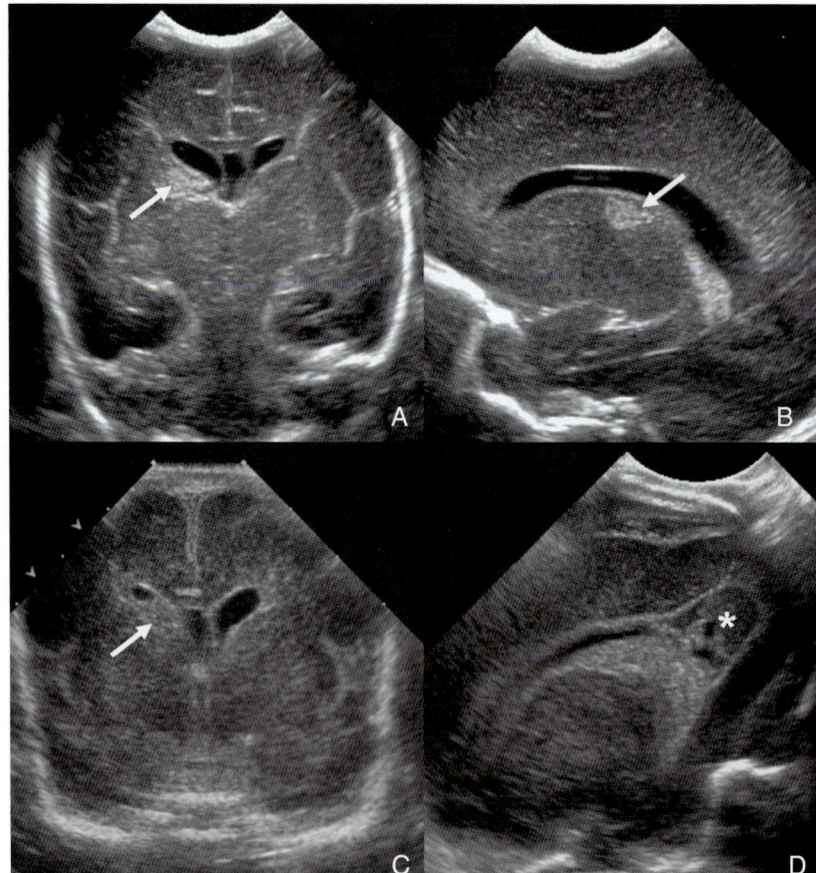

Figure 16-7 Grade 1 and 2 GMH. Coronal (**A**) and sagittal (**B**) cranial US demonstrates nodular hyperechogenicity *(arrows)* in the right caudothalamic groove consistent with grade 1 GMH. Coronal (**C**) and sagittal (**D**) cranial US images of a different preterm neonate demonstrate extension into the frontal *(arrows)* and occipital *(*)* horns of right lateral ventricle without significant hydrocephalus, consistent with grade 2 GMH.

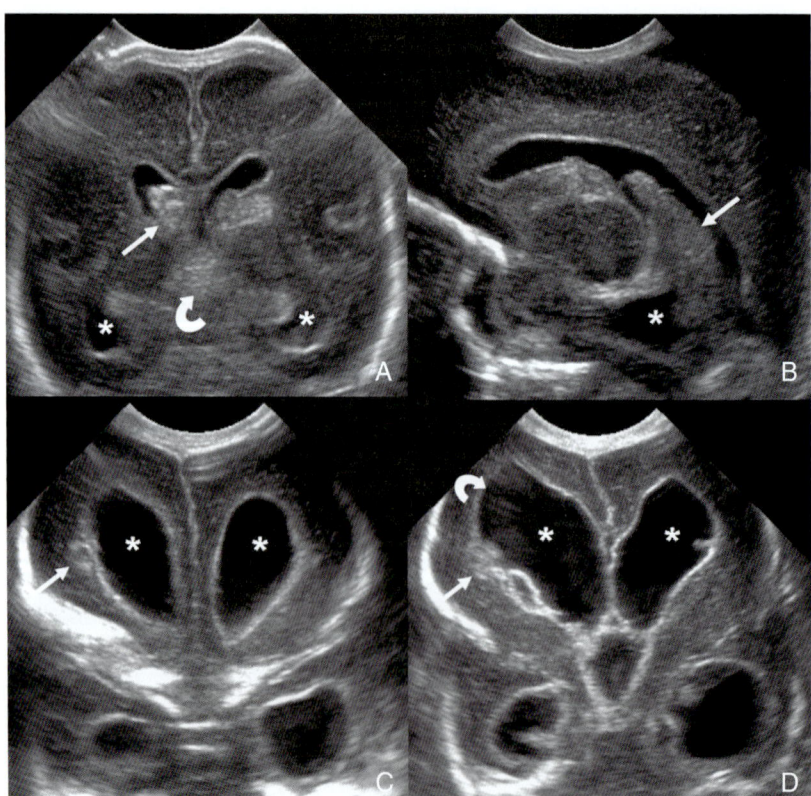

Figure 16-8 Grade 3 and 4 GMH. Coronal (**A**) and sagittal (**B**) cranial US images demonstrate nodular hyperechogenicity extending into lateral *(arrows)* and third *(curved arrow)* ventricles with associated hydrocephalus *(*)*, consistent with grade 3 GMH. Coronal (**C** and **D**) cranial US images of a different preterm neonate demonstrate intraparenchymal hemorrhage *(arrows)*, consistent with grade 4 GMH. Note that besides the hydrocephalus *(*)*, the right lateral ventricle is irregularly shaped *(curved arrow)*, suggestive of porencephalic cyst secondary to intraparenchymal hemorrhage.

Chapter 16 Neuroimaging of Pediatric Hypoxic–Ischemic Injury

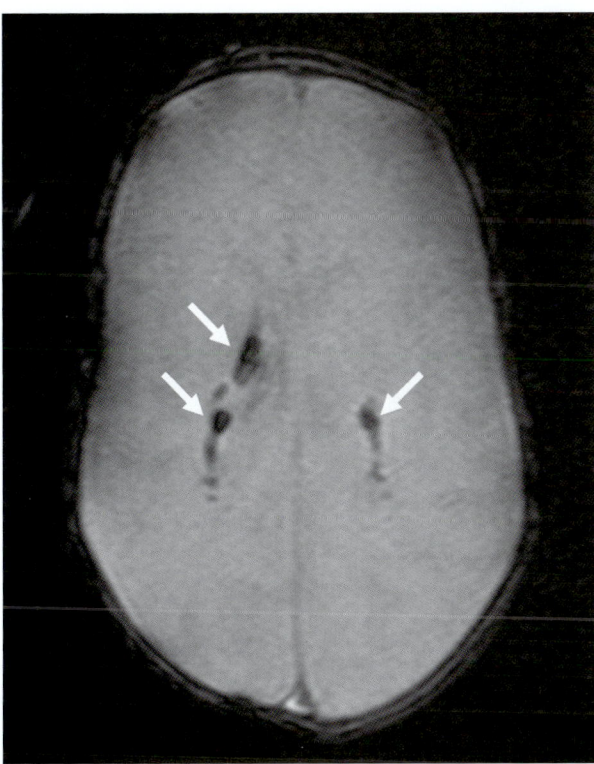

Figure 16-9 Intraventricular hemorrhage. Axial gradient-recalled echo (1770/3.9; flip angle = 30°) image demonstrates susceptibility effect from blood products in the choroid plexuses bilaterally *(arrows)*.

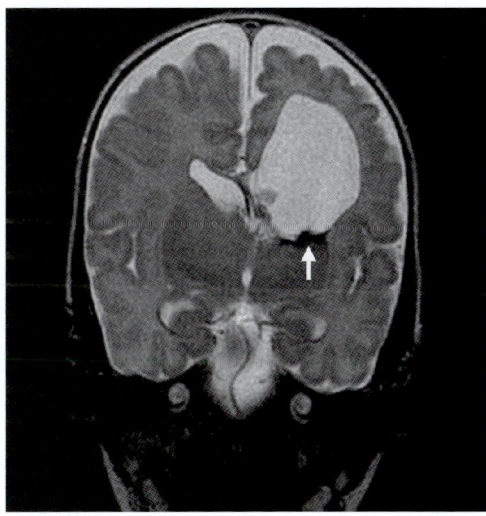

Figure 16-10 Porencephalic cyst secondary to intraparenchymal hemorrhage in a 5-year-old boy with history of 27-week premature birth. Coronal T2 (5000/1127.2) image demonstrates ex vacuo dilatation of the left lateral ventricle due to grade 4 GMH *(arrow)*. Note lack of midline shift, mass effect, or transependymal edema, which would be seen in unilateral hydrocephalus.

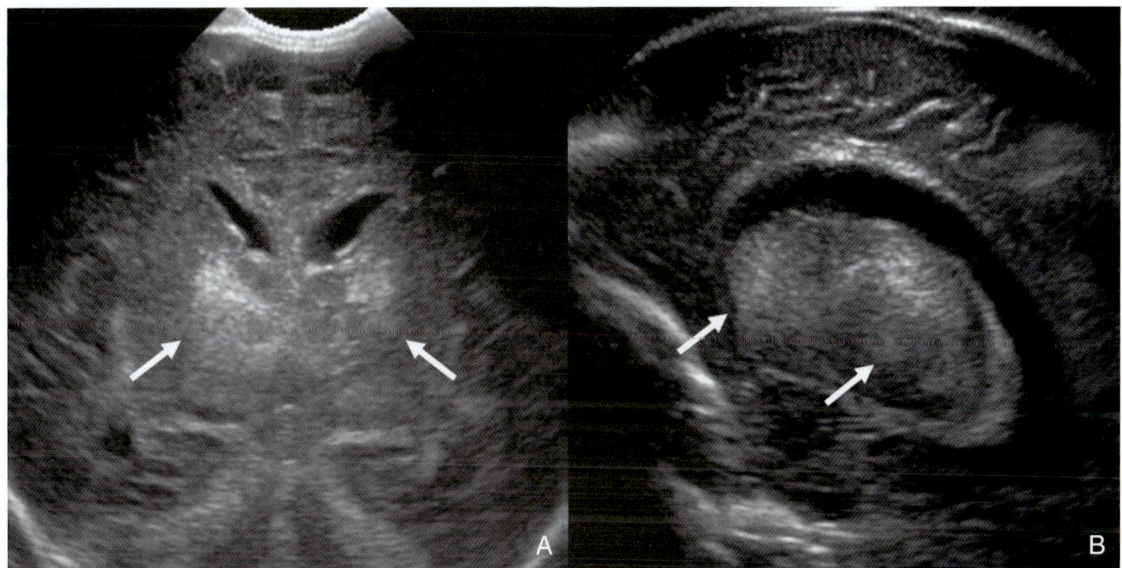

Figure 16-11 Profound asphyxia in a full-term neonate. Coronal **(A)** and sagittal **(B)** cranial US demonstrates hyperechogenicity in the basal ganglia and thalami *(arrows)*.

CT in Profound Asphyxia

Although CT is less sensitive than US and particularly RM, low attenuation related to edema or high attenuation related to blood or calcium may be appreciated in the thalami, basal ganglia, and brainstem.

MRI in Profound Asphyxia

MRI typically shows increased signal intensity on T1-weighted images, involving the ventral lateral thalami (Figure 16-12), posterolateral lentiform nuclei (Figure 16-13), posterior mesencephali (Figure 16-14),

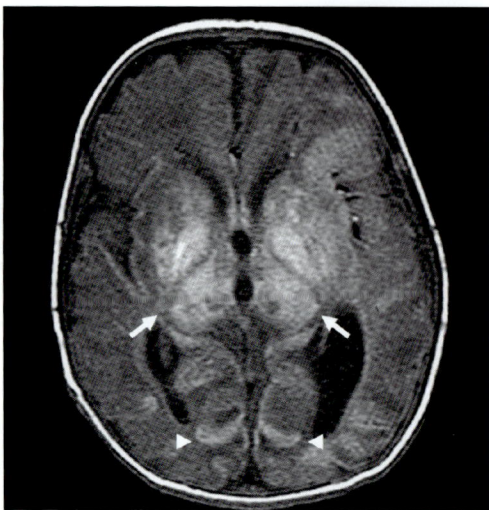

Figure 16-12 Profound hypoxic–ischemic injury in a 1-day-old full-term neonate. Axial T1 (433/9) image showing area of signal hyperintensity involving the basal ganglia and thalami bilaterally *(arrows)*. Note some cortical involvement in the occipital lobes *(arrowheads)*.

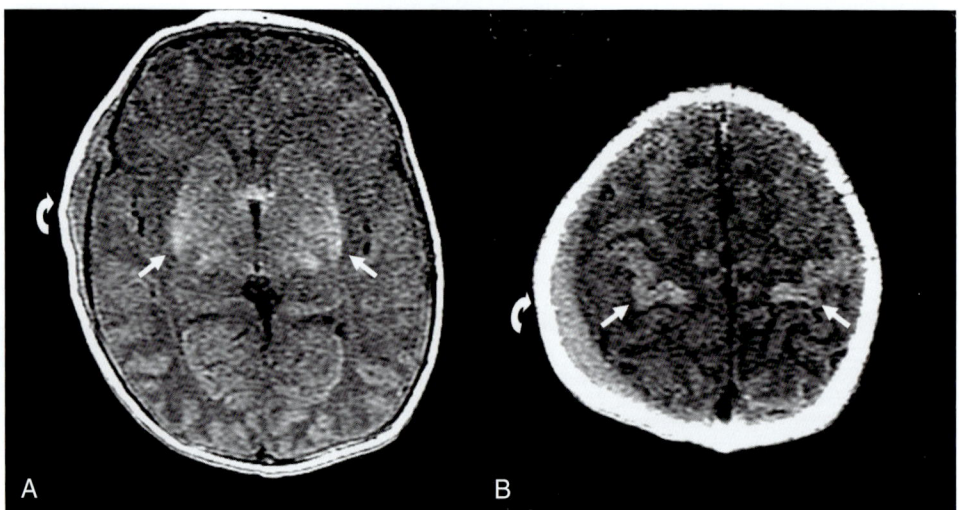

Figure 16-13 Profound hypoxic-ischemic injury in a 5-day-old full-term neonate. Axial T1 (400/9) image showing area of signal hyperintensity *(arrows)* involving the lentiform nucleus and thalami bilaterally **(A)** and central gyri bilaterally **(B)**. Note right temporoparietal cephalohematoma *(curved arrows)*.

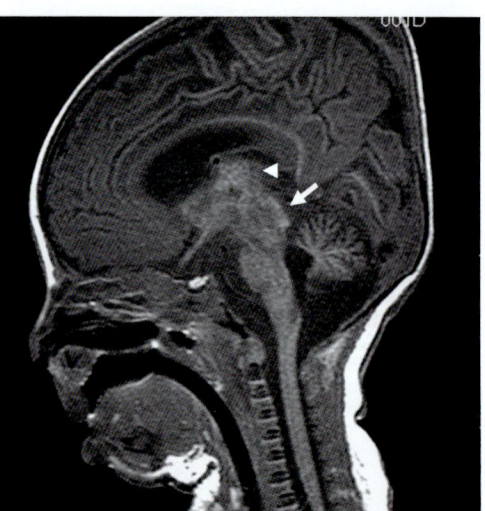

Figure 16-14 Profound hypoxic–ischemic injury in a 1-day-old full-term neonate. Sagittal T1 (450/9) image showing area of signal hyperintensity involving the posterior brainstem *(arrow)* and thalami *(arrowhead)*.

and hippocampi. Cavitation may be present. Progression with involvement of the lateral geniculate nuclei and perirolandic cerebral cortex may occur. MR may show no abnormality if imaging is performed to early, particularly in the first 6 hours.

MRS in Profound Asphyxia

Although some authors have documented a minimally elevated Lactate/Choline ratio (<0.15) in normal term neonates, others have advocated that differently from preterm infants and infants that are small for gestational age, MRS performed in the first 24 hours is sensitive to hypoxia–ischemia in term neonates. It has been reported that the lactate peak rises during hypoxia–ischemia, is rapidly cleared on resuscitation, and after 12 to 24 hours a secondary lactate peak appears. Depending on the severity of the insult, elevated lactate and diminished NAA tends to worsen in the first 5 days and then normalize. Persistent elevated lactate for more than 48 hours may be a sign of adverse prognosis.

DWI in Profound Asphyxia

DWI performed on day 3 of life, in term newborns with neonatal encephalopathy, is considered the most sensitive technique for assessing hypoxic-ischemic brain injury. DWI may be abnormal in the cortex, basal nuclei, or white matter before conventional MRI. It has been that DWI may not reveal the extent of the injury or late neuronal damage, related at least in part to cellular apoptosis (Figure 16-15).

Multicystic Encephalomalacia

Multicystic encephalomalacia represents the result of widespread brain necrosis that develops into cystic lesions (Figure 16-16). Multicystic encephalomalacia usually results from severe hypoxic–ischemic brain damage, particularly late in the third trimester of gestation and birth. It is generally due to severe asphyxia or hypotension in term or near-term neonates. Less frequently, it is due to infection, trauma, or other injuries.

Partial Prolonged Hypoxia–Ischemia

In partial prolonged hypoxia, vital brain areas, such as the brainstem, thalami, basal ganglia, hippocampus, and cerebellum are preserved at the expense of less metabolically active areas, such as the cerebral cortex and white matter. The watershed zones are particularly vulnerable because they are relatively hypoperfused when blood is shunted to the vital, more central areas. Similar findings can also result as a consequence of hypotension.

The subcortical white matter almost always undergoes atrophy and gliosis. As a result, the most typical imaging finding in these patients is ulegyria ("mushroom-shaped gyri"), which sometimes becomes an epileptogenic focus. This finding is most frequently seen in the triple watershed zone at the border zone of the anterior, middle, and posterior cerebral arteries.

Transcranial US in Partial Prolonged Hypoxia–Ischemia

US is particularly insensitive in infants with prolonged hypoxic-ischemic injury because of its limited visualization of the posterior parasagittal regions of the parietal lobes, where most of the abnormalities related to partial prolonged hypoxia-ischemia occur. It may show effacement of the gray–white junction from cytotoxic edema or volume loss from chronic gliosis in the anterior watershed zones.

CT in Partial Prolonged Hypoxia–Ischemia

It is possible to appreciate hypoattenuation with volume expansion from edema (Figure 16-17, A) or with volume loss from chronic gliosis involving the watershed distribution.

MRI in Partial Prolonged Hypoxia–Ischemia

MRI shows decreased signal intensity on T1-weighted images and increased signal intensity on T2-weighted images with volume expansion from edema (Figure 16-17, B and C), or with volume loss from chronic gliosis.

MRS in Partial Prolonged Hypoxia–Ischemia

Patients with partial prolonged hypoxia-ischemia may have elevated Lactate/Choline ratios in the white matter.

DWI in Partial Prolonged Hypoxia–Ischemia

In the acute phase, DWI may demonstrate areas of restricted diffusion with low ADC values in the parasagittal watershed zones (Figure 16-17, D).

ISCHEMIC STROKE DURING INFANCY AND CHILDHOOD

Arterial strokes in children can be attributed to a variety of causes including cardiac anomalies, intracranial vasculopathies, arterial dissection, migrainous vasospasm, mitochondriopathy, and hypercoagulable states, such as factor V Leiden, protein C, protein S, anticardiolipin antibody, polycythemia, sepsis, tumor, trauma, disseminated intravascular coagulation, and metabolic disorders. Imaging is usually used to differentiate ischemic versus hemorrhagic stroke, assess the extension of the infarct, and sometimes suggest a specific cause. Vascular imaging can display arterial dissection or venous thrombosis. Uni- or bilateral thalamic infarcts can occur in meningitis. Multiple infarcts involving predominantly the anterior circulation can be related to embolic storm (Figure 16-18) and multiple infarcts not strict to a vascular distribution involving predominantly the posterior lobes can be related to mitochondrial myopathy, encephalopathy, lactic acidosis, and stroke (MELAS) syndrome. Leigh's disease, also known as subacute necrotizing encephalomyelopathy, predominantly involves the basal nuclei, thalami, dorsal mesencephalon, pons and medulla bilaterally.

Cranial US in Ischemic Stroke During Infancy and Childhood

In infants with open fontanelle, US demonstrates loss of gray–white differentiation seen in early strokes. Edema appears as hyperechogenicity in the basal ganglia and cortex with signs of volume expansion. Hemorrhage

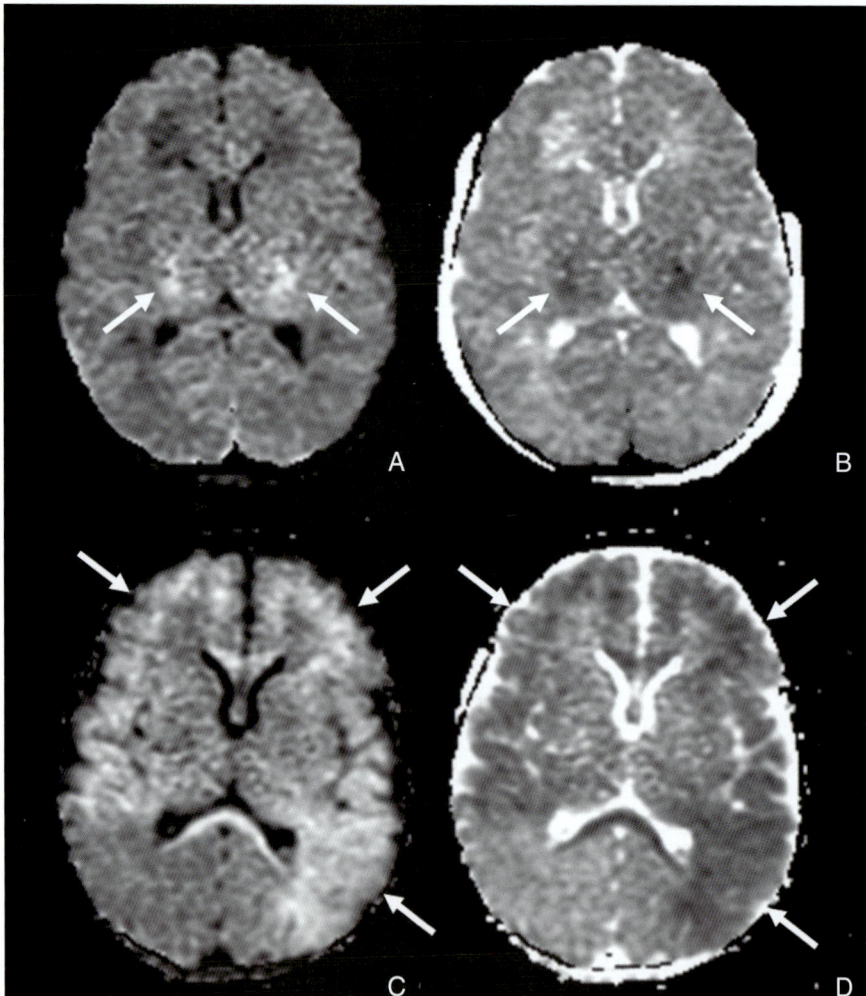

Figure 16-15 Late hypoxic–ischemic brain damage in a full-term neonate. Axial DWI (A) and ADC (B) images obtained in the first 24 hours after profound hypoxia–ischemia shows reduced diffusion and decreased ADC values in the ventral lateral thalami bilaterally *(arrows)*. Axial DWI (C) and ADC (D) images 72 hours after the hypoxic–ischemic event demonstrate widespread abnormality involving the cortex and white matter of both hemispheres *(arrows)*.

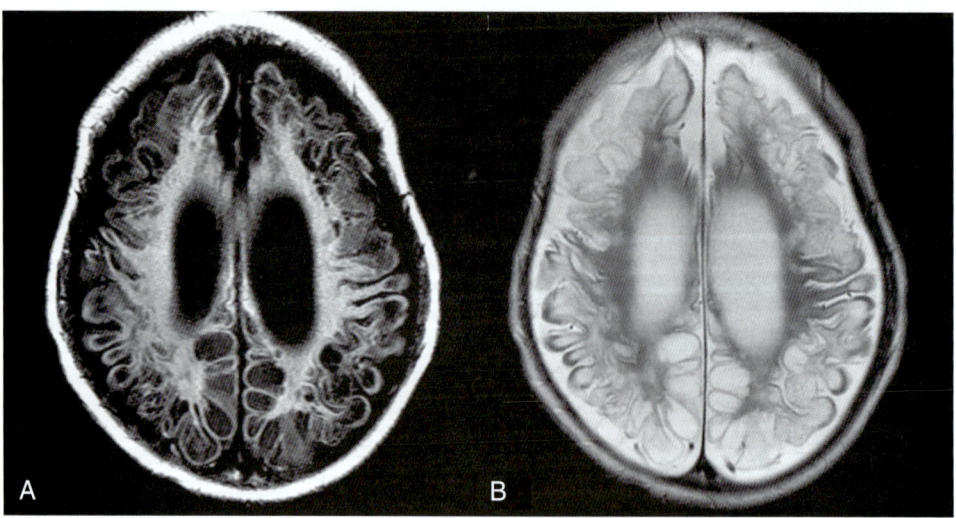

Figure 16-16 Multicystic encephalomalacia in a 1-year-old boy full-term neonate. Axial T1-weighted (433/9) (A) and T2 (5500/131.5) (B) images showing diffuse cystic transformation of the cortex and subcortical white matter.

should be suspected if foci or focal areas with increased hyperechogenicity are noted. US is not sensitive for small and peripheral strokes. On follow-up studies, US shows hyperechogenicity with volume loss and possible cystic areas.

CT in Ischemic Stroke During Infancy and Childhood

A low-dose radiation protocol is generally warranted. The temporal and occipital poles are particularly sensitive to artifact formation during low-dose radiation protocols.

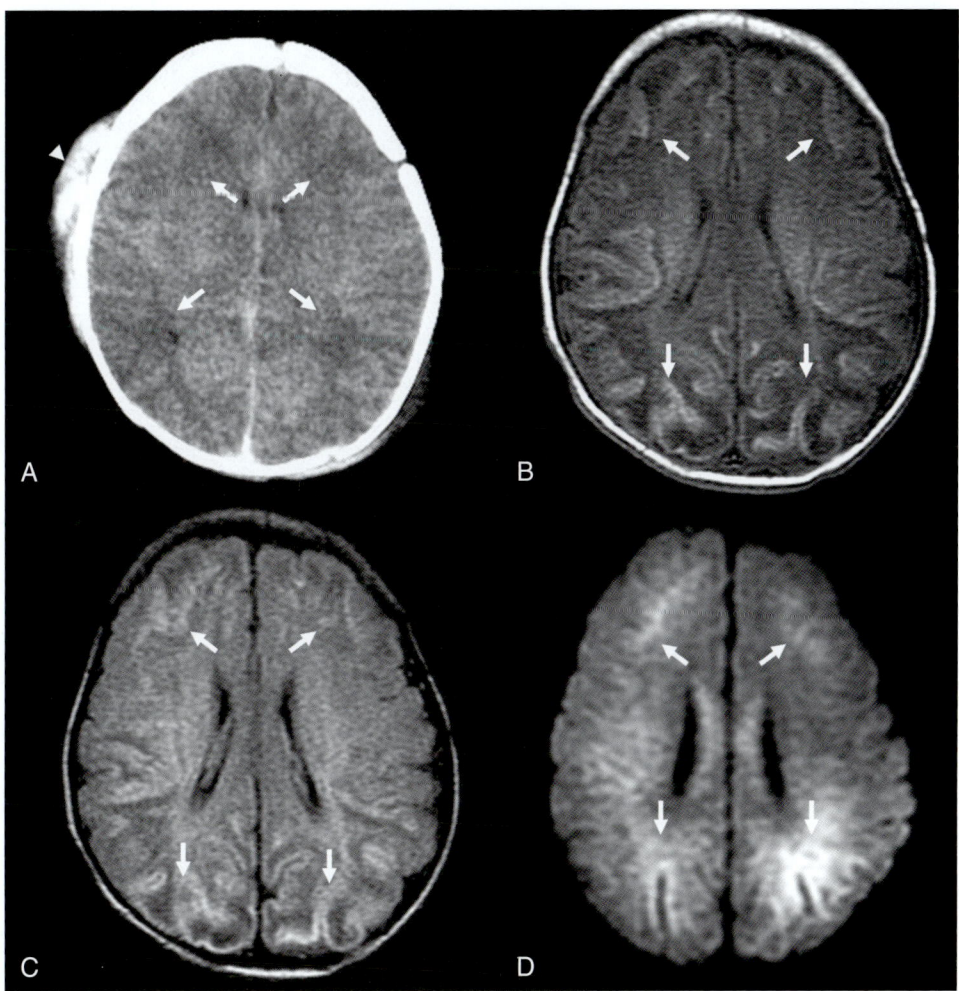

Figure 16-17 Partial prolonged hypoxic–ischemic insult in a 1-day-old girl. Noncontrast computed tomography axial image (**A**) demonstrating areas of hypoattenuation and some loss of gray–white matter differentiation in the parasagittal watershed zones bilaterally *(arrows)*. Note right temporal cephalohematoma *(arrowhead)*. T1-weighted (**B**) and T2 fluid-attenuated inversion recovery (**C**) images of a different 1-day-old girl who suffered partial prolonged hypoxic–ischemic injury showing signal hyperintensity and involving the cortex in the parasagittal watershed zones bilaterally. **D:** Diffusion-weighted imaging displaying high signal.

CT carries lower sensitivity to ischemic changes compared with MRI but has good sensitivity and specificity for ruling out intracranial hemorrhage. CT findings are similar to those of stroke in adults. Effacement of lentiform nucleus or insular ribbon, hypoattenuation in a vascular territory, tissue swelling, loss of gray–white matter differentiation, and dense thrombosed vessels may be found.

MRI in Ischemic Stroke During Infancy and Childhood

MRI is an alternative to CT to avoid ionizing radiation exposure in pediatric patients. A few hours after stroke onset, a loss of arterial signal void is sometimes observed. After 1 to 2 hours, patients with ischemic strokes generally demonstrate T1-weighted subtle effacement of the sulci due to cytotoxic edema. Around 4 to 8 hours, T2-weighted imaging shows hyperintense signal due to both cytotoxic and vasogenic edema. In complete infarction, cortical laminar necrosis enhances 5 to 7 days after the stroke and persists for several months. In incomplete infarction, cortical luxury perfusion may enhance within 2 to 4 hours after the stroke.

DWI in Ischemic Stroke During Infancy and Childhood

In general, high signal on DWI with corresponding low ADC values may be found as early as 30 minutes after stroke onset. Transition from decreasing to increasing ADC is estimated at 18 hours after stroke onset. Pseudonormalization is estimated to occur around 8 days after infarct.

PWI in Ischemic Stroke During Infancy and Childhood

PWI using first-pass contrast bolus injection or spin tagging of protons in the water in blood reveals reductions of cerebral blood flow and cerebral blood volume and an increased mean transit time of blood. Matched between the diffusion and perfusion abnormalities correlate with the region of infarction and are indicative of permanent neuronal death. Mismatched

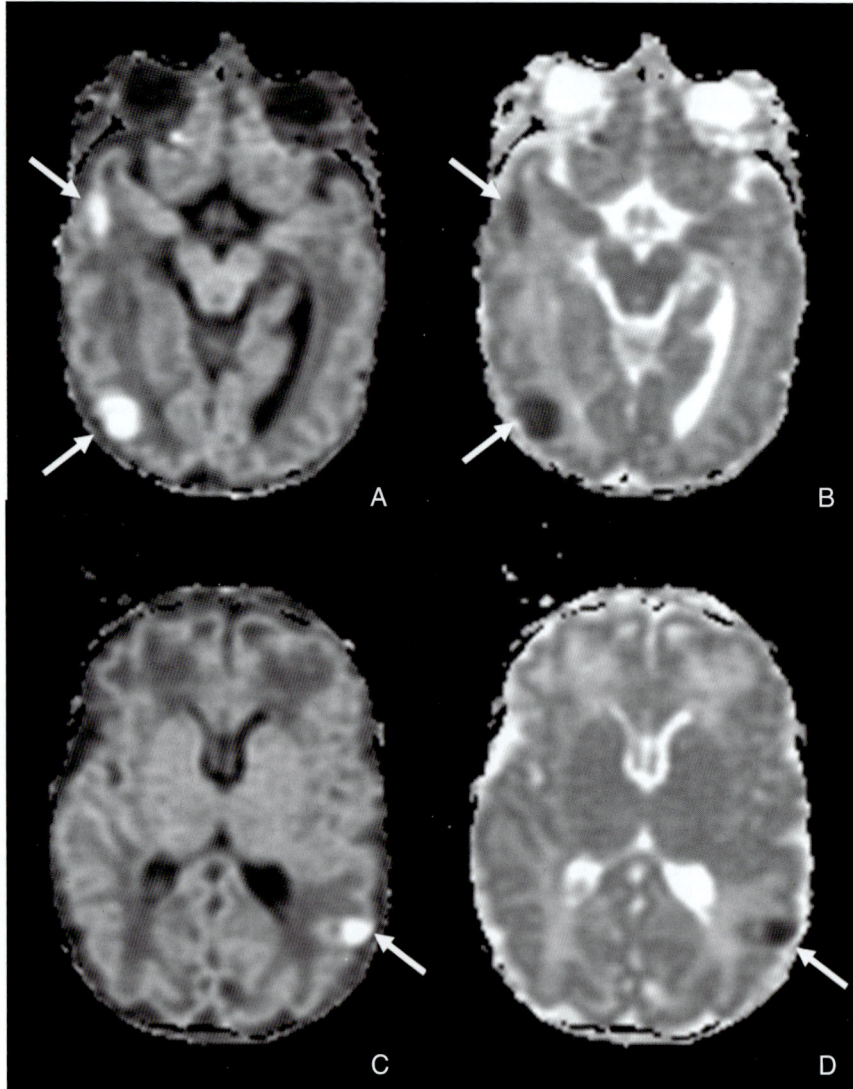

Figure 16-18 Multiple cortical infarcts in a newborn with atrioventricular septal defect. DWI (**A** and **B**) and ADC (**C** and **D**) demonstrate multiple cortical areas with reduced diffusion and decreased ADC values.

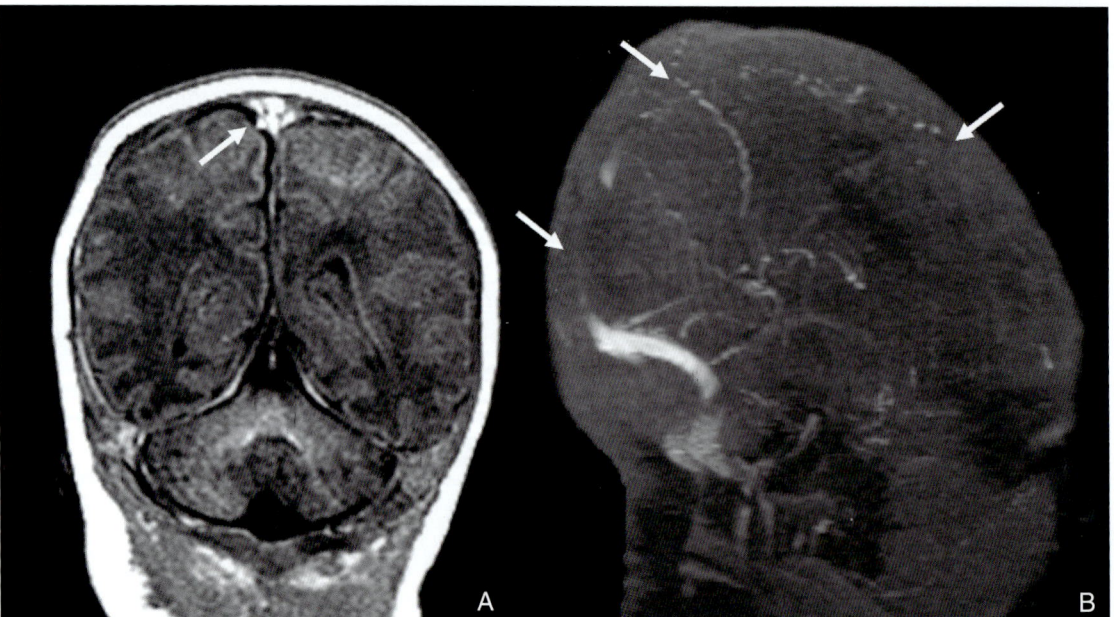

Figure 16-19 Superior sagittal sinus thrombosis in a newborn with sepsis. Coronal T1 (433/9) shows abnormal increased signal in the superior sagittal sinus *(arrow)* and MR venography without contrast demonstrates lack of flow *(arrows)*.

diffusion and perfusion abnormalities with the perfusion abnormality larger than the diffusion abnormality may be indicative of a region of reversible ischemic penumbra.

Magnetic Resonance Angiography in Ischemic Stroke During Infancy and Childhood

Magnetic resonance angiography is useful in cases of thrombosis to localize the site of occlusion and for cases of severe underlying vasculopathy.

Venous Thrombosis During Infancy and Childhood

Pediatric patients frequently present to the hospital with dehydration, which is a major risk factor of intracranial venous thrombosis. Other hypercoagulable states that may cause venous thrombosis include factor V Leiden, protein C, protein S, anticardiolipin antibody, polycythemia, sepsis, tumor, trauma, disseminated intravascular coagulation, and metabolic disorders.

Cranial US in Venous Thrombosis During Infancy and Childhood

Color Doppler US of the superior sagittal sinus should always be obtained as part of the cranial US in neonate infants. Although, color Doppler cannot rule out venous thrombosis in other venous sinuses, it is a simple and inexpensive way to detect thrombosis of the superior sagittal sinus that could be unnoticed on routine grayscale cranial US.

CT in Venous Thrombosis During Infancy and Childhood

Hyperattenuation in the venous sinus or in the cortical or deep intracranial veins on noncontrast CT should be concerning for venous thrombosis even in the absence of other imaging findings. Focal areas of hypoattenuation representing edema adjacent to the thrombosed sinus or vein may be present. These areas of edema from venous congestion typically do not respect an arterial distribution. CT venography demonstrates a filling defect representing the thrombus in a venous sinus or vein. Lack of contrast in a thrombosed cortical vein may be difficult to appreciate.

MRI in Venous Thrombosis During Infancy and Childhood

Loss of normal flow void sometimes with increased signal on T1-weighted image in the thrombosed sinus (Figure 16-19 B) or vein is one of the early signs and may be the only imaging finding on a noncontrast MR exam. Focal areas of hyperintense signal on T2-weighted imaging representing edema are typically seen in the brain parenchyma adjacent to the thrombosed sinus. Initially these areas may have little or no reduced diffusion; however, prolonged venous occlusion may impair arterial flow and cerebral infarcts with reduced diffusion may ensue. Lack of flow may also be observed on phase-contrast or Time-of-Flight MR venography without utilization of contrast (Figure 16-19 B). MR with contrast usually demonstrates a filling defect representing the thrombus in thrombosed vein or venous sinus.

Suggested Readings

Auld KL, Ashwal S, Holshouser BA, et al. Proton magnetic resonance spectroscopy in children with acute central nervous system injury. *Pediatr Neurol.* 1995;12:323-334.

Barkovich AJ. Techniques and methods in pediatric magnetic resonance imaging. *Semin Ultrasound CT MR.* 1988;9:186-191.

Barkovich AJ. The encephalopathic neonate: choosing the proper imaging technique. *AJNR Am J Neuroradiol.* 1997;18:1816-1820.

Barkovich AJ. *Pediatric Neuroradiology.* 4th ed. Philadelphia: Lippincott Williams & Wilkins; 2005.

Barkovich AJ. MR imaging of the neonatal brain. *Neuroimaging Clin N Am.* 2006;16:117-135:viii-ix.

Barkovich AJ, Sargent SK. Profound asphyxia in the premature infant: imaging findings. *AJNR Am J Neuroradiol.* 1995;16:1837-1846.

Barkovich AJ, Truwit CL. Brain damage from perinatal asphyxia: correlation of MR findings with gestational age. *AJNR Am J Neuroradiol.* 1990;11:1087-1096.

Barkovich AJ, Good WV, Koch TK, Berg BO. Mitochondrial disorders: analysis of their clinical and imaging characteristics. *AJNR Am J Neuroradiol.* 1993;14:1119-1137.

Barkovich AJ, Westmark K, Partridge C, Sola A, Ferriero DM. Perinatal asphyxia: MR findings in the first 10 days. *AJNR Am J Neuroradiol.* 1995;16:427-438.

Barkovich AJ, Westmark KD, Bedi HS, Partridge JC, Ferriero DM, Vigneron DB. Proton spectroscopy and diffusion imaging on the first day of life after perinatal asphyxia: preliminary report. *AJNR Am J Neuroradiol.* 2001;22:1786-1794.

Bartha AI, Yap KR, Miller SP, et al. The normal neonatal brain: MR imaging, diffusion tensor imaging, and 3D MR spectroscopy in healthy term neonates. *AJNR Am J Neuroradiol.* 2007;28:1015-1021.

Cady EB, Penrice J, Amess PN, et al. Lactate, N-acetylaspartate, choline and creatine concentrations, and spin-spin relaxation in thalamic and occipito-parietal regions of developing human brain. *Magn Reson Med.* 1996;36:878-886.

Copen WA, Schwamm LH, Gonzalez RG, et al. Ischemic stroke: effects of etiology and patient age on the time course of the core apparent diffusion coefficient. *Radiology.* 2001;221:27-34.

Detre JA, Wang ZY, Bogdan AR, et al. Regional variation in brain lactate in Leigh syndrome by localized 1H magnetic resonance spectroscopy. *Ann Neurol.* 1991;29:218-221.

Enzmann D, Murphy-Irwin K, Stevenson D, Ariagno R, Barton J, Sunshine P. The natural history of subependymal germinal matrix hemorrhage. *Am J Perinatol.* 1985;2:123-133.

Forbes KP, Pipe JG, Bird R. Neonatal hypoxic-ischemic encephalopathy: detection with diffusion-weighted MR imaging. *AJNR Am J Neuroradiol.* 2000;21:1490-1496.

Frigieri G, Guidi B, Costa Zaccarelli S, et al. Multicystic encephalomalacia in term infants. *Childs Nerv Syst.* 1996;12:759-764.

Fullerton HJ, Wu YW, Zhao S, Johnston SC. Risk of stroke in children: ethnic and gender disparities. *Neurology.* 2003;61:189-194.

Greene MF. Outcomes of very low birth weight in young adults. *N Engl J Med.* 2002;346:146-148.

Hill A, Volpe JJ. Pathogenesis and management of hypoxic-ischemic encephalopathy in the term newborn. *Neurol Clin.* 1985;3:31-46.

Hill A, Melson GL, Clark HB, Volpe JJ. Hemorrhagic periventricular leukomalacia: diagnosis by real time ultrasound and correlation with autopsy findings. *Pediatrics.* 1982;69:282-284.

Huang BY, Castillo M. Hypoxic-ischemic brain injury: imaging findings from birth to adulthood. *Radiographics.* 2008;28:417-439:quiz 617.

Kwong KL, Wong YC, Fong CM, Wong SN, So KT. Magnetic resonance imaging in 122 children with spastic cerebral palsy. *Pediatr Neurol.* 2004;31:172-176.

Lawn JE, Cousens S, Zupan J. 4 million neonatal deaths: when? Where? Why? *Lancet.* 2005;365:891-900.

Leth H, Toft PB, Pryds O, Peitersen B, Lou HC, Henriksen O. Brain lactate in preterm and growth-retarded neonates. *Acta Paediatr.* 1995;84:495-499.

Liauw L, van der Grond J, van den Berg-Huysmans AA, Laan LA, van Buchem MA, van Wezel-Meijler G. Is there a way to predict outcome in (near) term neonates with hypoxic-ischemic encephalopathy based on MR imaging? *AJNR Am J Neuroradiol.* 2008;29:1789-1794.

Low JA, Lindsay BG, Derrick EJ. Threshold of metabolic acidosis associated with newborn complications. *Am J Obstet Gynecol.* 1997;177:1391-1394.

Maalouf EF, Duggan PJ, Counsell SJ, et al. Comparison of findings on cranial ultrasound and magnetic resonance imaging in preterm infants. *Pediatrics.* 2001;107:719-727.

Mercuri E, He J, Curati WL, Dubowitz LM, Cowan FM, Bydder GM. Cerebellar infarction and atrophy in infants and children with a history of premature birth. *Pediatr Radiol.* 1997;27:139-143.

Norman MG. Perinatal brain damage. *Perspect Pediatr Pathol.* 1978;4:41-92.

Penrice J, Cady EB, Lorek A, et al. Proton magnetic resonance spectroscopy of the brain in normal preterm and term infants, and early changes after perinatal hypoxia-ischemia. *Pediatr Res.* 1996;40:6-14.

Penrice J, Lorek A, Cady EB, et al. Proton magnetic resonance spectroscopy of the brain during acute hypoxia-ischemia and delayed cerebral energy failure in the newborn piglet. *Pediatr Res.* 1997;41:795-802.

Riikonen R, Santavuori P. Hereditary and acquired risk factors for childhood stroke. *Neuropediatrics*. 1994;25:227-233.

Robertson RL, Ben-Sira L, Barnes PD, et al. MR line-scan diffusion-weighted imaging of term neonates with perinatal brain ischemia. *AJNR Am J Neuroradiol*. 1999;20:1658-1670.

Roze E, Kerstjens JM, Maathuis CG, ter Horst HJ, Bos AF. Risk factors for adverse outcome in preterm infants with periventricular hemorrhagic infarction. *Pediatrics*. 2008;122:e46-e52.

Sie LT, van der Knaap MS, van Wezel-Meijler G, Taets van Amerongen AH, Lafeber HN, Valk J. Early MR features of hypoxic-ischemic brain injury in neonates with periventricular densities on sonograms. *AJNR Am J Neuroradiol*. 2000;21:852-861.

Soul JS, Robertson RL, Tzika AA, du Plessis AJ, Volpe JJ. Time course of changes in diffusion-weighted magnetic resonance imaging in a case of neonatal encephalopathy with defined onset and duration of hypoxic-ischemic insult. *Pediatrics*. 2001;108:1211-1214.

Steinman KJ, Gorno-Tempini ML, Glidden DV, et al. Neonatal watershed brain injury on magnetic resonance imaging correlates with verbal IQ at 4 years. *Pediatrics*. 2009;123:1025-1030.

Villani F, D'Incerti L, Granata T, et al. Epileptic and imaging findings in perinatal hypoxic-ischemic encephalopathy with ulegyria. *Epilepsy Res*. 2003;55:235-243.

Wang ZJ, Vigneron DB, Miller SP, et al. Brain metabolite levels assessed by lactate-edited MR spectroscopy in premature neonates with and without pentobarbital sedation. *AJNR Am J Neuroradiol*. 2008;29:798-801:Epub 2008 Jan 2009.

Williams LS, Garg BP, Cohen M, Fleck JD, Biller J. Subtypes of ischemic stroke in children and young adults. *Neurology*. 1997;49:1541-1545.

Yuh WT, Crain MR, Loes DJ, Greene GM, Ryals TJ, Sato Y. MR imaging of cerebral ischemia: findings in the first 24 hours. *AJNR Am J Neuroradiol*. 1991;12:621-629.

CHAPTER 17
Intrauterine and Perinatal Infections

Andre D. Furtado, Saulo Lacerda, and Thomas P. Naidich

■ IMAGING: WHY, WHO, AND HOW?

Why Imaging?
Perinatal infections are a group of infections caused by bacteria, viruses, or parasites that are transmitted from a mother to her baby during pregnancy or childbirth. Brain damage is the most serious complication. Imaging provides important diagnostic and prognostic information.

Who Needs Imaging?
Imaging should be performed in all patients with suspected perinatal infection. Clinical presentation includes fever, maculopapular rash, hepatosplenomegaly, microcephaly, seizures, jaundice, thrombocytopenia, and generalized lymphadenopathy.

How to Image/Which Imaging?
Cerebral US is usually performed as the first imaging modality. Monthly obstetric ultrasound may be performed to evaluate brain abnormalities, calcifications, and growth retardation. Postnatally, US can be as good as computed tomography (CT) to detect intracranial calcifications with the advantages of no radiation use, cost effectiveness, and less stress for the neonate. US may demonstrate echogenic vasculature in the basal ganglia of neonates with cytomegalovirus (CMV), rubella, or congenital syphilis infections, but this finding is not specific and may also be seen in cases of chromosomal abnormality, such as trisomy 13 syndrome.

CT scanning is a useful modality for investigating calcification in patients with neonatal infections. During the perinatal period, CT should be performed with a low-dose protocol.

Magnetic resonance imaging (MRI) is the modality of choice for evaluating the fetal brain providing diagnostic and prognostic information in neonates with neonatal infection. Sedation of the mother is especially important for fetuses younger than 28 weeks of gestational age, when the head is not yet engaged in the pelvis and moves considerably.

■ GENERAL CONSIDERATIONS
Perinatal infections are most commonly caused by agents included in the acronyms TORCH (*T*oxoplasmosis, *O*thers, which is mainly syphilis, *R*ubella, *C*ytomegalovirus, *H*erpes simplex) and HIV (human immunodeficiency virus). Bacterial infections are most commonly transmitted from the cervix during delivery, whereas toxoplasmosis, syphilis, rubella, CMV, and most viruses are transmitted via the placenta. Herpes simplex virus (HSV) infection with active vaginal vesicles and HIV can also be transmitted during delivery. In such cases, cesarean section should be performed.

The most common imaging findings in infected fetuses include abnormal amniotic fluid volume, fetal growth restriction, hyperechogenic bowel, ascites, intrahepatic or intracranial calcifications, and ventricular dilatation. Ventricular dilatation may be secondary to malformation or brain damage. White matter injury on prenatal brain MRI has been associated with increased risk of premature birth.

■ COMMON IMAGING FINDINGS

Ventriculomegaly
Although ventriculomegaly is one of the most common imaging findings in fetuses with intrauterine infection, only approximately 5% of cases of fetal ventriculomegaly can be attributed to intrauterine infection. Most cases are attributed to neural tube defects.

Two criteria for fetal ventriculomegaly have been proposed: the lateral ventricular width and the lateral ventriculo-hemispheric ratio (VR).

The lateral ventricular width is measured at the atrium of the lateral ventricles using the choroid plexus as a landmark. This measurement typically ranges from 4 to 8 mm from 15 weeks to term. An upper limit of 10-12 mm is most commonly used (Figure 17-1). It is a very useful criterion during the second trimester.

VR is the distance from the midline to the lateral ventricular wall divided by the distance from the midline to the inner table of the parietal bone on the same image. This ratio is usually constant from 24 weeks to term, with

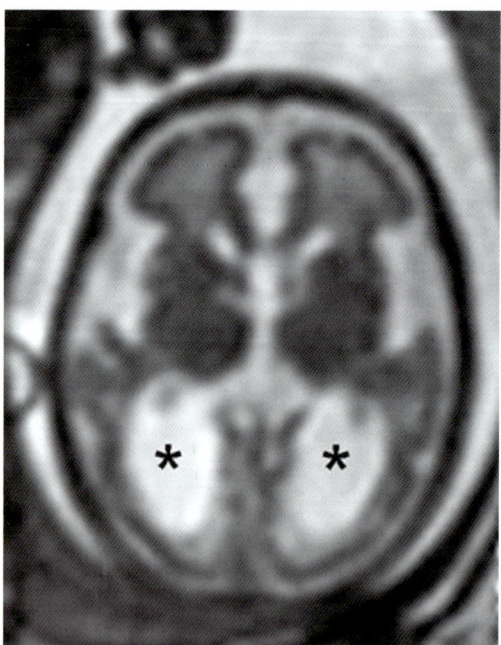

Figure 17-1 Ventriculomegaly. Axial T2-weighted HASTE (1000/144) image of a fetus at 30 weeks of gestation demonstrating enlarged lateral ventricles measured at the level of the atria (>10 mm).

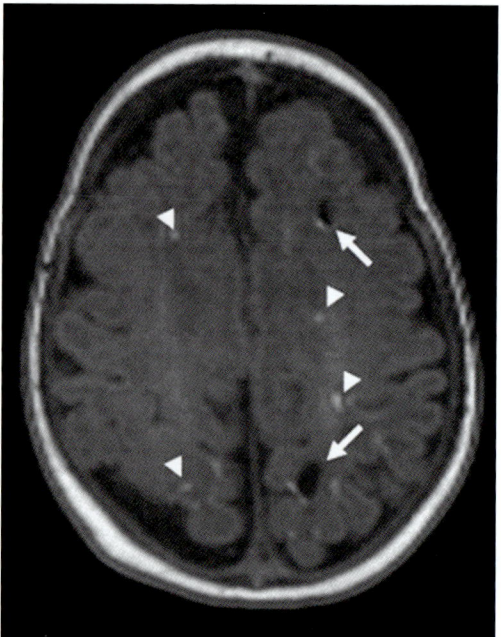

Figure 17-2 Calcifications. Axial reformatted three-dimensional spoiled gradient-recalled T1-weighted (1940/2) image of a 3-month-old boy with congenital toxoplasmosis demonstrating multiple foci of high signal (*arrowheads*) suggestive of calcifications. Also note a few cyst lesions (*arrows*).

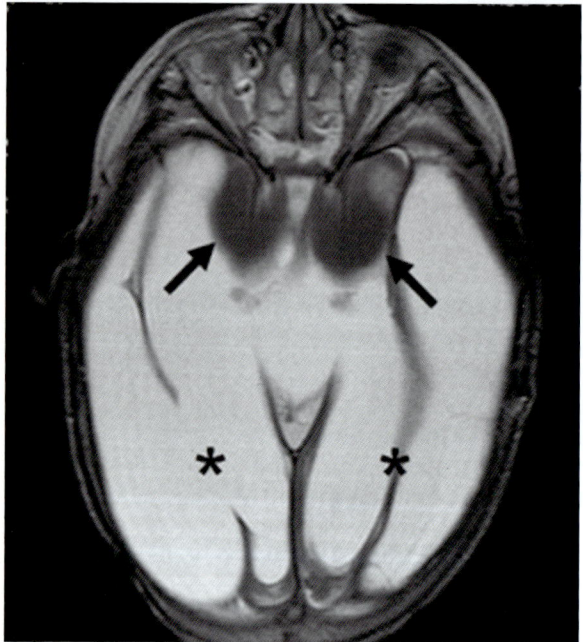

Figure 17-3 Hydranencephaly. Axial T2-weighted (4300/102.7) image demonstrating of no discernible brain parenchyma, which is replaced by cerebrospinal fluid–filled sac spaces (*asterisk*). The thalami typically are preserved (*arrows*).

an upper limit of 50%, but is normally much higher during early pregnancy and variable from 15 to 24 weeks.

Intracranial Calcifications

Intracranial calcifications are typically small and often do not exhibit the acoustic shadowing on cranial US. CT is considered the best imaging modality for detecting and characterizing intracranial calcifications. On MRI, calcifications usually present low T2 signal but variable T1 signal (low, intermediate, high, and mixed signal intensity) (Figure 17-2).

Intracranial calcifications may be difficult to detect, particularly during the second trimester and are most frequently seen in cases of fetal CMV and toxoplasmosis infections, but have been reported with congenital varicella, HSV, and rubella.

Hydranencephaly

Hydranencephaly is considered the most severe manifestation of the brain damage. The cerebral hemispheres are almost entirely replaced by fluid, but the brainstem, thalami, and posterior fossa structures are usually preserved. US demonstrates fluid-filled intracranial cavity with no discernible cerebral hemispheres. The falx is typically present but in some cases it may be absent. Hydranencephaly is more common in cases of congenital HSV infection and unusual in cases of toxoplasmosis and CMV (Figure 17-3).

Microcephaly

Microcephaly (small head size) is a result of poor cerebral development or arrested cerebral growth. It is often associated with chromossomal syndromes, fetal alcohol syndrome, cerebral malformations, and congenital infections. There are several measurements to assess microcephaly such as biparietal diameter, head circumference, abnormal head circumference to abdominal circumference, head circumference to femur length ratios, and poor fetal head growth on serial examinations. Head circumference of 2 standard deviations below the mean for gestational age is considered microcephaly. Isolated microcephaly has been documented in cases of congenital CMV, HSV, and rubella virus. It is less common in cases of congenital toxoplasmosis infection.

■ DIFFERENTIAL DIAGNOSTIC

The differential diagnostic of congenital infection includes fetal alcohol syndrome, teratogens, tuberous sclerosis, venous malformation, arteriovenous fistula, chronic venous ischemia, post natal neurocysticercosis, Fahr disease, idiopathic familial basal ganglia calcifications, and pseudo-TORCH syndromes, such as Baraister-Reardon, Aicardi-Goutieres, progressive cerebral and cerebellar demyelination. Metabolic disorders should always be ruled out, because early diagnosis and treatment of metabolic disorders can prevent further brain damage.

Overviews of the most common intrauterine and perinatal infections are discussed separately.

Cytomegalovirus

CMV is considered the most common serious congenital infection in the United States, affecting approximately 40,000 newborns each year. Most infants exposed to CMV before birth develop normally and do not show any symptoms; however, as many as 6,000 are born with serious complications. CMV infection in the newborn is usually diagnosed by urine culture. Treatment is basically supportive; however, ganciclovir and foscarnet may have some utility in selected cases.

The brain is the most commonly affected organ. Congenital CMV infection has been associated with microcephaly, cerebral calcifications, lissencephaly, polymicrogyria, cerebellar hypoplasia, dysplastic white matter, porencephaly, and ventricular dilatation.

Cranial Ultrasound
Cranial US can demonstrate calcifications, which are usually periventricular, ventriculomegaly, and microcephaly. Other findings that may be seen on US include intrauterine growth restriction, hepatosplenomegaly, cardiomyopathy, echogenic bowel, and hydrops.

Computed Tomography
CT is a valuable modality for detecting and characterizing diminutive periventricular and subependymal calcifications. CT can also show ventriculomegaly and microcephaly.

Magnetic Resonance Imaging
MRI is excellent for evaluating white matter volume loss with subsequent enlargement of lateral ventricles (Figures 17-4 and 17-5). MRI may also shows enlargement of the subarachnoid spaces, focal areas of dysplastic cortex, delayed myelination, paraventricular cysts, and some intracerebral calcification. MRI is not sensitivity for diminutive calcifications.

Toxoplasmosis

It is estimated that 400 to 4,000 cases of congenital toxoplasmosis occur per year in the United States. Most cases of acquired *Toxoplasma gondii* in immunocompetent pregnant women are mild. Cats are the definitive hosts and the three principal ways of transmission are ingestion of inadequately cooked infected meat, ingestion from contaminated soil or water, or transplacental.

Congenital toxoplasmosis infection typically causes meningoencephalitis, which may result in hydrocephalus, microcephaly, calcifications, porencephaly, or hydranencephaly. Congenital toxoplasmosis may not be apparent until late in infancy. The prognosis for normal neurologic outcome is good in the absence of brain abnormalities.

Cranial Ultrasound
Nonshadowing intracranial are the most typical imaging finding, which may be periventricular or random in distribution. US may miss small calcifications. Intrauterine growth restriction and ventriculomegaly can also occur. Echogenic bowel, hydramnios, enlarged placenta, hepatosplenomegaly, ascites, and fetal may be present.

Other less specific imaging findings are subependymal or white matter cysts, and echogenic striothalamic arteries ("candlestick sign").

Computed Tomography
CT demonstrates periventricular or random intracerebral calcifications, ocular calcifications, hydrocephaly, and microcephaly (Figure 17-6). The ocular calcifications may be similar to retinoblastoma.

Magnetic Resonance Imaging
MRI is routinely utilized to assess brain lesions, even when the US exam is normal. MRI may also be used serially during pregnancy for detection of development of brain abnormalities. In the acute phase, the white matter abnormality may manifest as effacement of the intermediate zone layer. Leukomalacia with parenchymal calcifications and cortical malformations occur later (Figure 17-7). The typically imaging finding is cystic lesions with calcified nodules (Figure 17-8).

Congenital Syphilis

Syphilis can also be transmitted from the mother to the fetus before birth. It is estimated that up to 50% of infants born with syphilis are premature, stillborn, or die shortly after birth. Symptoms of syphilis may develop as late as 2 years of age. Hepatosplenomegaly is a very sensitive sign but is nonspecific.

Leptomeningeal enhancement, particularly involving the basal meninges and extending into the brain parenchyma via the Virchow-Robin spaces may result in enhancing intraparenchymal lesions, known as gumma. Neonates with congenital syphilis may develop syphilitic endarteritis, which can cause ischemic or hemorrhagic strokes predominantly involving unilateral periventricular white matter.

Congenital Rubella (German Measles)

Rubella is extremely rare because of vaccination and prenatal screening. Rubella is the virus that causes German measles. When rubella infection occurs during early

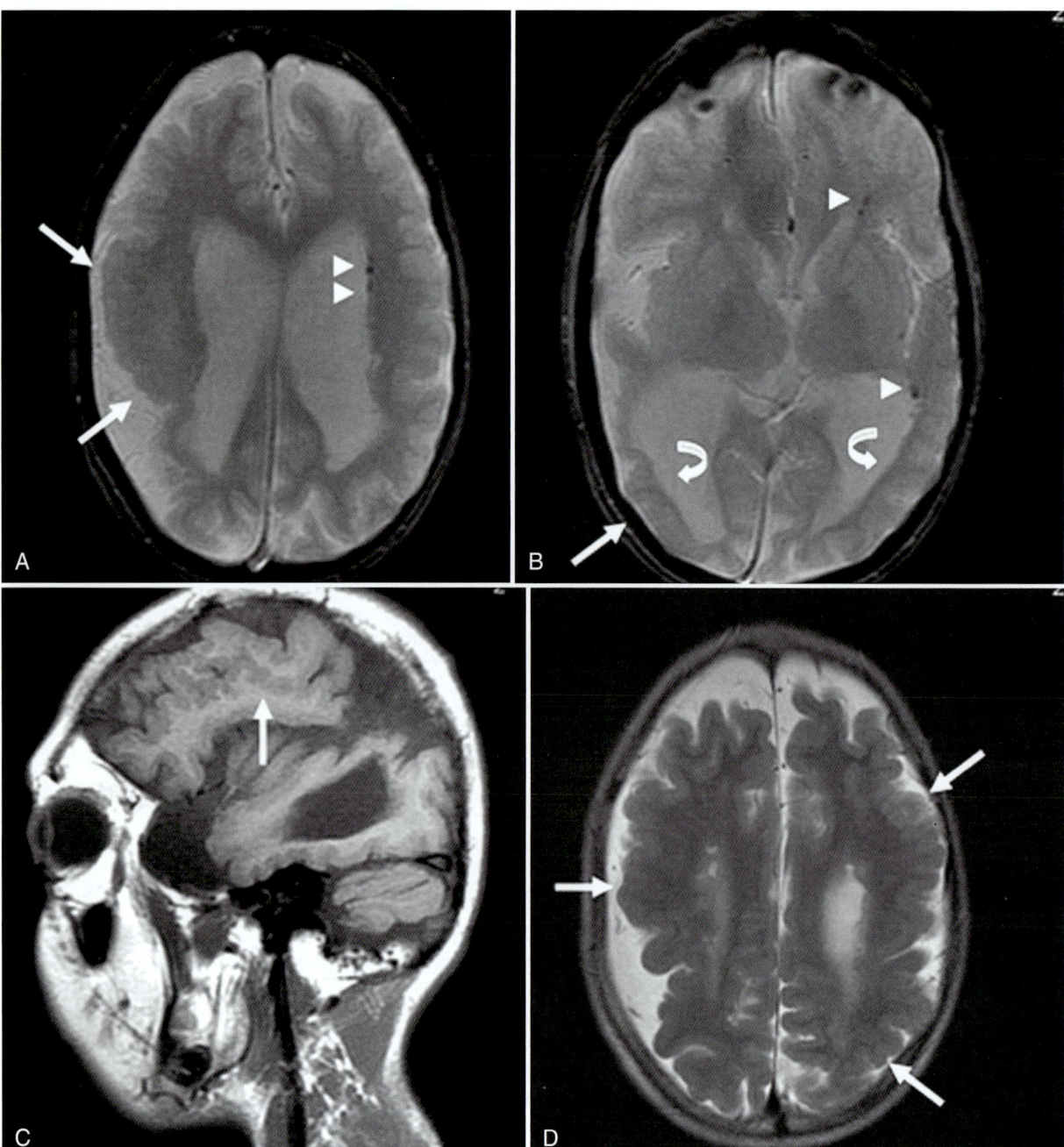

Figure 17-4 Congenital cytomegalovirus infection in a 15-year-old boy. Axial T2 (4700/111.6), gradient-echo (650/25), and sagittal T1 (350/9) images demonstrating dysplastic white matter *(curved arrows)*, periventricular calcifications *(arrowheads)*, and multiple areas of cortical malformations *(arrows)*, most commonly polymicrogyria.

pregnancy, it can be transmitted to the fetus, resulting in serious birth defects, including heart abnormalities, mental retardation, blindness, and deafness. Imaging demonstrates nonspecific findings such as microcephaly, leukoencephalopathy, and calcifications, particularly in the basal ganglia.

Congenital Varicella

Transplacental transmission of varicella following maternal chickenpox infection carries low risk of birth defects. The incidence of congenital varicella syndrome after maternal varicella during the first two trimesters is less than 1%.

Intrahepatic and intracranial calcifications are the most common imaging findings. Although rare, intrauterine encephalitis with atrophy and porencephaly have been reported. Calcifications may be seen in many organs, such as liver, heart, and kidney. Polyhydramnios due to neurologic impairment of swallowing, limb hypoplasia, and diaphragmatic paralysis are other imaging findings. Autonomic nervous system dysfunction may cause neurogenic bladder, hydroureter, esophageal dilatation with aspiration pneumonia.

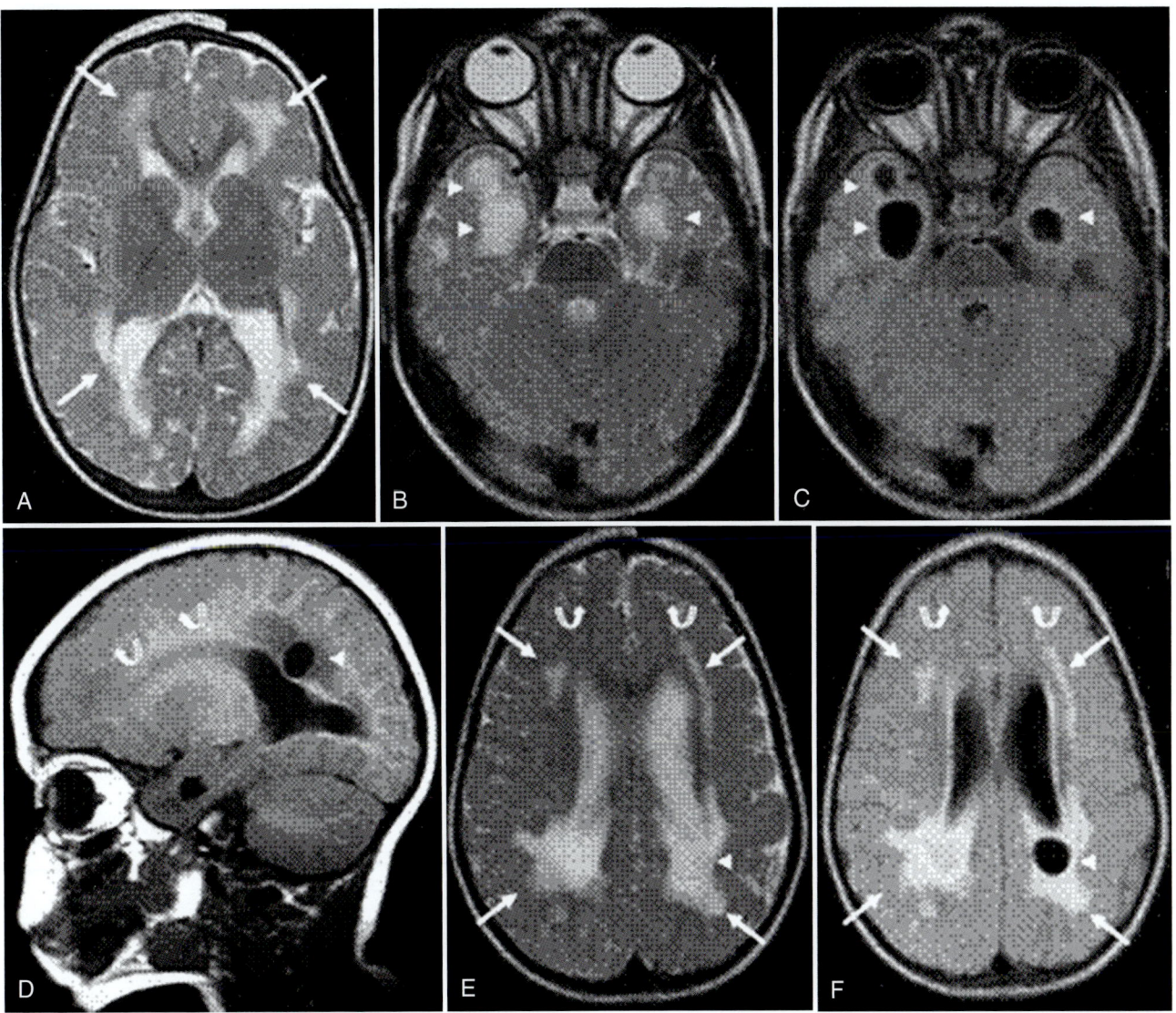

Figure 17-5 Congenital cytomegalovirus (CMV) infection in a 6-month-old girl. Axial T2 (2460.2/110) **(A, B, E)**, T2 FLAIR (11000/140) **(C, F)**, and sagittal T1 (406/12) **(D)** images demonstrating dysplastic white matter *(arrows)* with periventricular cysts *(arrowheads)* and multiple areas of cortical malformations, polymicrogyria *(curved arrows)*.

Cutaneous lesions in dermatomal distribution may also be seen.

Lymphocytic Choriomeningitis Virus

Lymphocytic choriomeningitis virus (LCMV) usually infects wild mice, but humans and a few other animals can also be infected. The virus is not transmitted from person to person; however, transplacental transmission may occur. For most healthy people, the disease is mild and recovery is complete. LCMV infection can have serious consequences in pregnant women and immunosuppressed individuals.

Congenital LCMV infection can result in miscarriage or birth defects, including severe brain damage. Therefore, pregnant women should avoid contact with rodents, including pet hamsters.

LCMV causes chorioretinitis, ependymitis, ependymal calcifications, polymicrogyria, microcephaly, and hydrocephalus. Brain imaging findings in fetus and neonates with congenital LCMV infection may be similar to those of toxoplasmosis and CMV. Of note, hepatosplenomegaly is infrequent in LCMV but is very common in toxoplasmosis and CMV.

Parvovirus B19

Parvovirus B19 infection during pregnancy can result in adverse fetal outcome. The risk of congenital defects is increased if maternal infection occurs during the first two trimesters, but may also occur during the third trimester. Infection during pregnancy can cause severe fetal anemia and nonimmune hydrops fetalis, myocarditis, and cardiac failure. Serial middle cerebral artery peak systolic flow velocity evaluation may be used to predict severe fetal anemia and guide the treatment with cordocentesis transfusion. Parvovirus infected fetuses with severe anemia treated with multiple cordocentesis transfusions may develop polymicrogyria, heterotopia, or cerebellar hemorrhage.

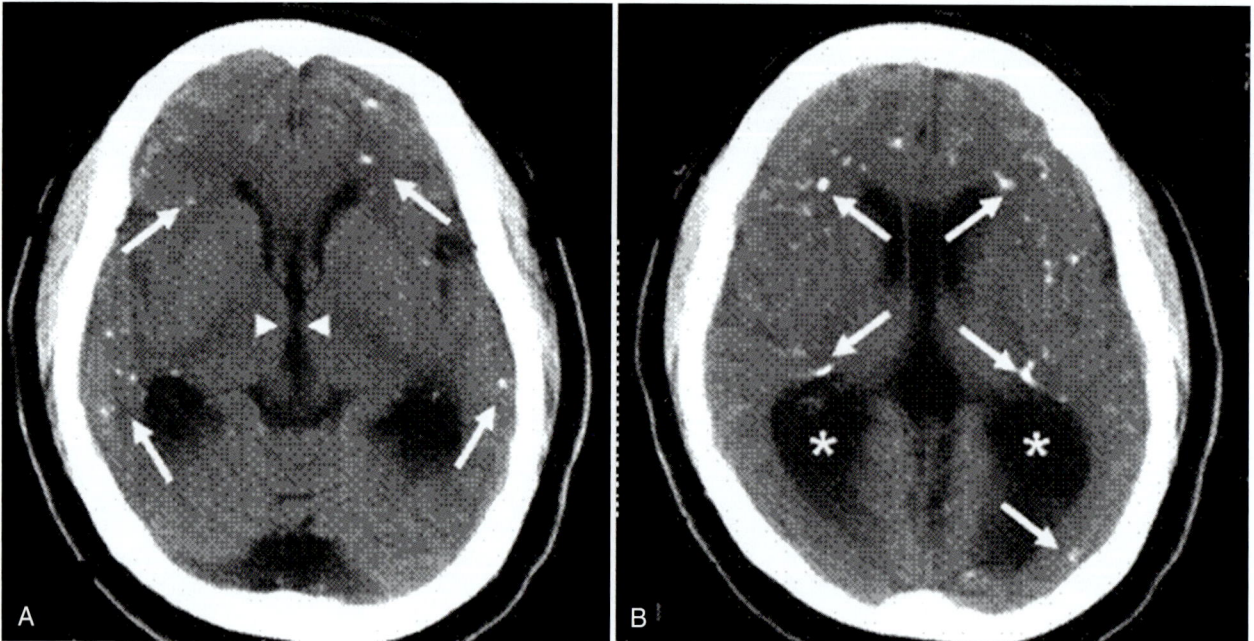

Figure 17-6 Axial noncontrast computed tomography showing dysplastic white matter bilaterally with secondary dilatation of the ventricles *(arrows)*. A normal third ventricle *(arrowheads)* helps to rule out acute hydrocephalus in this group of patients.

West Nile Virus

Population studies have not demonstrated that infants who were exposed to West Nile virus in utero have a higher risk of major birth defects. Rare anecdotal cases of cortical malformations, such as microcephaly and lissencephaly, or cystic white matter changes have been reported.

INTRAUTERINE AND PERINATAL INFECTION

Intrauterine and Perinatal HIV Infection

HIV infection can be transmitted in utero or during birth. Without treatment, the transmission rate of pregnant women infected with HIV to infect their newborn infants is approximately 30%. With treatment, it is possible to decrease the transmission rate to less than 2%. Elective cesarean section can prevent vertical transmission.

Congenital HIV infection rarely manifests acute neonatal symptoms. It most commonly causes developmental delay. The most common imaging findings are brain atrophy and basal ganglia calcifications. Neck lymphadenopathy and benign lymphoepithelial cysts in the parotid glands may also be seen.

With highly active antiretroviral therapy, patients with HIV live longer and HIV-related encephalopathy is becoming more common. Children with acquired immunodeficiency syndrome (AIDS) may develop cerebral aneurysms, central nervous system lymphoma, or extraaxial leiomyoma or leiomyosarcoma. HIV myelopathy with corticospinal tract degeneration and preservation of the posterior columns is not uncommon in children with AIDS.

Toxoplasmosis, CMV, and progressive multifocal leukoencephalomalacia caused by JC virus are the most common opportunistic infections in children with AIDS and low CD4 cell count.

Intrauterine and Perinatal HSV Type 2 Infections

HSV Type 2 infection can also be transmitted in utero or during birth. Pregnant women with genital herpes are at high risk for miscarriage or delivering a low-birthweight baby. Infection can be passed to the infant at the time of delivery if active genial herpes lesions are present. Diagnosis can be made via viral culture or polymerase chain reaction. HSV Type 2 infection early in pregnancy can cause hydranencephaly, intracranial calcifications, and microphthalmia. If the infection occurs late in pregnancy or during delivery, white matter and cortical involvement may rapidly affect the whole brain. There are often multiple hemorrhagic foci, cortical or leptomeningeal enhancement, and restricted diffusion. HSV-2 encephalitis usually develops in 5 to 15 days after birth. Later development of areas of cystic white matter changes is common.

NEONATAL INFECTION

Bacterial Infection

Pregnant women with vaginitis or urinary tract infection caused by Group B streptococcus can infect their infants in utero or during delivery. Group B streptococcus can cause premature birth, neonatal pneumonia, and neonatal meningitis. Other less common causes of neonatal bacterial meningitis are *Escherichia coli, Streptococcus pneumoniae, Haemophilus influenzae* type B, and *Listeria*

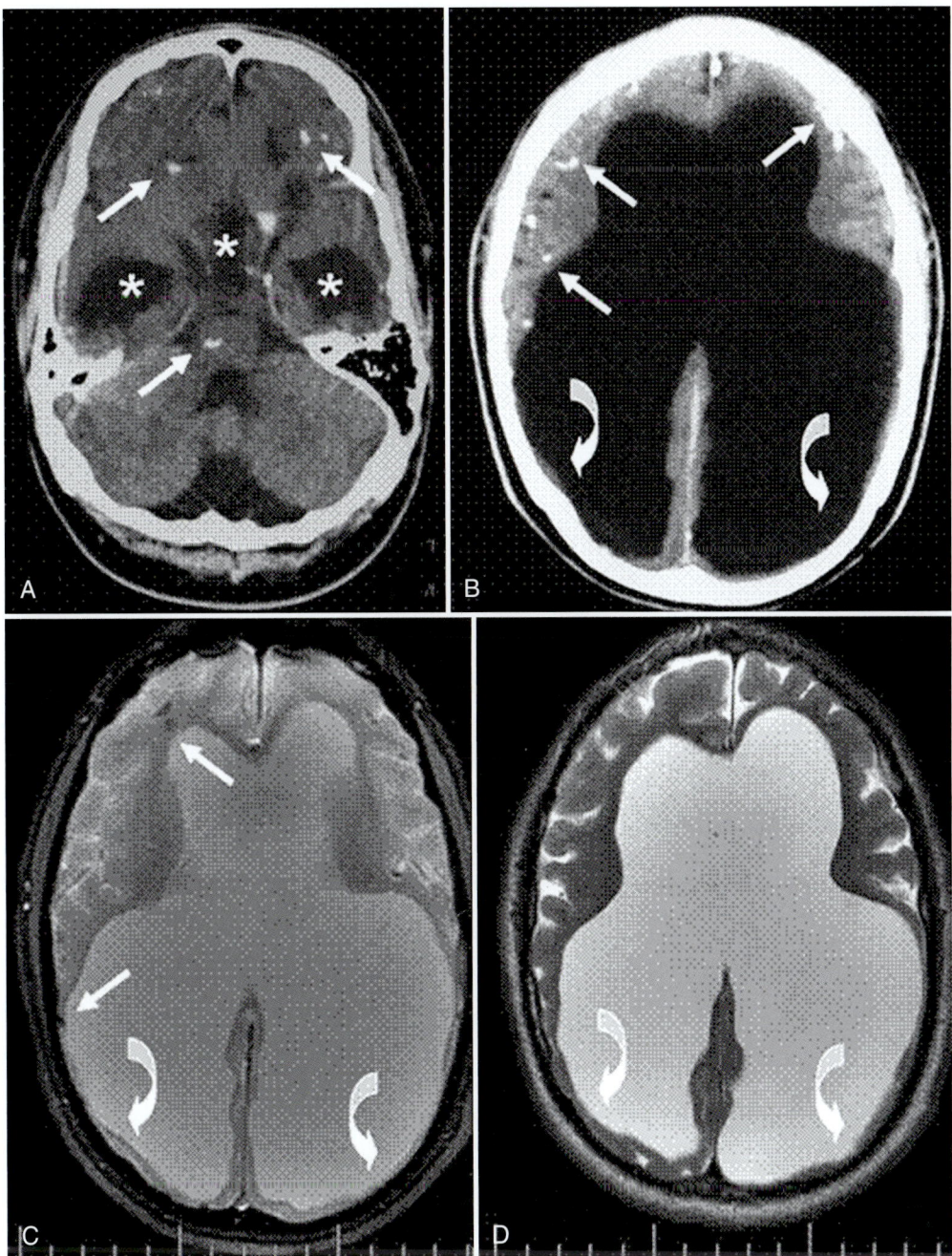

Figure 17-7 Congenital toxoplasmosis in a 21-year-old patient. Axial noncontrast computed tomography, T2 (5000/107.7), and gradient-echo (717/25) images showing marked dilatation of the ventricles in part due to dysplastic white matter *(curved arrows)*. Note there is also a component of hydrocephalus with dilatation of the temporal horns of the lateral ventricles and third ventricle *(asterisk)*. A pattern of multiple random calcifications is frequently seen in severe cases of congenital toxoplasmosis *(arrows)*.

monocytogenes. The most common imaging finding in neonatal meningitis is hydrocephalus, which occurs late in the course of the disease. Imaging should always be performed in patients with bacterial meningitis if they do not have a rapid response to treatment or develop focal neurologic deficit. In such patients, imaging is very helpful in investigating for occlusive venous thrombosis, arterial infarcts, cerebritis, empyema, and brain abscess.

Although neonatal *Citrobacter koseri (diversus)* meningitis is rare, it is often complicated by the formation of brain abscesses, which seem to have a predilection for the frontal lobes. Diffuse neonatal pneumocephalus has been reported in a neonate with *Citrobacter koseri* meningitis. Citrobacter meningitis usually carries poor neurologic outcome, with seizures, mental retardation, and paresis.

Fungal Infection

Candida
Candida as a commensal fungus is frequent in the intestine and other locations in neonates. Most infections do not occur by maternal infection. Vaginal infection is not an indication for cesarean section. The key risk

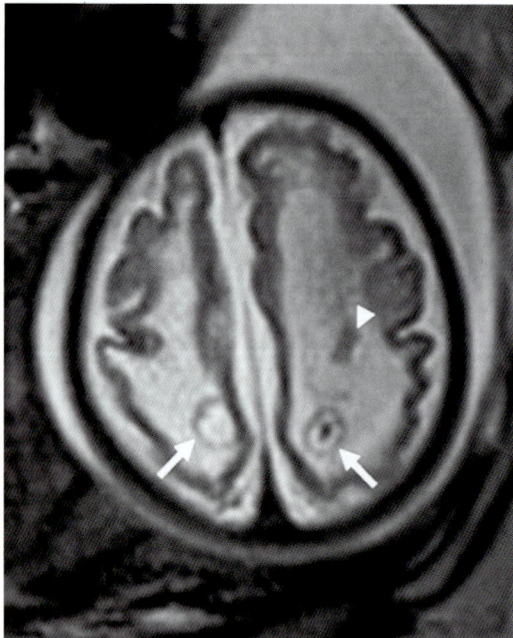

Figure 17-8 Congenital toxoplasmosis. Axial T2-weighted HASTE (1000/144) image of a fetus at 34 weeks of gestation demonstrating cyst lesions, some with calcified nodules *(arrows)* and solid nodules in the cerebral parenchyma.

factors are catheters and antibiotics. Candida infection can cause meningitis, multiple enhancing hemorrhagic microabscesses, or extensive brain necrosis. A case of intraventricular fungus ball has been reported in an immunocompetent neonate with refractory intracranial candidiasis.

Suggested Readings

Alviedo JN, Sood BG, Aranda JV, Becker C. Diffuse pneumocephalus in neonatal Citrobacter meningitis. *Pediatrics*. 2006;118:e1576-1579:Epub 2006 Sep 1525.
Barkovich AJ. *Pediatric Neuroimaging*. 4th ed., Philadelphia: Lippincott Williams & Wilkins; 2005.
Barkovich AJ, Girard N. Fetal brain infections. *Childs Nerv Syst*. 2003;19:501-507:Epub 2003 Jun 2019.
Barkovich AJ, Lindan CE. Congenital cytomegalovirus infection of the brain: imaging analysis and embryologic considerations. *AJNR Am J Neuroradiol*. 1994;15:703-715.
Belman AL. Acquired immunodeficiency syndrome and the child's central nervous system. *Pediatr Clin North Am*. 1992;39:691-714.
Berrebi A, Bardou M, Bessieres MH, et al. Outcome for children infected with congenital toxoplasmosis in the first trimester and with normal ultrasound findings: a study of 36 cases. *Eur J Obstet Gynecol Reprod Biol*. 2007;135:53-57:Epub 2006 Dec 2026.
Binning MJ, Lee J, Thorell EA, Riva-Cambrin JK. Intraventricular fungus ball: a unique manifestation of refractory intracranial candidiasis in an immunocompetent neonate. *J Neurosurg Pediatr*. 2009;4:584-587.
Boyer KM, Holfels E, Roizen N, et al. Risk factors for Toxoplasma gondii infection in mothers of infants with congenital toxoplasmosis: Implications for prenatal management and screening. *Am J Obstet Gynecol*. 2005;192:564-571.
Boyer KM, Remington JS, McLeod RL. Textbook of Pediatric Infectious Diseases. In: Feigin RD, Cherry JD, Demmler GJ, Kaplan SL, eds. 5th ed. Philadelphia: Saunders; 2004. p. 2755. *Pediatr Neurol*. 1995;12:323-334.
Cardoza JD, Filly RA, Podrasky AE. The dangling choroid plexus: a sonographic observation of value in excluding ventriculomegaly. *AJR Am J Roentgenol*. 1988;151:767-770.
Chervenak FA, Jeanty P, Cantraine F, et al. The diagnosis of fetal microcephaly. *Am J Obstet Gynecol*. 1984;149:512-517.
Coakley FV, Glenn OA, Qayyum A, Barkovich AJ, Goldstein R, Filly RA, Fetal MRI: a developing technique for the developing patient. *AJR Am J Roentgenol*. 2004;182:243-252.
Collins AT, Cromwell LD. Computed tomography in the evaluation of congenital cerebral toxoplasmosis. *J Comput Assist Tomogr*. 1980;4:326-329.
Crino JP. Ultrasound and fetal diagnosis of perinatal infection. *Clin Obstet Gynecol*. 1999;42:71-80:quiz 174-175.
Dubrovsky T, Curless R, Scott G, et al. Cerebral aneurysmal arteriopathy in childhood AIDS. *Neurology*. 1998;51:560-565.
Elective caesarean-section versus vaginal delivery in prevention of vertical HIV-1 transmission: a randomised clinical trial. The European Mode of Delivery Collaboration. *Lancet*. 1999;353:1035-1039.
Fakhry J, Khoury A. Fetal intracranial calcifications. The importance of periventricular hyperechoic foci without shadowing. *J Ultrasound Med*. 1991;10:51-54.
Filippi L, Serafini L, Dani C, et al. Congenital syphilis: unique clinical presentation in three preterm newborns. *J Perinat Med*. 2004;32:90-94.
Gavin P, Yogev R. Central nervous system abnormalities in pediatric human immunodeficiency virus infection. *Pediatr Neurosurg*. 1999;31:115-123.
Glenn OA, Bianco K, Barkovich AJ, Callen PW, Parer JT. Fetal cerebellar hemorrhage in parvovirus-associated non-immune hydrops fetalis. *J Matern Fetal Neonatal Med*. 2007;20:769-772.
Interim guidelines for the evaluation of infants born to mothers infected with West Nile virus during pregnancy. *MMWR Morb Mortal Wkly Rep*. 2004;53:154-157.
Lago EG, Baldisserotto M, Hoefel Filho JR, Santiago D, Jungblut R. Agreement between ultrasonography and computed tomography in detecting intracranial calcifications in congenital toxoplasmosis. *Clin Radiol*. 2007;62:1004-1011:Epub 2007 Jul 1020.
Lai PH, Lin SM, Pan HB, Yang CF. Disseminated miliary cerebral candidiasis. *AJNR Am J Neuroradiol*. 1997;18:1303-1306.
Leung AK, Sauve RS, Davies HD. Congenital cytomegalovirus infection. *J Natl Med Assoc*. 2003;95:213-218.
Marques Dias MJ, Harmant-van Rijckevorsel G, Landrieu P, Lyon G. Prenatal cytomegalovirus disease and cerebral microgyria: evidence for perfusion failure, not disturbance of histogenesis, as the major cause of fetal cytomegalovirus encephalopathy. *Neuropediatrics*. 1984;15:18-24.
Mitchell CD. HIV-1 encephalopathy among perinatally infected children: Neuropathogenesis and response to highly active antiretroviral therapy. *Ment Retard Dev Disabil Res Rev*. 2006;12:216-222.
Morel O, Chagnaud S, Laperrelle J, et al. [Parvovirus B19 in pregnancy: literature review]. *Gynecol Obstet Fertil*. 2007;35:1095-1104:Epub 2007 Nov 1019.
Nyberg Da MBSPDH. *Cerebral malformations. Diagnostic Ultrasound of Fetal Anomalies: Text and Atlas*. Chicago, IL: Year Book Medical Publishers; 1990, 83-145.
O'Leary DR, Kuhn S, Kniss KL, et al. Birth outcomes following West Nile Virus infection of pregnant women in the United States: 2003-2004. *Pediatrics*. 2006;117:e537-e545.
Pistorius LR, Smal J, de Haan TR, et al. Disturbance of cerebral neuronal migration following congenital parvovirus B19 infection. *Fetal Diagn Ther*. 2008;24:491-494:Epub 2008 Dec 2005.
Pratt RD, Nichols S, McKinney N, Kwok S, Dankner WM, Spector SA. Virologic markers of human immunodeficiency virus type 1 in cerebrospinal fluid of infected children. *J Infect Dis*. 1996;174:288-293.
Resnick L, Berger JR, Shapshak P, Tourtellotte WW. Early penetration of the blood-brain-barrier by HIV. *Neurology*. 1988;38:9-14.
Rogers MF, Shaffer N. Reducing the risk of maternal-infant transmission of HIV by attacking the virus. *N Engl J Med*. 1999;341:441-443.
Rose SJ. Neonatal meningitis due to Citrobacter koseri. *J Perinat Med*. 1979;7:273-275.
Sensini A. Toxoplasma gondii infection in pregnancy: opportunities and pitfalls of serological diagnosis. *Clin Microbiol Infect*. 2006;12:504-512.
Smith CK, Arvin AM. Varicella in the fetus and newborn. *Semin Fetal Neonatal Med*. 2009;14:209-217:Epub 2008 Dec 2019.
Straussberg R, Harel L, Amir J. Long-Term outcome of neonatal Citrobacter koseri (diversus) meningitis treated with imipenem/meropenem and surgical drainage. *Infection*. 2001;29:280-282.
Tortori-Donati P, Rossi A. *Pediatric Neuroradiology*, Germany: Springer; 2005.
Whitley R. Neonatal herpes simplex virus infection. *Curr Opin Infect Dis*. 2004;17:243-246.

SECTION IV

PROBLEM SOLVING: ANATOMIC REGIONS

CHAPTER 18
Head and Neck Radiology
Girish M. Fatterpekar and Peter M. Som

This chapter on head and neck radiology follows a slightly different format than the rest of the textbook. Instead of a problem-solving approach, a case-based approach is used. Toward this end, the discussion in this chapter is divided into seven subsections. Each subsection deals with a particular part of the head and neck: temporal bone; orbit; sinonasal cavities; salivary glands; masticator space, oral cavity including floor of mouth, and pharynx; thyroid, larynx; and other regions of the neck. In each of these subsections, the most common, clinically important cases are discussed. In a few of the pathologies outlined, the discussion is boosted by including relevant images of the differential diagnosis, allowing illustration of key distinguishing features.

■ TEMPORAL BONE

Eleven cases are discussed in this section. They include congenital anomalies involving the external ear, middle ear and inner ear, including large vestibular aqueduct syndrome, trauma (e.g., fractures), vascular anomalies (e.g., aberrant carotid artery), infectious and inflammatory conditions (e.g., mastoiditis, cholesteatoma, Bell's palsy), and tumors (e.g., cholesterol granuloma, glomus tumor, acoustic schwannoma).

Congenital External and Middle Ear Anomalies

Anomalies of the external and middle ear usually occur together due to the common embryologic origin from the first and second branchial arches. Isolated anomalies occur occasionally. An atretic pinna and hearing loss are common presenting features. Characteristic radiologic features include an atretic, ectopically placed pinna, absent or hypoplastic external auditory canal, hypoplastic tympanic cavity, and malformed ossicles, which are frequently attached to the lateral attic wall (Figure 18-1). Associated radiologic features can include an anomalous course of the facial nerve as it traverses the tympanic cavity and inner ear anomalies.

Congenital Inner Ear Anomalies

Anomalies of the inner ear result from partial or complete failure of development of the otic cyst during the first few weeks of embryonic life. Michel and Mondini malformations are some of the more common inner ear anomalies seen. Michel deformity refers to complete labyrinthine aplasia and represents arrest correlating with the third gestational week. Mondini anomaly refers to incomplete partition of the cochlea resulting in 1½ turns instead of the normal 2½ to 2¾ turns and represents arrest correlating with the seventh gestational week. Most patients present with congenital sensorineural hearing loss. Characteristic radiologic findings are variable depending on the gestational age at arrest of the developing otocyst. Thus, radiologic manifestations include complete labyrinthine aplasia, common cavity, incomplete partition of the cochlea, and various other dysplasias involving the cochlea, vestibule, and semicircular canals (Figure 18-2). Different classification systems have been proposed based on the anomalies seen. However, it is best to describe the anomalies without delving much into the classification system because of the lack of consensus on any one of them. Of note, in some inner ear anomalies, such as Alexander and Scheibe aplasia, the membranous labyrinth including the organ of Corti are affected. Radiologic assessment for such membranous abnormalities is beyond the resolution of current imaging modalities.

Large Vestibular Aqueduct Syndrome

Large vestibular aqueduct syndrome results from abnormal congenital enlargement of the membranous endolymphatic duct and sac. Most patients present with congenital sensorineural hearing loss. Characteristic radiologic findings include an enlarged vestibular aqueduct (>1.5 mm in diameter) in its midportion. A simpler way to diagnose this entity is to correlate the caliber of the vestibular aqueduct to the adjacent posterior semicircular canal. The posterior semicircular canal is approximately 1.5 mm in diameter. Thus, a vestibular aqueduct caliber greater than that of the adjacent posterior semicircular canal is suggestive of large vestibular aqueduct syndrome (Figure 18-3).

Temporal Bone Trauma

Temporal bone fractures usually occur secondary to blunt trauma. Three kinds of temporal bone fractures are known based on their orientation to the long axis of the temporal bone: *longitudinal variety*, with the fracture line along the long axis of the temporal bone; *transverse variety*, with the fracture line perpendicular to the long axis of the temporal bone; and *mixed variety*, which is a combination of the two fractures. The longitudinal variety causes disruption of the ossicles and trauma to the

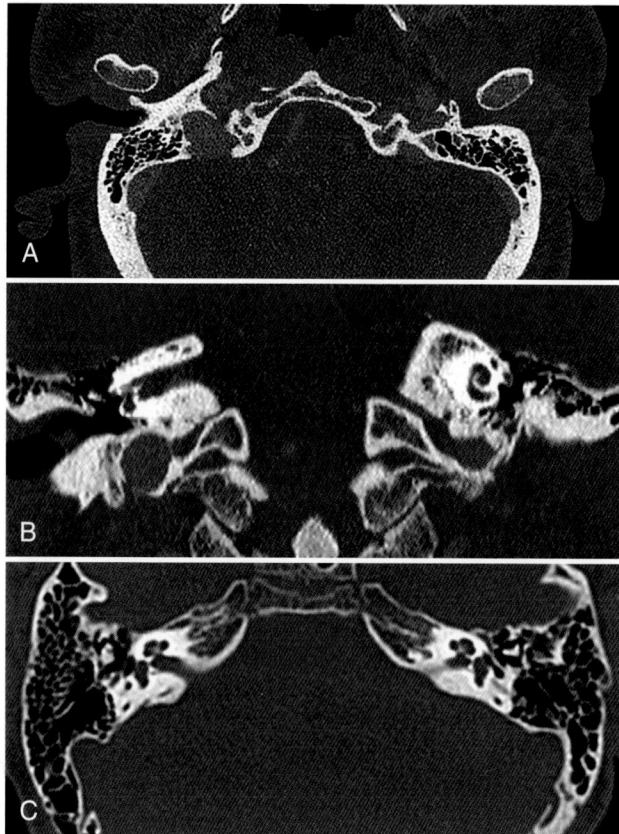

Figure 18-1 A: High-resolution axial computed tomographic (CT) scan through the temporal bones demonstrating a dysplastic left pinna and an absent external auditory canal. **B:** High-resolution coronal reformatted CT scan demonstrating a hypoplastic left tympanic cavity and malformed ossicles attached to the lateral tympanic cavity. **C:** In a different patient, axial CT scan demonstrating malformed ossicles on the left side and a hypoplastic tympanic cavity. On the right side, the anomaly is more subtle. The ice-cream cone appearance of the ossicles (produced by the head of the malleus and body of incus) is normally seen. However, close observation reveals that the ossicles are attached to the lateral wall of the tympanic cavity.

facial nerve. The transverse variety is more often associated with fractures of the inner ear structures. Swelling and tenderness to the ear following temporal bone trauma are common clinical features. Depending on the underlying structures affected, patients can present with conductive or sensorineural hearing loss and facial paresis or paralysis. A characteristic radiologic feature is demonstration of linear nonserrated lucencies consistent with fractures traversing the temporal bone. The course of the fracture line should be carefully evaluated to assess for fractures involving the ossicles and their associated dislocation, for fractures involving the inner ear structures, which can result in perilymph fistula, and for fractures involving the tegmen tympani, which can result in cerebrospinal fluid otorrhea. Hemotympanum as suggested by opacification of the mastoid air cells is a common associated finding (Figure 18-4). Very rarely, laceration of the adjacent venous sinus, such as the sigmoid sinus, is seen. Cerebrospinal fluid otorrhea or rhinorrhea and meningitis are delayed complications of temporal bone trauma.

Aberrant Carotid Artery

Aberrant carotid artery represents an enlarged inferior tympanic artery anastomosing with an enlarged caroticotympanic artery, when the vertical portion of the petrous segment of the internal carotid artery is underdeveloped or regresses during embryogenesis. It is essential to recognize this entity and not mistake it for a "mass" so as to avoid biopsy, which can otherwise result in catastrophic hemorrhage. Most patients are asymptomatic. Pulsatile tinnitus and conductive hearing loss are symptoms that have otherwise been described. Characteristic radiologic findings include an absent normal vertical petrous portion of the carotid canal. Instead, the carotid artery is seen to course upward and slightly laterally through an enlarged inferior tympanic canaliculus. It protrudes variably into the tympanic cavity, positioned lateral to the promontory of the middle ear, and

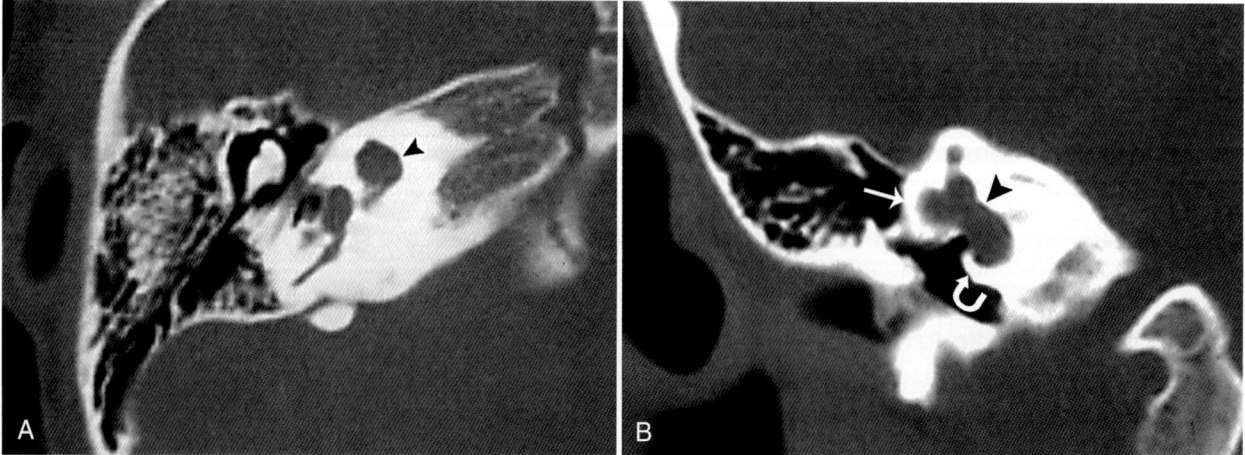

Figure 18-2 A: Axial computed tomographic (CT) scan demonstrating congenital cystic dilatation of the cochlea (arrowhead) with incomplete partitioning. **B:** In a different patient, high-resolution coronal CT scan demonstrating a dilated dysplastic vestibule (*arrowhead*) and lateral semicircular canal (*arrow*). There is mild dysplasia of the basal turn of cochlea (*curved arrow*).

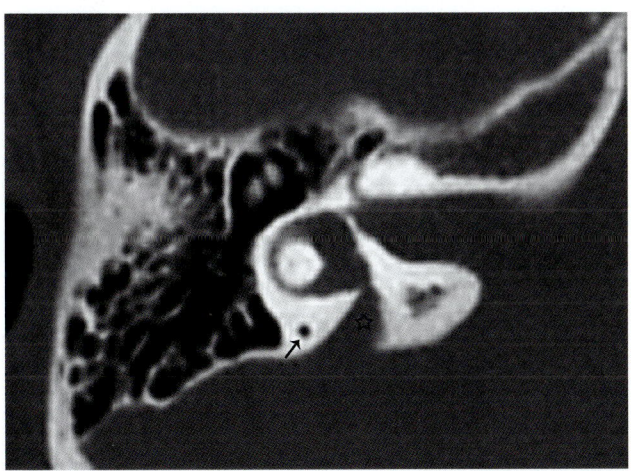

Figure 18-3 Axial computed tomographic scan demonstrating enlarged caliber (> 1.5 mm) of the vestibular aqueduct (*star*). *Arrow* points to posterior semicircular canal whose caliber can be used as a rough reference guide to determine the presence or absence of an enlarged vestibular aqueduct. A vestibular aqueduct caliber greater than that of the posterior semicircular canal is suggestive of large vestibular aqueduct syndrome.

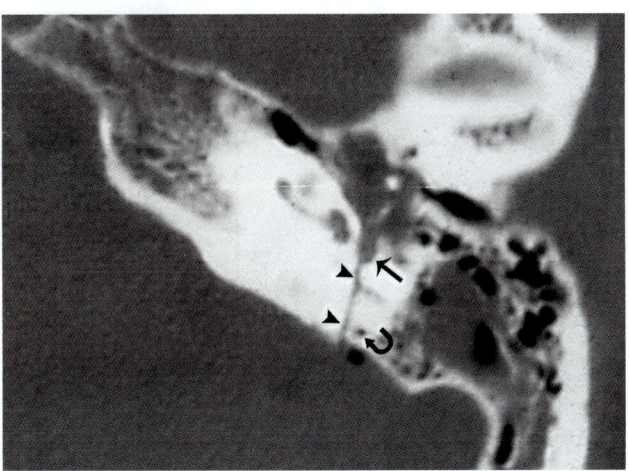

Figure 18-4 Axial computed tomographic scan demonstrating a transverse fracture (*arrowheads*) extending through the inner ear involving the posterior semicircular canal (*curved arrow*) and the vestibule (*arrow*). Opacified tympanic cavity and mastoid air cells reflect hemotympanum.

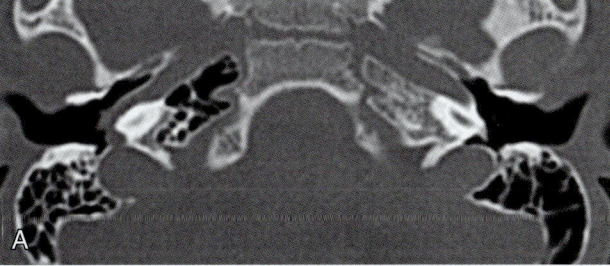
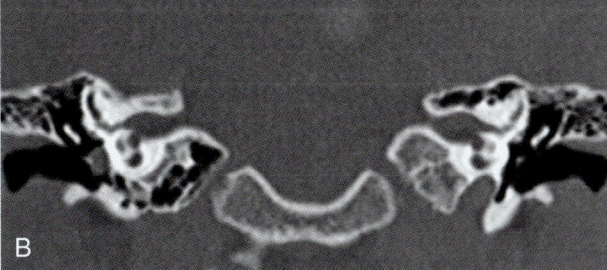
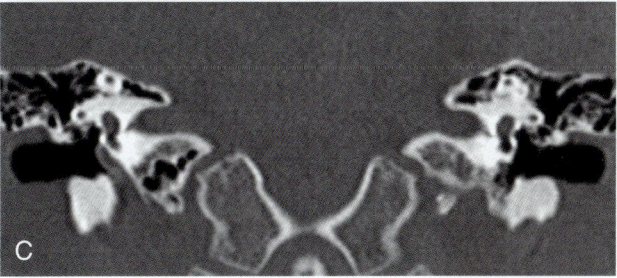

Figure 18-5 A: Axial computed tomographic scan demonstrating a curvilinear structure coursing through the medial wall of the right tympanic cavity, which appears contiguous with the vertical portion of the petrous internal carotid artery (ICA) posteriorly and with the horizontal portion of the petrous ICA anteriorly. **B:** Coronal reformatted CT scan demonstrating the same lesion to be in close proximity to the cochlear promontory. **C:** More posteriorly in the coronal plane, this lesion is contiguous with the vertical segment of the petrous ICA. The diagnosis is aberrant carotid artery.

courses further anteriorly through a normal horizontal petrous portion of the carotid canal (Figure 18-5). Differential diagnosis includes glomus tympanicum and persistent stapedial artery. Glomus tympanicum will be seen as a focal, intensely enhancing lesion overlying the cochlear promontory. Persistent stapedial artery will be seen as a curvilinear enhancing structure coursing along the medial wall of the tympanic cavity, with an absent foramen spinosum on the ipsilateral side.

Acute Mastoiditis

Acute otitis media is seen most often in the pediatric population. It refers to inflammation of the middle ear and mastoid air cells with resultant fluid collections. In most patients, the condition resolves with antibiotics. However, if not controlled, secondary complications can occur. Most patients present with fever and otalgia following a bout of upper respiratory tract infection. Imaging in acute otitis media is not routinely obtained. However, in patients who do not respond to antibiotic treatment or in whom complications are suspected, contrast-enhanced computed tomographic (CT) scans or magnetic resonance imaging (MRI) studies can be obtained. Typically, opacified mastoid air cells and tympanic cavity will be seen. Destruction of the mastoid air septae is suggestive of coalescent mastoiditis. Erosion of the cortex and extension of the infection into the adjacent soft tissues or intracranial compartment can result in abscess formation (Figure 18-6). Labyrinthitis, otitic hydrocephalus, venous sinus thrombosis, venous infarction, and meningitis are other complications that can be seen.

Cholesteatoma

Cholesteatoma is a collection of keratinous debris seen typically within the tympanic cavity. Such a collection commonly occurs following ingrowth of stratified squamous epithelium from the external auditory canal into the tympanic cavity, secondary to external otitis and perforation of the ear drum. Less commonly, such collections develop from congenital rests. Most patients present with painless otorrhea and hearing loss. CT scan is the imaging modality of choice to evaluate of cholesteatoma. It demonstrates a nonenhancing soft tissue lesion within the tympanic cavity with characteristic erosion of scutum and ossicles. Widening of the Prussak space will also be seen (Figure 18-7). Less commonly, erosion of the otic capsule is seen, resulting in perilymph fistula. Differential diagnosis includes glomus tympanicum and granulation tissue within tympanic cavity. Glomus tympanicum will be seen as a focal enhancing soft tissue mass overlying the cochlear promontory. There is no erosion of the adjacent ossicles or otic capsule. Granulation tissue will be seen as an enhancing soft tissue mass within the tympanic cavity. No erosion of the ossicles or scutum or otic capsule will be seen.

Bell's palsy

Bell's palsy is an acute, idiopathic, unilateral, peripheral, lower motor neuron facial nerve paralysis that gradually resolves over time. Most patients present with an acute onset of facial weakness. MR is the imaging modality of choice. The typical imaging appearance is asymmetric enhancement of some segments of the facial nerve or of the entire course of the facial nerve as it traverses the temporal bone (Figure 18-8). No obvious thickening of the facial nerve is seen. Differential diagnosis includes perineural extension of the tumor and facial nerve schwannoma. Usually with perineural extension, there will be an associated known high-grade malignant tumor. Enhancement along the course of the facial nerve will be seen. The nerve can also appear to be

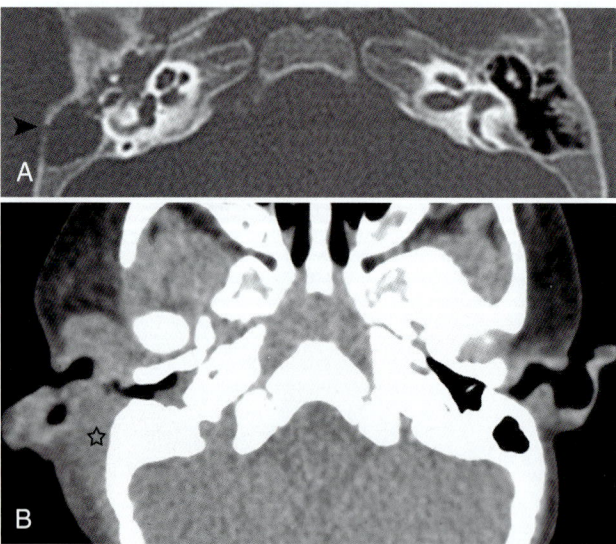

Figure 18-6 A: Axial computed tomographic (CT) scan demonstrating opacified right mastoid air cells and tympanic cavity. There is a suggestion of destruction of mastoid cortex (*arrowhead*). **B:** Axial CT scan, soft tissue window demonstrating soft tissue swelling (*star*) suggestive of phlegmonous change or early abscess formation. The diagnosis is acute coalescent mastoiditis with an early abscess in the overlying soft tissues.

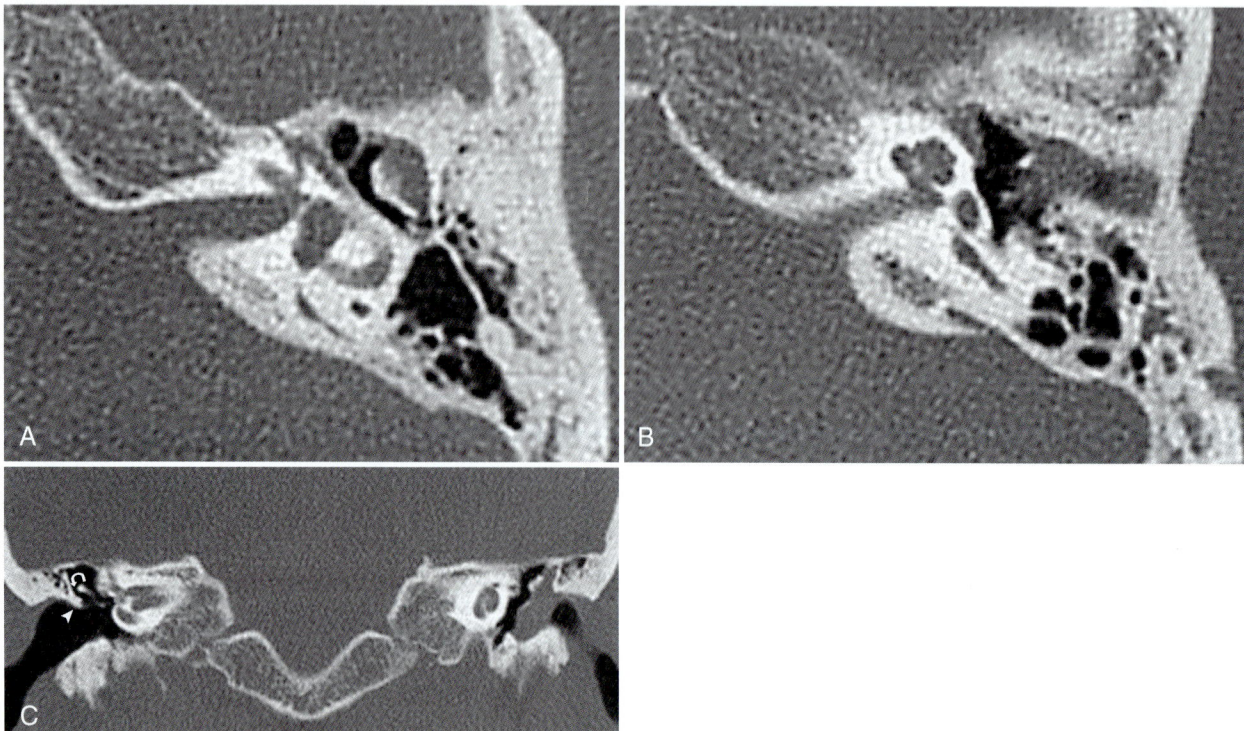

Figure 18-7 A: Axial computed tomographic (CT) scan demonstrating a soft tissue mass within the left lateral tympanic cavity eroding malleus and incus. **B:** At a slightly caudal level, axial CT scan demonstrating the soft tissue mass eroding the long process of incus. Extension of this soft tissue mass into the external auditory canal is also seen. **C:** Coronal reformatted CT scan demonstrating erosion of the ossicles and scutum, and widening of the Prussak space. The normal right scutum (*arrowhead*) and Prussak space (*curved arrow*) are shown for comparison. The diagnosis is cholesteatoma.

thickened. Facial nerve schwannoma will demonstrate fusiform thickening of the facial nerve. Variable degrees of enhancement will be seen.

Cholesterol Granuloma

Cholesterol granuloma is the most common petrous apex lesion. Most patients are young adults who present with tinnitus, hearing loss, and hemifacial spasms. On imaging, CT scan demonstrates an expansile lytic lesion involving the petrous apex. The lesion appears hyperintense on T1-weighted imaging (T1-WI), hyperintense on T2-WI, and does not demonstrate any enhancement. The characteristic hyperintense signal seen on T1-WI is highly suggestive of cholesterol granuloma (Figure 18-9, A and B). Occasionally, fluid–fluid level secondary to intralesional hemorrhage can be seen. Differential diagnosis includes chondrosarcoma, aneurysm of the petrous internal carotid artery, congenital cholesteatoma, and mucocele. Chondrosarcoma will demonstrate rings and arcs of calcification within the lytic lesion (Figure 18-9, C). The lesion will appear hypointense on T1-WI and exhibit heterogeneous enhancement following contrast administration. An aneurysm can be seen as an expansile lytic lesion within the temporal bone demonstrating peripheral calcification. Flow-related artifact can be seen on MRI. Contrast-enhanced MR angiogram and CT angiogram are diagnostic (Figure 18-9, D). Congenital cholesteatoma will appear hypointense on T1-WI and will not exhibit any enhancement. Depending on its protein content, mucocele can demonstrate variable signal intensity characteristics on T1-WI and T2-WI. It can sometimes be difficult to distinguish a cholesterol granuloma from a mucocele.

Glomus Jugulare

Glomus jugulare is a paraganglioma that arises in the jugular fossa from paraganglia located within the adventitia of the jugular bulb. Most patients present with dysphagia and hoarseness of voice. Cross-sectional imaging demonstrates an intensely enhancing lesion centered in the jugular foramen. The demonstration of an irregularly marginated lesion on CT and "salt-and-pepper" appearance on T2-weighted MRI are highly suggestive of glomus jugulare (Figure 18-10, A–D). "Salt" refers to the hemorrhage and "pepper" to the flow voids seen in most such lesions. Differential diagnosis includes schwannomas, meningiomas, and metastasis. Typically, schwannomas will demonstrate a lesion with smooth, rounded borders. No irregular bone destruction will be seen. Also, schwannomas appear more homogeneous on MRI and do not demonstrate the salt-and-pepper appearance of glomus tumors (Figure 18-10, E–H). Meningiomas will be associated with hyperostosis. An enhancing dural tail, although not specific, is more often seen with meningiomas than with glomus tumors. A primary tumor will be known in most patients with metastasis.

Acoustic Schwannoma

Acoustic schwannomas account for 60% to 80% of all cerebellopontine angle tumors. Most acoustic schwannomas arise from the vestibular division of the vestibulocochlear (VIII) nerve. Typically, patients present with unilateral sensorineural hearing loss. Large acoustic schwannomas can be evaluated by both CT and MR. An enhancing lesion widening the internal auditory canal and extending into the cerebellopontine angle cistern producing an "ice cream cone" appearance will be seen. Some such acoustic schwannomas are associated with cysts, typically along the medial margin of the lesion. Intracanalicular schwannomas are best evaluated by high-resolution MRI of the internal auditory canal. CT imaging can be limited in evaluation. Bilateral acoustic schwannomas are diagnostic of neurofibromatosis type 2 (NF2) (Figure 18-11). Differential diagnosis includes meningiomas, epidermoids, and arachnoid cysts. Meningiomas in the cerebellopontine angle cistern will be associated with hyperostosis of the petrous pyramid. A dural tail, although not specific, is more often seen with meningiomas than with glomus tumors. Epidermoids in the cerebellopontine angle cistern will be seen as nonenhancing cystic lesions that will typically demonstrate restricted diffusion. Arachnoid cysts in the cerebellopontine angle cistern will be seen as nonenhancing cystic lesions that will not demonstrate any restricted diffusion.

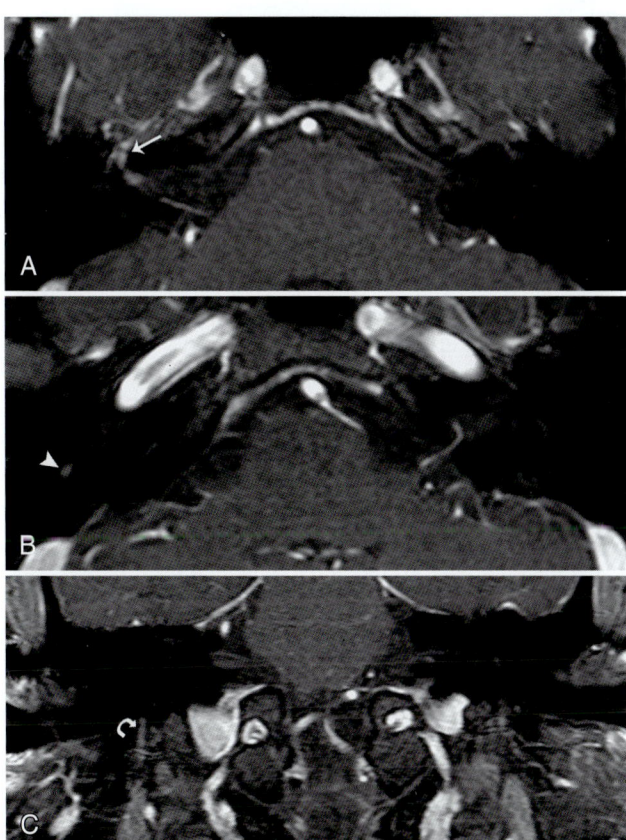

Figure 18-8 A, B: High-resolution, fat-suppressed, contrast-enhanced axial T1-weighted imaging through the temporal bones demonstrating asymmetric enhancement of the labyrinthine segment (*arrow*) and posterior tympanic segment (*arrowhead*) of the right facial nerve. **C:** High-resolution, fat-suppressed, contrast-enhanced coronal T1-weighted imaging demonstrating asymmetric enhancement of the mastoid segment (*curved arrow*) of the right facial nerve. The diagnosis is Bell's palsy.

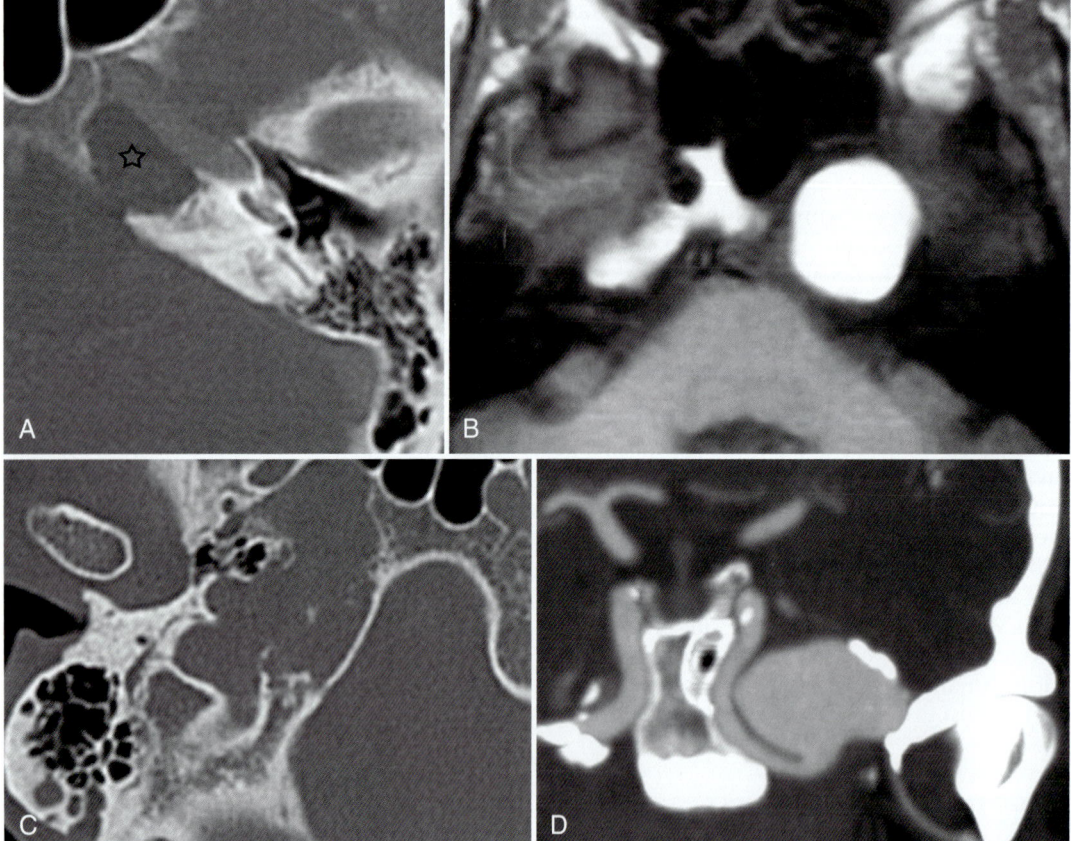

Figure 18-9 A: Axial computed tomographic (CT) scan demonstrating an expansile lytic lesion (*star*) in the left petrous apex. **B:** In a different patient, axial T1-weighted imaging demonstrating a rounded homogeneously hyperintense lesion at the petrous apex. The diagnosis in both of these patients is cholesterol granuloma. **C:** In another patient, axial CT scan demonstrating an expansile lytic lesion at the right petrous apex showing faint rings and arcs of calcification. The diagnosis in this patient is a chondrosarcoma. **D:** In yet another patient, coronal reformatted CT angiogram demonstrating a saccular aneurysm at the left petrous apex (Image courtesy: Shyamsunder Sabat, University of Alabama, Birmingham).

■ ORBIT

Eight cases are discussed in this section, including congenital vascular malformations (e.g., hemangiomas), orbital venous varix, trauma (e.g., orbital blowout fractures), infectious and inflammatory conditions (e.g., orbital cellulitis, Sjögren syndrome, Graves disease), tumors (e.g., lymphoma), and optic nerve gliomas.

Vascular Malformations: Hemangiomas

There are two types of hemangiomas: capillary and cavernous hemangiomas. Capillary hemangiomas typically are absent at birth but demonstrate rapid growth during infancy and spontaneous involution later in life. In contrast, cavernous hemangiomas typically are seen in middle-aged adults. Most often unilateral, these lesions are classically located in the retrobulbar compartment and demonstrate slow progressive enlargement. Most patients with capillary hemangioma are brought in by parents who notice a red periorbital area that blanches on pressure. Most patients with cavernous hemangioma present with ocular discomfort. Both lesions are seen on CT as relatively well-defined lesions that demonstrate intense enhancement following contrast administration. Less commonly, mild to moderate enhancement has been reported. MR demonstrates a well-defined, lobulated lesion hypointense on T1-WI and hyperintense on T2-WI, which demonstrates avid contrast enhancement (Figure 18-12). Flow voids and calcification are sometimes seen. Differential diagnosis of capillary hemangioma includes lymphangioma and rhabdomyosarcoma. Lymphangiomas typically are transspatial and do not demonstrate obvious enhancement. Rhabdomyosarcomas are seen as destructive lesions, eroding and not just scalloping the bones. Differential diagnosis of cavernous hemangioma includes schwannoma and hemangiopericytoma. Schwannomas typically occur along the course of cranial nerves III, IV, and VI. These lesions appear as well-defined soft tissue lesions hypointense on T1-WI and hyperintense on T2-WI, and demonstrate mild to moderate contrast enhancement. Hemangiopericytomas are rare intraorbital lesions that demonstrate intense early enhancement following contrast administration.

Orbital Venous Varix

Orbital varix is the most frequently encountered primary orbital venous abnormality. Patients usually are asymptomatic, but some may complain of intermittent proptosis, especially with a Valsalva-type maneuver. On imaging, a focal or segmental dilation of the superior

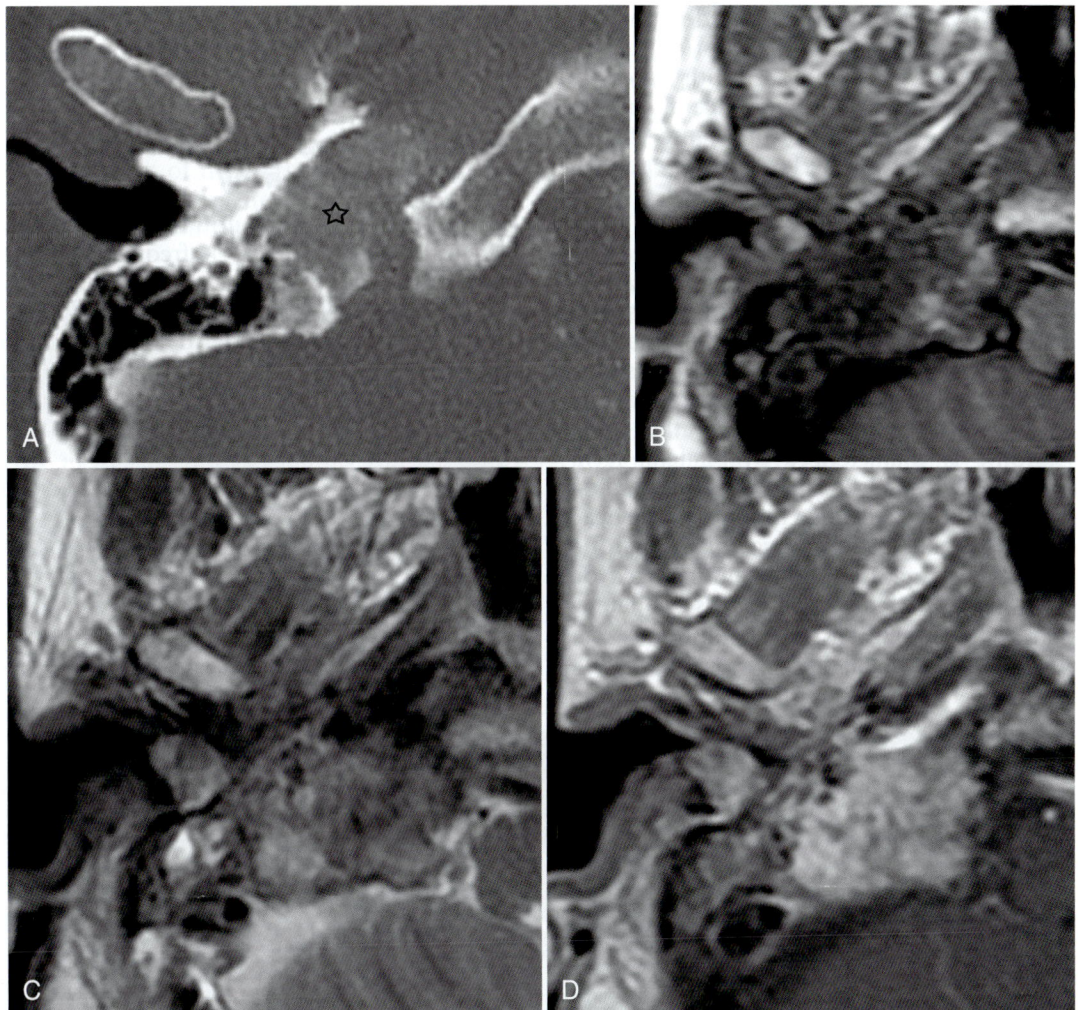

Figure 18-10 **A:** Contrast-enhanced axial computed tomographic (CT) scan demonstrating an irregularly marginated lytic lesion (*star*) in the right jugular foramen. Axial T1-weighted imaging **(B)**, axial T2-weighted imaging **(C)**, and contrast-enhanced axial T1-weighted imaging **(D)** demonstrating a heterogeneously enhancing lesion within the jugular foramen. The lesion demonstrates hypointense foci representing flow voids and hyperintense foci representing hemorrhage, producing the characteristic salt-and-pepper appearance of a glomus tumor. The diagnosis in this patient is glomus jugulare.

Continued

ophthalmic vein will be seen. Occasionally, the entire superior ophthalmic vein will be seen to be asymmetrically enlarged. Further dilation of the superior ophthalmic vein can occur following a Valsalva-type maneuver (Figure 18-13). Differential diagnosis includes carotid cavernous fistula, cavernous sinus thrombosis, and orbital vascular malformation. In direct carotid–cavernous fistula, an enlarged ipsilateral cavernous segment of the ipsilateral carotid artery will be seen. In indirect carotid–cavernous fistula, an arteriovenous fistula can be demonstrated on an angiogram. Also, reversal of flow will be seen in the superior ophthalmic vein. Cavernous sinus thrombosis will be seen as a filling defect in the cavernous sinuses. Orbital vascular malformation will demonstrate arterial feeders and a nidus.

Orbital Blowout Fracture

Orbital blowout fracture results from direct blunt trauma to the orbit. The sudden increase in intraorbital pressure from such an injury results in a fracture involving the inherently weak floor of the orbit, typically along the infraorbital foramen. The orbital rim classically remains intact. Fracture involving the floor of the orbit will be seen on CT studies (Figure 18-14). Enophthalmos is an ocular emergency and therefore should be evaluated. Inferior rectus entrapment is also a medical emergency; however, it is a clinical diagnosis. Thus, although entrapment of the inferior rectus can be suggested, it can never be diagnosed solely on imaging. Associated fractures, including those of the nasal bones and maxilla, are common and should be assessed.

Ocular Cellulitis

Ocular cellulitis can be broadly classified into preseptal cellulitis and postseptal (orbital) cellulitis. Of the two, postseptal cellulitis has a higher morbidity and therefore requires more aggressive treatment. The most common cause of orbital cellulitis is sinusitis. Most patients will present with orbital pain and swelling. Occasionally, patients complain of reduced

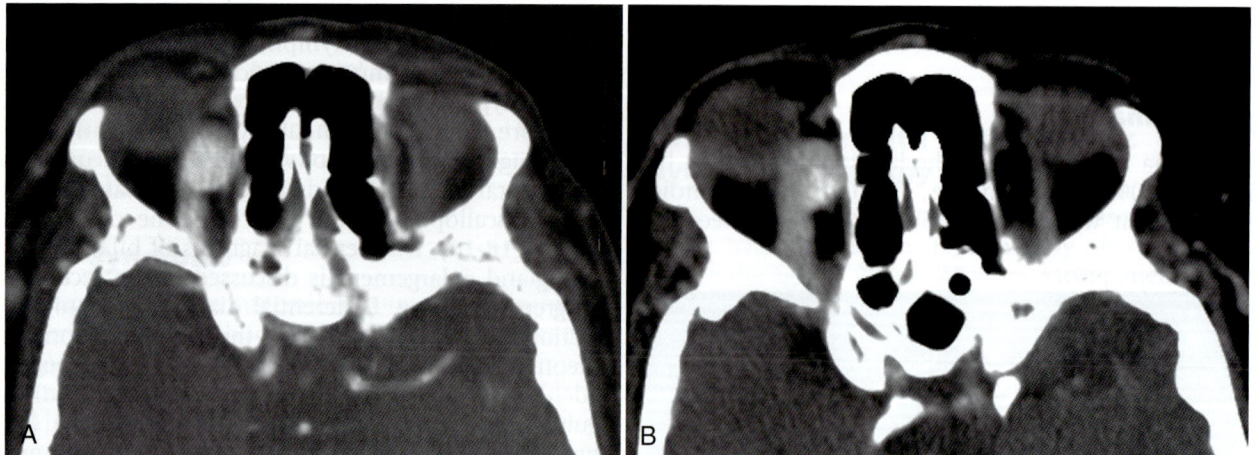

Figure 18-13 A: Contrast-enhanced axial computed tomographic (CT) scan demonstrating a dilated tortuous right superior ophthalmic vein. **B:** Contrast-enhanced axial CT scan following Valsalva maneuver demonstrating further increase in the caliber of the dilated superior ophthalmic vein. The cavernous sinuses do not demonstrate any filling defect (ruling out cavernous sinus thrombosis) or any asymmetric prominence (ruling out carotid cavernous fistula). The diagnosis is orbital venous varix.

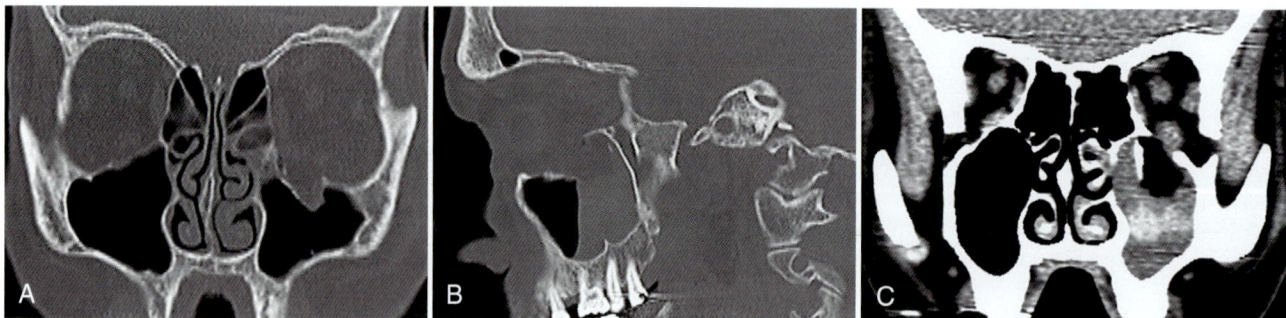

Figure 18-14 A: Coronal computed tomographic (CT) scan, bone window demonstrating a fracture involving the floor of the left orbit. **B:** Reformatted sagittal CT scan, bone window demonstrating the fracture involving the midportion of the floor of the orbit. The orbital rim is intact. **C:** Coronal CT scan, soft tissue window demonstrating the inferior rectus is adjacent to the fracture site, raising the possibility of inferior rectus entrapment. However, it should be noted that inferior rectus entrapment is a clinical diagnosis and can only be suggested but not diagnosed on imaging. Hyperdensity seen within the maxillary sinus represents hemorrhage. The diagnosis is orbital blowout fracture.

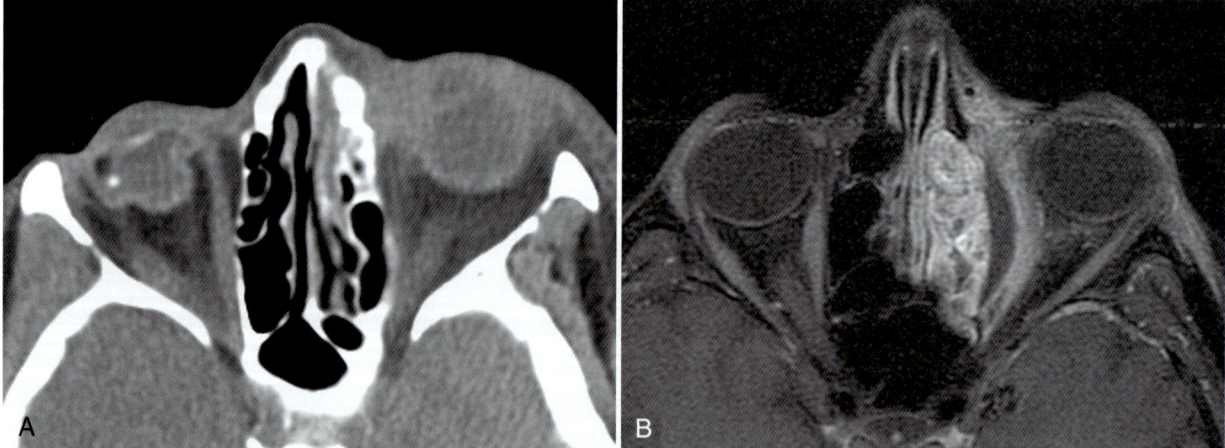

Figure 18-15 A: Axial computed tomographic scan demonstrating ill-defined soft tissue and stranding of periorbital fat predominantly within the preseptal compartment of the left orbit. Extension into the postseptal compartment is also seen. Shrunken right globe demonstrates dystrophic calcification. The diagnosis in this patient is left orbital cellulitis and right phthisis bulbi. **B:** Contrast-enhanced, fat-suppressed, axial T1-weighted imaging demonstrating left ethmoid sinusitis, a peripherally enhancing collection in the subperiosteal compartment, enhancement and thickening of the left medial rectus, and stranding of the retrobulbar fat. The diagnosis in this patient is left ethmoid sinusitis with subperiosteal abscess, myositis, and postseptal cellulitis.

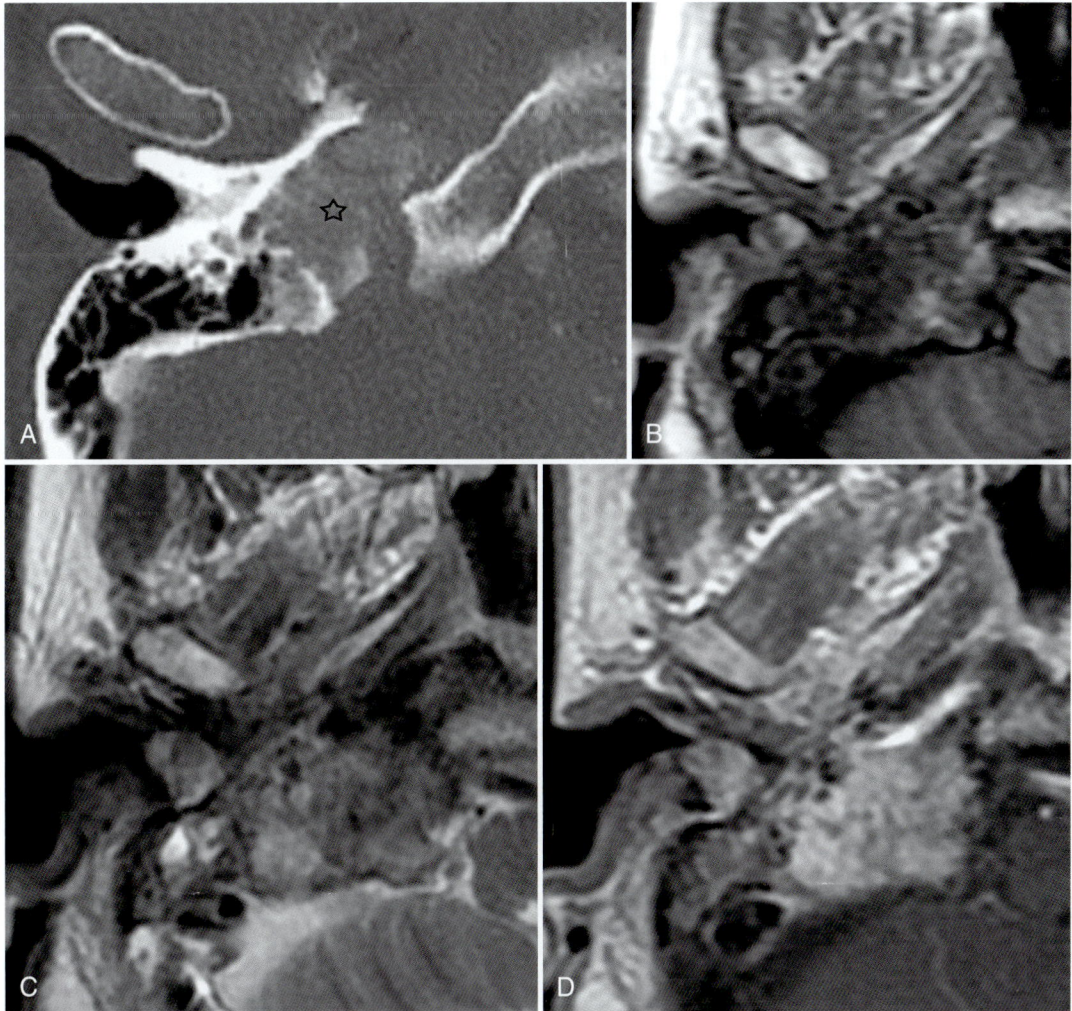

Figure 18-10 A: Contrast-enhanced axial computed tomographic (CT) scan demonstrating an irregularly marginated lytic lesion (*star*) in the right jugular foramen. Axial T1-weighted imaging (**B**), axial T2-weighted imaging (**C**), and contrast-enhanced axial T1-weighted imaging (**D**) demonstrating a heterogeneously enhancing lesion within the jugular foramen. The lesion demonstrates hypointense foci representing flow voids and hyperintense foci representing hemorrhage, producing the characteristic salt-and-pepper appearance of a glomus tumor. The diagnosis in this patient is glomus jugulare.

Continued

ophthalmic vein will be seen. Occasionally, the entire superior ophthalmic vein will be seen to be asymmetrically enlarged. Further dilation of the superior ophthalmic vein can occur following a Valsalva-type maneuver (Figure 18-13). Differential diagnosis includes carotid cavernous fistula, cavernous sinus thrombosis, and orbital vascular malformation. In direct carotid–cavernous fistula, an enlarged ipsilateral cavernous segment of the ipsilateral carotid artery will be seen. In indirect carotid–cavernous fistula, an arteriovenous fistula can be demonstrated on an angiogram. Also, reversal of flow will be seen in the superior ophthalmic vein. Cavernous sinus thrombosis will be seen as a filling defect in the cavernous sinuses. Orbital vascular malformation will demonstrate arterial feeders and a nidus.

Orbital Blowout Fracture

Orbital blowout fracture results from direct blunt trauma to the orbit. The sudden increase in intraorbital pressure from such an injury results in a fracture involving the inherently weak floor of the orbit, typically along the infraorbital foramen. The orbital rim classically remains intact. Fracture involving the floor of the orbit will be seen on CT studies (Figure 18-14). Enophthalmos is an ocular emergency and therefore should be evaluated. Inferior rectus entrapment is also a medical emergency; however, it is a clinical diagnosis. Thus, although entrapment of the inferior rectus can be suggested, it can never be diagnosed solely on imaging. Associated fractures, including those of the nasal bones and maxilla, are common and should be assessed.

Ocular Cellulitis

Ocular cellulitis can be broadly classified into preseptal cellulitis and postseptal (orbital) cellulitis. Of the two, postseptal cellulitis has a higher morbidity and therefore requires more aggressive treatment. The most common cause of orbital cellulitis is sinusitis. Most patients will present with orbital pain and swelling. Occasionally, patients complain of reduced extraocular motility. CT and MRI will demonstrate stranding of the periorbital fat. It is important to distinguish preseptal from postseptal cellulitis based on the infiltration of the fat and the presence of soft tissue with respect to the orbital septum (Figure 18-15). It also is imperative to evaluate for sinusitis and for associated abscess.

Sjögren Syndrome

Sjögren syndrome is a systemic autoimmune disorder characterized by lymphocytic infiltration of the exocrine glands. Most patients present with sicca symptoms (e.g., xerophthalmia [dry eyes], xerostomia [dry mouth], parotid gland enlargement). In the orbit, Sjögren syndrome is characterized by bilateral lacrimal gland enlargement, which can be demonstrated on both CT and MRI. Other associated findings in the head and neck include small cystic changes in the parotid glands. Such cystic changes are best demonstrated on T2-WI (Figure 18-16). Differential diagnosis of bilateral lacrimal gland enlargement includes lymphoma, sarcoidosis, and pseudotumor. Based on imaging, distinguishing these different clinical entities can be difficult, but clinical and laboratory correlation can help to establish the diagnosis.

Graves Disease with Characteristic Thyroid Orbitopathy

Graves disease is an autoimmune disease characterized by hyperthyroidism. It frequently affects women between the ages of 20 and 45 years. Most patients present with signs and symptoms of hyperthyroidism with diffuse enlargement of the thyroid gland and infiltrative orbitopathy. On imaging, bilateral enlargement of the muscle bellies of the extraocular muscles sparing the tendinous insertions will be seen (Figure 18-17). Although any extraocular muscle can be involved, the inferior rectus is most often affected. Associated orbital findings include increased deposition of retrobulbar fat, which results in proptosis. Differential diagnosis of enlarged extraocular muscles includes myositis, pseudotumor, and metastasis. In each of these clinical entities, unilateral orbital involvement is more common. Also, both the muscle bellies and the tendinous insertions

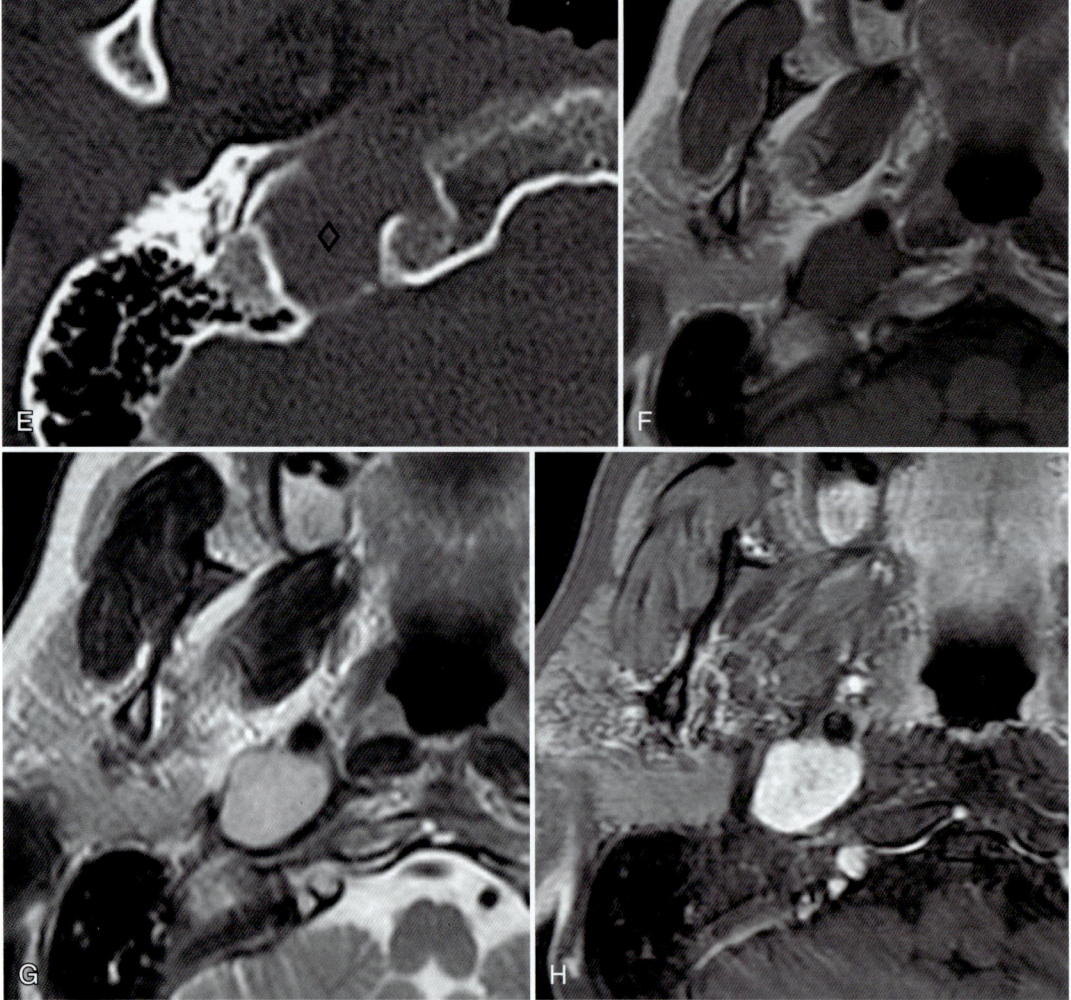

Figure 18-10, cont'd E: In a different patient, contrast-enhanced axial CT scan demonstrating a smoothly marginated lytic lesion (*diamond*) in the right jugular foramen. Axial T1-weighted imaging **(F)**, axial T2-weighted imaging **(G)**, and contrast-enhanced fat-suppressed axial T1-weighted imaging **(H)** demonstrating a homogeneously enhancing lesion. No abnormal flow voids or hemorrhages are associated with this lesion. The diagnosis in this patient is vagal schwannoma.

tend to become involved, a key distinguishing feature from Graves disease.

Lymphoma

Lymphoma involvement of the lacrimal glands can be primary (20%) in origin (i.e., from native lymphoid tissue present within the lacrimal glands) or secondary (80%) to lymphoid involvement from extraorbital origins. Most primary lymphomas affecting the lacrimal gland are of mucosa-associated lymphoid tissue (MALT) type. These tumors carry a better prognosis than the more common secondary lymphoma of the orbit. On imaging, homogeneous enlargement of unilateral or bilateral lacrimal glands is seen. Associated proptosis and scalloping of the adjacent bone can be seen (Figure 18-18). Differential diagnosis of bilateral lacrimal gland enlargement is discussed in the section on Sjögren syndrome. Differential diagnosis of unilateral lacrimal gland enlargement includes pseudotumor, pleomorphic adenoma, and malignant tumors such as adenoid cystic carcinoma. It can be difficult to distinguish pseudotumor and pleomorphic adenoma from lymphoma. Adenoid cystic carcinoma will appear more heterogeneous and can demonstrate bone destruction.

Optic Nerve Glioma

Optic nerve gliomas are low-grade neoplasms that can affect any portion of the optic nerve. They can be unilateral or bilateral. When bilateral, they are highly suggestive of neurofibromatosis type 1 (NF1). They are often seen in the first decade of life. Most often patients present with proptosis and progressive decrease in visual acuity. MR is better than CT in evaluating for optic nerve gliomas. Typically, enlargement of the involved portion of the optic nerve is seen. Variable degrees of enhancement have been noted following contrast administration (Figure 18-19, A–C). Differential diagnosis includes optic nerve sheath meningioma and optic neuritis. Optic nerve sheath meningioma is characterized by enhancement and thickening of the optic nerve sheath. The optic nerve itself is spared. This results in the classic tram-track sign of enhancement on contrast-enhanced MR studies (Figure 18-19 D). Optic neuritis is characterized by an enhancing optic nerve with no evidence of any obvious thickening (Figure 18-19 E). Most patients with optic neuritis have an acute presentation of a painful eye, with sudden loss of vision.

■ SINONASAL CAVITIES

Six cases are discussed in this section. They include trauma (e.g., Le Fort I fractures), infectious and inflammatory conditions (e.g., sinonasal polyposis, mucocele,

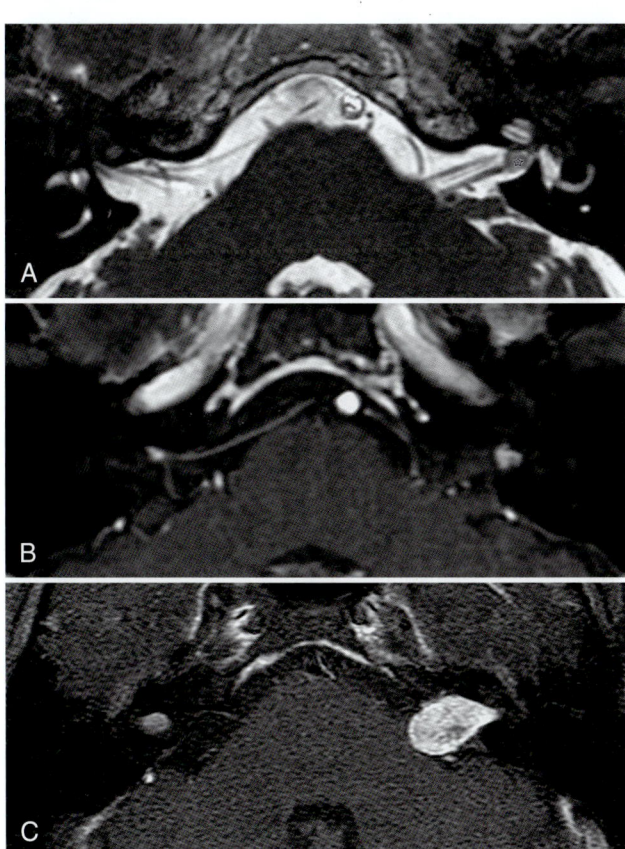

Figure 18-11 **A:** High-resolution constructive interference in steady-state (CISS) image demonstrating a focal soft tissue lesion within the left internal auditory canal. **B:** High-resolution contrast-enhanced fat-suppressed axial T1-weighted imaging demonstrating enhancement of the lesion. The diagnosis in this patient is an intracanalicular acoustic schwannoma. **C:** In a different patient, high-resolution, contrast-enhanced, fat-suppressed axial T1-weighted imaging demonstrating focal enhancing lesions (left larger than right) within both internal auditory canals. The diagnosis in this patient is bilateral acoustic schwannomas diagnostic of neurofibromatosis type 2 (NF2).

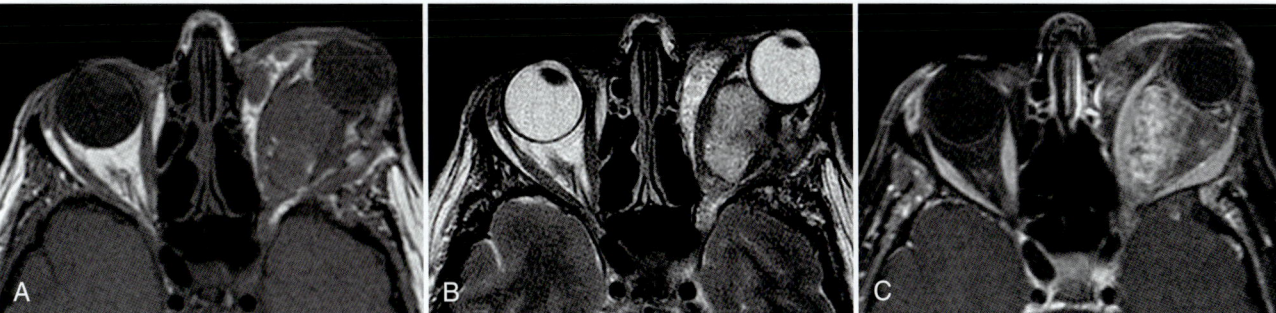

Figure 18-12 Axial T1-weighted imaging (**A**), axial T2-weighted imaging (**B**), and contrast-enhanced fat-suppressed axial T1-weighted imaging (**C**) demonstrating left-sided proptosis with a large multilobulated lesion in the retrobulbar compartment of the left orbit appearing hypo- to isointense on T1-weighted imaging and hyperintense on T2-weighted imaging, and demonstrating moderate heterogeneous enhancement. Smaller components of this large lesion showing similar imaging characteristics are seen medial to the medial rectus. The diagnosis is cavernous hemangioma.

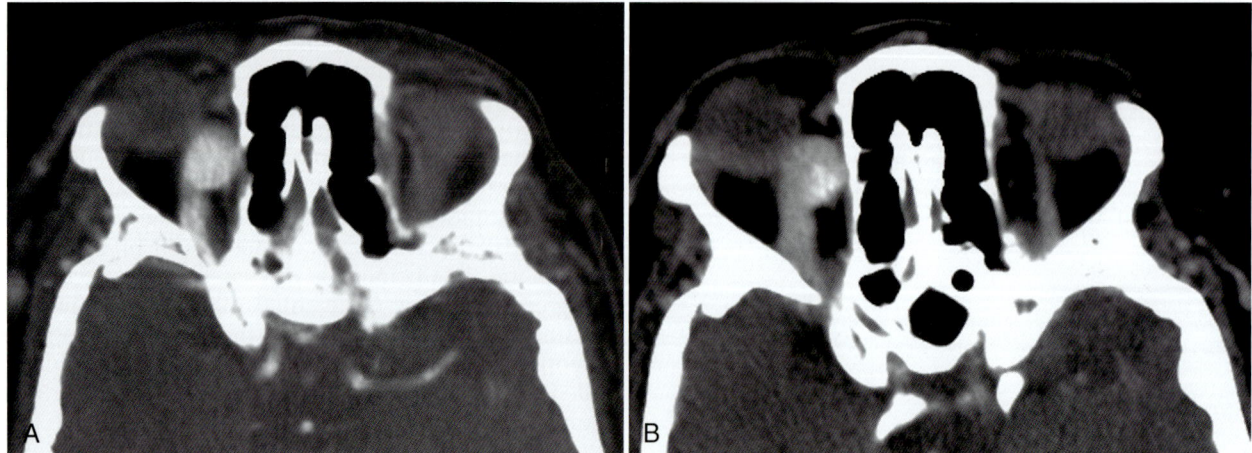

Figure 18-13 A: Contrast-enhanced axial computed tomographic (CT) scan demonstrating a dilated tortuous right superior ophthalmic vein. B: Contrast-enhanced axial CT scan following Valsalva maneuver demonstrating further increase in the caliber of the dilated superior ophthalmic vein. The cavernous sinuses do not demonstrate any filling defect (ruling out cavernous sinus thrombosis) or any asymmetric prominence (ruling out carotid cavernous fistula). The diagnosis is orbital venous varix.

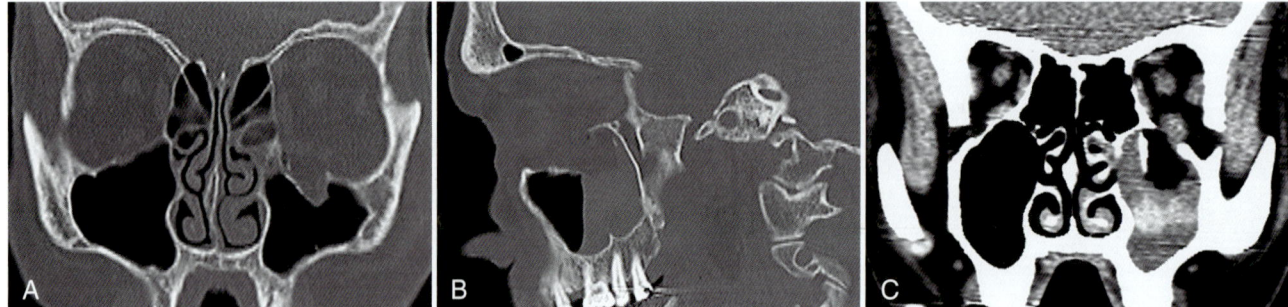

Figure 18-14 A: Coronal computed tomographic (CT) scan, bone window demonstrating a fracture involving the floor of the left orbit. B: Reformatted sagittal CT scan, bone window demonstrating the fracture involving the midportion of the floor of the orbit. The orbital rim is intact. C: Coronal CT scan, soft tissue window demonstrating the inferior rectus is adjacent to the fracture site, raising the possibility of inferior rectus entrapment. However, it should be noted that inferior rectus entrapment is a clinical diagnosis and can only be suggested but not diagnosed on imaging. Hyperdensity seen within the maxillary sinus represents hemorrhage. The diagnosis is orbital blowout fracture.

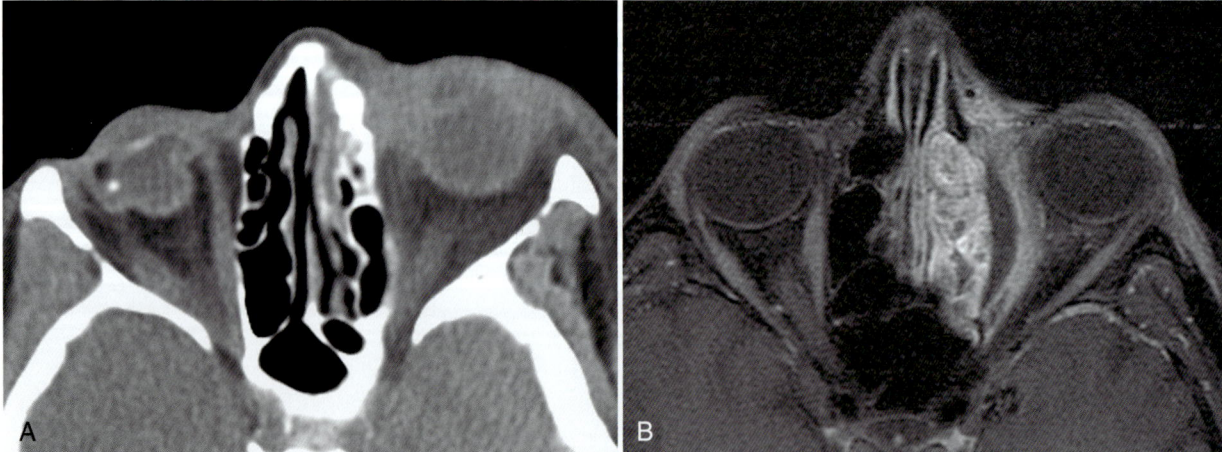

Figure 18-15 A: Axial computed tomographic scan demonstrating ill-defined soft tissue and stranding of periorbital fat predominantly within the preseptal compartment of the left orbit. Extension into the postseptal compartment is also seen. Shrunken right globe demonstrates dystrophic calcification. The diagnosis in this patient is left orbital cellulitis and right phthisis bulbi. B: Contrast-enhanced, fat-suppressed, axial T1-weighted imaging demonstrating left ethmoid sinusitis, a peripherally enhancing collection in the subperiosteal compartment, enhancement and thickening of the left medial rectus, and stranding of the retrobulbar fat. The diagnosis in this patient is left ethmoid sinusitis with subperiosteal abscess, myositis, and postseptal cellulitis.

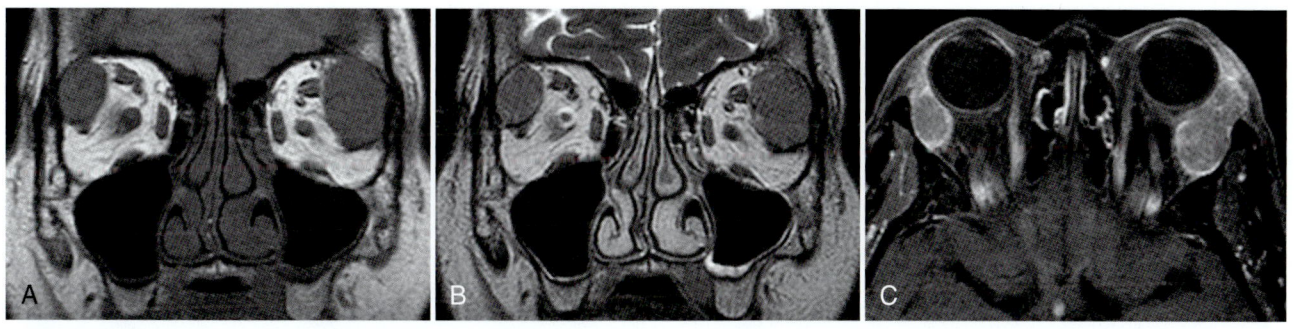

Figure 18-16 Coronal T1-weighted imaging (A), coronal T2-weighted imaging (B), and contrast-enhanced, fat-suppressed, axial T1-weighted imaging (C) through both orbits demonstrate enlarged, enhancing lacrimal glands bilaterally. The diagnosis is Sjögren syndrome.

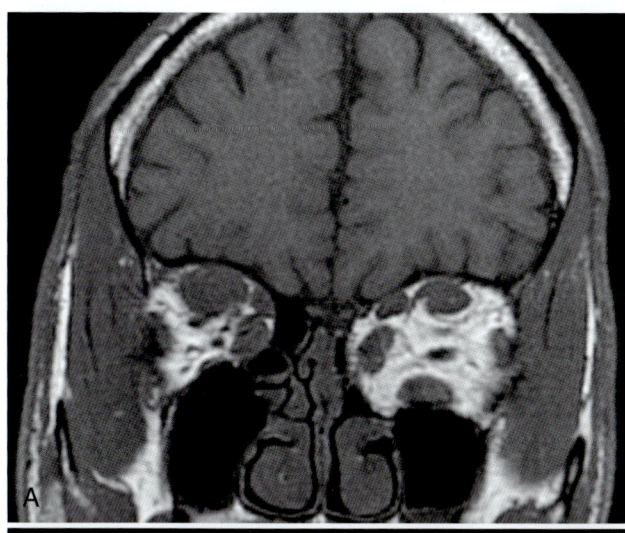

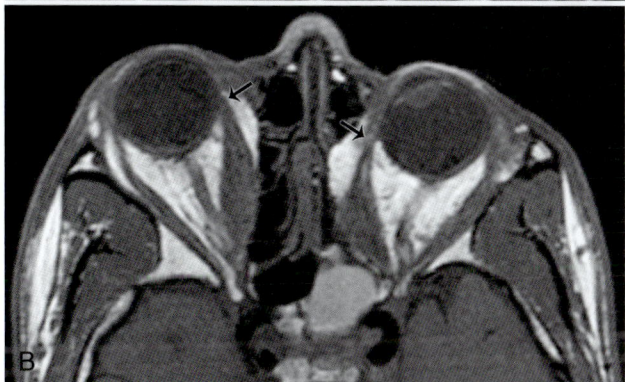

Figure 18-17 Coronal T1-weighted imaging (A) and axial T1-weighted imaging (B) demonstrating enlargement of muscle bellies of most of the extraocular muscles bilaterally. Sparing of the tendinous insertions (*arrows*) can be appreciated on the axial image. The diagnosis is Graves disease with characteristic thyroid orbitopathy.

fungal sinusitis), and tumors (e.g., olfactory neuroblastoma, squamous cell carcinoma).

Le Fort I Fractures

Le Fort fractures account for 10% to 20% of all facial fractures. There are three types of Le Fort fractures. Le Fort I fracture results from a blow delivered low on the maxillary alveolar rim. The fracture extends through the lower nasal septum, the maxillary alveolar rim above the teeth apices, and the zygomaticomaxillary junction, to involve the pterygoid plates. Le Fort II fracture results from a blow delivered to the central facial region. It is one of the most severe of the facial fractures. The fracture extends through the root of the nose to involve the frontal processes of the maxilla, the lacrimal bones, the inferior orbital floor, to extend under the zygoma, across the pterygomaxillary fissure to involve the pterygoid plates. Le Fort III fracture results from a blow to the central to upper midface. It is regarded as the most severe of all facial fractures. This fracture starts at the root of the nose and extends posteriorly along the lacrimal bones and the medial wall of the orbit, to involve the floor of each orbit. The fracture then continues superolaterally through the lateral orbital wall and the zygomatic arch to involve the pterygoid plates and the base of the sphenoid. Most patients present with facial swelling, bleeding, and crepitus. Reduced visual acuity, paresthesia along the infraorbital nerve distribution, loose teeth, and malocclusion are other common symptoms. Facial fractures are best evaluated with CT scans complemented with three-dimensional reconstructions. Typically, Le Fort I fractures are seen to extend through the lower nasal septum, across the maxillary alveolar rim and the zygomaticomaxillary junction, to involve the pterygoid plates (Figure 18-20).

Sinonasal Polyposis

Sinonasal polyposis is inflammatory polypoidal change involving the paranasal sinuses and nasal cavity. The most common underlying etiology is seasonal pollinosis, most commonly associated with ragweed allergy. Other causes of pansinusitis include cystic fibrosis, immotile cilia syndrome, and unusual allergens such as aspirin intolerance. Most patients present with nasal obstruction, running nose, and headache. Common radiologic manifestations include near-complete to complete opacification of the paranasal sinuses and nasal cavities with mucosal inflammatory change and polyps (Figure 18-21). Bony scalloping of the sinus walls is occasionally seen.

Mucocele

Mucoceles are cystic expansile lesions of the paranasal sinuses, which are formed due to ostial obstruction. The frontal and ethmoid sinuses are often involved. Most

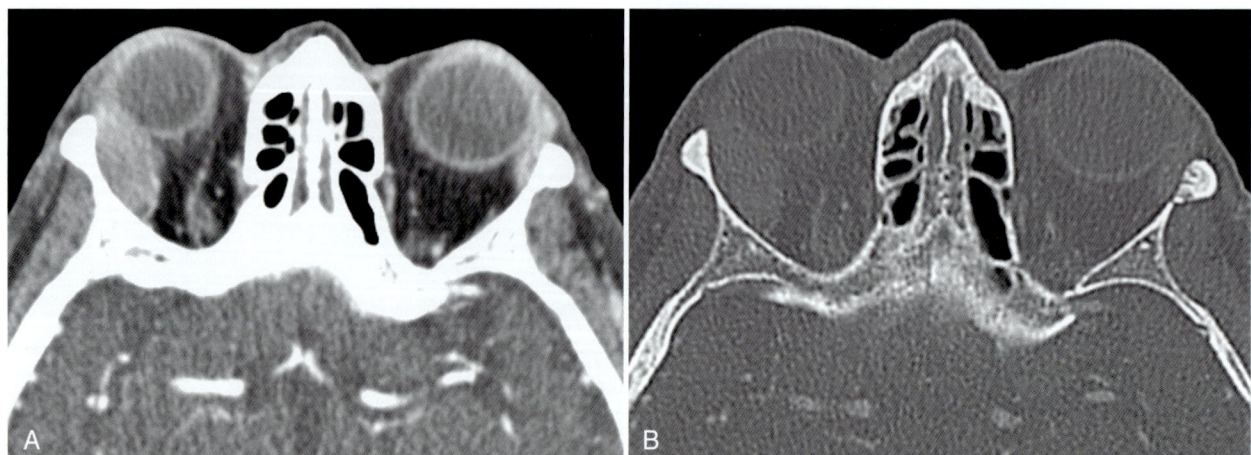

Figure 18-18 A: Contrast-enhanced axial computed tomographic (CT) scan, soft tissue window demonstrating asymmetrically enlarged, enhancing right lacrimal gland. **B:** Corresponding axial CT scan, bone window demonstrating mild scalloping of the adjacent superolateral orbital wall. The diagnosis is primary orbital (mucosa-associated lymphoid tissue) lymphoma.

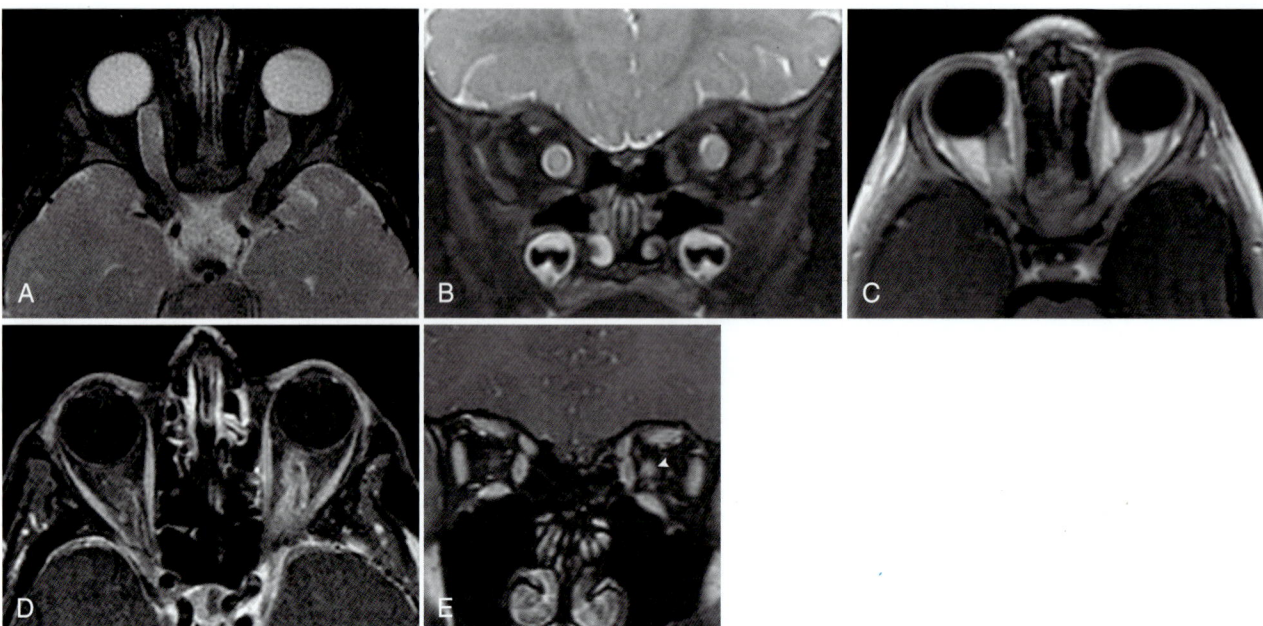

Figure 18-19 Axial T2-weighted imaging (**A**), coronal T2-weighted imaging (**B**), and contrast-enhanced axial T1-weighted imaging (**C**) demonstrating enlarged enhancing optic nerves bilaterally. The diagnosis is bilateral optic nerve gliomas in this child with neurofibromatosis type 1 (NF1). **D:** In a different patient, contrast-enhanced, fat-suppressed, axial T1-weighted imaging demonstrating thickened, enhancing left optic nerve sheath surrounding the optic nerve producing the tram-track sign diagnostic of optic nerve sheath meningioma. **E:** In another patient, contrast-enhanced, fat-suppressed, coronal T1-weighted imaging demonstrating asymmetric enhancement of the left optic nerve. The diagnosis in this patient is optic neuritis.

patients present with nasal obstruction, facial discomfort, and headache. Common radiologic manifestations include an expansile cystic lesion involving the paranasal sinuses. Thinning of the walls of the paranasal sinuses with occasional pressure deossification and erosion can be seen. Most such cystic lesions are hypointense on T1-WI and hyperintense on T2-WI, and do not exhibit any contrast enhancement. Variable signal intensity within the mucocele can be seen due to variability in the hydration state and protein content of these lesions (Figure 18-22). The differential diagnosis includes sinonasal polyposis, and benign and aggressive sinonasal neoplasms. Typically, sinonasal polyposis involves almost all the paranasal sinuses. Benign sinonasal neoplasms (e.g., retention cysts, focal polyps) appear as focal cystic lesions within the paranasal sinuses. They typically do not expand the paranasal sinuses. Other benign polyps (e.g., antrochoanal polyps) will demonstrate a soft tissue component. The typical growth pattern of antrochoanal polyp expanding the maxillary sinus and extending into the nasal cavity helps distinguish it from other lesions (Figure 18-22, *E*). Aggressive sinonasal neoplasms will demonstrate an enhancing soft tissue mass with associated destruction of the sinus walls.

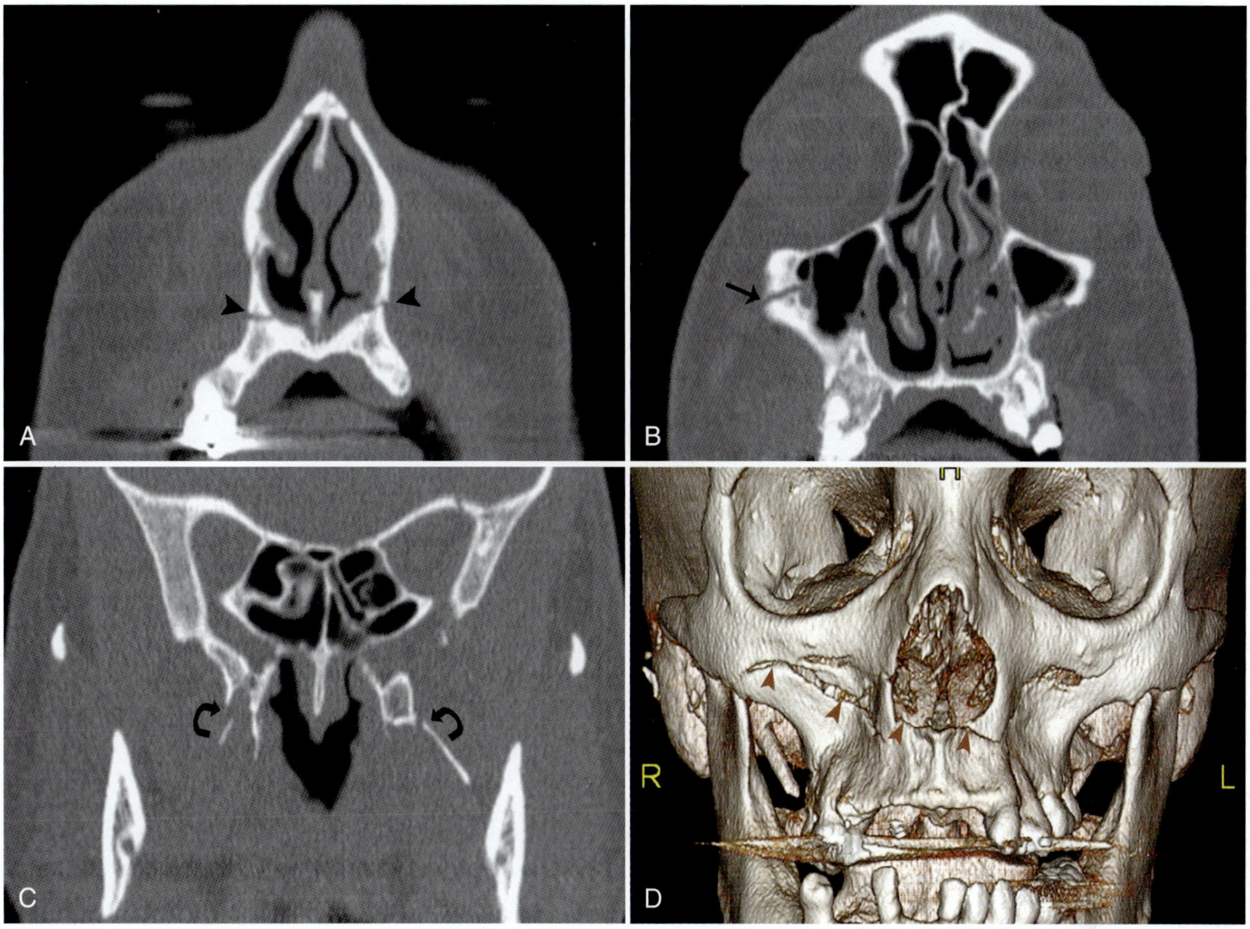

Figure 18-20 A–C: Coronal reformatted computed tomographic scans demonstrating a fracture line traversing through the frontal processes of the maxillae (*arrowheads*), the right zygomaticomaxillary junction (*arrow*), and the pterygoid plates (*curved arrows*). Three-dimensional surface-shaded display (3D-SSD) demonstrates the fracture line (*arrowheads*) coursing through the nasal septum, across the frontal processes of the maxillae to extend further laterally to involve the region adjacent to the right zygomaticomaxillary junction. The diagnosis is Le Fort I fracture.

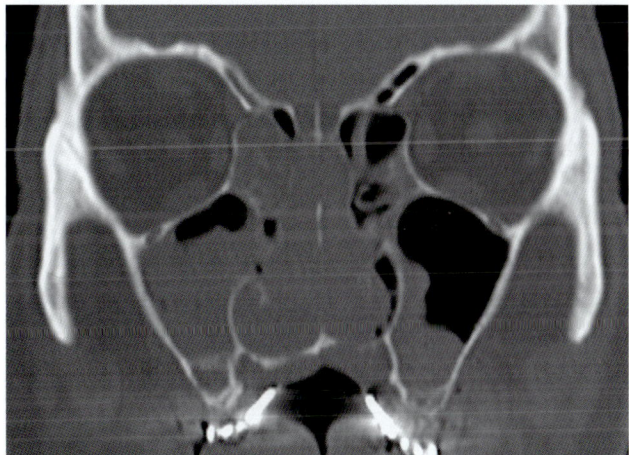

Figure 18-21 Coronal reformatted computed tomographic scan demonstrating polypoid mucosal thickening involving all the visualized paranasal sinuses and the nasal cavity. There is mild bowing of the bony walls of the nasal cavity. The diagnosis is sinonasal polyposis.

Fungal Sinusitis

Fungal diseases of the paranasal sinuses can be categorized into noninvasive and invasive varieties. The noninvasive form seen in immunocompetent individuals can be classified into fungal ball (or mycetoma) or allergic fungal sinusitis. The invasive form is typically seen in immunocompromised patients and has been classified as acute fulminant fungal sinusitis, granulomatous invasive fungal sinusitis, and chronic invasive fungal sinusitis. The noninvasive form is more indolent in presentation. Headache, facial pain, and numbness are typical presenting features. The invasive form is more acute in presentation. Fever and headache are typical presenting features. CT scan is the imaging modality of choice. However, in patients with the invasive form of fungal sinusitis, MRI with contrast may be obtained to evaluate for intracranial involvement and extension into the adjacent soft tissues. Fungal concretions are typically seen as hyperdense foci within the abnormal soft tissue seen within the paranasal sinuses. More specifically, a fungus ball or mycetoma will be seen as either a hyperdense area within the sinus cavity or as a focus of calcific density of varying size within the inflammatory soft tissue mass in the paranasal sinuses. Allergic fungal sinusitis has nonspecific imaging findings such as polypoid mucosal thickening. Invasive fungal sinusitis presents as inflammatory mucosal thickening completely opacifying the involved paranasal sinuses. Spread to adjacent regions

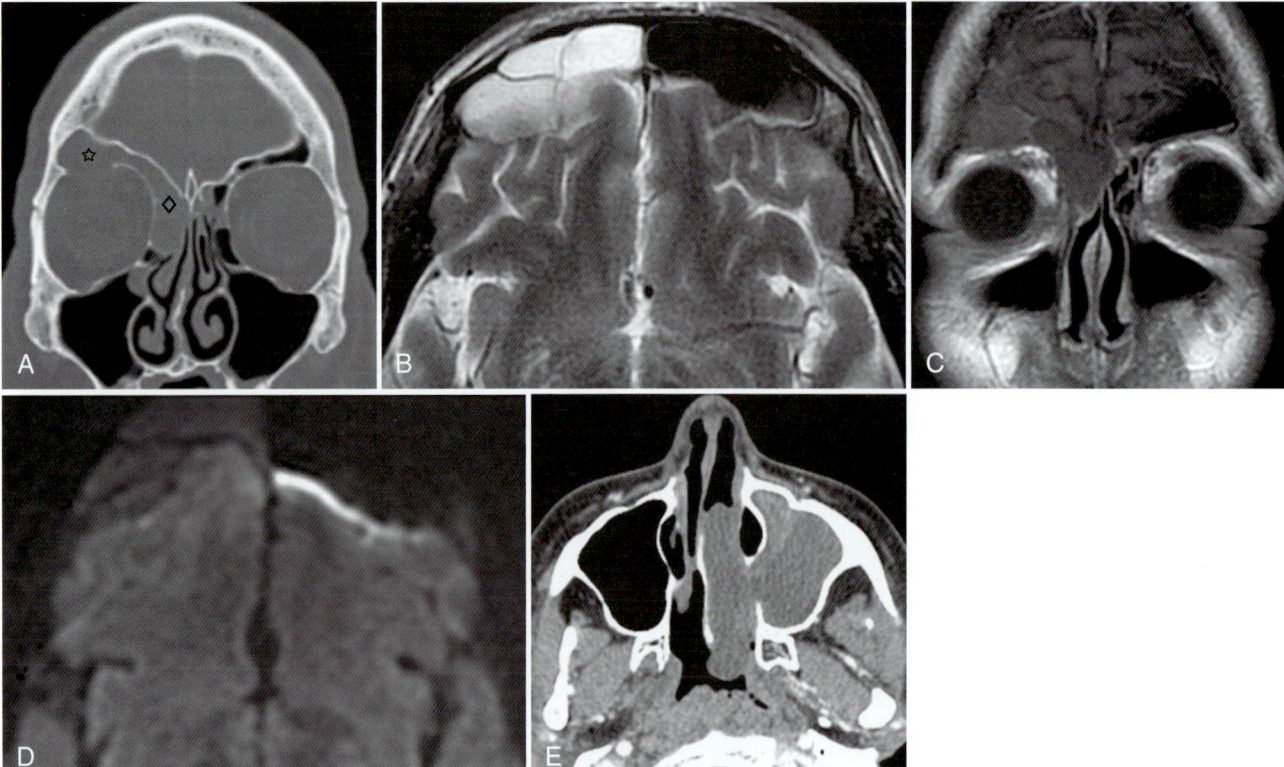

Figure 18-22 A: Coronal reformatted computed tomographic scan demonstrating an expansile cystic-appearing lesion involving the right supraorbital ethmoid sinus (*star*) with pressure de-erosion of its inferior wall and inferior displacement of right ocular globe. Complete opacification of the right frontal sinus is seen (*diamond*). **B:** Axial T2-weighted imaging demonstrating predominantly hyperintense signal within the right supraorbital ethmoid sinus with fluid–fluid level suggestive of variability in the protein content of the lesion. Near-complete opacification of right frontal sinus is seen. **C:** Contrast-enhanced coronal T1-weighted imaging demonstrating no obvious enhancement. **D:** Axial diffusion-weighted imaging does not demonstrate any restricted diffusion. The diagnosis is right supraorbital ethmoid mucocele with right frontal sinusitis. **E:** Axial CT scan through the maxillary sinuses demonstrates soft tissue lesion extending from one left maxillary sinus extending into the nasal cavity. The lesion demonstrates a polypoidal configuration suggestive of an antrochoanal polyp.

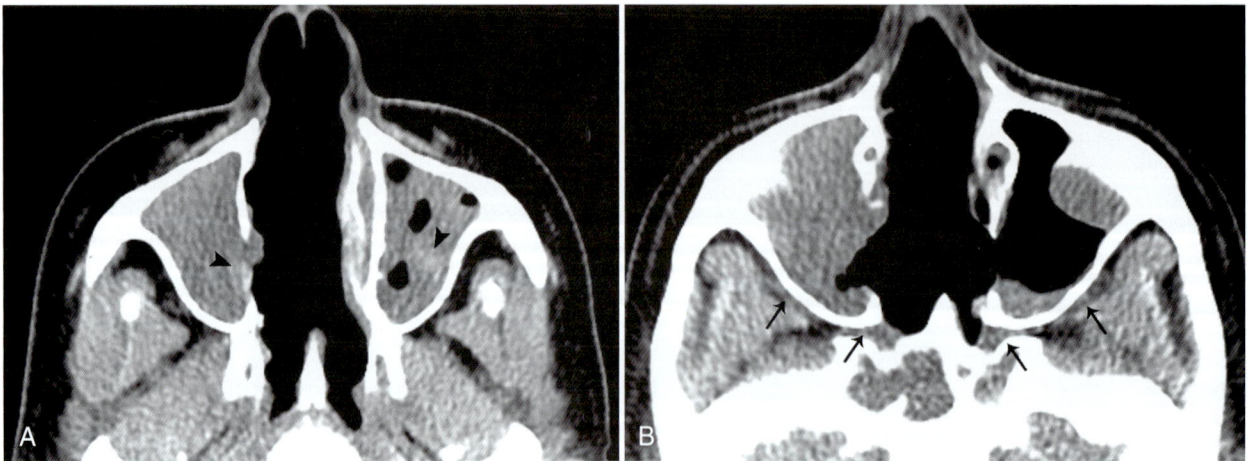

Figure 18-23 A 25-year-old man with a known case of bone marrow transplant and paranasal sinus surgery in the recent past presented with fever, headache, and sinusitis. **A:** Axial computed tomographic (CT) scan demonstrating evidence of prior paranasal sinus surgery. Hyperdense foci (*arrowheads*) are seen within nearly completely opacified bilateral maxillary sinuses. **B:** Axial CT scan at a more caudal level demonstrating infiltration of fat in the region of the pterygomaxillary fissures (*arrows*) bilaterally. Completely opacified sphenoid sinuses are seen. The diagnosis is fungal sinusitis.

can be suspected when there is infiltration of fat in the adjacent soft tissues including the cheek, orbit, and infratemporal fossa (Figure 18-23). In immunocompromised patients, such spread with *intact* sinus walls should raise a red flag for invasive fungal sinusitis. Occasionally, reactive sclerosis alternating with areas of bony destruction is seen on the affected sinus walls. Intracranial extension is better assessed with MRI. Dural thickening, empyema, intracranial abscess, and mycotic aneurysms can occur.

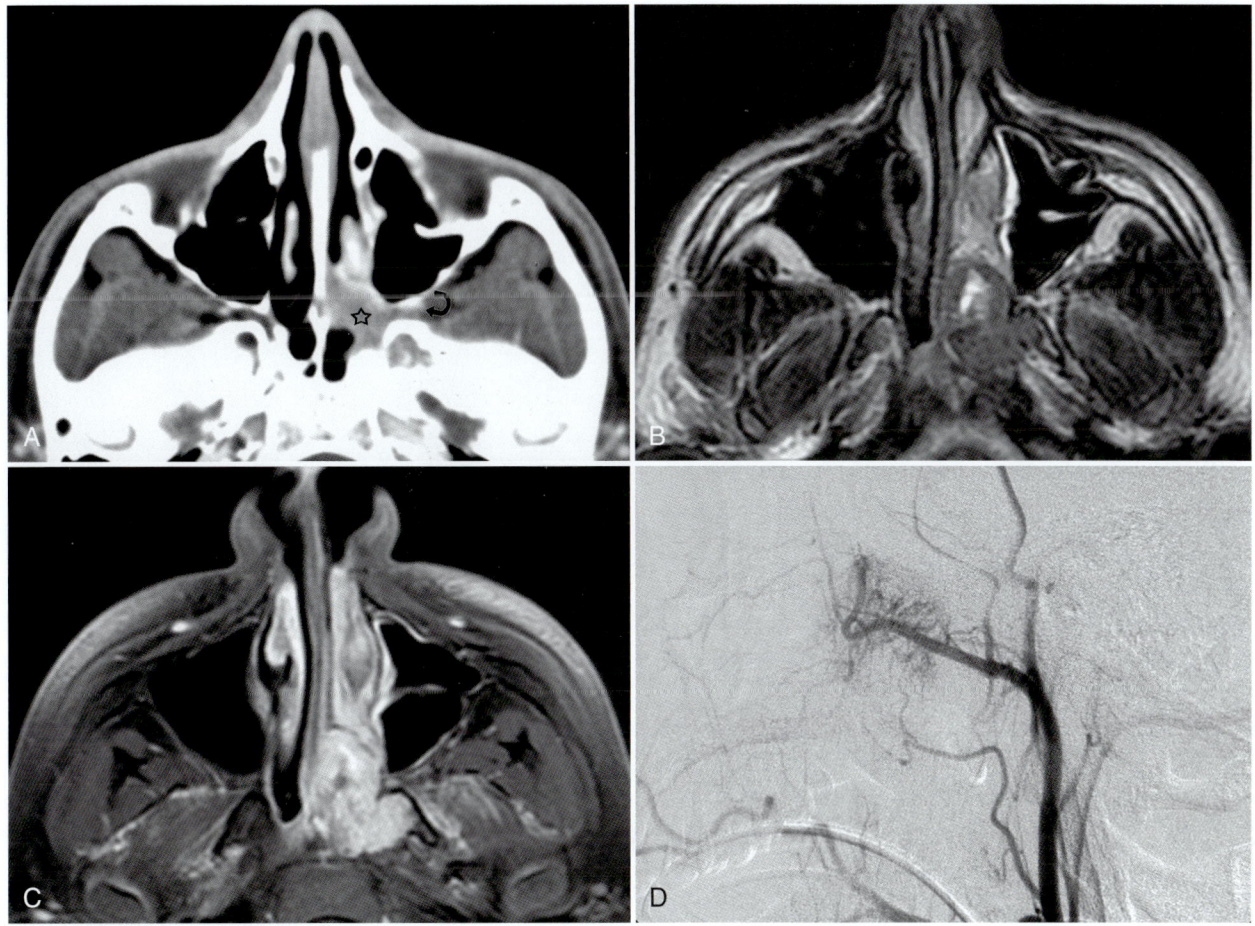

Figure 18-24 A: Contrast-enhanced axial computed tomographic scan demonstrating a lobulated enhancing mass (*star*) in the posterior nasal cavity. The mass extends into the left pterygomaxillary fissure (*curved arrow*). Subtle anterior bowing of the posterior wall of the left maxillary sinus is seen. B: Axial T2-weighted imaging demonstrating a lobulated heterogeneous mass in the posterior nasal cavity. C: Contrast-enhanced fat-suppressed axial T1-weighted demonstrates intense enhancement of this mass is seen following contrast administration on the contrast-enhanced, fat-suppressed, axial T1-weighted image. D: Digital subtraction angiogram demonstrating tumor blush from arterial feeders arising from the left internal maxillary artery. The diagnosis is juvenile nasopharyngeal angiofibroma.

Juvenile Nasopharyngeal Angiofibroma

Juvenile nasopharyngeal angiofibroma is a locally aggressive, benign hypervascular tumor found exclusively in adolescent males. Most patients present with nasal stuffiness and epistaxis. Imaging demonstrates an intensely enhancing mass centered in the region of the sphenopalatine foramen (posterior nasal cavity region). Extension contiguously anteriorly into nasal cavity, posteriorly and inferiorly into the nasopharynx, laterally via the pterygomaxillary fissure into the infratemporal fossa, and posterosuperiorly into the sphenoid sinus is typically seen. Extension into the middle cranial fossa is rarely seen. Juvenile nasopharyngeal angiofibroma typically scallops adjacent bony structures and widens fissures through which it extends (Figure 18-24). Erosion is seen, but later in the disease process. Differential diagnosis includes rhabdomyosarcoma and angiomatous polyp. Rhabdomyosarcoma is seen in children about 6 to 8 years of age or in the late second decade of life. Mild to moderate enhancement is seen. Bone destruction can be seen.

Angiomatous polyp is an uncommon soft tissue lesion, typically seen in adult males. Although it is typically located in the posterior nasal cavity, it does not exhibit extension into the infratemporal fossa or sphenoid sinus. The lesion does not cause anterior bowing of the posterior wall of the maxillary sinus, which is typically seen in cases of juvenile nasopharyngeal angiofibroma.

Olfactory Neuroblastoma

Olfactory neuroblastoma (historically referred to as *esthesioneuroblastoma*) is a rare malignant tumor of the nasal cavity. It accounts for up to 6% of all malignant tumors of the nasal cavity. It arises from the olfactory neuroepithelium, which extends from the roof of the nasal cavity into the adjacent superior turbinates. Most patients present with nasal obstruction and occasional epistaxis. A homogeneously enhancing nasal cavity mass is seen (Figure 18-25, *A* and *B*). Extension into the adjacent paranasal sinuses is occasionally seen. Intracranial extension can be identified by the presence of focal enhancing

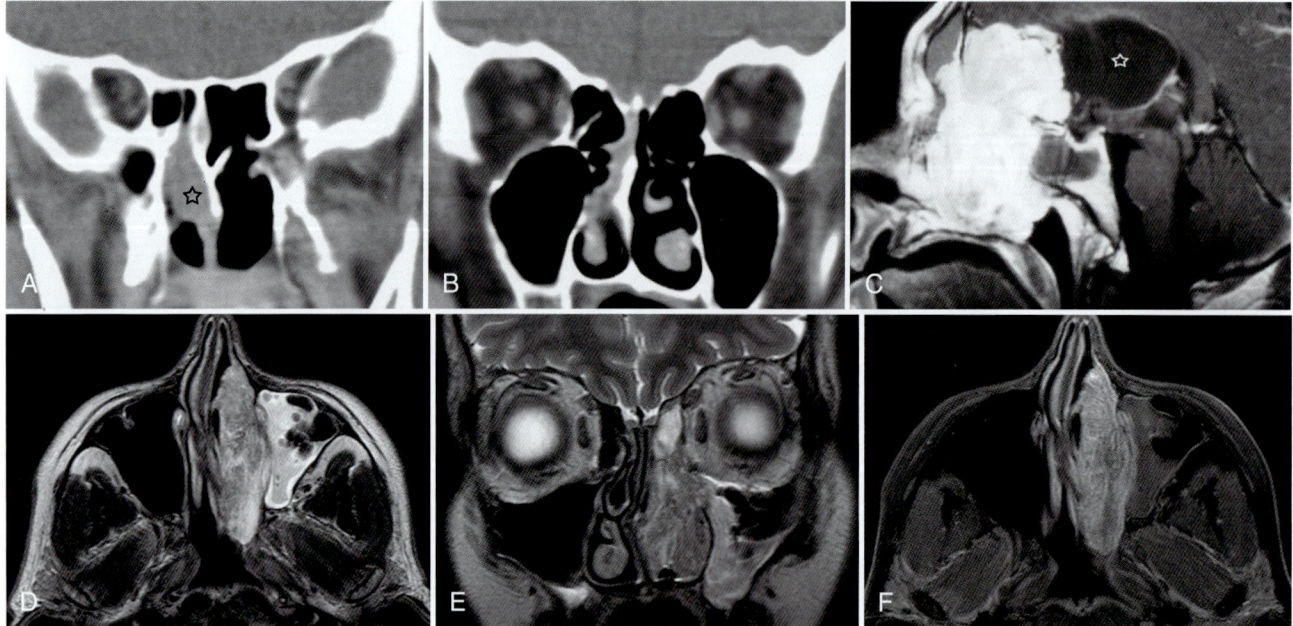

Figure 18-25 A: Contrast-enhanced coronal reformatted computed tomographic (CT) scan demonstrating an enhancing polypoidal soft tissue mass (*star*) in the right nasal cavity. **B:** More anteriorly, coronal reformatted CT scan demonstrating the polypoid soft tissue mass is attached to the right cribriform plate. The diagnosis in this patient is olfactory neuroblastoma. **C:** In a different patient, contrast-enhanced sagittal T1-weighted imaging demonstrating an enhancing homogeneously enhancing mass in the sinonasal cavities with intracranial extension. The lesion demonstrates a cystic component (*star*) along the posterior aspect of its intracranial component. Obstructive sphenoid and frontal sinusitis is seen. The diagnosis in this patient is also an olfactory neuroblastoma. In another patient, axial (**D**) and coronal (**E**) T2-weighted imaging demonstrate an expansile left nasal cavity mass. This mass demonstrates heterogeneous signal with alternating bands of hyperintense and hypointense signal producing a "cerebriform-like appearance." Obstructive left maxillary sinusitis is seen. **F:** Contrast-enhanced, fat-suppressed, axial T1-weighted imaging demonstrating heterogeneous enhancement. The diagnosis in this patient is inverted papilloma.

dura. Sometimes, intracranial extension is associated with a cyst that occurs along the margins of the tumor. Presence of such an associated intracranial cyst is highly suggestive of olfactory neuroblastoma (Figure 18-25, C). Differential diagnosis includes inverted papilloma, pleomorphic adenoma, lymphoma, and melanoma. Based on imaging, it can be difficult to distinguish a completely intranasal olfactory neuroblastoma from these different clinical entities. However, inverted papilloma demonstrates a cerebriform-like appearance on T2-WI, which can help distinguish it from other polypoidal nasal cavity masses (Figure 18-25, D–F).

Squamous Cell Carcinoma

Squamous cell carcinoma is the most common type of malignancy arising in the nasal cavity and paranasal sinuses. These carcinomas constitute over 80% of neoplasms of the paranasal sinuses. About 70% occur in the maxillary sinus, 12% in the nasal cavity, and the remainder in the remaining sinuses and nasal vestibule. Most patients present during the fifth to sixth decade of life. Clinical presentation varies and includes rhinorrhea, epistaxis, and pain. CT, positron emission tomography/CT, and MR can be used to evaluate squamous cell carcinoma. An enhancing aggressive mass lesion causing bone destruction is seen (Figure 18-26). Differential diagnosis includes sinonasal undifferentiated carcinoma, adenocarcinoma, melanoma, malignant lymphoma, Wegener granulomatosis, and metastasis. Based on imaging, it is difficult to distinguish these different clinical entities.

■ SALIVARY GLANDS

Three cases are discussed in this section. They include infectious and inflammatory disorders (e.g., sialadenitis), acquired immunodeficiency syndrome (AIDS)-related parotid cysts, and tumors (e.g., pleomorphic adenoma).

Sialolithiasis and Sialadenitis

Sialolithiasis most commonly affects the submandibular gland, less commonly the parotid gland, and uncommonly the sublingual gland. Most patients present with pain, swelling, and tenderness of the involved salivary gland. CT scan is the imaging modality of choice. Sialoliths are typically seen as well-defined hyperdense foci within the main drainage duct of the gland or within the gland itself (Figure 18-27). Secondary sialectasis (dilation of the ducts and ductules) and sialadenitis (enlarged involved salivary gland) are seen. Stranding can be seen in the adjacent soft tissues. Rarely, secondary infection occurs, resulting in abscess formation.

AIDS-Related Parotid Cysts

AIDS-related parotid cysts are benign lymphoepithelial cysts that occur in patients who are positive for human immunodeficiency virus. Most patients present with painless swelling in the region of the parotid glands. Imaging demonstrates nonenhancing cystic lesions involving both parotid glands. Rarely, unilateral involvement is seen. AIDS-related parotid cysts are usually accompanied by enlarged nasopharyngeal lymphoid

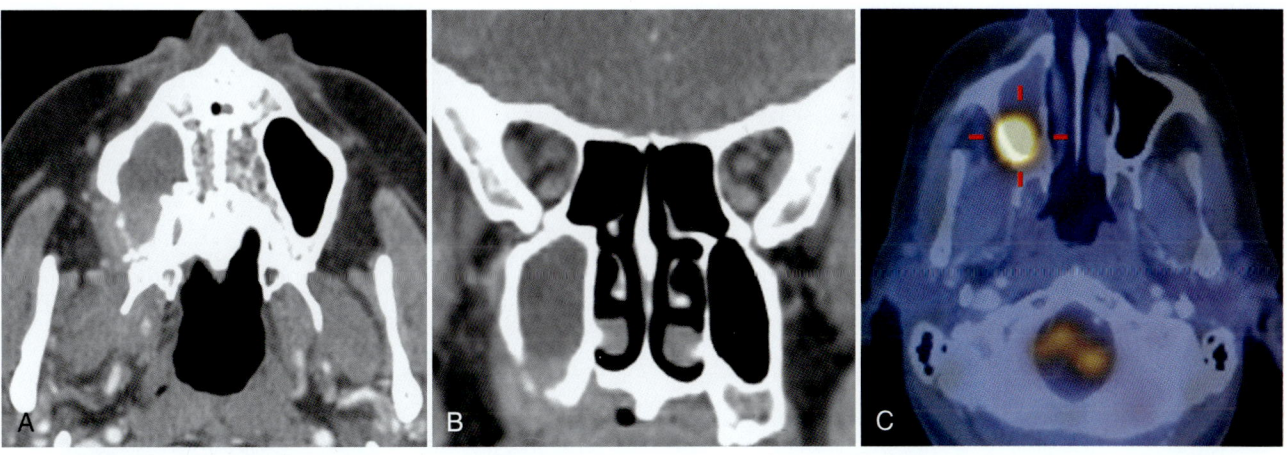

Figure 18-26 Contrast-enhanced axial (**A**) and reformatted coronal (**B**) computed tomographic scans demonstrating an aggressive destructive lesion involving the right maxillary sinus. **C:** Positron emission tomographic-computed tomographic imaging demonstrating increased uptake by the mass seen in the right maxillary sinus. The diagnosis is squamous cell carcinoma involving the maxillary sinus.

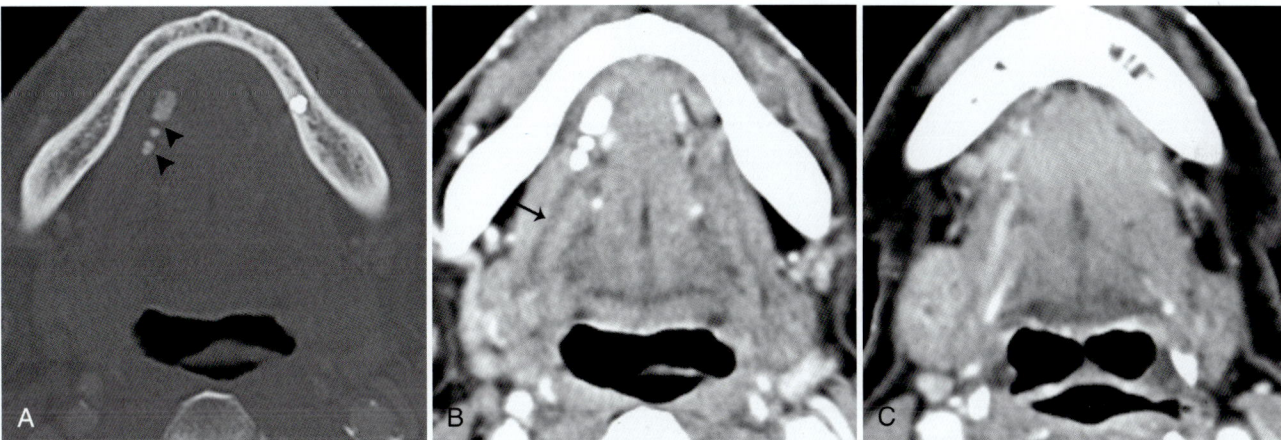

Figure 18-27 A: Axial computed tomographic (CT) scan, bone window demonstrating multiple hyperdense foci (*arrowheads*) in the region of the right floor of mouth suggestive of sialolithiasis. **B:** Axial CT scan, soft tissue window at a corresponding level demonstrating dilatation of the right Wharton duct (*arrow*). **C:** Axial CT scan at more caudal level demonstrating an asymmetrically enlarged right submandibular gland suggestive of sialadenitis.

tissue and cervical lymphadenopathy (Figure 18-28, *A*). Differential diagnosis includes Warthin tumor, intraparotid lymph nodes, and Sjögren syndrome. Warthin tumor is typically associated with an enhancing nodule along the periphery of the cyst (Figure 18-28, *B*). Intraparotid lymph nodes are more solid appearing. The intraparotid cysts in Sjögren syndrome are much smaller than those of AIDS-related parotid cysts (Figure 18-28, *C*).

Pleomorphic Adenoma

Pleomorphic adenoma is the most common benign salivary gland tumor. They most often involve the parotid glands and less commonly involve the submandibular glands and minor salivary glands. Most patients present with a slow-growing mass. Both CT and MR can be used to evaluate pleomorphic adenomas. CT will demonstrate a well-defined ovoid lesion with a slightly higher attenuation than the surrounding parotid parenchyma. Occasionally, the tumors have a more cystic appearance due to areas of necrosis. On MR, these tumors typically appear hypointense on T1-WI and hyperintense on T2-WI. Occasionally, a low-signal-intensity "capsule" is seen. Variable degrees of contrast enhancement are seen following contrast administration (Figure 18-29). When large, they tend to have a lobulated contour that is highly suggestive of their diagnosis. Differential diagnosis includes Warthin tumor and other low-grade or high-grade neoplasms of the salivary glands. Warthin tumor will typically demonstrate an enhancing nodule along the periphery of the cyst. It can be difficult to distinguish a low-grade malignant neoplasm from pleomorphic adenoma. Most high-grade malignant neoplasms, such as mucoepidermoid carcinomas, will demonstrate an irregular margin and appear hypointense on T2-WI.

■ MASTICATOR SPACE, ORAL CAVITY INCLUDING FLOOR OF MOUTH, AND PHARYNX

Six cases are discussed in this section. They include trauma (e.g., foreign body), infectious and inflammatory conditions (e.g., peritonsillar abscess), Ludwig angina, and tumors (e.g., lingual tonsil squamous cell carcinoma, retromolar trigone carcinoma, rhabdomyosarcoma, ameloblastoma).

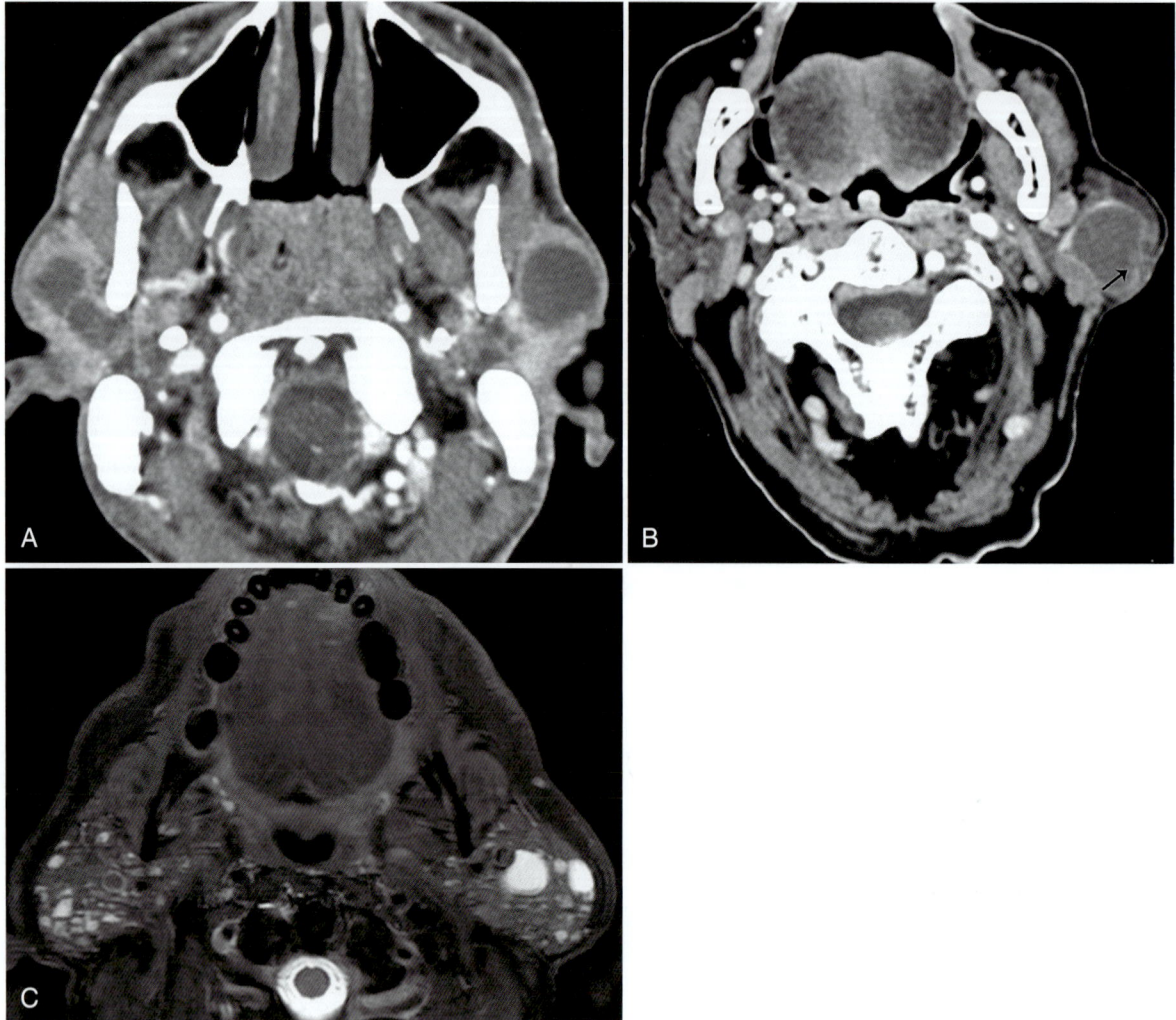

Figure 18-28 A: Contrast-enhanced axial computed tomographic (CT) scan demonstrating multiple, nonenhancing cystic lesions within both parotid glands. Note prominence of nasopharyngeal soft tissue. The diagnosis in this patient is AIDS-related parotid cysts and prominent nasopharyngeal soft tissue. **B:** In a different patient, contrast-enhanced axial CT scan demonstrating enhancing nodule (*arrow*) along the periphery of the left parotid cyst. The diagnosis in this patient is Warthin tumor. **C:** In another patient, fat-suppressed axial T2-weighted imaging demonstrating multiple subcentimeter cystic lesions within both parotid glands. The diagnosis in this patient is Sjögren syndrome.

Peritonsillar Abscess

Peritonsillar abscesses are more commonly seen in the pediatric population. The most common organisms associated with peritonsillar abscess are group A beta-hemolytic streptococcus and fusobacterium. Most patients present with fever, sore throat, odynophagia, and occasionally otalgia. Contrast-enhanced CT will demonstrate a predominantly necrotic peripherally enhancing lesion in the region of the tonsil, typically in the (presumed) space between the tonsil and its capsule (Figure 18-30). An enlarged retropharyngeal lymph node is a common associated finding.

Ludwig Angina

Ludwig angina is a serious, potentially life-threatening infection of the floor of mouth, which most commonly occurs secondary to dental caries or manipulation. Most patients present with fever, pain, and tenderness at the floor of mouth. With more extensive spread of infection, the patient may experience a sensation of strangling as the inflammatory change pushes the tongue posteriorly, which can potentially block the oropharynx. Contrast-enhanced CT scan is the imaging modality of choice. It demonstrates a peripherally enhancing, predominantly necrotic lesion suggestive of an abscess involving the floor of mouth. Stranding of fat in the floor of mouth and inflammatory change in the adjacent soft tissues are common (Figure 18-31). Reactive cervical lymphadenopathy is also common. Rarely, osteomyelitis of the mandible is seen. An accompanying history of dental caries, recent dental manipulation, or, less commonly, history of sialolithiasis and sialadenitis involving the submandibular gland helps establish the diagnosis. Differential diagnosis includes necrotic lymph node, lymphangioma, and ranula. A known primary tumor or other enlarged cervical lymph nodes will be seen with a necrotic level I (floor mouth) lymph node. Lymphangioma classically presents as a nonenhancing multiloculated, transspatial lesion. No inflammatory changes

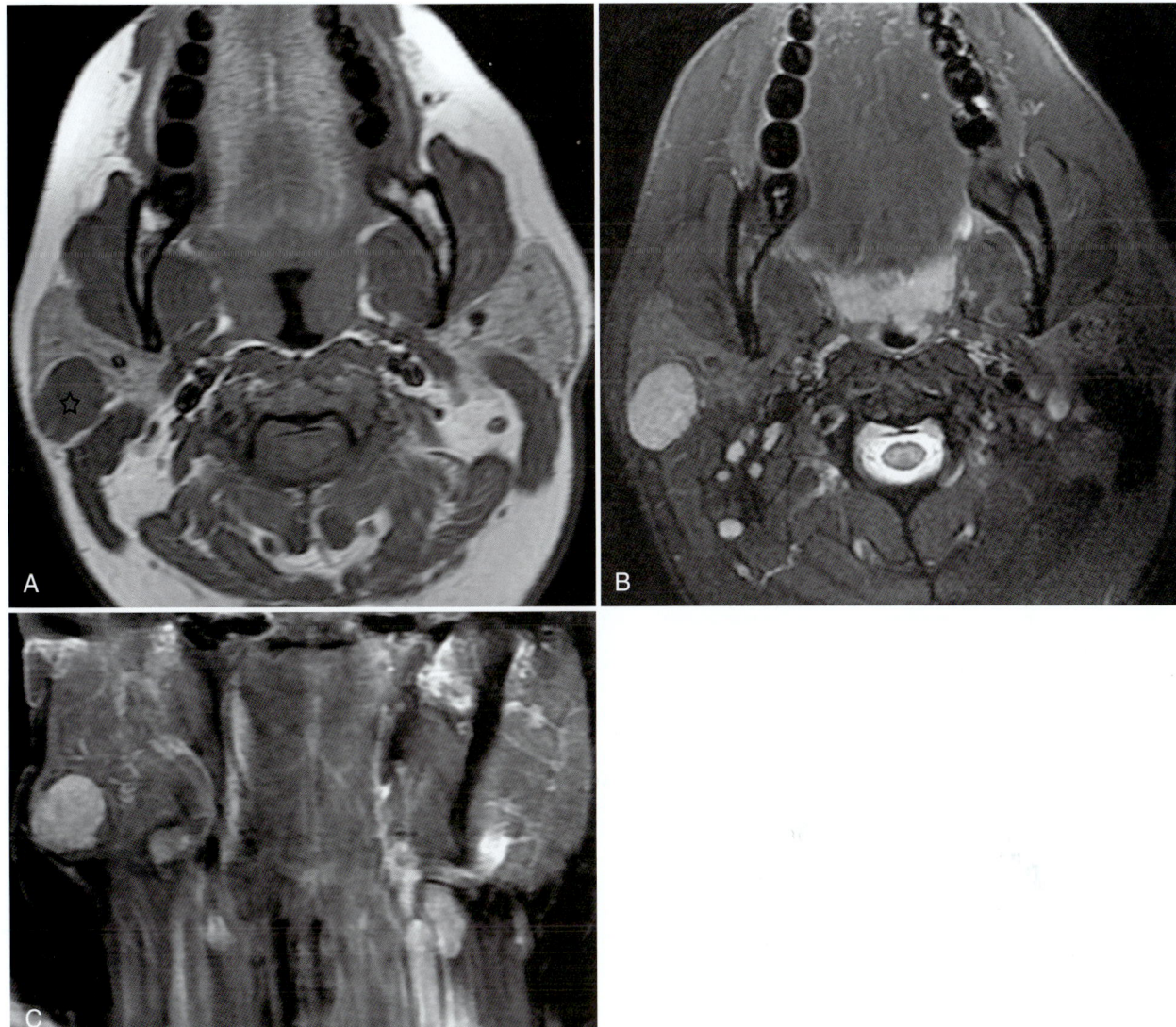

Figure 18-29 A: Axial T1-weighted imaging demonstrating a well-defined, ovoid, predominantly hypointense lesion (*star*) within the right parotid gland. B: Fat-suppressed axial T2-weighted imaging demonstrating the lesion is minimally hyperintense to the rest of the visualized parotid gland. C: Contrast-enhanced, fat-suppressed, coronal T1-weighted imaging demonstrating near-homogeneous enhancement of this lesion. The diagnosis is pleomorphic adenoma.

are seen. A ranula classically presents as a thin-walled, unilocular, well-defined, nonenhancing, cystic-appearing lesion in the lateral floor of the mouth arising from the sublingual gland. Typically this cystic lesion remains above the mylohyoid muscle sling. No inflammatory changes are seen.

Lingual Tonsil Squamous Cell Carcinoma

Lingual tonsil squamous cell carcinoma, also known as *base of tongue carcinoma*, is seen as a mass lesion posterior to the circumvallate papilla, extending inferiorly to the vallecula. Most such tumors remain clinically indolent for a long time and are seen only when they are large. Patients typically have cervical lymphadenopathy at the time of presentation. On imaging, an asymmetrically enhancing mass lesion is seen at the tongue base (Figure 18-32). It is critical to evaluate the spread of tumor for better staging and treatment planning (i.e., anteriorly into the oral tongue and sublingual space, posterolaterally into palatine tonsil, and inferiorly into supraglottic larynx). Also, cervical lymphadenopathy should be evaluated. Differential diagnosis includes lingual tonsil hyperplasia and minor salivary gland malignancy. Asymmetric lingual tonsil hyperplasia can sometimes mimic base of tongue carcinoma. However, the enhancing mass lesion seen with base of tongue carcinoma is not noted with lingual tonsil hyperplasia. Based on imaging, it can be difficult to distinguish minor salivary gland malignancy from base of tongue carcinoma.

Retromolar Trigone Carcinoma

Usually retromolar trigone carcinomas are squamous cell carcinomas. Excessive alcohol and tobacco abuse are the most common risk factors. Most patients

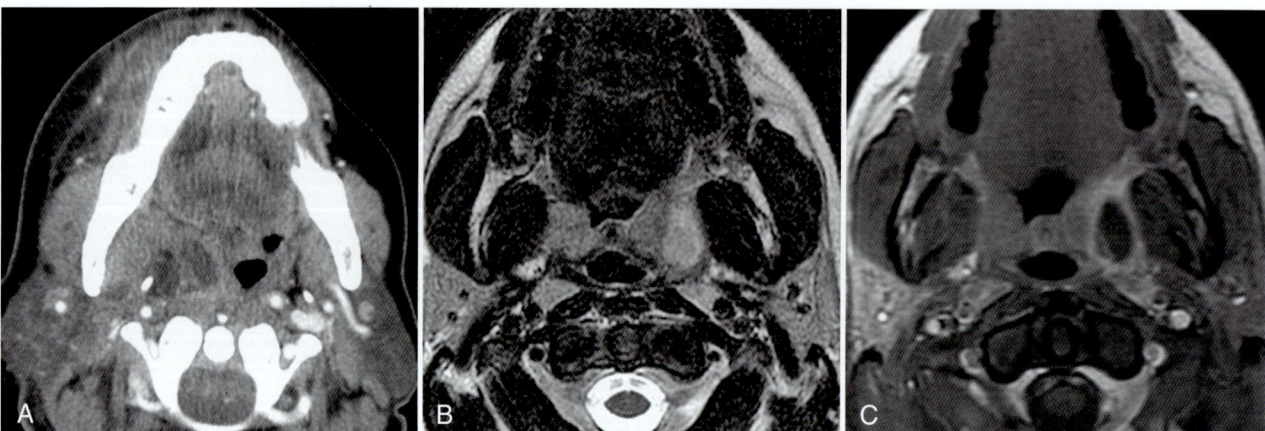

Figure 18-30 A: Contrast-enhanced axial computed tomographic scan demonstrating a predominantly necrotic lesion involving the right tonsil. Inflammatory change is seen involving the adjacent right parapharyngeal space. Mass effect on the airway and midline shift to the left is seen. The diagnosis in this patient is right peritonsillar abscess. **B:** In a different patient, axial T2-weighted imaging demonstrating a predominantly necrotic lesion in the left peritonsillar region. **C:** Contrast-enhanced, axial T1-weighted imaging demonstrating peripheral enhancement of this predominantly necrotic lesion suggestive of a peritonsillar abscess.

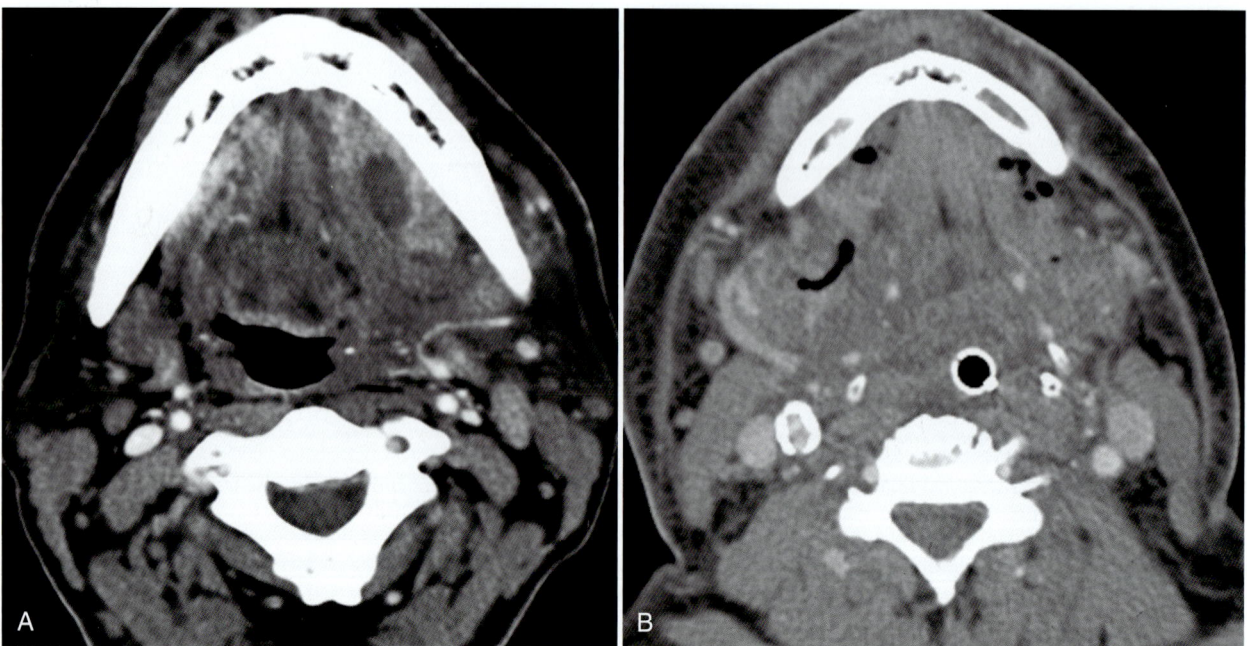

Figure 18-31 A: Contrast-enhanced axial computed tomographic (CT) scan demonstrating a well-defined necrotic lesion in the left floor of the mouth with adjacent inflammatory change. Note reactive thickening of the left oropharyngeal wall. The diagnosis in this patient is Ludwig angina. **B:** In a different patient, contrast-enhanced axial CT scan demonstrating ill-defined inflammatory change, predominantly involving the right floor of mouth adjacent to the submandibular gland. Pockets of air are seen scattered throughout the floor of mouth. Extensive reactive edematous changes extend to involve the tongue base and oropharynx, resulting in near-complete occlusion of the airway. An endotracheal tube is seen in situ. The diagnosis in this patient is also Ludwig angina. Purulent material obtained from an ill-defined collection in the right floor of mouth demonstrated a mixture of aerobic and anaerobic flora, with gas-forming organisms (*Klebsiella* and anaerobic streptococci).

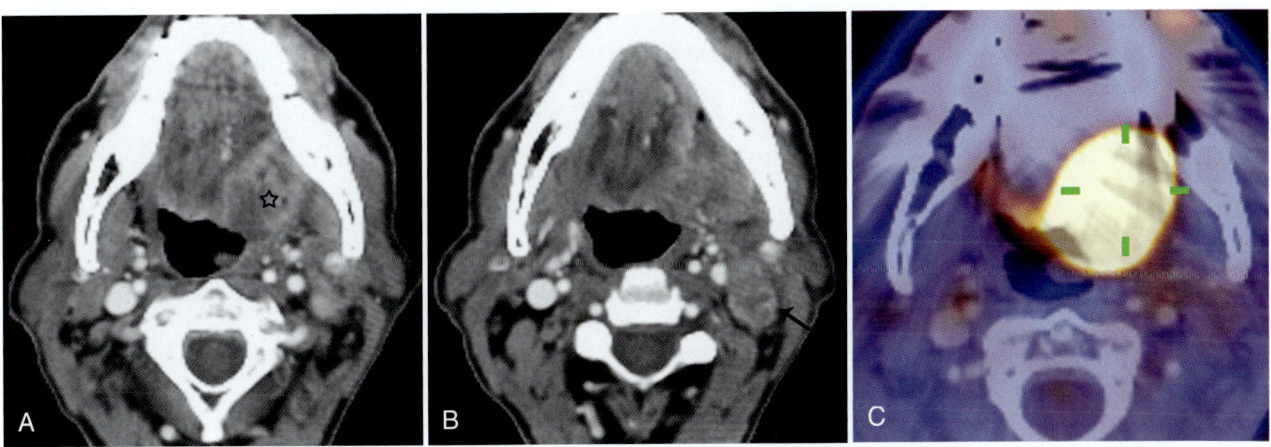

Figure 18-32 A: Contrast-enhanced axial computed tomographic (CT) scan demonstrating an ill-defined heterogeneous lesion (*star*) involving the left tongue base. Extension anteriorly into the oral tongue and posteriorly into the left oropharynx is seen. There is no extension of the lesion across the midline. **B:** Contrast-enhanced axial CT scan demonstrating a predominantly necrotic left level IIA lymph node (*arrow*) with extracapsular spread. **C:** Positron emission tomography/CT study demonstrates increased uptake at the left tongue base. The diagnosis is left tongue base carcinoma with cervical lymphadenopathy.

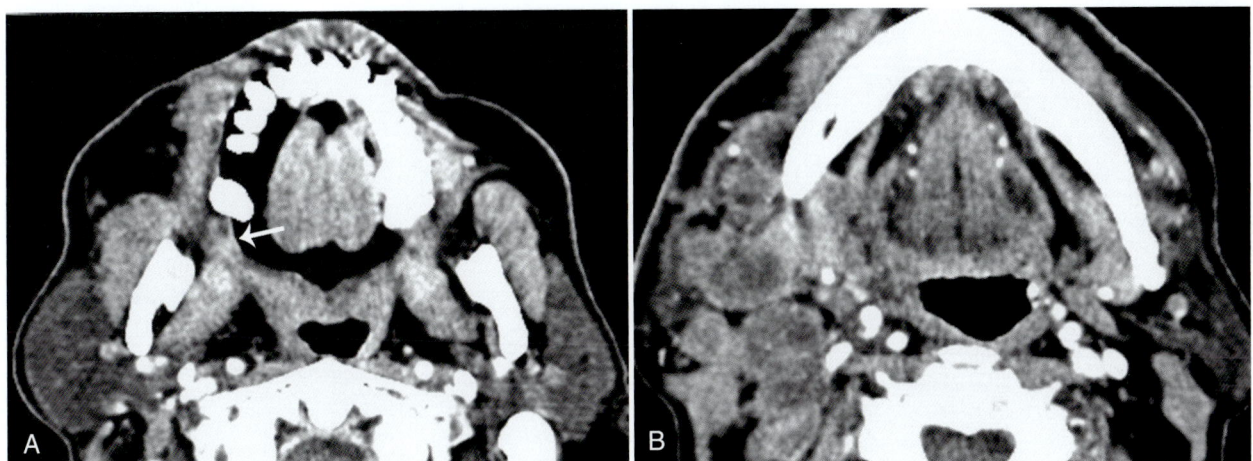

Figure 18-33 A: Contrast-enhanced axial computed tomographic (CT) scan at the level of the oral cavity demonstrating an ill-defined soft tissue mass (*arrow*) in the right retromolar trigone. **B:** Contrast-enhanced axial CT scan at the level of the floor of the mouth demonstrating possible contiguous extension of the mass along the right oropharyngeal region. Extensive, necrotic right level I and II lymphadenopathy is seen. The diagnosis is right retromolar trigone carcinoma and cervical lymphadenopathy.

present with discomfort in the region of the oral cavity or painless bleeding. On imaging, a mass lesion will be seen in the region of the retromolar trigone. It is essential to map the tumor on imaging for better staging and treatment planning. Spread of the tumor into the masticator space usually portends a poor prognosis (Figure 18-33). Cervical lymphadenopathy is seen in 20% to 30% of cases and should also be assessed.

Rhabdomyosarcoma

Rhabdomyosarcoma is the most common soft tissue sarcoma in children. It shows a bimodal peak age presentation, at 2 to 5 years, and again at 15 to 20 years. It is uncommonly seen in adults. Most patients present with a slowly growing mass lesion. Occasionally trismus is noted, especially when the temporomandibular joint is involved. Imaging demonstrates a heterogeneously enhancing soft tissue mass with poorly defined margins. Bone remodeling and destruction are also noted (Figure 18-34). Differential diagnosis includes plexiform neurofibroma and juvenile nasopharyngeal angiofibroma. Plexiform neurofibroma will demonstrate multiple serpiginous or ovoid soft tissue lesions causing scalloping of the bone. Other features of NF1 may be seen. Juvenile nasopharyngeal angiofibroma is seen as an intensely enhancing mass in the region of the posterior nasal cavity, extending into adjacent spaces. The lesion typically extends into the infratemporal fossa, widening the pterygomaxillary fissure and bowing the posterior wall of the maxillary sinus.

Ameloblastoma

Ameloblastoma accounts for 10% of all odontogenic tumors. It is the most common epithelial odontogenic tumor and is typically seen in young adults. The lesion

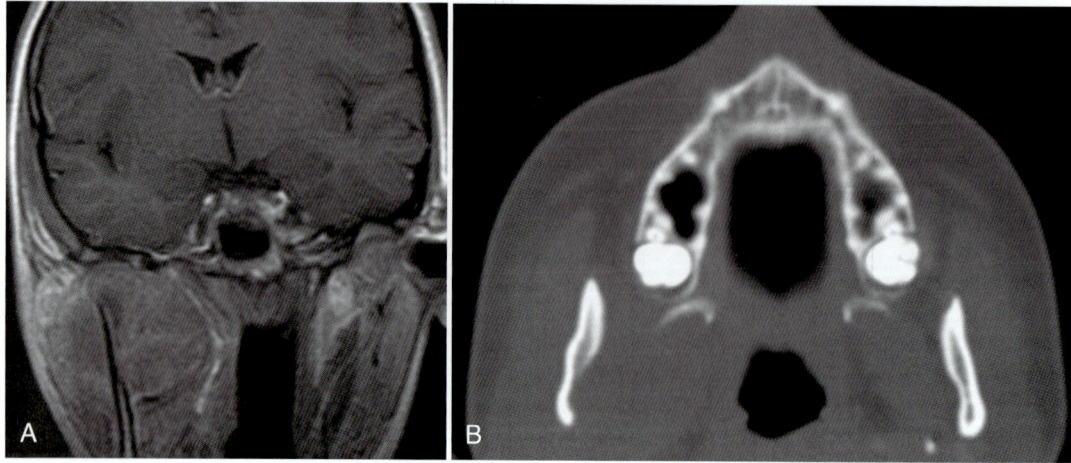

Figure 18-34 **A:** Contrast-enhanced coronal T1-weighted imaging demonstrating an enhancing lesion in the right masticator space with possible involvement of the ramus and condyle of the mandible. **B:** Axial computed tomographic scan demonstrating scalloping and erosion of the ramus of the mandible. The diagnosis is rhabdomyosarcoma.

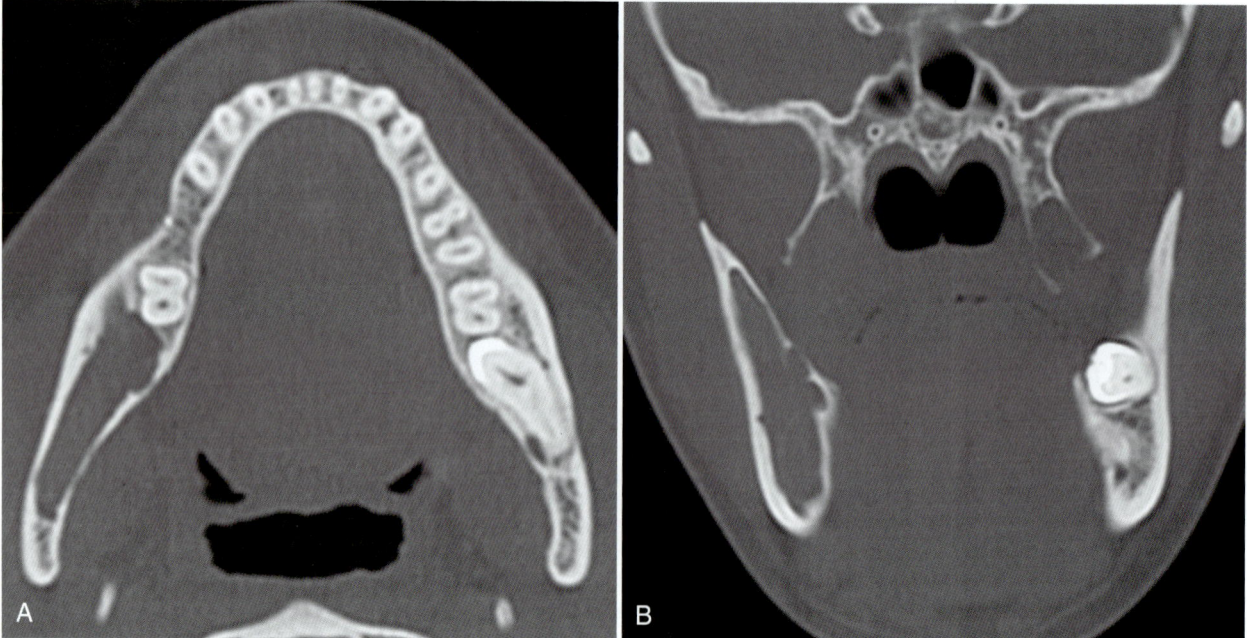

Figure 18-35 Axial computed tomographic (CT) scan **(A)** and coronal reformatted CT scan **(B)** demonstrating predominantly lytic lesion showing mild scalloping and thinning of the cortex involving ramus of right mandible. The diagnosis is ameloblastoma.

can involve the mandible or the maxilla, although the most common site is the posterior body or ramus of the mandible. Most patients present with a slow-growing painless mass. Imaging demonstrates an expansile, unilocular lesion seen in the posterior body or ramus of the mandible (Figure 18-35). Sometimes a multilocular lesion is seen. Differential diagnosis includes odontogenic keratocyst, dentigerous cyst, metastasis, and multiple myeloma. Odontogenic keratocyst is usually a solitary lesion and can have the same imaging appearance as ameloblastoma. However, a lesion located in the posterior body or the ramus of the mandible is more likely to represent an ameloblastoma.

A dentigerous cyst usually has a tooth associated with the cyst wall. Metastasis and multiple myelomas are usually seen as multiple lytic lesions, unlike typical, solitary, more well-defined ameloblastomas. Of these two clinical entities, metastasis only rarely involves the mandible.

■ THYROID AND LARYNX

Six cases are discussed in this section. They include congenital anomalies (e.g., lingual thyroid, thyroglossal duct cyst), inflammatory conditions (e.g., Hashimoto thyroiditis, goiter), and neoplastic conditions (e.g., anaplastic thyroid carcinoma, laryngeal carcinoma).

Lingual Thyroid

Ectopic thyroid tissue most commonly is located at the tongue base but can be found anywhere along its embryonic course (i.e., from the foramen cecum at the junction of the anterior two thirds and posterior one third of the

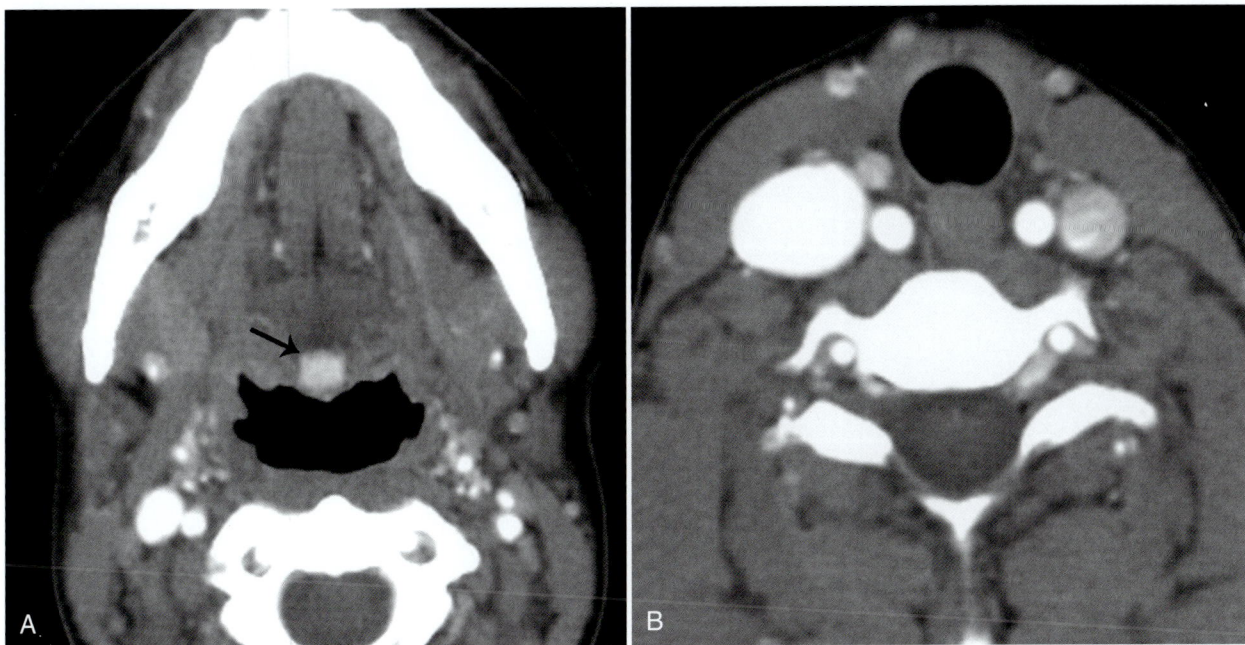

Figure 18-36 A: Contrast-enhanced axial computed tomographic (CT) scan at the level of the floor of the mouth demonstrating an enhancing lesion (*arrow*) in the midline base of tongue. **B:** Contrast-enhanced axial CT scan at the level of the thyroid bed does not demonstrate any evidence of normal native thyroid tissue. The diagnosis is ectopic thyroid with absent normal native thyroid tissue.

tongue up to its normal location in the neck). It is imperative to scan the thyroid bed in the neck for normal thyroid tissue if ectopic thyroid tissue is found. Most patients are asymptomatic. Some patients present with hypothyroidism. CT scan shows a well-defined, high-density lesion, which demonstrates intense enhancement at the tongue base (or anywhere along the embryonic course of thyroid) (Figure 18-36). MR study demonstrates lingual thyroid as a well-defined mass, hyperintense on both T1-WI and T2-WI. In such cases, a nuclear medicine scan should be obtained to evaluate for any other ectopic thyroid tissue sites and for any evidence of functioning thyroid tissue at its normal location.

Thyroglossal Duct Cyst

The thyroglossal duct cyst is the most common congenital neck mass. It is classically seen as a cystic lesion in or just off the midline. The cysts result from failure of normal involution of the thyroglossal duct with subsequent cyst formation. Most patients present with a slow growing, nontender midline neck mass. Imaging demonstrates thyroglossal duct cyst as a midline, unilocular cystic lesion, at or just below the level of the hyoid bone (Figure 18-37, *A*). In the lower neck, the thyroglossal duct cyst is seen just outside the thyroid cartilage, in the midline or just off midline, and tends to insinuate itself between the strap muscles (Figure 18-37, *B* and *C*). The presence of solid tissue within a thyroglossal duct cyst could represent residual thyroid tissue (Figure 18-37, *D*). However, coexistent thyroid carcinoma (usually papillary) merits consideration (Figure 18-37, *E*). Differential diagnosis includes necrotic lymph node, lymphangioma, and branchial cleft cyst. A necrotic lymph node typically demonstrates a slightly thick enhancing wall. Associated additional cervical lymphadenopathy with or without a primary mass lesion will be seen. Lymphangiomas typically appear as multiloculated, transspatial, nonenhancing cystic lesions. Branchial cleft cysts are typically seen more laterally, typically in the posterior triangle of the neck.

Hashimoto Thyroiditis

Hashimoto thyroiditis (chronic lymphocytic thyroiditis) is an autoimmune form of thyroiditis. Most patients are women in their third to fifth decade of life who present with signs and symptoms of hypothyroidism. An association with lymphoma has been described. In fact, a small percentage of patients with Hashimoto thyroiditis develop malignant lymphoma of the thyroid gland, and most patients with thyroid lymphoma have coexistent Hashimoto thyroiditis. Diagnosis of Hashimoto thyroiditis is generally based on clinical presentation and laboratory analysis of thyroid function. Imaging does not play a critical role in making the diagnosis. However, three distinct patterns have been described on imaging: a large solitary nodule, multiple small nodules, and diffuse infiltration of the gland (Figure 18-38). Violation of the thyroid capsule or presence of cervical lymphadenopathy suggests an underlying lymphoma. Differential diagnosis includes de Quervain thyroiditis and goiter. Based on imaging, it can be difficult to distinguish these clinical entities. Clinical and laboratory correlation is helpful in establishing the diagnosis.

Goiter

Enlargement of the thyroid gland due to any cause is known as *goiter*. Patients can present with a neck mass and signs and symptoms of hyperthyroidism or

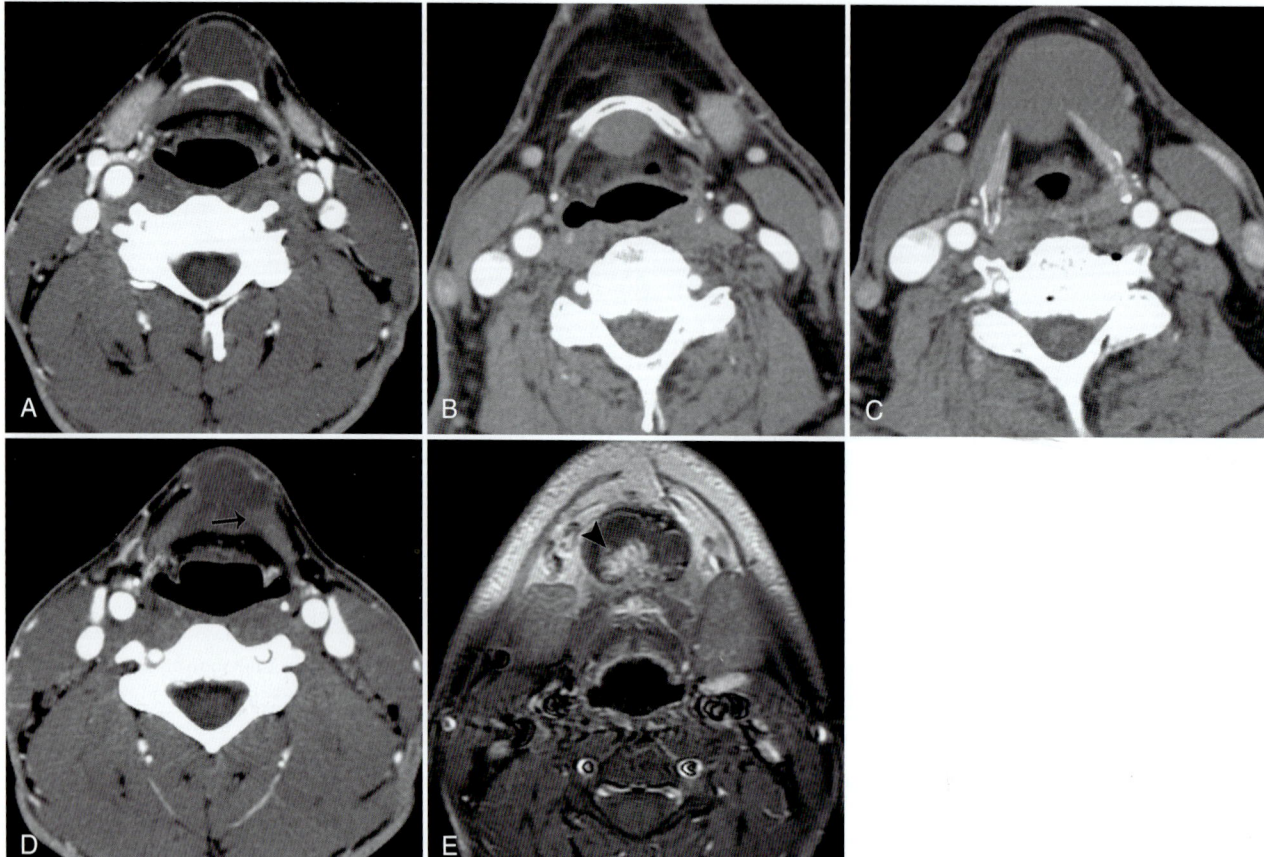

Figure 18-37 **A:** Contrast-enhanced axial computed tomographic (CT) scan demonstrating a predominantly cystic lesion attached to the hyoid bone in the midline neck. The diagnosis in this patient is thyroglossal duct cyst. **B, C:** In a different patient, contrast-enhanced axial CT scans demonstrating a well-defined abnormal density lesion in the midline neck, attached to hyoid bone and insinuating itself between the strap muscles. The slightly higher density seen within this lesion suggests a more proteinaceous content of the thyroglossal duct cyst. **D:** In another patient, contrast-enhanced axial CT scan demonstrating soft tissue (*arrow*) along the margins of a cyst in midline neck. This soft tissue was proven to be normal thyroid tissue within thyroglossal duct cyst. **E:** In yet another patient, contrast-enhanced, fat-suppressed, axial T1-weighted imaging demonstrating irregularly marginated, heterogeneous enhancing lesion (*arrowhead*) within the cyst in midline neck. This enhancing soft tissue was proven to be mixed papillary and follicular carcinoma within thyroglossal duct cyst.

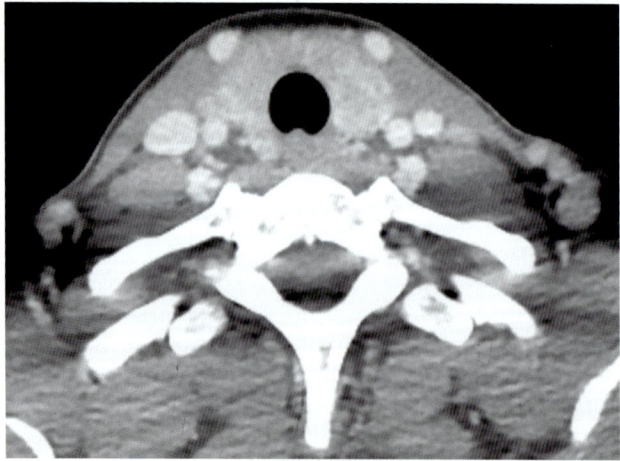

Figure 18-38 Contrast-enhanced axial computed tomographic scan demonstrating heterogeneous enhancement of the thyroid gland. The thyroid gland enhances less than normal. The diagnosis is Hashimoto thyroiditis.

hypothyroidism. Rarely, patients present with dysphagia and dyspnea due to esophageal and tracheal compression. Of note, hoarseness does not occur in benign enlargement of thyroid gland. In fact, presence of hoarseness suggests underlying malignant transformation and recurrent laryngeal nerve paralysis. Heterogeneous enlargement of the thyroid gland is seen. Such enlargement can affect a single lobe or can diffusely involve the whole gland. Such enlargement can be focal and remain confined to the vicinity of the thyroid bed, or it can be more widespread, extending for a variable distance along the pharynx superiorly or to a retrosternal location inferiorly (Figure 18-39). There is no violation of the thyroid capsule or cervical lymphadenopathy. Narrowing and displacement of the trachea are seen and should always be evaluated.

Anaplastic Thyroid Carcinoma

Anaplastic thyroid carcinoma is the most aggressive variety of thyroid malignancy. It accounts for less than 2% of all thyroid cancers but is responsible for up to 40% of deaths

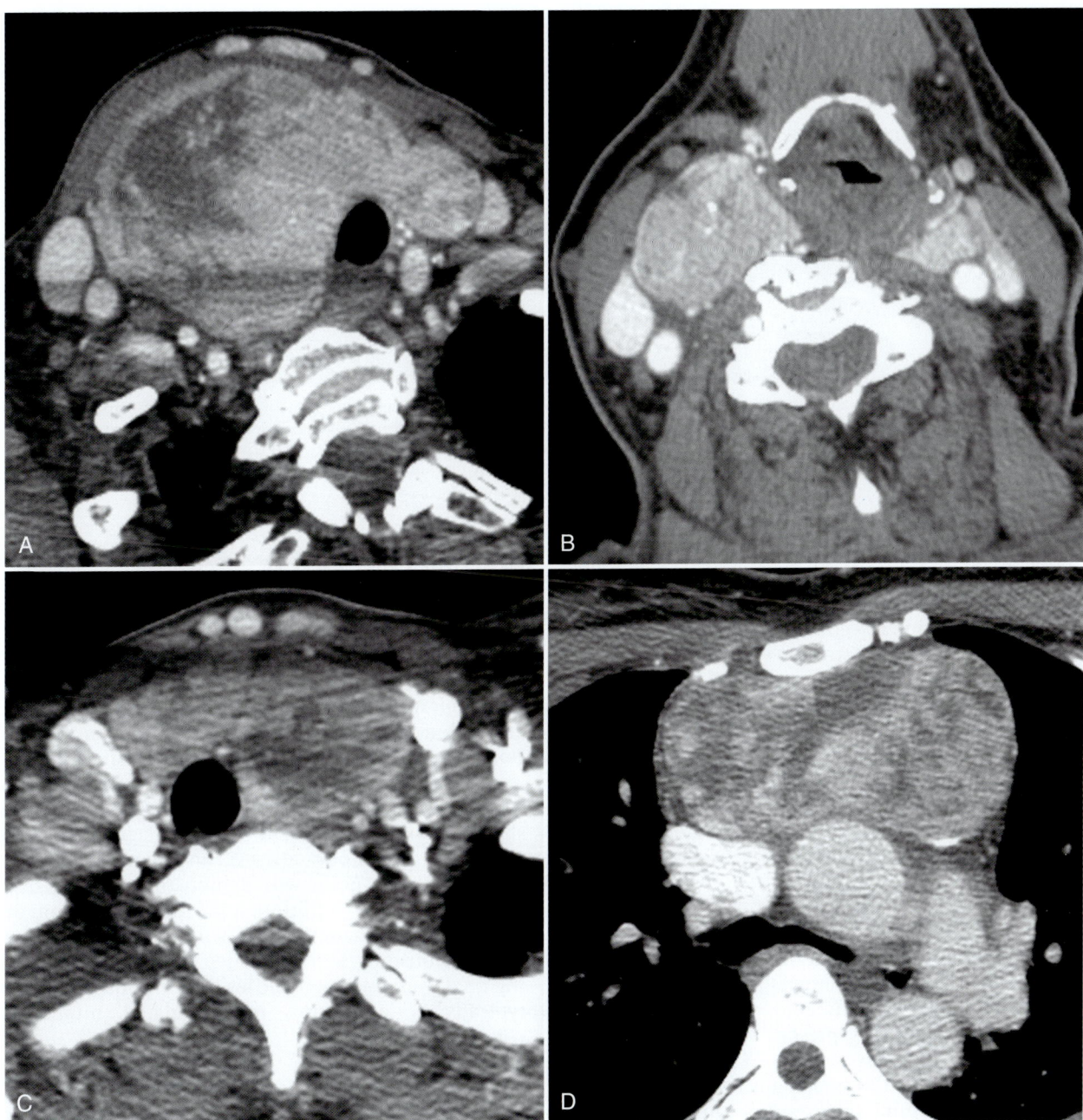

Figure 18-39 A: Contrast-enhanced axial computed tomographic (CT) scan demonstrating diffuse heterogeneous enlargement of the entire thyroid gland including the isthmus (right lobe > left lobe). There is no violation of the thyroid capsule. Displacement of the trachea to the left is seen with mild tracheal luminal compromise. **B:** Axial CT scan at a more cranial level demonstrating superior extension of the enlarged lobes of the thyroid gland along the pharynx up to the level of the supraglottic larynx. The diagnosis in this patient is goiter. **C:** In a different patient, contrast-enhanced axial CT scan demonstrating heterogeneous enlargement of the thyroid gland suggestive of goiter. Displacement of the trachea to the right is seen with mild tracheal luminal compromise. There is no violation of the thyroid capsule. **D:** Caudally, axial CT scan demonstrating retrosternal extension of goiter.

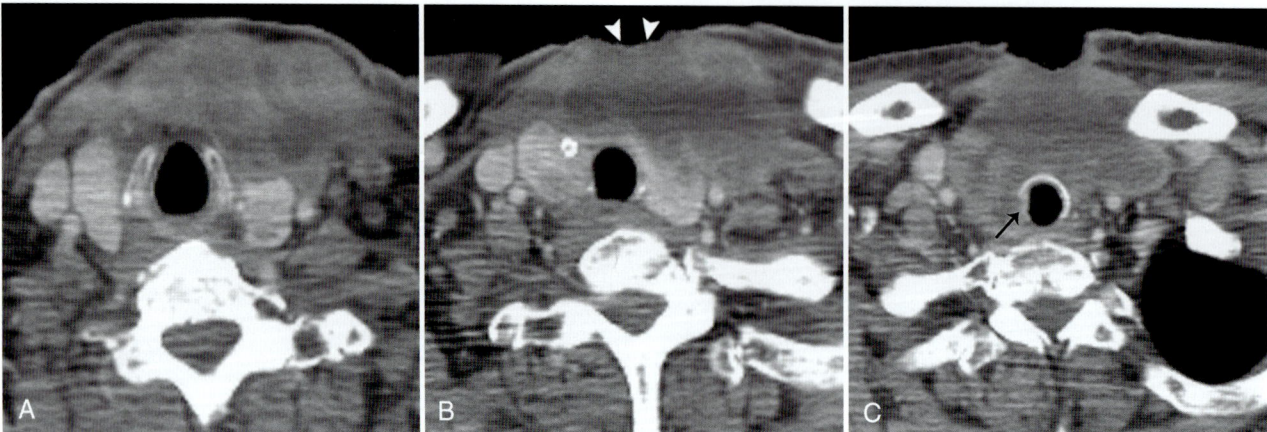

Figure 18-40 A: Contrast-enhanced axial computed tomographic (CT) scan demonstrating a heterogeneous mass lesion involving the left lobe of the thyroid gland and extending through its capsule to involve the left sternocleidomastoid. **B:** Axial CT scan at a caudal level demonstrating the mass to extend up to the skin surface with associated ulceration (*arrowheads*) along its margins. **C:** Axial CT scan at a more caudal level demonstrating marginal extension into the trachea (*arrow*). The diagnosis is anaplastic thyroid carcinoma.

from thyroid cancers. Most patients are elderly women, who present with a rapidly growing neck mass, hoarseness, dyspnea, and dysphagia. An aggressive heterogeneous thyroid-based mass lesion is seen violating its capsule, extending into adjacent soft tissue structures including the trachea and larynx (Figure 18-40). Cervical lymphadenopathy is common. Lung metastasis is not uncommon. Rarely, invasion of vascular structures occurs. Hematogenous metastasis and brain metastasis are known. Differential diagnosis includes other primary thyroid cancers, such as papillary, follicular, and medullary thyroid cancer. However, these thyroid cancers are not as aggressive in spreading to adjacent structures as is anaplastic thyroid cancer.

Squamous Cell Carcinoma of Larynx

Squamous cell carcinoma accounts for the overwhelming majority of all malignancies of the larynx. Risk factors include alcohol, tobacco, and human papillomavirus. Most patients present with hoarseness of voice. An enhancing mass lesion will be seen on imaging. However, the goal of imaging is not to identify the tumor but to determine the extent of tumor and evaluate for metastasis. In particular, evaluation should be performed to determine the presence of cartilage invasion and transglottic spread of tumor (Figure 18-41). This finding can have significant surgical implications, including voice conservation surgery and choice of treatment protocol. In addition, extension of tumor across the anterior commissure to involve more than one third of the contralateral larynx precludes vertical hemilaryngectomy. Evaluation for cervical lymphadenopathy and metastasis should also be performed.

■ NECK MISCELLANEOUS

Six cases are discussed in this section. They include congenital anomalies (e.g., branchial cleft cyst, cystic hygroma), trauma (e.g., foreign body), infectious and inflammatory conditions (e.g., Lemierre syndrome), and tumors (e.g., carotid body tumor, lymphoma).

Brachial Cleft Cyst II

Branchial cleft cysts are congenital anomalies arising from anomalous embryogenesis of the branchial arches. Depending on the arch involved, four such branchial cleft cysts are seen in the neck. Of these, the type 2 branchial cleft cyst is the most common. Most patients present with a neck mass or some discomfort in the neck. Imaging demonstrates a uniform thin-walled cyst posterolateral to the submandibular gland, anteromedial to the sternocleidomastoid and anterolateral to the carotid sheath (Figure 18-42). Differential diagnosis includes necrotic lymph node, abscess, and lymphangioma. A necrotic lymph node will demonstrate some peripheral thickening. In addition, a primary mass lesion and additional lymphadenopathy will be seen. An abscess will demonstrate a thick-walled peripherally enhancing predominantly necrotic lesion. Lymphangiomas are typically nonenhancing, multiloculated, multispatial congenital lesions.

Cystic Hygroma

Cystic hygroma is the most common form of lymphangioma. The other less common varieties include cavernous lymphangioma, capillary lymphangioma, and vasculolymphatic malformations. Cystic hygromas can occur anywhere in the neck, but most are located in the posterior triangle of the neck. Most patients present with a growing neck mass. Nonenhancing, multiloculated, occasionally transspatial cystic lesion, sometimes demonstrating fluid–fluid level suggestive of intralesional hemorrhage, is seen (Figure 18-43). Differential diagnosis includes thyroglossal duct cyst and branchial cleft cysts. Thyroglossal duct cyst is typically seen in the midline neck. These cysts are attached to, or are in close proximity to, the hyoid bone and typically insinuate themselves between the strap muscles. The unilocular, nonseptated appearance of the branchial cleft cysts and their specific locations in the neck help distinguish branchial cleft cysts from lymphangiomas.

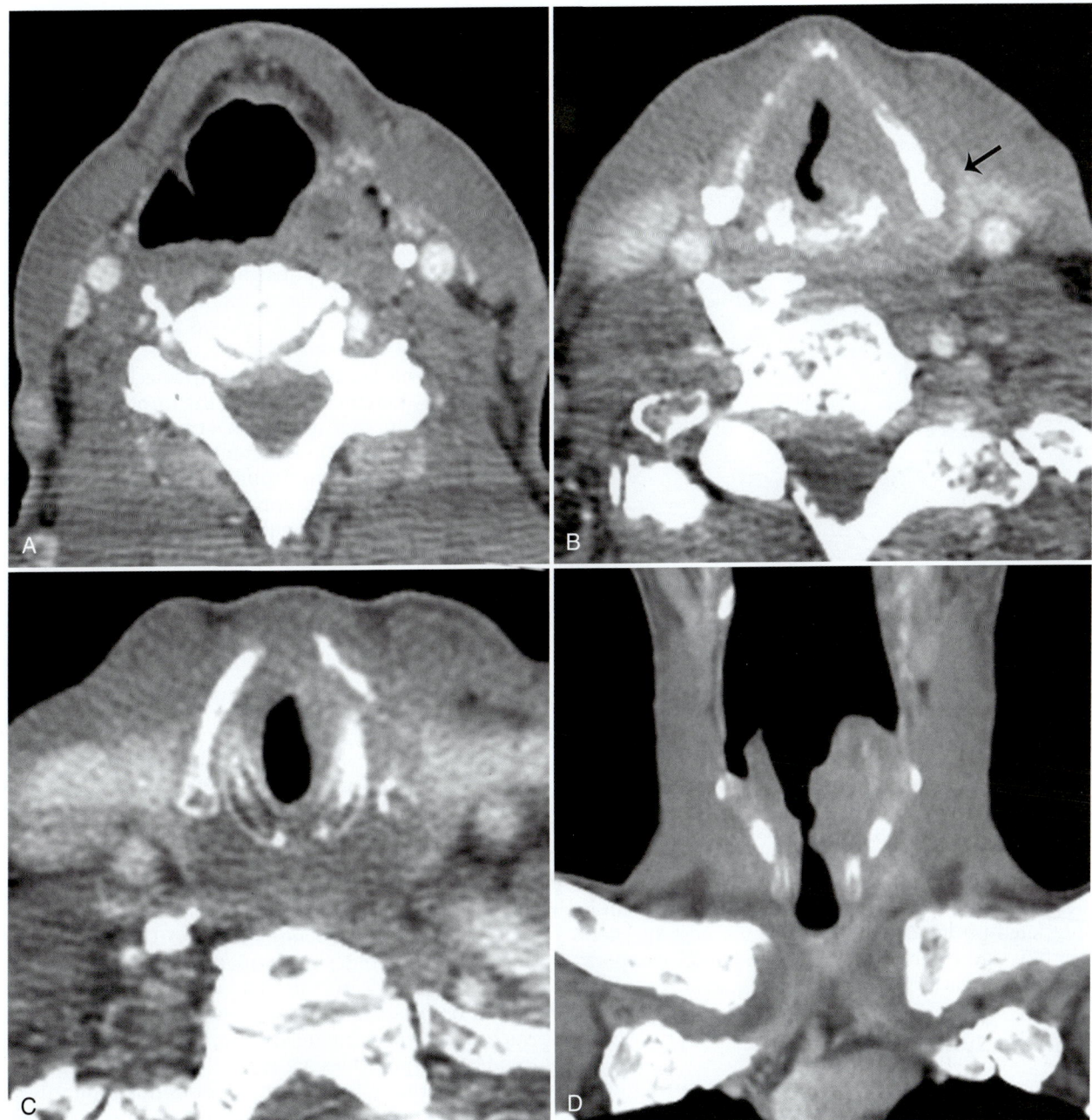

Figure 18-41 **A:** Contrast-enhanced axial computed tomographic (CT) scan demonstrating irregularly marginated soft tissue mass obliterating the left pyriform sinus. **B:** Axial CT scan at a caudal level demonstrating mass lesion extending contiguously along the left true cord. There is a hint of extension of this mass lesion across the left thyroid cartilage into the adjacent strap muscles (*arrow*) suggestive of cartilage invasion. **C:** Axial CT scan at a more caudal level demonstrating irregularity along the left lateral aspect of the subglottis. **D:** Coronal reformatted CT scan confirms findings demonstrated on axial scans of a heterogeneous mass (carcinoma) seen in the left supraglottic region with transglottic spread.

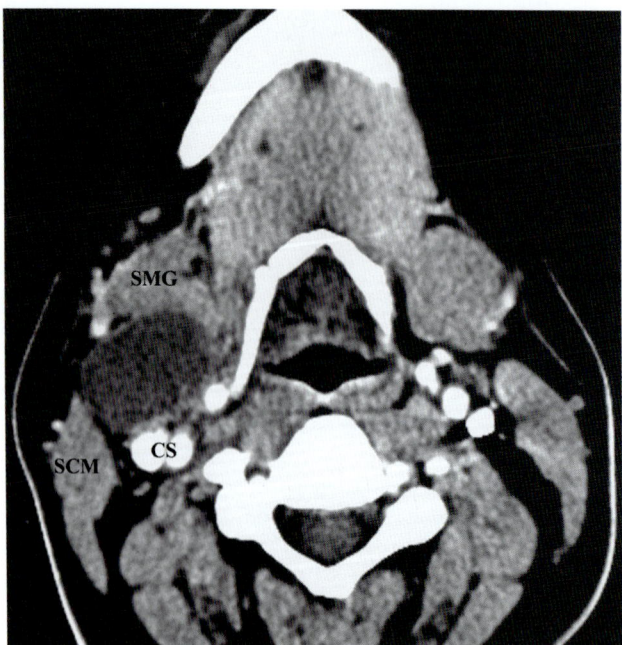

Figure 18-42 Contrast-enhanced axial computed tomographic scan demonstrating a nonenhancing cystic lesion posterior to the submandibular gland (*SMG*), anterior to the carotid sheath (*CS*), and anteromedial to the sternocleidomastoid (*SCM*) suggestive of a type 2 branchial cleft cyst.

Foreign Body

Most foreign bodies seen in the neck result from accidental ingestion. Patients present with a foreign body sensation in the throat. Occasionally, dysphagia and dyspnea are also present. Most foreign bodies are identified as hyperdensities of varying shapes. Associated retropharyngeal soft tissue swelling is seen, and can be appreciated on lateral scout film of the neck or lateral plain film of the neck. The foreign body is best appreciated on CT scans (Figure 18-44).

Lemierre Syndrome

Lemierre syndrome is an anaerobic suppurative thrombophlebitis of the internal jugular vein, occurring most commonly secondary to pharyngeal, dental, or mastoidal infection. Most patients present with fever, sore throat, neck pain, and tenderness. Color Doppler ultrasound demonstrates a distended internal jugular vein, which does not demonstrate any flow within. Contrast-enhanced CT scan demonstrates an enlarged jugular vein, with filling defect within the vein. Stranding of the adjacent fat will be seen. Asymmetrically thickened ipsilateral oropharyngeal wall is often seen (Figure 18-45).

Carotid Body Tumor

Carotid body tumor is a type of paraganglioma. Most paragangliomas are sporadic. Occasionally, they are familial with autosomal dominant inheritance and incomplete penetrance. In the head and neck, based on their anatomic location, four types of paragangliomas have been described. Paragangliomas that arise at the nodose ganglion of the vagus nerve are known as *glomus vagale*; those at the carotid body bifurcation are known as *carotid body tumors*; those at the jugular foramen are known as *glomus jugulare*; and those at the cochlear promontory are known as *glomus tympanicum tumors*. Most patients with carotid body tumor present with a slowly growing pulsatile mass in the neck. On imaging, an intensely enhancing mass at the carotid bifurcation, splaying the internal and external carotid arteries, is seen (Figure 18-46, A–D). Differential diagnosis includes schwannoma and lymph nodes. A vagal schwannoma is seen as a moderately enhancing lesion that typically displaces the internal jugular vein posterolaterally and internal carotid artery anteromedially (Figure 18-46, E and F). Lymph nodes are uncommonly seen in the carotid sheath. Typically, such lymphadenopathy will be associated with lymphadenopathy elsewhere in the neck.

Lymphoma

Lymphoma is the second most common primary malignancy that occurs in the head and neck. It occurs as either Hodgkin disease or non-Hodgkin lymphoma. Hodgkin disease (HD) predominantly affects adolescents and young adults, and it typically involves the lymph nodes. Extranodal disease is rare in head and neck. The diagnosis is established by the presence of Reed-Sternberg cells. Non-Hodgkin lymphoma (NHL) is most commonly seen in older patients. Extranodal involvement is seen in 60% cases of NHL, with areas rich in lymphoid tissue such as the Waldeyer ring, more prone to such occurrence. Enlarged, homogeneously enhancing cervical lymph nodes are typically seen, although non-homogeneous, necrotic lymph nodes uncommonly can occur (Figure 18-47). Differential diagnosis includes tumors (e.g., leukemia, metastasis, posttransplant lymphoproliferative disorder), infectious etiologies (e.g., cat-scratch disease, tuberculosis), and inflammatory conditions (e.g., sarcoidosis, Kimura disease, Castleman disease). Presence of necrosis and calcification raises the possibility of metastasis and infectious etiologies such as tuberculosis. However, it can sometimes be difficult to establish the diagnosis on imaging. Therefore, lymph node biopsy is indicated in most cases.

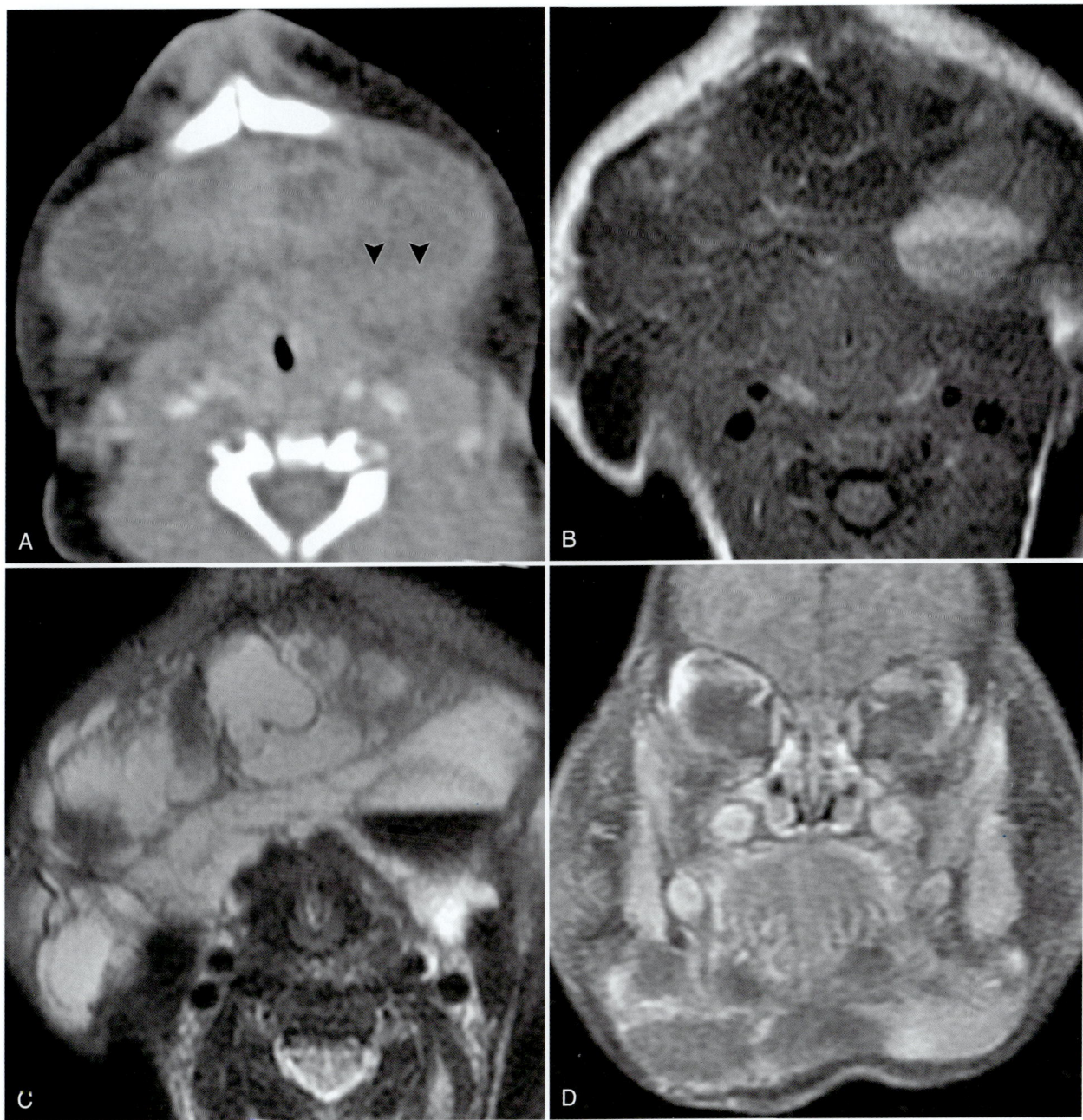

Figure 18-43 **A:** Contrast-enhanced axial computed tomographic (CT) scan demonstrating nonenhancing, multiloculated, transspatial cystic lesion in the region of the floor of mouth. Fluid level (*arrowhead*) seen within one of these loculations suggests intralesional hemorrhage. Axial T1-weighted imaging (**B**), axial T2-weighted imaging (**C**), and contrast-enhanced fat-suppressed coronal T1-weighted imaging (**D**) confirm the morphologic appearance of the lesion seen on CT study. The diagnosis is cystic hygroma.

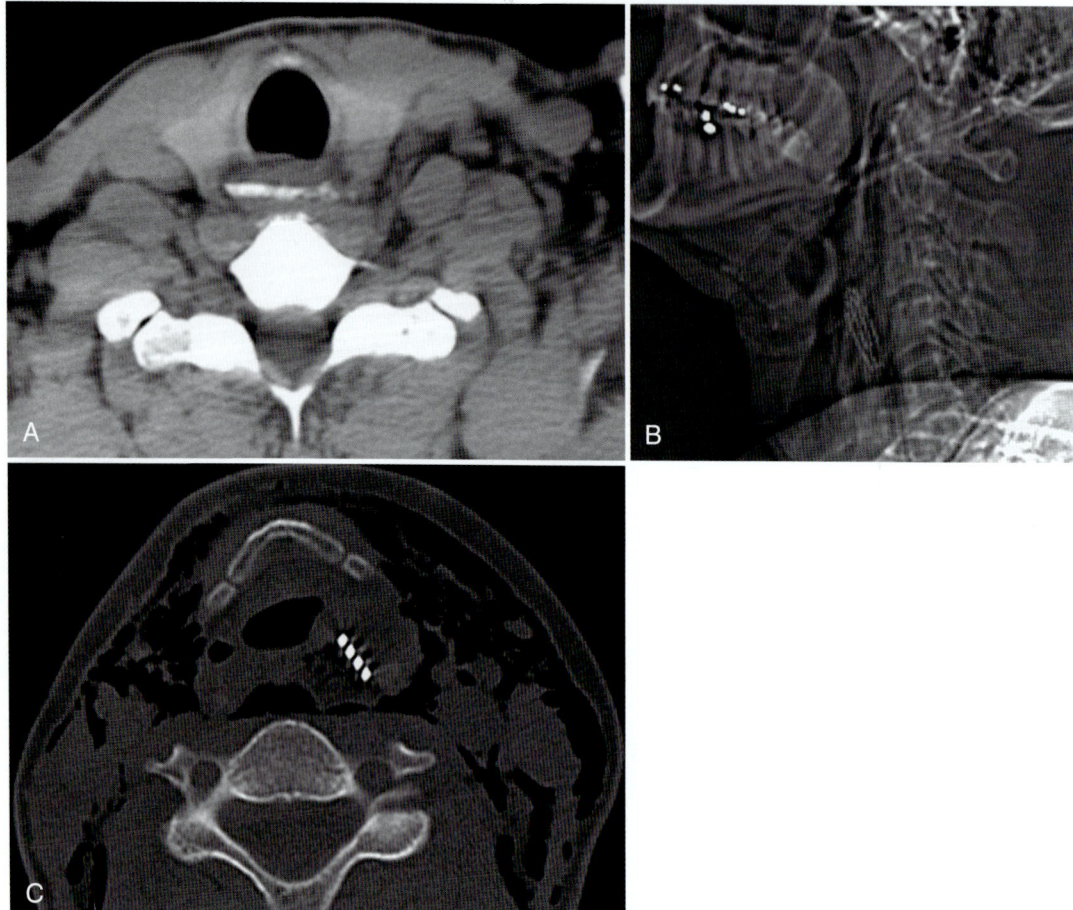

Figure 18-44 A: Noncontrast axial computed tomographic (CT) scan of the neck demonstrating a linear hyperdensity within the cervical esophagus. The diagnosis in this patient is a swallowed chicken bone. **B:** In a different patient, lateral scout film demonstrating a toothbrush in the hypopharynx with extensive heterogeneity of the soft tissues suggestive of emphysema. **C:** Noncontrast axial CT scan of the neck demonstrating bristles of the toothbrush in the region of the left pyriform sinus with extensive emphysematous changes.

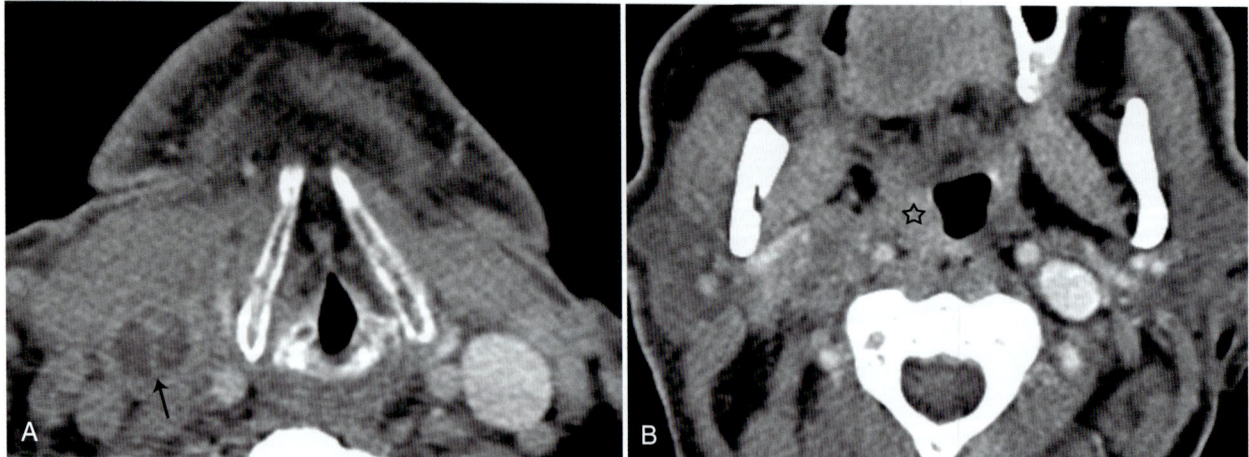

Figure 18-45 A: Contrast-enhanced axial computed tomographic (CT) scan at the level of the true cords demonstrating a filling defect within the right internal jugular vein (*arrow*) with adjacent inflammatory changes. **B:** Axial CT scan at the level of the oral cavity demonstrating asymmetric thickening of the right oropharyngeal wall (*star*). The diagnosis is Lemierre syndrome.

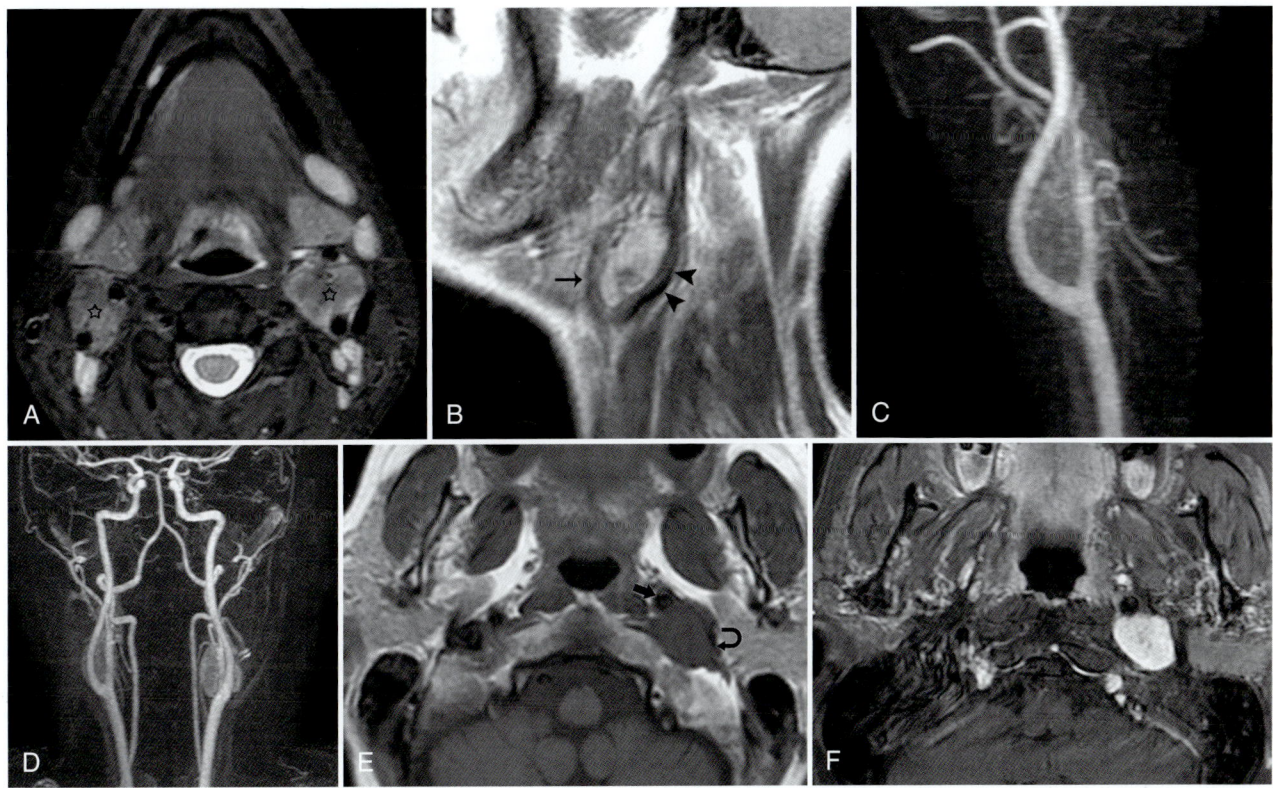

Figure 18-46 A: Fat-suppressed axial T2-weighted imaging just distal to the carotid bifurcation demonstrating mass lesions (*stars*) displacing the internal carotid arteries posteriorly and external carotid arteries anteriorly. B: Contrast-enhanced sagittal T1-weighted imaging demonstrating an intensely enhancing lesion splaying the internal carotid artery posteriorly (*arrowheads*) and external carotid artery anteriorly (*arrow*). C: Contrast-enhanced time-resolved imaging of contrast kinetics (TRICKS) magnetic resonance angiography (MRA) image reconstructed in the sagittal plane demonstrating tumoral blush at the carotid bifurcation. D: TRICKS MRA image in the coronal plane demonstrating tumoral blush at the carotid bifurcation bilaterally. The diagnosis in this patient is bilateral carotid body tumors. E: In a different patient, axial T1-weighted imaging demonstrating a soft tissue lesion displacing the left internal carotid artery anteromedially (*black arrow*) and internal jugular vein posteriorly (*curved arrow*). F: Contrast-enhanced, fat-suppressed, axial T1-weighted imaging demonstrating enhancement of the mass. The diagnosis in this patient is vagal schwannoma.

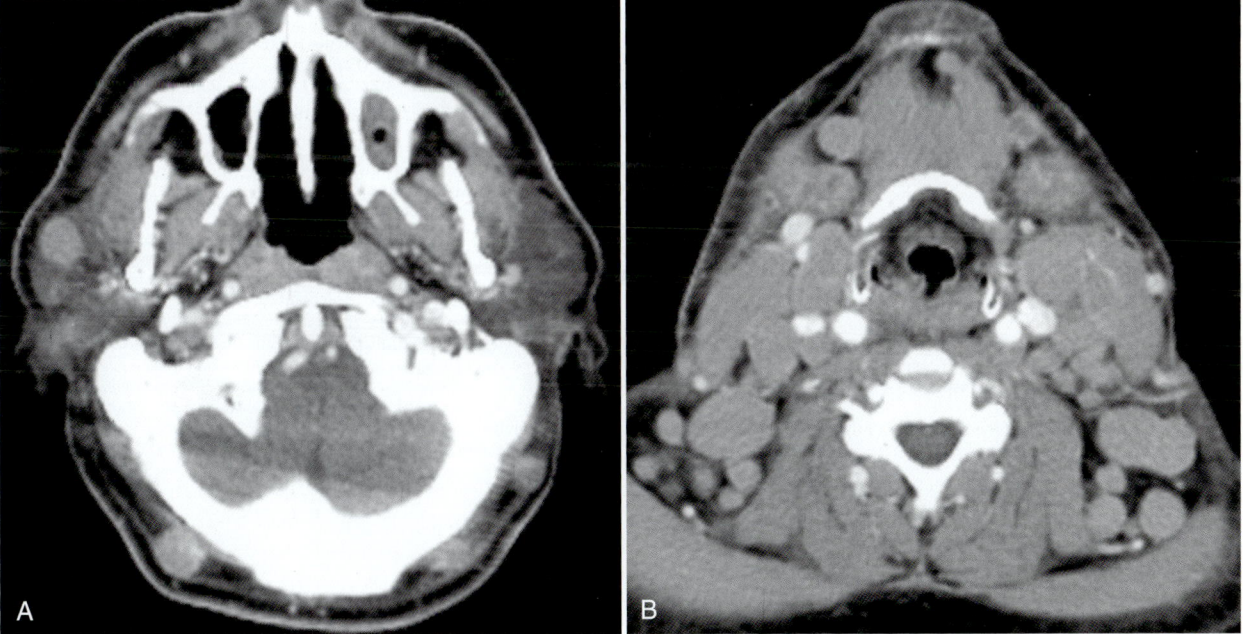

Figure 18-47 A: Contrast-enhanced axial computed tomographic (CT) scan at the skull base demonstrating enlarged suboccipital and intraparotid lymph nodes. There is no obvious prominence of the nasopharyngeal soft tissue. B: Contrast-enhanced axial CT scan at the supraglottic level demonstrating multiple, homogeneously enlarged cervical lymph nodes bilaterally. The diagnosis is Hodgkin lymphoma.

Suggested Readings

Anderson GJ, Tom LW, Womer RB, et al. Rhabdomyosarcoma of the head and neck in children. *Arch Otolaryngol Head Neck Surg.* 1990;116:428-431.

Arcand P, Desrosiers M, Dube J, Abela A. The large vestibular aqueduct syndrome and sensorineural hearing loss in the pediatric population. *J Otolaryngol.* 1991;20:247-250.

Berrettini S, Forli F, Bogazzi F, et al. Large vestibular aqueduct syndrome: audiological, radiological, clinical, and genetic features. *Am J Otolaryngol.* 2005;26:363-371.

Bilanuik LT. Orbital vascular lesions: role of imaging. *Radiol Clin North Am.* 1999;37:169-83.

Burm JS, Chung CH, Oh SJ. Pure orbital blowout fracture: new concepts and importance of medial orbital blowout fracture. *Plast Reconstr Surg.* 1999;103:1839-1849.

Caldemeyer KS, Mathews VP, Azzarelli B, Smith RR. The jugular foramen: A review of anatomy, masses and imaging characteristics. *Radiographics.* 1997;17:1123-1139.

Chin SC, Rice H, Som PM. Spread of goiters outside of the thyroid bed: a review of 190 cases and analysis of the incidence of the various extensions. *Arch Otoloaryngol Head Neck Surg.* 2003;129:1198-1202.

Connor S. Laryngeal cancer: How does the radiologist help? *Cancer Imag.* 2007;7:93-103.

Curtin HD, Sanelli PC, Som PM. Temporal bone: embryology and anatomy. In: Som PM, Curtin HD, eds. *Head and neck imaging.* St Louis: Mosby; 2003:1057-1092.

Drutman J, Harnsberger HR, Babbel RW, et al. Sinonasal polyposis: investigation by direct coronal CT. *Neuroradiol.* 1994;36:469-472.

Eustis HS, Mafee MF, Walton C, Mondonca J. MR imaging and CT of orbital infections and complication in acute rhinosinusitis. *Radiol Clin North Am.* 1998;36:1165-1183.

Fatterpekar GM, Doshi AH, Dugar M, et al. Role of 3D CT in evaluation of the temporal bone. *Radiographics.* 2006;26:S117-S132.

Fatterpekar GM, Mukherji SK, Arbelaez A, Maheshwari S, Castillo M. Fungal diseases of the paranasal sinuses. *Semin Ultrasound CT MR.* 1999;20:391-401.

Greenberg JJ, Oot RF, Wismer GL, et al. Cholesterol granuloma of the petrous apex: MR and CT evaluation. *AJNR Am J Neuroradiol.* 1988;9:1205-1214.

Gullane PJ, Davidson J, O'Dwyer T, Forte V. Juvenile angiofibroma: a review of the literature and a case series report. *Laryngoscope.* 1992;102:928-933.

Guneri A, Ceyan K, Igci E, Kovanlikaya A. Lingual thyroid: The diagnostic value of magnetic resonance imaging. *J Laryngol Otol.* 1991;105:493-495.

Holliday RA. Inflammatory diseases of the temporal bone: evaluation with CT and MR. *Semin Ultrasound CT MR.* 1989;10:213-235.

Holliday RA, Cohen WA, Schinella RA, et al. Benign lymphoepithelial parotid cysts and hyperplastic cervical adenopathy in AIDS-risk patients: a new CT appearance. *Radiology.* 1988;168:439-441.

Hopper RA, Salemy S, Sze RW. Diagnosis of midface fractures with CT: What the surgeon needs to know. *Radiographics.* 2006;26:783-793.

Hughes GK, Miszkiel KA. Imaging of the lacrimal gland. *Semin Ultrasound CT MR.* 2006;27:476-91.

Izumi M, Eguchi K, Uetani M, et al. MR features of the lacrimal gland in Sjogren's syndrome. *AJR Am J Roentgenol.* 1998;170:1661-6.

Jackson A, Patankar T, Laitt RD. Intracanalicular optic nerve meningioma: a serious diagnostic pitfall. *AJNR Am J Neuroradiol.* 2003;24:1167-70.

Jahrsdoerfer RA, Yeakley JW, Aguilar EA, et al. Grading system for the selection of patients with congenital aural atresia. *Am J Otol.* 1992;13:6-12.

Kakimoto N, Gamoh S, Tamaki J, et al. CT and MR images of pleomorphic adenoma in minor and major salivary glands. *Eur J Radiol.* 2009;69:464-72.

Kirsch C. Oral cavity cancer. *Top Magn Reson Imaging.* 2007;18:269-80.

Koeller KK, Alamo L, Adair CF, Smirniotopoulos JG. Congenital cystic lesions of the neck: Radiologic-pathologic correlation. *Radiographics.* 1999;19:121-146.

Kornreich L, Blaser S, Schwarz M, et al. Optic pathway glioma: correlation of imaging findings with the presence of neurofibromatosis. *AJNR Am J Neuroradiol.* 2001;22:1963-9.

LeBlang SD, Nunez DB. Helical CT of the cervical spine and soft tissue injuries of the neck. *Radiol Clin North Am.* 1999;37:515-32.

Lo WWM, Solti-Bohman LG, McElveen JT. Aberrant Carotid artery: Radiologic diagnosis with emphasis on high resolution computed tomography. *Radiographics.* 1985;5:985-994.

Loevner L, Sonners A. Imaging of the neoplasms of the paranasal sinuses. *Neuroimag Clin North Am.* 2004;14:625-646.

Loevner LA. Thyroid and parathyroid glands: anatomy and pathology. In: Som PM, Curtin HD, eds. *Head and Neck Imaging.* 4th ed. St Louis, Missouri: Mosby; 2003:2134-2171.

Mafee MF. Imaging of the orbit. In: Valvassori GE, Mafee MF, Carter B, eds. *Imaging of the Head and Neck.* Stuttgart: Georg Thieme; 1995:248-327.

Mafee MF, Putterman A, Valvassori GE, et al. Orbital space-occupying lesions: role of computed tomography and magnetic resonance imaging. An analysis of 145 cases. *Radiol Clin North Am.* 1987;25:529-559.

Mafee MF, Lachenauer CS, Kumar A, et al. CT and MR imaging of intralabyrinthine schwannoma: report of two cases and review of the literature. *Radiology.* 1990;174:395-400.

Meriot P, Veillon F, Garcia JF, et al. CT appearance of ossicular injuries. *Radiographics.* 1997;118:827-829.

Moret J, Delvert JC, Lasjaunias P. Vascularization of the ear: Normal variants, glomus tumors. *J Neuroradiol.* 1982;9:209-260.

Mukherji SK, Fatterpekar GM, Castillo M, et al. Imaging of congenital anomalies of the branchial apparatus. *Neuroimaging Clin N Am.* 2000;10:75-93.

Nemzek WR, Swartz JD. Temporal bone: inflammatory disease. In: Som PM, Curtin HD, eds. *Head and neck imaging.* St Louis, Mo: Mosby; 2003:1173-1230.

Ohnishi T, Noguchi S, Murakami N, et al. Extraocular muscles in Graves ophthalmopathy: usefulness of T2 relaxation time measurements. *Radiology.* 1994;190:857-862.

Parker GD, Harnsberger HR. Clinical-radiologic issues in perineural tumor spread of malignant diseases of the extracranial head and neck. *Radiographics.* 1991;11:283-399.

Rabinov JD. Imaging of salivary gland pathology. *Radiol Clin North Am.* 2000;38:1047-1057.

Rao VM, El-Noueam KI. Sinonasal imaging. *Radiol Clin North Am..* 1998;36:921-939.

Romo LV, Casselman JW, Robson CD. Temporal bone: Congenital anomalies. In: Som PM, In: Som PM, Curtin HD, eds. *Head and neck imaging.* St Louis, Mo: Mosby; 2003:1057-1092.

Sakaguchi M, Sato S, Asawa S, Taguchi K. Computed tomographic findings in peritonsillar abscess and cellulites. *J Laryngol Otol.* 1995;109:449-451.

Sando I, Shibahara Y, Takagi A, et al. Frequency and localization of congenital anomalies of the middle and inner ears: a human temporal bone histopathological study. *Int J Pediatr Otorhinolaryngol.* 1988;16:1-22.

Sando I, Akahara T, Ogawa A. Congenital anomalies of the inner ear. *Ann Otol Rhino Laryngol.* 1984;93(suppl 112):110-118.

Scholl RJ, Kellett HM, Neumann DP, Lurie AJ. Cysts and cystic lesions of the mandible: Clinical and Radiologic-Histopathologic review. *Radiographics.* 1999;19:1107-1124.

Smoker WR, Harnsberger HR. Differential diagnosis of head and neck lesions based on their space of origin. 1. The infrahyoid part of the neck. *AJR Am J Roentgenol.* 1991;157:145-59.

Som P, Lidov M, Brandwein M, et al. Sinonasal esthesioneuroblastoma with intracranial extension: marginal tumoral cysts as a diagnostic MR finding. *AJNR Am J Neuroradiol.* 1994;15:1259-1262.

Som PM, Brandwein MS. Lymph nodes. In: Som PM, Curtin HD, eds. *Head and neck imaging.* 4th ed. St Louis, Mo: Mosby; 2003:1865-1934.

Stuckey SL, Harris AJ, Mannolini SM. Detection of acoustic schwannoma: use of constructive interference in the steady state three-dimensional MR. *AJNR Am J Neuroradiol.* 1996;17:1219-1225.

Tien R, Dillon WP, Jackler RK. Contrast-enhanced MR imaging of the facial nerve in 11 patients with Bell's palsy. *AJNR Am J Neuroradiol.* 1990;11:735-741.

Tong KA, Harnsberger HR, Swartz JD. The vestibulocochlear nerve, emphasizing the normal and diseased internal auditory canal and cerebellopontine angle. In: Swartz JD, Harnsberger HR, eds. *Imaging of the temporal bone.* 3rd ed. New York: Thieme; 1998:394-473.

Valvassori GE, Naunton RF, Lindsay JR. Inner ear anomalies: clinical and histopathological considerations. *Ann Otol Rhino Laryngol.* 1969;78:929-938.

Valvassori GE, Clemis JD. The large vestibular aqueduct syndrome. *Laryngoscope.* 1978;88:723-728.

Vazquez E, Castellote A, Piqueras J, et al. Imaging of complications of acute mastoiditis in children. *Radiographics.* 2003;23:359-372.

Venkatesh YS, Ordonez NG, Schultz PN, et al. Anaplastic carcinoma of the thyroid. A clinicopathologic study of 121 cases. *Cancer.* 1990;66:321-330.

Yuh W, Buehner L, Kao S. Magnetic resonance of pediatric head and neck cystic hygromas. *Ann Otol Rhinol Laryngol.* 1991;100:737-742.

CHAPTER 19
Spine: Tumors and Infection
Paul E. Kim, Johan W.M. Van Goethem, and Alyssa T. Watanabe

PROBLEMS IN SPINAL TUMOR IMAGING

This chapter elucidates a few relatively common problems encountered in imaging of spinal tumors and infections. It should be kept in mind that the primary tasks of diagnostic imaging can be summarized, largely in order of importance, as follows: (1) detection of the pathological lesion, (2) localization of the lesion, and (3) characterization of the lesion to make the most specific diagnosis possible.

The first and second issues, detection and localization of pathology, have been largely resolved since the development of cross-sectional imaging, particularly magnetic resonance imaging (MRI), which is generally quite sensitive as well as capable of highly specific anatomic localization. The third issue, specific diagnosis, has been elusive in an absolute sense for all but a few entities; however, ever-evolving technological advancements over the past several decades have resulted in an increasing ability to better characterize lesions and generate more specific differential diagnoses with higher probabilistic certainty.

LESION DETECTION AND LOCALIZATION PROBLEM SOLVING: IMAGING MODALITIES

The first task of imaging is detection of pathology, which is primarily a function of the *sensitivity* of an imaging modality. This is a complex issue that requires distinguishing pathology from surrounding normal tissue, which involves spatial resolving capacity when the pathology is a mass lesion and atomic, molecular, biochemical, physiologic, magnetic, or electrochemical properties for non–space-occupying pathologies. The second task is localization of the pathology, a relatively simple function of an imaging modality's anatomic resolving power, which necessitates high spatial resolution as well as tissue contrast.
- MRI versus computed tomography (CT) versus other (plain x-ray, nuclear medicine, positron emission tomography): Practically speaking, the best combination of sensitivity, spatial localization, and specificity for the spine is afforded by MRI. Although some modalities can surpass MRI in sensitivity for certain processes (e.g., technetium-99m [Tc-99m] bone scintigraphy for detection of bone metastases), spatial/contrast resolution and specificity are typically much less robust. CT provides generally less precise localization information because of relatively poor tissue contrast despite excellent spatial resolution, and plain radiography significantly provides even less so in both respects. However, in the spine, both are capable of specifying the anatomic compartment involved if myelographic contrast is used, based on the filling defect pattern of contrast displacement (Figure 19-1, *A*).
- Localization of a lesion in the spine means delineation of (1) spine segment level involved; (2) which of three principal anatomic compartments from which the lesion originated— intramedullary, intradural–extramedullary, or extradural (Figure 19-1, *B*); and (3) "subcompartment" site of origin (e.g., distinguishing site of origin among disc, vertebral body, facets, etc., for an extradural process).
- MRI should be the initial and principal modality of choice for evaluation of tumors of the spine. The protocol should include a T2-weighted fat-suppression sequence (fat saturation or inversion recovery) in the sagittal plane as well as contrast-enhanced T1-weighted images in both sagittal and transverse planes, with fat suppression.
- Other considerations:
  - CT, plain x-ray, and angiography: Despite some of the limitations noted previously, these modalities often have adjunctive roles in the workup of spinal tumors. CT, in particular, can show bony detail not assessed by MRI. Angiography is reserved for evaluation of vascular lesions.
  - Advanced imaging techniques: Diffusion tensor imaging (DTI), spectroscopy, and multimodality imaging could play significant roles in lesion characterization under certain circumstances and are likely to play greater roles in the future. Additionally, because of recent and ongoing advances in MR angiography and CT angiography, a viable noninvasive alternative to conventional angiography likely will be realized in the near future.

DETECTION AND LOCALIZATION TO CHARACTERIZATION AND DIFFERENTIAL DIAGNOSIS

Lesion Localization for Differential Diagnosis

The differential diagnostic process should initially begin with anatomic localization. A broad anatomically based differential diagnosis is created by identifying the site

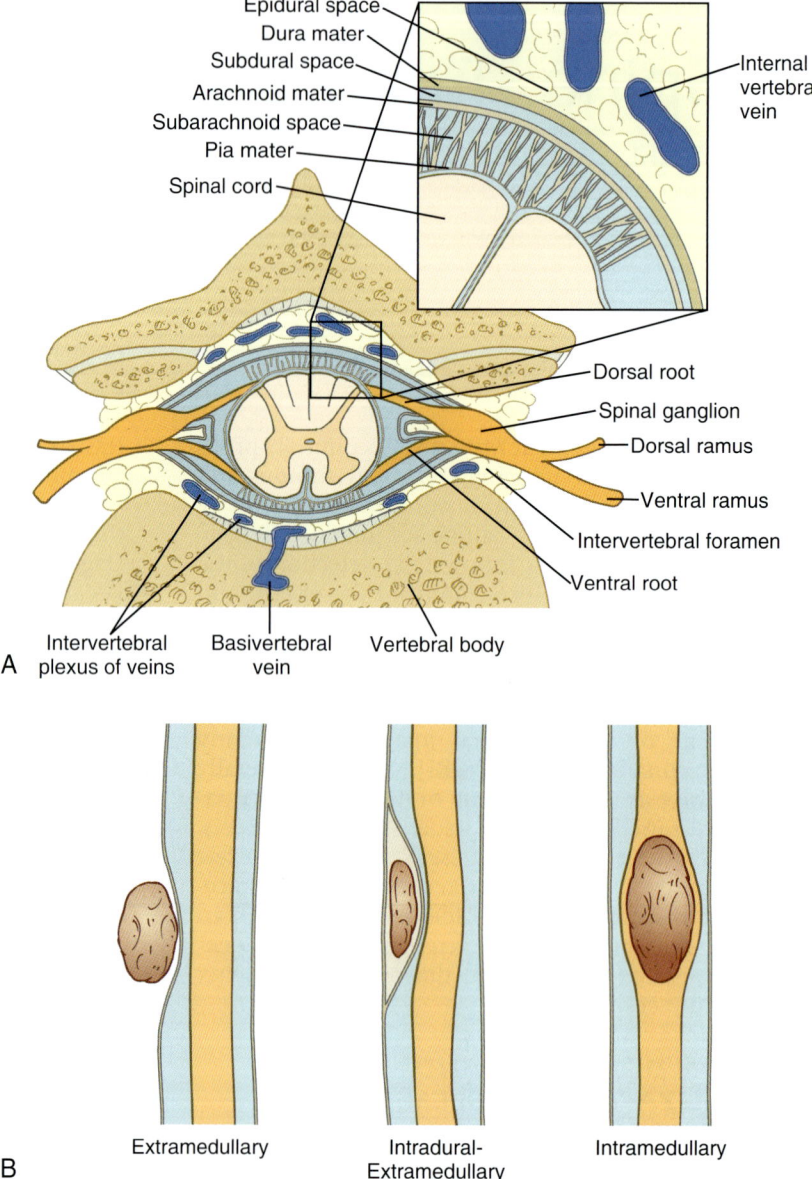

Figure 19-1 **A:** Anatomic diagram detailing meningeal layers of the spinal canal that delineate the epidural, subdural, subarachnoid, and intramedullary spaces. **B:** Schematic diagram of myelographic contrast patterns reflecting lesion space of origin.

of origin of the lesion as one of three specific anatomic compartments (Table 19-1):
- Intramedullary (Figure 19-2, A)
- Intradural–extramedullary (Figure 19-2, B)
- Extradural (Figure 19-2, C)

Caveat: The larger the lesion, the more difficult it may be to identify the site of origin as the mass of the lesion extends into more than one compartment. Consideration of more than one anatomic category of differential diagnosis may then be required.

Narrowing the Differential Diagnosis: Moving Beyond a Broad Anatomically Specific Tabulation

How specific can imaging be in problem solving? With the exception of lesions that have nearly pathognomonic imaging features (so-called "Aunt Minnies" of Felson) (Table 19-2 and Figures 19-3 through 19-5), most lesions overlap significantly in appearance with one or more other diagnoses, and specific imaging features per se merely promote a higher probability diagnosis rather than an absolute one. Thus, once the anatomic site of the lesion has been determined, the differential diagnostic equation requires consideration of both clinical information and specific imaging characteristics to further narrow the differential diagnosis (Table 19-3):

- Clinical information: Demographics, clinical presentation, and laboratory studies. For example, spinal cord ependymomas are more common in adults, whereas astrocytomas are more common in pediatric patients.
- Specific imaging features that are more characteristic of certain tumor types: Some features are relatively idiosyncratic to a specific diagnosis and thus have a greater impact on diagnostic probability, for example, the classic appearance of a spinal cord hemangioblastoma presenting as an enhancing nodule

Table 19-1 Differential Diagnosis of Spinal Lesions by Compartment

Intramedullary	Intradural–Extra-medullary	Extradural
Astrocytoma	Meningioma	Metastasis*
Ependymoma	Schwannoma	Epidural hematoma
Hemangioblastoma	Myxopapillary ependymoma	Epidural abscess
Metastasis*	Drop metastasis	Schwannoma
Lymphoma*	Dural metastasis*	Disc herniation
Multiple sclerosis	Lymphoma*	Lymphoma*
Infarct	Arachnoid cyst	Chordoma
Arteriovenous malformation	Cysticercosis	Granulomatous*: Fungal, sarcoid, TB
Syringomyelia	Granulomatous*: Fungal, sarcoid, TB	
Rare: Neuronal–glial tumors		
Granulomatous*: Fungal, sarcoid, TB		

TB, Tuberculosis.
*Metastases, lymphoma, and granulomatous processes occur in all three compartments.

abutting the pial surface of the cord with extensive cord edema (Figure 19-6). Other characteristics may have only slightly greater prevalence in one tumor type compared to another. For example, the common diagnostic dilemma of ependymoma versus astrocytoma, in which the findings of cyst formation, heterogeneity, and greater and more homogeneous contrast enhancement and blood products can be found in both tumor types but are somewhat more prevalent in ependymoma than astrocytoma.

Caveat: Absolute differentiation frequently is not possible, but differentiating relative probabilities among ependymoma, astrocytoma, metastasis, and hemangioblastoma still may be clinically important because treatment differs among these lesions. Ependymoma may be a surgically resectable lesion, whereas astrocytoma typically is not. In this regard, advanced imaging techniques such as DTI may be of additional value. Ependymomas being of ependymal cell origin will grow concentrically from the central canal displacing fiber tracts, whereas astrocytomas typically will have an eccentric location and will tend to infiltrate the fiber tracts.

Common Problems of Differential Diagnosis in Spinal Tumor Imaging

Neoplasm versus Atypical (Lipid-Poor) Hemangioma (Figure 19-7)

The typical hemangioma within the vertebral body or neural arch contains enough fat to be pathognomonic on imaging, but a minority, probably less than 15%, lack significant fatty components and thus demonstrate high signal intensity on T2-weighted images and low signal intensity on T1-weighted images. Contrast enhancement also is common. These findings can be a difficult mimic of metastatic disease. The following considerations should be made:

- Plain x-ray or CT correlation: Classic coarse trabecular "corduroy" appearance of hemangioma.
- Nuclear medicine: Tc-99m bone scintigraphy and fluorodeoxyglucose-positron emission tomography typically do not show increased activity in hemangiomas and increased activity with tumor. In addition, Tc-99m red blood cell pool scans can show radiotracer accumulation in hemangiomas with low fat content.
- Confirmation of long-term stability with prior comparison studies.
- Biopsy: Last resort.

Neoplasm versus Modic 1 Changes

Modic 1 degenerative end plate changes and vertebral metastases demonstrate the same T1, T2, and contrast enhancement characteristics: hypointense on T1, hypointense on T2, and significant contrast enhancement with gadolinium (Figure 19-8). The distinction usually is readily made by noting the configuration of the lesion. Modic 1 degenerative end plate changes usually extend along the vertebral end plate adjacent to a disc showing varying degrees of degenerative change. Metastases involving the vertebral bodies are typically circumscribed geographic lesions. However, rarely a metastasis attains a configuration that mimics Modic 1 changes along an end plate. Signs of adjacent degenerative disc disease may be unhelpful because it is so prevalent in the patient demographic with metastases. The problem-solving algorithm should include the following:

- Comparison with prior imaging studies: This is not an absolute because inflammatory Modic 1 changes can develop during a follow-up interval.
- Bone scan: Modic 1 changes do not typically accumulate significant radiotracer activity. In addition, identification of metastatic lesions elsewhere in the skeleton by scintigraphy can mitigate the dilemma.
- Biopsy: Last resort.

Neoplasm versus Infection

Spinal infections usually begin at the osteocartilaginous end plate and thus typically involve the intervertebral disc. Neoplasms such as metastases do not typically involve the disc space. However, in some instances, particularly when a granulomatous process is in consideration, neoplastic and inflammatory processes exhibit similar imaging features: (1) Infection presenting primarily as vertebral osteomyelitis without discitis. This is particularly the case with tuberculous spondylitis, in which multiple vertebral bodies may be involved with sparing of the disc spaces (Figure 19-9). (2) Neoplasm breaking through the end plate to involve the disc (Figure 19-9, *C*). The approach to this problem include consideration of the following:

- Clinical factors: Fever, leukocytosis, history of intravenous drug use, etc., all are nonspecific associations of infection. Known history of cancer may raise consideration for metastasis.
- Nonenhancing paraspinous fluid versus enhancing solid paraspinous mass: Nonenhancing fluid favors infection, whereas enhancing solid mass favors neoplasm. Again, this is not absolute because granulomatous inflammatory masses may appear solid, and a pathologic fracture

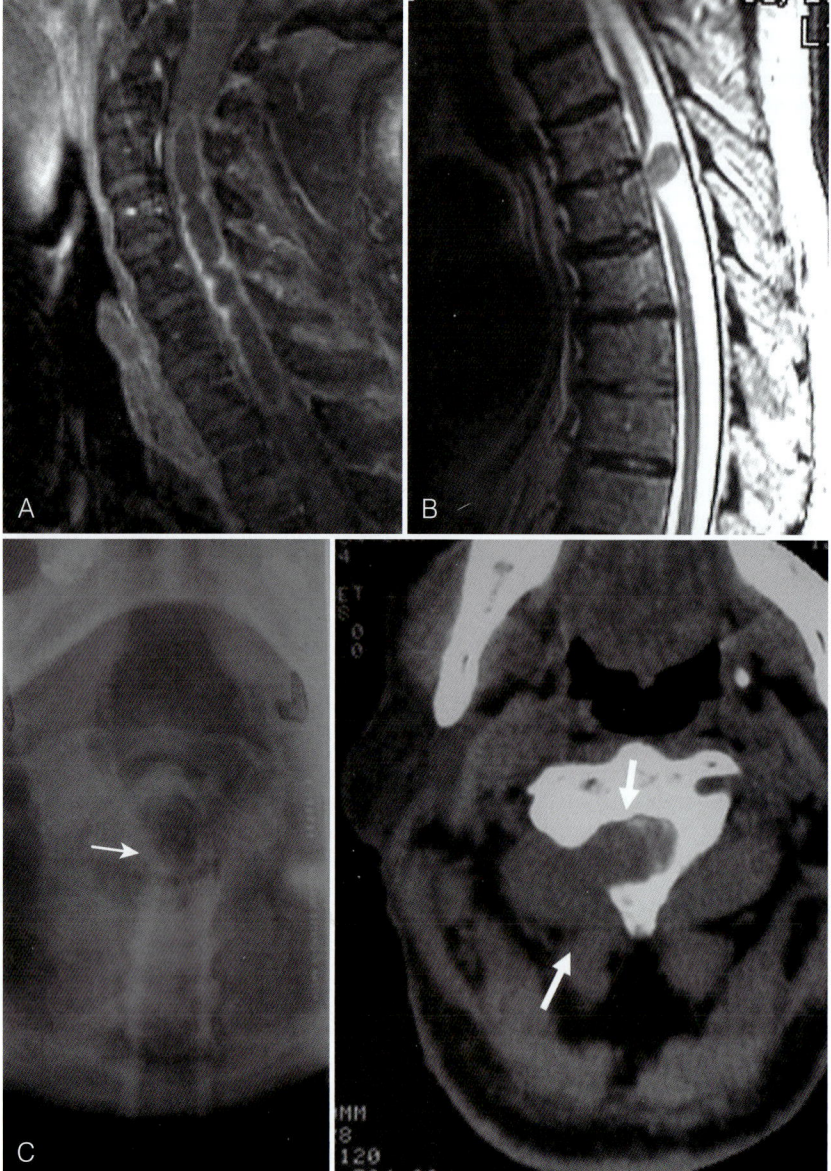

Figure 19-2 A: Intramedullary process. Sagittal T1-weighted contrast-enhanced image of the cervical spine demonstrating a circumscribed peripherally enhancing, lobulated, cystic lesion arising within the cervical cord. The imaging appearance initially was thought to be most consistent with an ependymoma; this was subsequently believed to be unlikely given a history of very acute onset and rapidly progressive course. Diagnosis was intramedullary abscess due to *Staphylococcus aureus*. **B:** Intradural–extramedullary process. Sagittal T2-weighted image of the thoracic spine demonstrating an intermediate/low-signal-intensity circumscribed lesion dorsal to the thoracic cord with mass effect. Meningioma. **C:** Extradural process. Conventional myelography *(left)* and computed tomography myelography *(right)* demonstrating a lobulated extradural mass extending through the right C2/3 neural foramen with mass effect on the right side of the thecal sac and cervical cord. This lesion demonstrates the classic "dumbbell" appearance of a schwannoma.

Table 19-2 "Aunt Minnies"

- Cavernous malformation
- Typical cavernous hemangioma of spine
- Disc herniation
- Modic 2 and 3 changes

may rarely develop a paraspinous hematoma forming a nonenhancing fluid collection.

- Nuclear medicine: Tc-99m bone scans have an accuracy of about 90% in patients with more than 2 days of symptoms, and gallium scans may be positive even before the technetium scan. The combined accuracy of technetium and gallium scans has been reported to be as high as 94%. Indium white blood cells scans probably are useful only if antibiotic therapy has not been administered.
- Biopsy: Last resort.

Metastases versus Cellular Marrow Proliferation

Cellular marrow conversion, whether diffuse or heterogeneous and patchy, appears as diffuse or patchy areas of hypointensity on T1-weighted images and thus can be concerning for infiltrative metastases. This problem

Chapter 19 Spine: Tumors and Infection

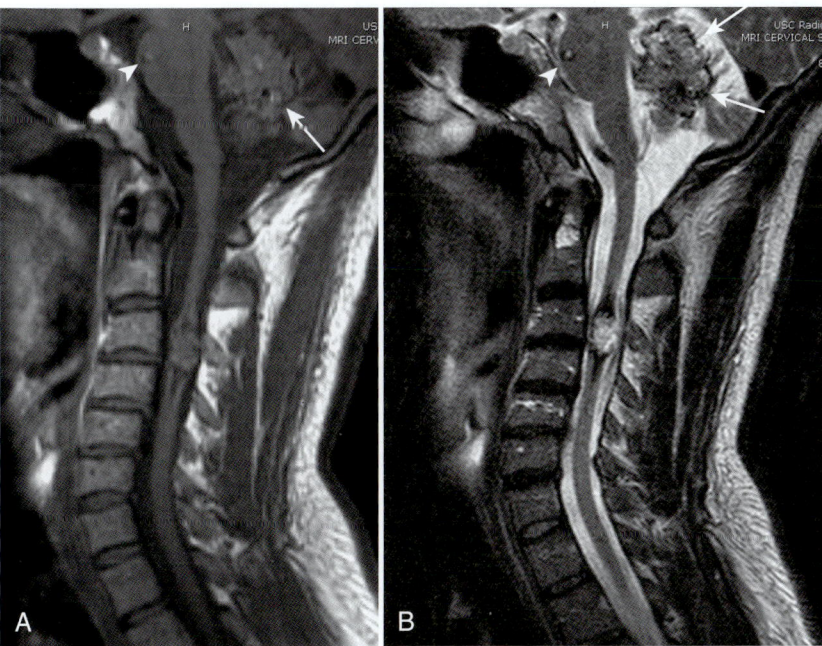

Figure 19-3 Cavernous malformation. Patient with multiple cavernous malformations of the brain and spinal cord. Sagittal T1-weighted **(A)** and T2-weighted **(B)** images of the cervical spine demonstrating classic appearance of cavernous malformation and "popcorn"-like appearance with heterogeneous high and low signal areas corresponding to variegated blood products (methemoglobin, hemosiderin, and serous fluid resulting from multiple prior hemorrhages). In addition to the cervical cord lesion at C3, a small pontine lesion *(arrowhead)* and a large lesion in the cerebellar vermis *(small arrows)* are seen.

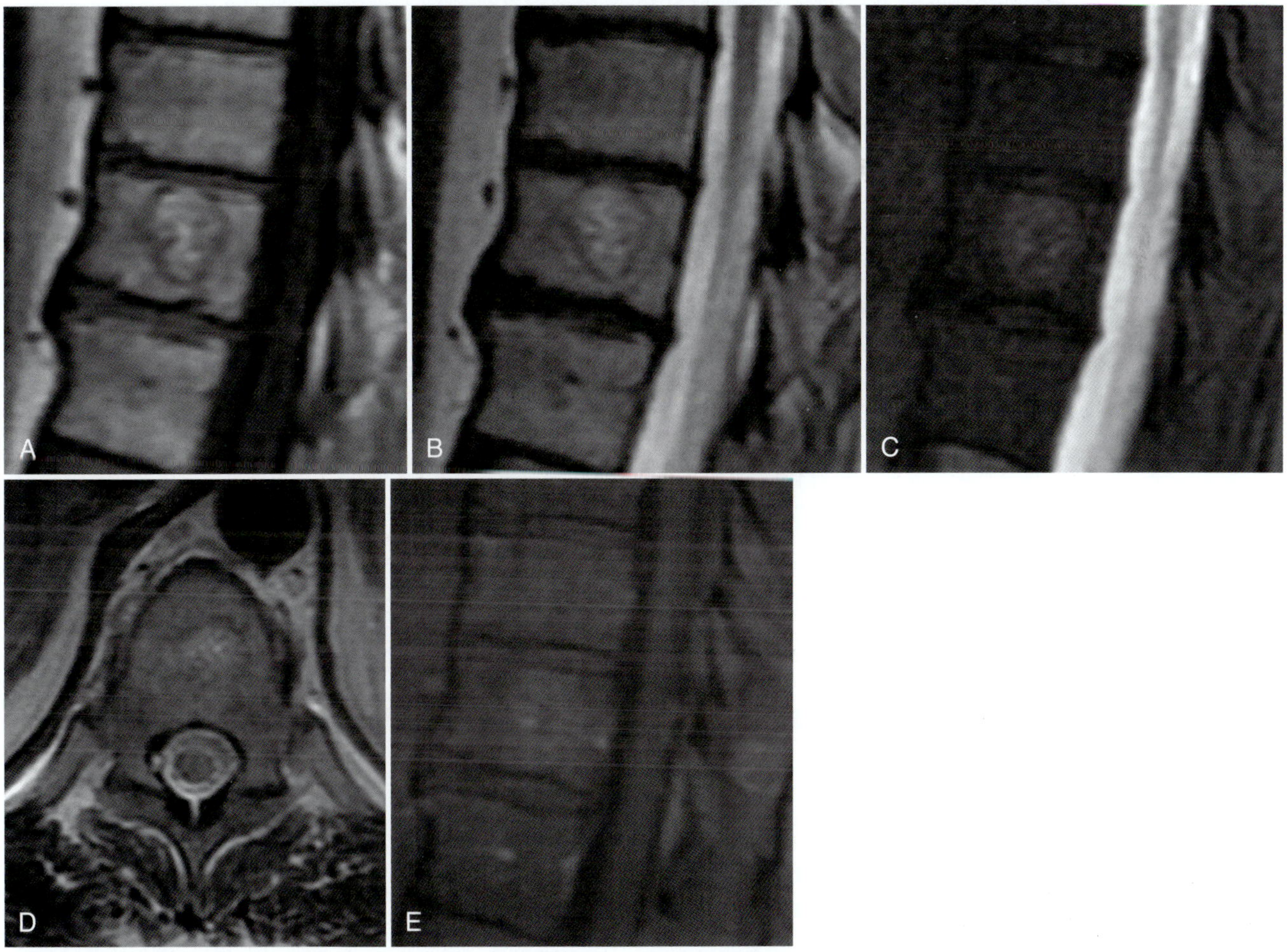

Figure 19-4 Hemangioma. Typical osseous hemangioma of the vertebral body. Sagittal T1 **(A)**, sagittal T2 **(B)**, sagittal T2 with fat saturation **(C)**, transverse T2 **(D)**, contrast-enhanced T1 with fat saturation **(E)** images. Note signal characteristics corresponding to fat within much of the lesion, demonstrating high signal on T1 and good suppression on both T1 and T2 fat suppression sequences. The suggestion of "corduroy"-type appearance on sagittal images and dot-like appearance on transverse images are characteristic. Contrast enhancement may be minimal to mild, as shown in **E**.

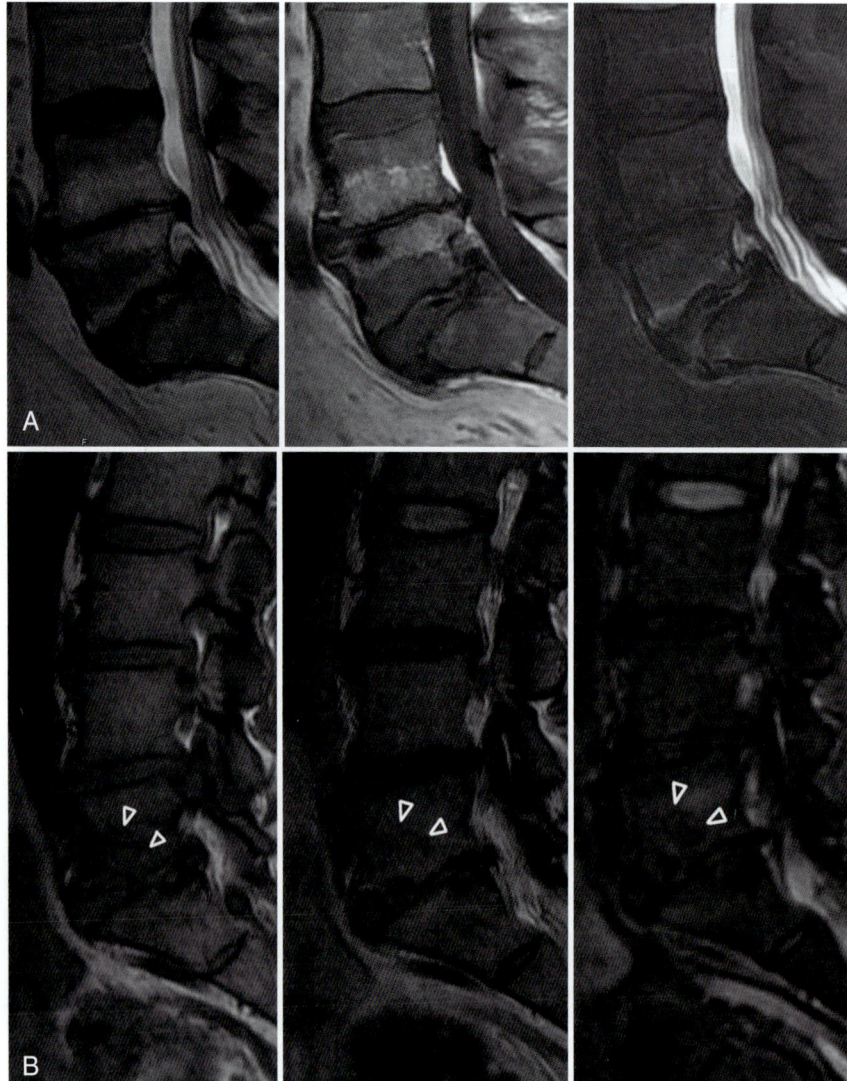

Figure 19-5 Modic 2 **(A)** and Modic 3 **(B)** changes. Sagittal T1-weighted *(left)*, T2-weighted *(middle)*, and T2 fat suppression *(right)* images. **A:** Modic 2 changes show hyperintense marrow adjacent to the L4–5 end plates on T1-weighted images due to increased fat content that characterizes Modic 2 changes. Note hyperintensity of these fatty changes on fast spin-echo T2-weighted sequence due to suppression of J-coupling effects and diffusion-mediated susceptibility dephasing. Fat saturation sequence shows effective fat suppression and hypointensity of Modic 2 fatty marrow changes. Note mild Modic 1 changes at the L5–S1 level. **B:** Modic 3 changes at the L5–S1 level demonstrating hypointensity on all sequences *(arrowheads)*. This example demonstrates a mixed pattern as well, with small areas of Modic 1 change.

usually is readily resolved by observation of two key features (Figure 19-10):

- Fat-suppressed T2 weighted images: Signal intensity remains relatively hypointense with cellular marrow, whereas metastases are typically hyperintense unless osteoblastic.
- Contrast enhancement: Does not occur with cellular marrow.

Pathologic Fracture versus Benign Osteoporotic Compression Fracture

Benign osteoporotic compression fractures are hypointense on T1, hyperintense on T2 due to edema, may have small to moderate amounts of paraspinous mass-like blood/edema/bone fragments (in the case of burst fractures), and show significant contrast enhancement, all features of pathologic fracture due to underlying neoplasm or infection.

- Configuration of posterior vertebral fracture margin: A smooth rounded convex posterior vertebral body retropulsion is seen with much greater frequency in pathologic compression fractures (Figure 19-9, C) than in benign fractures, which typically show a more sharply angulated and fractured or retropulsed contour (Figure 19-11). In addition, a well-delineated hypointense fracture line may be identified in a benign fracture.
- Significant extension of abnormal signal into the posterior arch is seen in metastatic disease but not typically with benign fractures.
- Signal changes in metastatic disease tend to be somewhat more homogeneous and diffuse than in benign fractures.

Table 19-3 Potentially Differentiating Features of Common Spinal Mass Lesions*

Astrocytoma	*Age:* Children/young adults *Gender:* M > F = 3:1 *Presentation:* ■ Slow-onset myelopathy ■ May cause painful scoliosis	*Imaging:* ■ <4 segments ■ ±Cyst/syrinx ■ Hemorrhage uncommon ■ Low T1, high T2, relatively homogeneous ■ +Enhancement: Usually mild/moderate
Ependymoma	*Age:* 35–45 years *Gender:* F ≥ M *Presentation:* ■ Neck/back pain ■ Progressive paraparesis, paresthesias	*Imaging:* ■ Circumscribed mass with hemorrhagic foci ■ Low T1, high T2; more inhomogeneous than astrocytoma due to hemorrhagic foci ■ +Enhancement: Usually moderate/intense
Cord metastasis	*Age:* Any with known primary *Gender:* Depends on primary *Presentation:* ■ Rapidly progressive paraparesis ■ Pain, hyperesthesia, Brown-Séquard syndrome	*Imaging:* ■ Usually <1.5 cm ■ Always enhances ■ Spherical or oval ■ Key differentiation from hemangioblastoma: Usually not subpial ■ Syrinx rare
Meningioma	*Age:* Middle age, elderly *Gender:* F > M = 4:1 *Presentation:* ■ Pain ■ Myelopathy from extrinsic compression: motor/sensory deficit, gait disturbance	*Imaging:* ■ Broad base against dural sac ■ Intermediate/low signal on both T1 and T2 ■ Prominent contrast enhancement ± "dural tail"
Schwannoma	*Age:* Middle age, 30–60 years *Gender:* M = F *Presentation:* ■ Radicular pain most common	*Imaging:* ■ Classic: "Dumbbell" tumor extending through neural foramen frequently not seen ■ 70% intradural, 15% dumbbell intra/extradural, 15% completely extradural ■ Enlarged neural foramen ■ T1: Intermediate/low T2: Extremely variable 75% hyperintense, remainder mixed areas of high and low signal, usually peripherally hyperintense and hypointense centrally ■ Intense contrast enhancement ■ Cysts 40% ■ Hemorrhage 10%
Myxopapillary ependymoma	*Age:* All ages (peak 30–40 years) *Gender:* M > F = 2:1 *Presentation:* ■ Back pain ■ Paraparesis ■ Lower-extremity radiculopathy	*Imaging:* ■ Almost exclusively conus, filum terminale, cauda equina ■ May fill entire thecal sac ■ Medial pedicle erosion and posterior vertebral body scalloping ■ Low T1, high T2; often with heterogeneous foci of hemorrhage ■ +Enhancement: Intense, homogeneous

*Features listed are typical, not exclusive.
F, Female; *M*, male.

■ Volume of extraspinous mass: Neoplasm or infection can result in relatively voluminous paraspinous mass or fluid. This is rarely the case with benign fractures, which typically show only paraspinous edema and/or small hematomas.

"Pseudohypointense" Vertebral Body Lesion in Fast Spin-Echo T2-Weighted Images

A small pathologic lesion such as a metastasis can be mistaken for a benign osteoma or enostosis because it appears hypointense on both T1-weighted and T2-weighted images acquired with fast spin-echo technique. This is a common pitfall among trainees due to the hyperintense appearance of marrow fat on the fast spin-echo sequence, an effect of multiple 180-degree refocusing pulses, which eliminate diffusion-mediated susceptibility dephasing and suppress J-coupling modulation of the echo train. Because window width and level are user defined, bright fatty marrow appears as a hypointense vertebral body lesion. Because most metastatic neoplasms are hyperintense on T2-weighted images, this high signal can only be appreciated with a fat suppression sequence such as short tau inversion recovery (STIR) (Table 19-4). Contrast enhancement is also a differentiating feature, so gadolinium-enhanced imaging should be performed if necessary (Figure 19-12). One caveat is blastic metastasis, which will be hypointense on *all* sequences and may not show appreciable contrast enhancement if sufficiently sclerotic.

In all of the instances discussed in which the problem was metastasis versus other, one should always search for the presence of other more typical metastatic lesions. Although this does not specify the nature of any given

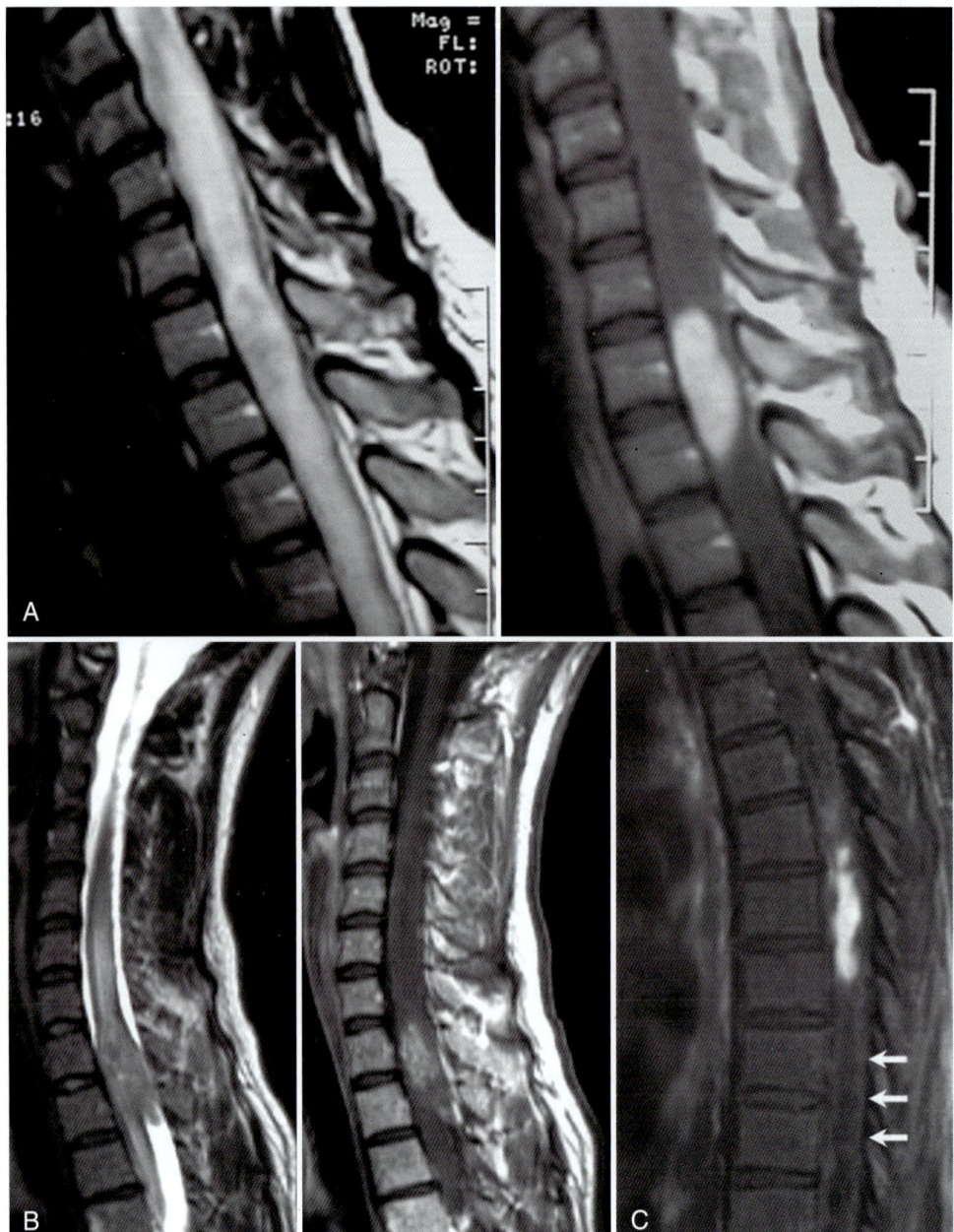

Figure 19-6 A: Hemangioblastoma. Sagittal T2 *(left)* and contrast-enhanced T1 *(right)* images of spinal cord hemangioblastoma with common characteristic features: relatively small nodular homogeneously enhancing mass, subpial in location, with extensive cord edema out of proportion to size of the mass. **B:** Ependymoma. Sagittal T2 *(left)* and contrast-enhanced T1 *(right)* images of ependymoma showing more central location of the lesion and less prominent edema. (Courtesy M. Law.) **C:** Astrocytoma. T1 contrast-enhanced image showing solid enhancing lesion and large distal cord syrinx. Note relative homogeneity of the enhancing portion of the mass compared to ependymoma.

Chapter 19 Spine: Tumors and Infection

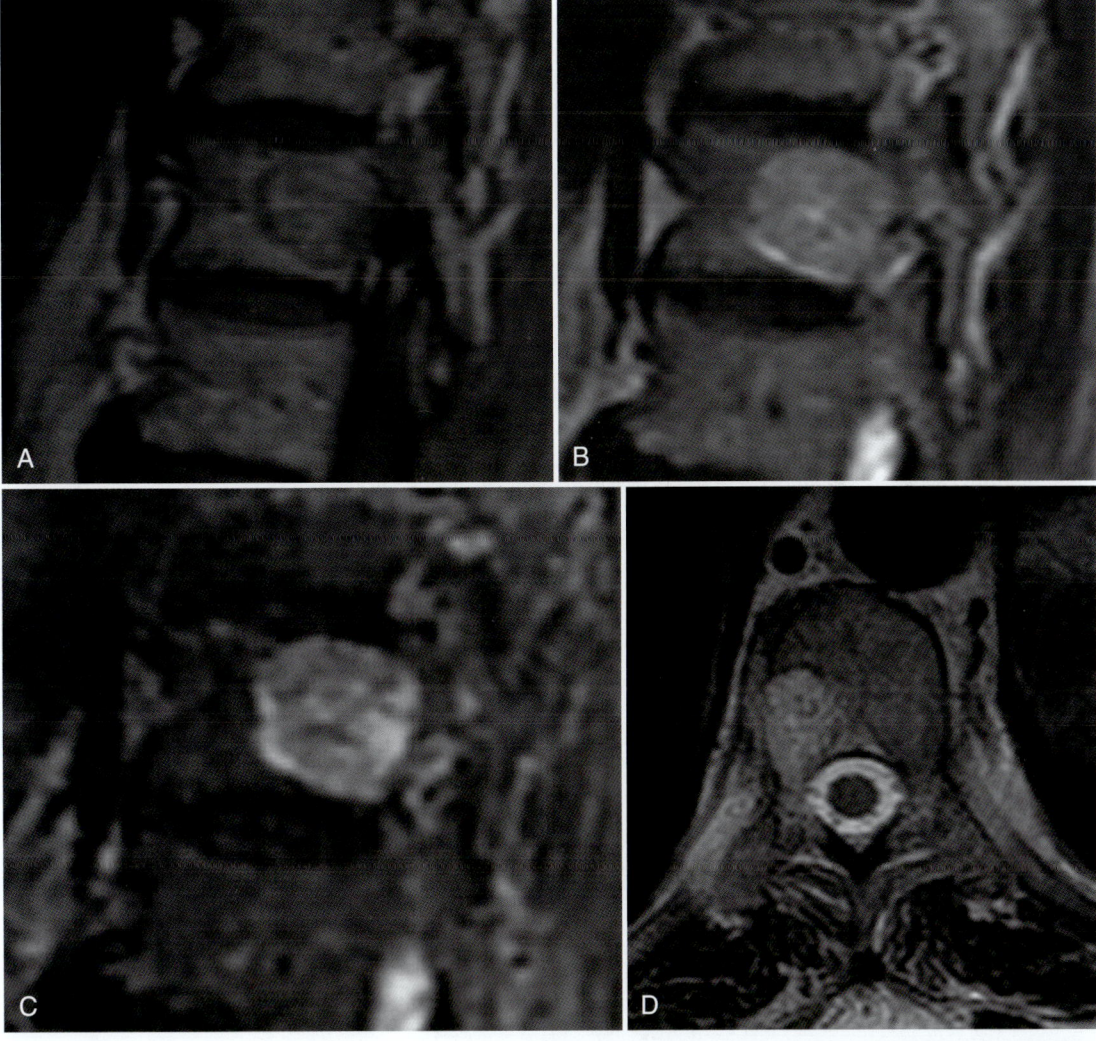

Figure 19-7 Atypical hemangioma of the spine. Sagittal T1 (**A**), sagittal T2 (**B**), sagittal T2 with fat saturation (**C**), and transverse T2 (**D**) images. This lesion demonstrates low lipid content characterized by primarily low signal intensity on T1-weighted and high signal intensity on T2-weighted images that does not suppress with fat saturation. This lesion continues to demonstrate findings of trabecular coarsening seen as a dot-like appearance on transverse images (**D**), but these lesions are often difficult to differentiate from metastases in patients with known cancer. Technetium-99m–labeled red blood cell studies can be helpful for these atypical lipid-poor lesions.

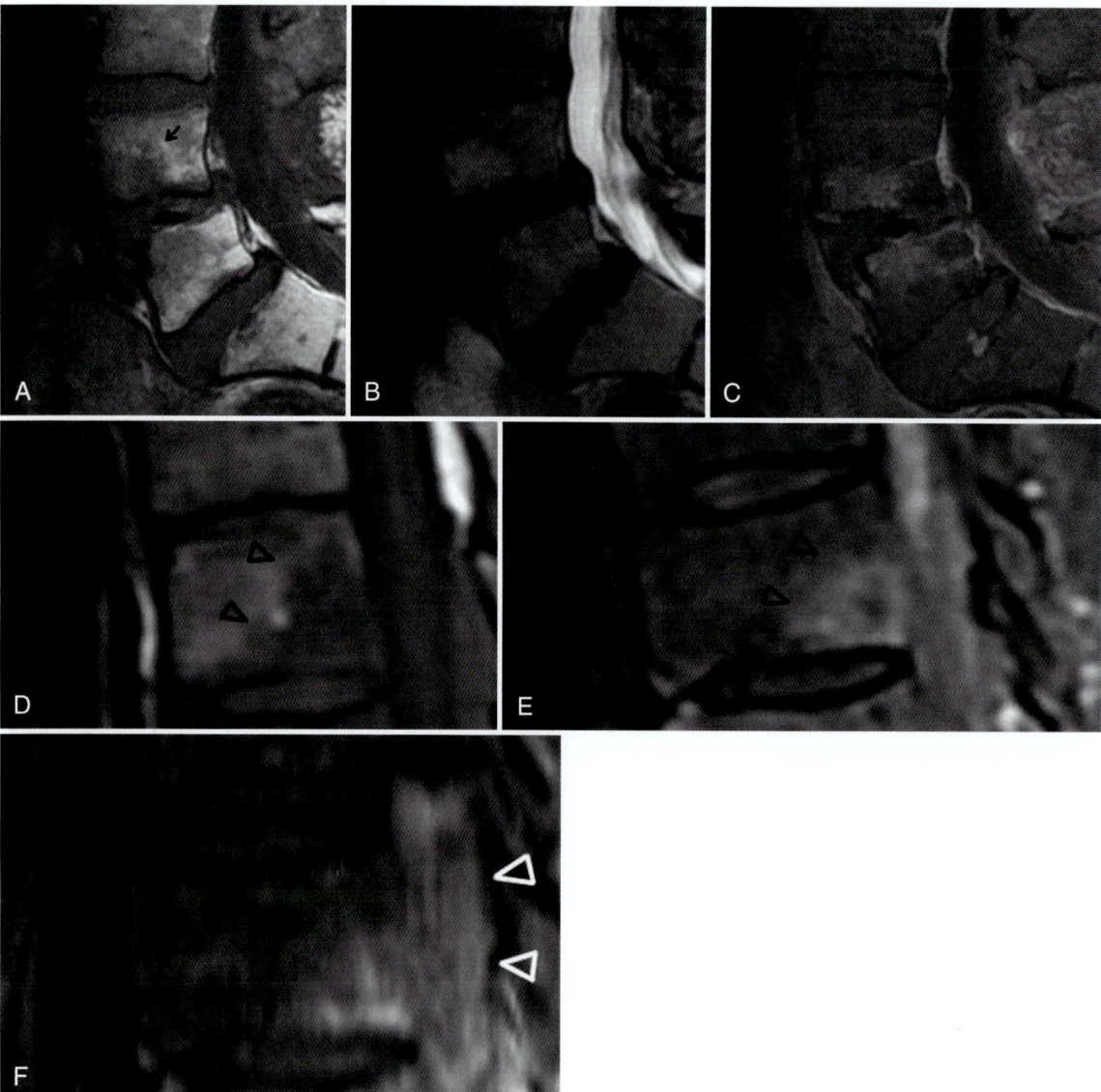

Figure 19-8 **A–C:** Modic type 1 degenerative marrow changes. **D–F:** Vertebral metastasis. **A:** Sagittal T1-weighted images showing typical wedge-shaped area of hypointensity along anteroinferior corner of the L4 vertebral body *(arrows)*. **B:** T2-weighted image with fat saturation showing hyperintensity reflecting marrow edema in Modic 1. **C:** Contrast enhancement after gadolinium administration is common. **D–F:** Corresponding image sequences in a patient with metastatic breast carcinoma along the posteroinferior corner of L1 *(arrowheads)*. Note intraspinal extension of tumor in **F** *(white arrowheads)* facilitates distinction from Modic 1 changes.

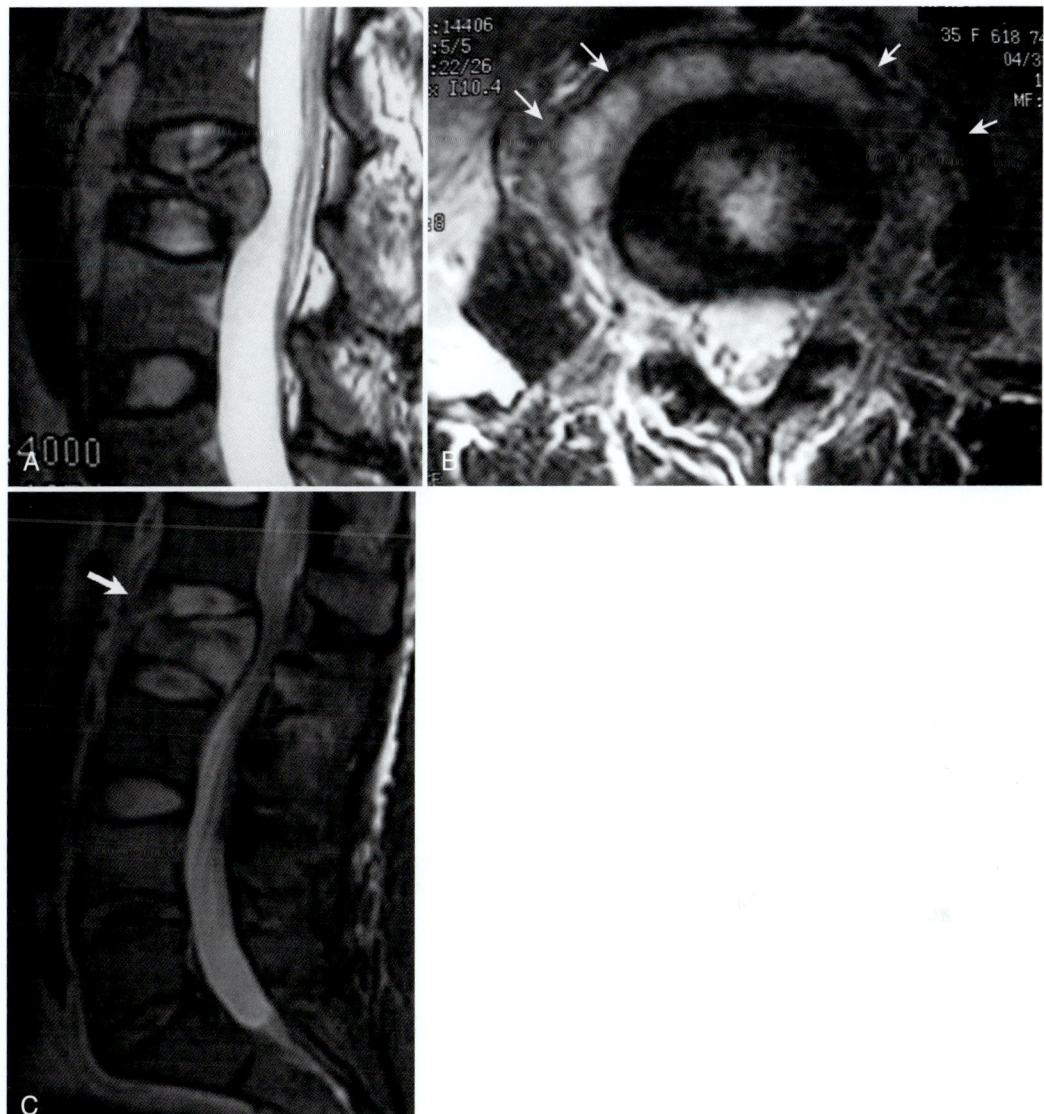

Figure 19-9 **A, B:** Tuberculous spondylitis. **C:** Breast carcinoma metastases. Sagittal **(A)** and transverse **(B)** T2-weighted images of tuberculous spondylitis at L3. Characteristic features include sparing of disc spaces, severe vertebral body collapse/deformity, and relatively large paraspinous abscesses *(arrows)*. Similar features are seen in T2 weighted image of metastatic breast carcinoma at L2 in **(C)**. Similar features are seen in T2-weighted image of metastatic breast carcinoma at L2, but note relatively modest paraspinous soft tissue abnormality consisting of small amounts of tumor and perhaps hemorrhage, but no large fluid collections. Note additional metastasis at L4, skipping the L3 level, that is also less characteristic of tuberculous spondylitis, which more often demonstrates contiguous involvement. Note focal breakthrough of the end plate with disc involvement, a feature more commonly associated with infection (**C,** *white arrow*).

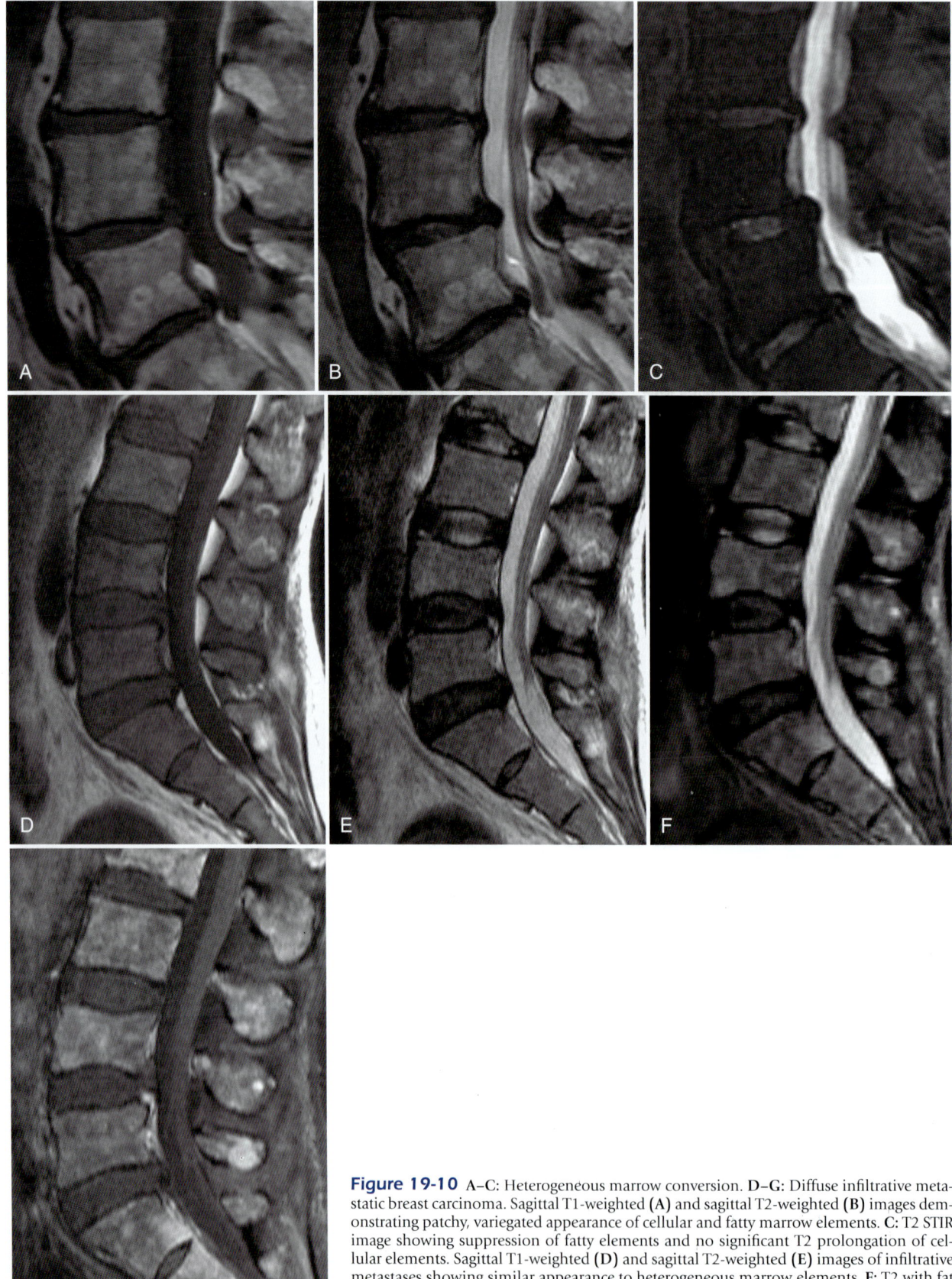

Figure 19-10 A–C: Heterogeneous marrow conversion. D–G: Diffuse infiltrative metastatic breast carcinoma. Sagittal T1-weighted (A) and sagittal T2-weighted (B) images demonstrating patchy, variegated appearance of cellular and fatty marrow elements. C: T2 STIR image showing suppression of fatty elements and no significant T2 prolongation of cellular elements. Sagittal T1-weighted (D) and sagittal T2-weighted (E) images of infiltrative metastases showing similar appearance to heterogeneous marrow elements. F: T2 with fat saturation showing T2 prolongation and hyperintensity of infiltrative metastatic elements. G: Contrast-enhanced T1 with fat saturation showing enhancement of metastatic elements after gadolinium administration.

Chapter 19 Spine: Tumors and Infection

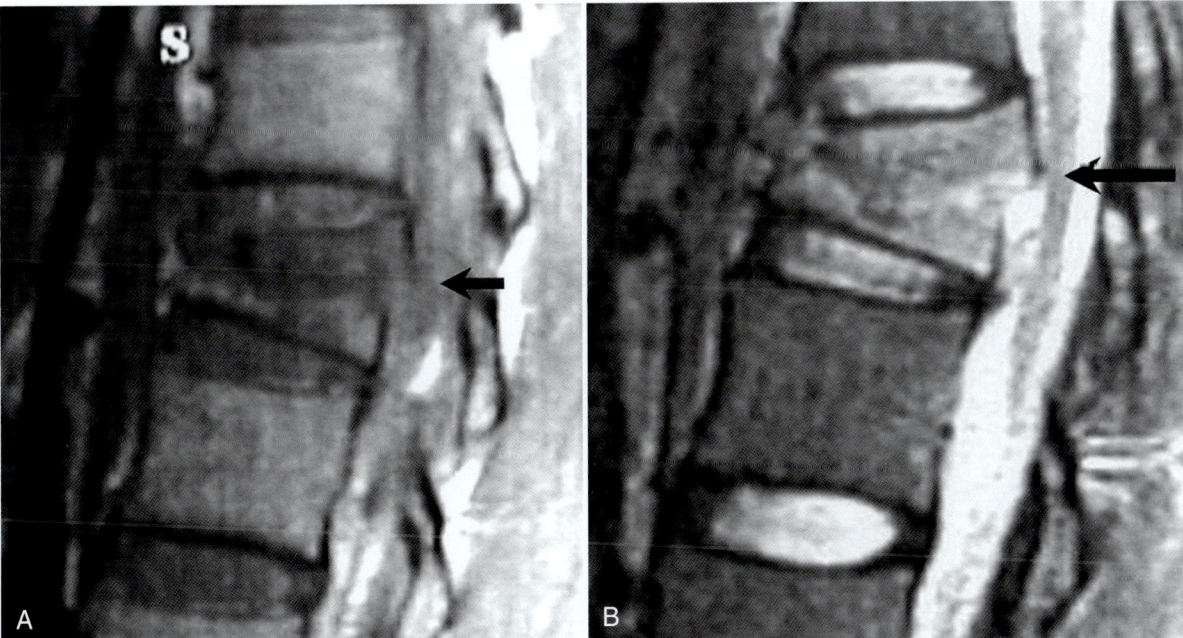

Figure 19-11 Benign vertebral body fracture. Sagittal T1-weighted **(A)** and T2-weighted STIR **(B)** images. Features suggestive of benign fracture are discrete linear fracture line and irregular, interrupted linear or jagged retropulsion contour *(arrows)*. Note features of pathologic fractures depicted in Figure 19-9, C, of indistinct fracture line and smoother convex retropulsion contour.

Table 19-4 Vertebral Body Lesions

High T1, High T2, Low STIR	Low T1, Low T2, High STIR	Low T1, Low T2, Low STIR
■ Hemangioma ■ Modic 3	■ Neoplasm (metastasis, lymphoma) ■ Lipid-poor hemangioma ■ Osteomyelitis ■ Modic 1	■ Blastic metastasis ■ Osteoma ■ Paget disease ■ Chronic osteomyelitis ■ Bone infarct

STIR, Short tau inversion recovery.

lesion, it does tilt the probability toward a metastatic etiology. It should be relatively uncommon to encounter a vertebral body lesion that remains indeterminate after all imaging considerations are addressed. For these lesions, biopsy remains the last resort.

■ PROBLEM SOLVING WITH ADVANCED IMAGING: SPECTROSCOPY, DIFFUSION, DTI, AND TRACTOGRAPHY

DTI of the spinal cord has been studied for a number of conditions, including trauma, multiple sclerosis, and transverse myelitis. With respect to spinal tumor imaging, DTI may have the ability to differentiate between ependymoma and metastases or fibrillary astrocytomas, which are typically infiltrating lesions, whereas ependymomas are typically well-circumscribed lesions (Figure 19-13).

MR spectroscopy of spinal cord lesions has shown some promise for differentiating neoplastic and inflammatory or demyelinating lesions. Currently it is an investigational tool, but some useful results have been obtained, such as elevated myoinositol levels in spinal cord astrocytomas compared to multiple sclerosis. As could be expected, the primary limitation of the technique is overcoming the technical limitations associated with the small tissue volumes inherent to the spinal cord.

■ PROBLEM SOLVING: COMMON PROBLEMS IN SPINAL INFECTION IMAGING

As with spinal tumors, the principal role of imaging in spinal infection is twofold: first, localizing the lesion; and second, suggesting a diagnosis or a differential diagnosis. Scanning protocols are essentially identical to those for tumor imaging, consisting of routine noncontrast sagittal T1, sagittal T2, sagittal T2 with fat suppression such as STIR or fat saturation, transverse T1 and transverse T2, and contrast-enhanced T1-weighted imaging with fat suppression in the sagittal and transverse planes.

Localization

As with tumor imaging, differential diagnosis is best approached using the same anatomic categorization: extradural, intradural–extramedullary, and intramedullary (Table 19-5).

■ PROBLEM: INFECTION VERSUS NONINFECTIOUS/INFLAMMATORY PROCESSES

Clinical and imaging mimics of infection can make the diagnosis of infection challenging both clinically and radiographically. Common presenting symptoms, such

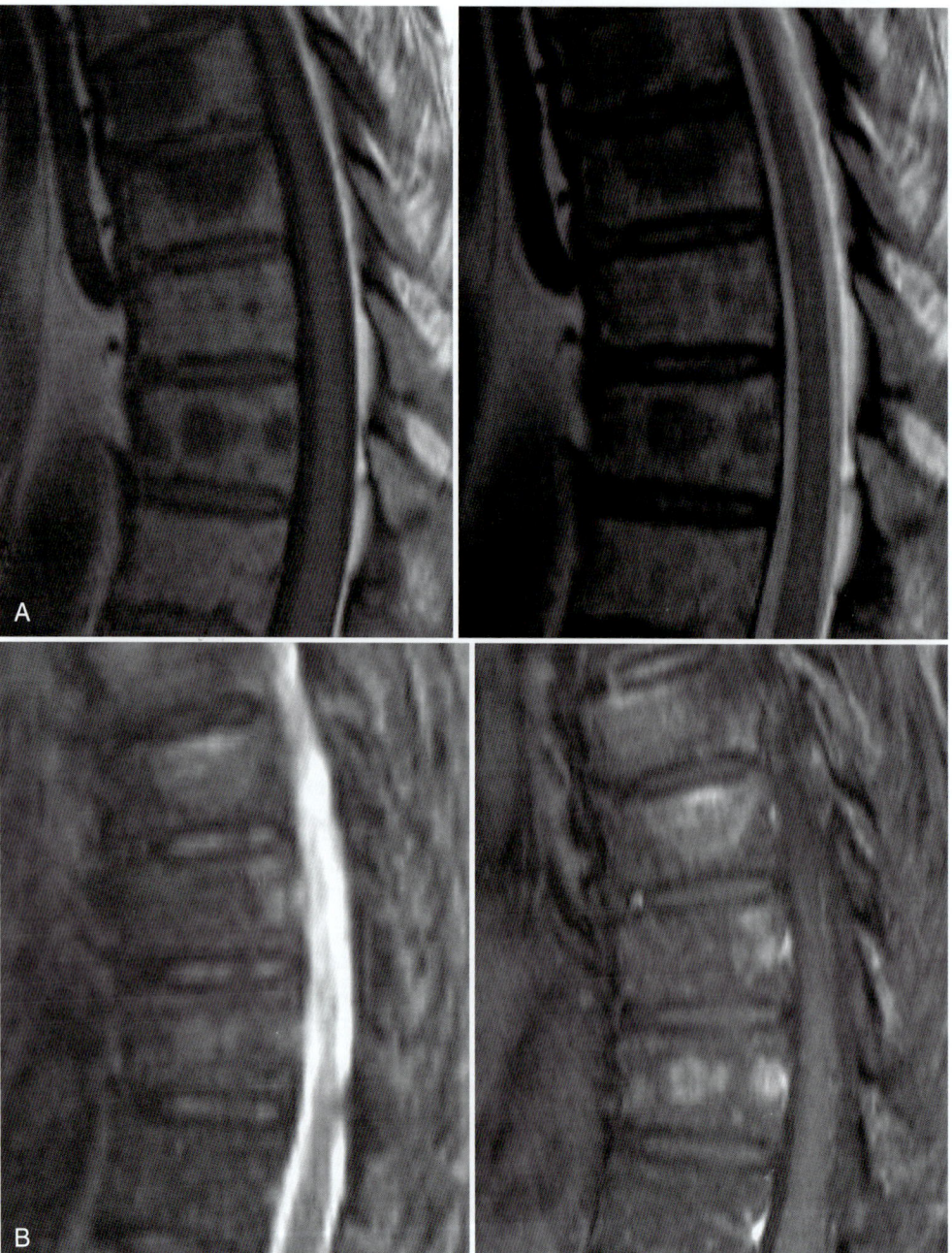

Figure 19-12 A: Sagittal T1 *(left)* and fast spin-echo T2 *(right)* images both apparently demonstrating apparently hypointense focal vertebral lesions. **B:** T2 STIR image *(left)*, however, more accurately depicting the relatively long T2 relaxivity of the lesions as T2 hyperintensity when surrounding marrow fat is suppressed. Contrast-enhanced T1 with fat saturation *(right)* showing prominent enhancement of these metastatic lesions.

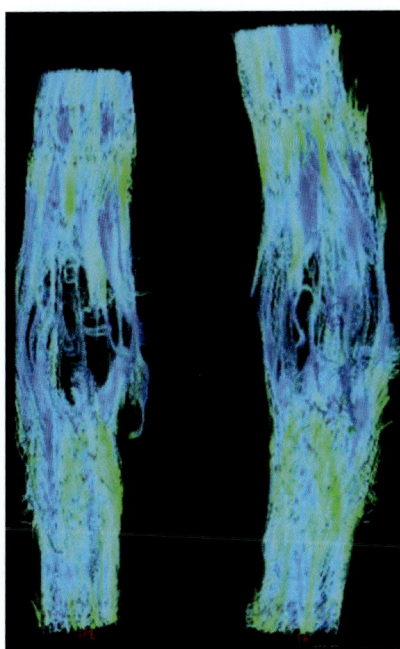

Figure 19-13 Tractography obtained from diffusion tensor imaging dataset demonstrating displacement of fibers around the central cord lesion, consistent with ependymoma. Astrocytic tumors are more likely to demonstrate disruption or infiltration of fiber tracts rather than displacement. (Courtesy M. Thurnher and M. Law.)

Table 19-5 Infections Considered by Compartment

Intramedullary	Intradural–Extramedullary	Extradural
Viral myelitis Cord abscess Granulomatous: TB, fungal	Granulomatous: TB, fungal Spinal meningitis Parasitic: Cysticercosis, echinococcus, schistosomiasis	Granulomatous: TB, fungal Spondylodiscitis and osteomyelitis Epidural abscess and phlegmon Facet joint septic arthritis

TB, Tuberculosis.

as simple back pain, can occur with or without fever and leukocytosis, which themselves are nonspecific when present and thus are only indirectly helpful. Likewise, antecedent history, such as intravenous drug use, raises suspicion for but does not specify the diagnosis.

Infectious Spondylodiscitis versus Spondylosis

The inflammatory component of degenerative disc disease is typically manifested on MRI as Modic 1 changes. Occasionally degenerative changes, particularly when associated with mixed or persistent inflammatory Modic 1 changes, can be quite severe, showing bony erosion, edema, and inflammation and are virtually indistinguishable from infection (Figure 19-14). Plain radiographs and even nuclear medicine studies may show findings similar to infection. Problem-solving considerations are as follows:

- Vacuum disc: Although common in advanced degenerative disc disease, it is virtually never seen in infection and is probably the most reassuring imaging finding in establishing the absence of infection.
- Erythrocyte sedimentation rate and C-reactive protein: These levels should not be significantly elevated in spondylosis.
- Comparison with prior and follow-up examinations: The time course is typically much shorter than for spondylosis.

Septic Arthritis of Facet Joint versus Aseptic Facet Synovitis (Figure 19-15)

Mild inflammatory changes normally associated with facet osteoarthritis is not typically a diagnostic problem. However, inflammatory changes occasionally are so acutely severe that they very closely mimic the appearance of septic arthritis. Like septic arthritis, the MRI appearance of aseptic facet inflammation is characterized by varying amounts of joint effusion, erosive change, and edema in the subarticular bone and periarticular soft tissues, and prominent contrast enhancement. The following must be considered:

- Clinical history: Fever, leukocytosis, clinical setting, and laboratory studies.
- Erythrocyte sedimentation rate and C-reactive protein: C-reactive protein is somewhat more specific and generally more helpful.
- Aspiration: Should be last resort.
- Treatment: Facet synovitis can be treated by injection of corticosteroids, which is contraindicated in case of infection.

Infectious Spondylodiscitis versus Neuropathic Spondyloarthropathy

Like some cases of spondylosis, neuropathic spondyloarthropathy can exhibit all characteristics of infection (edema, hyperemia, inflammatory and erosive changes on plain x-ray and MRI). Diagnostic considerations should include the following:

- Clinical factors: Medical history of a neuropathic condition is significant.
- Nuclear medicine: Indium-111 white blood cell scan may be the most reliable in differentiating these entities. Tc-99m bone scans are likely to be falsely positive.
- Biopsy: Last resort.

Infectious Spondylodiscitis versus Dialysis Spondyloarthropathy (Figure 19-16)

Dialysis spondyloarthropathy is a virtual mimic of infection on plain radiographs only. It is not usually a diagnostic problem for MRI because MRI will be negative for typical imaging features of infection.

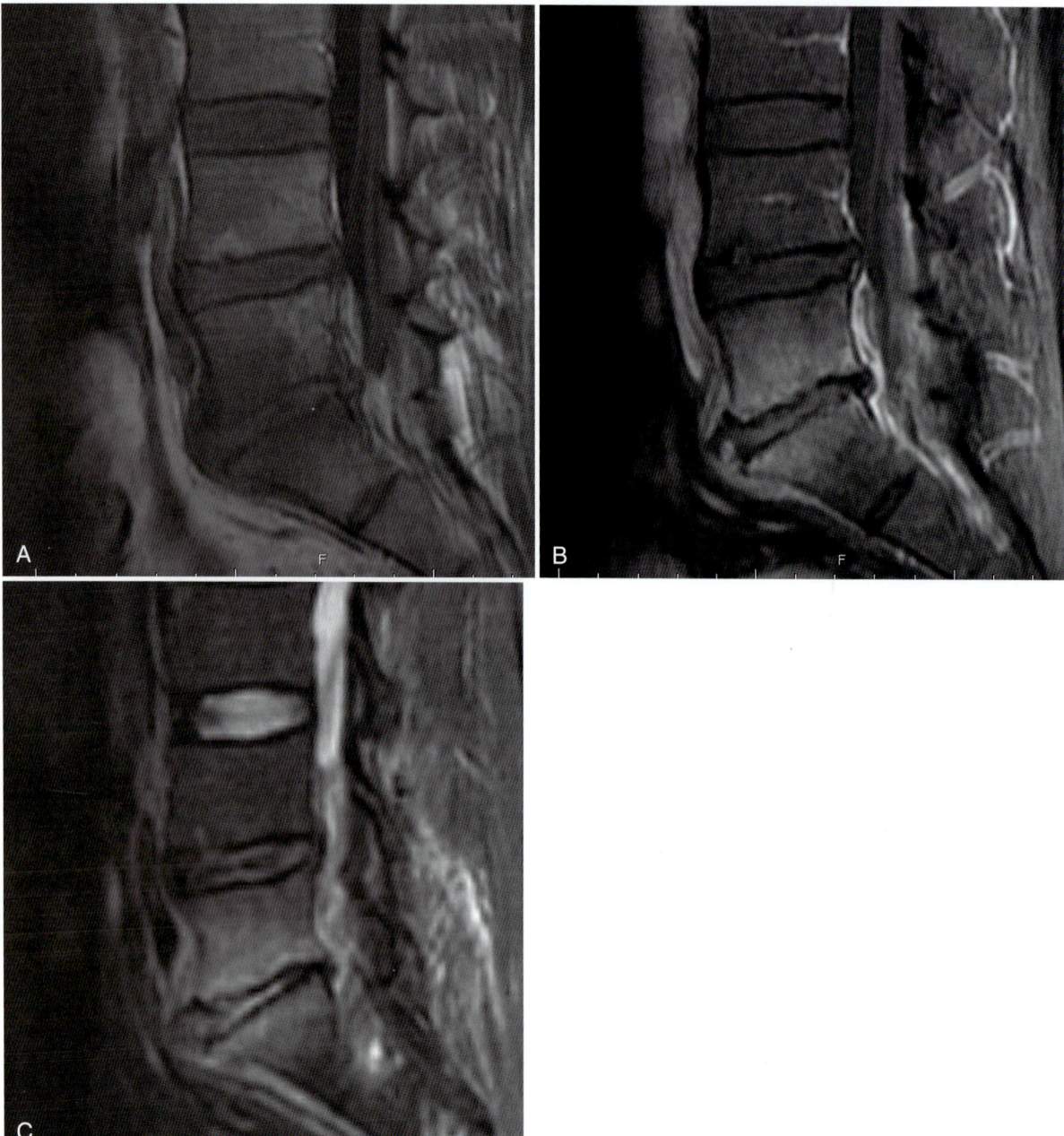

Figure 19-14 Aseptic inflammatory degenerative changes. Sagittal T1 **(A)**, contrast-enhanced T1 with fat saturation **(B)**, and T2 STIR **(C)** images. Inflammatory changes associated with degenerative spondylosis may be a close mimic of infection, occasionally with relatively prominent contrast enhancement and edema. When inflammatory changes are this pronounced, infection should be favored until excluded by correlation with C-reactive protein and/or biopsy if necessary.

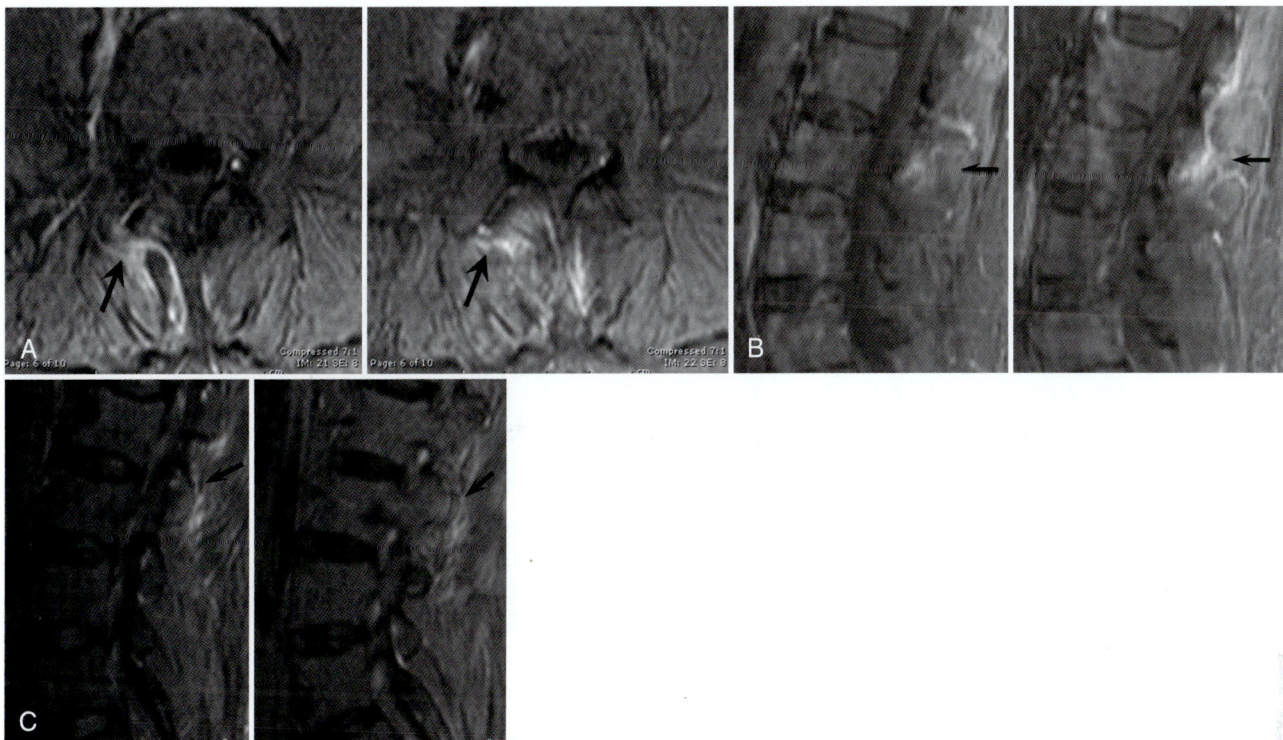

Figure 19-15 Inflammatory changes of facet osteoarthritis. Contrast-enhanced T1 with fat saturation **(A, B)** and T2 with fat saturation **(C)** images. Like aseptic inflammatory changes of the disc, inflammatory changes associated with degenerative changes of the facet may sometimes approach the appearance of infection. Bone edema, increased joint space fluid, and periarticular inflammation are all depicted here.

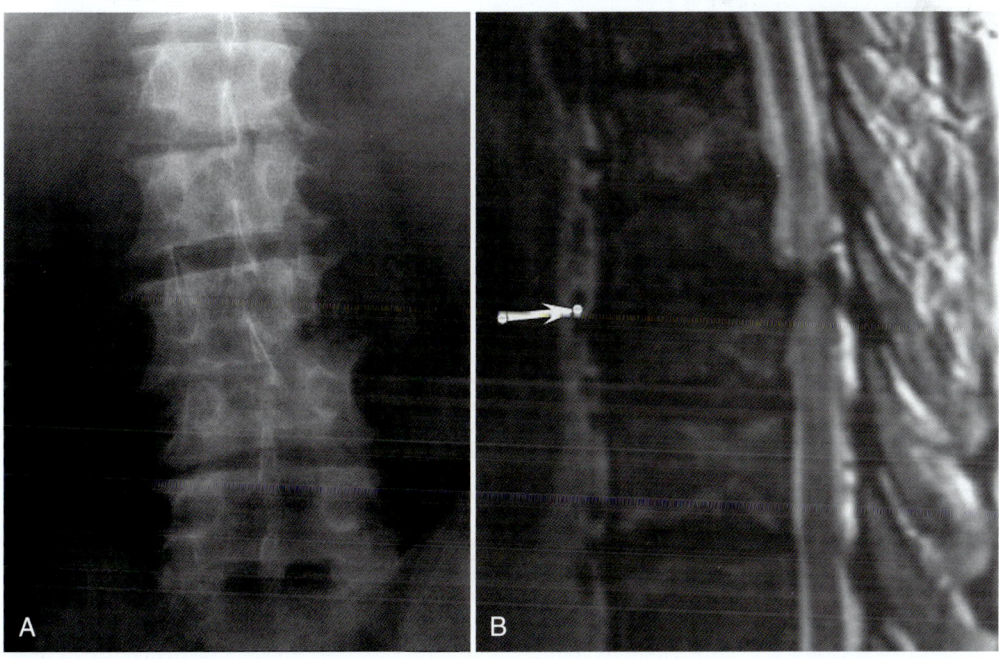

Figure 19-16 Dialysis spondyloarthropathy. **A:** Plain x-ray film showing loss of disc height and erosive changes at L3–4, mimicking infection. **B:** Sagittal T2 STIR magnetic resonance image in a different patient demonstrating chronic changes of end plate sclerosis with no active edema or inflammatory changes *(arrow)*. (Courtesy D.M. Forrester.)

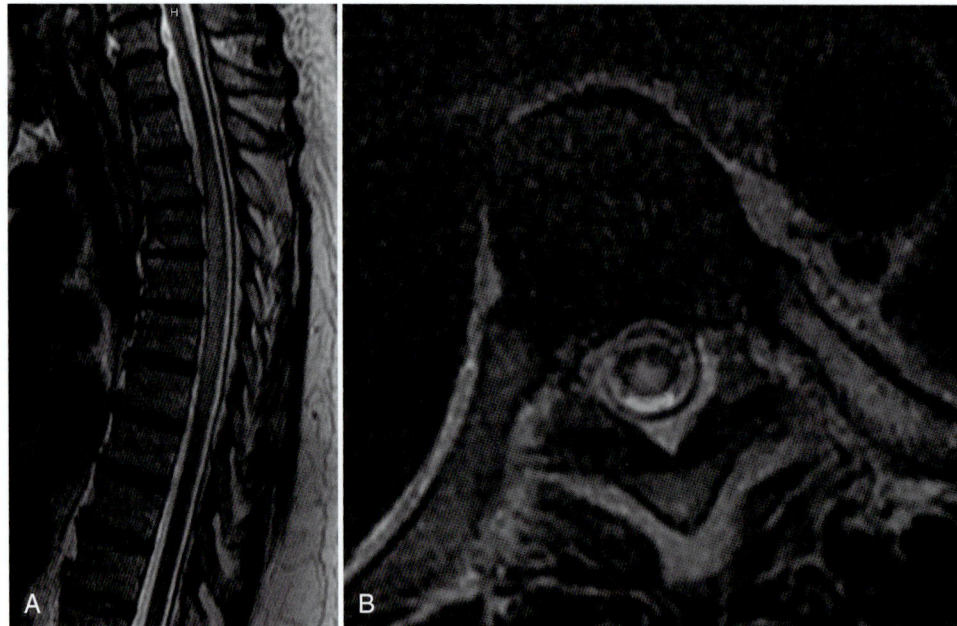

Figure 19-17 T2-weighted sagittal (A) and axial (B) images of the thoracic spinal cord. Human immunodeficiency virus (HIV) myelopathy. Although the appearance may be nonspecific, the tendency for involvement primarily within the posterior and lateral aspects of the cord, as seen here, is highly suggestive in a patient with known HIV.

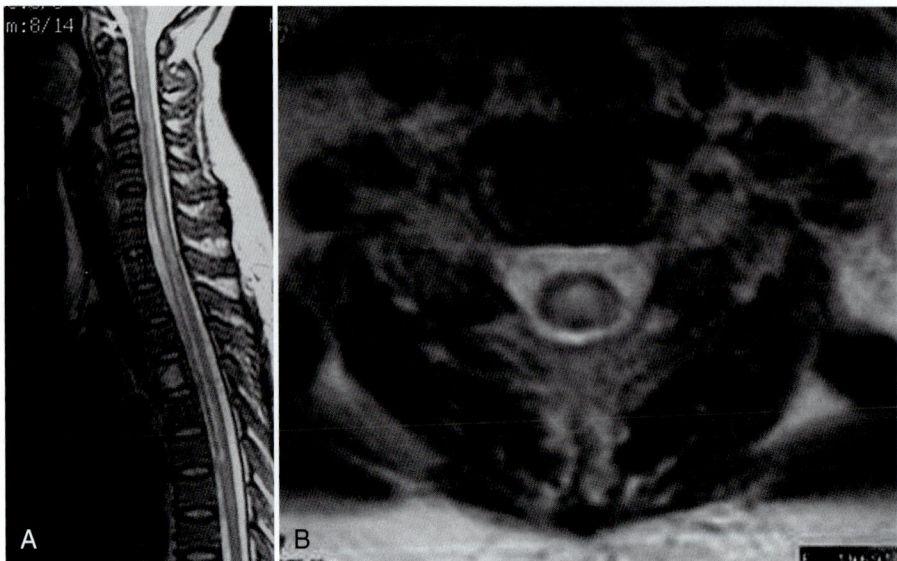

Figure 19-18 T2-weighted sagittal (A) and axial (B) images of the thoracic spinal cord. Herpes simplex virus (HSV) myelitis. The appearance is a nonspecific transverse myelitis, overlapping with other entities such as HIV. In this case, note the more central location of the lesion within the cord. Additionally, HSV may be necrotizing and demonstrate characteristic involvement of the nerve roots of the cauda equina.

Infectious Myelitis versus Demyelinating Disease or Tumor

Intramedullary pyogenic or granulomatous infection is extremely rare. Infectious myelitis is usually of viral origin, most commonly human immunodeficiency virus (HIV), herpes simplex virus (HSV), and cytomegalovirus. Typical reported imaging features are not always present, and all entities can present with a nonspecific appearance that could mimic tumor or multiple sclerosis. Cord volume probably is helpful only if a discrete mass is clearly present, which favors tumor. Mild cord expansion is not a helpful distinguishing feature because it can occur in infection and multiple sclerosis if active inflammation is present, and some tumors can present without significant cord expansion. Diagnostic considerations include the following:

- Clinical features: Known systemic infection with specific agents tilts diagnostic probability significantly.
- HIV: HIV can present as a myelitis or as a subacute process known as *vacuolar myelopathy*. Vacuolar myelopathy is seen as T2 hyperintensity along the dorsal and lateral aspects of the cord (Figure 19-17), reminiscent of myelopathy associated with vitamin B_{12} deficiency. Because there is no inflammatory component in subacute vacuolar myelopathy, no contrast enhancement is seen.
- Cytomegalovirus and HSV: Although these entities can present as a typical myelitis (Figure 19-18), a characteristic presentation is polyradiculitis, with

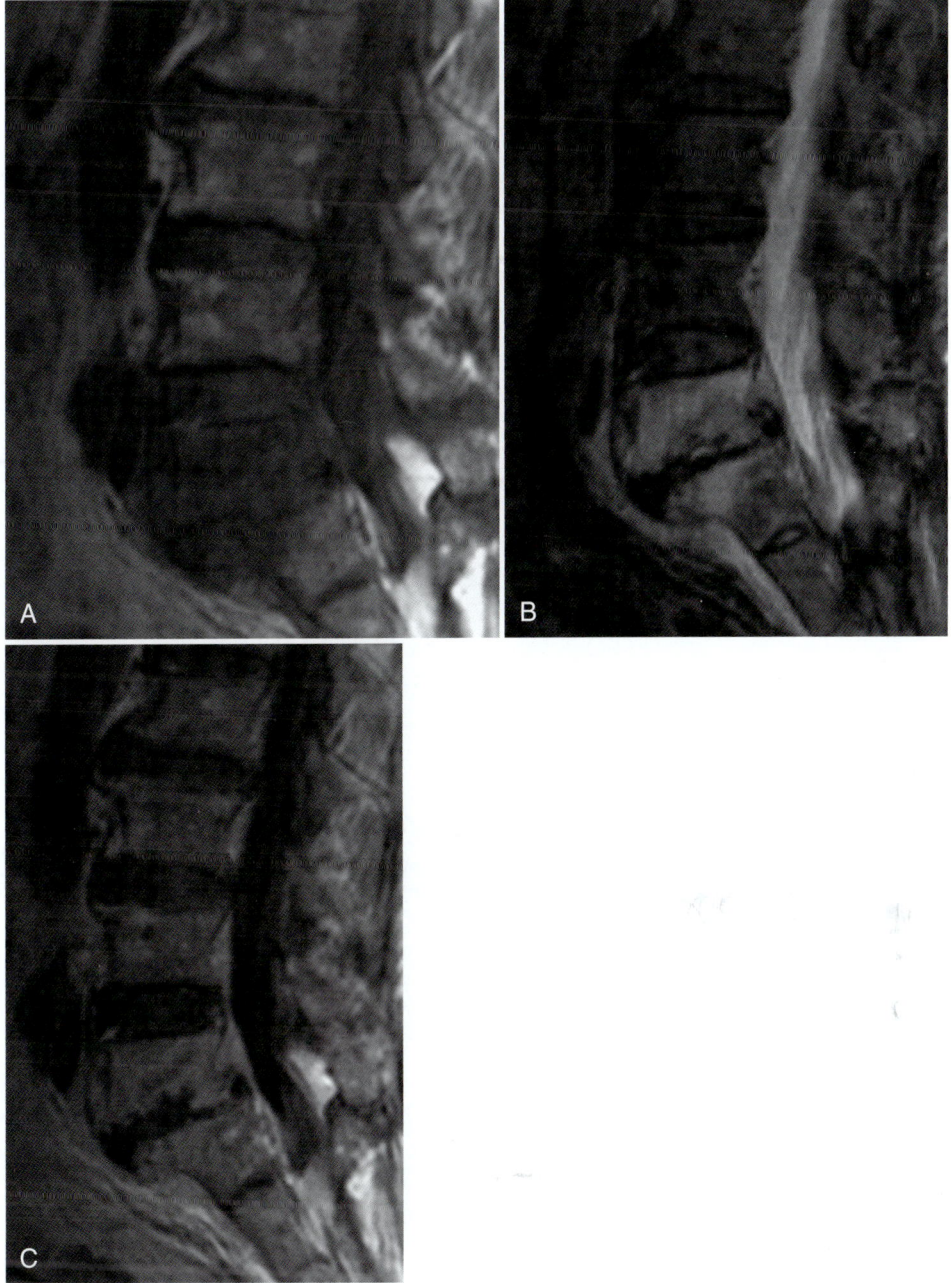

Figure 19-19 Pyogenic spondylodiscitis at L5–S1 in an intravenous drug abuser. T1 (**A**), T2 STIR (**B**), and contrast-enhanced T1 (**C**) images showing characteristic appearance of end plate/disc space involvement, relatively small epidural/paraspinous abscess formation, and relatively little bony deformity/collapse compared to tuberculous spondylitis.

prominent enhancement and clumping of nerve roots of the cauda equina and enhancement of the leptomeninges of the cord. Because HSV is also encountered in HIV patients, differentiation from HIV myelopathy by imaging may be made when contrast enhancement, necrosis, and/or hemorrhage is seen, in addition to nerve root clumping and enhancement.

Infectious Spondylodiscitis Suspected Radiographically

Determination of Type of Infection

Once infection is suspected radiographically, the next diagnostic consideration is whether the infection is pyogenic or granulomatous. Each entity demonstrates features that are more characteristic of one over the other:

- Primary involvement of disc space, mild or moderate destruction of end plates or vertebral bodies, and variable but usually small- to moderate-sized paraspinous fluid collections (abscesses), fever, leukocytosis, and history of intravenous drug abuse are more typical of pyogenic spondylodiscitis (Figure 19-19).
- Relative sparing of the disc spaces with extensive vertebral body involvement including severe vertebral body collapse and deformity, large paraspinous fluid collections ("cold" abscesses), clinical presentation primarily of back pain without significant fever and leukocytosis favor tuberculous spondylitis (Figure 19-20).

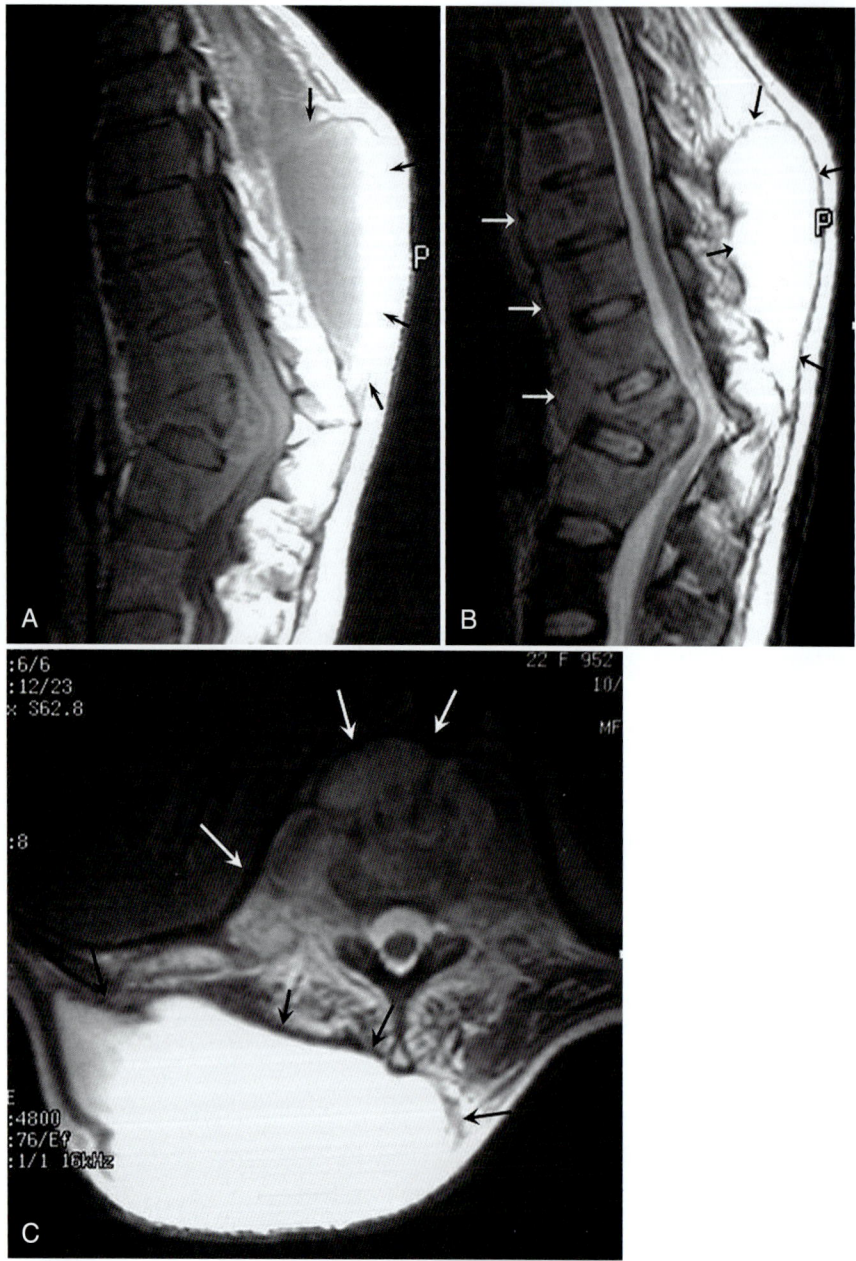

Figure 19-20 Typical features of tuberculous (TB) spondylitis. Sagittal T1 **(A)**, T2 STIR **(B)**, and axial T2-weighted **(C)** images demonstrating many hallmarks of TB spondylitis: relative sparing of discs; subligamentous spread to multiple contiguous levels *(white arrows)*; extensive vertebral body destruction and deformity, including gibbus deformity; and large paraspinous "cold abscesses" *(black arrows)*.

Suggested Readings

An HS, Seldomridge JA. Spinal infections: diagnostic tests and imaging studies. *Clin Orthop Relat Res.* 2006;444:27-33

Casey B. AuntMinnieTV: What's an Aunt Minnie? Interview with Dr. Maurice Reeder. AuntMinnie.com, 2004. www.youtube.com/watch?v=FsCcnkkMovU

Czervionke LF, Fenton DS. Fat-saturated MR imaging in the detection of inflammatory facet arthropathy (facet synovitis) in the lumbar spine. *Pain Med.* 2008;9(4):400-6.

Choi YY, Seong JY, Yang SO, Lee SR, Cho S. Tc-99m RBC SPECT demonstrating vertebral hemangioma. *Clin Nucl Med.* 1998;23(9):632-4.

Cuénod CA, Laredo J-D, Chevret S, et al. Acute vertebral collapse due to osteoporosis or malignancy: appearance on unenhanced and gadolinium-enhanced MR images. *Radiology.* 1996;199(2):541-549.

D'Aprile P, Tarantino A, Jinkins JR, Brindicci D. The value of fat saturation sequences and contrast medium administration in MRI of degenerative disease of the posterior/perispinal elements of the lumbosacral spine. *Eur Radiol.* 2007;17(2):523-31.

Ducreux D, Lepeintre JF, Fillard P, Loureiro C, Tadié M, Lasjaunias P. MR diffusion tensor imaging and fiber tracking in 5 spinal cord astrocytomas. *AJNR Am J Neuroradiol.* 2006;27(1):214-6.

Fenton DS. Treatment of facet synovitis. Presented at the American Society of Spine Radiology 2007 Annual Symposium, Marco Island, Florida, February 22-25, 2007.

Forrester DM. Infectious spondylitis. *Semin Ultrasound CT MR.* Dec. 2004;25(6):461-73.

Han BK, Ryu JS, Moon DH, et al. Bone SPECT imaging of vertebral hemangioma: correlation with MR imaging and symptoms. *Clin Nucl Med.* 1995;20:916.

Henkelman RM, Hardy PA, Bishop JE, Poon CS, Plewes DB. Why fat is bright on fast spin-echo imaging. *J Magn Reson Imaging.* 1992;2(5):533-40.

Henning A, Schär M, Kollias SS, Boesiger P, Dydak U. Quantitative magnetic resonance spectroscopy in the entire human cervical spinal cord and beyond at 3T. *Magn Reson Med.* 2008;59(6):1250-8.

Kolsi I, Dubois C, Berthelot JM, Maugars Y, Desal H, Prost A. Super-acute aseptic spondylitis as the first manifestation of round calcifying nucleopathy in a 77-year-old man. A case report. *Spine.* 1997;22(15):1784-6.

Koyanagi I, Iwasaki Y, Hida K, Sawamura Y, Abe H, Miyasaka K. Diagnosis of spinal cord ependymoma and astrocytic tumours with magnetic resonance imaging. *J Clin Neurosci.* 1999;6:128-132.

Laredo JD, Assouline E, Gelbert F, Wybier M, Merland JJ, Tubiana JM. Vertebral hemangiomas: fat content as a sign of aggressiveness. *Radiology.* 1990;177(2):467-72.

Marliani AF, Clementi V, Albini-Riccioli L, Agati R, Leonardi M. Quantitative proton magnetic resonance spectroscopy of the human cervical spinal cord at 3 Tesla. *Magn Reson Med.* 2007;57(1):160-3.

Modic MT, Feiglin DH, Piraino DW, et al. Vertebral osteomyelitis: Assessment using MR. *Radiology.* 1985;157:157-166.

Modic MT, Steinberg PM, Ross JS, Masaryk TJ, Carter JR. Degenerative disk disease: assessment of changes in vertebral body marrow with MR imaging. *Radiology.* 1988;166:193-199.

Nakajima H, Furutama D, Kimura F, et al. Herpes simplex virus myelitis: clinical manifestations and diagnosis by the polymerase chain reaction method. *Eur Neurol.* 1998;39:163-167.

Norris S, Ehrlich MG, McKusick K. Early diagnosis of disk space infection with 67 Ga in an experimental model. *Clin Orthop.* 1979;144:293-298.

Sartoretti-Schefer S, Blattler T, Wichmann W. Spinal MRI in vacuolar myelopathy, and correlation with histopathological findings. *Neuroradiology.* 1997;39:865-869.

Scutellari PN, Rizzati R, Antinolfi G, Malfaccini F, Leprotti S, Campanati P. The value of computed tomography in the diagnosis of low back pain. A review of 2,012 cases. *Minerva Med.* 2005;96(1):41-59.

Smith AS, Weinstein MA, Mizushima A, et al. MR imaging characteristics of tuberculous spondylitis vs vertebral osteomyelitis. *AJR Am J Roentgenol.* 1989;153(2):399-405.

Thrush A, Enzmann D. MR imaging of infectious spondylitis. *AJNR Am J Neuroradiol.* 1990;11(6):1171-80.

Thurnher MM, Post MJD, Jinkins JR. MRI of infections and neoplasms of the spine and spinal cord in 55 patients with AIDS. *Neuroradiology.* 2000;42:551-563.

Vargas MI, Delavelle J, Jlassi H, et al. Clinical applications of diffusion tensor tractography of the spinal cord. *Neuroradiology.* 2008;50(1):25-9.

Varma R, Lander P, Assaf A. Imaging of pyogenic infectious spondylodiskitis. *Radiol Clin North Am.* 2001;39(2):203-13.

Whalen JL, Brown ML, McLeod R, Fitzgerald Jr RH. Limitations of indium leukocyte imaging for the diagnosis of spine infections. *Spine.* 1991;16(2):193-7.

Wukich DK, Abreu SH, Callaghan JJ, et al. Diagnosis of infection by preoperative scintigraphy with indium-labeled white blood cells. *J Bone Joint Surg Am.* 1987;69(9):1353-60.

Zhang YH, Zhao CQ, Jiang LS, Chen XD, Dai LY. Modic changes: a systematic review of the literature. *Eur Spine J.* 2008;17(10):1289-99.

CHAPTER 20
Spine and Lower Back Pain
Johan W.M. Van Goethem, Paul E. Kim, and Alyssa T. Watanabe

■ LOW BACK PAIN

Low back pain (LBP) is a common complaint in Western society, with a prevalence ranging from 5% to 65% and a mean of 18.7%. Estimates of total costs per capita per year for LBP in Europe range from €116 to €399. Most occurrences of LBP are believed to be benign and self-limiting. The real challenge to the clinician is to distinguish serious spinal pathology or nerve root pain from nonspecific LBP. Clinical, anamnestic, and laboratory findings may help in differentiating these causes. In cases where either serious spinal pathology and/or treatable causes of LBP are not ruled out, imaging can be very valuable.

Low Back Pain

Acute Low Back Pain
Acute LBP is limited to 6 to 12 weeks in duration before it is considered chronic. In general, imaging is not recommended for first episodes of acute LBP without leg pain unless specific findings are present. These specific findings, called *red flags*, are indicators of possible underlying serious disease. In acute LBP, these findings include trauma, cauda equina syndrome, progressive neurologic deficit, infection, and/or malignancy. In chronic LBP, these red flags are more elaborate.

Trauma
Spinal trauma is covered more extensively in Chapter 13. In summary, in acute traumatic LBP, clinical criteria allow reliable patient triage of those who need or do not need be imaged. Two large prospective studies on C-spine trauma determined simple clinical criteria that can be used to exclude fractures safely without imaging in many low-risk subjects. The recommendations of the older National Emergency X-Radiography Utilization Study (NEXUS) are largely surpassed by the newer Canadian C-Spine Rule study. The criteria of the Canadian C-Spine Rule are listed in Table 13-1. In subjects in whom imaging is indicated and are high-risk subjects, cost-effectiveness analysis suggests that computed tomography (CT) is the preferred initial strategy. To appropriately identify these high-risk subjects, the Harborview criteria are very useful. Compared with radiography, the higher short-term costs of CT are counterbalanced by the decreased need for further imaging in patients without injury and the increased sensitivity for fractures or other significant lesions.

Cauda Equina Syndrome
Cauda equina syndrome is typically characterized by LBP, sciatica, lower-extremity sensorimotor loss, and bowel and bladder dysfunction. Classically, the full-blown syndrome includes urinary retention, saddle anesthesia of the perineum, bilateral lower-extremity pain, numbness, and weakness. The pathophysiology remains unclear but may be related to damage to the nerve roots composing the cauda equina, usually from direct mechanical compression but also less frequently from venous congestion and/or ischemia. Early diagnosis is often challenging because the initial signs and symptoms frequently are subtle. Because treatment is urgent surgical decompression of the spinal canal, imaging is a cornerstone in the workup of these patients. Frequent causes of cauda equina syndrome include disc herniation, trauma, and/or vertebral metastasis with secondary spinal stenosis and compression of the cauda equina. Because of the diversity of the potential causes of compression and the uncertain thoracolumbar level of compression, magnetic resonance (MR) is the preferred imaging technique for cauda equina syndrome.

Infection
Spinal infections are covered more extensively in Chapter 19. Spinal infections can occur in the bone of the vertebral column, the intervertebral disc space, the spinal canal, or any combination of these. Spinal infections are most frequently caused by bacteria and cause significant LBP.

Aspecific Acute LBP
From 80% to 90% of cases of LBP are considered *aspecific* because the anatomic origin of the pain remains elusive. Intervertebral discs, facet and sacroiliac joints, and, to a lesser degree, ligaments and muscles all can play a role as pain generator in acute LBP. It is usually impossible to assign acute LBP to a structural or functional correlate using anamnestic, clinical, or imaging findings.

Intervertebral disc pathology is thought to be one of the causative factors of LBP. Studies demonstrating innervation to the intervertebral disc provide evidence that may account for instances of discogenic LBP. Innervation of the inner disc was observed only in painful discs, not in normal control discs. Based on these observations, nerve ingrowth into the inner disc may be a cause of nonspecific discogenic LBP. Magnetic resonance imaging (MRI) findings that correlate with painful discs on discography are those typical for disc degeneration, mainly signal loss of the disc on T2-weighted imaging (T2-WI),

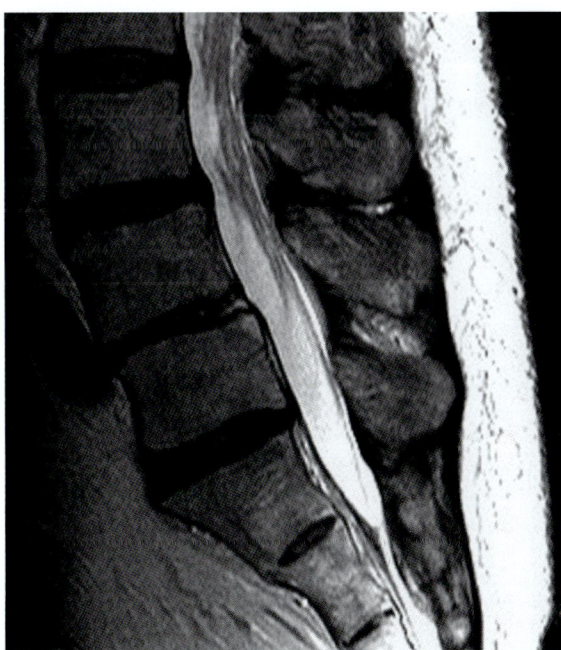

Figure 20-1 Tear in the annulus fibrosus (now referred to as hyperintensity zones). Tears in the annulus fibrosus are best seen on T2-weighted imaging where they appear as bright zones in the intervertebral disc. They are also noted on T1-weighted imaging after gadolinium because they tend to enhance. Tears are classified as radial, transverse, or concentric, involving one or many layers of the annular lamellae.

Table 20-1 Modic Changes According to Magnetic Resonance Signal Intensity Changes of Adjacent Vertebral End Plates

Modic Classification	T1–SI	T2–SI	Represents
1	–	+	Vascularized bone marrow and/or edema
2	+	+	Proliferation of fatty tissue
3	–	–	Sclerotic bone

but also loss of disc height, presence of a hyperintensity zone, and bone marrow changes.

The *hyperintensity zone* is a localized region of high signal intensity on T2-WI at the midline within the posterior annulus fibrosus. Histopathologically these lesions represent replacement of the normal lamellar structure by a disorganized, vascularized granulation tissue consisting of small round cells, fibroblasts, and newly formed blood vessels around tears that extend from the nucleus pulposus to the outer region of the annulus fibrosus. Originally the presence of a hyperintensity zone was strongly correlated with a painful disc on discography. This correlation was confirmed in multiple later studies but also was questioned in a few other studies. In general, the association between an annular tear on MRI and LBP is unclear (Figure 20-1).

Modic changes in the vertebral end plates adjoining a degenerative disc were first described in 1988 (Table 20-1). Modic et al. reported two types of changes: *Modic type 1* (Figure 20-2), histopathologically corresponding to vascular granulation tissue, and *Modic type 2*, representing fatty degeneration (Figure 20-3). *Modic type 3* changes representing bone sclerosis were added later (Figure 20-3). Some groups also use the term *Modic type 0* for normal vertebral bone marrow. Modic type 1 changes are dark on T1-WI and bright on T2-WI, Modic type 2 changes are bright on both sequences, and Modic type 3 changes are dark on both sequences.

In general, Modic type 2 changes are the most frequent (60%–90%), followed by type 1 changes (10%–40%). Type 3 changes are rare. Mixed types are recognized but are also less frequent. The prevalence of Modic changes in asymptomatic patients is reported between 0% and 10%, with Modic type 1 changes being very uncommon (<0.1%). The prevalence of Modic changes increases with age. In patients with LBP, the prevalence of Modic changes is reported between 20% and 60%. Modic changes are a common finding in patients with nonspecific LBP (median prevalence 43%) and are less common in nonclinical populations (median prevalence 6%). Modic changes are associated with LBP, with estimated odds ratios between 2.0 and 19.9. There is no statistical difference in the association between LBP and the type of Modic changes. The reasons why Modic changes are associated with LBP are not known. The lumbar vertebral end plate contains immunoreactive nerves, and it has been reported that an increased number of tumor necrosis factor immunoreactive nerve cells and fibers are present in end plates that have Modic changes, especially type 1 changes.

Chronic LBP

Although the differential diagnosis is extensive, most cases of chronic LBP have biomechanical causes. Diagnostic imaging should be ordered only when necessary because of the high incidence of radiologic abnormalities in asymptomatic persons. Therefore, history and physical examination are important in distinguishing potential causes and identifying red flags for more serious conditions. The presence of red flags calls for imaging, and an overview is given in Figure 20-4. Some conditions (listed in bottom half of Figure 20-4) warrant prompt MRI of the spine.

Known Malignancy and Systemic Disease
The spine is recognized as the most common site for bony metastases in patients with known malignancy and are found in 10% of patients with malignant neoplasms. Suspicion for vertebral metastatic disease is especially high in these patients with (chronic) LBP. Spinal metastases most often originate from carcinomas of the breast (21%), lung (14%), prostate (7.5%), kidney (5%), and gastrointestinal tract (5%). These tumors generally involve the bones of the vertebrae or the surface of the spinal cord, and less than 5% of all metastatic spine tumors are intradural (either intramedullary or extramedullary). The sensitivity for detecting, and especially for ruling out, vertebral metastases is much higher for MRI than for plain film, warranting MRI as a first examination technique in these patients. MRI is also more accurate than radionuclide bone scan and is

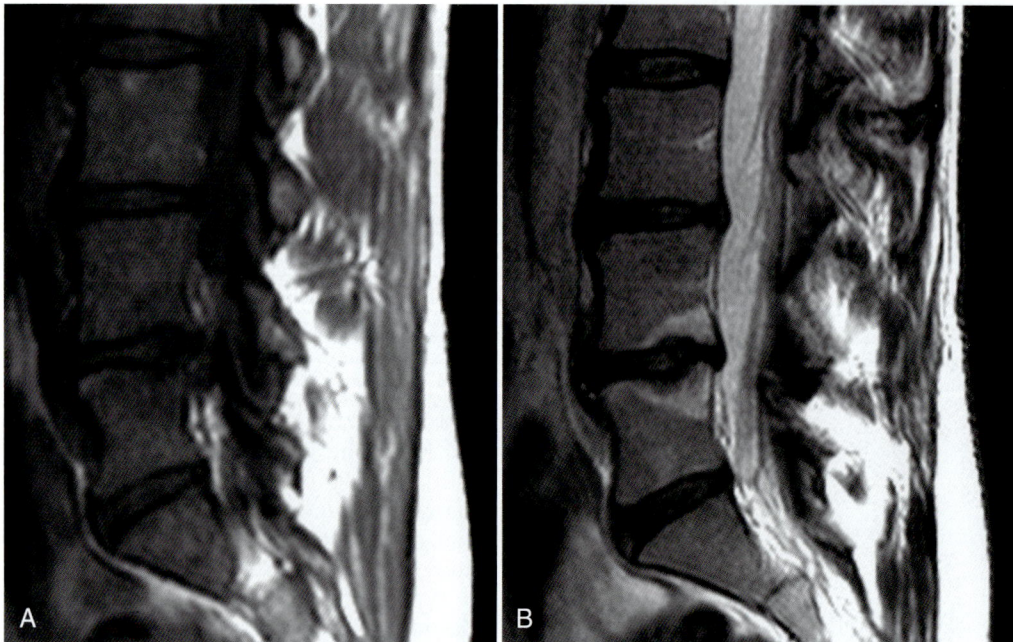

Figure 20-2 Modic type 1 changes. Reactive vertebral body modifications associated with disc inflammation and degenerative disc disease as seen on magnetic resonance images. Type 1 refers to decreased signal intensity on T1-weighted spin-echo images (**A**) and increased signal intensity on T2-weighted images (**B**), indicating bone marrow edema associated with acute or subacute inflammatory changes.

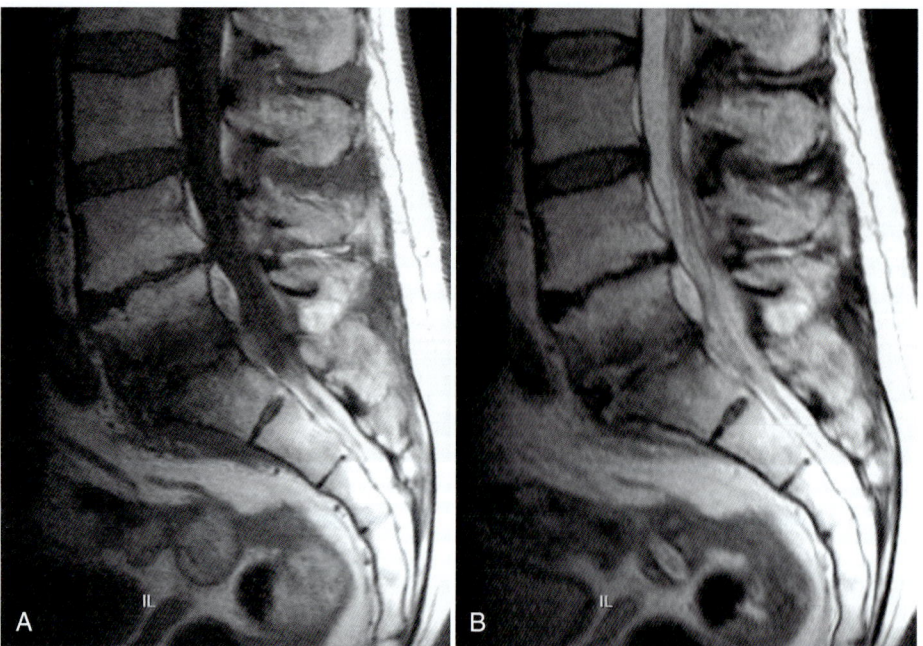

Figure 20-3 Modic type 2 and type 3 changes. Types 2 and 3 indicate chronic changes. Type 2 refers to increased signal intensity on T1-weighted image (**A**, level L4–5) and isointense or increased signal intensity on T2-weighted image (**B**, level L4–5), indicating replacement of normal bone marrow by fat. Type 3 refers to decreased signal intensity on both T1-weighted and T2-weighted images (**A** and **B**, level L5–S1), indicating reactive osteosclerosis classification of lumbar disc abnormalities.

advocated as a screening tool in patients with a high risk of metastatic disease in breast, lung, and prostate carcinoma.

When screening for vertebral metastases, sagittal (T) spin-echo (SE) T1-WI and T2-WI should be performed (Figure 20-5). In addition, a sagittal gradient-recalled echo (GRE) (so-called out-of-phase) sequence can be used. This is a sequence with a specific echo time (TE) corresponding to the time it takes for water and fat protons to move exactly 180 degrees out of phase. This time depends on the field strength of the magnet and is approximately 7 ms for a 1.5-T imager and 11 ms for a 1.0-T machine. In the normal adult human, the medullary bone of the vertebral bodies contains approximately equal amounts of water and fat protons. In out-of-phase conditions, the signal of both will cancel out, leaving the vertebrae completely black. In the case of vertebral pathology, the signal will increase, and, as such, vertebral metastases (or other lesions) will clearly stand out. If a metastasis extends into the spinal canal or neural foramen, additional axial T1-WI after gadolinium injection should be performed.

Besides metastatic disease, many other systemic diseases may affect the spine, including multiple myeloma, lymphoma, and leukemia.

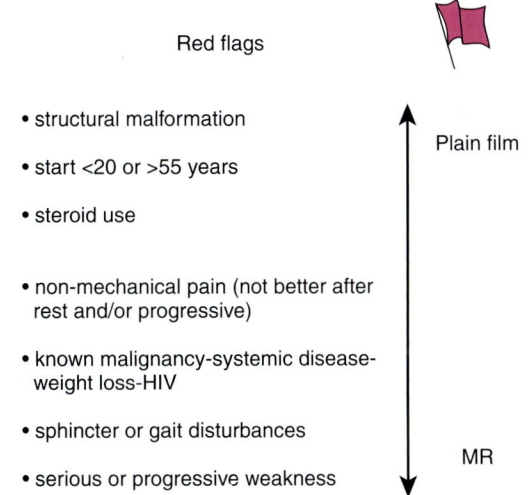

Figure 20-4 Red flags in chronic low back pain. The presence of any of these findings warrants further investigation with imaging. Depending on the possible underlying cause, a gradient among these red flags exists in which plain film imaging can be performed before deciding whether further imaging (magnetic resonance [MR] imaging and/or computed tomography) is necessary in the first group and MR imaging is mandatory in the last group. *HIV*, Human immunodeficiency virus.

Structural Malformation: Scoliosis

The normal human spine has a series of curves in the sagittal plane, including a cervical lordosis that averages (depending on the endpoints) 20 to 50 degrees (C2–7) or 30 to 70 degrees (C1–T1), a thoracic kyphosis averaging 30 to 35 degrees (T5–T12), and a lumbar lordosis averaging 50 to 60 degrees (T12–S1). The normal cervical lordosis is a circular arc. In the frontal plane, the normal load-bearing spine is straight. *Scoliosis* is defined as a deviation from the midline in a frontal plane. A small deviation (<10 degrees) is sometimes called *spinal asymmetry*, whereas "true" scoliosis has a deviation 10 degrees or greater. This deviation is accompanied by a rotation that is maximal at the apex of the curve. Imaging in scoliosis is very important. Most cases of scoliosis are idiopathic, and imaging is used routinely for monitoring the changes of the deformity that take place during growth. In addition, imaging is crucial in determining the underlying etiology in nonidiopathic cases of scoliosis. Finally, imaging is used in preoperative and postoperative monitoring. Most frequently scoliosis is idiopathic (80%). Substantial research efforts have identified several factors that contribute to the development of idiopathic scoliosis. Genetic factors are a potential etiologic component in the development of scoliosis. Studies suggest a multigene dominant inheritance pattern with variable phenotypic expression, although no specific genes have been identified so far. Family members of affected individuals have an increased incidence of scoliosis. Studies in families with twins have identified 73% to 92% concordance in monozygotic twins and only 36% to 63% concordance in dizygotic twins. The prevalence of scoliosis increases seven times in individuals with affected siblings and three times in those with affected parents.

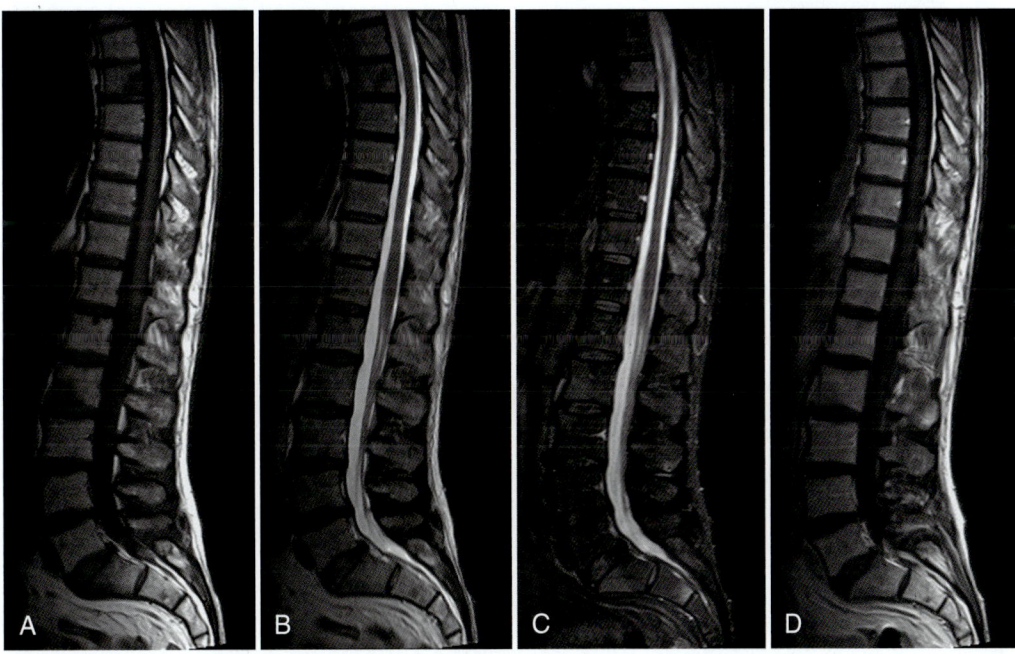

Figure 20-5 Vertebral metastases. **A:** Sagittal T1-weighted imaging (T1-WI) without gadolinium usually shows the most contrast between normal bone marrow and invasive pathology such as metastatic disease. **B:** Lesions are clearly less conspicuous on T2-WI because of high signal of fat containing bone marrow and equally high signal of lesions. **C:** This is partly overcome with fat-saturated T2-WI. **D:** Note hypointense bone marrow lesions on T1-WI (such as most metastases) become less conspicuous after administration of gadolinium because enhancement of lesions renders them isointense to normal marrow.

There is no difference in the prevalence of back pain or mortality between patients with untreated adolescent idiopathic scoliosis and the general population. Patients with mild idiopathic scoliosis (<25 degrees) usually have no or only very little discomfort. Cardiopulmonary complications are almost exclusively seen in early-onset scoliosis (<5 years old). Patients presenting with severe pain, neurologic symptoms, or rapidly progressing scoliosis require thorough further examination.

The ideal imaging modality for screening in scoliosis is the upright posteroanterior radiograph of the entire spine (Figure 20-6). The head and pelvis should be on the same film. The patient must be standing, but in young patients or patients with severe neuromuscular disorders a sitting or even supine radiograph may be the only possibility. In general, no attempt should be made to equalize differences in leg length. A lateral film is not required as part of the screening examination. Radiographic techniques should be used to minimize radiation of sensitive organs (most importantly breast, thyroid, ovaries, bone marrow and lens. It is imperative that radiation-lowering techniques are used judiciously to minimize the radiation burden.

Leg Pain

Leg pain can occur following a particular dermatome, also called *radicular pain* or *sciatica*, or in an aspecific region, known as *nonradicular pain*.

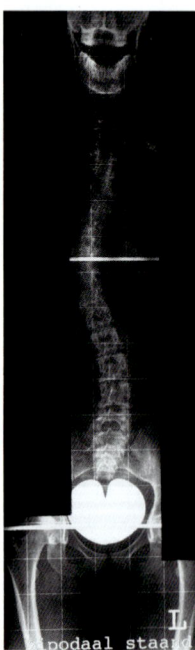

Figure 20-6 Scoliosis. An upright posteroanterior film of the complete spine that includes the head and pelvis is the standard screening examination in the diagnosis and follow-up of scoliosis. Meticulous radiation dose reduction is important because these patients usually are adolescents who have highly radiation-sensitive organs, including the breasts, thyroid, and reproductive organs. Patients having scoliosis with a Cobb angle less than 25 degrees do not have a significantly higher prevalence of back pain.

Radicular Pain

Acute lumbar disc herniations are the most common cause of acute radicular leg pain. After excluding emergent causes, such as cauda equina syndrome, epidural abscess, fracture, and malignancy, a 6-week trial of conservative management is indicated. Patients should be advised to stay active. If symptoms persist after 6 weeks or neurologic function worsens, imaging and invasive procedures may be considered. Most patients with lumbar disc herniations improve over 6 weeks.

If a disc herniation is identified that correlates with physical findings, surgical discectomy may improve symptoms more quickly than continued conservative management. Epidural steroid injections can also provide short-term relief.

Herniated discs are more easily detected with MRI than with CT for a number of reasons (Figure 20-7). First, MRI allows visualization of the complete lumbar (or cervical or thoracic) spine in one examination. Second, sagittal images also depict the spinal canal in between intervertebral disc spaces. It is not unusual for a disc fragment to migrate (or extend) into the area behind the vertebral body (Figure 20-8). Some of these migrated discs can be missed on CT if axial slices are limited to the intervertebral disc spaces examined. Finally, intrinsic tissue contrast is usually better on MR. The cervicothoracic and/or lumbosacral regions can be particularly hard to assess on CT due to beam hardening, especially in larger patients.

The terms used to describe or classify bulging or herniated discs are somewhat ambiguous and sometimes misused. The nomenclature project initiated by the American Society of Spine Radiology has found wide acceptance among radiologists, clinicians, and surgeons. In this nomenclature, *herniation* is defined as a localized displacement of disc material beyond the limits of the intervertebral disc space. The disc material may be nucleus, cartilage, fragmented apophyseal bone, annular tissue, or any combination thereof. The term *localized* contrasts to *generalized*, the latter being arbitrarily defined as greater than 50% (180 degrees) of the periphery of the disc. Localized displacement in the axial (horizontal) plane can be "focal," signifying less than 25% of the disc circumference, or "broad based," meaning between 25% and 50% of the disc circumference. The presence of disc tissue "circumferentially" (50%–100%) beyond the edges of the ring apophyses may be called *bulging* and is not considered a form of herniation, nor are diffuse adaptive alterations of the disc contour secondary to adjacent deformity, as may be present in severe scoliosis or spondylolisthesis. Herniated discs may take the form of protrusion or extrusion, based on the shape of the displaced material. Protrusion is present if the greatest distance, in any plane, between the edges of the disc material beyond the disc space is less than the distance between the edges of the base in the same plane. The base is defined as the cross-sectional area of disc material at the outer margin of the disc space of origin, where disc material displaced beyond the disc space is continuous with disc material within the disc space. In the craniocaudal direction, the length of the base cannot exceed, by definition, the height of the intervertebral space.

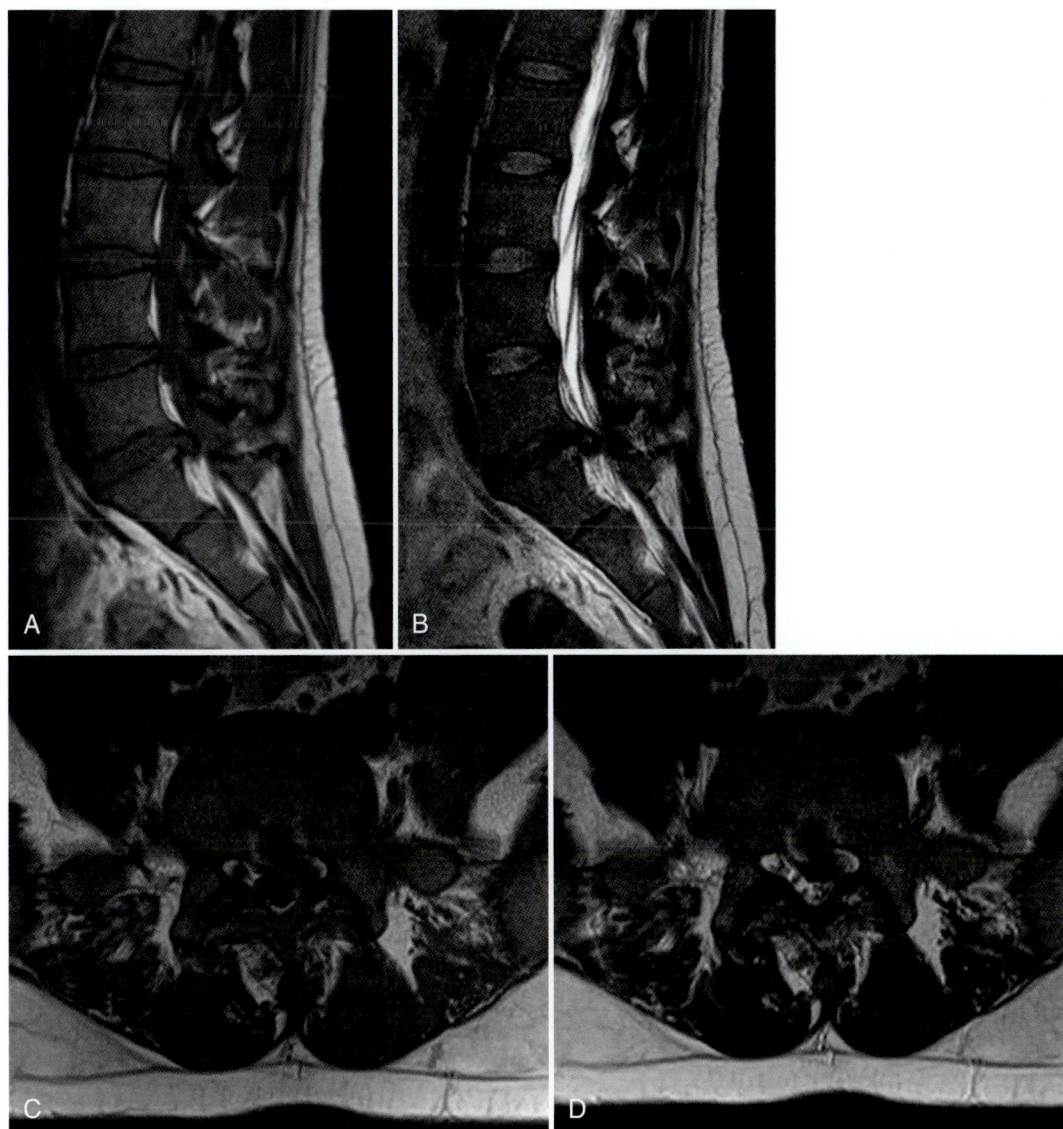

Figure 20-7 Lumbar disc herniation-type extrusion. Sagittal T1-weighted (**A**) and T2-weighted (**B**) imaging and axial T1-weighted (**C**) and T2-weighted (**D**) imaging of an L4–5 disc herniation. A disc herniation is defined as a localized displacement of disc material beyond the limits of the intervertebral disc space. Herniated discs may take the form of protrusion or extrusion, based on the shape of the displaced material. Protrusion is present if the greatest distance, in any plane, between the edges of the disc material beyond the disc space is less than the distance between the edges of the base, in the same plane. The base is defined as the cross-sectional area of disc material at the outer margin of the disc space of origin, where disc material displaced beyond the disc space is continuous with disc material within the disc space. In the craniocaudal direction, the length of the base cannot exceed, by definition, the height of the intervertebral space. Extrusion is present when, in at least one plane, any one distance between the edges of the disc material beyond the disc space is greater than the distance between the edges of the base, or when no continuity exists between the disc material beyond the disc space and that within the disc space.

Extrusion is present when, in at least one plane, any one distance between the edges of the disc material beyond the disc space is greater than the distance between the edges of the base in the same plane, or when no continuity exists between the disc material beyond the disc space and that within the disc space (Figure 20-7). Extrusion may be further specified as sequestration, if the displaced disc material has completely lost all continuity with the parent disc (Figure 20-8). The term *migration* may be used to signify displacement of disc material away from the site of extrusion, regardless of whether or not it is sequestrated. Because posteriorly displaced disc material is often constrained by the posterior longitudinal ligament, images may portray a disc displacement as a protrusion on axial sections and an extrusion on sagittal sections, in which cases the displacement should be considered an extrusion. Herniated discs in the craniocaudal (vertical) direction through a break in the vertebral body end plate are referred to as *intravertebral herniations*. Disc herniations may be further specifically described as *contained*, if the displaced portion is covered by the outer annulus, or *uncontained*, if any such covering is absent. Displaced disc tissues may also be described by location, volume, and content.

Chronic radicular pain can be caused by a disc herniation, but vertebral osteophytic spurs and degenerative foraminal stenosis are other important causes of nerve root irritation. Foraminal nerve root entrapment is best

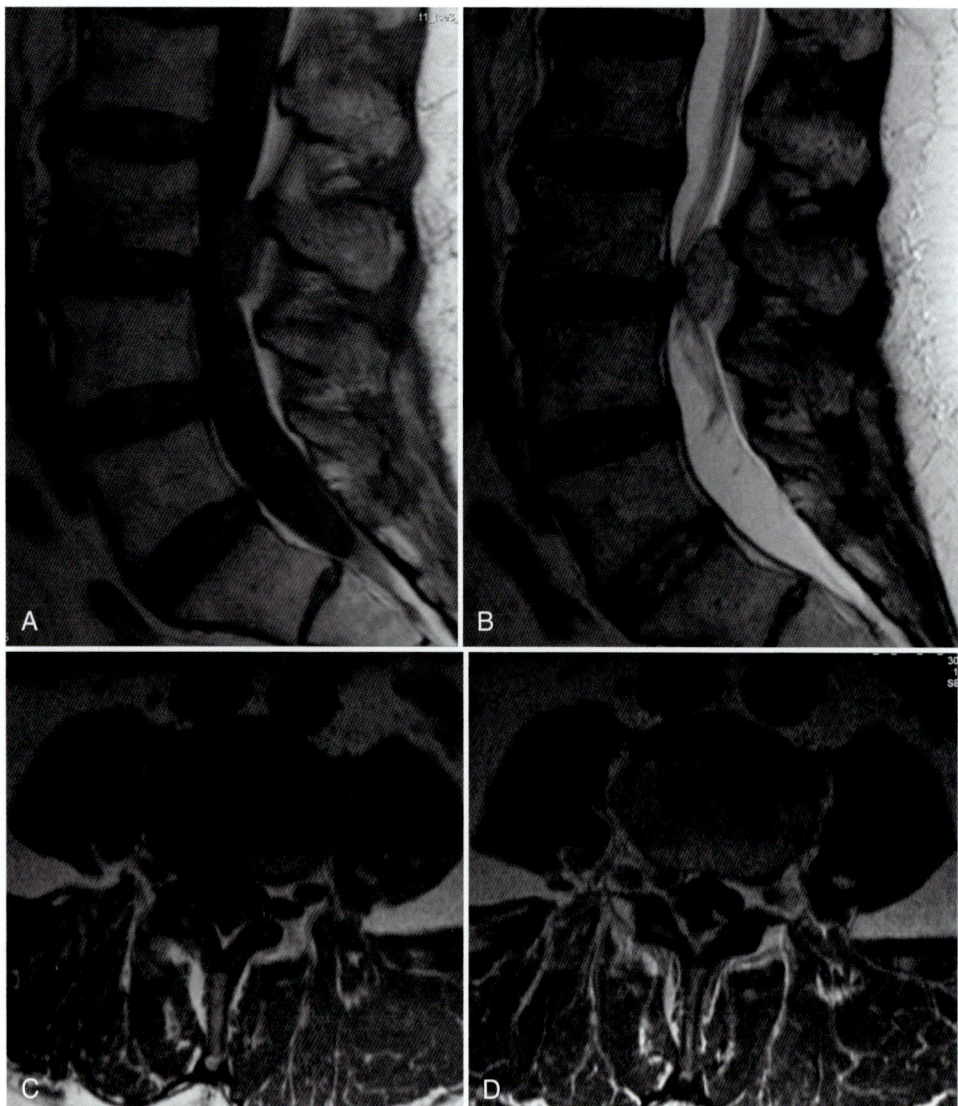

Figure 20-8 Lumbar disc herniation-type extrusion, sequestration and migration. Sagittal T1-weighted (**A**) and T2-weighted (**B**) imaging and axial T1-weighted imaging before (**C**) and after administration of gadolinium (**D**) of a surgically proven L3–4 disc herniation. Extrusion may be further specified as *sequestration* if the displaced disc material has lost completely any continuity with the parent disc. The term *migration* may be used to signify displacement of disc material away from the site of extrusion, whether sequestrated or not.

visualized on MRI where the high contrast between fat tissue and the nerve root sheath is of great help (Figure 20-9). Usually a combination of hypertrophic degenerative facets with osteophytic spurs posteriorly and vertebral osteophytes and/or disc herniation anteriorly diminishes the anteroposterior diameter of the foramen. Foraminal height is lessened by degenerative disc disease and subsequent disc height loss. Whenever the normal rounded (oval) appearance of the nerve root sheath is lost in combination with loss of the surrounding fat tissue, nerve root compression should be considered.

Nonradicular Pain

Nonradicular LBP may arise from changes of the posterior elements/perispinal tissues of the lumbar spine (i.e., the "posterior vertebral compartment"). This includes facet joint pathology (Figure 20-10) (e.g., osteoarthritis, joint effusion, synovitis, synovial cysts), spinal/perispinal ligamentous degenerative–inflammatory changes and perispinal muscular changes. MRI is the most sensitive imaging method for evaluation of spinal degenerative pathology, even in the initial stages of the disease. T2-weighted sequences with fat saturation and, when indicated, contrast-enhanced T1-WI with fat saturation permit visualization of degenerative–inflammatory changes of the posterior elements of the lumbar spine that in most cases would have been overlooked with conventional non–fat-suppressed imaging.

Pathology of the vertebral column, such as spondylosis, (osteoporotic) fractures, and vertebral metastases, are other possible causes of irradiating nonradicular spinal pain.

■ NEUROGENIC CLAUDICATION

Contrary to intermittent claudication, which is caused by poor blood circulation, neurogenic claudication is due to spinal cord or spinal nerve root compression

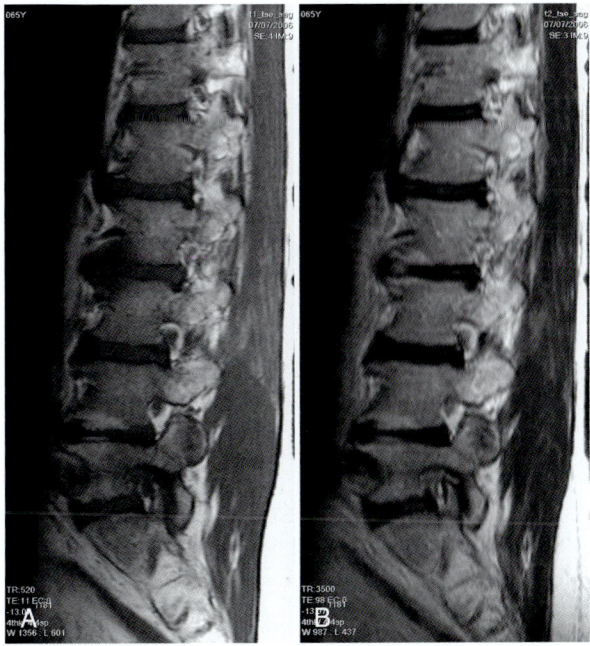

Figure 20-9 Foraminal stenosis by degenerative disease with intraforaminal facet joint cyst. Foraminal nerve root irritation/compression is fairly frequent in degenerative spinal disease. Usually a combination of disc degeneration with lessened foraminal height and facet degeneration with osteophytic spurs and/or hypertrophic changes causes the narrowing. In this case, an intraforaminal degenerative facet joint cyst further compresses the exiting nerve root. The cyst is difficult to distinguish on T1-weighted imaging (A) but is clearly visible on T2-weighted imaging (B).

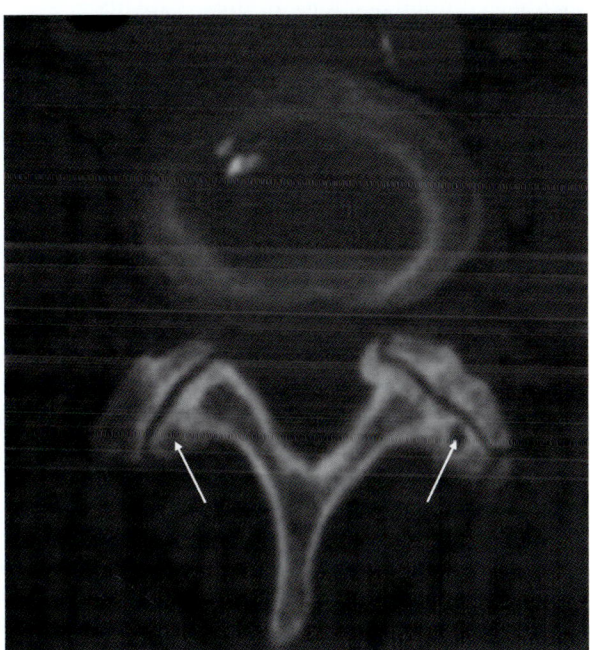

Figure 20-10 Degenerative facet disease. Computed tomographic image nicely depicting the different aspects of degenerative facet disease: narrowing of the joint space, formation of osteophytic spurs, subchondral bone sclerosis, and subchondral cyst formation *(arrows)*. Degenerative facet disease not only causes low back pain but also can be responsible for irradiating nonradicular leg pain.

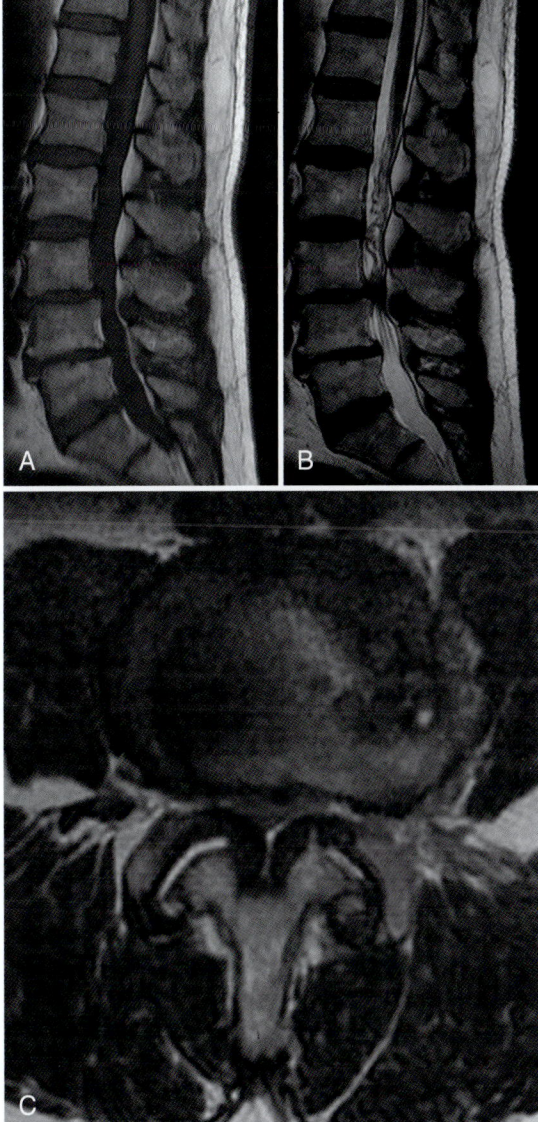

Figure 20-11 Spinal stenosis. Sagittal T1-weighted (A) and T2-weighted (B) imaging and axial T1-weighted imaging (C). Degenerative spinal stenosis mainly due to degenerative facet disease with anterolisthesis but also due to disc herniation. In severe stenosis, the nerve roots of the cauda equina can be pulled through the stenosis in flexion but remain above in a neutral position, causing the typical image of curly nerve roots above the stenosis known as *redundant nerve roots*.

and/or spinal stenosis. This compression most often occurs in the lumbar portion of the spine and clinically presents with pain and numbness in the low back, legs, and buttocks after walking or extension of the lumbar spine (Figure 20-11). The symptoms associated with lumbar spinal stenosis are usually relieved with flexion of the lower back. Spinal stenosis may be the result of narrowing of the spinal canal, which is the more common cause of neurogenic claudication, but sometimes multilevel lateral recess and/or foraminal stenosis produces comparable symptoms.

Several imaging criteria in diagnosing spinal stenosis have been established. Spinal stenosis can be evaluated by measuring the diameter of the spinal canal or by looking at the relative space that is available for the nerves of the cauda equina. In radiologic evaluation of spinal stenosis, remember that not all patients with a narrow spinal canal have neurogenic claudication. Also keep in mind that the diameter of the spinal canal usually is maximal during CT and/or MR examinations when the patient is in supine unloaded position. In performing absolute measurements of the spinal canal, 10 mm is the accepted minimal anteroposterior diameter of the dural sac at the lumbar level. Any measurement less than 10 mm is interpreted as a spinal stenosis. Looking at the relative space available, absence of cerebrospinal fluid (CSF) around the roots of the cauda equina (i.e., only nerve roots are seen in the dural sac and no fluid is detected) is a frequently used criterion to diagnose relevant spinal stenosis on imaging, both cross-sectional and on plain film myelography.

■ POSTOPERATIVE LUMBAR SPINE

Postoperative Acute Recurring Pain

Postoperative Acute Recurring LBP

Acute recurring LBP in the immediate postoperative period should raise the suspicion of a surgical complication, including bleeding, malplacement or disengagement of instrumentation, and severe inflammatory reaction. Severe recurring pain several days to a few weeks after surgery is typical for a postoperative infection (e.g., postoperative spondylodiscitis).

Plain film is an appropriate technique to check the placement and integrity of spinal instrumentation immediately after surgery. Misplacement of pedicle screws, especially in the upper lumbar or thoracic level, is sometimes easier appreciated on CT. For all other surgical complications, including hemorrhage, inflammation, and infection, MR is the imaging technique of choice.

Malplacement of pedicle screws is not always clinically significant. Only screws (or cages) that encroach on the spinal canal, and especially the neuroforamen, and correlate with the clinical picture by their position relative to the possibly affected neural structures are significant in acute recurring leg pain. Pedicle screws that penetrate the anterior vertebral border, especially at the S1 level, are usually not clinically significant and even are sometimes placed there on purpose to have better screw fixation (bicortical placement).

Hemorrhage and/or fluid in the posterior soft tissues along the surgical tract in the first days after surgery is a normal finding, unless the mass effect causes significant compression of surrounding structures (Figure 20-12). Although uncommon, occurring in less than 1% of patients, symptomatic postoperative hemorrhage typically presents hours to days following the spinal surgical procedure.

Inflammation depicted by Modic type 1-like changes in the vertebral bodies and/or enhancement in the intervertebral and epidural space is normal in the first 6 months after surgery. Separating abnormal inflammation and normal postoperative changes on imaging alone can be impossible. Severe postoperative inflammatory changes without infection is also sometimes called *sterile spondylodiscitis*.

Comparably, diagnosing *postoperative spondylodiscitis* and differentiating it from the normal inflammatory postoperative changes can be very difficult, if not impossible, in some cases. Postoperative spondylodiscitis occurs in about 0.4% of patients in the cervical spine and between 0.1% to 3% in the lumbar spine. Although the incidence of postoperative infection may be progressively decreasing due to better technical and prophylactic measures, it has not been completely eliminated. The infection is mostly due to direct intraoperative contamination, although a preoperative or perioperative infection at another anatomic site or an underlying immunocompromising condition can also predispose. The organisms involved are usually *Staphylococcus epidermidis* or *Staphylococcus aureus*. Patients with postoperative spondylodiscitis usually present with severe recurrent LBP 7 to 28 days after surgery. Imaging is mostly important in excluding a suspected postoperative spondylodiscitis. Patients without high signal of the intervertebral space on T2-WI or without Modic type 1-like changes in the vertebral bodies of the affected level or without enhancement of at least part of the intervertebral space and/or vertebral bodies are very unlikely to have postoperative spondylodiscitis. In general, the diagnosis of postoperative spondylodiscitis is based on a combination of clinical, laboratory, and imaging findings (Figure 20-13).

Postoperative Acute Recurring Leg Pain

Acute recurring leg pain, if radicular, is in principle due to nerve root irritation. In almost all cases, MRI is the imaging technique of choice in these patients.

MRI in the early postoperative phase (first 6 weeks) in asymptomatic patients shows a residual disc herniation with mass effect in about 1 of 4 cases. This number reduces significantly 6 months after surgery. Diagnosing a clinically significant early recurrent disc herniation is therefore very challenging. On the other hand, abnormal postoperative findings, including hemorrhage and failure or misplacement of instrumentation, with nerve root irritation are easier to diagnose.

The normal epidural fat in the lumbar spine is very bright on T1-WI and contrasts well with the dural sac and the adjacent normal or pathologic intervertebral disc. This explains why axial T1-WI is of high value in the lumbar region. Furthermore, the high signal of normal epidural fat contrasts well with postoperative epidural fibrosis, which is dark. On unenhanced images immediately after surgery, postdiscectomy changes can mimic the preoperative appearance of disc herniation in the epidural space because of disruption of the annulus fibrosus and edema of the epidural tissues. These render the outline of the dural sac and the posterior margin of the intervertebral disc and may efface the anterior border of the thecal sac. Additional axial T1-WI after intravenous gadolinium are mandatory in patients who have undergone prior disc surgery. Use of contrast medium is important in differentiating scar tissue (fibrosis) from recurrent disc herniation, which is essential because the

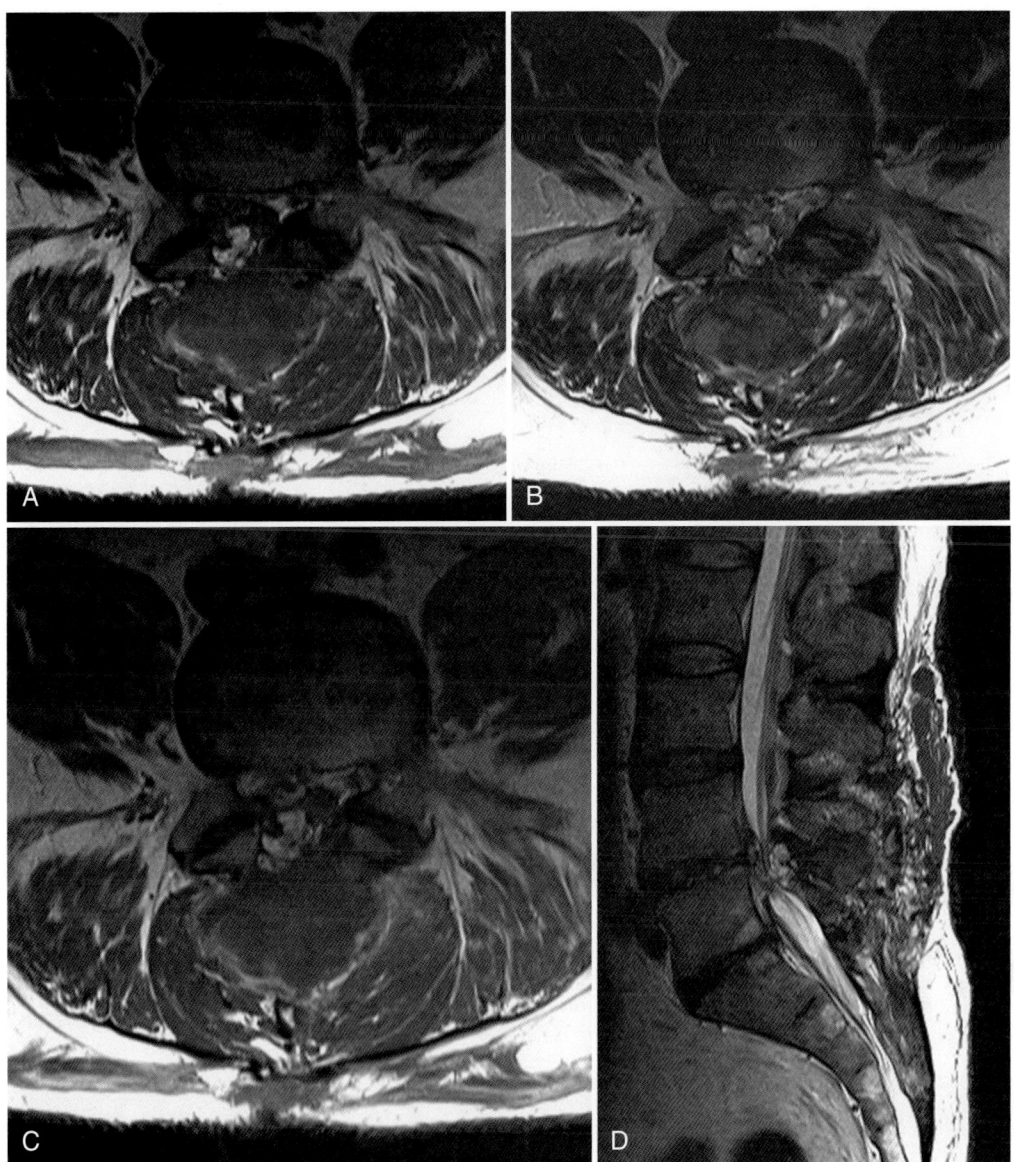

Figure 20-12 Postoperative hemorrhage in same patient as shown in Figure 20-15, 1 week later, 2 days after surgery. Patient experienced numbness in both legs and back pain. Partial resection of the L4 spinous process with an inhomogeneous mass posterior on the midline. Both axial T1-weighted imaging before gadolinium (**A**) and axial T2-weighted imaging (**B**) show a bright polylobular lesion posterior intraspinal representing a hemorrhage. **C:** T1-weighted imaging after gadolinium showing enhancement in the anterior right epidural space representing postoperative granulomatous changes with a small nonenhancing region: resection of the large herniation shown in Figure 20-15. **D:** Sagittal T2-weighted imaging showing the hemorrhage as bright (posterior intraspinal) and granulomatous changes as intermediate (anterior intraspinal). Compression of the dural sac. Reintervention was deemed unnecessary based on clinical findings.

latter is generally accepted to be a possible indication for further surgery.

A recurrent disc herniation can be differentiated from epidural scar formation on the basis of existing criteria. Epidural fibrosis shows early enhancement after gadolinium injection (Figure 20-14). A recent recurrent disc herniation initially shows no enhancement because it has no vascularization (Figure 20-15). However, it is surrounded by epidural fibrosis that does show enhancement. Contrast medium diffuses from this epidural fibrosis into the disc material, causing mild enhancement from the outside in, late after contrast injection. Therefore, images after gadolinium injection should be acquired as quickly as possible after injection.

Postoperative Chronic Recurrent Pain

Chronic recurrent postoperative pain may have many causes. It is a frequent finding that even has its own name: *failed back surgery syndrome*. The incidence of failed back surgery syndrome is estimated between 10% and 40%. Degenerative disease (accelerated or not), spinal stenosis, recurrent disc herniation, meningocele, and arachnoiditis are frequent causes. However, the main reason for failed back surgery syndrome is surgery that was performed on a structure that was not responsible for the symptoms in the first place. The best way to prevent failed back surgery syndrome is to not perform surgery

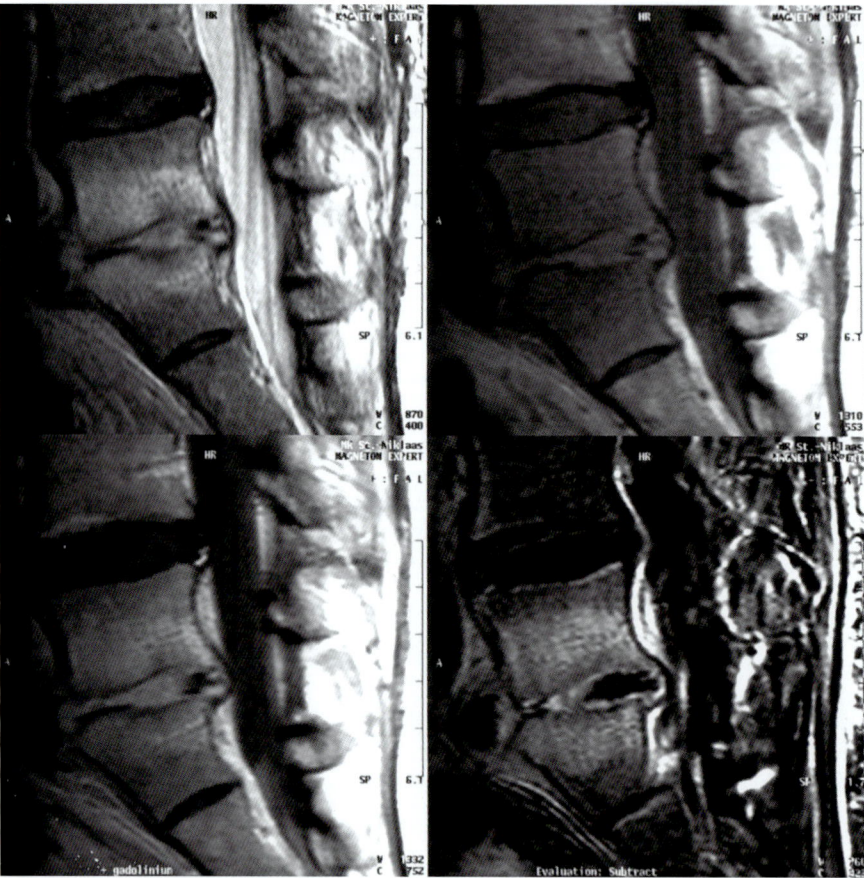

Figure 20-13 Postoperative spondylodiscitis. Sagittal T2-weighted imaging (T2-WI), T1-WI, gadolinium enhanced T1-WI, and subtraction of T1-WI after and before contrast administration. Typical inflammatory changes seen in spondylodiscitis are edematous changes in the end plates, bright signal on T2-WI in the disc space, and enhancement in both the disc space and the end plates. Unfortunately, the same changes can be observed in both infectious postoperative spondylodiscitis and in noninfected ("sterile") severe inflammatory postoperative changes. Therefore, the value of imaging mostly lies in the exclusion of infection in case of absence of these changes.

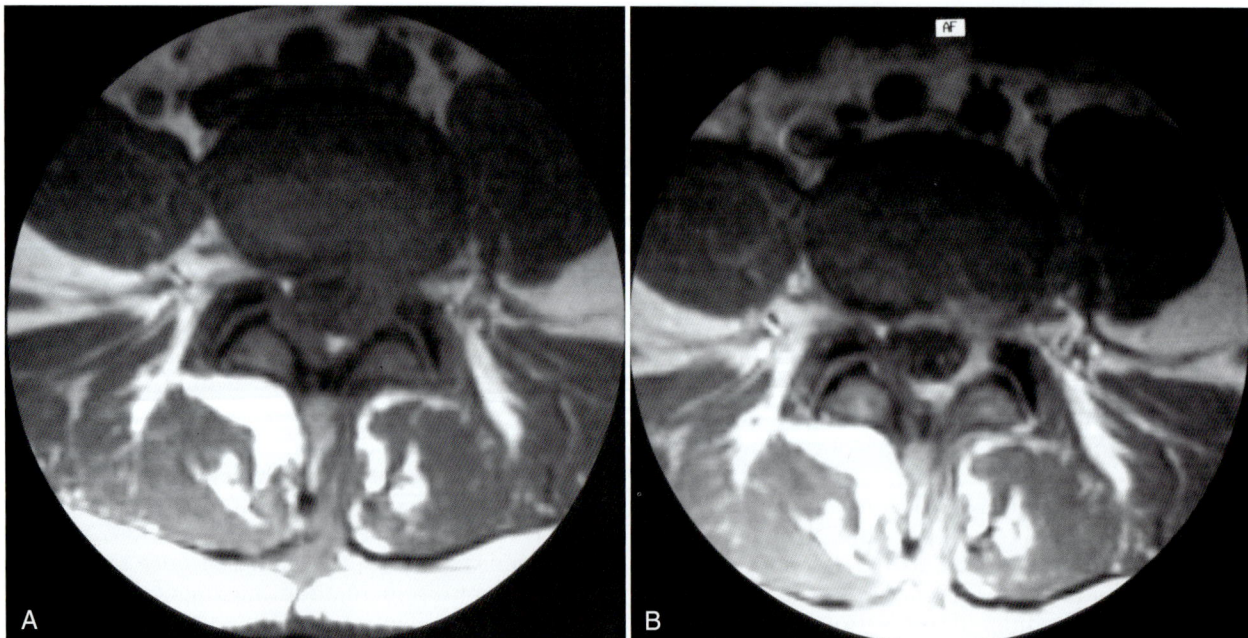

Figure 20-14 Postoperative epidural fibrosis. Axial T1-weighted imaging before **(A)** and after gadolinium enhancement **(B)**. In this typical example of (normal) epidural fibrosis, the nonenhanced image shows effacement of the bright fat signal in the left epidural space, marking the operative changes. This epidural region enhances brightly and completely after gadolinium administration with normal lining of the dural sac and the nerve roots, which is the expected postoperative image.

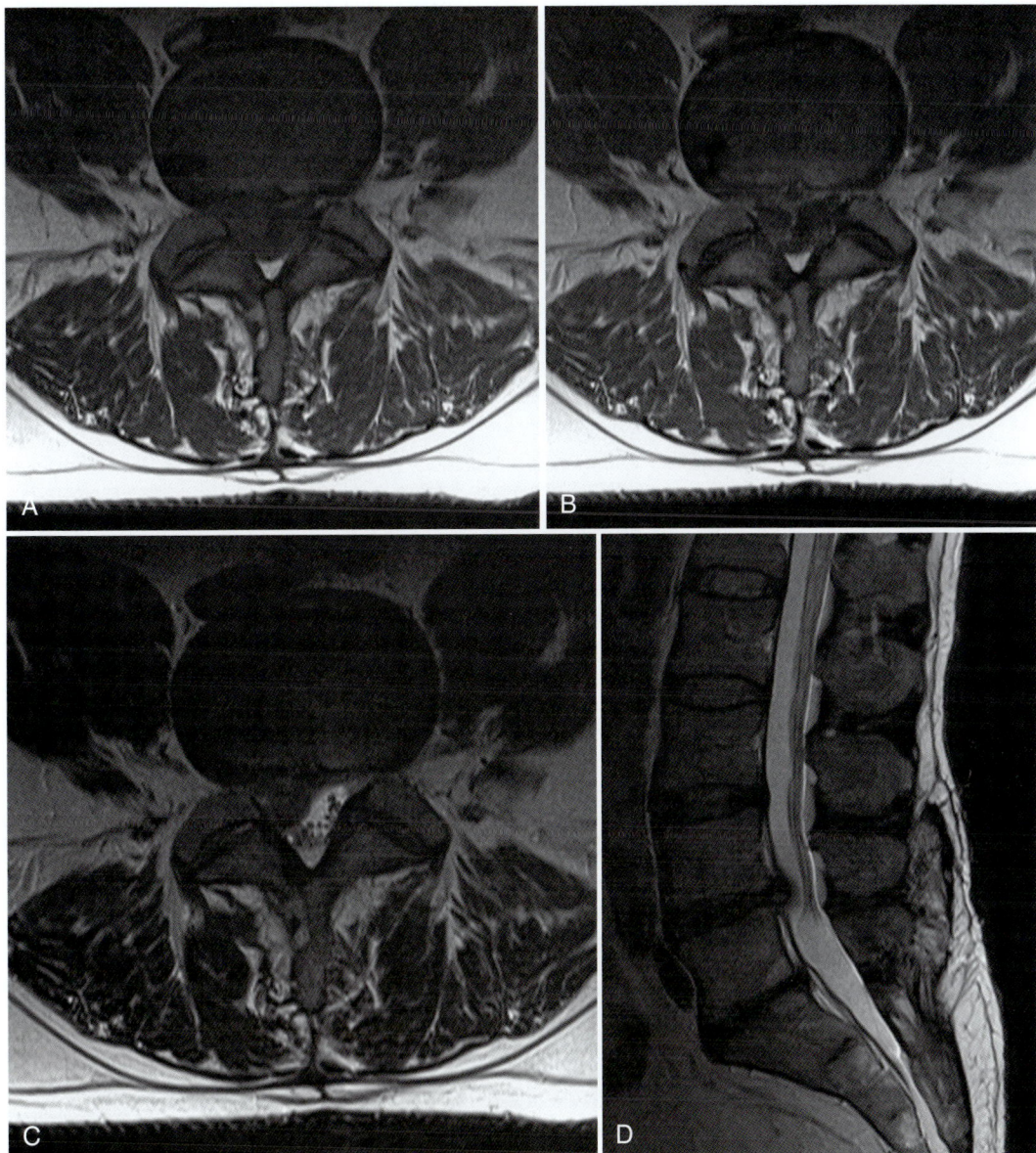

Figure 20-15 Postoperative recurrent disc herniation. **A:** Axial T1-weighted imaging before gadolinium showing effacement of the normal bright epidural fat on the right. To differentiate between scar and/or a recurrent herniation, intravenous gadolinium is used. **B:** After gadolinium, there is subtle peripheral enhancement demonstrating expected postoperative fibrosis. However, centrally in the anterior epidural space is a large nonenhancing mass corresponding to a large recurrent disc herniation. Axial **(C)** and sagittal **(D)** T2-weighted imaging showing the important mass effect.

that is apt to lead to an unsatisfactory result, hence the critical importance of thorough preoperative imaging evaluation. Besides the classic discectomy/herniectomy, fusion surgery is becoming more popular, also in the lumbar spine. The main difference in imaging the failed spine after fusion surgery is the importance of differentiating fusion from nonfusion. This topic is discussed in the section on Fusion versus Pseudoarthrosis.

Postoperative Spinal Stenosis

Removing (part of) an intervertebral disc biomechanically alters the operated segment. Height loss due to either accelerated degeneration or removal of disc material is a typical complication late after discectomy. The main consequence of disc height loss is foraminal narrowing with possible nerve root impingement. However, altered biomechanics may lead to accelerated degeneration of the discovertebral and zygapophyseal joints at the operated segment with consequent spinal narrowing. This process of altered biomechanics ultimately may affect the adjacent levels with accelerated degeneration at other levels and consequent spinal stenosis.

Postoperative Meningocele

Pseudomeningoceles are CSF-filled collections extending from the central spinal canal into the perispinal soft tissues. It is an uncommon complication, often an incidental finding, that causes no symptoms. They are not true meningoceles because they have no true

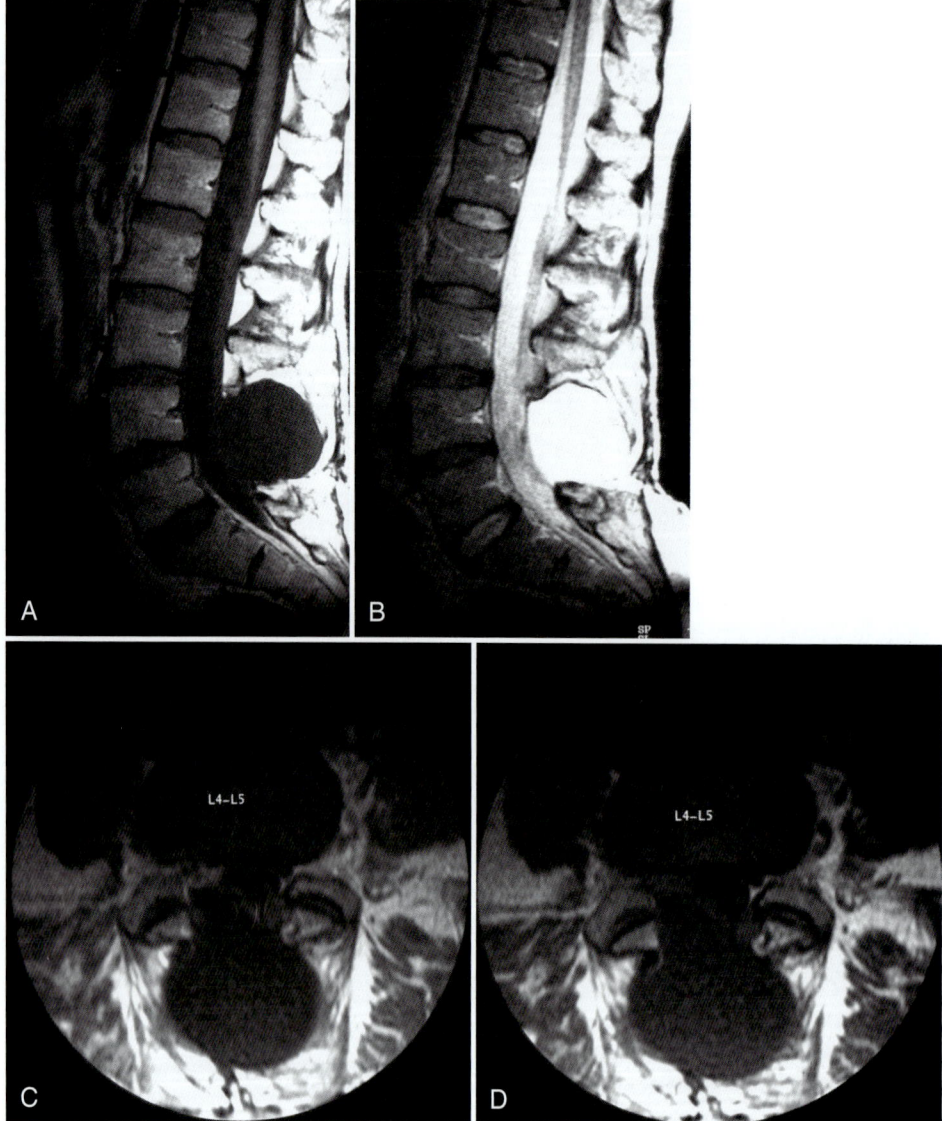

Figure 20-16 Postoperative meningocele. Sagittal T1-weighted **(A)** and T2-weighted **(B)** imaging and axial T1-weighted imaging before **(C)** and after gadolinium enhancement **(D)**. A large cystic mass is visible in the laminectomy defect. It has signal intensities identical to cerebrospinal fluid (CSF) and shows no enhancement. These postoperative meningoceles develop after inadvertent tears of the meninges with subsequent collection of CSF. Because they are not lined with meninges, they would be more appropriately called *pseudomeningoceles*.

arachnoidal lining but instead have walls of reactive fibrous tissue.

Pseudomeningoceles typically develop after inadvertent surgical laceration of the dural sac during surgery or following incomplete closure of the dural sac in cases of intradural surgery. Usually they protrude through a surgical bony defect of the posterior spinal elements to form a cystic lesion with imaging characteristics comparable to CSF on both CT and MRI (Figure 20-16). In the cervical spine, it mostly develops after an anterior approach, and here it may present a difficult challenge to treat. Patients with ossification of the posterior longitudinal ligament are especially prone to dural leaks and resultant pseudomeningocele formation. In some cases, compression of nerve roots and/or spinal cord may occur, causing symptoms. Spinal cord herniation in the pseudomeningocele is a rare but serious condition that requires urgent intervention.

Postoperative Arachnoiditis

Potential factors inciting chronic sterile spinal arachnoiditis are much debated but include the surgical procedure itself, the presence of intradural blood following surgery, diagnostic lumbar puncture, treated perioperative spinal infection, previous use of myelographic contrast media (especially older oil-based preparations), prior intraspinal injection of anesthetic, and antiinflammatory or chemotherapeutic agents (e.g., steroids, methotrexate). Chronically persistent lumbosacral signs and symptoms in 6% to 16% of postsurgical patients have been attributed to sterile arachnoiditis. The three MRI patterns described in adhesive arachnoiditis are (1) scattered groups of matted or "clumped" nerve roots; (2) an "empty" thecal sac caused by adhesion of the nerve roots to its walls; and (3) an intrathecal soft tissue "mass" with a broad dural base, representing a large group of matted roots, which may obstruct the CSF

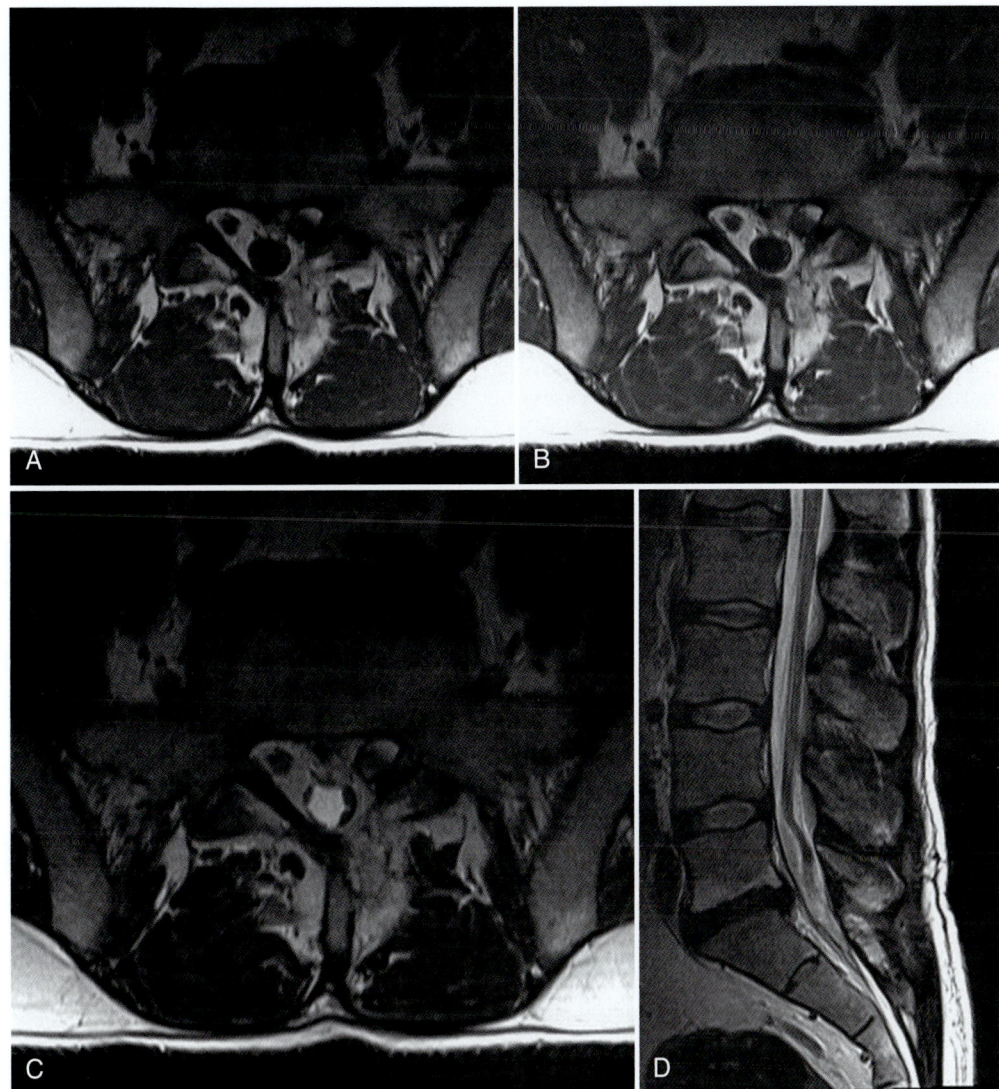

Figure 20-17 Postoperative arachnoiditis. Axial T1-weighted imaging before (**A**) and after gadolinium (**B**), and axial (**C**) and sagittal T2-weighted imaging (**D**). Axial images demonstrate the small laminectomy defect on the left. Discrete enhancement in the epidural space representing normal postoperative fibrosis, no residual disc herniation. **C:** Axial T2-weighted imaging showing clumped nerve roots in the periphery of the dural sac that is centrally empty. **D:** Sagittal image showing the thickened nerve roots regionally in the lower lumbar spine excluding other, systemic, causes of thickened nerve roots in this case of postoperative arachnoiditis.

pathways (Figure 20-17). These changes may be focal or diffuse. Contrast enhancement of the thickened meningeal scarring and underlying intrathecal roots may or may not be observed.

■ NECK PAIN

Although pathology of the cervical spine resembles that of the lumbar spine in many ways, there are some significant differences. One notable dissimilarity is based on an anatomic difference: besides discovertebral and zygapophyseal joints, the cervical vertebrae also articulate in the uncovertebral joints. Uncovertebral degenerative disease may cause spinal and/or foraminal narrowing. Strangely enough, investigations into the role of the uncovertebral articulations in cervical pain are almost nonexistent. Another important difference occurs due to a different surgical approach of cervical pathology. Most cervical surgery is performed from anterior in order to avoid manipulation of the spinal cord. Therefore, fusion surgery is relatively more frequent, and the problem of differentiating epidural fibrosis from recurrent disc herniation is nonexistent in imaging of the postoperative cervical spine.

Uncovertebral Degenerative Disease

Uncovertebral degenerative disease or short uncarthrosis is an important cause of cervical and/or irradiating shoulder/arm pain. Besides pain due to the degenerative process itself, the formation of osteophytes with secondary narrowing of the neuroforamen is especially significant. This foraminal narrowing is well visualized on oblique plain film and CT but is sometimes more difficult to quantify on MR due to the susceptibility artifacts in this region, which contains fat, water, and bone. This is most pronounced on gradient-echo sequences that are often used in the cervical spine. These osteophytic spurs may extend medially, giving rise to narrowing of the lateral recess and sometimes the spinal canal. Even compression of the cervical cord can be seen in severe cases of uncovertebral degeneration.

Postoperative Cervical Spine

Because of the vulnerability of the spinal cord, most cervical spine surgery for degenerative disease usually is performed by an anterior approach. The posterior approach is mainly reserved for decompression in cases of spinal stenosis or for surgery of the intradural compartment, mainly for dural or medullary lesions.

Fusion versus Pseudarthrosis

The main goal in the anterior approach is to fuse the painful segment and sometimes to widen the neuroforamen. In order to reach fusion, either bone or an artificial intervertebral cage is used. Bone can be obtained from cadavers or can be hosted from the patient, usually from the iliac crest. Bony fusion can be assessed using CT or MR. Continuity of bone between both vertebrae is the most reliable imaging sign of successful fusion. Although successful cartilage bridging occurs earlier, bone continuity may sometimes be visible only 12 months or later after surgery. On imaging 6 months or later after fusion surgery, persistent bone edema (on MRI) and/or a lucency around the cage (on plain film or CT) are signs suggestive for nonfusion or pseudarthrosis. Subsidence or migration of the cage is often accompanied by nonfusion. Although fusion is the final goal in this kind of surgery, not all cases of nonfusion are symptomatic. Most notably, a *locked-in cage*, although technically nonfused, may provide a mechanically stable situation comparable to fusion.

Adjacent Segment Degeneration

A typical complication of cervical spinal fusion is accelerated degeneration of the adjacent, especially superior, segment. A new disc herniation above the successful fused segment is a relatively common problem. Its origin is a mechanically altered situation wherein the segment above the fusion undergoes significantly higher forces after, rather than before surgery, possibly leading to accelerated degeneration. To prevent this complication, artificial discs are implanted in order to relieve pain caused by degeneration while maintaining spinal mechanics as normal as possible.

Artificial Discs

Artificial discs have their own typical complications that usually are easily identifiable on plain films. They include migration (usually anterior), fusion, sagittal

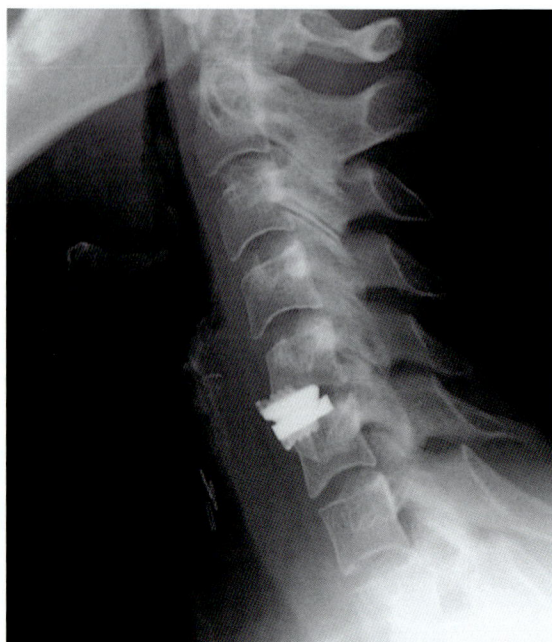

Figure 20-18 Dislodged cervical artificial disc. Anterior displacement/dislodgement of a cervical artificial disc. The most anterior part of the artificial disc should never protrude more than 3 mm anterior of the intervertebral space. Dislodgement gives subsequent abnormal motion and loads and usually leads to cervical pain and stiffness.

imbalance, and mechanical wear and/or breakdown. The most anterior part of the artificial disc can sometimes protrude anterior of the intervertebral space, but anything more than 3 mm has to be considered abnormal (Figure 20-18). Fusion of the vertebral segment after artificial disc placement can be considered a complication but is almost always asymptomatic. Abnormal sagittal alignment, especially cervical kyphosis, is usually due to abnormal placement and loading of the artificial disc. It may cause significant cervical pain, spinal and foraminal narrowing, and abnormal secondary degeneration. Finally, mechanical breakdown or abnormal wear of the artificial disc presents differently depending on the type used and usually requires reintervention.

Suggested Readings

Bircher MD, Tasker T, Crawshaw C, Mulholland RC. Discitis following lumbar surgery. *Spine*. 1988;13:98-102.
Blackmore CC. Evidence-based imaging evaluation of the cervical spine in trauma. *Neuroimaging Clin N Am*. 2003 May;13(2):283-291.
Dall BE, Rowe DE, Odette WG, Batts DH. Postoperative discitis. Diagnosis and management. *Clin Orthop Relat Res*. 1987:138-146.
Milette PC. The proper terminology for reporting lumbar intervertebral disk disorders. *AJNR Am J Neuroradiol*. 1997;18:1859-1866.

Index

A
ABCD 1 gene mutations, 385b
Abscess
    bacterial
        dental intervention-related, 95f
        differentiated from other conditions, 107, 110f-111f
        diffusion-weighted MRI of, 85-97, 107, 110f-111f
        MRI of, 107-112
        relative cerebral blood volume within, 95f-96f
    cerebral, 373-380
        aspergillosis-related, 374-378, 378f
        fungal, 374-378, 378f-379f
        pyogenic, 374, 375f-376f
        tuberculous, 374, 377f
    epidural, 31-32, 363
    fungal, 379f
    paraspinal, 31
    peritonsillar, 574, 576f
    pyogenic, 31-32
    retropharyngeal, 49-51, 52f
    subperiosteal, 45, 48f
    tuberculous, 107-112, 112f-113f
Acceleration-deceleration injuries, 438-439, 453
N-Acetylaspartate (NAA), 119, 121f, 123, 124f, 408, 408t
Acidemia, 383t
    methylmalonic, 401
    propionic, 401, 409
Aciduria, glutaric, 405
Acoustic meatus, external, 45f
Acquired immunodeficiency syndrome (AIDS). See also Human immunodeficiency virus (HIV) infection
    dementia complex of, 345
    parotid cysts associated with, 572-573
    toxoplasmosis-related brain abscess associated with, 373
    tuberculous meningitis associated with, 363-364, 364f
Adenocarcinoma, metastatic, 299f, 306f
Adenoid cystic carcinoma, 133-134, 134f
    of the lacrimal gland, 46-47
    of the soft palate, 141
Adenoma
    pleomorphic, 193t, 202, 203f, 573, 575f
    thyroid, 202
Adrenoleukodystrophy, 384f, 404-405, 408
    X-linked, 384-385, 385b
Adrenoleukomyeloneuropathy, 385b
Adrenomyeloneuropathy, 385f, 385b
Aging, successful, 334
Agraphia, 337
Air bubbles, in catheters, 354
Alcohol use, as cognitive dysfunction cause, 345
Alexander disease, 384-388, 388f, 388b, 404-405, 408-409
Alpers syndrome, 393, 398f, 398b, 401
ALS. See Amyotrophic lateral sclerosis
Alzheimer disease
    clinical diagnosis of, 336
    clinical subtypes of, 336

Alzheimer disease (Continued)
    dementia of, 333, 336
        differential diagnosis of, 119, 121f
    differentiated from
        dementia with Lewy bodies, 352, 353f
        mild cognitive impairment, 348-351, 349f-351f
        Parkinson disease with dementia, 340, 352, 353f
        semantic dementia, 346f
        vascular dementia, 352
    frontal variant of, 351
    Lewy body variant of, 339
    pathophysiology of, 336
    rapidly progressive variants of, 336
    temporal lobe atrophy in, 337f
Ameloblastoma, 577-578, 578f
American College of Radiology, 76
Amino acidurias, 383t
Amnestic syndrome, 345
Amyloid deposits, 337, 338f, 351f
Amyotrophic lateral sclerosis, 123, 123f, 333, 336, 343-344, 345f
    corticospinal tract abnormalities in, 387-388
    differentiated from atypical motor neuron disease, 354
    T2 white matter hyperintensities in, 355
    with or without dementia, 343-344
Anastomoses
    carotid-basilar, 218, 220f, 220t, 221, 226f, 236
    extracranial and/or intracranial, 264t
Aneurysm clips, as artifact cause, 13
Aneurysms, 237f
    angiographic evaluation of, 245-247
        delineation of aneurysm neck in, 245-246, 246f
        optimal angiographic views of, 245-247
        2D vs. 3D rotational views of, 234f, 237f, 245-247
    arteriovenous malformation-associated, 286, 286f
    of basilar artery, 232f
    of carotid cave, 221-224
    characteristics of, 238
    classification of, 238
    clinical presentation of, 242-243
    common locations of, 242-243
    computational fluid dynamics (CFD) model of, 242f
    computed tomography angiography of, 9, 11f, 247, 248f
    correlation with subarachnoid hemorrhage distribution, 246
    with "daughter" blebs, 241-242, 246
    deconstruction of, 277
    dissecting, 238, 272
    endovascular treatment (coil embolization) of, 276-281, 278f
        angiographic follow-up of, 235f, 249
        assist techniques for, 279f, 286f
        balloon test occlusion in, 277, 278f
        balloon-assisted, 279, 279f
        complications of, 280-281

Aneurysms (Continued)
        detachable balloon risk of, 277-278
        general method of, 278-279, 278f
        limitations of, 286f
        stent-assisted, 280
    familial intracranial, 241
    flow-related, 225f, 239
    fusiform, 238, 239f
        giant serpentine, 238
    giant, 246-247
    high aspect ratio for, 241-242, 245f
    of internal carotid artery, 278f
    middle cerebral artery branch dissecting, 277f
    multiple, 237f, 246
    mycotic, 239
    neoplastic (oncotic), 239
    noninvasive evaluation of, 247-249
    pediatric, 295-296
    related to vascular malformations, 225f, 239
    rupture of
        angiographic evaluation of, 246
        clinical outcome after, 243-245
        risk of, 238, 241-242
    saccular ("berry"), 238
    small, 247
    surgical ligation of, 277, 277f
    traumatic, 239, 240f-241f, 269-271
    untreated, 243-245
Angiitis, hypersensitivity (allergic), 258
Angiofibroma, juvenile nasopharyngeal, 571, 571f
Angiofibroma, nasopharyngeal, 266
    juvenile, 47-49, 51f
Angiogenesis, antiangiogenic agents and, 116-118
Angiography. See Diagnostic cerebral angiography
Angioma, cavernous, 253
Annulus fibrosus, tears in, 611, 611f
Anosmia, posttraumatic, 466, 468f
Anterior cerebral artery, 232, 233f
    absent A1 segment of, 236
    aneurysm of, 237f
    azygos, 236, 238f
    brain herniation-related compression of, 443
    fenestration of, 236
    infraoptic origin of, 236
    ischemic infarction of, 447f
    stroke-related infarcts in, 352
    subfalcine brain shift-related compression of, 451
Anterior communicating artery, 232, 233f
    absent, 234-236
    aneurysm of, 238f
    normal variants of, 234-236
    single, 234-236
Anterior inferior cerebellar artery, angiogram of, 214f
Anterior thalamoperforating arteries, 214f, 233-234
Antiangiogenic agents, novel, biomarkers for, 116-118, 120f
Antibiotic therapy, biopsy prior to, 321, 321f

Note: "b" following an entry indicates a box, "f" indicates a figure, and "t" indicates a table.

Antiphospholipid syndrome, 258
Antiretroviral therapy, 367
　highly-active (HAART), 345
Aortic arch
　angiographic imaging of, 211
　bovine, 216–217, 337f
Aphasia
　logopenic progressive, 339
　primary progressive, 339, 351
　progressive nonfluent, 339
Aplasia, cochlear, 33
Apparent diffusion coefficient (ADC)
　in fungal abscess, 374–378
　in glioblastoma multiforme, 120f
　in progressive multifocal leukoencephalopathy, 371f
　in subdural empyema, 361
Arachnoiditis
　postoperative, 622–623, 623f
　posttraumatic, 494, 495f
Argyrophilic grain disease, 333–334
Arterial dissections, 269, 270f
Arterial fenestrations, 232f, 241
Arteriovenous lesions, of the central nervous system, 286–289
Arteriovenous malformations, 286–288
　as aneurysm cause, 239
　angiographic evaluation of, 250–253, 251f–252f
　angiographically occult, 253
　as arterialized venous malformations, 252–253
　cryptic, 253
　embolic agents for, 287
　endovascular (embolization) treatment for, 287–288
　pediatric, 294, 294f
　Spetzler-Martin grading of, 250, 250t, 251f
　spinal, 289–291
　with stagnating arteries, 253
　in temporooccipital lobe, 252f
　thrombosis of, 253
　transdural arterial supply of, 252–253, 252f
　unusual variants of, 252–253
Artery of Adamkiewicz, inadvertent embolization of, 326f–327f
Artery of cervical enlargement, 289, 289f
Artery of Percheron, 233–234
Artifacts
　in FDG PET/CT, 191
　metallic
　　in computed tomography, 30–31
　　in magnetic resonance imaging, 30–31
　　in noncontrast computed tomography, 13
　in MRI, 66–67, 67–75, 68f
Artificial discs, cervical, 624, 624f
ARUBA (A Randomized Trial of Unruptured Brain AVMs), 250
Aspergillosis
　as brain abscess cause, 374–378, 378f–379f
　of the central nervous system, 399
　periorbital and orbital, 43
Aspergillus fumigatus, 239
Asphyxia, profound, in neonates, 537–541, 539f–540f
Astrocytic tumors, 417
Astrocytoma, 412
　anaplastic, 88f, 418f
　　recurrent, 423f
　choline-to-N-acetylaspartate ratio in, 417, 422f

Astrocytoma (*Continued*)
　differential diagnosis of, 591t
　fibrillary, 91f
　low-grade, 417f
　pilocytic, 25, 27f
Asymptomatic Carotid Atherosclerosis Study (ACAS), 284–285
Ataxia, progressive, 336
Atelectasis, of left maxillary sinus, 48f
Atherosclerosis
　angiographic evaluation of, 262–263
　extracranial carotid, 284–286
　as vasculitis-like angiographic pattern cause, 257
Atherosclerotic plaques, dual-energy computed tomography of, 55
Atlantoaxial dislocations, 477, 478f
Atlantoaxial rotations, 477, 478f
Atlantooccipital dislocations, 477, 477f
Atrioventricular septal defects, 544f
Atrophy
　asymmetric, 355
　cortical
　　dominant, 355
　　posterior, 337, 339f
　multisystem, 333, 341
　neurodegenerative disease-related, 354–355
　nonselective diffuse, 355
　progressive, 336
　selective diffuse, 355
　selective *versus* nonselective, 336–344
　side dominant, 355
　subcortical, dominant, 355
　volume loss, 335
Auditory canal, left, absence of, 40f
"Aunt Minnies," 592t
Autosomal polycystic kidney disease, 241
Avastin (bevacizumab), 116–117, 120f
Axonal fibers, three-dimensional representations of, 80
Axonal shearing injury, 70f

B

Bacteroides infections, 373
Balint syndrome, 337
Balloon catheterization, of endovascular aneurysm occlusion, 276
Basal ganglia
　arteriovenous malformation of, 286f
　calcification of, 335
　iron deposition in, 335
Basilar artery
　angiogram of, 212–213, 214f
　anomalies of, 232, 232f
　as circle of Willis component, 232, 233f
　fenestrated, 232f
　megadolichobasilar anomaly of, 238
　ranches and common variants of, 228–232
Beading, 260
Bell palsy, 560–561, 561f
Benson's syndrome, 337, 339f
Bevacizumab (Avastin), 116–117, 120f
Binswanger disease, 355
Biomarkers, for novel antiangiogenic agents, 116–118
Biometric analysis, 336
Biopsy, spinal, 299–330
　biopsy needles for, 316–321, 317f–319f
　cervical, 305, 310f–314f
　complication rate of, 321
　considerations prior to, 299–305
　drainage catheters for, 318–321, 320f
　expected results in, 321

Biopsy, spinal (*Continued*)
　of hypervascular neoplasms, 321, 322f–327f
　intradural, 314, 314f–315f
　lumbar, 300–301, 301f–308f
　MRI-guided, 316
　of multiple targets, 310f, 314, 315f
　needle safety in, 321, 328f
　pitfalls in, 321
　post-biopsy patient care, 314–316
　thoracic, 301, 308f–309f
Bladder cancer, metastatic, 47, 50f
Blake pouch, 503
　persistent, 504, 504f
Blood flow, craniocervical collateral, in arterial occlusion, 264, 264t
Blood-brain barrier, 112–113, 266, 414–417, 420f
Bone contusions, spinal, 485, 488f
Bone island, 33
Bone marrow, edema of, 474–475
Bone marrow transplantation patients, brain abscesses in, 374, 378
Bone tumors, preoperative embolization of, 291
Borrelia infections, 372–373
Brachial plexus, traumatic injuries to, 492f
Bradyzoites, encysted, 378–380
Brain
　atrophy of, HIV infection-related, 367, 370f
　congenital abnormalities of, 496–506
　　categories of, 496
　　cerebellum malformations, 503–504
　　cerebral cortex malformations, 500–503
　　Chiari malformations, 504–506
　　of corpus callosum, 496–497
　　holoprosencephalies, 497–500
　　of telencephalic fissures, 496–497
　normal aging of, 334–335, 334f
Brain herniation, 443–446
　central, 444
　complications of, 464f
　subfalcine, 443, 445f–446f
　through the craniectomy, 445
　tonsillar, 445, 445f–446f
　transtentorial ascending, 444
　transtentorial descending (uncal), 443–444, 445f–446f
Brain shift, brain herniation-related, 464f
Brain swelling, 442–443
　after hematoma drainage, 459
　"dense cerebellum sign" of, 463f
　hyperemia-related, 461
Brain trauma, 427. *See also* Head trauma
　facial and/or orbital trauma associated with, 454–458, 457f–458f
Brain tumor imaging, 412–426. *See also specific types of brain tumors*
　of chemoradiation-induced pseudoprogression, 101–106, 106f
　for differential diagnosis, 416t
　of disrupted blood-brain barrier, 414–417
　key questions for problem-solving in, 412
　MRI-based multiparametric approach to, 85–97, 85f–96f
　　alternate approach in, 97–99, 98f–106f
　　Cho-Cho/Cho(n)/relative cerebral blood flow relationship in, 92f, 97, 98f
　　differential diagnoses in, 85
　　perfusion and tumor vascularity assessment in, 85

Brain tumor imaging (Continued)
  of post-therapy necrosis, 99–101, 101f
  presurgical angiographic, 264–266
  proposed MRI protocol, 413t
  of recurrent tumors, differentiated from therapeutic-induced changes, 99–101, 101f, 417
  tumor classification and, 412
Brainstem
  in cortical gray matter diseases, 399–400
  injuries to, 437–442
Breast cancer, metastatic, 92f, 310f, 315f–316f, 598f–600f, 611–612
Bridging veins, subdural hematoma and, 433f
Brooks, B., 276
Brucellosis, spinal, 30–31, 372–373
Buccal squamous cell carcinoma, FDG PET/CT of, 129–133, 133f
  of possible bony metastases, 164f
  post-surgical, 195f
Burst (Jefferson) fractures, 479, 479f, 483–484, 486f
N-Butyl cyanoacrylate, 276

C

CADASIL (cerebral autosomal dominant arteriopathy with subcortical infarcts and leukoencephalopathy), 355
Calcification
  in basal ganglia, 335
  cerebral, 419f
  distribution within neoplastic mass, 25, 27f
  of the globe, 566f
  intracranial, pediatric, 548, 548f
  susceptibility weighted MRI of, 414
Call (Call-Fleming) syndrome, 260
Callosohippocampal commissure, 496
  agenesis of, 496, 497f
  hypoplasia of, 496–497
  interhemispheric cysts of, 497, 498f
  lipoma of, 497, 498f
Canadian C-Spine Rule, 473, 474t, 610
Canavan disease, 123, 124f, 388–389, 391f, 391b, 401, 404b, 405, 408
Candidiasis
  differentiated from tuberculosis, 300f
  neonatal, 553–554
Caput succedaneum, 469
Carbon monoxide poisoning, 401
Cardiac implants, implication for MRI, 75–76
Caroticotympanic artery, 218–220
  hypertrophied, 222f
Carotid arteries. See also External carotid artery; Internal carotid artery
  aberrant, 558–559, 559f
  in oral squamous cell carcinoma, 157–159
  stenosis of, 261–262, 261f
Carotid artery stenosis, 284–286
  endarterectomy of, 284–285
  stenting of, 285
    complications of, 285
    follow-up to, 285–286
    technique of, 285
Carotid body tumors, 49, 52f, 266, 584, 587f
Carotid cave, 221–224
Carotid endarterectomy, 284–285
  diagnostic angiography prior to, 261–262
Carotid Revascularization Endarterectomy vs. Stenting Trial (CREST), 262, 285
Carotid sinus, 217–218, 217f
Carotid siphon, 219f, 221–224

Carotid-basilar anastomoses, 218, 220f, 220t, 221, 226f
  persistent, 236
Carotid-cavernous fistula, traumatic, 271f, 271–272
Carotidynia, 269
Catheterization
  intracranial, 460
  intraventricular, 448
  subdural, 448
Catheters, angiographic, safety procedures with, 213, 215–216
Cauda equina syndrome, 610
Caudate nucleus, in deep gray matter disease, 397, 399–400
Cavernoma, 253–254
Cavernous malformation, 592t, 593f
Cavernous sinus, right, 223f
Cavernous sinus syndrome, 239
CBD. See Corticobasal degeneration
Cellular marrow proliferation, versus metastases, 592–594, 600f
Cellulitis
  ocular, 563–564, 566f
  orbital, 48f
  post-septal (orbital), 45, 47f
    differentiated from preseptal, 43–45
  preseptal, 43–45, 47f
Central nervous system infections, 361–382
Cephalohematoma, 469
Cerebellar arteries
  anterior, 230
  anterior inferior, 214f, 230
  superior, 214f, 230, 231f
Cerebellar peduncles, superior, atrophy of, 390, 394f, 394b
Cerebellitis, cytomegalovirus-related, 370, 370f
Cerebello-oculo-renal syndrome spectrum, 504
Cerebellum
  malformations of, 503–504
    Dandy-Walker malformation, 503–504, 503f
    mega cistern magna, 504, 504f
    molar tooth malformation, 504, 505f
Cerebral autosomal dominant arteriopathy with subcortical infarcts and leukoencephalopathy (CADASIL), 355
Cerebral contusions, 448
  routine serial follow-up of, 460–461
Cerebral cortex
  malformations of, 500–503
    embryology and classification of, 500
    focal cortical dysplasia, 500, 501f
    hemimegalocephaly, 500, 500f
    lissencephaly spectrum, 500–501, 501f
Cerebral infarction, acute, 73–74, 73f
Cerebritis, 373f
  brain abscess-related, 373f, 374
  as brain tumor mimic, 112–113
Cerebrospinal fluid
  blood in, 436–437
  infected subdural, 361–362
Cerebrospinal fluid analysis, in HIV-related encephalopathy, 370f
Cerebrospinal fluid space, 449, 451f
CereTom scanners, 57–59, 59f
Cervical artery, dissection of, 269–272, 272f
Cervical spine
  fractures of, 28–30, 35f
  masses and infections of, 47–51
  postoperative, 624, 624f
  tumors of, 47–51
  uncovertebral degenerative disease of, 623–624

Chance fractures, 482, 486f
Chemical shift artifacts, 66–67, 68f
Chemodectoma, 49, 52f
Chemotherapy
  effect on central white matter, 392, 396f
  effect on gray matter, 401
  as pseudoprogression cause, 101–106, 106f
Chiari malformations, 504–506
  Chiari I, 504, 505f
  Chiari II, 504–505, 505f
Child abuse, as head trauma cause, 471–472, 471f
Childhood cerebral adrenoleukodystrophy (CCALD), 385b
Children. See also Intrauterine and perinatal infections; Neonates; Premature neonates
  aneurysms in, 295–296
  carotid bifurcation in, 217–218
  cerebellar brain abscess in, 375f
  dural sinus malformations in, 294, 294f
  head trauma in, 466–472
    child abuse-related, 471–472, 471f
    postnatal, 469–471
  hypothyroidism in, 400
  hypoxic-ischemic injury in, 533–546
  intracranial aneurysms in, 243
  meningitis in, 361
  mycotic aneurysms in, 239
  traumatic aneurysms in, 239
  tuberculomas in, 377f
  tuberculous meningitis in, 365f
  vascular lesions in, 292–296
  vein of Galen varix in, 253
Cholesteatoma, 33–34, 559–560, 560f
Choline, elevated levels of, 79, 408, 408t
Chondronecrosis, 182f
Chondrosarcoma, 33
Chordoma
  as skull base erosion cause, 28, 32f
  spinal, 33
Choristoma, orbital, 46
Choroid plexus tumors
  as extraaxial tumor, 417
  perfusion metrics of, 82–85
Choroidal arteries
  anterior, 219f, 224–227
    prominent, 236f
  in vein of Galen aneurysmal malformations (VGAMs), 253
Cingulate gyrus, posterior, in Alzheimer's disease, 336
Circle of Willis
  anatomic diagram of, 233f
  aneurysms of, 242–243, 245, 245f
  angiographic imaging of, 74, 232–236, 233f–238f
  common variants of, 232–236
  location of aneurysms on, 245f
  selective catheterization of, 276
CJD. See Creuztfeldt-Jakob disease
Claudication
  intermittent, 616–617
  neurogenic, 616–618
Clay shoveler's fractures, 482
Clivus, defect in, 478f
CLOTBUST trial, 284
Coats disease, 47, 50f
Cochlea
  aplasia of, 34
  congenital cystic dilatation of, 558f
Cochlear aqueduct, 35–36, 44f
Cockayne disease, 405
Cockayne syndrome, 400, 404b

Cognitive disorder, vascular. *See* Dementia, vascular
Cognitive impairment, mild
 amnestic, 337f, 348–351
  differentiated from Alzheimer's disease, 337f, 348–351
Colon cancer, with intracranial metastases, 12–13
Commissural agenesis, 496, 497f
Commissural hypoplasia, 496–497
Common carotid arteries, angiographic imaging of, 216–217, 217f
 of common variants, 216–217, 217f
 imaging landmarks for, 217–218, 217f
 of stenosis, 261f
 technique in, 211–212
Computed tomography
 dynamic volumetric, 56
 flat-panel volume (fpVCT), 35–40, 43f–44f, 56–57, 58f
  dynamic mode, 56
  fluoroscopy mode, 57
  ultra-high resolution mode, 56, 58f
 noncontrast
  for stroke management, 9–13, 12f–13f
  of subarachnoid hemorrhage, 9
 portable scanners, 57–59, 59f
 of pyogenic meningitis, 361
 of tuberculous meningitis, 363–364, 365f
Computed tomography angiography, 13–15
 in acute stroke, 9, 14–15
 of aneurysms, 9, 11f
  post-endovascular treatment, 249
 of carotid disease, 262
 comparison with magnetic resonance imaging, 13–14
 contrast-enhanced, 61
  of aneurysms, 11f
 conversion to CTV, 15
 dynamic intraarterial, 255f, 257
 of hematoma contrast extravasation, 7–9
 of intracranial atherosclerotic arterial stenosis, 263
 of intracranial dissection, 272–273
 of ischemic stroke, 263–264
 of spine trauma, 474
 of traumatic cervical artery dissection, 269
 of vascular cerebral malformations, with arteriovenous shunting, 255–257
Computed tomography myelography, of spinal trauma, 475
Computed tomography perfusion imaging, in acute stroke, 15–21, 18f–20f, 22f
Congenital conditions
 heart disease, 241
 orbital, 46
  masses and neoplastic conditions, 46–47
  vascular and lymphatic malformations, 46
Contusions
 bone, 485, 488f
 cerebral, 13, 448
  routine serial follow-up of, 460–461
 cortical, 453
 "hot spots" for, 454f
Corpus callosum
 congenital abnormalities of, 496–497
 infarction of, 75f
 posterior, in central white matter disorders, 384–385
 shearing injuries to, 441f–442f
Corpus striatum, in deep gray matter diseases, 399–400

Cortex
 in deep gray matter diseases, 400
 zones and lesions of, 508t
Cortical contusions, 453
 "hot spots" for, 454f
Cortical contusions, head trauma-related, 437–442, 438f
Cortical gray matter metabolic disorders, 393
Corticobasal degeneration, 343, 344f
 definition of, 333
 dementia of, 336
 differentiated from progressive supranuclear palsy, 354
Corticosteroids, effect on brain perfusion estimations, 82–85
Coumadin, discontinuation prior to biopsy, 299–300
Coup injuries, 438–439
Coup-contrecoup injuries, 438–439, 439f, 453
Crack-like vessels, 254
Cranial nerves
 eighth
  anomalous course of, 33
  branching into vestibular part, 35, 43f
  vestibular branching of, 43f
 seventh
  anomalous course of, 33
  involvement in mastoid fractures, 42f
Craniectomy, brain herniation through, 445
Craniocervical collateral blood flow, 264, 264t
Craniofacial malformations, congenital, 5f
Craniopharyngioma, 25, 27f
Creatine, 408, 408t
Creatine deficiency, 401
Crescent sign, 269
CREST (Carotid Revascularization Endarterectomy *vs.* Stenting Trial), 262, 285
Cretinism, endemic neurologic, 400
Creutzfeldt-Jakob disease, 333, 345–348
 deep gray matter abnormalities in, 400, 403f
 mimics of, 336
 MRI in, 62f
 variants of, 345, 348f
  Heidenhain variant, 336, 345–348
Cricoarytenoid joint, anatomy of, 142
Cryptococcoma, 378, 380f
Cryptococcus neoformans infections, 366
Cystic hygroma, 582, 585f
Cysticercosis, 258
Cysts/cystic lesions
 aneurysmal bone, 33, 311f
 arachnoid, differentiated from epidermoid cysts, 67–70, 423, 425f
 brachial cleft, 582, 584f
 colloid, 24f, 25
 dermoid, 61
 epidermoid, 21–25, 24f
  differentiated from arachnoid cysts, 67–70, 423, 425f
 interhemispheric, 497, 498f
 lymphoepithelial, 54f
 parotid, AIDS-related, 572–573, 574f
 porencephalic, 539f
 Scheiderian, 193t, 202, 202f
 Thornwaldt, 202
 thyroglossal duct, 579, 580f
 toxoplasmosis-related, 378–380
 white matter disorders-related, 388
Cytochrome oxidase deficiency, 399–400
Cytomegalovirus infections, 370, 370f

D

Dandy-Walker malformation, 503–504, 503f
DAT ligands, 355
Dawborn, James, 276
Deep gray matter disease, 393–401
Deep gray matter metabolic disorders, 393–401
Defibrillators, implication for MRI, 75–76
Delta sign, of thrombus, 15, 17f
Dementia
 advanced MRI technique use in, 118–123
 alcoholic, 345
 cortical, 333
 definition of, 333
 frontotemporal, 339, 340f–341f, 350f
  behavioral variant, 339
  clinical diagnosis of, 336
  differentiated from Alzheimer disease, 122f, 351–352, 351f
  onset age of, 351
  rapidly progressive variants of, 336
 HIV-associated, 367
 infectious, 345
 with Lewy bodies, 340f, 333, 339, 350f
  clinical diagnosis of, 336
  differentiated from Alzheimer disease, 351f, 352, 353f
  differentiated from Parkinson disease with dementia, 352, 353f
  rapidly progressive variants of, 336
 metabolic abnormalities in, 350f
 mixed, 352
 presenile, 333
 rapidly progressive, 336
 reversible *versus* irreversible, 344–348
 semantic, 339, 346f
 senile (late-onset)
  argyrophilic grain disease-related, 333–334
  definition of, 333
 stroke-related, 352
 subcortical, 333
 subtypes, differentiation among, 118–123
 vascular, 339, 342f, 350f
  clinical diagnosis of, 336
  differentiated from Alzheimer disease, 338f, 350f, 352
 with visual symptoms, 336
Dementia paralytica, 345
Demyelination disorders. *See also* Myelinopathies
 spectroscopic metabolite patterns in, 408
"Dense cerebellum sign," 463f
Dental interventions
 as artifact cause, 133f, 163f
 as bacterial abscess cause, 95f
 as false-positive result cause, 191, 195f
 as subdural empyema cause, 363f
Dentures, as false-positive result cause, 191, 195f–196f
Developmental venous anomalies (DVAs), 253–254
Dexamethasone, effect on brain perfusion estimations, 82–85
Diagnostic cerebral angiography, 211–275. *See also* Computed tomography angiography; Magnetic resonance angiography
 of aneurysms, 245–247
  comparison with computed tomography angiography, 247
  delineation of aneurysm neck in, 245–246, 246f
  optimal angiographic views of, 245–247

Diagnostic cerebral angiography *(Continued)*
    post-endovascular treatment, 235f, 249
    2D *vs.* 3D rotational views of, 234f, 237f, 245–247
    angiographic technique in, 211–213
      aortic arch imaging, 211
      common carotid arteries imaging, 211–212
      internal carotid artery imaging, 212
      vertebral arteries imaging, 212–213, 214f
    of brain tumors, 264–266
    of carotid disease, 261–262, 261f
    of cerebral vascular malformations
      arteriovenous fistulae, 253
      arteriovenous malformations, 218f, 250–253
      classification of, 249, 250t
      developmental venous anomalies (DVAs), 253–254
      dural arteriovenous fistulas, 254–255, 256f
      with arteriovenous shunting, 250–253, 250t
      without arteriovenous shunting, 250t, 253–254
    of cerebrovascular trauma and dissection, 266–269
    complications and risk factors associated with, 213–216
      neurologic, 215
      nonneurologic, 213–215
      relationship to operator's experience, 216
      silent emboli, 216
      transient and permanent neurologic deficits, 215–216
    for cranial vasculature evaluation, 216–236
      circle of Willis, 232–236
      of common carotid arteries, 217–218, 217f
      of great supraaortic arteries, 216–217, 217f
      of internal carotid arteries, 218–227, 218f–227f
      of vertebrobasilar system, 227
    development of, 211
    of intracranial atherosclerosis, 262–263
    of intracranial dissection, 272–273
    of ischemic stroke, 263–264
    safety procedures in, 213
    of subarachnoid hemorrhage, 247
    of traumatic arterial injuries, 266
Diffuse axonal injuries, 4, 437–442, 441f–443f, 448, 453–454
    appearing after acute admission imaging, 464
    routine serial follow-up of, 460–461
Disc herniation, 474–475
Disc injuries, traumatic, 484, 487f
Discitis, 309f
Dislocations, spinal
    atlantoaxial, 477, 478f
    atlantooccipital, 477, 477f
    hyperextension, 483
    injury mechanisms of, 476
Djindjian, D., 276
DLB. *See* Dementia, with Lewy bodes
DNA, mitochondrial, mutations of, 393–397
Doppman, J. L., 276
"Dragging" artifacts, 449–451, 452f
Dural sinus malformations, 294, 294f
Dural tail sign, 424f

Dural tears, 461–464
Duraplasty, 445, 459
Dynamic contrast-enhanced magnetic resonance imaging (DCE MRI), 82
Dynamic susceptibility contrast perfusion magnetic resonance imaging (DSC MRI), 82–85, 82
    of bacterial abscess, 95f–96f
    of bacterial and tuberculous infections, 106f
    of brain tumors
      fibrillary astrocytoma, 91f
      glioblastoma, 104f
      high-grade glioma, 84f, 89f–90f, 98f
      limitations in, 80, 84f
      low-grade oligodendroglioma, 80–82
      medulloblastoma, 105f
      post-therapy necrosis, 99–106, 101f, 106f
      pseudoprogression, 106f
      recurrent tumors, 99–106, 102f, 104f–105f
      vasogenic edema, 92f
    of tumefactive demyelinating lesions, 94f, 99f
Dysplasia
    focal cortical, 500, 501f
    septooptic, 499–500

E

Ear
    external, anomalies of, 557, 558f
    inner
      anomalies of, 557, 558f
      virtual endoscopy of, 36–40, 45f
    middle
      anomalies of, 557, 558f
      virtual endoscopy of, 36–40, 45f
ECASS II (European Cooperative Acute Stroke Study II), 263
Edema
    of bone marrow, 474–475
    cerebral, intracranial pressure in, 449–451
    intramedullary, 256f
    vasogenic, 92f, 95f, 109f
      cerebral hematoma-related, 440f
Ehlers-Danos syndrome, 241
    type IV, 241, 257–258, 257t
Embolic agents, 276, 287
    as artifact cause, 13
Embolism
    diagnostic angiography-related, 215
    silent, diagnostic angiography-related, 216
Embolization
    of cerebral arteriovenous malformations, 287–288
    preoperative, of hypervascular neoplasms, 321, 322f–327f
    preoperative, of vascular tumors, 291–292
Emergency department, multidetector computed tomography use in, 3–9
    for foreign body evaluation, 4, 7f–8f
    for intracranial hemorrhage evaluation, 4–9, 8f–9f
    for skull fracture evaluation, 3–4, 5f–6f
EMI Central Research Laboratories, 3
Empyema
    epidural, 363
    subdural, 361–362, 363f
Encephalitis
    autoimmune limbic, 336
    brainstem, 372–373, 372f
    as brain tumor mimic, 112–113
    diffuse micronodular, 370

Encephalitis *(Continued)*
    toxoplasmosis-related, 378–380
    viral, 366t
      cytomegalovirus-related, 370
      herpes simplex virus-related, 366–367, 366t, 367f
      HIV-related, 367, 370f
Encephalomalacia, multicystic, 541, 542f
Encephalomalacic supratentorial lesions, 465
Encephalomyelopathy, subacute necrotizing (Leigh disease), 402b
Encephalopathies
    bilirubin, 401
    as brain tumor mimic, 112–113
    hepatic, 401
    Leigh-like, 389
    mitochondrial, 393–397, 399t
    neonatal, 533
Endoscopy, virtual, of middle and inner ear, 36–40, 45f
Enophthalmos, 48f
Enterobacter infections, 313f
Enterovirus infections, 366t
Ependymoma
    differential diagnosis of, 591t
    myxopapillary, differential diagnosis of, 591t
Epidermoid tumor, 21–25, 24f
Epiglottis
    anatomy of, 142
    in tongue base, squamous cell carcinoma, 134–135, 136f
Epilepsy, 507–532
    causes of, 510–528, 511t
      cerebral neoplasms, 512–517, 514f–515f
      dysembryonic neuroepithelial tumors, 512, 516f
      gangliomas, 512
      gliosis, 524, 526f
      herpes simplex encephalitis, 524–527, 527f–528f
      infection and inflammatory causes, 524–528, 527f
      limbic encephalitis, 527–528, 528f–529f
      malformations of cortical development, 517–524, 519f–523f
      mesial temporal sclerosis, 510–511, 512f, 530f
      pilocytic astrocytomas, 512, 516f
      pleomorphic xanthoastrocytomas, 517
      Rasmussen encephalitis, 528, 529f
      tuberous sclerosis, 523–524, 525f
      vascular malformations, 517, 517f–519f
    hippocampus anatomy in, 510
    limbic system anatomy in, 507–508
    MRI imaging of, 507–532
      protocol, 507, 508f
    Papez circuit in, 508
    pitfalls in imaging of, 528–530, 530f
    supplementary and complementary tests for, 530–532, 532f
    temporal lobe anatomy in, 510
    traumatic, 465
Epilepsy, myoclonus, with ragged red fibers (MERRF), 390, 394f, 394b, 399t
Epistaxis, exsanguinating, 239
Escherichia coli infections, 312f
Esthesioneuroblastoma, 571–572
Esthesioneuroblastoma, preoperative embolization of, 291
Ethmoid arteries, anterior, 226f–227f
Ethmoid bone, fractures of, 456

European Cooperative Acute Stroke Study II (ECASS II), 263
European Organization for Research and Treatment of Cancer, 101–106
Exophthalmos, 40, 43
External carotid artery, squamous cell carcinoma of, 239
"Extraaxial compartment," 450f, 448–449
Extraaxial tumors
    common, 417, 423f
    relative cerebral blood flow levels in, 114–116

F

"Face of the giant panda" sign, 356, 356f
Facet joints
    biopsy of, 301, 301f–302f
    degenerative disease of, 617f
    dislocation of, 480
    septic arthritis of, 603, 605f
    synovitis of, 603, 605f
Facial nerve, multiple segments of, 35–36, 43f
Failed back surgery syndrome, 619–621
False-localizing sign, 443–444
Falx artery, anterior, 219f, 224, 227f
Fat, preepiglottic, 134–135
Fat pads, buccal, 129–133, 133f
Fat saturation, frequency-selective, 71, 71f
Fibrosis, epidural, postoperative, 619, 620f
Fick's law, 79
Fistula
    arteriovenous, 253
        traumatic, 266–269, 271–272
    carotid-cavernous, 239, 454, 455f
    cerebrospinal, 448
    dural arteriovenous, 288–289, 288f
        angiographic evaluation of, 254–255, 255f, 257
        venous drainage classification in, 254–255, 254t, 255f–256f
    perilymph, 34–35
    posttraumatic cerebrospinal fluid, 467f
    spinal arteriovenous, 290, 290f–291f
    trigeminal-cavernous, 221
Focal cortical dysplasia, 500, 501f
Foraminal stenosis, 617f
Foreign bodies
    multidetector computed tomography of, 4, 7f–8f
    in the neck, 584, 586f
    orbital, 457–458
Fossa of Rosenmüller, in squamous cell carcinoma of the tongue, 130f–131f
Fractures
    benign vertebral, 601f
    Chance, 482, 486f
    clay shoveler's, 482
    facial, brain injury-associated, 454–458, 457f–458f
    frontal eminence, 5f
    Le Fort I, 567, 569f
    mastoid, 449f, 42f, 448
    maxillary, 569f
    odontoid, 480f–481f
    parietal bone, 5f–6f
    pathologic, differentiated from benign osteoporotic compression fractures, 594–595
    skull
        basal, 239
        depressed, 429, 430f
        epidural hematoma associated with, 432f
        multidetector computed tomography evaluation of, 3–4, 5f–6f

Fractures (Continued)
    multiple, 441f–442f
    pediatric, 469, 470f
    "ping-pong," 431f, 470
    semicircular canal involvement in, 42f
    spinal, 28–30
        injury mechanisms of, 476
    teardrop, 482–483, 485f
    temporal bone, 34–35, 42f, 557–558, 558f–559f
    wedge, 482f–483f
Free induction decay, 61
Frontal eminence, fractures of, 5f
Frontal lobe, contusions to, 13
Frontal sinus, fractures of, 457
Frontoparietal operculum, vasogenic edema of, 92f
Frontotemporal lobar degeneration. See Dementia, frontotemporal
FTD. See Dementia, frontotemporal
Fungal balls, 569–570
Fungal infections
    periorbital and orbital, 43
    sinusitis, 569–570, 570f
Fusion, versus pseudoarthrosis, 624

G

Gadolinium-based contrast agents
    contraindications to, 76
    as nephrogenic systemic fibrosis cause, 76
    as paramagnetic material, 67
    use of, 67
Galactitol, 409
Galactosemia, 388–389, 391b, 409
Gastrointestinal cancer, metastatic, 611–612
Gelfoam, 321, 322f–325f
Genioglossus muscles
    in buccal mucosa squamous cell carcinoma, 133f
    in tongue squamous cell carcinoma, 128f–131f, 129
Genu, anterior and posterior, 220–221
Gerstmann syndrome, 337
"Ghosts." See Motion/ghost artifacts
"Giant panda" sign, 356, 356f
Glasgow Coma Scale, 427, 427t
Glioblastoma multiforme, 98f, 412
    differentiated from bacterial abscess, 114
    methylguanine-DNA methyltransferase (MGMT) promoter methylation status of, 106
    perfusion metrics of, 82–85
    recurrent, 117–118, 119f
    therapeutic response biomarkers for, 116–117
Glioma
    anaplastic, recurrent, 116–117
    blood-brain barrier in, 416
    differentiated from
        lymphoma, 417
        metastases, 97
    disrupted blood-brain barrier in, 414–416
    high-grade
        Cho/Cho(n)/relative cerebral bloodflow relationship in, 97, 98f
        choline elevation in, 89f
        differentiated from lymphoma, 85, 90f
        differentiated from metastases, 85
        mortality rate in, 116–117
        perfusion MRI of, 421f
        recurrent, 102f
        relative cerebral blood volume within, 88f, 90f
        tumor cellularity of, 85, 90f
        untreated, 116–117

Glioma (Continued)
    infiltrating, 85
    low-grade, vascular permeability of, 86f
    malignant, 420f
    mixed, 412
    MRI FLAIR imaging of, 414
    1p 19q chromosomal deletion in, 114
    of optic nerve, 565, 568f
    of optic pathway, 46–47
    recurrent malignant, 415f
    therapeutic response biomarkers for, 116–117
    well-circumscribed, 85
Gliotic supratentorial lesions, 465
Globe
    calcification of, 566f
    proptosis of, 49f
Globus pallidus, in deep gray matter diseases, 400–401
Glomerular filtration rate (GFR), gadolinium-based contrast agents and, 76
Glomus jugulare, 561, 563f–564f
Glomus jugulare tumors, 266
Glomus tumors, 49, 52f
Glossectomy, 177f–178f, 193, 198f
Glottic squamous cell carcinoma, 142–149, 145f, 147f–148f, 150f, 152–156
Glottis, anatomy of, 142
Glutamate, 408–409, 408t
Glutamine, 408–409, 408t
GM_2 gangliosidosis, 401, 406f, 406b, 408–409
Goiter, 579–580, 581f
Granuloma
    aspergillosis-related, 374
    cholesterol, 561, 562f
    eosinophilic, 25, 27f
    tuberculous, 107–112, 374, 374
Granulomatosis, Churg-Strauss, 258
Granulomatous diseases, orbital, 40–41
Graves disease, 41–43, 47f, 564–565, 567f
Gray matter metabolic disorders
    cortical, 393
    deep, 393–401
Great supraaortic arteries
    angiographic evaluation of, 216–217, 217f
    common variants of, 216–217, 217f
Guglielmi, Guido, 276–277

H

Hallervorden-Spatz syndrome, 401, 405f, 405b
Hamartoma, orbital, 46
Hangman's fracture, 481f
Hard palate squamous cell carcinoma, FDG PET/CT of, 133–134, 134f–135f
    artifacts in, 195f–196f
    metastatic, 136, 152
    of recurrent disease, 190f
Hashimoto thyroiditis, 579, 580f
Head and neck radiology
    case-based approach in, 557–588
    masticator space and oral cavity pathology, 573–578
        ameloblastoma, 577–578, 578f
        lingual tonsil squamous cell carcinoma, 575, 577f
        Ludwig angina, 574–575, 576f
        peritonsillar abscess, 574, 576f
        retromolar tongue carcinoma, 575–577, 577f
        rhabdomyosarcoma, 577, 578f
    miscellaneous conditions of the neck, 582–584

Head and neck radiology *(Continued)*
  brachial cleft cysts, 582, 584f
  carotid body tumor, 584, 587f
  cystic hygroma, 582, 585f
  foreign bodies, 584, 586f
  Lemierre syndrome, 584, 586f
  lymphoma, 584, 587f
  multidetector computed tomography, 33–47
    of congenital orbital conditions, 46–47
    of inflammatory and metabolic conditions, 40–43
    of orbital pathologies, 40
    of orbital trauma, 40
    of periorbital and orbital infections, 43–45
    of temporal bone pathology, 33–34
  orbital pathology, 562–565
    Graves disease, 564–565, 567f
    hemangiomas, 562, 565f
    lymphoma, 565, 568f
    ocular cellulitis, 563–564, 566f
    optic nerve glioma, 565, 568f
    orbital blowout fractures, 563, 566f
    orbital venous varix, 562–563, 566f
    Sjögren syndrome, 564, 567f
  salivary gland pathology, 572–573
    AIDS-related parotid cysts, 572–573, 574f
    pleomorphic adenoma, 573, 575f
    sialolithiasis and sialadenitis, 572, 573f
  sinonasal cavity pathology, 565–572
    fungal sinusitis, 569–570, 570f
    juvenile nasopharyngeal angiofibroma, 571, 571f
    Le Fort I fractures, 567, 569f
    mucocele, 567–568, 570f
    olfactory neuroblastoma, 571–572, 572f
    sinonasal polyposis, 567, 569f
    squamous ell carcinoma, 572, 573f
  temporal bone pathology, 557–561
    aberrant carotid artery, 558–559, 559f
    acoustic schwannoma, 561, 565f
    acute mastoiditis, 559, 560f
    Bell palsy, 560–561, 561f
    cholesteatoma, 559–560, 560f
    cholesterol granuloma, 561, 562f
    congenital external and middle ear anomalies, 557, 558f
    congenital inner ear anomalies, 557, 558f
    fractures, 34–35, 42f, 557–558, 558f–559f
    glomus jugulare, 561, 563f–564f
    large vestibular aqueduct syndrome, 557, 559f
    multidetector computed tomography of, 33–34
    right, three-dimensional view of, 44f
    three-dimensional model of, 36, 44f
  thyroid and larynx pathology, 578–582
    anaplastic thyroid carcinoma, 580–582, 582f
    goiter, 579–580, 581f
    Hashimoto thyroiditis, 579, 580f
    lingual thyroid, 578–579, 579f
    squamous cell carcinoma of the larynx, 582, 583f
    thyroglossal duct cysts, 579, 580f
Head and neck squamous cell carcinoma, FDG PET/CT of, 126–208
  after neoadjuvant chemoradiotherapy, 140f, 155f, 170, 172f–174f

Head and neck squamous cell carcinoma, FDG PET/CT of *(Continued)*
  benign tumor FDG uptake and, 170, 193t, 202, 202f–203f
  of bone metastases, 161–166, 161f, 163f–164f
  of buccal mucosa, 129–133, 133f
  of carcinoma of unknown primary origin (CUP), 154f–155f, 169, 169–170
  of cervical lymph node metastases, 127t, 137f–138f, 149f, 152–161, 152f
    in combination with contrast-enhanced CT, 137f, 149f, 152f, 157–159, 157f
    occult metastases, 160–161
    with reactive lymphoid hyperplasia, 137f, 149f, 152f, 159
    with semiquantitative PET methods, 137f–138f, 149f, 159–160, 159f–160f
    SUV_{max} cutoff values in, 137f–138f, 149f, 159–160, 159f–160f
  contrast-enhanced CT of, 126
  of distant metastases, 166, 182–184
  effect of surgically-induced changes on, 191–193, 194f
  effect on management at initial stage, 137f, 149f, 152f, 166f, 168, 168f
  false-positive results in, 138f, 157–161, 160f, 170, 191
    cervical lymph node-related, 202
  imaging characteristics of, 192t
  of mediastinal lymph node metastases, 166, 168f
  pitfalls in, 191–193
  of post-reconstructive defects, 193, 197f
  for post-therapy surveillance, 184–191
  of post-therapy vocal cord changes, 193, 200f–201f
  for primary tumor response prediction, 170, 172f–174f
  of pulmonary metastases, 166, 166f
  of radiation-induced changes, 183f, 193, 199f–200f
  for recurrent tumor detection, 170–191, 175f–178f, 187f–190f
  staging of, 126, 127t
    misinterpretation in, 193t
  of synchronous malignancies, 166–168
  tonsillar carcinoma, 127f
  for treatment response evaluation, 170
Head and neck trauma, cerebrovascular vessel injury in, 266–269
Head trauma, 427–428
  acute admission imaging, 428–458
    brain swelling, 442–443
    brainstem injuries, 437–442
    cerebral hematoma, 437–442
    cerebrospinal fluid blood, 436–437
    cortical contusions, 437–442, 438f
    diffuse axonal injuries, 437–442, 441f–443f
    of epidural hematoma, 429, 431f
    extraaxial collection, 429
    primary lesions, 429
    primary and secondary lesions, 429, 429t
    secondary lesions, 442–448
    of subarachnoid hemorrhage, 434–437, 436f
    of subdural hematoma, 429–434, 433f
    "The Container," 448, 449f
    "The Content," 449–454, 451f
    "The Extraaxial Compartment," 448–449, 450f
    of vascular complications, 446–448, 447f

Head trauma *(Continued)*
  as brain herniation cause
    central, 444
    subfalcine, 443, 445f–446f
    through the craniectomy, 445
    tonsillar, 445, 445f–446f, 451–453
    transtentorial ascending, 444
    transtentorial descending (uncal), 443–444, 445f–446f
  chronic imaging of, 464–466
  indications for imaging in, 427t, 427–428
  as ischemic infarct cause, 461
  minor, 427, 428t
  optimal techniques and protocols, 427–428
  pediatric
    child abuse-related, 471–472, 471f
    labor and delivery-related, 466–472
    postnatal, 469–471
    primary lesions, routine serial follow-up of, 460–461, 461f
    secondary lesions, follow-up imaging of, 461–464
  subacute imaging, 458–464
    postsurgical, 458–460, 459f
    routine serial follow-up, 460–464
Headaches
  subarachnoid hemorrhage-related, 242–243
  "thunderclap," 260
Hemangioblastoma, 291
  spinal, atypical, 597f
  of spinal cord, 596f
Hemangioma
  capillary, of the orbit, 46–47
  cavernous, 46
  orbital, 562, 565f
  vertebral, 33
  of vertebral body, 593f
Hemangiopericytoma, 268f
  preoperative embolization of, 291
Hematoma
  cerebral
    appearing after acute admission imaging, 464
    posttraumatic, 437–442, 440f
    routine serial follow-up of, 460–461
  epidural, 4, 7, 429, 431f
    postsurgical follow-up of, 459f
    size increase in, 448
    spinal, 488–489, 491f
    spinal trauma-related, 474–475
    surgical treatment of, 448
  extraaxial, 4, 7
  groin, 212–213
  intraaxial, 7
  intracranial
    expansion of, 7–9, 10f
    posttraumatic, 4–7
  subdural, 429–434, 433f
    brain herniation associated with, 447f
    isodense, 7, 9f
    post-drainage, 462f
    rebleeding in, 429–434, 434f–435f
    ruptured posterior communicating artery aneurysm-related, 244f
    small right temporoparietal, 8f
    spinal, 488–489
    subgaleal, 469
Hemimaxillectomy, 134f, 163f
Hemimegalocephaly, 500, 500f
Hemochromatosis, chronic, 400

Hemorrhage, 414
  arteriovenous malformation-related, 250
  basal ganglia arteriovenous malformation-related, 286f
  Duret, 454, 459, 460f, 464
  extraaxial, pediatric, 469
  germinal matrix, 536–537, 537t, 538f
  gradient-recalled echo (GRE) sequence MRI detection of, 69f
  intracranial
    in emergency department setting, 4–9
    iodine extravasation in, 55, 55f
    multidetector computed tomography evaluation of, 4–9, 8f–9f
  intraparenchymal, 55f
  intraventricular, 434–437, 436f, 539f
  iron-containing, as paramagnetic material, 67
  nonaneurysmal perimesencephalic, 247
  postoperative, 618, 619f
  subarachnoid, 434–437, 436f
    adverse effects of, 448
    angiogram-negative, 247
    appearing after acute admission imaging, 464
    cerebral vasospasm following, 260–261, 261f
    cerebrospinal fluid hyperintensity in, 436–437, 437f
    cerebrospinal fluid spaces in, 449
    computed tomography angiographic evaluation of, 247, 248f
    correlation with aneurysm sites, 246
    cortical contusion-associated, 438–439
    diagnostic angiography-related, 215
    as headache cause, 242–243
    Hunt and Hess clinical classification system for, 243, 245t
    MRI FLAIR imaging of, 67–70
    multidetector computed tomography of, 7
    multiple aneurysms associated with, 238
    noncontrast computed tomography of, 9
    rebleeding risk of, 238
    routine serial follow-up, 460
    small subtle, 13
    surgical treatment of, 448
    traumatic aneurysm-related, 239
Hepatolenticular degeneration (Wilson disease), 399, 400b, 405
Hereditary spastic paresis, 354
Herniations, cerebral, 266
Herpes simplex virus infections, 366–367, 366t, 367f
Heteroplasmy, 393–397
Heterotopia
  subcortical band, 501
  subependymal, 502, 502f
Highly-active antiretroviral therapy (HAART), 345, 367
Hirayama disease, 354
"Hockey-stick" sign, 345–348, 355–356, 400
Holoprosencephalies, 497–500
  alobar, 497–500
  lobar, 499
  middle interhemispheric, 499, 499f
  semilobar, 499, 499f
Horner syndrome, 269
"Hot cross bun" sign, 343f, 352–353, 355
Hounsfield, Godfrey, 3

Human immunodeficiency virus (HIV) infection, of the central nervous system, 367, 370f
  conditions associated with
    cryptococcal meningitis, 366
    cryptococcoma, 378, 380f
    encephalitis, 367, 370f
    intracranial vasculopathy, 258
    mesenrhombencephalitis, 372–373
    myelopathy, 606, 606f
    progressive multifocal leukoencephalopathy, 114f, 370–371
"Hummingbird silhouette" sign, 344f
Hunter syndrome, 397f, 397b
Huntington disease, 333, 343, 345f, 399b, 408–409
  caudate nuclei atrophy in, 397, 489f
  dementia of, 333
Hurler syndrome, 396f, 397b
Hurler-Scheie syndrome, 397b
Hydranencephaly, 548, 548f
Hydrocephalus
  craniopharyngioma-related, 25
  normal pressure, 346f, 350f
  obstructive, 361
  tuberculoma-associated, 377f
  tuberculous meningitis-related, 363–364, 365f
Hydroxymethylglutaryl (HMG)-CoA lyase deficiency, 409
Hygroma
  cystic, 582, 585f
  subdural, 465f
Hyoglossus muscle, in squamous cell carcinoma of the tongue, 129
Hyperemia, 442
  as brain swelling cause, 461
  intracranial pressure in, 449–451
Hyperextension injuries, spinal, 476, 482–483, 487f
Hyperflexion injuries, spinal, 476, 480–482, 482f–483f
  levels of, 482–486
Hyperglycemia, nonketotic, 392, 409
Hyperintense putaminal rim sign, 343f, 355
Hyperintensity zone, 611
Hyperpharyngeal squamous cell carcinoma, recurrent, 185f
Hypertension, intracranial, cerebrospinal fluid space in, 451f
Hypoglossal artery, persistent, 220t
Hypoglottic squamous cell carcinoma, postsurgical, 194f
Hypoglycemia, 401
Hypometabolism, cerebral
  in neurodegenerative diseases, 355
  selective versus nonselective, 336–344
Hypoperfusion, cerebral
  in neurodegenerative diseases, 355
  selective versus nonselective, 336–344
Hypopharyngeal tumors, 142
  squamous cell carcinoma, 149, 151f, 156, 157f
Hypophyseal artery, inferior, 220–221
Hypothyroidism, in children, 400
Hypoxic-ischemic injuries, prenatal and neonatal, 533–541, 533–546, 534f–540f, 534t
  ischemic stroke, 541–545, 544f
  multicystic encephalomalacia, 541, 542f
  partial prolonged hypoxia-ischemia, 541, 543f
  profound asphyxia, 537–541, 539f–540f
  venous thrombosis, 545

I
ICSS (International Carotid Stenting Study), 262
Immunocompromised patients. See also Acquired immunodeficiency syndrome (AIDS); Human immunodeficiency virus (infection)
  cryptococcomas in, 378, 380f
  cytomegalovirus-related cerebellitis in, 370, 370f
  necrotic lymphoma in, 93f
Incus, 45f
Infarction, cerebral
  in anterior cerebral artery, 352
  cortical, neonatal, 544f
  infarct fogging of, 12
  in middle cerebral artery, 352
  restricted diffusion in, 405
  in tuberculous meningitis, 363–364, 365f
  in vascular dementia, 339
Infections
  cerebral, 361–382
  intrauterine and perinatal, 547–554
    common imaging findings in, 547–549
    congenital rubella (German measles), 549–550
    congenital syphilis, 549
    congenital varicella, 550–551
    cytomegalovirus, 549, 550f–551f
    differential diagnosis of, 549–552
    general considerations in, 547
    herpes simplex virus infections, 552
    human immunodeficiency virus (HIV) infection, 552
    hydranencephaly, 548, 548f
    intracranial calcifications, 548, 548f
    lymphocytic choriomeningitis virus, 551
    microcephaly, 548–549
    parvovirus B19, 551
    toxoplasmosis, 549, 553f–554f
    ventriculomegaly, 547–548, 548f
    West Nile virus, 552
  neonatal
    bacterial infections, 552–554
    fungal infections, 553–554, 553f–554f
  orbital, 43
  periorbital and orbital, 43
  spinal, 31–32, 47–51
Inferolateral trunk, 220–221, 225f
Inflammatory disorders
  of the brain, 361–382
  as brain tumor mimic, 112–113
  orbital, 40–43
Informed consent, for biopsy, 300
Innominate artery, as left common carotid artery origin site, 216–217
Intercostal artery, embolization of, 326f–327f
Intermediate injuries, 441f–442f
Internal carotid artery
  aneurysm of, 11f
  angiographic imaging of, 217–227
    anatomic segments, 218–227, 218f
    branches, 218–227
    C1 (cervical) segment, 217f, 218, 219f
    C2 (petrous) segment, 218–220, 219f, 222f
    C3 (lacerum) segment, 219f, 220
    C4 (cavernous) segment, 219f, 220–221, 223f, 225f
    C5 (clinoid) segment, 219f, 221
    C6 (communicating) segment, 219f, 224–227

Internal carotid artery *(Continued)*
　　C6 (ophthalmic) segment, 219f, 221–224, 226f
　　　carotid-basilar anastomoses, 218, 220f, 220t
　　　common variants, 218–227
　　　technique in, 212
　　cavernous, hyperdense mass on, 25, 29f
　　as circle of Willis component, 232, 233f
　　isolated, 234–236
　　left
　　　A1 segment fenestration of, 236f
　　　angiogram of, 233f
　　　dissection of, 17f
　　　occlusion of, 21, 23f
　　　pseudoaneurysm of, 16f
　　　stenosis of, 16f
　　occlusion of, 282f
　　posterior
　　　aneurysm of, 245
　　　angiographic evaluation of, 214f, 245
　　right, 234f–235f
　　　occlusion of, 265f
　　traumatic dissection of, 269
International Carotid Stenting Study (ICSS), 262
International Study of Unruptured Intracranial Aneurysms, 241–242
International Subarachnoid Aneurysm Trial (ISAT), 243
Interventional Management of Stroke (ISM) trials, 281–282
Intervertebral disc pathology, as low back pain cause, 610–611, 611f
Intraaxial injuries, pediatric, 469
Intraaxial tumors, common, 416–417
Intracranial dissection, 272–273, 272f
Intracranial pressure elevation
　　brain swelling-related, 442
　　cerebral edema-related, 449–451
　　hyperemia-related, 449–451
　　localized supratentorial, 451
　　Monro-Kellie hypothesis of, 4–7
　　in posterior fossa, 451–453, 453f
　　serial subacute imaging in, 464
Intramedullary process, 592f
Intraosseous disc, 307f
Intrauterine and perinatal infections
　　common imaging findings in, 547–549
　　congenital rubella (German measles), 549–550
　　congenital syphilis, 549
　　congenital varicella, 550–551
　　cytomegalovirus, 549, 550f–551f
　　differential diagnosis of, 549–552
　　general considerations in, 547
　　herpes simplex virus infections, 552
　　human immunodeficiency virus (HIV) infection, 552
　　hydranencephaly, 548, 548f
　　intracranial calcifications, 548, 548f
　　lymphocytic choriomeningitis virus, 551
　　microcephaly, 548–549
　　parvovirus B19, 551
　　toxoplasmosis, 549, 553f–554f
　　ventriculomegaly, 547–548, 548f
　　West Nile virus, 552
Iron deposition
　　in basal ganglia, 335
　　with neurodegeneration (NBIA), 400–401, 401, 400–401, 405b, 409
ISAT (International Subarachnoid Aneurysm Trial), 243
Ischemia, cerebral, acute *vs.* chronic, 73–74, 74f

ISM (Interventional Management of Stroke) trials, 281–282
Isotropic maps, 72, 72f

J
Jefferson (burst) fractures, 479, 479t, 483–484, 486f

K
Kearns-Sayre syndrome, 397, 399t, 400, 403f, 404b
Kennedy disease, 354
Kernicterus, 401, 404f
Kernohan notch syndrome, 443–444
Kidney cancer, metastatic, 611–612
Krabbe disease, 387–388, 389f, 401, 404–405
Kricheff, 276
KSS. *See* Kearns-Sayre syndrome
Kyphoscoliotic deformity, 37f

L
Labor and delivery, as pediatric head trauma cause, 466–469
Labyrinth, ossified, 34–35
Labyrinthine arteries, 228–230
Lacrimal artery, 224, 226f–227f
Lacrimal gland, adenoid cystic carcinoma of, 46–47
Lactate, 408–409, 408t
Lactate, elevated levels of, 79
Large vestibular aqueduct syndrome, 557, 559f
Larmor frequency, 61
Laryngeal squamous cell carcinoma, FDG PET/CT of
　　anatomic subsites in, 142–149
　　of cartilage involvement, 142, 145f–147f
　　glottic subtype of, 142–149, 145f, 147f, 150f, 152–156
　　metastases risk in, 166
　　post-treatment, 191
　　of primary tumor involvement, 142, 143f–145f
　　of recurrent disease, 182–184, 185f, 191, 196f
　　subglottic subtype of, metastatic, 154–156
　　subtypes of, 142–149
　　supraglottic subtype of, 142, 148f–150f, 149
　　　metastatic, 143f, 149f, 154–156, 156f–157f
　　　post-treatment, 173f
　　of tracheostomy site, 196f
　　transglottic subtype of, 142–149, 148f, 150f
　　　metastatic, 148f, 154–156
Laryngectomy, supraglottic, 134–135, 136f
Larynx
　　anatomic levels of, 142
　　squamous cell carcinoma of, 582, 583f
　　supraglottic, in tongue base squamous cell carcinoma, 134–135, 136f
Lathyrism, 354
Le Fort classification, of midface fractures, 456–457, 457f
Le Fort I fractures, 567, 569f
Leber hereditary optic neuropathy, 388–389, 392f, 397
Leg pain, 614–616
　　acute, postoperative, 618–619
　　chronic, postoperative, 619–623
　　nonradicular, 614, 616
　　radicular, 614–616
Leigh disease, 402f, 402b, 541
　　infantile-type, 402f

Leigh syndrome, 397, 399–400, 402f, 404b
Lemierre syndrome, 51, 53f, 584, 586f
Lens, subluxation of, 40
Leptomeningeal disease, 67–70
Leukemia
　　acute lymphoblastic, 379f
　　acute myelocytic, 378f
　　chronic lymphocytic, 315f
Leukodystrophies, 383–393, 383t
　　with bilateral caudothalamic groove involvement, 385
　　with bilateral optic nerve involvement, 389
　　with cystic white matter lesions, 388
　　with dense thalami and basal ganglia, 387–388
　　with diffuse hypomyelination, 390, 395f
　　with early predilection for anterior white matter, 386–387
　　with early predilection for posterior white matter, 386
　　with early subcortical white matter involvement, 388–389
　　fibrinoid, 386–387, 388f, 388b
　　globoid cell, 387–388, 388b, 389f
　　globus pallidus in, 401
　　with macrocephaly, 389
　　metachromatic, 385–386, 387f, 387b, 405, 409
　　with peritrigonal involvement, 384–388
　　spectroscopic metabolite patterns in, 408
　　with subcortical U fiber involvement, 389
　　with symmetric anterior and posterior distribution, 385–386
　　with tigroid-pattern perivascular white matter, 387f, 389–390
　　with white matter abnormalities, 384t
Leukoencephalopathies
　　facilitated diffusion in, 404–405
　　hereditary, 383–384
　　megaloencephalic, 388, 390b
　　　with subcortical cysts, 390b
　　posttraumatic bifrontal, 468f
　　progressive multifocal, 370–372, 371f
　　　HIV infection-associated, 114f
　　radiation, 100
Ligamentous injuries, spinal, 485, 488f
Lipids, elevated levels of, 79
Lipoma, 61
　　as chemical shift artifact cause, 68f
　　of the corpus callosum, 497, 498f
Lissencephaly, 500–501, 501f
　　classical, 500–501, 501f
　　cobblestone, 501, 502f
Listeria monocytogenes infections
　　meningitis, 361
　　mesenrhombencephalitis, 372–373, 372f
Liver disease, Zellweger syndrome-related, 385
Locked-in cages, 624
Lou Gehrig disease. *See* Amyotrophic lateral sclerosis
Low back pain, 610–616
　　acute, 610–614
　　　aseptic, 610–611
　　　cauda equina syndrome-related, 610
　　　infection-related, 610
　　　postoperative, 618
　　　trauma-related, 610
　　chronic, 611–614
　　　metastases-related, 611–613
　　　nonradicular, 616
　　　radicular, 614–616
　　　scoliosis-related, 613–614
　　　systemic disease-related, 613
　　red flags in, 613f

Lowe syndrome (oculocerebrorenal syndrome), 21, 388, 390f, 390b, 409
Luessenhop, A. J., 276
Lumbar disc herniation, as leg pain cause, 614–616, 615f–616f, 619, 621f
Lumbar spine, postoperative, 618–623
　acute recurring leg pain and, 618–619
　acute recurring low back pain and, 618
Lung cancer, 110f, 166–168
　metastatic, 611–612
Lyme disease, 258
Lymphadenitis, human immunodeficiency virus infection-related, 54f
Lymphangioma, 46–47, 49f
Lymphatic malformations, orbital, 46, 49f
Lymphoma, 25–28, 30f, 85
　Burkitt, 25, 29f
　cerebral
　　differentiated from bacterial abscess, 107
　　differentiated from cerebral toxoplasmosis, 374–378
　　differentiation from glioma, 417
　　perfusion values in, 422f
　of the neck, 584, 587f
　necrotic, in immunocompromised patients, 93f
　orbital, 46–47, 565, 568f
　perfusion values in, 417, 422f
　spinal, 33
　　anaplastic, 38f
Lysosomal storage disorders, 383t
　globoid cell leukodystrophy, 387–388, 388b, 389f
　metachromatic leukodystrophy, 385–386, 387f, 387b

M

Macrocephaly, 389
Magnetic resonance angiography (MRA)
　for aneurysm follow-up, 249
　of carotid disease, 262
　contrast enhanced, 74, 76f
　of intracranial dissection, 272–273
　of ischemic stroke, 263
　time-of-flight (TOF), 74, 76f
　　flow-related enhancement in, 74
　of vascular cerebral malformations, with arteriovenous shunting, 255–257
Magnetic resonance imaging (MRI)
　advanced, 79–125. See also Dynamic contrast susceptibility perfusion magnetic resonance imaging (DCS MRI); Magnetic resonance spectroscopy (MRS); Magnetic resonance imaging (MRI), perfusion imaging
　　for bacterial and tuberculous infections imaging, 107–112
　　as biomarker for antiandrogenic agents, 116–118
　　for brain tumor imaging, 85–106
　　of conditions which mimic brain tumors, 112–113
　　of developmental diseases, 123
　　imaging techniques in, 79–85
　　of metabolic diseases, 123
　　of neurodegenerative diseases, 118–123
　　pitfalls in, 113–114
　　of white matter diseases, 123
　artifacts in, 66–67, 66–67, 68f
　basic sequences in, 63
　　fluid-attenuated inversion recovery (FLAIR), 64f, 65
　　gradient refocused echo, 63–65, 64f

Magnetic resonance imaging (MRI) (Continued)
　　inversion recovery, 64f, 65
　　spin echo, 63, 64f
　　spoiled or incoherent GRE, 63–64
　　unspoiled or coherent GRE, 64–65
　of brain tumors
　　key questions in, 412
　　practical aspects of, 414–423
　comparison with multidetector computed-tomography, 3, 4t
　current research and future directions in, 76–78
　diffusion tensor, 74, 79–82
　　of aging brain, 335
　　of amyotrophic lateral sclerosis, 123
　diffusion-weighted, 71–74, 73f, 79–82
　　of abscess, 107, 107f–111f, 373f, 375f–376f
　　in acute stroke, 15
　　apparent diffusion coefficient maps in, 73
　　of brain tumors, 101, 105f
　　of glioblastoma multiforme, 120f
　　isotropic maps in, 71, 72f
　　of metabolic disorders, 404–405
　　of subdural empyema, 361–362, 363f
　　in therapeutic follow-up, 101
　　of tuberculomas, 374, 377f
　　as tumor cellularity indicator, 85–97, 90f
　false positive/false negative results in, 66–67
　fast imaging techniques in, 65
　　comparison among, 66f
　　echo planar imaging (EPI), 65
　　fast spin-echo (FSE), 65, 66f
　　half-Fourier acquisition single-shot turbo spin echo (HASTE), 65
　　rapid acquisition with refocused echo (RARE), 65
　　single-shot RARE, 65
　　turbo spin-echo (TSE), 65, 66f
　fat saturation, frequency-selective, 71, 71f
　fluid-attenuated inversion recovery (FLAIR), 63, 65, 67–70
　　in herpes simplex encephalitis, 366–367, 367f
　　of high-grade glioma, 88f
　　of progressive multifocal leukoencephalopathy, 371f
　　of pyogenic meningitis, 361, 362f
　　of toxoplasmosis, 112f–113f
　　of tuberculous abscess, 112f–113f
　free induction decay in, 61
　frequency-encoding gradient in, 61–62
　gradient echo, 67
　gradient-recalled echo, 69f
　high-field strength in, 76, 77f
　　specific absorption rate (SAR) of, 77
　image generation in, 61–62
　image quality in, 63
　inversion recovery, 64f, 65
　　short tau (STIR), 65
　Larmor frequency in, 61
　normal image appearance in, 65–67
　perfusion, 82–85. See also Dynamic susceptibility contrast perfusion magnetic resonance imaging (DSC MRI); Dynamic contrast-enhanced magnetic resonance imaging (DCE MRI)
　　alternate multiparametric algorithmic approach in, 97–99
　　multiparametric algorithmic approach in, 85–97
　　for therapeutic monitoring, 99–106

Magnetic resonance imaging (MRI) (Continued)
　　phase-encoding gradient in, 61–62
　　physical basis of, 61
　　pitfalls and limitations of, 75–76
　　as problem-solving tool, 61
　　proton density parameter of, 62–63
　　RF coils in, 62, 62f
　　slice-select gradient in, 61–62
　　specific uses for, 67
　　spin echo, 67
　　of spine trauma, 474–475
　　systems for image analysis with, 67–74
　　T1-weighted, 62
　　T2-weighted, 62–63
　　　comparison with CT, 69f
　　time to echo in, 63
　　time to repetition in, 63
　　tissue contrast in, 62–65
　　in tuberculous meningitis, 363–364, 365f
　　turbo spin echo, 67
　　two-dimensional, image generation in, 62
　　volumetric, of brain volume loss "atrophy," 335
Magnetic resonance spectroscopy (MRS), 79
　advanced techniques in, 79
　of aging brain, 335
　of metabolic disorders, 405–409
　of white matter diseases, 123
Mandible
　fractures of, 456, 456f
　squamous cell carcinoma of, 133f, 136, 161
Mandibular reconstructions, 191
Maple syrup urine disease, 390–392, 395f, 395b, 405, 409
Marfan syndrome, 241
Masticator space and oral cavity pathology, 129–133, 573–578
　ameloblastoma, 577–578, 578f
　lingual tonsil squamous cell carcinoma, 575, 577f
　peritonsillar abscess, 574, 576f
　retromolar tongue carcinoma, 575–577, 577f
　rhabdomyosarcoma, 577, 578f
Mastoid bone, fractures of, 42f, 448, 449f
Mastoiditis, acute, 559, 560f
Maxilla
　fractures of, 569f
　squamous cell carcinoma invasion of, 161, 162f
Maxillary sinus
　foreign body in, 7f
　silent sinus syndrome of, 45, 48f
　sinonasal oncocytic Scheiderian papilloma of, 202f
McLeod, Allan, 3
Mechanical embolus retrieval in cerebral ischemia (MERCI) device, 282f–283f, 284
Medial lenticulostriate arteries, 233–234
Median prosencephalic vein, in vein of Galen aneurysmal malformations (VGAMs), 253
Medical implants, implication for MRI, 75–76
Medulla, perforating arterial supply to, 230
Medulloblastoma, recurrent, 101, 105f
Mega cistern magna, 504, 504f
Megadolichobasilar anomaly, 238
Melanoma, 413f
　ocular, 46–47
MELAS (mitochondrial myopathy, encephalopathy, lactic acidosis, and stroke-like episodes), 25, 399, 404–405, 407f, 407b, 541

Index

Melting brain syndrome, 254
Memory loss, 335-336
Meningeal arteries
  anterior, 228
  hypertrophied, "sunburst" pattern of, 266, 267f-268f
  middle, 227f
  posterior, 228, 230f
  recurrent, 227f
Meningioma, 25, 25f-26f, 412
  atypical, 117f-118f
  blood-brain barrier in, 416
  differential diagnosis of, 591t
  differentiated from
    acoustic neuroma, 116
    schwannoma, 425f, 423, 424f
  as extraaxial tumor, 417, 423f
  falcine, 117f-118f
  optic nerve sheath, 46-47
  perfusion metrics of, 82-85
  preoperative angiographic evaluation of, 266, 267f
  preoperative embolization of, 291
  relative cerebral blood flow levels in, 114-116
Meningitis, 361-366
  aspergillosis-related, 374
  bacterial, 361
  cryptococcal, 366
  as neurosyphilis risk factor, 345
  pyogenic, 361, 362f
  tuberculous, 363-364, 364f-365f
Meningocele, postoperative, 621-622, 622f
Meningohypoglossal artery, 220-221, 224f
Meningohypophyseal artery/trunk, 224f
Menkes kinky hair disease, 398b
Menkes syndrome, 393, 399t
MERCI (mechanical embolus retrieval in cerebral ischemia) device, 282f-283f, 284
MERRF (myoclonus epilepsy with ragged red fibers), 390, 393-397, 394f, 394b, 399t, 408
Mesenrhombencephalitis, 372-373, 372f
Metabolic disorders, 383-411
  classification of, 383t, 389-390
  of cortical gray matter, 393-401
  of deep gray matter, 393-401
  diffusion-weighted imaging of, 404-405
  magnetic resonance spectroscopy of, 405-409
  orbital, 40-43
  of white matter (myelination disorders), 383-393
    central disorders, 384-388, 384f-385f, 385b
    peripheral disorders, 388-389
    progressive multifocal leukoencephalopathy, 370-371
Metallic artifacts
  in computed tomography, 30-31
  in magnetic resonance imaging, 30-31
  in noncontrast computed tomography, 13
Metastases
  versus cellular marrow proliferation, 592-594, 600f
  cerebral
    as brain tumor mimic, 416-417
    differentiated from bacterial abscess, 110f
    with edema, 421f
    extracranial, preoperative embolization of, 291

Metastases (Continued)
  intracranial, preoperative embolization of, 291
  vertebral
    as leg pain cause, 616
    as low back pain cause, 611-613, 613f
Methylguanine-DNA methyltransferase (MGMT) promoter methylation status, 106
"Mickey Mouse" sign, 344f, 355
Microcatheters, flow-guided or guidewire-directed, 276
Microcephaly, 548-549
Microfractures, spinal, 485
Microhemorrhage, 70f
Microhemosiderin deposits, multifocal, 335
Middle cerebral artery
  aneurysms of, 242-243, 245f
    angiographic evaluation of, 245
    ruptured, 261f
  occlusion of, 226f, 282f
  perfusion imaging of, 19-21, 20f
  stroke-related hyperdensity of, 12-13, 13f
  stroke-related infarcts in, 352
Middle cranial fossa, venous epidural hematoma of, 432f
Midface, fractures of, 456-457, 457f
Mitochondrial disorders, 383t
  maple syrup urine disease, 390-392, 395f, 395b, 405, 409
  myoclonus epilepsy with ragged red fibers (MERRF), 390, 394f, 394b
Mitochondrial myopathy, encephalopathy, lactic acidosis, and stroke-like episodes (MELAS), 25, 397, 399, 399t, 404-405, 407f, 407b
Mitochondrial respiratory chain insufficiency theory, 400
Modic changes, in vertebral end plates, 611, 611t, 612f, 618
  differentiated from spinal tumors, 591, 594f, 598f
Molar tooth malformation, 504, 505f
Mondini malformation, 33, 41f
Moniz, Egas, 211, 276
Mononeuritis multiplex, cytomegalovirus-related, 370
"Moose sign," 468f
Morquio syndrome, 397b
"Mother-in-law" sign, 266
Motion/ghost artifacts, in MRI, 66
Motor neuron diseases, atypical, differentiated from amyotrophic lateral sclerosis, 354
Mount Sinai Medical Center, epilepsy imaging protocol at, 510t
Mouth floor, squamous cell carcinoma of, 128f, 129, 132f
Movement disorders. See also Huntington disease; Parkinson disease
  definition of, 333
  nonparkinson, 336
Moyamoya disease, 258, 295f, 296
Moyamoya-like angiographic pattern, 257-258
MR RESCUE trial, 284
Mucocele, 567-568, 570f
  nasolacrimal, 456
Mucoepidermoid carcinoma, 133-134
  of the soft palate, 141
Mucopolysaccharidoses, 388, 392-393, 396f, 404-405, 408
  metabolite patterns in, 409
  type IH (Hurler syndrome), 396f
  type IIA (Hunter syndrome), 397f, 397b

Mucormycosis, periorbital and orbital, 43
Multidetector computed tomography, 3-60
  of cervical spinal masses and infections, 47-51
  comparison with magnetic resonance imaging, 3, 4t
  in the emergency department, 3-9
    of foreign bodies, 4, 7f-8f
    of intracranial hemorrhage, 4-9, 8f-9f
    of skull fractures, 3-4, 5f-6f
  of head and neck pathologies, 33-47
    of congenital orbital conditions, 46-47
    of inflammatory and metabolic conditions, 40-43
    of orbital pathologies, 40
    of orbital trauma, 40
    of periorbital and orbital infections, 43-45
    of temporal bone pathology, 33-34
  in intracranial neoplastic conditions, 21-28
  spinal, 28-33
    for preoperative and postoperative evaluations, 30-31
    of spinal infections, 31-32
    of spinal trauma, 28-30
    of spinal tumors, 32-33
  of spine trauma, 473-475, 475f
  state of the art and future trends in, 51-59, 54f
    contrast resolution, 52
    dual-source and dual-energy computed tomography, 53-56, 55f
    spatial resolution, 51-52
    temporal resolution, 52-53
    wide-coverage scanners, 56
  in stroke management, 9-21, 11f-13f
Multiple myeloma, 33, 39f
Multiple sclerosis, T2 white matter hyperintensities in, 355
Multisystem atrophy, 343f
  differentiated from Parkinson disease, 354f
  with parkinsonism symptoms, 352-353
Muscular atrophy, postpolio, 354
Mycetoma, 569-570
Mycobacterium tuberculosis infections, 372-373
Myelinolysis, central pontine, 392, 395f
Myelinopathies, 383-393, 384t
Myelitis
  cytomegalovirus-related, 370
  human immunodeficiency virus (HIV) infection-related, 606
Myelohyoid muscles, in squamous cell carcinoma of the tongue, 130f-131f
Myeloma, multiple, 31f
Myelopathy, human immunodeficiency virus (HIV) infection-related, 606f
Myoclonus epilepsy with ragged red fibers (MERRF), 390, 393-397, 394f, 394b, 399t, 408
Myoinositol, 408-409, 408t
  in Alzheimer disease dementia, 119, 121f
Myopathy, mitochondrial, 541
Myositis, orbital, 41, 46f

N

Nasopharynx
  in palate squamous cell carcinoma, 134f
  in tongue squamous cell carcinoma, 130f-131f
National Cancer Institute of Canada, 101-106

National Emergency X-Radiography Utilization Study (NEXUS), 610
National Institutes of Neurological Disorders and Stroke (NINDS) trial, 281
NBCS embolic agent, 287
Neck
 blunt vascular injuries to, 474
 lymphoma of, 584, 587f
Neck pain, 623–624
Neck squamous cell carcinoma. *See* Head and neck squamous cell carcinoma
Necrosis, therapy-induced, 99–106, 101f, 106f
Needlestick injuries, 321, 328f
Neisseria meningitides infections, 361
Neonates
 bacterial infections in, 552–554
 fungal infections in, 553–554, 553f–554f
 hypoxic-ischemic injuries in
  ischemic stroke, 541–545, 544f
   multicystic encephalomalacia, 541, 542f
   partial prolonged hypoxia-ischemia, 541, 543f
   profound asphyxia, 537–541, 539f–540f
   venous thrombosis, 545
Neovascularity, 266
Nerve sheath tumors, 417
Neuritis, optic, 40–41
Neuroblastoma, 33f, 46
 as bone erosion cause, 28, 33f
 olfactory, 571–572, 572f
Neurocutaneous syndromes, angiographic evaluation of, 257, 257t
Neurodegeneration with brain iron accumulation (NBIA), 356, 401, 409
Neurodegenerative disorders, 333–360. *See also* Dementia
 characteristic imaging features in, 354–356
 clinical diagnosis of, 335–336
 definitions of, 333–354
 hypometabolism in, 355
 hypoperfusion in, 355
 specific imaging signs in, 355–356
 specific radiotracer uptake in, 355
Neuroepithelial tumors, 412
Neurofibrillary tangles, in Alzheimer's disease, 336
Neurofibroma, 49f
 orbital, 46–47
Neurofibromatosis, type 1, 46, 49f, 241, 257–258, 257t
Neurointerventional radiology, 276–298
 of acute stroke
  aggressive mechanical clot disruption techniques, 284
  intravenous thrombolysis, 281–284, 282f, 283f
 brief historical background of, 276
 of central nervous system arteriovenous lesions, 286–289
 of extracranial carotid atherosclerotic disease, 284–286
 of pediatric cerebral arteriovenous malformations, 294, 294f
 of pediatric vascular lesions, 292–296
 preoperative vascular tumor embolization, 291–292
 of spinal vascular malformations, 289–291
Neuroma, acoustic, differentiated from meningioma, 116

Neuronal ceroid lipofuscinosis (NCL), 393, 398b
NEUROSTAT, 336–337
Neurosyphilis, 345, 348f
NEXUS (National Emergency X-Radiography Utilization Study), 610
North American Symptomatic Carotid Endarterectomy Trial (NASCET), 261–262, 284–285

O

Occipital bone, fractures of, 6f
Oculocerebrorenal syndrome (Lowe syndrome), 21, 388, 390f, 390b, 409
Odontoid fractures, 480f–481f
Oligoastrocytoma, 414f
Oligodendroglioma, 412
 calcified, 419f
 grade II, 416f
 low-grade, 87f, 113–114
  cerebral blood volume within, 87f
  choline elevation in, 87f
  perfusion of, 85, 87f
 1p 19q chromosomal deletion in, 114, 115f–116f
Onyx embolic agent, 276, 287, 287f
 as artifact cause, 13
Ophthalmic artery, 219f, 224, 226f–227f
 anomalous origin of, 227f
Ophthalmic vein
 dilated tortuous right superior, 566f
 superior, in carotid-cavernous fistula, 454, 455f
Ophthalmology, thyroid-associated. *See* Graves disease
Ophthalmoplegia, chronic progressive external (CPEO), 404b
Optic nerve
 fracture-related compression of, 457
 in Krabbe disease, 387–388
 in Leber optic neuropathy, 389
 in Zellweger syndrome, 385
Optic nerve glioma, 565, 568f
Optic nerve sheath, meningioma of, 46–47
Oral and oropharyngeal squamous cell carcinoma, FDG PET/CT evaluation of, 126–141
 anatomic subsites in, 126
 genioglossus muscles in
  in buccal mucosa squamous cell carcinoma, 133f
  in squamous cell carcinoma of the tongue, 128f–129f, 129
  in tongue squamous cell carcinoma, 130f–131f
 hyoglossus muscle in, 129f
 metastatic, 128f, 137f, 153–154, 156f
 of mouth floor, 128f, 129, 132f
 myelohyoid muscles in, 130f–131f
 nasopharynx in
  in palate squamous cell carcinoma, 134f
  in tongue squamous cell carcinoma, 130f–131f
 osteotomy-related FDG uptake in, 193
 pharyngeal recess in, 130f–131f
 with possible bone metastases, 149f
 post-surgical, 198f–199f
 recurrent, 170–182
 streak artifacts in, 129–133, 133f
 of subtypes, 134–141
Orbital pathology, 562–565
 congenital conditions, 46
 congenital tumors, 46–47
 fractures, 457, 566f
  orbital blowout, 13, 457, 458f, 563, 566f

Orbital pathology (*Continued*)
 Graves disease, 564–565, 567f
 hemangiomas, 562, 565f
 infections, 43
 inflammatory and metabolic conditions, 40–43
 lymphoma, 565, 568f
 masses and neoplasms, 46–47
 multidetector computed tomography of, 40, 43–45
 oblique sagittal section through, 45f
 ocular cellulitis, 563–564, 566f
 optic nerve glioma, 565, 568f
 orbital venous varix, 562–563, 566f
 sagittal section through, 45f
 Sjögren syndrome, 564, 567f
 traumatic injuries, 40, 454–458
 vascular and lymphatic malformations, 46
Orbitopathy, thyroid-associated, 40–41
Osmotic demyelination syndrome, 392, 395f
Ossicular chain, 44f
Osteochondroma, 33
Osteoid osteoma, 33
Osteomyelitis, 309f
Osteotomy, FDG uptake in, 193
Otic artery, persistent, 218–220, 220t
Otic capsule, mineralization/demineralization of, 35
Otosclerosis, 33
Overlap syndromes, 354
Oxygen therapy, effect on MRI scans, 67–70

P

Pacemakers, implication for MRI, 75–76
Palate cell carcinoma, with bone metastases, 161, 163f
Pantothenate kinase-associated neurodegeneration (PKAN), 401, 405f, 405b
Papez circuit, 508
Papilloma, choroid plexus, 47
Paraganglioma, intercarotid, 49, 52f
Paraglottic fat plane, laryngeal tumor invasion of, 148f
Paramagnetic materials, 67
Paramyxovirus infections, 366t
Parapharyngeal space, tonsillar squamous cell carcinoma invasion of, 136
Paraplegia, spastic, without amyotrophy, 336
Parietal bone, fractures of, 5f–6f
Parkinson disease
 with amyotrophic lateral sclerosis, 333
 with dementia, 340, 350f
 dementia of, 333
 differentiated from
  corticobasal degeneration, 354
  multisystem atrophy, 352–353
  progressive supranuclear palsy, 353–354, 354f
 idiopathic, 340, 342f
Parkinson disorders, atypical, definition of, 333
Parkinson plus disorders, 333, 336
Parkinson plus syndromes, 352
Parkinsonian symptoms, 336
Parkinsonian syndromes, clinically uncertain (CUPS), 353
PD. *See* Parkinson disease
"Pearl and string" sign, 238, 272
Pearson syndrome, 404b
Pedicle screws, malplacement of, 618
Pelizaeus-Merzbacher disease, 385–386, 390, 393f, 393b

"Penguin silhouette" sign, 344f, 353–355
Penumbra system, 281–282, 284
Perfusion studies, of acute stroke, 15–21, 18f–20f, 22f
Perinatal infections. See Intrauterine and perinatal infections
Periodontal disease, effect on FDG uptake, 191, 195f–196f
Perivascular spaces, mucopolysaccharidosis-related dilation of, 392–393, 396f
Periventricular leukoencephalomalacia, 533, 535f–536f
    cystic, 535f, 537f
Periventricular white matter
    in premature neonate, 534f
Peroxisomal disorders, 383t, 383–384
    adrenoleukodystrophy, 384f
    X-linked, 384–385, 385b
    adrenoleukomyeloneuropathy, 385b
    Zellweger syndrome (cerebrohepatorenal syndrome), 385, 386f, 386b, 404–405
Pharyngeal recess, in tongue squamous cell carcinoma, 130f–131f
Pharyngeal wall, in tongue squamous cell carcinoma, 136f
Pharyngoepiglottic folds, in tongue squamous cell carcinoma, 134–135
Phenylketonuria, 386, 387b, 405, 409
Pick disease, 339
Picture Archiving and Communication System (PACS), 13
Pilocytic tumors, 417
Piriform sinus
    hypopharyngeal tumors of, 142, 149, 151f
    squamous cell carcinoma of, 202f
Pittsburgh B compound, 355
Pituitary adenoma, presurgical angiographic evaluation of, 266
Pituitary blush, posterior, 224f
Pituitary macroadenoma, 25, 28f
Plasmacytoma, 33
Pneumocephalus, 15–19, 28, 32f, 448
Pneumorbit, tension, 457
Poliodystrophies. See also Cortical gray matter disorders
    progressive cerebral (Alpers syndrome), 393, 398f, 398b, 401
Polyarteritis nodosa, 258
Polymicrogyria, 502–503, 502f
Polyomavirus, 370–371
Polyposis, sinonasal, 567, 569f
Polyradiculopathy, cytomegalovirus-related, 370
Pons, perforating arterial supply to, 230
Pontine perforating arteries, 228–230, 230f
Pöschl plane, 33–35, 39f
Positron emission tomography (PET)
    of Alzheimer's disease, 336–337, 337f
    amyloid, 337, 338f, 351f
Posterior cerebral artery, 232–233, 233f
    fetal, 234–236
    ischemic infarction of, 447f
Posterior communicating artery, 219f, 220t, 224, 232–236, 233f–234f
    absent, 234–236
    aneurysm of, 234f–235f, 244f, 245, 247
    fetal-type, 232
    infundibulum of, 224
    small, 234–236
Posterior fossa
    intracranial pressure elevation in, 451–453, 453f
    MRI FLAIR imaging of, 70
Posterior inferior cerebellar artery, 214f, 228, 229f–230f

Posterior reversible leukoencephalopathy syndrome (PRES), 260
Posterior thalamoperforating arteries, 214f, 233–234
Preepiglottic fat plane, laryngeal tumor invasion of, 148f
Pregnancy
    MRI during, 76
    reversible cerebral vasoconstriction syndromes of, 221f, 260
Premature neonates, hypoxic-ischemic injuries in, 533–536, 534f, 534t
    computed tomography of, 534
    diffusion-weighted resonance spectroscopy of, 536
    germinal matrix hemorrhage, 536–537, 537t, 538f
    magnetic resonance imaging of, 534
    magnetic resonance spectroscopy of, 536
    periventricular leukoencephalomalacia, 533, 535f–536f
Prion disease, 336
PROACT II trial, 284
Proatlantal intersegmental artery, 220t
Probst bundles, 496
Progressive supranuclear palsy, 333, 342, 344f, 353–354, 354f
Proptosis
    of the globe, 49f
    orbital, 49f
Prostate cancer, 309f
    metastatic, 311f, 611–612
Pseudoaneurysms
    oncotic, 239
    traumatic, 266–271
Pseudocysts, gelatinous, 366
Pseudomeningocele, 621–622, 622f
Pseudomeningocele, posttraumatic, 30, 36f
Pseudoprogression, of brain tumors, 101–106, 106f
Pseudotumor, orbital, 40–43, 46f
PSP. See Progressive supranuclear palsy
Pterygoid muscles, in squamous cell carcinoma of the tongue, 130f–131f
"Pulvinar" sign, 345–348, 355–356
Putamen, in deep gray matter diseases, 399–400
Putaminal rim sign, 343f, 355

R
Radiation therapy
    effect on central white matter, 392, 396f
    as pseudoprogression cause, 101–106, 106f
Radicular pain, low back, 614–616
Radiotracer uptake, in neurodegenerative diseases, 355
Ragged red fibers, 399t
Rectus muscle, medial, central deviation of, 48f
Recurrent artery of Heubner, 233–234
Renal cell carcinoma, metastatic, 304f
Renal failure
    acute, diagnostic angiography-related, 215
    chronic, as contraindication to gadolinium-based contrast agents, 76
Retinitis, cytomegalovirus-related, 370
Retinoblastoma, 47, 50f
    orbital, 46–47
Reversible cerebral vasculopathy syndromes (RCVS), 260, 260t
Rhabdomyosarcoma, 577, 578f
    alveolar-type, 47, 50f
    differentiated from lymphangiomas, 46
Rheumatoid disease, 258

Rhinorrhea, posttraumatic, 466
Right subclavian artery, angiogram of, 213f

S
Sacral mass, hypervascular, 322f–325f
Salivary gland pathology, 572–573
    AIDS-related parotid cysts, 572–573, 574f
    pleomorphic adenoma, 573, 575f
    sialolithiasis and sialadenitis, 572, 573f
    tumors, 141, 152
Sandhoff disease, 401, 406b, 409
Sanfilippo syndrome, 397b
Sarcoidosis, 258
    orbital, 40–41
Scheie syndrome, 397b
Schizencephaly, 503, 503f
Schwannoma
    acoustic, 561, 565f
    angiographic evaluation of, 266
    differential diagnosis of, 591t
    differentiated from meningioma, 423, 424f–425f, 425f
    relative cerebral blood flow levels in, 114–116
    sympathetic chain, 49
SCIWORA ("spinal cord injury without radiographic abnormalities"), 488, 490f
Scleroderma, 258
Sclerosis
    primary lateral, 336, 354
    of the skull, 32f
    spinal, 38f
Scoliosis, 30, 37f
    as low back pain cause, 613–614, 614f
Segmental callosal hypoplasia, 496–497
Seizures, 507
Sella tumors, as extraaxial tumor, 417
Sella turcica-sphenoid sinus complex, fractures of, 266–269
Semicircular canals
    involvement in mastoid fractures, 42f
    superior
        dehiscence syndrome of, 33–34, 39f
        Stenvers and Pöschl orientation planes of, 33, 39f
Sepetka, Ivan, 276–277
Septooptic dysplasia, 499–500
Serbinenko, F. A., 276
Shermna, F. E., 276
Shunts
    arteriovenous, 266
    dural arteriovenous. See Fistula, dural arteriovenous
    ventricular, 448
Shy-Drager syndrome, 341, 343f
Sialadenitis, 572, 573f
Sialolithiasis, 572, 573f
Sickle cell disease, 241, 257–258, 257t
Silent sinus syndrome, 45, 48f
Sinonasal cavity pathology, 565–572
    fungal sinusitis, 569–570, 570f
    juvenile nasopharyngeal angiofibroma, 571, 571f
    Le Fort I fractures, 567, 569f
    mucocele, 567–568, 570f
    olfactory neuroblastoma, 571–572, 572f
    sinonasal polyposis, 567, 569f
    squamous cell carcinoma, 572, 573f
Sinusitis, fungal, 569–570, 570f
Sjögren syndrome, 258, 564, 567f
Skull base tumors, presurgical angiographic evaluation of, 266
Skull fractures, 429, 430f
    basal, 239
    depressed, 429, 430f

Skull fractures *(Continued)*
  epidural hematoma associated with, 432f
  multidetector computed tomography evaluation of, 3–4, 5f–6f
  multiple, 441f–442f
  pediatric, 469, 470f
  "ping-pong," 470, 470f
  semicircular canal involvement in, 42f
Small perforating arteries, 228, 230f
"Soap bubbles," 366
Soft palate squamous cell carcinoma, 141, 141f
  metastatic, 136, 141f, 154
SOMATOM Definition dual-source computed tomography scanners, 53
Spence, W. T., 276
Spetzler-Martin Grading System, for arteriovenous malformations, 250, 250t, 251f
Sphenoid bone
  eosinophilic granuloma of, 25, 27f
  fibrous dysplasia of, 31f
  neuroblastoma of, 33f
Sphenoid bone, fractures of, 457
Spinal artery
  anterior, 228, 229f, 289, 289f
  posterior, 228, 290
Spinal asymmetry, 613
Spinal canal, meningeal layers of, 590f
Spinal cord
  in deep gray matter diseases, 399–400
  diffusion tensor imaging of, 601, 603f
  hemangioblastoma of, 596f
  magnetic resonance spectroscopy of, 601, 603f
  normal blood supply to, 289–290
Spinal cord injuries, 486–490, 489f
Spinal cord injury without radiographic abnormalities (SCIWORA), 488
Spinal cord metastases, differential diagnosis of, 591t
Spinal infections, 31–32, 589–609, 601, 610
  differential diagnosis of
    infectious myelitis *versus* demyelinating disease or tumor, 606–607, 606f
    infectious spondylodiscitis *versus* dialysis spondyloarthropathy, 603, 605f
    infectious spondylodiscitis *versus* spondylosis, 603, 604f
    noninfectious/inflammatory processes, 601–607
    septic arthritis of facet joints *versus* aseptic facet synovitis, 603, 605f
    versus spinal tumors, 591–592, 599f
    suspected infectious spondylodiscitis, 607, 607f–608f
  localization of, 601
Spinal muscular atrophy, type IV, 354
Spinal nerve root injuries, 486–490, 492f
Spinal pain
  leg pain and, 614–616
    nonradicular, 614, 616
    radicular, 614–616
  low back, 610–616
    acute, 610–614
    cauda equina syndrome–related, 610
    chronic, 611–614
    infection-related, 610
    metastases-related, 611–613
    nonradicular, 616
    radicular, 614–616
    scoliosis-related, 613–614, 614f
    systemic disease–related, 613
    trauma-related, 610

Spinal stenosis, 616–618, 617f
  postoperative, 621
Spinal trauma
  as low back pain cause, 610
  triage of, 474t
Spinal trauma imaging, 28–30, 473
  acute, 475–476, 490–491
    three-column stability concept of, 475, 476f
  atlantoaxial dislocations, 477, 478f
  atlantoaxial rotations, 477, 478f
  atlantooccipital dislocations, 477, 477f
  bone contusions, 485, 488f
  C2 fractures, 479, 480f–481f
  at craniovertebral junction, 477, 479, 481f
  of craniovertebral junction, 477
  delayed findings in, 493–494, 494f
  disc injuries, 484, 487f
  epidural hematoma, 488–489, 491f
  indications for, 473–475
  ligamentous injuries, 485, 488f
  microfractures, 485
  pitfalls in, 491–493, 493f
  SCIWORA ("spinal cord injury without radiographic abnormalities"), 488, 490f
  spinal cord injuries, 494f
  subdural hematoma, 488–489
  vertical compression injuries, 483–484
  whiplash injuries, 485–486
Spinal tumors, 32–33, 589–609
  advanced imaging of, 601
  detection of, 589
    for differential diagnosis, 589–591, 591t
  differential diagnosis of, 591t
    versus atypical hemangioma, 591, 597f
    versus infection, 591–592, 599f
    metastases *versus* cellular marrow proliferation, 592–594, 600f
    versus Modic changes, 591, 594f, 598f
    pathologic fractures *versus* benign osteoporotic compression fractures, 594–595, 601f
    "pseudohypointense" vertebral body lesions, 595–601, 602f
  localization of, 589
    for differential diagnosis, 589–591, 591t
Spine
  multidetector computed tomography of, 28–33
    for preoperative and postoperative evaluations, 30–31
    of spinal infections, 31–32
    of spinal trauma, 28–30
    of spinal tumors, 32–33
  vascular malformations of, 289–291
Spondylitis, tuberculous, 599f, 608f
Spondyloarthropathy, dialysis, 603, 605f
Spondylodiscitis
  infectious, 31, 38f, 607, 607f
    versus dialysis spondyloarthropathy, 603, 605f
    versus spondylosis, 603, 604f
    suspected radiographically, 607, 607f–608f
  tuberculous, 31–32
  postoperative, 618, 620f
  pyogenic, 607f
  sterile, 618
Spondylolisthesis, 37f
Spondylolysis, traumatic C2, 481f
Spondylosis
  degenerative, 604f
  as leg pain cause, 616
Sporadic olivopontocerebellar atrophy, 341

"Spot" sign, 7–9, 10f, 55
Squamous cell carcinoma
  of external carotid artery, 239
  of the head and neck. *See* Head and neck squamous cell carcinoma
  of the larynx, 582, 583f
  lingual tonsil, 575, 577f
  metastatic, 308f
  sinonasal, 572, 573f
  of the soft palate, 141
Stapedial artery, persistent, 218–220, 223f
Staphylococcus aureus infections, 373, 618
Staphylococcus epidermidis infection, 320f–321f, 618
Stein, B. M., 276
Stents
  carotid artery, 285
    complications of, 285
    follow-up to, 285–286
    technique of, 285
  as intracranial stenosis treatment, 263
  self-expanding nitinol, 280
Stenvers plane, 33–35
Stereotactic surgery, as arteriovenous malformation thrombosis cause, 253
Streptococcus infections, 373
Streptococcus pneumoniae infections, 361
Streptococcus viridans infections, 239
Striatonigral degeneration, 341
"String" sign, 212
Stroke
  aggressive mechanical clot disruption techniques for, 284
  atherosclerosis-related, 262
  brain tumor–related, 266
  cardiogenic, 14–15, 16f–17f, 487f
  computed tomography angiography of, 9, 11f, 14–15
  computed tomography perfusion studies of, 15–21, 18f–20f, 22f
  intravenous thrombolysis for, 281–284, 282f, 283f
    benefits of, 281–282
    inclusion and exclusion criteria for, 282
    technique of, 282–283
  ischemic
    angiographic evaluation of, 263–264
    normalized Cho/Cho(n) in, 99, 100f
    pediatric, 541–545, 544f
    thrombolytic therapy for, 263
  multidetector computed tomography–based management of, 9–13, 11f–13f, 92f
  noncontrast computed tomography in, 9, 482f
  pediatric, 533
  systemic necrotizing vasculitides–related, 258
  therapy for, 281–284
  as vascular dementia cause, 352
Subcortical band heterotia, 501, 501f
Subependymal heterotopia, 502
Subglottis, anatomy of, 142
Superior cerebellar artery, left, aneurysm of, 239f
Superior sagittal sinus
  meningioma near, 26f
  thrombus in, delta sign of, 15, 17f
Supraglottic squamous cell carcinoma, FDG PET/CT of, 142, 148f–150f, 148f
  metastatic, 143f, 149f, 154–156, 156f
  post-therapy, 173f, 199f
SURF1 gene mutations, 399–400
Susceptibility, 67, 68f
Syncleinopathies, definition of, 333

Syntelencephaly, 499, 499f
Syphilis, 33–34
  meningovascular, 258
Syrinx, 314f
Systemic lupus erythematosus, 258

T

"Target sign," 374
Target Therapeutics, 276
Tau protein, in Alzheimer's disease, 336
Tauopathies, definition of, 333–334
Tay-Sachs disease, 401, 406f, 406b, 409
TDP-43 proteinopathy, 354
Teardrop fractures, 482–483, 485f
Tegmentum, perforating arterial supply to, 230
Telangiectasia
  arteriovenous-capillary, 252–253
  capillary, 253
Telencephalic fissures, congenital abnormalities of, 496–497
Temozolomide, 101–106
Temporal bone pathology, 557–561
  aberrant carotid artery, 558–559, 559f
  acoustic schwannoma, 561, 565f
  acute mastoiditis, 559, 560f
  Bell palsy, 560–561, 561f
  cholesteatoma, 559–560, 560f
  cholesterol granuloma, 561, 562f
  congenital external and middle ear anomalies, 557, 558f
  congenital inner ear anomalies, 557, 558f
  fractures, 34–35, 42f, 557–558, 558f–559f
  glomus jugulare, 561, 563f–564f
  large vestibular aqueduct syndrome, 557, 559f
  multidetector computed tomography of, 33–34
  right, three-dimensional view of, 44f
  three-dimensional model of, 36, 44f
Temporal lobe, anterior, contusions to, 13
Temporal squama, fracture of, 431f
Thalamus, in deep gray matter diseases, 401
Thalidomide, 117–118
Thiamine deficiency, 399, 401f
Thoracolumbar spine
  hyperextension injuries to, 482–483
  hyperflexion injuries to, 480–482
  vertical compression injuries of, 483–484
Thoracolumbar spine, kyphoscoliotic deformity of, 37f
Thrombolytic therapy, 281–284, 282f, 283f
  benefits of, 281–282
  inclusion and exclusion criteria for, 282
  technique of, 282–283
  therapeutic time windows for, 263
Thrombosis
  superior sagittal, 544f
  venous
    deep, noncontrast computed tomography of, 14f
    pediatric, 545
    sinus, 15, 15
    sinus dural, 15, 18f
Thrombus
  formation in catheters, 213
  intravascular, 263–264
  left atrial appendage, 15, 17f
  in superior sagittal sinus, delta sign of, 15, 17f
Thyroid carcinoma, anaplastic, 580–582, 582f
Thyroid cartilage
  involvement glottic tumors, 146f–147f, 149
  involvement in laryngeal cancer, 145f
Thyroid gland, subglottic squamous cell carcinoma invasion of, 149
Thyroiditis, Hashimoto, 579, 580f
Thyroid pathology, 578–582
  anaplastic thyroid carcinoma, 580–582, 582f
  goiter, 579–580, 581f
  Hashimoto thyroiditis, 579, 580f
  lingual thyroid, 578–582, 579f
  thyroglossal duct cysts, 579, 580f
"Tiger-eye" sign, 356, 356f
Tissue plasminogen activator (tPA), intravenous, 281–284, 282f–283f
Titanium rods, 198f–199f
Tongue, lymphatic drainage of, 152
Tongue carcinoma, retromolar, 575–577, 577f
Tongue/tongue base squamous cell carcinoma, FDG PET/CT of, 128f–131f
  effect of periodontal disease on, 195f–196f
  metastatic, 128f, 136, 136f–137f, 153, 153f, 160f
    bone metastases, 161, 162f
    cervical lymph node metastases, 128f, 136f–137f, 153, 153f, 160f, 189f
    distant metastases, 167f, 179f
    pulmonary metastases, 166f
  with necrotic lymph nodes, 130f–131f
  post-therapy, 171f–172f, 175f–181f, 183f, 195f–196f, 198f, 199f
  with radiation-related inflammatory changes, 164f–165f
  of recurrent tumors, 175f, 179f, 183f, 186f–189f
Tonsillar squamous cell carcinoma
  FDG PET/CT of, 127f, 136–141, 138f–139f
  effect of surgical metallic clips on, 194f
  false-positive result in, 142
  of metastases, 127f, 137f, 153–154, 155f, 185f
  of metastases, in combination with contrast-enhanced CT, 166–168
  post-therapy, 174f, 183f, 197f
  recurrent, 183f, 185f, 194f
  vocal cord FDG uptake in, 201f
  treatment for, 141
Tonsillitis, misdiagnosed as tonsillar squamous cell carcinoma, 140f, 169
Tooth extractions. See Dental interventions
Toxoplasmosis, 107
  in AIDS patients, 378–380, 381f
  as brain abscess cause, 373
  of the central nervous system, 378–380, 381f
  differentiated from
    cerebral lymphoma, 374–378
    tuberculous abscess, 112f–113f
Tracheostomy site, 191, 196f
Tractography, three-dimensional fiber, 80
Transglottic squamous cell carcinoma, 142–149, 148f, 150f
  metastatic, 148f, 154–156, 168f
Transitional cell carcinoma, 308f
Trauma
  arterial, 269–272
  cerebrovascular, 266–269
  orbital, 40, 46f, 454–458
  spinal, 28–30
Treponema pallidum, 345
Trichopoliodystrophy, 398b
Trigeminal artery
  persistent, 220t, 221, 226f
  primitive, 220t
Trigeminal-cavernous fistula, 221
Tuberculoma, 107–112, 374–378, 377f
Tuberculosis
  AIDS-related, 363–364, 364f
  differentiated from candidiasis, 300f
  as meningitis cause, 363–364, 364f–365f
  orbital, 40–41
Tufts University, 3
Tullio phenomenon, 33–34
Tumefactive demyelinating lesions (TDLs), 94f, 97–99, 97f, 99f
Tumor "blush," 266
  differentiated from vascular blush, 224f
Tympanic artery, inferior, enlarged, 222f
Tympanosclerosisf, 33, 35, 42f

U

Uncovertebral degenerative disease, 623–624
Urea cycle disorders, 392

V

Vacuolization, spectroscopic metabolite patterns in, 408
Vallecula, in tongue squamous cell carcinoma, 134–135, 136f
van der Knaap disease, 404–405
Varices, venous, 46
Vascular "blush," 224f
  choroidal, 219f, 224, 226f
Vascular cerebral malformations
  aneurysms related to, 225f, 239
  with arteriovenous shunting, 255–257
  classification of, 249, 250t
  orbital, 46, 49f
Vascular endothelial growth factor (VEGF), 85–97, 107–112, 107f–108f
Vascular endothelial growth factor (VEGF) receptor, monoclonal antibody against, 117
Vascular lesions/tumors
  embolization of, 291–292
  pediatric, 292–296
Vasculitis, cerebral
  angiographic evaluation of, 257–259, 257t
  noninvasive imaging alternatives for, 258–259
  primary, 259f
Vasculopathies, cerebral
  inherited, 257, 257t
  intracranial nonatheromatous, 257t
  reversible syndromes of, 221f, 260
Vasospasm, cerebral, 260–261
Vein of Galen
  aneurysmal malformations (VGAMs) of, 253
  dilatation of, 253
  dural, 253
  malformations of, 292–294, 293f
  varix of, 253
Ventricles, cerebral
  effect of brain edema on, 461
  trauma-related enlargement of, 465, 466f
Ventriculomegaly, 547–548, 548f
Vertebral arteries
  diagnostic angiographic evaluation of, 227–228
    anatomic segments, 227–228
    branches, 228, 229f–230f
    common variants, 227–228

Vertebral arteries *(Continued)*
  technique, 212–213, 214f
    V1 (extraosseous) segment, 227
    V3 (extraspinal) segment, 227, 228f
    V2 (foraminal) segment, 227, 228f
    V4 (intradural) segment, 228, 228f
  left, 289f
  traumatic dissection of, 16f, 269
Vertebral bodies
  hemangioma of, 593f
  infection of, 31
  necrosis of, 38f
  "pseudohypointense" lesions of, 595–601, 602f
Vertebral end plates, Modic changes in, 611, 611t, 618
  differentiated from spinal tumors, 591, 598f
Vertebral fractures, benign, 601f
Vertebrobasilar system, diagnostic angiographic evaluation of, 227
Vertical compression injuries, spinal, 483–484
Vessel occlusion, 263–264
Vidian artery, 218–220

Virchow-Robin spaces
  aging-related enlargement of, 335
  cryptococcal cystic lesions of, 366
Vocal cords
  FDG uptake in, 201f
  post-therapy-related changes in, 193, 200f–201f
  squamous cell carcinoma of, FDG PET/CT of, 191f
    post-laser excision, 200f
    post-radiation therapy, 200f–201f
Volumetric analysis, of cerebral volume loss, 336

W

Warfarin, discontinuation prior to biopsy, 299–300
Warthin tumor, 193t, 202, 203f
Wedge fractures, 482f–483f
Wegener granulomatosis, 40–41
Wernicke-Korsakoff syndrome, 345
Wernicke's encephalopathy, 347f
Whiplash injuries, 485–486

White matter
  aging-related changes in, 335
  fiber tractography of, 80, 80–82
  HIV infection-related abnormalities of, 367
  magnetic resonance spectroscopy of, 123
  metabolic disorders of (myelination disorders), 383–393
    central disorders, 384–388, 384f–385f, 385b
    peripheral disorders, 388–389
    progressive multifocal leukoencephalopathy, 370–371
  in neurodegenerative diseases, 355
Wilson disease (hepatolenticular degeneration), 399, 400b, 405
Wolpert, S. M., 276

Z

Zanetti, P. H., 276
Zellweger syndrome (cerebrohepatorenal syndrome), 385, 386f, 386b, 404–405
Z-score imaging, in Alzheimer's disease, 336–337, 338f